THE ORTHOMOLECULAR TREATMENT OF CHRONIC DISEASE

65 Experts on Therapeutic and Preventive Nutrition

Edited by

Andrew W. Saul, PhD

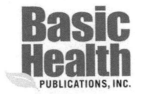

Basic Health
PUBLICATIONS, INC.

DISCLAIMER: The information in this book is not in any way offered as prescription, diagnosis, nor treatment for any disease, illness, infirmity, or physical condition. Any form of self-treatment or alternative health program necessarily must involve an individual's acceptance of some risk, and no one should assume otherwise. Persons needing medical care should obtain it from a physician. Consult your doctor before making any health decision.

Neither the author nor the publisher has authorized the use of their names or the use of any material contained within in connection with the sale, promotion, or advertising of any product or apparatus. Such use is strictly prohibited.

The opinions offered in this book are those of the author, who is not a physician, and are not necessarily the views of the publisher.

Basic Health Publications, Inc.
28812 Top of the World Drive
Laguna Beach, CA 92651
949-715-7327 • www.basichealthpub.com

Library of Congress Cataloging-in-Publication Data
Saul, Andrew W.
    The orthomolecular treatment of chronic disease : 65 experts on therapeutic and preventive nutrition / edited by Andrew W. Saul, PhD.
        pages cm
    Includes bibliographical references and index.
    ISBN 978-1-59120-370-4 (pbk)
    ISBN 978-1-59120-392-6 (hc)
    1. Chronic diseases—Treatment. 2. Orthomolecular therapy.
    3. Chronic diseases—Nutritional aspects. I. Saul, Andrew W.

    RC108.O78   2014
    616^1.044—dc23

                                                                    2014016229

Editor: Cheryl Hirsch
Typesetting/Book design: Theresa Wiscovitch
Cover design: Mike Stromberg

*To Abram Hoffer and Linus Pauling,
the innovative founders and great teachers
of orthomolecular medicine*

CONTENTS

PART ONE: FOUNDATIONS OF ORTHOMOLECULAR THERAPY

PART TWO: PIONEERS OF ORTHOMOLECULAR MEDICINE

PART THREE: ORTHOMOLECULAR TREATMENT

APPENDICES

FOREWORD

HEALTH IS UNDENIABLY A REQUIREMENT for our happiness, as well as for our family, friends, and children of the coming generation, yet I consider this era to be the most difficult time in history to maintain our health. In the past, we had a hope that all diseases would disappear with advancements in medicine. It turns out that we are seeing increases in the number of patients with stroke, cardiovascular diseases, cancer, allergic diseases, psychiatric diseases, and various other health issues.

We live in an environment stressed by pollution, poisonous food additives, and low-nutrition junk foods. This environment puts our health in jeopardy and vulnerable to various chronic diseases.

As scientists and journalists confirm, the number of sick people should decrease if medicine has really evolved as much as we are told. The unfortunate fact is that modern standard medicine, which centers on pharmacotherapy, has difficulty treating, let alone curing, chronic diseases; it may even create new diseases due to adverse effects of conventional treatments.

Healthcare professionals and the public are becoming aware of the limits of standard medicine. Orthomolecular medicine can surpass these limits and bring hope to the future by providing what is really good for people's physical and mental health. Orthomolecular medicine prevents and treats diseases by providing optimal amounts of substances that are natural to the body. This means that we can prevent and treat illness and maintain ideal health through proper diet with the supplemental addition of vitamins, minerals, essential fats, and amino acids. Orthomolecular medicine has been proven to be effective, with considerable medical evidence from the leaders and pioneers, including Dr. Abram Hoffer and Dr. Linus Pauling, the two-time Nobel Prize winner.

Orthomolecular medicine provides effective treatments without adverse effects, unlike synthetic medicine, by enhancing the body's natural healing power to fight chronic diseases. Our colleagues and other healthcare professionals have successfully treated thousands of patients with chronic diseases utilizing orthomolecular medicine and nutritional therapy.

Nutritional therapy should be the first choice for treatment and prevention of diseases. We should choose standard medicine only when nutritional treatment has proven ineffective, because it is a doctor's duty to choose a safe treatment with the least adverse effects. Nutritional treatment has evolved in the long history of humankind, proving its safety and effectiveness. Orthomolecular medicine has been established as a scientific way of treatment. Our second choice—the standard treatment—uses pharmaceutical drugs as the lead option. The reason for its placement as the second choice is that tens of millions of people suffer every year from the adverse effects of drugs, and hundreds of thousands are dying from them. This simple fact is surely enough for us to realize that our first choice should be nutritional treatment.

Unfortunately, it has become the norm in the last 20 to 30 years for doctors and patients to choose drugs as soon as they spot a disease. What we consider as a "dangerous drug" is their first choice. Behind this trend are the pharmaceutical giants, who grow rich from people choosing the dangerous products. Magazines, newspapers, and television do not seem to hesitate when advertising the drugs that may be harmful for the patients. We have to give a cautious look at how we treat diseases, and take a lead in spreading the safe way of medicine with nutritional treatment.

For that purpose, Dr. Andrew W. Saul has compiled *The Orthomolecular Treatment of Chronic Disease*. Dr. Saul is an educator on orthomolecular medicine for doctors, as well as an evangelist to enlighten the public with the excellence of nutritional treatment. He has made a global contribution by establishing www.DoctorYourself.com where the correct medical information is communicated. He has long served as an editorial board member for the *Journal of Orthomolecular Medicine*, and also as the editor-in-chief of the *Orthomolecular Medicine News Service*. The International Society for Orthomolecular Medicine (ISOM) chose him as an inductee for Orthomolecular Medicine Hall of Fame in 2013 for his contribution to the field for many years. I, as the president of ISOM, deeply appreciate his friendship and support as a great advisor.

Dr. Saul has reviewed numerous studies by nutritional pioneers published in the *Journal of Orthomolecular Medicine*, the *Orthomolecular Medicine News Service*, and other publications. In editing this book, he has carefully chosen papers and reviews written by 65 experts. Part One of this book focuses on orthomolecular medicine's history, philosophy, and logic; Part Two introduces pioneers who established the field of orthomolecular medicine; and Part Three discusses treatment for chronic diseases.

Numerous discoveries and new evidence have driven the evolution of orthomolecular medicine. One recent example is high-dose vitamin C treatment of health issues related to radioactive contamination from the March 2011 accident in the Fukushima nuclear plant in my native Japan. Orthomolecular medicine, as you will read in this book, can be considered as the most effective tool in defending our bodies from radiation.

As the president of ISOM, representing 23 organizations from 20 nations around the globe, I would like to express my deepest gratitude to Dr. Saul for publishing this remarkable book, *The Orthomolecular Treatment of Chronic Disease*. The book brilliantly and successfully captures what we need to know about orthomolecular medicine now. Its information should be viewed as a comprehensive seminal standard that has been long awaited by healthcare professionals worldwide who practice, or are planning to practice, orthomolecular medicine and nutrition. We know that there are doctors and scholars who have skepticism towards this field of medicine. This book will convey the scientific truth about orthomolecular medicine that will remove their suspicion.

Orthomolecular medicine is a science, philosophy, and an art that is beneficial to people's physical and mental health. I truly believe that this book will contribute to save many people who are suffering from chronic diseases, by encouraging the world to know what good orthomolecular medicine can do for their health.

— Atsuo Yanagisawa, MD, PhD
President, International Society for Orthomolecular Medicine

ACKNOWLEDGMENTS

I AM GRATEFUL FOR the work and the memory of the great orthomolecular pioneers. Most of all, thanks to all the authors whose articles are incorporated into this book. I would like to also thank Steven Carter, Executive Director of the International Schizophrenia Foundation, the editors of the *Journal of Orthomolecular Medicine*, and the editorial board of the *Orthomolecular Medicine News Service*. I thank Dr. Atsuo Yanagisawa for kindly providing this book's foreword, and I thank Dr. Jonathan Prousky for the preface.

Grateful appreciation is expressed to the Riordan Clinic for permission to publish their complete intravenous vitamin C protocol, with my special thanks to Paul R. Taylor, Mike Stewart, Nina Mikirova, PhD, James A. Jackson, PhD, Neil Riordan, PhD, Joseph Casciari, PhD, and Ron Hunninghake, MD.

My personal thanks are due to Colleen, Jason, Helen, Justine, John I. Mosher, Robert G. Smith, and Norman Goldfind.

I wish to express my unreserved appreciation to my editor, Cheryl Hirsch, whose professionalism and dedication were absolutely essential to this project.

Also, a special thank you to all critics of orthomolecular medicine. Their decades of marginalization of successful nutritional treatments for chronic disease have made this book possible, and necessary.

— ANDREW W. SAUL

PREFACE

THE ORTHOMOLECULAR TREATMENT OF CHRONIC DISEASE presents an opportunity to empower yourself with information about how to improve not only your life span (how long you live), but your health span (how well you live) as well.

People with chronic disease face a psychological and medical conundrum. Modern treatment of chronic illness often involves the use of one or more prescription drugs. These medications can cause medical mayhem within the body, which in turn can increase chronic disease susceptibility (e.g., hypertension, obesity, and immune dysfunction) as well as premature death (e.g., diabetes, heart disease, and infectious disease). What would happen if, instead of being drugged for life, such people had an opportunity to mostly use orthomolecular medicine based on the information in this book?

Orthomolecular medicine relies on natural substances normally present in the human body and brain (e.g., vitamins, minerals, amino acids, essential fatty acids, and hormones). These natural substances support the physiological and biochemical processes that the body and brain use to function normally, enabling people to reap tremendous psychological and physical benefits. In fact, the consistent use of orthomolecular medicine would mitigate other risks that increase chronic disease susceptibility as well as premature death.

Given the fact that many "modern" treatments make well people sick or sick people sicker, it makes sense to use this information to change your life and your future. For every health condition in *The Orthomolecular Treatment of Chronic Disease*, there are reasonable orthomolecular alternatives that can lessen the burden of drug therapies, or perhaps replace drug therapies altogether. Why wait any longer? Go for it, and help you and your family to live long, healthy lives.

— JONATHAN E. PROUSKY, ND
Editor, *Journal of Orthomolecular Medicine*

ABRAM HOFFER: AN APPRECIATION

SOME YEARS AGO, AS I SAT at lunch with Dr. Abram Hoffer, I took some vitamin pills. Dr. Hoffer leaned toward me and said, "You know, you're going to live a lot longer if you take those." As I looked at him, he added, "I guarantee it. If you don't, come back and tell me." So said the founding father of orthomolecular medicine.

It was 60 years ago that Dr. Abram Hoffer and his colleagues began curing schizophrenia with niacin. While some physicians are still waiting, those who have used niacin with patients and families know the immense practical value of what Dr. Hoffer discovered. Dr. Abram Hoffer's life has not merely changed the face of psychiatry; he changed the course of medicine for all time. His 30 books, 600 scientific papers, and thousands of cured patients have yet to convince orthodox medicine. Dr. Hoffer has said that it takes about two generations before a truly new medical idea is accepted. Perhaps in the case of high-dose nutrient therapy, maybe it's three generations. Great ideas in medicine, or anywhere else, are never self-evident. That is why this book was published.

Over the years, I was honored to ultimately write four books with Abram and to work with him when I was assistant editor of the *Journal of Orthomolecular Medicine*. Abram taught me much, as he taught so many. He was a prompt responder and enthusiastic. Hardly a day went by without an email from Abram, and typically there were several. They were both wide-ranging and frequent, answering my questions and then some. He led by example. Once a speaker at a medical conference made two factual errors about niacin. I was sitting next to Abram, and he was, to all appearances, dozing off. He was not. He gave me a nod and, during the question session, got up to take the microphone. He complimented the speaker on his presentation, mentioned a few additional things about niacin, made another supportive remark, and sat down. The speaker was delighted. And he never knew he had just been corrected. This was Abram Hoffer.

Thanks to him, medicine will never be the same. That may be the best of legacies.

— A.W.S.

INTRODUCTION

DECADES OF PHYSICIANS' REPORTS and laboratory and clinical studies support the therapeutic use of large doses of vitamins and other nutrients. Effective doses are high doses, often tens or hundreds of times higher than the U.S. Recommended Dietary Allowance (RDA) or Dietary Reference Intakes (DRI). A cornerstone of medical science is that dosage affects treatment outcome. This premise is accepted with pharmaceutical drug therapy, but not with vitamin therapy. Most vitamin research has used inadequate, low doses. Low doses do not get clinical results. Investigators using vitamins in high doses have consistently reported excellent results. The medical literature has ignored nearly 75 years of laboratory and clinical studies on high-dose nutrient therapy.

High doses of vitamins were advocated shortly after they were first isolated. Claus Jungeblut, MD, prevented and treated polio in the mid-1930s using a vitamin. Chest specialist Frederick Klenner, MD, was curing multiple sclerosis and polio back in the 1940s using vitamins. William Kaufman, MD, cured arthritis similarly in the 1940s. In the 1950s, Drs. Wilfrid and Evan Shute were curing various forms of cardiovascular disease with a vitamin. At the same time, psychiatrist Abram Hoffer, MD, PhD, was using niacin to cure schizophrenia, psychosis, and depression. In the 1960s, Robert F. Cathcart, MD, cured influenza, pneumonia, and hepatitis. In the 1970s, Hugh D. Riordan, MD, was obtaining cures of cancer with intravenous vitamin C. Dr. Harold Foster and colleagues arrested and reversed full-blown AIDS with nutrient therapy, and, in just the last few years, Atsuo Yanagisawa, MD, PhD, has shown that vitamin therapy can prevent and reverse sickness caused by exposure to nuclear radiation. All of these doctors used very high doses, and all consistently reported striking success rates. And all these doctors reported great patient safety.

Much medical knowledge has come from physician reports, which are neither double-blind nor placebo-controlled. They are the valuable experiences of qualified observers. They are valid: just ask the patients who got better. Yet doctors' reports, as well as those of their patients, are typically marginalized by the medical establishment as mere "anecdotes." But how can they be ignored when they show results?

Nutritional supplementation is not the answer to every health problem, but it does not have to be. Nutrient therapy, properly dosed and administered, is the answer to many chronic medical problems. The list is far longer than the deficiency diseases. A drug in either low or high doses cannot act as a vitamin. However, vitamins in large doses can act as drugs, and with far greater safety.

Years ago, Dr. Hugh Riordan observed, "Orthomolecular is not an answer to any question posed in medical school." That statement is still substantially true: not only do medical schools fail to teach students how to effectively utilize nutrition therapy, they don't even discuss it. But the public is learning that orthomolecular medicine is the answer to an ever more pharmaceutical-based, ever more dangerous, ever more costly disease-care system. Dr. Hoffer has said that the worst fate that could befall opponents of orthomolecular medicine is for them to never, ever use it.

High doses of vitamins have been known to cure serious illnesses for nearly 80 years now. But, unlike other books, this book is not about simple "deficiency" diseases. Instead, *The Orthomolecular Treatment of Chronic Disease* targets often severe ailments that are generally not believed to be treatable with nutrition therapy. We will discuss which nutrients can be used in place of drug treatment, with dosage specifics and case stories of how this approach has worked so well for so many. You will learn the real story about how vitamins cure disease inexpensively, safely, and effectively.

Some topics have not been included because of relatively less available orthomolecular medical research. Some are excluded because they have already been addressed elsewhere. Basic Health Publication's Vitamin Cure series covers many illness topics quite well. No single volume can encompass them all. Intentionally, there is no specific nutrients section in this book. Many good books already discuss individual nutrients. A recommended reading list is provided at the end of the book to serve as a resource guide.

Orthomolecular (nutritional) medicine is based on physicians' reported experiences as well as laboratory study. Since 1967, much of this research has been published in the *Journal of Orthomolecular Medicine (JOM)*, formerly known as the *Journal of Schizophrenia* (1967), *Schizophrenia* (1968), and *Orthomolecular Psychiatry* (1971). This book provides important material selected from more than 47 years of *JOM* for the general reader and the general reader's doctor. In so doing, we have chosen to include some classic (old but very important) papers. Dr. Hoffer and other leaders in the field strongly felt, and still feel today, that this is timeless material. While articles were carefully chosen for inclusion in this book, the reader will note that some have been abridged or otherwise edited for this publication.

The Orthomolecular Treatment of Chronic Disease is a very large book, but it is also a very practical book. As you read it, you will see that it takes a problem-based approach, not an encyclopedic one. If you want to know which illnesses best respond to nutrition therapy, and how and why that therapy works, this is the book for you. Part One presents the principles of orthomolecular medicine and the science behind them. Part Two is devoted to orthomolecular pioneers, introducing maverick doctors and nutrition scientists in a reader-friendly way that brings the subject to life. Part Three brings together extraordinary clinical and experimental experiences with vitamins by experts in such major chronic illnesses as Alzheimer's disease, AIDS, addiction (alcohol and drug), depression, cancer, heart disease, radiation illness, and schizophrenia and other mood disorders. Physician reports and patient case histories appear throughout to illustrate safe, successful nutrition-based treatment.

Safety of high doses is often addressed within the *JOM* papers we have selected. There is further discussion of vitamin safety in the Appendix. The online archive of the *Orthomolecular Medicine News Service*, another peer-reviewed publication, contains dozens of recent reviews on supplement safety.

If the word "cure" intrigues you, this book will also. Inside you'll find a body of knowledge that you and your doctor have likely never been exposed to before. Many people have heard their doctor say, "I have never seen any evidence that nutrient therapy cures disease." Those doctors are telling the truth: they personally have never seen the evidence. But that is not because it doesn't exist. It does, and *The Orthomolecular Treatment of Chronic Disease* shows exactly how innovative physicians have gotten outstanding clinical results with high-dose nutrient therapy. Their work is here for you to see and decide for yourself.

— A.W.S.

PART ONE

FOUNDATIONS OF ORTHOMOLECULAR THERAPY

MEDICAL INNOVATION FALLS into two main classes: 1) major discoveries, which create a paradigm shift in medical philosophy and treatment; and 2) minor discoveries, which expand upon and exploit the new paradigm. Inevitably, there are few major discoveries and a large number of minor ones. The leading role played by the new paradigm is bolstered at first by the host of minor discoveries, but eventually these destroy the major paradigm, which is replaced by a new and better one. Unfortunately, the major paradigm (generally accepted theories and hypotheses) may rule long after it has served its usefulness. It then becomes a major impediment to newer discoveries.

It may take anywhere from 40 to 60 years or more after the first major assault on the old paradigm before it is replaced by a newer one. A current example is the slow pace in which the vitamin paradigm of nutrition (vitamins as prevention of deficiency) is being replaced by the orthomolecular paradigm (vitamins as treatment of disease). Vitamins have never been embraced warmly by the medical profession. The vitamin deficiency paradigm began in the late 19th century and by the late 1940s was firmly established, meaning that they were useful only for preventing the classical deficiency diseases such as pellagra, scurvy, and beriberi, and were needed only in small vitamin doses.

Information follows a growth curve, well known in biology. If one seeds a glass of sterile milk with 1 million lactobacilli that will eventually turn it sour, nothing appears to happen for a long time, perhaps for days, depending upon the temperature. Then suddenly it curdles. What has happened is that the bacteria have been dividing at a rapid pace, but only when enough lactic acid has been generated by that colony will the milk curdle. The phase where nothing appears to be happening (but in fact the bacteria are growing rapidly) is called the lag phase. Just before and during the curdling process the growth appears to accelerate, and after that growth diminishes as the bacteria run out of food. The growth curve has a slowly ascending lag phase, then a rapidly ascending phase followed by a phase where growth levels off and stops.

Information growth follows a similar pattern of growth. The orthomolecular paradigm has been in the lag phase for about 40 to 60 years, but we are now entering the phase of rapid growth. It may take another 5 to 10 years before we reach the stage of maturation, except of course in psychiatry, which is many years backward. I believe the ascending phase begins when about 10 percent of the professional population is convinced there is merit to the new ideas. By then perhaps 50 percent of the general population is convinced.

The vitamin paradigm has resisted stoutly using every means, fair and foul, at its disposal, including lies manufactured by its stoutest defenders who generate toxicity of vitamins where none have ever been shown to exist. The establishment press has provided the defenders of the paradigm ample space in which to promote their views, and has been equally assiduous in rejecting information from the orthomolecular camp who are attacking the paradigm.

It is time we gave the vitamin paradigm a decent and honorable funeral. An enormous number of patients would have benefited from the newer paradigm. It is impossible to estimate the enormous cost we have had to pay, because of the inertia and the ability of a deadly paradigm to suppress the development of a newer, more helpful one. It should not be beyond the wit of science and the public to devise a system by which this enormously long delay in the examination of new ideas can be reduced, from the usual 40 to 60 years to perhaps 10 or so years. This will be the only way by which the enormous healthcare costs are ever going to be decreased and unnecessary loss of lives saved.

— ABRAM HOFFER, *JOM* 1993

TERMS OF ORTHOMOLECULAR THERAPY

ASCORBIC ACID. Ascorbic acid is a weak acid, far weaker than stomach hydrochloric acid. For oral administration, orthomolecular physicians tend to specify ascorbic acid rather than the nonacidic vitamin C salts (calcium ascorbate, magnesium ascorbate, sodium ascorbate) because ascorbic acid seems to get better clinical results than the salts do. Intravenous administration of vitamin C requires either sodium ascorbate or carefully buffered ascorbic acid.

AVITAMINOSIS. A lack of one or more essential vitamins.

HYPOASCORBEMIA. A population-wide, genetically based deficiency of ascorbic acid.

IATROGENIC. Physician-caused.

NUTRIENT DEFICIENCY. An inadequate supply of essential vitamins and minerals in the diet, resulting in malnutrition or disease.

NUTRIENT DEPENDENCY. Nutrient dependency is not the same as nutrient deficiency. A nutrient-dependent person has unusually high needs that diet alone cannot meet.

ORTHOMOLECULAR. The term means the right or the correct molecule. It was coined by Linus Pauling in 1968.

OXIDATION-REDUCTION REACTIONS. Also called redox reactions. Refers to the transfer of electrons; oxidation involves the loss of electrons, while reduction involves the gain of electrons. Antioxidants prevent oxidation damage by donating electrons to replace those lost to oxidation.

PHARMACOKINETICS. The study of how a substance is absorbed, distributed, and excreted in the body.

RECOMMENDED DIETARY ALLOWANCE (RDAS). Guidelines that recommend how much of each vitamin and mineral most people should get each day. The recommendations are based on the assumption that individual requirements do not vary.

VITAMIN C. Also called ascorbic acid or ascorbate. Vitamin C was the first vitamin to be identified and isolated by Albert Szent-Györgyi in 1927. The human body is unable to synthesize vitamin C.

VITAMINS-AS-PREVENTION PARADIGM. Vitamins in minimal (small) doses will prevent deficiency diseases such as beriberi (vitamin B1), pellagra (vitamin B3), rickets (vitamin D), and scurvy (vitamin C). Sufficient amounts of vitamin are assumed to be found in a well-balanced diet.

VITAMINS-AS-TREATMENT PARADIGM. Also called the orthomolecular paradigm. Vitamins in optimum (large) doses can be used to prevent and treat a variety of conditions not considered to be vitamin deficiency diseases. Higher doses provide more optimal health.

WHEN EVIDENCE IS A CHOICE
by Andrew W. Saul, PhD

It is a cornerstone of medical science that dose affects treatment outcome. This premise is accepted with pharmaceutical drug therapy but not with nutrient therapy. In nutritional therapy, dose is very important. That hardly seems a provocative statement. Investigators using nutrients in high doses have consistently reported success. Dr. Frederick Klenner wrote, "If you want results, use adequate ascorbic acid."[1] Drs. Evan and Wilfrid Shute said the same of vitamin E, and Dr. Abram Hoffer spoke similarly about niacin. The medical literature has ignored such "anecdotal" physician reports and nearly 80 years of well-controlled, but not strictly double-blind placebo-controlled clinical studies on high-dose nutrient therapy.

> "The modern church of medicine does not relish alerting the press when the news is good about vitamins. There is no money in it and potentially a loss if vitamins displace drugs, as they should. I sometimes harbor a silent wish for all our critics: that is, that they should never under any circumstances ever take any supplemental nutrients, and must be restricted to only eating modern high-tech food. Can you think of a more severe punishment?" —ABRAM HOFFER

Evidence-based anything is only as good as the evidence collected. You can set up any experiment to fail. One way to ensure failure is to make a meaningless test. A meaningless test is guaranteed if you make the choice to use insufficient quantities of the substance to be investigated. Randomized controlled trials (RCTs) of high vitamin doses are very rare. (RCTs are considered the gold standard for measuring an intervention's impact.) RCTs with low doses of nutrients are plentiful. Low doses don't work. Performing meta-analyses (statistical syntheses of related studies) of many low-dose studies teaches nothing worth knowing. The first rule of building a brick wall is that you have got to have enough bricks.

Obstacles to Megadose Research

Some twenty years ago Dr. Robert F. Cathcart wrote:

As evidence of the value of nutrients, especially vitamin C . . . becomes more and more evident to the public, researchers produce a mass of articles on minute aspects of vitamin C. I have been consulted by many researchers who proposed bold studies of the effects of massive doses of ascorbate. Every time the university center, the ethics committee, the pharmacy committee, or some other board deny permission for the use of massive doses of ascorbate and render the study almost useless. Seasoned researchers depending upon government grants do not even try to study adequate doses. All of this results in a massive accumulation of knowledge about very little, which gives the impression that there is no more of real importance to be learned. This accumulation of minutia hides the great effects of ascorbate already known by some . . . As you read these learned papers, you will realize that they seem to be completely unaware of the uses of massive doses of ascorbate. One of the most amusing aspects of this research are the speculations and research into the toxicity and other adverse reactions of tiny doses of ascorbate when many have used for years 20 to 100 times the amounts being discussed.[2]

Dosage is set by the researcher. In terms of experimental design, it is not much harder to use 2,000 international units (IU) of vitamin E than to

From the *J Orthomolecular Med* 2010;25(4):164–165.

use 200 IU. Investigators may choose to test only low nutrient doses because of arbitrary "Safe Upper Limits." Such limits, largely theoretical, effectively keep Institutional Review Boards (IRBs) from allowing megadose research. I have colleagues who serve on IRBs. None of them knew that, in the entire United States, there was not even one death caused by a dietary supplement in 2008.[3] Zero reported deaths from vitamins, minerals, herbs, and amino acids does not mean that they are unconditionally safe. It does, however, strongly suggest that nutrients in large doses are safer than pharmaceuticals at any dose. A good case could be made that nutrient Safe Upper Limits are themselves not evidence-based.

Investigators may choose to employ low nutrient doses because they are unaware, or choose to be unaware, of established high-dose benefits. Or, investigators may claim that they are in fact using high doses and editorialize as such in their conclusions. Linus Pauling specifically warned against this in his first orthomolecular book, *Vitamin C and the Common Cold* (1970). Forty years later, we still see new nutritional research presenting 500 milligrams (mg) or 1,000 mg of ascorbate as if it were a lot. With an arbitrary governmental Safe Upper Limit set at 2,000 mg, where is the surprise?

What Constitutes Evidence?

The majority of medical interventions have never been rigorously tested. A mere 11 percent have been shown to be beneficial and another 23 percent are "likely to be beneficial."[4] Conventional chemotherapy for cancer contributes only 2.1 percent in the United States.[5] It would be difficult to make a case that such treatment is evidence-based. Indeed, some oncologists will recommend chemotherapy for patients with a cancer against which chemotherapy is known to be ineffective.

If you think medical research may allow for some flexible truth, you should consider nutrition. For example, the U.S. Department of Agriculture (USDA) states that "the guinea pig's vitamin C requirement is 10–15 mg per day under normal conditions and 15–25 mg per day if pregnant, lactating, or growing."[6] An adult guinea pig weighs about 1 kilogram (kg), so guinea pigs need between 10 and 25 mg of vitamin C per kilogram. An average American adult human weighs (at least) 82 kg (180 lbs). That means the USDA's standards, if fairly applied to us, would set our vitamin C requirement somewhere between 820 mg and 2,000 mg vitamin C per day. The U.S. Recommended Dietary Allowance (RDA) for vitamin C is 90 mg for men; 75 mg for women. For smokers, they allow an additional 35 mg a day.

Shooting beans at a charging rhinoceros is not likely to influence the outcome. If you were to give every homeless person you met on the street 25 cents, you could easily prove that money will not help poverty. The public and their doctors look to scientific researchers to test and confirm the efficacy of any nutritional therapy. As long as such research continues to use small doses of vitamins, doses that are too small to work, orthomolecular medicine will be touted as "unproven."

REFERENCES

1. Saul AW. Hidden in plain sight: the pioneering work of Frederick Robert Klenner, MD. *J Orthomolecular Med* 2007;22:31–38.

2. Cathcart RF. Delay by intellectualization. Available at: www.orthomed.com/index2.htm.

3. Bronstein AC, Spyker DA, Cantilena LR, et al. 2008 Annual Report of the American Association of Poison Control Centers' National Poison Data System (NPDS): 26th Annual Report. *Clin Toxicol* 2009;47:911–1084.

4. BMJ Clinical Evidence. Available at: www.clinicalevidence.bmj.com/ceweb/about/knowledge.jsp.

5. Morgan G, Ward R, Barton M. The contribution of cytotoxic chemotherapy to 5-year survival in adult malignancies. *Clinical Oncol* 2004;16:549–560.

6. U.S. Department of Agriculture Animal Care Resource Guide, Animal Care, 12.4.2. Available at: www.aphis.usda.gov/animal_welfare/downloads/manuals/dealer/feeding.pdf.

LINUS PAULING AND THE ADVENT OF ORTHOMOLECULAR MEDICINE
by Stephen Lawson

The journal *Science* published a revelatory article in its April 19, 1968, issue.[1] The author, Dr. Linus Pauling, was no stranger to the pages of *Science*, but his article, "Orthomolecular Psychiatry," heralded a dramatically new direction in his thinking and research. Dr. Pauling had enjoyed widespread fame as the world's greatest chemist and tireless peace advocate for many decades, but his venture into the field of nutrition, especially concerning micronutrients and their role in maintaining mental and physical health, attracted new attention and ignited controversy. In a letter published in the June 14 issue of *Science*, Donald Oken, a psychiatrist at the National Institutes of Health (NIH), wrote:

> The article 'Orthomolecular Psychiatry' illustrates elegantly the pitfalls which occur when an expert in one field enters another area. With his characteristic brilliance, Linus Pauling describes a biochemical mechanism which *could* be responsible for some forms of mental illness (or, indeed, for illness of many other types). Remote plausibility, however, no matter how intriguing and creative its nature, should not be confused with evidence. Unfortunately for Pauling's thesis, there is no adequate evidence to back up his view.[2]

In response, Pauling noted that he had been working for 12 years on the molecular basis of mental illness with his research supported by the NIH, the Ford Foundation, and private donors, implying that he was not a newcomer to the field of brain chemistry. Indeed, he had published his theory on the molecular mechanism of anesthetic agents, particularly the inert gases, in 1959 and had begun working on biological molecules in the late 1930s. Those efforts culminated in the discovery of the structural themes of proteins, including the alpha-helix and pleated sheet, and the cause of sickle-cell anemia—the first disease to be characterized as a molecular disease—and established Pauling as the major founder of molecular biology. Pauling also remarked that psychiatrists had a

duty, in his view, to employ the techniques of orthomolecular psychiatry in addition to the standard therapies.[3]

Oken was certainly justified in his praise of Pauling's brilliance but missed entirely the point of his genius: the ability to span diverse scientific and medical fields and synthesize original, compelling perspectives into perplexing issues. Pauling, the only person to have won two unshared Nobel Prizes, was one of history's greatest embodiments of the interdisciplinary approach, decades before it became considered essential. In the "Millennium Essay" published in *Nature* in 2000, the Indian chemist Gautam Desiraju characterized Pauling as "one of the great thinkers and visionaries of the millennium," ranking him alongside Galileo, Da Vinci, Faraday, Newton, and Einstein. Dr. Desiraju noted that "Pauling's ingenuity and awesome intuition permeated quantum mechanics, crystallography, biology, medicine and, above all, structural chemistry" and that modern chemistry, unlike biology or physics, is utterly dependent on the work of a single scientist: Linus Pauling.[4]

A Revolutionary Concept

What, then, was Pauling's paper "Orthomolecular Psychiatry" about, and why did it generate such criticism? Written while Pauling was a professor in the chemistry department in the University of California at San Diego, "Orthomolecular Psychiatry" established the theoretical basis for treating cerebral avitaminosis by "the provision of the optimum molecular environment for the mind, especially the optimum concentrations of substances normally present in the human body." Somewhat later, Pauling broadly defined orthomolecular medicine as preserving good health and treating disease by "varying the concentrations in the human body of substances that are normally present in the body and are required for health."[5] Drawing on evidence

From the *J Orthomolecular Med* 2008;23(2):62–76.

from microbial genetics and molecular reaction rates, Pauling suggested that the brain's sensitivity to its biochemistry affects the mind. While this concept seems as intuitive and obvious as some of Pauling's other discoveries like biological specificity or the molecular clock, it was very controversial when first introduced. Many nutritionists and psychiatrists like Oken felt that Pauling was trespassing on their domains and adopted an almost reactionary stance. Pauling's encyclopedic knowledge and awesome memory, as well as his great personal charm, served him extremely well in debates with his detractors over the next decades.

In 1945 Pauling had postulated the cause of sickle-cell anemia as an abnormal hemoglobin that combines with itself in deoxygenated blood, forming long rods that distort the shape of red blood cells into the characteristic sickle shape observed in the disease. Four years later, he and colleagues published a paper in *Science* that confirmed this mechanism and heralded the new era of molecular medicine.[6] Pauling returned to the concept of molecular disease in "Orthomolecular Psychiatry," noting that phenylketonuria is a molecular disease in which phenylalanine (an amino acid) accumulates in the tissues of afflicted children because of a genetic defect in the enzyme that catalyzes the conversion of phenylalanine to tyrosine (another amino acid). The resultant pathology includes mental manifestations and physical problems, such as severe eczema, but can be attenuated by replacing a normal diet with one that is limited in phenylalanine—an example of orthomolecular medicine.

In "Orthomolecular Psychiatry," Pauling noted the mental manifestations of the B vitamin deficiency diseases that produce physical pathology, supporting his thesis that these vitamins play crucial roles in mental health. He explained that evolution may favor the loss of certain functions, such as the synthesis of vitamin C, if the environment supplies sufficient amounts of the critical substance. A mutant that synthesizes an adequate but suboptimum amount of a vital substance may also outcompete the wild-type organism if the energy saved by diminished synthesis can be applied advantageously elsewhere. To support this point,

Pauling discussed the *Neurospora* work of his friends, Nobel Prize winners George Beadle and Edward Tatum. They showed that the growth rate of a pyridoxine (vitamin B6) requiring mutant strain, produced by irradiation, actually increased to about 7 percent greater than the parental strain when large amounts of pyridoxine were supplied in the medium. Similar results were obtained for a para-aminobenzoic-acid-requiring strain, another B-vitamin dependent mold.

Pauling then discussed the dependence of reaction rates on molecular concentrations. Echoing his interest in the 1950s on the potential role of abnormal enzyme function in mental illness, Pauling noted that enzyme-catalyzed reaction rates are proportional to the concentration of the reactant, assuming that there are no enzyme inhibitors present. The rate decreases as the enzyme becomes saturated. If the enzyme is defective, as may be the case with those involved in abnormal brain function, the saturating concentration is larger because the enzyme has less affinity for its substrate. However, the rate may be normalized by increasing the concentration of the substrate. This provides the rationale for supplying high-dose vitamins to treat biogenic (biologically caused) mental illness. Building on this concept, in a paper published in the *American Journal of Clinical Nutrition* in 2002, biochemist Bruce Ames discussed the remediation of about 50 human genetic diseases caused by defective enzymes with high-dose B vitamins and other micronutrients.[7]

To illustrate his hypothesis, Pauling focused on cobalamin (vitamin B12,) niacin (vitamin B3), vitamin C, and glutamic acid (an amino acid). He cited a Norwegian study that found abnormally low levels of B12 in the blood of about 15 percent of patients admitted to a mental hospital, compared to values observed in the general population. He then recounted the successful application of niacin in the southeastern United States that alleviated psychosis in thousands of patients with pellagra (a condition caused by niacin deficiency). Citing the work of Virgil Sydenstricker and Hervey Cleckley, and the work of Abram Hoffer and Humphry Osmond, he discussed the use of high-dose niacin and, in the case of Drs. Hoffer and Osmond, the combination of high-dose niacin and vitamin C, to treat schizophrenia without the side effects typically seen with drugs. Vitamin C deficiency in schizophrenics has often been reported and is also associated with depression in patients with scurvy. Dr. Pauling briefly noted that Irwin Stone (the biochemist who first got him interested in vitamin C) estimated the optimum intake of vitamin C at 3,000–15,000 milligrams (mg) per day, based on cross-species comparisons and other arguments. A few years later, the first paper from the newly founded Linus Pauling Institute of Science and Medicine, "Results of a Loading Test of Ascorbic Acid, Niacinamide, and Pyridoxine in Schizophrenic Subjects and Controls," reported that almost all of the schizophrenic patients examined excreted abnormally low amounts of one or more of the orally administered vitamins given in doses over 1,000 mg each, compared to controls.[8] Pauling explained that several investigators in the 1940s reported that large doses of glutamic acid had beneficial effects in subjects with convulsive disorders or mental retardation. The effective dosage was found to be 10,000–20,000 mg per day, higher than the estimated intake from food of about 5,000–10,000 mg per day.

In the penultimate section of "Orthomolecular Psychiatry" on Localized Cerebral Deficiency Diseases, Pauling argued that a simple model of fluid dynamics in the body leads to calculations demonstrating that localized deficiencies of vital substances could occur in specific reservoirs. The steady-state concentration of a vital substance in the brain could be much less than its concentration in blood. In schizophrenia the situation would be aggravated by genes affecting the regulation of vitamin metabolism or other critical functions so that massive doses of certain vitamins may be required to normalize cerebral concentrations and, therefore, mental function.

"All attacks on supplement safety are really attacks on supplement efficacy."
—ABRAM HOFFER

Pauling elaborated on and extended the concept of orthomolecular psychiatry and medicine in many publications over the next decades. In the article "Some Aspects of Orthomolecular Medicine," published in 1974, he introduced new examples of orthomolecular medicine, such as the treatment of diabetes with injected insulin, the use of iodine to prevent goiter, and the management of methylmalonic aciduria, which is treated by supplying large amounts of vitamin B12 (1,000 times the normal concentration) to normalize the conversion of methylmalonic acid to succinic acid.[9] *In How to Live Longer and Feel Better*, published a dozen years later, he added another example: the treatment of galactosemia—a genetic disease characterized by a deficiency of an enzyme that metabolizes galactose in lactose—by the provision of a diet free of milk sugar.[10] Pauling stressed that he used the adjective "orthomolecular" to "express the idea of the right molecules in the right concentrations" and contrasted orthomolecular medicine with the use of potentially dangerous drugs used in conventional allopathic medicine. Pauling believed that the biological plausibility of his arguments was evident and that the available evidence was supportive. Of course, as is the case with many revolutionary ideas, "orthomolecular psychiatry" was not greeted with universal acclaim. The American Psychiatric Association (APA), in particular, was skeptical and dismissive.

In the fall of 1974, Pauling contributed an article, "On the Orthomolecular Environment of the Mind: Orthomolecular Therapy," to the *American Journal of Psychiatry*, which provided an opportunity to comment on the American Psychiatric Association's *Task Force Report: Megavitamin and Orthomolecular Therapy in Psychiatry*, issued in 1973.[11] He was clearly dismayed with the negative reaction of conventional psychiatry to his ideas and the scientific evidence and criticized what he considered to be specious arguments and fallacies in the report.

After discussing the probability that abnormal enzyme function may cause mental illness and listing examples of successful orthomolecular treatment with vitamins, Pauling faulted the APA report for ignoring evidence on vitamin C and pyridoxine; misunderstanding simple biochemistry, including the nature of vitamins and how a population of molecules can easily serve several functions—they don't all have to be committed to one reaction as implied by the task force; and intentional or unintentional bias, resulting in "a sort of professional inertia that hinders progress."

Setting the Stage

Several childhood experiences and later episodes set the stage for Pauling's codification of orthomolecular medicine and his fascination with vitamin C. His father was a druggist and, in the era before the Food and Drug Administration (FDA), concocted many medicines in his store, where Linus was exposed to this medicinal chemistry as a youngster. Later, he set up a laboratory in his basement where he carried out exciting chemical reactions. He was deeply impressed by the transformation of substances during reactions, and those early experiments stimulated an intense desire to learn more about chemistry, which was fulfilled as an undergraduate in Oregon Agricultural College (now Oregon State University) and in graduate work in the California Institute of Technology (Caltech). When Pauling and his wife were in Europe on a Guggenheim Fellowship in 1926, after earning his doctorate in chemistry and mathematical physics, his mother, Belle, died from pernicious anemia in a hospital for the insane in Salem, Oregon. Pernicious anemia, caused by a deficiency of vitamin B12, is characterized by neurological problems and loss of normal mental function, resulting in delusions known as "megaloblastic madness" and, ultimately, death. In the year that Belle Pauling died, George Minot and William Murphy discovered that eating raw liver reversed pernicious anemia. In 1934, they won the Nobel Prize in Medicine or Physiology for their work, and 14 years later, vitamin B12 was isolated independently by Pauling's friends, Karl Folkers and Alexander Todd. Another of Pauling's friends, Dorothy Hodgkin, won the Nobel Prize in Chemistry in 1964 for elucidating the molecular structure of B12 by x-ray crystallography in 1956.

In 1938 Pauling gave a speech at the dedication of the Crellin Laboratory at Caltech in which he said: "There is, however, a related field of knowledge of transcendent significance to mankind which has barely begun its development. This field deals with the correlation between chemical structure and physiological activity of those substances, manufactured in the body or ingested in foodstuffs, which are essential for orderly growth and the maintenance of life, as well as of the many substances which are useful in the treatment of disease."[12]

Pauling remarked on the structural complexity of many vitamins and predicted that, given the rapid progress in the synthesis of vitamins in the preceding decade, "success will soon reward the men who are now carrying on the attack on vitamin E." Clearly, in the heyday of vitaminology, Pauling was thinking about the virtues of these vital substances. Indeed, the early part of the 20th century, especially the 1930s, was the prime time for the discovery of vitamins and their use to correct and prevent associated deficiency diseases. For example, vitamin A was identified as a vitamin in 1914 and structurally characterized in 1930. Vitamins D2 and D3 were chemically characterized in 1932 and 1936, respectively. Vitamin E was discovered in 1922 but not isolated until 1936. Vitamin K was discovered in the early 1930s and identified in 1939. Pauling's friend Albert Szent-Györgyi, first isolated vitamin C in 1928. Thiamine was isolated in 1911 by Casimir Funk, who coined the term "vitamine," and structurally characterized in 1936 by Robert R. Williams.

Williams's brother, Roger J. Williams, first identified the structure of pantothenic acid (vitamin B5) in 1940 and later proposed important concepts about biochemical individuality that greatly influenced Pauling. In his classic book *Biochemical Individuality*, Roger Williams described significant anatomical and biochemical variations due to genetic polymorphisms (variations) among humans and postulated, "practically every human being is a deviate in some respects."[13] He noted that if 95 percent of the population is normal with respect to one measured value, only 0.59 percent of the population would be normal with respect to 100 uncorrelated measured values. In December 2007, the journal *Science* heralded human genetic variation and its implication for disease risk and personal traits as the "Breakthrough of the Year."[14] Riboflavin (vitamin B2), the first vitamin to be recognized as a coenzyme, was isolated in 1933. Vitamin B6 (pyridoxine and related forms) was isolated in 1938, and its structure was determined a year later. Niacin (vitamin B3) was isolated in 1867 but not identified as the anti-pellagra factor until 1937. As mentioned previously, vitamin B12 was not isolated until 1948, five years after another group of pharmaceutical scientists isolated folic acid. Biotin was first isolated in 1936, and its structure was elucidated in 1942. Many early vitamin pioneers won accolades for their work that spared millions of people from the ravages of debilitating and fatal deficiency diseases. From the 1920s until the mid-1960s,[16] Nobel Prizes were awarded to scientists who discovered, isolated, synthesized, or structurally characterized vitamins.

While Pauling was well aware of these developments in biochemistry and nutrition in the 1930s, his only relevant research in that era concerned the molecular structures of some carotenoids and the flavonoid anthocyanidin. In 1939, the year in which he published papers on hemoglobin, the structures of benzene and proteins, and *The Nature of the Chemical Bond*—the most cited scientific book of the 20th century and work for which he was awarded the 1954 Nobel Prize in Chemistry—Pauling published a quantum-mechanical explanation of the intense colors in flavonoids, carotenoids, and dyes,[15] as well as a discussion of the use of resonance theory to understand anthocyanidin and carotenoid structures.[16]

"A Theory of the Formation of Antibodies" followed in 1940, after which Pauling published papers with László Zechmeister on the structure of prolycopene, an isomer of lycopene obtained from the tangerine tomato, with comments on the structural characteristics of lutein, zeaxanthin, and the carotenes, among other isomers.[17,18] However, Pauling's interest in these carotenoids and flavonoids was confined to their chemical structures and the influence of structure on optical properties; he did not address their health functions.

In 1941 Pauling was diagnosed with Bright's disease, or glomerulonephritis, which was at the time an often-fatal kidney disorder. On the advice of physicians at the Rockefeller Institute, he went to San Francisco for treatment by Thomas Addis, an innovative Stanford nephrologist. Addis prescribed a diet low in salt and protein, plenty of water, and supplementary vitamins and minerals that Pauling followed for nearly 14 years and completely recovered. This was dramatic firsthand experience of the therapeutic value of the diet.

Revelations

When Pauling cast about for a new research direction in the 1950s, he realized that mental illness was a significant public health problem that had not been sufficiently addressed by scientists. Perhaps his mother's megaloblastic madness and premature death caused by B12 deficiency underlay this interest. At about this time, Pauling's eldest son, Linus Jr., began a residency in psychiatry, which undoubtedly prompted Pauling to consider the nature of mental illness. Thanks to funding from the Ford Foundation, Pauling investigated the role of enzymes in brain function but made little progress. When he came across a copy of *Niacin Therapy in Psychiatry* (1962) by Abram Hoffer in 1965, Pauling was astonished to learn that simple substances needed in minute amounts to prevent deficiency diseases could have therapeutic application in unrelated diseases when given in very large amounts. This serendipitous and key event was critically responsible for Pauling's seminal paper in his emergent medical field. Later, Pauling was especially excited by Hoffer's observations on the survival of patients with advanced cancer who responded well to his micronutrient and dietary regimen, originally formulated to help schizophrenics manage their illness.[19,20] The regimen includes large doses of B vitamins, vitamin C, vitamin E, beta-carotene, selenium, zinc, and other micronutrients. About 40 percent of patients treated adjunctively with Hoffer's regimen lived, on average, five or more years, and about 60 percent survived four times longer than controls. These results were even better than those achieved by Scottish surgeon Ewan Cameron, Pauling's close clinical collaborator, in Scotland.

After a long and extremely productive career at Caltech, Pauling left under political pressure in late 1963 after winning the Nobel Peace Prize for his efforts to ban the atmospheric testing of nuclear weapons. Following a short tenure in the Center for the Study of Democratic Institutions in Santa Barbara, California, Pauling became professor of chemistry at the University of California, San Diego, in 1967. Two years later, he accepted an appointment as professor of chemistry in Stanford University in Palo Alto, where he remained through 1973. His ideas about orthomolecular medicine had been incubated at a number of institutions over the course of over 15 years, but it wasn't until he and two colleagues founded the independent Institute of Orthomolecular Medicine, shortly renamed the Linus Pauling Institute of Science and Medicine, in 1973 that they began to flourish. Stanford had provided an academic base while Pauling continued to develop his arguments for supplemental vitamin C, culminating in an important paper, "Evolution and the Need for Ascorbic Acid," published in the *Proceedings of the National Academy of Sciences USA* in 1970 and a book, *Vitamin C and the Common Cold*, also published in 1970, that won the Phi Beta Kappa Award as the best science book of the year and sold well. The Institute remained his base until his death in 1994.

Pauling's fascination with his favorite molecule —vitamin C—led to numerous papers and was the focus of hundreds of his speeches from the 1960s until his death. Pauling was stimulated to think deeply about vitamin C after being contacted by Irwin Stone in 1966. Stone had been in the audience in 1966 when Pauling gave a talk at the reception for his acceptance of the Carl Neuberg Society for International Scientific Relations Medal in New York City.[21] In his speech, Pauling remarked that he hoped and expected to live a long time. Stone wrote to Pauling about hypoascorbemia and suggested that he might well live for a longtime, perhaps enjoying another 50 years of good health, by taking supplemental vitamin C. In his reply to Stone, Pauling cited his 1962 paper with Austrian-American biologist Emile Zuckerkandl on molecular diseases in which they argued that the loss of the endogenous synthesis of a vitamin can be considered to be a molecular disease, corrected by a palliative diet.[22]

Pauling reviewed the evidence supplied by Stone and decided to take 3,000 mg of vitamin C per day, partly for optimum health and partly to prevent the serious colds that had afflicted him for many years, seriously interfering with his work. His wife, Ava Helen, also began to take supplemental vitamin C, and both reported better health and a greatly reduced incidence of colds, in accord with the scant clinical literature. Pauling was so impressed that he decided to write a book on the use of vitamin C to prevent and treat the common cold. The book was also a response to a letter from a critic, Victor Herbert, who complained about "vitamin hucksters" and challenged Pauling on statements he made in a talk at the dedication of the Mt. Sinai Medical School in 1968 on the efficacy of vitamin C in preventing and ameliorating colds.[23] Herbert asked for evidence from properly controlled trials, and Pauling discussed evidence from four such trials in his book.

In a new edition of that book, *Vitamin C, the Common Cold, and the Flu*, published in 1976, Pauling added material on influenza, especially concerning the work of Claus Jungeblut and Akira Murata on the inactivation of viruses by vitamin C and the work of Murata, Frederick Klenner, Fukimi Morishige, and others on the prophylactic and therapeutic effect of vitamin C in viral diseases.[24] Pauling noted that in 1935 Jungeblut was the first to report that high-dose vitamin C inactivates polio, and he was intrigued by Klenner's use of very high-dose vitamin C, usually given intravenously, to treat viral diseases like hepatitis, poliomyelitis, and pneumonia, and toxicological conditions like venomous snake bites. Klenner had published his work in regional medical journals since 1948.

In the late 1980s, Pauling's attention returned to infectious disease and vitamin C. On the basis of in vitro and clinical evidence, he and his associates argued that vitamin C should be used in conjunction with newly introduced antiviral drugs like AZT (azidothymidine), which prevents the de novo (repeat) infection of cells, to inhibit replication of HIV and prevent the formation of abnormal giant T lymphocytes called syncytia, which are markers of viral infectivity and cytopathology.[25] Pauling and Cameron completed a draft of a new book, never published, on vitamin C and AIDS.

Szent-Györgyi and Pauling shared the opinion that the optimum intake of vitamin C is much larger than the RDA, the daily amount set by the Food and Nutrition Board to prevent scurvy. Pauling wrote to Szent-Györgyi in 1970, asking about Stone's ideas. Szent-Györgyi replied:

> As to ascorbic acid, right from the beginning I felt that the medical profession misled the public. If you don't take ascorbic acid with your food you get scurvy, so the medical profession said that if you don't get scurvy you are all right. I think that this is a very grave error. Scurvy is not the first sign of the deficiency but a premortal syndrome, and for full health you need much more, very much more . . . there is an enormous scattering in the need of vitamins and it is quite easily believable that many diseases which have not been connected until now with vitamins are really expressions of a lack of vitamins.[26]

Robert F. Cathcart, an orthopedic surgeon in California, read Pauling's book on vitamin C and the common cold in 1971 and began taking large doses of vitamin C to prevent colds from developing. Based on his success, he treated patients with high-dose oral vitamin C and observed the "bowel tolerance" threshold effect, which refers to a laxative function of high-dose vitamin C that depends on the health status of the subject.[27] Cathcart used this observation to titrate the therapeutic dose of vitamin C. A study suggested that vitamin C, by stimulating the cystic fibrosis transmembrane conductance regulator (CFTR), increases fluid secretion in epithelial cells, such as those found in the lung and intestine.[28] This may account for the observed laxative effect and could be variable depending on the individual's health status.

Pauling's public celebrity became increasingly associated with the advocacy of high-dose vitamin C to prevent and treat infectious diseases, even though he continued to work productively for the rest of his life on theoretical problems in chemistry and physics, notably his closed-pack spheron theory of atomic nuclei, as well as on solving chemical structures of organic and inorganic substances. Of course, he also continued to honor a commitment to his wife and himself to advocate for peace among nations at every opportunity.

A collaboration with Cameron on the adjunctive use of high-dose oral and intravenous vitamin C in advanced cancer that began in 1971 continued until Cameron's death in 1991. Cameron had written a book, *Hyaluronidase and Cancer,* in 1966 about the quest for a physiological hyaluronidase inhibitor (PHI) that would interfere with the action of the enzyme hyaluronidase in attacking hyaluronic acid in the ground substance that permits the growth of tumors.[29] Such a strategy might enhance "host resistance" to cancer and slow the growth of solid tumors, making cancer a manageable disease. Cameron read about Pauling's statements on the putative value of vitamin C in controlling cancer and wrote to him in 1971.[30] Cameron began to give his patients hospitalized with advanced cancer about 10,000 mg of vitamin C per day for about 10 days or longer, typically by slow-drip intravenous administration followed by oral dosage. Pauling and Cameron argued that vitamin C benefits cancer patients by stimulating the synthesis of a PHI or by being incorporated into one, augmenting the immune system, and optimizing collagen synthesis, thus encapsulating tumors and enhancing tissue integrity.[31] Pauling also thought about the cytotoxicity (cell-killing ability) of vitamin C, involving copper and redox chemistry, as early as 1975[32] and in 1983 published a paper with Japanese colleagues implicating hydrogen peroxide as the cytotoxic molecular species, based on in vitro and animal studies. Despite repeated denials of federal grant requests over eight years, Pauling and his colleagues managed to publish scores of papers on vitamin C and cancer encompassing in vitro research, animal experiments, and clinical work. In 1979, he and Cameron published *Cancer and Vitamin C,* which remains in print in an expanded and updated edition.

"I am really impressed with the concern some scientists share over those 'dangerous' vitamins. I wish they were as worried over those dangerous poisons called drugs."
—ABRAM HOFFER

With funding from the National Cancer Institute, the Mayo Clinic conducted two randomized controlled trials of high-dose vitamin C and advanced cancer.[34,35] Both studies failed to demonstrate any benefit of supplemental vitamin C, which was given only orally and for a short period. Pauling, Cameron, and others noted serious methodological flaws in the Mayo studies, which have been amply discussed elsewhere.[36] In recent years, Mark Levine and colleagues in the NIH have studied the pharmacokinetics of vitamin C in young, healthy men and women.[37,38] Based on their results demonstrating dramatic differences in plasma concentration of vitamin C depending on the mode of administration—intravenous administration produces plasma levels of 14,000 micromoles per liter (umol/L) compared to about 220 umol/L with oral dosing—Levine considered the anticancer role of intravenous vitamin C,[39] extensively used by Cameron, and by Hugh Riordan and colleagues.[40] He published several papers showing that, with high concentrations attained by intravenous infusion, the ascorbate radical is formed in the extracellular milieu around cancer cells, helping to generate hydrogen peroxide that then diffuses into malignant cells, inducing apoptosis (cell death) and pyknosis (cell degeneration), and disrupting mitochondrial function (the energy-producing function of the cell).[41] This activity is selective—normal cells are unaffected—and appears to be dependent on the presence of an unidentified small molecular weight protein. Other recent papers have reported that vitamin C modulates hypoxia-inducible factor-1 (HIF-1), a transcription factor induced by hypoxia in cancer cells.[42,43] Vitamin C inhibits HIF-1 induction and related gene expression, resulting in decreased growth of tumor cells. It's possible that multiple mechanisms are involved in the anticancer effect of vitamin C and, based on Cameron's results with oral vitamin C, that some types of cancer may be more therapeutically sensitive to vitamin C. Fortunately, interest in this area has been renewed.[44]

In the late 1980s, Pauling's renewed friendship with a German cardiologist led to the formulation of a novel hypothesis on the possible cause of atherosclerosis: lipoprotein(a), a major constituent of atherosclerotic plaque, serves as a surrogate for vitamin C in chronic vitamin C insufficiency.[45] A number of related concepts were derived from this putative surrogacy, including the role of lysine and vitamin C in ameliorating exercise-induced severe angina pectoris in patients with advanced heart disease. Indeed, Pauling wrote three case reports in the early 1990s that discussed such relief associated with the use of 3,000–6,000 mg per day each of lysine and vitamin C.[46–48]

Clinical studies in recent years have repeatedly demonstrated that high-dose vitamin C promotes relaxation of the arteries and improves blood flow—reversing endothelial dysfunction (poor blood vessel tone) in patients with heart disease or diabetes[49,50] probably by stabilizing or increasing tetrahydrobiopterin, a molecule involved in nitric oxide synthesis.[51] Other clinical studies have shown that high-dose vitamin C reduces systolic blood pressure in hypertensive subjects by about 10 points.[52] Of course, none of these beneficial effects are directly related to the classic role of vitamin C as a vitamin in preventing scurvy by promoting collagen synthesis.

The Work Continues—A Brief Survey

We have witnessed an explosion in research in orthomolecular medicine in the last 40 years. Nutritional epidemiological studies, mainly observational studies, have reported associations between many dietary factors and the risk for disease, and these initial associations have been followed up by biochemical and molecular biological studies to determine the substances and molecular mechanisms responsible for the putative benefits. While nutritional epidemiological studies do not prove a causal relationship, they do suggest possibly fruitful areas for further research. Foremost among epidemiological studies in the United States are the Nurses' Health Study I, organized in 1976 with 122,000 women; the Nurses' Health Study II, established in 1989 with 117,000 women; and the Health Professionals Follow-up Study, organized in 1986 with about 51,500 men. Subjects report periodically on their diet and health using food-frequency and health-status questionnaires, and some biological samples such as toenail clippings, blood, and urine have been collected. Compliance has been extremely good, with about a 90 percent response rate, and the value of the food frequency and health questionnaires has been generally verified,[53] although many scientists remain skeptical of associations derived from observational studies. One of the outcomes of the Nurses' Health Study has been the discovery of the strong association between the intake of trans fat and coronary heart disease, which has led to the reduction of trans fat in the American diet through labeling and food industry practices. In the Netherlands, the work of Martijn Katan, has been equally important in this area.[54] Other large nutritional epidemiological studies have been organized, including the Netherlands Cohort Study (121,000 men and women, begun in 1986) and the European Prospective Investigation into Cancer and Nutrition (EPIC) study (440,000 men and women, begun in 1993), which found a link between the consumption of red meat and colorectal cancer, as well as myriad other findings, such as impressive inverse relationships between plasma vitamin C and all-cause mortality[55] or risk of stroke.[56]

Reports from these large-scale studies and others have identified associations between the consumption or avoidance of certain foods and supplements with disease risk, and scientific reductionism and biological plausibility have prompted the investigation of dietary constituents putatively responsible for the observed effects. Ellagic acid and anthocyanidins in berries; flavonoids like catechins in tea and chocolate and others in fruit and vegetables; isothiocyanates, including sulforaphane and indole-3-carbinol from cruciferous vegetables; resveratrol in wine, grapes, and peanuts; chlorophyll and its derivative, chlorophyllin; carotenoids like lutein and lycopene; allicin and its derivates from garlic; phytosterols; lignans; fiber; essential fatty acids; curcumin; and soy isoflavones are some of the dietary phytochemicals for which substantial literature has emerged in recent years. Research on the role of fish-derived omega-3 fatty acids in attenuating cardiovascular disease, inflammatory diseases, and mental illness has also been robust. The antioxidant function of flavonoids has been emphasized, but their poor absorption and rapid metabolism has led to the suggestion that fructose, not flavonoids, in ingested fruit increases the antioxidant capacity of plasma by stimulating the synthesis of uric acid, a strong physiological antioxidant, in the liver.[57] A new focus on the cell-signaling properties of flavonoids and transient antioxidants like alpha-lipoic acid has emerged.[58] The Micronutrient Information Center on the Linus Pauling Institute website provides a resource for updated and comprehensive information on micronutrients, phytochemicals, and other dietary substances, and their roles in health and disease (http://lpi.oregon state.edu/infocenter).

Interest in improving health span by dietary strategies has also accelerated, leading to remarkable studies with acetyl-L-carnitine and lipoic acid. Supplementation with these compounds has increased ambulatory activity and cognitive performance in old rats and old dogs, suggesting that they may be useful in slowing or even reversing age-related deficits inhumans.[59,60] Mitochondrial dysfunction, caused partly by oxidative damage and inflammation, has been implicated in neurodegenerative diseases, such as Parkinson's, amyotrophic lateral sclerosis (ALS), and Alzheimer's, as well as in age-related decline, and therapeutic efficacy for coenzyme Q10, lipoic acid, and other antioxidants has been suggested.[61,62]

Vitamin D is critical for cell differentiation, immune function, calcium utilization, and bone health, and it is required to prevent rickets and osteomalacia. A number of conditions, such as skin color, advanced age, fat malabsorption syndromes, obesity, and inflammatory bowel disease, are associated with increased risk for vitamin D deficiency. Concern about chronic suboptimum levels of vitamin D in northern latitudes, implicated in increased cancer risk, autoimmune disease, and osteoporosis, has prompted discussion of increasing the Adequate Intake, or AI (the recommended daily average intake when no RDA has been established). Clinical studies have also been conducted to determine if intervention with supplements identified by observational studies will attenuate disease risk.

In 1993, two prospective studies from the aforementioned epidemiological research showed that the intake of vitamin E supplements significantly reduced the risk for coronary heart disease in men and women.[63–64] While this had been common knowledge among those familiar with the Shute brothers' work in Canada and with Pauling's writings, the papers stimulated much clinical interest in high-dose vitamin E and heart disease, leading to several randomized controlled trials. Results have been inconsistent, possibly owing to insufficient dose and/or duration, inadequate instructions about how to take vitamin E with fat-containing food for sufficient absorption, and the polypharmacy of patients with heart disease. For example, investigators have speculated that vitamin E may induce drug-detoxifying enzymes in the liver that could interfere with the therapeutic efficacy of certain drugs.[65–66] Additionally, one recent study in hypercholesterolemic subjects found that oxidative stress, as measured by plasma F2-isoprostanes, was significantly suppressed (by 35 and 49 percent) only by daily doses of d-alpha-tocopherol of 1,600 international units (IU) or 3,200 IU, respectively, for at least 16 weeks.[67] Smaller daily doses (400 IU or 800 IU) resulted in non-statistically significant reductions in plasma F2-isoprostanes.

Recent studies have also identified in vitro and in vivo anti-inflammatory roles for gamma-tocopherol in alleviating oxidative and nitrative stress,[68,69] despite the more rapid metabolism and clearance of gamma-tocopherol compared to alpha-tocopherol,[70] for which a transport protein has been discovered. About 70 percent of the vitamin E intake in the United States is in the form of gamma-tocopherol. One recent review of the role of gamma-tocopherol in the prevention of heart disease and cancer noted that the results of prospective studies of gamma-tocopherol and the risk for heart disease are inconsistent, but some evidence suggests that high plasma gamma-tocopherol levels are associated with a decreased risk for prostate cancer.[71] The media have compounded confusion about vitamin E and heart disease by not carefully distinguishing primary prevention trials in which subjects at baseline have not manifested heart disease from secondary prevention trials in which patients with heart disease have been supplemented with micronutrients to determine if supplementation decreases clinical events like myocardial infarction, stroke, or death.

Cellular transport mechanisms for vitamin C— the sodium vitamin C transporters (SVCT 1 and 2)—have been discovered in recent years.[72] Dehydroascorbic acid (DHA) and glucose are facilitatively transported by GLUT1, GLUT3, and GLUT4.[73,74] DHA has a half-life of only about seven minutes, and its levels in plasma are about a thousandfold less than circulating glucose, so its uptake is likely to be competitively inhibited by glucose.[75] Ascorbic acid, on the other hand, is actively transported by the SVCT proteins, and the activity of one, SCVT1, declines with age,[75] suggesting that older people need higher intakes to maintain a plasma status similar to young people at lower intakes of vitamin C.[76] New biochemical functions have been reported for vitamin C, such as the ascorbylation reaction in which vitamin C combines with reactive aldehydes, potentially protecting biomolecules from damage.[77] Mechanistic and pharmacokinetic studies on vitamin C and vitamin E and their roles in disease prevention and treatment will continue to be further explored in the near future.

Nutritionally essential minerals, such as selenium, zinc, and magnesium, have also garnered attention after inverse associations with risk for disease, especially cancer, emerged from epidemiological studies. Deficiencies of selenium or zinc impair immune function and increase susceptibility to infectious diseases, including HIV/AIDS.[78–79] A long-term intervention trial found that daily supplementation with selenium-enriched yeast was associated with about a 50 percent reduction in prostate cancer incidence,[80] although the risk for non-melanoma skin cancer was increased by 25 percent.[81] In a large-scale randomized controlled trial, daily zinc supplements alone or in combination with antioxidant vitamins significantly reduced the risk for age-related macular degeneration by about 25 percent or more.[82] In another large-scale, long-term study, high-serum magnesium levels were associated with substantial decreases in all-cause mortality (40 percent), cardiovascular disease mortality (40 percent), and cancer mortality (50 percent), compared to low-serum magnesium.[83]

Over half of Americans appear to ingest less than the daily Estimated Average Requirement (EAR) for magnesium, and a significant percentage of premenopausal American women ingest less than the daily EAR for iron, which increases vulnerability for heme deficiency (a part of hemoglobin used to transport oxygen in blood) and anemia.[84] [Note: The EAR is considerably lower than the RDA; EAR intake is estimated to satisfy the needs of 50 percent of the people; the RDA, 97 percent.] From these studies we can ascertain with certainty that relationships between micronutrients are complex and, in many cases, poorly understood. It is also clear that many people do not have adequate intakes of vital micronutrients, resulting in poor health and increased risk for disease. There is much to learn about the optimum intake of specific micronutrients or combinations of micronutrients, and new emphasis on translational research and evidence-based medicine will continue to stimulate research. Uncertainties propel research forward, and the future of orthomolecular medicine is bright.

REFERENCES

1. Pauling L. Orthomolecular psychiatry. *Science* 1968;160:265–271.

2. Oken D. Vitamin therapy: treatment for the mentally ill. *Science* 1968;160:1181.

3. Pauling L. Letter. *Science* 1968;160:1181.

4. Desiraju G. The all-chemist. *Nature* 2000;408:407.

5. Pauling L. *Vitamin C and the Common Cold.* San Francisco: W. H. Freeman, 1970.

6. Pauling L, Itano H, Singer S, et al. Sickle cell anemia, a molecular disease. *Science* 1949; 110:543–548.

7. Ames B, Elson-Schwab I, Silver E. High-dose vitamin therapy stimulates variant enzymes with decreased coenzyme binding affinity (increased Km): relevance to genetic disease and polymorphisms. *Am J Clin Nutr* 2002;75:616–658.

8. Pauling L, Robinson A, Oxley S, et al. Results of a loading test of ascorbic acid, niacinamide, and pyridoxine in schizophrenic subjects and controls. In: Hawkins D and Pauling L, eds. *Orthomolecular Psychiatry.* San Francisco: W.H. Freeman, 1973, 18–34.

9. Pauling L. Some aspects of orthomolecular medicine. *J Intern Acad Prev Med* 1974;1:1–30.

10. Pauling L. *How to Live Longer and Feel Better.* New York: W.H. Freeman, 1986.

11. Pauling L. On the orthomolecular environment of the mind: orthomolecular theory. *Am J Psychiatry* 1974;131:1251–1257.

12. Pauling L. The future of the Crellin Laboratory. *Science* 1938;87:563–566.

13. Williams R. *Biochemical Individuality.* New York: John Wiley & Sons, 1956; 3.

14. Breakthrough of the year: human genetic variation. *Science* 2007;318:1842–1843.

15. Pauling L. A theory of the color of dyes. *Proc Natl Acad Sci* 1939;25:577–582.

16. Pauling L. Recent work on the configuration and electronic structure of molecules; with some applications to natural products. *Fortschr Chem organis Naturstoffe* 1939;3:203–235.

17. Zechmeister L, LeRosen A, Went F, et al. Prolycopene, a naturally occurring stereoisomer of lycopene. *Proc Natl Acad Sci* 1941;27:468–474.

18. Zechmeister L, LeRosen A, Schroeder W, et al. Spectral characteristics and configuration of some stereoisomeric carotenoids including prolycopene and pro-gamma-carotene. *J Am Chem Soc* 1943;65:1940–1951.

19. Hoffer A, Pauling L. Hardin Jones biostatistical analysis of mortality data for cohorts of cancer patients with a large fraction surviving at the termination of the study and a comparison of survival times of cancer patients receiving large regular oral doses of vitamin C and other nutrients with similar patients not receiving those doses. *J Orthomolecular Med* 1990;5:143–154.

20. Hoffer A, Pauling L. Hardin Jones biostatistical analysis of mortality data for a second set of cohorts of cancer patients with a large fraction surviving at the termination of the study and a comparison of survival times of cancer patients receiving large regular oral doses of vitamin C and other nutrients with similar patients not receiving those doses. *J Orthomolecular Med* 1993;8:157–167.

21. Stone I. Letter to L. Pauling, 4 April 1966.

22. Pauling L. Letter to I. Stone, July 1966.

23. Herbert V. Letter to L. Pauling, 11 November 1968.

24. Pauling L. *Vitamin C: The Common Cold, and the Flu.* San Francisco: W.H. Freeman & Co., 1976

25. Harakeh S, Jariwalla R, Pauling L. Suppression of human immunodeficiency virus replication by ascorbate in chronically and acutely infected cells. *Proc Natl Acad Sci USA* 1990;87:7245–7249.

26. Szent-Györgyi A. Letter to L. Pauling, 15 April 1970.

27. Cathcart R. Vitamin C, titrating to bowel tolerance, anascorbemia, and acute induced scurvy. *Med Hypotheses* 1981;7:1359–1376.

28. Fischer H, Schwarzer C, Illek B. Vitamin C controls the cystic fibrosis transmembrane conductance regulator chloride channel. *Proc Natl Acad Sci USA*, 2004;101:3691–3696.

29. Cameron E. *Hyaluronidase and Cancer.* Oxford: Pergamon Press, 1966.

30. Cameron E. Letter to L. Pauling, 30 November 1971.

31. Cameron E, Pauling L. Ascorbic acid and the glycosaminoglycans. *Oncology* 1973; 27:181–192.

32. Pauling L. *Letter to E. Cameron,* 19 August 1975.

33. Kimoto E, Tanaka H, Gyotoku J, et al. Enhancement of antitumor activity of ascorbate against Ehrlich ascites tumor cells by the copper: glycylglycylhistidine complex. *Cancer Res* 1983; 43:824–828.

34. Creagan E, Moertel C, O'Fallon J, et al. Failure of high-dose vitamin C (ascorbic acid) therapy to benefit patients with advanced cancer. A controlled trial. *N Engl J Med* 1979;301:687–690.

35. Moertel C, Fleming T, Creagan E, et al. High-dose vitamin C versus placebo in the treatment of patients with advanced cancer who have had no prior chemotherapy: a randomized double-blind comparison. *N Engl J Med* 1985;312:137–141.

36. Richards E. *Vitamin C and Cancer: Medicine or Politics?* New York: St. Martin's Press, 1991.

37. Levine M, Conry-Cantilena C, Wang Y, et al. Vitamin C pharmacokinetics in healthy volunteers: evidence for a recommended dietary allowance. *Proc Natl Acad Sci USA* 1996;93:3704–3709.

38. Levine M, Wang Y, Padayatty S, et al. A new recommended dietary allowance of vitamin C for healthy young women. *Proc Natl Acad Sci USA* 2001;98:9842–9846.

39. Padayatty S, Sun H, Wang Y, et al. Vitamin C pharmacokinetics: implications for oral and intravenous use. *Ann Intern Med* 2004;140:533–537.

40. Riordan H, Hunninghake R, Riordan N, et al. Intravenous ascorbic acid: protocol for its application and use. *P R Health Sci J* 2003;22:287–290.

41. Chen Q, Espey M, Sun A, et al. Ascorbate in pharmacologic concentrations selectively generates ascorbate radical and hydrogen peroxide in extracellular fluid in vivo. *Proc Natl Acad Sci USA* 2007;104:8749–8754.

42. Vissers M, Gunningham S, Morrison M, et al. Modulation of hypoxia-inducible factor-1 alpha in cultured primary cells by intracellular ascorbate. *Free Radic Biol Med* 2007;42:765–772.

43. Gao P, Zhang H, Dinavahi R, et al. HIF-dependent antitumorigenic effect of antioxidants in vivo. *Cancer Cell* 2007;12:230–238.

44. Riordan H, Casciari J, Gonzalez M, et al. A pilot clinical study of continuous intravenous ascorbate in terminal cancer patients. *P R Health Sci J* 2005;24:269–276.

45. Rath M, Pauling L. Hypothesis: lipoprotein(a) is a surrogate for ascorbate. *Proc Natl Acad Sci USA* 1990;87:6204–6207.

46. Pauling L. Case report: lysine/ascorbate-related amelioration of angina pectoris. *J Orthomolecular Med* 1991;6:144–146.

47. McBeath M, Pauling L. A case history: lysine/ascorbate-related amelioration of angina pectoris. *J Orthomolecular Med* 1993;8:77–78.

48. Pauling L. Third case report on lysine-ascorbate amelioration of angina pectoris. *J Orthomolecular Med* 1993;8:137–138.

49. Frei B. On the role of vitamin C and other antioxidants in atherogenesis and vascular dysfunction. *Proc Soc Exp Biol Med* 1999;222:196–204.

50. Gokce N, Keaney J, Frei B, et al. Long-term ascorbic acid administration reverses endothelial vasomotor dysfunction in patients with coronary artery disease. *Circulation* 1999;99:3234–3240.

51. Huang A, Vita J, Venema R, et al. Ascorbic acid enhances endothelial nitric-oxide synthase activity by increasing intracellular tetrahydrobiopterin. *J Bio Chem* 2000;275:17399–17406.

52. Duffy S, Gokce N, Holbrook E, et al. Treatment of hypertension with ascorbic acid. *Lancet* 1999;354:2048–2049.

53. Willett W, Sampson L, Browne M, et al. The use of a self-administered questionnaire to assess diet four years in the past. *Am J Epidemiol* 1988;127:188–199.

54. Mensink R, Katan M. Effect of dietary trans fatty acids on high-density and low-density lipoprotein cholesterol levels in healthy subjects. *N Engl J Med* 1990;323:439–445.

55. Khaw K, Bingham S, Welch A, et al. Relation between plasma ascorbic acid and mortality in men and women in EPIC-Norwalk prospective study: a prospective population study. *Lancet* 2001;357:657–663.

56. Myint P, Luben R, Welch A, et al. Plasma vitamin C concentrations predict risk of incident stroke over 10 y in 20,649 participants of the European Prospective Investigation into Cancer–Norfolk prospective population study. *Am J Clin Nutr* 2008;87:64–69.

57. Lotito S, Frei B. The increase in human plasma antioxidant capacity after apple consumption is due to the metabolic effect of fructose on urate, not apple-derived antioxidant flavonoids. *Free Radic Biol Med* 2004;37:251–258.

58. Suh J, Shenvi S, Dixon B, et al. Decline in transcriptional activity of Nrf2 causes age-related loss of glutathione synthesis, which is reversible with lipoic acid. *Proc Natl Acad Sci USA* 2004;101:3381–3386.

59. Hagen T, Liu J, Lykkesfeldt J, et al. Feeding acetyl-L-carnitine and lipoic acid to old rats significantly improves metabolic function while decreasing oxidative stress. *Proc Natl Acad Sci USA* 2002;99:1870–1875.

60. Milgram N, Araujo J, Hagen T, et al. Acetyl-L carnitine and alpha-lipoic acid supplementation of aged beagle dogs improves learning in two landmark discrimination tests. *FASEB J* 2007;13:3756–3762.

61. Lin M, Beal M. Mitochondrial dysfunction and oxidative stress in neurodegenerative diseases. *Nature* 2006;443:787–795.

62. Rodriguez M, MacDonald J, Mahoney D, et al. Beneficial effects of creatine, CoQ10, and lipoic acid in mitochondrial disorders. *Muscle Nerve* 2007;35:235–242.

63. Stampfer M, Hennekens C, Manson J, et al. Vitamin E consumption and the risk of coronary disease in women. *N Eng J Med,* 1993;328:1444–1449.

64. Rimm E, Stampfer M, Ascherio A, et al. Vitamin E consumption and the risk of coronary disease in men. *N Eng J Med* 1993;328:1450–1456.

65. Brigelius-Flohe R. Vitamin E and drug metabolism. *Biochem Biophys Res Commun* 2003;305:737–740.

66. Traber M. Vitamin E, nuclear receptors and xenobiotic metabolism. *Arch Biochem Biophys* 2004;423:6–11.

67. Roberts II L, Oates J, Linton M, et al. The relationship between dose of vitamin E and suppression of oxidative stress in humans. *Free Radic Biol Med* 2007;43:1388–1393.

68. Jiang Q, Elson-Schwab I, Courtemanche, et al. gamma-Tocopherol and its major metabolite, in contrast to alpha-tocopherol, inhibit cyclooxygenase activity in macrophages and epithelial cells. *Proc Natl Acad Sci USA* 2000;97:11494–11499.

69. Devaraj S, Leonard S, Traber M, et al. Gamma-tocopherol supplementation alone and in combination with alpha-tocopherol alters biomarkers of oxidative stress and inflammation in subjects with metabolic syndrome. *FreeRadic Biol Med* 2008;44:1203–1208.

70. Leonard S, Paterson E, Atkinson J, et al. Studies in humans using deuterium-labeled alpha and gamma-tocopherols demonstrate faster plasma gamma-tocopherol disappearance and greater gamma-metabolite production. *Free Radic Biol Med* 2005;38:857–866.

71. Dietrich M, Traber M, Jacques P, et al. Does gamma-tocopherol play a role in the primary prevention of heart disease and cancer? A review. *J Am Coll Nutr,* 2006;25:292–299.

72. Daruwala R, Song J, Koh W, et al. Cloning and functional characterization of the human sodium-dependent vitamin C transporters hSVCT1 and hSVCT2. *FEBS Lett* 1999;460:480–484.

73. Rumsey S, Kwon O, Xu G, et al. Glucose transporter isoforms GLUT1 and GLUT3 transport dehydroascorbic acid. *J Biol Chem* 1997;272:18982–18989.

74. Rumsey S, Daruwala R, Al-Hasani H, et al. Dehydroascorbic acid transport by GLUT4 in Xenopus oocytes and isolated rat adipocytes. *J Biol Chem* 2000;275:28246–28253.

75. Michels A, Hagen T. Vitamin C status declines with age. In: Asard H, May J, and Smirnoff N, eds. *Vitamin C.* New York: Garland Science/BIOS Scientific Publishers, 2004;203–227.

76. Brubacher D, Moser U, Jordan P. Vitamin C concentrations in plasma as a function of intake: a meta-analysis. *Int J Vitam Nutr Res* 2000;70:226–237.

77. Sowell J, Conway H, Bruno R, et al. Ascorbylated4-hydroxy-2-nonenal as a potential biomarker of oxidative stress response. *J Chromatogr B Analyt Technol Biomed Life Sci* 2005;827:139–145.

78. Shankar A, Prasad A. Zinc and immune function: the biological basis of altered resistance to infection. *Am J Clin Nutr* 1998;68:447S-463S.

79. Baum M, Campa A. Role of selenium in HIV/AIDS. In: Hatfield D, Berry M, and Gladyshev V, eds. *Selenium: Its Molecular Biology and Role in Human Health.* 2nd ed. New York: Springer, 2006;299–310.

80. Duffield-Lillico A, Dalkin B, Reid M, et al. Selenium supplementation, baseline plasma selenium status and incidence of prostate cancer: an analysis of the complete treatment period of the Nutritional Prevention of Cancer Trial. *BJU Int* 2003;91:608–612.

81. Duffield-Lillico A, Slate E, Reid M, et al. Selenium supplementation and secondary prevention of nonmelanoma skin cancer in a randomized trial. *J Natl Cancer Inst* 2003;95:1477–1481.

82. A randomized, placebo-controlled, clinical trial of high-dose supplementation with vitamins C and E, beta carotene, and zinc for age-related macular degeneration and vision loss: AREDS report no. 8. *Arch Ophthalmol* 2001;119:1417–1436.

83. Leone L, Courbon D, Ducimetiere P, et al. Zinc, copper, and magnesium and risks for all-cause, cancer, and cardiovascular mortality. *Epidemiology* 2006;17:308–314.

84. Moshfegh A, Goldman J, Cleveland L. What we eat in America, NHANES 2001–2002: usual nutrient intakes from food compared to dietary reference intakes. USDA Agricultural Research Service, 2005.

SIDE EFFECTS OF OVER-THE-COUNTER DRUGS
by Abram Hoffer, MD, PhD

Every doctor has learned the Hippocratic oath, the most well-known and most important ethical rule in medicine: *Primum non nocere* ("Above all, do no harm"). This is the physician's first rule: a treatment prescribed to a patient must not harm the patient. It does not say harm should be relative, although that is how the rule is interpreted. It does make the point that the harm, ideally, should be as little as is humanly possible. Paracelsus, founder of the discipline of toxicology, wrote, *Sola dosis facit venenum* ("The dose makes the poison"). In other words, too much of anything will hurt you. For centuries, this has precipitated the question, How much is too much? Any discussion of side effects or of toxic reactions without specifying the doses is meaningless, for at zero levels nothing is toxic and at sufficiently high levels everything is toxic, including oxygen and water.

"Acceptable" Side Effects
Over-the-counter (OTC) drugs are considered much safer than prescription drugs. That is why they are more freely available. Acetylsalicylic acid, also called aspirin, is the most popular OTC drug and most often recommended by doctors. It is effective in dealing with heart disease, for arthritis, perhaps inhibiting colon cancer,

and for headaches. I have selected this OTC drug not because I disapprove of it but to illustrate what is considered acceptable for OTC drugs. Here are some of the official warnings from the medical literature and the drug companies that are listed for aspirin.[1]

- **Fluid and electrolyte effects.** Increased metabolic rate, pyrexia (fever), tachypnea (rapid breathing), and vomiting lead to fluid loss and dehydration. Compensation for respiratory alkalosis leads to increased renal excretion of bicarbonate and increased excretion of sodium and potassium. Because of significant water losses, hyponatremia (low blood sodium) might not be present; however, hypokalemia (low blood potassium) is prominent.

- **Central nervous system (CNS) effects.** Toxic effects in the CNS range from mild confusion to coma. The exact mechanism that produces CNS toxicity is not known, but the degree of CNS effects, as well as overall mortality, correlates with the concentration of salicylates in brain tissue. Acidemia (low blood pH) increases the non-ionized form of salicylates, allowing for movement across the blood-brain barrier and, therefore, increasing CNS toxicity.

- **Gastrointestinal (GI) effects.** Salicylate ingestion can cause nausea, vomiting, and abdominal pain. Vomiting is produced by salicylate stimulation of medullary chemoreceptors and by local irritation of the GI tract. Upper GI ulceration and bleeding can occur. Gastrointestinal effects are much more prominent in acute ingestion.

- **Ototoxicity.** Salicylate toxicity results in a reversible ototoxicity characterized by tinnitus, deafness, and dizziness.

- **Pulmonary effects.** Non-cardiogenic pulmonary edema is the most common cause of major morbidity and might be related to an increase in permeability of pulmonary vasculature caused by salicylates. Acute respiratory distress syndrome (ARDS) is more prominent in chronic ingestions than in acute ingestions.

- **Hematological effects.** Salicylates inhibit vitamin K-dependent synthesis of coagulation factors II, VII, IX, and X, leading to a prolonged prothrombin (clotting) time. Salicylates prolong bleeding time by inhibiting a prostaglandin-initiated sequence required for platelet aggregation.

- **Hepatic (liver) effects.** Dose-dependent hepatotoxicity can occur with salicylate poisoning. A small percentage of patients might develop hepatitis, but the majority will have asymptomatic elevation of transaminases (an indicator of liver damage).

- **Renal effects.** Acute renal failure has been reported rarely.

- **Mortality/morbidity.** Mortality rates vary with chronicity of exposure. Chronic toxicity carries a higher morbidity and mortality rate than acute toxicity and is more difficult to treat.

- **Acute overdose.** Mortality rate of less than 2 percent.

- **Chronic overdose.** Mortality rate as high as 25 percent.

Use with Caution

Azer and others[2] used more than 11 pages of printed material to describe the toxicity of aspirin including treatment information and medical care. And these are the side effects, toxic reactions, contraindications, and warnings that have to be studied before taking just this one very popular OTC drugs. None of the vitamins have side effects and toxic reactions remotely similar to this.

It is clear that drugs allowed to be sold over the counter have to be used with caution because they are xenobiotic (substances foreign to the body). Xenobiotics interfere with reactions in the body and often suppress some reactions, but because they are foreign they must be converted to less toxic substances and then excreted. If excretion is too slow the drug and its metabolic products will build up in the body. This is the reason they cause toxic reactions and within the recommended dose range can be, and often are, harmful. Within the recommended doses vitamins are safe.

REFERENCES

1. Medical Economics. *Physicians' Desk Reference 2002*. 56th ed. Oradell, NJ: Thomson, 2001.
2. Azer eMedicine.com. March 1, 2002.

From the *J Orthomolecular Med* 2003;18(3&4):169–172.

PANDEFICIENCY DISEASE
by Abram Hoffer, MD, PhD

Diagnosis classifies disease for two reasons: 1) to improve prognosis, and 2) to improve treatment. Prognosis is very important so patients and family can prepare for the future especially if the future is very dim. Estimating when a person will die may be extremely important for all sorts of reasons. Before specific treatment was discovered doctors were judged on their ability to prognose correctly. It would be very bad for the physician's reputation if his or her prognosis were wrong. Many years ago when I started to practice, some of my patients, while giving me their history, would tell me that their doctor had told them they would die but the doctor died before they did. Good doctors were good prognosticators and this depended upon accurate diagnosis. Diagnosis became even more important when specific treatment was discovered. Diagnosis advised the clinician what treatment to use. It was assumed that patients with the same diagnosis would respond to similar treatment, which had already been described by other doctors.

I had pneumonia in my early teens. Our friendly family doctor (he was also surgeon, emergency doctor, obstetrician, etc., as he was the only one in the community) told mother I had pneumonia and ordered mustard plasters (a poultice of mustard seed). It must have been very effective or else my pneumonia was very mild as I was well in a couple of days. That was standard treatment for a disease that killed a large proportion of its victims. This diagnosis was a descriptive diagnosis. By listening to my chest the doctor discovered something wrong and it was most likely pneumonia. No other diagnostic tests were available.

After it was discovered that many lung lesions were possible, it became necessary to distinguish one from another. Was it bacterial and if so which bacteria: staph or strep? Was it cancer or silica or tuberculosis? Specific laboratory tests are used. Diagnosis is now etiologic; it is based on the cause of the condition. Until the causal diagnosis is made, the treatment cannot be very successful. This is the pathway diagnosis has traveled, from description of the site, the organ, and later to the cause when known. If the cause remains unknown, the diagnosis remains descriptive. Psychiatric diagnosis is almost entirely descriptive.

Deficiency Disease

Clinical or descriptive diagnosis is not very accurate. It depends too much on the orientation and skill of the clinician, and surprises are common. Disease caused by one factor can take a variety of expressions. This means that the descriptive principle of classification cannot be used. A perfect example is pellagra.

Pellagra is a classical deficiency disease caused by a deficiency of niacin (vitamin B3) in food. But pellagra's expression is so varied that one can only with difficulty visualize it as one disease. Classical pellagra expresses itself in major skin lesions, gastrointestinal changes, mental changes, and death—known collectively as the four Ds. The pellagrous skin varies enormously and even today expert dermatologists fail to recognize it. It does not by itself point to the cause. The gastrointestinal symptoms might need the diagnostic skills of a gastroenterologist and the psychiatric manifestations might need the skills of a psychiatrist. During the great pellagra pandemic over 100 years ago in the United States, one-third of the patients in the southeast mental hospitals in some years were psychotic and could not be distinguished from schizophrenics. When niacin and/or niacinamide (both forms of vitamin B3) became available, it became simple: if one suspected pellagra (and that was natural in the pandemic areas), one needed only to give the patients niacin. If they were pellagrin they would recover, sometimes quickly, sometimes it would take much longer. For a physician not familiar with this major disease, it would be almost impossible to accept that these conditions could be caused by a lack of only one factor. Doctors specializing in pellagra

From the *J Orthomolecular Med* 2008;23(1):29–40.

were known as pellagrologists. We still do not have a laboratory test for it. Blood assays for this vitamin will not reveal it until patients are close to the fourth D of pellagra—death.

Saccharine Disease

During World War II, Surgeon Captain T. L. Cleave was concerned about the physical ill health of many of the sailors. From his studies, he concluded that most of them were suffering from one disease over all others, which he called "saccharine disease." In 1966, he wrote a book also called *The Saccharine Disease*. I had a copy of his original publication but it was worn out by constant use. This book turned my life around. Because of it, I became a full-time nutritionist. In it, Dr. Cleave showed convincing evidence that increases in diabetes, coronary disease, obesity, malabsorption of nutrients, peptic ulcer, constipation, hemorrhoids, varicose veins, kidney stones, dental caries, and many skin conditions and infections such as appendicitis, cholecystitis, pyelitis, and diverticulitis could be traced to the modern diet. This nutritional disease affected all the organs and systems, which were then diagnosed according to the organ or malfunction of that organ. The cause was a diet that was too rich in sugars and refined carbohydrates and too deficient in food containing its original fiber. The diet typically consisted of refined cereals devoid of their bran and germ such as white bread, polished rice, plus a heavy intake of sugar averaging about 125 pound per person each year. The diet is also deficient in vitamins, minerals, and essential fatty acids (EFAs), but Cleave did not consider the role played by the deficiency of essential nutrient factors. He emphasized an excessive intake of sugar and a deficiency of fiber as the two main problems.

The massive evidence Cleave discussed had little impact except for a sudden interest in bran, as if it were a drug especially designed for people with constipation. Cleave did give his sailors bran but he was much more concerned with the white flour they were eating. His message was clear that what was needed was the original whole-grain cereals as in whole wheat and rice. Just adding bran provided a partial answer. In 1972, Professor John Yudkin published his book *Sweet and Dangerous*. He presented the evidence that proved sugars were the culprit. His work was ignored.

In contrast, in 1953, Professor Ancel Keys, best known for the so-called Seven Countries study, found a negative correlation between fat intake and cardiovascular disease. Professor Keys had looked up the statistics of over 20 countries that had records of their fat intake and the incidence of heart disease. He selected a third (seven) of the countries that fit the correlation he had in mind, and showed that the countries with the highest fat intake had the highest incidence of heart disease. Later, however, when all the countries—including the ones he had not used—were looked at, the correlation disappeared. (Almost all the clinical studies show that the problem comes from the sugars and not from the fats.) But because Keys was so highly regarded and determined, his hypothesis swept the field. Food fats became the villains and medicine adopted a hypothesis that has been very detrimental ever since: the low-fat diet.

It was predicted with utmost confidence that switching away from meat and fats and replacing them with carbohydrates would solve most cardiovascular problems, such as heart disease, high cholesterol, obesity, and more. This view became the 10 commandments of modern nutrition and were enshrined in North America's food rules. However, the new diet and national food rules did not

"Each person must take an individualized program which they can discover if they are lucky to have a competent orthomolecular doctor. If they do not, they can read the literature and work out for themselves what is best for them. I believe the public is hungry for information. As more and more drugs drop by the wayside, the professions are going to become more and more dependent on safe ways of helping people, and using drugs is not the way to do that. Using nutrients is."—ABRAM HOFFER

eliminate disease. Instead, we have an even worse pandemic of obesity, cardiovascular disease, and a whole host of other conditions such as diabetes. The evidence is massive that the major villain was, and always will be, sugar and refined foods that are converted into sugar too quickly and absorbed too quickly. This is typically the modern high-tech diet, which is characterized by too much sugar and too little of all the other important nutrients. How could such a massive error be made and imposed on the whole world? In his book *Good Calories, Bad Calories* (2008), Gary Taube traces from the beginning the influences that led to this debacle.

How could this one explanation account for the amazing number of diseases? This is how: constipation is the main outcome of a diet deficient in fiber-rich foods, not in a simple deficiency of fiber. If it were a simple deficiency of fiber, one could eat fiber made from wood. This will certainly increase the fiber intake but will do little for one's health. Chronic constipation leads to other diseases of the intestines. In South Africa it was said you had be English to get appendicitis. The natives who still ate high-fiber foods did not. The remaining diseases came from the high-sugar intake. These are diabetes, coronary heart disease, and metabolic syndrome (a cluster of conditions including increased blood pressure, high blood sugar levels, excess belly, and high cholesterol levels).

Saccharine disease is also characterized by a deficiency in vitamins and minerals. The foods richest in these nutrients are not consumed. There is really no question about this, and it is well recognized by the government as well as by the public. If governments concluded that the diets were adequate, they would not have mandated the addition of nutrients to white flour. And I would not have gotten my first job as a control chemist in a flour mill. Vitamin C, thiamine (vitamin B1), riboflavin (vitamin B2), niacin (vitamin B3), vitamin D, iodine, and calcium are some of the nutrients that enrich our foods. The most striking example was the eradication of pellagra within two years in the United States after it mandated adding niacin to white flour in 1942.

In my book *Orthomolecular Nutrition* (1978), coauthored with Morton Walker, I describe some of the psychiatric symptoms associated with saccharine disease, with the excess sugar that helps to generate it, including anxiety and depression. The patients were referred to me by their family doctors because of these symptoms. When I first read about the role of hypoglycemia in causing mental disease, I was very skeptical but I was also curious. A young female was referred to me for depression. She told me that her main problem was that she was frigid. Psychoanalysis was riding high many years ago, and it occurred to me that she would be a perfect candidate for psychoanalysis or deep psychotherapy to explore why she was having this problem. However, since I felt it was unlikely that this was caused by hypoglycemia, she would be ideal to disprove its effect. I ordered the five-hour glucose tolerance test. The curve was typically hypoglycemic, to my surprise. Not expecting that it would help, I still advised her to avoid all sugar and to increase her intake of protein. To my amazement, she was normal in one month. I was now more interested than skeptical. I began to routinely have patients with anxiety and depression take the test, and found that over 75 percent had the typical abnormal glucose tolerance curves. I no longer remained skeptical. Since then I have placed every patient on a sugar-free and refined-carbohydrate-free diet without doing any more tests. The condition was present in every one of 300 alcoholics I treated. I did not realize it then, but sugar created disease by playing havoc with the metabolism of sugar, altering it up and down. Many patients are allergic to it. Other foods, like milk, to which patients are allergic, will also give the typical glucose tolerance curves. Over the years I concluded that if every doctor who referred their patients to me were to test them and treat them with the special diet first, I would lose half of my psychiatric practice.

Pandeficiency Disease

Cleave did not consider the fact that the saccharine disease diet was also deficient in the B vitamins. Nutritionists since then have ignored this, even though massive surveys have shown that it is impossible to obtain enough B vitamins with this diet. Nor did it occur to me until I had many more years of experience using large doses of the B vitamins. We treated schizophrenic patients with large doses of niacin and ascorbic acid. This treatment was based on our hypothesis that schizophrenia was caused by the excess conversion of adrenaline to adrenochrome, a toxic product of oxidation. We used niacin to decrease the formation of adrenaline and ascorbic acid to inhibit its oxidation. Other catecholamines could also be oxidized in the body due to superoxidative stress. Over the following years it became clear that many other diseases also responded to increased doses of some of the vitamins.

Eventually, my objective in treating patients changed. I no longer aimed at just curing their disease; I was now interested in much more. I planned on giving them a multinutrient program that would not only help them get well but would also keep them well until they died, as long as they remained on the program. Life extension also became an objective as it had already been shown that niacin would decrease death rate and increase longevity. Finally, I concluded that I would no longer adhere to the one disease, one drug concept that permeates medicine and the drug industry. Instead, I would do what I could using nutrition and relevant nutrients to help patients regain their ability to deal with stress and with disease. People heal themselves if they are given the right tools with which to do so.

I have been using the following program for many years and have seen a large number of patients recover from different physical and mental disorders using it. In the same way that added sugar and refined carbohydrates will cause saccharine disease, a multiple deficiency of vitamins will cause what I now call the pandeficiency disease. (The prefix "pan" is short for "pandemic.") Pandeficiency disease is a general disorder that can affect any organ, system, or function, or any combination of them. About half the population suffers from this chronic pervasive disease, caused by the overall deficiencies present in modern high-tech diets. If the psychiatric profession were to look carefully at the diagnostic system it now uses, it could eliminate hundreds of psychiatric disorders right along with their DSM numbers (*Diagnostic and Statistical Manual of Mental Disorders*, published by the American Psychiatric Association). Almost all of the attention-deficit hyperactivity disorder (ADHD) diagnoses of children could be eliminated.

Treatment of Pandeficiency Disease

The treatment of pandeficiency disease includes restoration of a nutritious diet and the following few nutrients. The doses depend on the state of the patient's health and his or her symptomatology.

- **Vitamin B3:** From 100 milligrams (mg) to several thousand milligrams three times daily after meals; in decreasing order of preference, try niacin, niacinamide, or non-flush preparations (the best and safest non-flush product is niacin as the flush generally goes away with continued use).

- **Vitamin C:** From 500 mg to several thousand milligrams three times daily after meals.

- **B complex:** 100 mg of each major B vitamin, one time daily with any meal, but up to 500 mg more of vitamin B6 (pyridoxine) a day may be needed.

- **Vitamin D:** 4,000 international units (IU) daily in the summer months; 6,000 IU per day in the winter months; if living in the far north with little sun exposure, take 6,000 IU daily all year.

Other nutrients that may also be needed include:

- **Vitamin B1 (thiamine):** 100–500 mg three times daily with meals for alcoholics and very heavy consumers of sugars.

- **Folic acid:** 25–50 mg (prescription needed) as an antidepressant, but less to lower elevated homocysteine levels.

- **Vitamin E:** 400–800 IU daily, but up to 4,000 IU for muscle-wasting diseases, including Huntington's disease and amyotrophic lateral sclerosis (ALS).

- **Essential fatty acids:** 1,000 mg from fish oil three times daily after meals.

- **Selenium:** 200–600 micrograms (mcg) one time per day with any meal; this is especially important when living in selenium-deficient areas.

- **Zinc citrate:** 50 mg (or 220 mg of zinc sulfate) one time per day with any meal.

- **Calcium-magnesium:** 1,000 mg of calcium with 500 mg of magnesium daily.

This program is compatible with any medication and has the major advantage that when used in combination the drug dose can be drastically reduced thus decreasing the toxic side effects. During my long career in treating schizophrenic patients with a combination of drugs and orthomolecular treatment, less than a handful of my patients developed tardive dyskinesia, a serious side effect of antipsychotic drugs that causes repetitive, involuntary movements of the face and limbs. It was never a problem and is easily treated. The basic medical injunction "First, do no harm" applies to drugs. With vitamins it has much less relevance since they do no harm.

The total cost of this program per month should be less than the cost of one pill of any antidepressant or antipsychotic drug. Ideally, we need specific laboratory tests that are cheap and will tell us exactly which nutrients are needed. With drugs it is far better to err on the side of too little as they are so toxic, but with vitamins it is better to err on the side of a little more as they are so safe, so free of side effects, and so cheap. Vitamins will have beneficial side effects. No one dies from vitamins.

Some Conditions That Benefit

Table 1 present some of the conditions that benefit from the multivitamin and mineral regimen described above. I've described case histories using these nutrients, beginning in 1960 in 30 books and in more than 600 orthodox and alternative medical journals. These conclusions are based upon my personal experience in treating many patients with these conditions.

Patients with these diagnoses will respond to the multivitamin and mineral regimen described here. Not all of these nutrients may be needed for a particular disease, but as there is no way of determining which ones are most needed for that person and since a deficiency of only one nutrient is very rare, it is better to use the whole regimen which is safe and can do no harm. Patient acceptance of this regimen is very high. After the patient has recovered, they may find out for themselves which ones are most important by eliminating one at a time to see if it makes any difference. Many patients after they have been well for a long time

will gradually modify the program and may go off it entirely. If they relapse, as many do, they will resume the program. The relapse may occur in weeks, months, or even after several years.

TABLE 1. SOME CONDITIONS THAT RESPOND TO THIS VITAMIN AND MINERAL REGIMEN		
PSYCHIATRIC DISORDER	**NUTRIENT EMPHASIZED**	**PATIENTS TREATED**
Alcoholism	Niacin	Over 500
Autism	Pyridoxine	Over 25
Fetal alcohol syndrome	Multiple nutrients	2
Huntington's disease	Niacin, vitamin E	2
Learning and behavioral disorders	Multiple nutrients	Over 2,000
Mood disorders	Niacin	Over 1,000
Schizophrenia	Niacin	Over 5,000
PHYSICAL DISORDER	**NUTRIENT EMPHASIZED**	**PATIENTS TREATED**
Aging	Niacin	Over 100
Arthritis	Niacin, vitamin B6, zinc	Over 50
Bacterial infections	Vitamin C	—
Cancer	Niacin, vitamin C, vitamin D, selenium	Over 1,500
Cardiovascular disease	Niacin, vitamin C	—
Diabetes	Niacin	10
Multiple sclerosis	Niacin, vitamin B1, vitamin D	Over 50
Obesity	B-complex vitamins	—
Skin problems	Niacin, EFAs	—
Viral infections, including HIV/AIDS	Vitamin C, selenium	—

Causes of Pandeficiency Disease

Here is a short list of causes that can trigger pandeficiency disease. It will be expanded when research physicians look at this condition more enthusiastically.

• **Diet.** This is the most common reason. During wars, drought, famine, and other catastrophes, the food supply is always jeopardized. This is so well known that in emergencies the first efforts are to provide food and clean water. Africa suffers from these catastrophes in many areas today. Her people will surely suffer permanent ill health even after the situation has been corrected. If the starvation and malnutrition are sustained too long and combined with stress, it can cause the afflicted to become vitamin dependent on one or more vitamins. This is what happened to those who survived concentration camps in Europe or prisoner-of-war camps in Asia. Many ex-prisoners of war suffered from permanent ill health, even after the situation had been corrected. Overall deficiencies present in the modern high-tech diet is another cause.

• **Allergies.** A strong association exists between food allergies and the need for vitamin and mineral supplements. I became aware of this connection when I started fasting my patients to determine what foods they were reacting to. I soon found that some patients who needed 12,000 mg of niacin in order to control partially their psychotic symptoms could not tolerate nearly that much when these foods were identified and removed. Patients needing this much would do even better on 3,000 mg; this puzzled me. I think the explanation is relatively simple: foods to which any person is allergic cause a chronic inflammation of the small intestine. The inflammation then allows polypeptides that have not been fully broken down to their basic amino acids to enter the bloodstream (from a leaky gut), which in turn decreases the adsorption of vitamins and minerals. When this continues for a long period of time, the mild chronic deficiency caused by the food allergy will become a dependency, especially for niacin and perhaps for other nutrients as well.

• **Diseases of the gastrointestinal tract.** Any disease of the gastrointestinal system (appendicitis, colitis, cancer, constipation, diarrhea, etc.) will interfere with absorption of nutrients, and if this becomes chronic will convert a deficiency to a dependency condition.

> *"There is a principle which is a bar against all information, which is proof against all argument, and which cannot fail to keep man in everlasting ignorance. That principle is condemnation without investigation."*
> —WILLIAM PALEY, 1794, often attributed to British philosopher Herbert Spencer

• **Iatrogenic treatment.** No attention to the nutritional needs of patients in hospitals under very severe stress. Vitamin deficiency occurs in hospitals if patients have to live there too long.

• **Viral infections.** The best example is HIV, which produces a selenium deficiency (the symptoms of AIDS are identical with the symptoms of selenium deficiency).

• **Deficiency and dependency.** A deficiency is present when the amount of any nutrient in the diet is below what the average person needs. Classically, it applies to the well-known deficiency diseases such as scurvy (vitamin C), beriberi (vitamin B1), pellagra (vitamin B3), and rickets (vitamin D). This was the basis of the old paradigm called vitamins-as-prevention, clearly developed about 100 years ago and reluctantly accepted by the medical profession about 50 years ago. Since then it has become so solidly established as if it were writ in stone even though it is totally out of date, wrong, and harmful to so many patients. The reason it is inadequate is that it assumes that everyone has the same nutritional needs. That is like assuming that everyone has the same fingerprints. A large number of our population have needs for vitamins that are much greater than can be obtained from our modern diets and if they depend upon the diet only they will never achieve optimum health. For these people, the correct term is dependency.

A deficiency will become a dependency if the deficiency is chronic. The risk of becoming dependent varies and the rapidity with which this occurs varies with malnutrition and its duration and intensity; with the presence of disease such as infection of the gastrointestinal tract, food allergies, and systemic infections and their duration and intensity; and with the level and duration of stress. When all these factors are operating at high levels, the time needed to become dependent will be shortened. Cleave found that it took 20 years before the saccharine disease developed in a person eating a high-sugar, high-refined carbohydrate, low-fiber diet, but without abnormal stress. Many prisoners of war became dependent in four years. But their malnutrition, presence of disease, and stress was much more severe.

Prevention and Treatment

The prevention and treatment of pandeficiency disease is, of course, very obvious. The diet must be improved, stress must be alleviated, and disease must be treated. In addition, niacin must be given in optimum amounts and other nutrients as well. It is no secret that stress should be relieved and that disease should be treated, but the medical profession and the nutritional professions have not yet learned that nutrients in high doses will also be needed. If one expects to endure stress and illness, it is wise to start on these few important nutrients immediately. Unfortunately, the poor will not be able to afford prevention and adequate treatment. Orthomolecular treatment, due to the ignorance of medicine, is available only to people who can afford to seek and find orthomolecular practitioners. To prevent and/or treat disease, the three most important principles are: 1) optimize the diet, 2) remove the trigger factors, and 3) use the correct nutrients in optimum doses.

REFERENCES

Cleave TL. *The Saccharine Disease*. New Canaan, CT: Keats Publishing, 1975.

Cleave TL, Campbell GD, Painter NS. *Diabetes, Coronary Thrombosis, and the Saccharine Disease*. 2nd ed. Bristol, England: John Wright & Sons, 1969.

Foster HD. New strategies for reversing vital pandemics: the role of nutrition. *Proceedings of International Forum for Public Health* Shanghai, 2007.

Foster HD. *What Really Causes AIDS*. Victoria, BC: Trafford Publishing, 2002. Available at: hdfoster.com/WhatReallyCausesAIDS.pdf.

Hoffer A. An orthomolecular look at obesity. Editorial. *J Orthomolecular Med* 2007;22(1):3–7.

Hoffer A. *Healing Children's Attention and Behavior Disorders*. Toronto, ON: CCNM Press, 2005.

Hoffer A. *Hoffer's ABC of Natural Nutrition for Children*. Kingston, ON: Quarry Press, 1999.

Hoffer A. Hong Kong veterans study. *J Orthomol Psychiat* 1974;3:34–36.

Hoffer A. *Mental Health Regained*. DVD. Toronto, ON: International Schizophrenia Foundation, 2007.

Hoffer A. *Orthomolecular Treatment for Schizophrenia and Other Mental Illnesses*. Toronto, ON: International Schizophrenia Foundation, 2007.

Hoffer A, Foster HD. *Feel Better, Live Longer with Vitamin B3*. Toronto, ON: CCNM Press, 2007.

Hoffer A, Prousky J. *Naturopathic Medicine. A Guide to Nutrient-Rich Food and Nutritional Supplements for Optimum Health*. Toronto, ON: CCNM Press, 2006.

Hoffer A, Walker M. *Orthomolecular Nutrition*. New Canaan, CT: Keats Publishing, 1978.

Prousky J. *Anxiety: Orthomolecular Diagnosis and Treatment*. Toronto, ON: CCNM Press, 2007.

Taubes G. *Good Calories, Bad Calories*. New York: Knopf, 2007.

Wald G, Jackson B. Activity and nutritional deprivation. *Proc Natl Acad Sci USA* 1944;30(9): 255–263.

Yudkin J. *Sweet and Dangerous*. New York: Bantam Books, 1972.

REFLECTIONS ON TWO MODERN MEDICAL RESEARCH IDEAS: DOUBLE-BLIND TRIALS AND PEER REVIEWS

by Abram Hoffer, MD, PhD

One of the main tenets of modern clinical therapeutic trials is that the double-blind method must be used. A double-blind trial compares one group of people who receive the "real treatment" with another supposedly similar group of people who receive a placebo. Anything else is called anecdotal, in a pejorative sense. One of the main tenets in evaluating research publications is that the methodology and the final manuscripts must be reviewed by peer committees. Although they have never been scientifically established, both these beliefs are politically correct, so correct that anyone who questions these beliefs immediately runs into massive opposition from the defenders of the faith.

Double-Blind Trials

Fortunately, double-blind methodology is facing more opposition recently, and it is about time. About 40 years ago Sir Lancelot Hogben, the English mathematician, exposed it as an inappropriate way of conducting human therapeutic trials. His analysis led him to conclude that the two fundamental prerequisites for randomized sampling were missing. These are 1) that it is possible to obtain representative samples from the human population that have to be tested, and 2) that the phenomenon being tested is invariant (unchanging). His first objection is that contrary to trials in agriculture in which millions of plants can be compared, large-scale human studies are so costly that they are not done and most trials are on a small scale. With such small samples, it is impossible to be sure that a trial truly is a representative sample of any larger population from which it is drawn. I have raised several objections to the double-blind randomized methods.[1,2]

My main objections are that 1) this method removes faith (a psychological healing benefit essential in treating anyone) from the therapeutic process. It creates an unreal situation that has no relevance to the clinical practice of good physician healers and is like studying the natural behavior of gorillas by observing them in a cage. 2) This method is dishonest and unethical. To be truly double-blind, the patients must be kept in the dark, that is, told lies. They are allowed to believe that they are being treated with some active compound, but at least temporarily they may be getting nothing, that is, a placebo. I must make clear I am not against controlled experiments. They are essential but they do not have to be double blind and they must take into account the many errors generated by sampling techniques.

A major criticism of the double-blind study, which is usually not discussed, is that it often shows compounds to be ineffective when in fact long usage has shown that they are effective. The best examples are the early double-blind experiments in the 1950s showing that the medication L-dopa, which is converted in the brain to dopamine, was not therapeutic for Parkinson's disease. It was not until decades of clinical use of L-dopa had shown symptomatic improvement in Parkinson's patients that the drug achieved a breakthrough. A more recent example has shown that the mood-elevator imipramine is no more effective than a placebo in treating depression. Physicians and psychiatrists know from long usage that this antidepressant does have antidepressant properties. Kapser, Moller, Montgomery, and Zondag[3] reported on a well-designed double-blind therapeutic trial comparing imipramine, fluvoxamine, and a placebo on 338 depressed patients. Their conclusion was that "Fluvoxamine but not imipramine was significantly superior to placebo in severely depressed patients" and that "No significant improvement was observed with imipramine."[3] Modern attempts are being made to bypass the double-blind method by using what is called meta-analysis. With this technique, single studies, which are considered inadequate standing alone, are simply lumped together into a large statistical table using mathematical formula and then conclusions are drawn from the data.

From the *J Orthomolecular Med* 1998;13(4):195–197.

An example of a recent major trial that in my opinion should never have been published is the Finnish double-blind controlled experiments using as subjects heavy drinkers and smokers. The effect of beta-carotene and vitamin E was studied using randomized groups. The randomization was not good: the group given beta-carotene had been smoking on average one more year than any of the other groups. The authors concluded that the beta-carotene group had slightly more patients with lung cancer. Actually, the fact that some subjects had been smoking one year more probably did make a difference since lung cancer is progressive and may take years to fully develop. They should have concluded only that the beta-carotene did not inhibit the development of cancer. Yet, they allowed the conclusion that beta-carotene had increased the incidence of lung cancer to be publicized widely. There were many other points about their design which have been severely criticized by others. The public—not being aware of the niceties of this statistical technique—assumed simply that beta-carotene increased the incidence of lung cancer. In my opinion, the double-blind method best serves not the interests of science or medicine, but the interests of editors of journals, and those who evaluate research grant applications, for the double-blind removes the need to really think about the subject matter. All is left to the holy $P < .05$ (meaning that the finding has only a 5 percent chance of not being true).

Peer-Review Committees

It is widely believed that peer-review committees maintain the purity of science and prevent bad science from penetrating into our medical journals or from obtaining research grants. I do not think there is much evidence that this is true. The orthodox journals who depend so heavily on peer-review committees published many fraudulent articles over and over. And any competent editor can manipulate his peers in such a way as to eliminate any paper with which he does not agree or which goes against the policy of that journal. For example, the *New England Journal of Medicine* had a firm policy of not publishing anything that provided evidence that vitamins in large doses were useful. If such a paper arrived, it would be simple to send it to peers who are part of the vitamins-as-prevention establishment, who would then automatically reject it. Linus Pauling could not get his vitamin C papers accepted by that journal.

Several years ago, a professor of medicine at McGill Medical School in Montreal found that all of eight patients with a bleeding disorder called idiopathic thrombocytopenic purpura were markedly benefited by vitamin C. There is no effective orthodox treatment for this disease. Here we have a disease that has a zero response rate to treatment, but when given vitamin C there was a 100 percent response rate. This paper was submitted to the *New England Journal of Medicine* and was rejected because it was not done double blind. The difference in results was so striking that anyone with any common sense would know that even given the study's small size, the therapeutic value of this vitamin was established. I have used it for three such patients with equally good results.

The term "peer" cannot be applied to a new science until it has had a chance to develop scientists who are familiar with it. They can then become the peers. Even then I do not think it is a good idea because, as I see it, the main function of peers is to maintain the purity of the current paradigm. I like Linus Pauling's definition of peers: "Peers," he said, "are people who pee together." I find that the best and most interesting journals are those where the editor is wide open to new ideas and does not send the manuscripts to any peers. This is why many physicians turn to the letters section of any journal, for only here will they find uncensored letters with ideas that may be good or bad but at least they are interesting.

Double-blind studies do not ensure that effective drugs will be found to be effective and that ineffective drugs will be ruled out as ineffective. They do not serve the needs of science or of patients. Peer-review committees do not serve the needs of science either. They serve the needs of editors and of grant evaluators. Their main function is to protect the status quo.

REFERENCES

1. Hoffer A, Osmond H. Double-blind clinical trials. *J Neuropathol* 1961;2:221–227.

2. Hoffer A. A theoretical examination of double-blind design. *Can Med Assoc J* 1967;97:123–127.

3. Kasper S, Moller HJ, Montgomery SA, et al. Antidepressant efficacy in relation to item analysis and severity of depression: a placebo controlled trial of fluvoxamine versus imipramine. *Int Clin Psychopharmacol* 1995;90(Suppl 4):3–12.

PHARMACEUTICAL ADVERTISING BIASES JOURNALS AGAINST VITAMIN SUPPLEMENTS

by Andrew W. Saul, PhD

It may be the worst-kept secret in medicine: pharmaceutical money buys journal influence. What the public has so long suspected has now been demonstrated in a recently published peer-reviewed study.[1] Researchers from Wake Forest University School of Medicine and the University of Florida found that "in major medical journals, more pharmaceutical advertising is associated with publishing fewer articles about dietary supplements." Furthermore, they found that more pharmaceutical company advertising resulted in the journal having more articles with "negative conclusions about dietary supplement safety."

This new study, the first of its kind, specifically looked at pharmaceutical advertising as compared with journal text about dietary supplements. The authors reviewed a year's worth of issues from each of 11 of the largest medical journals: the *Journal of the American Medical Association, New England Journal of Medicine, British Medical Journal, Canadian Medical Association Journal, Annals of Internal Medicine, Archives of Internal Medicine, Archives of Pediatric and Adolescent Medicine, Pediatrics and Pediatric Research*, and *American Family Physician*.

The results were statistically significant . . . and embarrassing. Medical journals carrying the most pharmaceutical ads "published significantly fewer major articles about dietary supplements per issue than journals with the fewest pharmads. Journals with the most pharmads published no clinical trials or cohort studies about supplements. The percentage of major articles concluding that supplements were unsafe was 4 percent in journals with fewest and 67 percent among those with the most pharmads." The authors concluded that "the impact of advertising on publications" is real, and said that "the ultimate impact of this bias on professional guidelines, health care, and health policy is a matter of great public concern."

Indeed it is. Health care costs are rising and drug profits are enormous. Canadian psychiatrist Abram Hoffer, MD, PhD, says: "We all have to work hard to educate the public about the merits of sane treatment for everyone, where the patient is primary, not Big Pharma." Bo H. Jonsson, MD, PhD, of the Karolinska Institute in Sweden, comments that "Positive reports about the effects of high-dose vitamins have long been ignored by the medical establishment instead of being further examined scientifically."

When patients ask about nutritional treatments, many a family physician has replied, "I've never seen any studies supporting the safety or efficacy of vitamin supplements in my professional journals. The research is simply not there."

Sadly, they are right. And now we know why.

Major medical journals, their editors, and their authors appear to be on the take. Harsh words? Perhaps, but only because the truth is harsh. "On the take" refers to receiving cash in exchange for influence. It is naive to assume that money does not corrupt. Promoting vested interests masquerading as science is wrong and it must be stopped. At the very least, accepting money carries an obligation to account for the source of that money. All medical journals should be compelled to print a full disclosure in every issue itemizing exactly how much money comes from exactly which sources.

Any medical journal that won't disclose has a reason to not disclose. And that reason has nothing to do with public health. It's about private cash. The cash that induces the journals to sway the doctors to persuade the public.

If the medical journals deny this, let them prove it with full disclosure. Now.

REFERENCES

1. Kemper KJ. *BMC Complement Altern Med*;8:11.

Excerpted from the *Orthomolecular Medicine News Service*, February 5, 2009.

MEGAVITAMINS
by Harvey M. Ross, MD

A few weeks ago a physician had his secretary call me to find out what megavitamins he should order for his patient. The next day when the physician himself called I explained to him that vitamins were only a part of the treatment called orthomolecular psychiatry. His suspicion was aroused. "Why can't you just give me a starting dosage? Why are you being so mysterious about the treatment? It can't be that complicated." He was assured that the treatment was not complicated at all, that I would challenge anyone to explain to me in a three-minute telephone conversation the "starting dosage" of the antipsychotic chlorpromazine (Thorazine) and how to use it effectively. I explained to him that if he was interested enough to try the orthomolecular approach, I was certain that he wanted to do it properly.

Too many physicians have attempted to use megavitamins by giving inadequate doses of a few vitamins to the wrong people for an insufficient amount of time only to achieve the failure that could have been predicted. Unfortunately, they conclude that megavitamin therapy is a fraud rather than recognizing that they have not really followed the method as practiced by the orthomolecular psychiatrists. The proper perspective on the use of megavitamins is necessary, since so many people feel that the treatment is a thoroughly simplistic approach of "take lots of vitamins and mental health will follow."

There are exceptions, of course, and we all can cite cases where the addition of only vitamins in large doses was instrumental in achieving a good result, but these are exceptions. In the majority of cases treated, vitamins are only a part of the treatment. What follows are some practical aspects of the practice of orthomolecular psychiatry and the proper use of megavitamins.

What Vitamins Are Used?

Vitamins are divided into two groups: water-soluble vitamins and fat-soluble vitamins. From a practical standpoint, water-soluble vitamins are easily discarded from the body through the kidneys; this makes it unlikely that they are stored in the body. Fat-soluble vitamins, on the other hand, are stored in the body, and there are cases of toxic effects from taking large doses of fat-soluble vitamins over prolonged periods of time. The only fat-soluble vitamin that is used with any regularity in orthomolecular treatment is vitamin E. All the other vitamins used in large doses are water-soluble (vitamin C and the B-complex vitamins).

For the beginner, there is always some confusion about terminology, especially with vitamin B3 (commonly referred to as niacin). Niacin and nicotinic acid are synonymous. The amide form is niacinamide, which is the same as nicotinamide. The other B vitamins used fairly regularly are pantothenic acid (vitamin B5) and pyridoxine (vitamin B6). Other B vitamins that may be used are thiamine (vitamin B1), riboflavin (vitamin B2), cobalamin (vitamin B12), and folic acid (sometimes referred to as vitamin B9).

What Medical Conditions Can These Vitamins Treat?

In the early 1950s, Drs. Abram Hoffer and Humphry Osmond used vitamins to treat schizophrenia. Just as the treatment has changed and expanded from those early days, so have the number of conditions treated changed. Not only is adult schizophrenia treated, but schizophrenia of childhood is also treated.

Anyone who has worked with the psychiatric disorders of childhood begins to recognize that there is a hodgepodge of diagnostic categories that run from learning disorders, hyperactivity, and minimal brain disorder to schizophrenia and autism. Graphically, these disorders may be visualized as a continuous wavy line, the peaks indicating each diagnostic category having its own specific criteria on which to base the diagnosis.

From the *J Orthomolecular Psych* 1974;3(4):254–258.

There will be a few pure cases falling neatly into place, but the majority have mixed features. The result is a diagnostic nightmare, especially for the bewildered parents who, after visiting five physicians, have six diagnoses. This is pertinent to the orthomolecular physicians since there are some cases of all the diagnostic categories of children who have been mentioned that respond to the orthomolecular approach. As one leaves the schizophrenic conditions and the disorders of children, there are other areas treated successfully by this method. Many of the so-called neurotic disorders, including depression, anxiety, even obsessive-compulsive disorders have responded successfully to the orthomolecular approach. Alcoholics and drug addicts are also treated.

How to Use the Vitamins?

Dosages sometimes vary between practitioners. What follows is the program I use. The dosage is different depending on the condition being treated and whether the patient is a child or an adult. For the discussion of how to use the vitamins, the following categories will be considered separately: adult schizophrenia and drug addiction, the neuroses and alcoholism, and the childhood disorders.

Adult Schizophrenia and Drug Addiction

These categories are classed together because it is my belief that addicts who benefit from this treatment are schizophrenics. I am not considering the treatment of an acute LSD reaction, but rather the hard drug addict. The observation has been made for a long time that many heroin addicts, when withdrawn from drugs, present a classic schizophrenic picture. It is this group of addicts who are benefited from the orthomolecular approach. A typical starting dose of vitamins includes the following three times a day after meals: ascorbic acid (1,000 mg), pantothenic acid (100 mg), pyridoxine (200 mg), vitamin E as d-alpha tocopherol (400 IU), B complex (50 mg of each major B vitamin), and niacin or niacinamide (1,000 mg).

A special word needs to be mentioned about vitamin B3. If niacin is used, I start with a divided dose three times a day for three days, and then increase it after the third day. In doing this, I find that the patient is usually able to withstand the flush that occurs when niacin is first started. I have preferred niacin over niacinamide because I do not know what the final dose for the patient will be and there is a greater tolerance for large doses of niacin than there is for niacinamide.

Subsequent doses are determined by clinical course and physical response. Vitamin B3 is raised on subsequent office visits if there is no improvement. The usual maintenance dosage is between 6,000 and 12,000 mg, rarely higher. The most notable exception to this is the group of alcoholic schizophrenic patients who seem to need and tolerate dosages sometimes in the 20,000- to 30,000-mg level. Ascorbic acid may also need to be raised but I seldom go over 6,000 mg a day. The physician needs to monitor, evaluate, and tailor the dose to the individual.

There are some specific indications for use of other vitamins. Sometimes I check vitamin B12 and folic acid levels, and if they are low normal or below normal, I use these vitamins. I prefer to give the B12 by injection, 1,000 microgram (mcg) up to three times a week; folic acid is usually prescribed at 2 to 3 mg, three times a day. When depression is significant, 1,000 mg of thiamine is given three times a day.

Neuroses and Alcoholism

People with neuroses and alcoholics are considered separately for in these conditions the vitamins take a secondary position in relation to the diet because it is the hypoglycemia that has resulted, in many instances, in the neurotic symptoms of depression, anxiety, and, in other cases, alcoholism. In case this is misunderstood, it should be stated in another way: not every neurotic and alcoholic is hypoglycemic, but low blood sugar should be considered as a possible contributory cause to those conditions. Vitamins are used in the treatment of hypoglycemia, especially the B complex, which are involved in the metabolism of glucose. In a simple case of hypoglycemia, I usually prescribe a B complex (50 mg of each major B vitamin), vitamin C (1,000 mg), and vitamin E (400 IU) to be taken two to three times a day.

Childhood Disorders

Typical starting levels for treating childhood psychotic conditions or learning disabilities are determined by child's body weight. For children of 35 pounds or more, the starting daily level is: niacin or niacinamide (1,000 mg), ascorbic acid (1,000 mg), pyridoxine (200–400 mg), and pantothenic acid (200–400 mg). If the child is under 35 pounds, the vitamin B3 and vitamin C are started at a lower dosage and increased within two weeks if the vitamins are tolerated without nausea. For those children over 45 pounds, the optimum daily dose is usually around 3,000 mg of vitamins B3 and C a day. It may be preferable to divide the doses; often this improves absorption and therefore results. One third of each of the above nutrients with each meal is the simplest way to do so.

Are There Precautions to Know About?

After this moderately detailed description of the dosage of vitamins, I would warn that when the vitamins are used to treat an illness, it should be done under the supervision of a qualified physician. If, on the other hand, vitamins are used simply as a nutritional supplement, medical advice is not necessary, since there is enough literature available for an individual to learn what supplements are advisable for his particular needs.

That said, some precautions must be observed in using vitamins to supplement the diet or treat a condition. For example, for patients with high blood pressure or a history of rheumatic heart disease, the fat-soluble vitamin E should be cautiously introduced in low dosages (under 100 IU a day). Niacin may cause an elevation of the glucose-tolerance curve, which resembles diabetes; it may also cause an elevation of uric acid as seen in gout. Niacinamide does not cause these reactions, so in a patient with a history of gout or diabetes I prefer to use niacinamide. Pyridoxine can adversely affect the benefit of L-dopa, a common medication given for parkinsonism. Vitamins in megadoses should be used with caution if there is a history of gastric or duodenal ulcer.

Are There Any Side Effects?

The above are some of the precautions to be observed, but there are also some side effects. The non-serious side effects from the vitamins mentioned are the very common niacin flush, along with a sensation of heat, and occasionally itching and headache. Since these effects usually happen with the small initial dose and diminish or disappear with a larger dose, they rarely require special consideration other than warning the patient what to expect. If it is important for the patient to take niacin and he or she cannot tolerate the flush, an antihistamine may be given before the vitamin is taken. No-flush niacin, such as inositol hexaniacinate, is readily available and an inexpensive option. It does not work quite as well as niacin, but it is generally very well tolerated by people who would otherwise refuse to take it due to the flush.

One common side effect of vitamin B3 is nausea and vomiting. Some orthomolecular psychiatrists suggest pushing the dose of niacin up to a point of vomiting that might indicate the tolerance of the body, and then reducing it to a lower dosage. The vomiting that occurs is a persistent vomiting over several hours. If this occurs after a small, insufficient dose of niacin, then it is best to switch to niacinamide and vice versa. Management of persistent vomiting should include a history to make certain that the vitamins are taken after meals. If a history is obtained indicating that the nausea and vomiting are most often present on awakening, then the last dose of vitamins should be taken late in the afternoon. The use of 500 mg of inositol (part of the B complex, even though it is not officially recognized as a vitamin), taken with the vitamins, is effective sometimes in alleviating the nausea and vomiting. Also to be considered is a change in the brand of vitamin since at times the excipients (materials that hold the active vitamin material together) are the cause of the nausea. Another possibility in management is the use of long-acting or sustained-release vitamins. There have been a few reports of gastrointestinal ulcers occurring during megavitamin therapy.

There are also reports of abnormal liver tests when niacin is used in large doses. While most of the time there is no evidence by physical examination that the liver is malfunctioning, I have had one case of a child who became jaundiced during each of two trials with vitamins.

Other reported side effects are blurring of vision, which may be a result of edema or fluid getting into the optic nerve. Sometimes a dark discoloration of the skin occurs, especially in the folds of the neck and arm, due to a fungus. This latter side effect happens with niacin and not niacinamide. The discoloration responds to changing from niacin to niacinamide and the use of an abrasive washcloth. Cases of water retention have also been seen, causing swelling of the extremities. A very few people respond to large doses of niacinamide by becoming depressed, and some respond to large doses of thiamine with an uncomfortable agitation. A common side effect of vitamin C is diarrhea and excessive urination. All of these side effects are resolved when a change is made in the dosage or vitamin given.

Much has been written about the need to balance the B vitamins, but I find that using a high-potency B complex seems to be enough to avoid relative deficiencies. However, on occasion, I see signs of a riboflavin deficiency manifested by the typical cracked corners of the mouth.

Anyone using the vitamins prescribed should also know that the urine becomes dark yellow in color; this change is not significant other than worrying some patients who do not realize that it is to be expected.

Positive Side Effects

Side effects are most often thought of in terms of negative side effects. In observing the treatment of thousands of patients with large doses of vitamins, I have been impressed with some positive side effects, or bonuses, of the treatment, which I had not expected. In a true sense, these should not be classed as "side effects" but as actions of the vitamins. We are all aware of the use of vitamin C for the common cold. There have been several studies done with the announced intention of disproving Linus Pauling's claims. However, most of the studies found that either the incidence of colds was decreased and/or the severity and number of sick days were decreased. Many women who have suffered with severe menstrual cramps are amazed with the absence of pain, especially on large doses of pyridoxine. Persistent diseases of the skin have cleared. Vague, long-standing aches and pains have disappeared. This may be as much the result of improved diets as of the vitamins. It is obvious that when the psychiatrist begins to treat a patient to provide the optimum environment for the nervous system, he or she is also changing the environment of the rest of the cells of the body. While most of the time this seems to be for the improvement of the individual, negative side effects can and do occur. This is another reason why using large doses of vitamins to treat disease should not be self-prescribed.

Do Brands of Vitamins Differ?

In using vitamins the physician should be aware of some of the practical matters of vitamin manufacture. Most tablets are at least 50 percent excipients. One of the best excipients from the standpoint of effectiveness and low cost is starch or sugar. For orthomolecular treatment which may involve 30 to 60 tablets a day, the excipients are more likely to cause stomach distress than the pure nutrients. However, the excipients are there for a reason: most vitamins do not taste good, and tablets have to be held together somehow.

Capsules, chewables, powders, or liquid preparations may be appropriate options, especially for children. Reading the label carefully is a must. Also, allergist Ben Feingold has implicated

> "Let the opponents of vitamin therapy cite the double-blind, placebo-controlled studies upon which they have based their toxicity allegations. They can't because there aren't any."
> —ABRAM HOFFER

food coloring and flavoring in hyperactivity in children, so it is especially important that vitamins for children and probably adults do not contain artificial coloring and additives. The ideal vitamin would be pure powder but, in addition to unpalatability, the use of powder is more likely to lead to inexact measurement of dose. For example, 500 mg is only about an eighth of a teaspoon. The best solution is the use of vitamin tablets in large dosage that are sugar and starch free, and that have no artificial coloring or flavoring. Technical departments of vitamin manufacturers usually supply this information to interested persons on request. If they do not, choose another brand.

■ CONCLUSION

Now, if that physician who asked me over the phone to tell him what vitamins to give his patient hears this or reads it, I hope he understands as you do that the use of vitamins in the treatment of psychiatric conditions is only part of the orthomolecular treatment. Orthomolecular psychiatry takes knowledge, skill, and experience to apply, and just as other medical treatments, it will have a greater chance of being successful if managed by the experienced and careful physician.

REFERENCES

Adams R, Murray F. *Megavitamin Therapy*. New York: Larchmont Books, 1973.

Cott A. Megavitamins: the orthomolecular approach to behavioral disorders and learning disabilities. *Academic Therapy Quarterly* 1972;7:3.

Cott A. Treatment of schizophrenic children. *Schizophrenia* 1969;1:44–59.

Hawkins D, Pauling L, eds. *Orthomolecular Psychiatry*. San Francisco: W.H. Freeman & Co, 1973.

Mosher LR. Nicotinic acid side effects and toxicity: a review. *Am J Psychiatry* 1970;126:9.

Winter SL, Boyer JL. Hepatic toxicity from large doses of vitamin B3 (nicotinamide). *N Engl J Med* 1973; 289:1180–1182.

Wohl MG, Goodhart RS, eds. *Modern Nutrition in Health and Disease*. 4th ed. Philadelphia: Lea & Febiger, 1968.

VITAMIN C AND SHINGLES
by Thomas E. Levy, MD, JD

The pharmaceutical industry—and many doctors—appear to be making great efforts to get as many people as possible vaccinated against shingles. Even if such an intervention was highly effective in preventing shingles, which certainly has not been shown to be the case, the information below should make it clear that such vaccinations are unnecessary.

Shingles is an infection resulting from the varicella zoster virus, usually manifesting in areas supplied by spinal nerves, known as dermatomes. More commonly known in medical circles as herpes zoster, the infection is typically characterized by a blistering skin rash of extraordinary pain for most individuals. The initial infection with the virus is usually remote from the shingles outbreak, typically occurring in childhood when chickenpox is contracted. For years the virus remains latent in nerve cell bodies or autonomic ganglia. It is when the virus, for unclear reasons, breaks out of these storage sites and travels down the nerve axons that shingles occurs.

Left to itself along with mainstream therapies that include analgesics, antiviral agents like acyclovir (Zovirax), and corticosteroids, the rash will generally resolve in two to four weeks. The pain is generally lessened little by analgesics. Some unfortunate individuals can experience post-herpetic neuralgia, a syndrome of residual nerve pain that can continue for months or years following a shingles outbreak.

Treatment with Vitamin C

The clinical response of shingles to vitamin C therapy is decidedly different from its response to traditional therapies. While there are not many reports in the literature on vitamin C and shingles, the studies that do exist are striking. Frederick Klenner, MD, who pioneered the effective use of vitamin C in a wide variety of infections and toxin exposures, published the results of his vitamin C therapy on eight patients with shingles. He gave 2,000–3,000 milligrams (mg) of vitamin C by injection every 12 hours, supplemented by 1,000 mg in fruit juice by mouth every two hours. In seven of the eight patients treated in this manner, complete pain relief was reported within two hours of the first vitamin C injection. All patients received a total of five to seven vitamin C injections. Having had shingles myself years before I knew of the efficacy of vitamin C therapy, I can assert that this is nothing short of a stunning result on what is usually a painful and debilitating disease.

Furthermore, the blisters on Dr. Klenner's patients were reported to begin healing rapidly, with complete resolution within the first 72 hours. As with other infectious conditions, Dr. Klenner hastened to add that treatment needed to continue for at least 72 hours, as recurrence could readily occur even when the initial response was positive. Dr. Klenner also found a similar regimen of vitamin C just as readily resolved the blistering lesions of chickenpox, with the recoveries usually complete in three to four days. Similar clinical response by chickenpox and shingles to vitamin C is further evidence, albeit indirect, that the chickenpox virus and the later appearing herpes zoster virus are the same pathogen (Klenner, 1949 & 1974).[1,2]

Even before Dr. Klenner's observations were published, another researcher reported results just as astounding when measured against today's mainstream therapies. Dainow[3] (1943) reported success with 14 shingles patients receiving vitamin C injections. In another study, complete resolution of shingles outbreaks was reported in 327 of 327 patients receiving vitamin C injections within the first 72 hours (Zureick, 1950).[4] While all of this data on vitamin C and shingles is quite old, there is an internal consistency among the report in how the patients responded. Until further clinical trials are conducted, these results stand. They clearly show that vitamin C should be an integral part of any therapeutic approach used on a patient presenting with shingles.

Vitamin C and Viruses

Vitamin C has a general virus-inactivating effect, with herpes viruses being only one of many types of virus that vitamin C has neutralized in the test tube or has eradicated in an infected person (Levy, 2002).[5] As with the inactivation seen with other viruses mixed with vitamin C in the test tube (in vitro), two early studies were consistent with the clinical results later seen with vitamin C in herpes infections. Vitamin C inactivated herpes viruses when mixed with them in the test tube (Holden and Resnick, 1936; Holden and Molloy, 1937).[6,7]

Vitamin C accumulating inside viral particles can rapidly destroy viruses by that approach. The spike of the bacteriophage virus is laden with iron, and the focal Fenton reaction is probably how it penetrates its host cell membrane (Bartual et al., 2010; Yamashita et al., 2011; Browning et al., 2012).[8-10] Viruses accumulate iron and copper, and these metals are also part of the surfaces of viruses (Samuni et al., 1983).[11] As such, wherever the concentrations are the highest, vitamin C will focally upregulate the Fenton reaction, and irreversible viral damage will generally ensue. Fenton activity and its upregulation is the only really well-documented way by which viruses, pathogens, and also cancer cells can be killed by vitamin C, and it is the stimulation of this reaction by vitamin C that makes it therapeutically effective in resolving many infections and cancers (Vilcheze et al., 2013).[12]

Vitamin C helps resolve infections of all varieties, but its effect on acute viral syndromes are especially dramatic and prompt. It should always be part of any treatment protocol for an infected patient. The most important factor in the treatment of any virus with vitamin C is to give enough, for a long enough period of time.

REFERENCES

1. Klenner F. Southern Medicine & Surgery 1949;111:209–214.
2. Klenner F. Journal of the International Academy of Preventive Medicine 1974;1:45–69.
3. Dainow I. Dermatologia 1943;68:197–201.
4. Zureick M. Journal des Praticiens 1950;64:586.
5. Levy T. Curing the Incurable: Vitamin C, Infectious Diseases, and Toxins. Henderson, NV: MedFox Publishing.
6. Holden M. Journal of Immunology 1936;31:455–462.
7. Holden M. Journal of Immunology 1937;33:251–257.
8. Bartual S. Proceedings of the National Academy of Sciences of the United States of America 2010;107:20287–20292.
9. Yamashita E. Acta Crystallographica. Section F, Structural Biology and Crystallization Communications 2011;67:837–841.
10. Browning C. Structure 2012;20:326–339.
11. Samuni A. European Journal of Biochemistry 1983;137:119–124.
12. Vilcheze C. Nature Communications 2013;4:1881.

Excerpted from the Orthomolecular Medicine News Service, August 27, 2013.

VITAMIN DEPENDENCY
by Andrew W. Saul, PhD

Dependency is a fact of life. The human body is dependent on food, water, sleep, and oxygen. Additionally, its internal chemistry is absolutely dependent on vitamins. Without adequate vitamin intake, the body will sicken; virtually any prolonged vitamin deficiency is fatal. Surely this constitutes a dependency in the generally accepted sense of the word. Nutrient deficiency of long standing may create an exaggerated need for the missing nutrient, a need not met by dietary intakes or even by low-dose supplementation.

Vitamin-Deficiency and Vitamin-Dependency Conditions

Recently,[1] Dr. Robert P. Heaney used the term "long-latency deficiency diseases" to describe illnesses that fit this description. He writes:

> Inadequate intakes of many nutrients are now recognized as contributing to several of the major chronic diseases that affect the populations of the industrialized nations. Often taking many years to manifest themselves, these disease outcomes should be thought of as long-latency deficiency diseases . . . Inadequate intakes of specific nutrients may produce more than one disease, may produce diseases by more than one mechanism, and may require several years for the consequent morbidity to be sufficiently evident to be clinically recognizable as "disease." Because the intakes required to prevent many of the long-latency disorders are higher than those required to prevent the respective index diseases, recommendations based solely on preventing the index diseases are no longer biologically defensible.

There are at least two key concepts presented here: The first is, "Inadequate intakes of specific nutrients may produce more than one disease." This exactly supports Dr. William Kaufman's statements to this effect 55 years ago, when he wrote that, in considering

> different clinical entities one cannot exclude the possibility that they may be caused by the same etiologic agent, acting in different ways. For example, in experimental animals, it has been shown that the lack of a single essential nutrient can produce a variety of dissimilar clinical disorders in different individuals of the same species . . . One might not suspect that the same etiologic factor, lack of a specific essential nutrient, was responsible for each of the various clinical syndromes of the same tissue deficiency disease which is permitted to develop at different rates in different individuals of the same species.[2]

While amyotrophic lateral sclerosis, progressive muscular atrophy, progressive bulbar palsy, and primary lateral sclerosis are not all the same illness, they and the other neuromuscular diseases may have a common basis: unacknowledged, untreated long-term vitamin dependency. Therefore, each may respond to an orthomolecular approach such as that successfully used by Dr. Frederick Klenner[3] for multiple sclerosis and myasthenia gravis, half a century ago.

The second key point Heaney makes is that vitamin "intakes required to prevent many of the long-latency disorders are higher than those required to prevent the respective index diseases." This confirms Dr. Abram Hoffer's observations to this effect some 40 years ago, when he treated prisoners of war presenting severe, protracted nutrient deficiencies. Hoffer wrote[4] that when released, after as long as 44 months of captivity,

> only 75 percent had survived. They had lost about one-third of their body weight. In camp they suffered from classical scurvy, beriberi, pellagra, many infections, and from protein and calorie deficiency. They were rehabilitated in hospitals and were given doses of vitamins that were then considered high. Since then these Hong Kong veterans have suffered from a variety of physical and psychiatric conditions. [However] the history of a small sample, about 12, is much different, for they have been taking nicotinic acid (niacin) 3 grams

From the *J Orthomolecular Med* 2004:19(2):67–70.

[3,000 milligrams (mg)] per day. These 12 have recovered and remain well as long as they take this quantity of vitamin regularly.

About 35 years ago (in the 1930s and 1940s) it was reported that some chronic pellagrins required at least 600 mg per day of vitamin B3 to prevent the return of pellagra symptoms. This was astonishing then and unexplainable since pellagra as a nicotinic acid deficiency disease should have yielded to vitamin (small) doses. Today the concept of vitamin-dependency disease has developed. It is based upon the realization that there is a much wider range of need for nutrients than was believed to be true then.

A person is said to be vitamin dependent if his requirements for that vitamin are much greater (perhaps 100-fold greater or more) than is the average need for any population. The optimum need is that quantity that maintains the subject in good health, not that quantity that barely keeps him free of pellagra. From this point of view, the Hong Kong veterans have become vitamin B3 dependent as a result of severe and prolonged malnutrition. It is likely that any population similarly deprived of essential nutrients for a long period of time will develop one or more dependency conditions.

Thirty years ago, in another paper,[5] Hoffer made this statement:

> The newer concept of vitamin-dependent disease changes the emphasis from simply dietary manipulation to consideration of the needs of the organism. It comes within the field of orthomolecular disease. The borderline between vitamin-deficiency and vitamin-dependency conditions is merely a quantitative one when one considers prevention and cure.

The Rebound Effect

The differentiation between deficiency and dependency is dose. Every patient that was ever helped by high-dose nutrient therapy lends support to the concept of vitamin dependency. By the same token, symptoms resulting from inappropriate and abrupt termination of large doses of nutrients provide equally good evidence for vitamin dependency. While deprivation of low doses of vitamin C causes scurvy, abrupt termination of high maintenance doses may cause its own set of problems. Called "rebound scurvy," this includes classical scorbutic symptoms, as well as a predictable relapse of illness that had already responded to high-dose therapy.

Writes Dr. Robert F. Cathcart:

> There is a certain dependency on ascorbic acid that a patient acquires over a long period of time when he takes large maintenance doses. Apparently, certain metabolic reactions are facilitated by large amounts of ascorbate and if the substance is suddenly withdrawn, certain problems result such as a cold, return of allergy, fatigue, etc. Mostly, these problems are a return of problems the patient had before taking the ascorbic acid. Patients have by this time become so adjusted to feeling better that they refuse to go without ascorbic acid. Patients do not seem to acquire this dependency in the short time they take doses to bowel tolerance to treat an acute disease. Maintenance doses of 4 grams [4,000 mg] per day do not seem to create a noticeable dependency. The majority of patients who take over 10–15 grams [10,000–15,000 mg] of ascorbic acid per day probably have certain metabolic needs for ascorbate which exceed the universal human species need. Patients with chronic allergies often take large maintenance doses. The major problem feared by patients benefiting from these large maintenance doses of ascorbic acid is that they may be forced into a position where their body is deprived of ascorbate during a period of great stress such as emergency hospitalization.
>
> Physicians should recognize the consequences of suddenly withdrawing ascorbate under these circumstances and be prepared to meet these increased metabolic needs for ascorbate in even an unconscious patient. These consequences of ascorbate depletion which may include shock, heart attack, phlebitis, pneumonia, allergic reactions, increased susceptibility to infection, etc., may be averted only by ascorbate. Patients unable to take large oral doses should be given intravenous ascorbate. All hospitals should have supplies of large amounts of ascorbate for intravenous use to meet this need.[6]

This need is especially serious for the cancer patient, whose exceptionally positive response to mega-ascorbate therapy, and dramatically negative response to ascorbate deprivation, is the very picture of vitamin dependency. Linus Pauling's colleague Dr. Ewan Cameron wrote:

> Ascorbate, however administered, is rapidly excreted in the urine, so that administration should be continuous or at very frequent intervals. Furthermore, exposure to high-circulating levels of ascorbate induces overactivity of certain hepatic enzymes concerned with its degradation and metabolism. These enzymes persist for some time after sudden cessation of high intakes, resulting in depletion of circulating levels of ascorbate to well below normal unsupplemented values. This is known as the rebound effect. It causes a sharp decrease in immunocompetence and must be avoided in the cancer patient. Clinical experience has shown that the best responses are observed when vitamin C is administered intravenously, so insuring a high plasma level. However, because long-term continuous intravenous administration is impractical, we recommend an initial intravenous course of 10 days duration, followed by continuous maintenance oral regimen.[7]

Positive Nutrient Dependencies

In short, the body only misses what it needs. That is dependency. The destructive consequences of alcohol and other negative drug dependencies are taught in elementary schools. At the same time, the consequences of ignoring our positive nutrient dependencies go largely undiscussed even in medical journals. Vitamin dependencies induced by genetics, diet, drugs, or illness are most often regarded as medical curiosities. The Hoffer-Osmond discovery that schizophrenics, forming about 2 percent of the population, are dependent on multi-gram doses of niacin, remains a psychiatric heresy. The Irwin Stone-Linus Pauling idea of population-wide, genetically based hypoascorbemia has received negative attention, when it has received any attention at all. Yet, writes Dr. Emanuel Cheraskin, "Hypovitaminosis C is a very real and common, probably epidemic, problem which clearly has not been properly viewed and surely not adequately reported."[8] This is not a total surprise. It took decades for medical acknowledgement that selenium and vitamin E are actually essential to health. Simple cause-and-effect micronutrient deficiency, a doctrine long held dear

by the dietetic profession, is not always sufficient to explain persistent physician reports of megavitamin cures of a number of diseases outside the classically accepted few. Perhaps it is a law of orthomolecular therapy that the reason one nutrient can cure so many different illnesses is because a deficiency of one nutrient can cause many different illnesses.

If nutrient deficiency is basically about inadequate intake, then dependency is essentially about heightened need. As a dry sponge soaks up more milk, so a sick body generally takes up higher vitamin doses. The quantity of a nutritional supplement that cures an illness indicates the patient's degree of deficiency. It is therefore not a megadose of the vitamin, but rather a megadeficiency of the nutrient that we are dealing with. Orthomolecular practitioners know that with therapeutic nutrition, you don't take the amount that you believe ought to work; rather, you take the amount that gets results. The first rule of building a brick wall is that you must have enough bricks.

A sick body has exaggeratedly high needs for many vitamins. We can either meet that need, or else suffer unnecessarily. Until the medical professions fully embrace orthomolecular treatment, "medicine" might well be said to be "the experimental study of what happens when poisonous chemicals are placed into malnourished human bodies."

REFERENCES

1. Heaney RP. Long-latency deficiency disease: insights from calcium and vitamin D. *Am J Clin Nutr* 2003;78(5):912–919.

2. Kaufman W. The common form of joint dysfunction: its incidence and treatment. Brattleboro, VT: E.L. Hildreth & Co, 1949.

3. Smith L. Vitamin C as a fundamental medicine: abstracts of Dr. Frederick R. Klenner's published and unpublished work. Tacoma, WA: Life Sciences Press, 1988.

4. Hoffer A. Editorial. *J Orthomolecular Psych* 1974;3(1):34–36.

5. Hoffer A. Mechanism of action of nicotinic acid and nicotinamide in the treatment of schizophrenia. In: Hawkins D and Pauling L: *Orthomolecular Psychiatry: Treatment of Schizophrenia.* San Francisco: W.H. Freeman & Co, 1973, 202–262.

6. Cathcart RF. Vitamin C, titration to bowel tolerance, anascorbemia, and acute induced scurvy." *Med Hypoth* 1981;7:1359–1376.

7. Cameron E. Protocol for the use of vitamin C in the treatment of cancer. *Med Hypoth* 1991;36:190–194. Also: Cameron E. Protocol for the use of intravenous vitamin C in the treatment of cancer. Palo Alto, CA: Linus Pauling Institute of Science and Medicine. Undated, c.1986.

8. Cheraskin E. Vitamin C and fatigue. *J Orthomolecular Med* 1994;9(1):39–45.

"Safe Upper Levels" for Nutritional Supplements: One Giant Step Backward

by Alan R. Gaby, MD

In May 2003, the Expert Group on Vitamins and Minerals (EVM), an advisory group originally commissioned in 1988 by the then Ministry of Agriculture Fisheries and Food, and subsequently reporting to the Food Standards Agency in England, published a report that set Safe Upper Levels (SULs) for the doses of most vitamin and mineral supplements. The establishment of SULs was based on a review of clinical and epidemiological evidence, as well as animal research and in vitro studies. For those nutrients for which the available evidence was judged insufficient to set an SUL, the EVM instead established Guidance Levels, which were to be considered less reliable than SULs.

This writer's analysis of the EVM report reveals that the dose limits were set inappropriately low for many vitamins and minerals, well below doses that have been used by the public for decades with apparent safety. While the release of this 360-page document would be of little import, were it to be used solely as a manifesto for the pathologically risk-averse, preliminary indications are that it could be used very actively to support the arguments of those who are seeking to ban the over-the-counter sale of many currently available nutritional supplements. If the report is used that way, then the public health could be jeopardized.

On May 30, 2002, the European Union adopted Directive 2002/46/EC, which established a framework for setting maximum limits for vitamins and minerals in food supplements. The EVM report is seen by the U.K. government as the basis for its negotiating position in the process of setting these pan-European limits.

The apparent anti-nutritional-supplement, anti-self-care bias that permeated the process of setting safety levels is evident both in the way in which the SUL was defined and in the fact that the benefits of nutritional supplements were purposely ignored. The SUL was defined as the maximum dose of a particular nutrient "that potentially susceptible individuals could take daily on a life-long basis, without medical supervision in reasonable safety." In other words, it is the highest dose that is unlikely to cause anyone any harm, ever, under any circumstance. Furthermore, the EVM was specifically instructed not to consider the benefits of any of the nutrients, and not to engage in risk/benefit analysis.[1]

There is little or no precedent in free societies for restricting access to products or activities to levels that are completely risk free. Aspirin causes intestinal bleeding, water makes people drown, driving a car causes accidents, and free speech may offend the offendable. Politicians and bureaucrats do not seek to ban aspirin or water or driving or free speech, because their benefits outweigh their risks. For vitamins and minerals, however, some authorities seem to believe that unique safety criteria are needed.

Moreover, the government's instructions to disregard the many documented benefits of nutritional supplements introduced a serious bias into the evaluation process. As the EVM acknowledged, determining safety limits involves an enormous degree of uncertainty and a fairly wide range of possible outcomes. The committee might have established higher safety limits than it did, had it been told to weigh benefits against risks. The government's instructions appeared to be an implicit directive to err on the side of excluding doses that are being used to prevent or treat disease. And that is what the EVM did, often by making questionable interpretations of the data, and doing so in what appears to have been an arbitrary and inconsistent manner.

Riboflavin Guidance Level

A typical example of the EVM's dubious approach to establishing safety limits is its evaluation of riboflavin (vitamin B2). The committee acknowledged that no

From the J Orthomolecular Med 2003;18(3–4):127–130.

toxic effects have been reported in animals given an acute oral dose of 10,000 milligrams per kilogram (mg/kg) of body weight, or after long-term ingestion of 25 mg/kg/day (equivalent to 1,750 mg/day for a 70-kg [154-lb] human). Moreover, in a study of 28 patients taking riboflavin for treatment of migraine, a dose of 400 mg/day for three months did not cause any adverse effects. Despite a complete absence of side effects at any dose in either humans or animals, the EVM set the Guidance Level for riboflavin at 40 mg/day. That level was established by dividing the 400 mg/day used in the migraine study by an "uncertainty factor" of 10, to allow for variability in the susceptibility of human beings to adverse effects.

A more appropriate conclusion regarding riboflavin would have been that no adverse effects have been observed at any dose, and that there is no basis at this time for establishing an upper limit. If the EVM's recommendation is used to limit the potency of riboflavin tablets to 40 mg, then migraine sufferers will have to take 10 pills per day, in order to prevent migraine recurrences.[2]

"Orthomolecular medicine restores natural metabolism with nutrients, such as vitamins and minerals, in optimum quantities. This means much more than the RDA or any other government standard. To overturn decades of error on the part of governments and the professions will take a good deal of effort and patience. Linus Pauling often spoke vigorously against the RDA in general and was ignored. These old, erroneous standards are part of the vitamins-as-prevention paradigm and will not yield until this old and stale paradigm is fully replaced by the vitamins-as-treatment paradigm. Pauling took 18,000 milligrams of ascorbic acid daily, which was 300 times the RDA. He loved to tell his audiences why he took so much." —ABRAM HOFFER

Vitamin B6 Safe Upper Level

Similar reasoning led to an SUL of 10 mg/day for pyridoxine (vitamin B6), even though this vitamin has been used with apparent safety, usually in doses of 50 to 200 mg/day, to treat carpal tunnel syndrome, premenstrual syndrome, asthma, and other common problems. The SUL for vitamin B6 was derived from an animal study, in which a dose of 50 mg/kg of body weight/day (equivalent to 3,000 mg/day for a 60-kg [132-lb] person) resulted in neurotoxicity. The EVM reduced that dose progressively by invoking three separate "uncertainty factors:" 1) by a factor of 3, to extrapolate from the lowest observed-adverse-effect-level (LOAEL) to a no observed-adverse-effect-level (NOAEL); 2) by an additional factor of 10, to account for presumed inter-species differences; and 3) by a further factor of 10, to account for individual variation in humans. Thus, the neurotoxic dose in animals was reduced by a factor of 300, to a level that excludes the widely used 50- and 100-mg tablets.

The decision to base the SUL for vitamin B6 on animal data (modified by a massive "uncertainty factor") was arbitrary, considering that toxicology data are available for humans.[3] Sensory neuropathy has been reported in some individuals taking large doses of vitamin B6.[4,5] Most people who suffered this adverse effect were taking 2,000 mg/day or more of pyridoxine, although some were taking only 500 mg/day. There is a single case report of a neuropathy occurring in a person taking 200 mg/day of pyridoxine, but the reliability of that case report is unclear. The individual in question was never examined, but was merely interviewed by telephone after responding to a local television report that publicized pyridoxine-induced neuropathy.[6]

Because pyridoxine neurotoxicity has been known to the medical profession for 20 years, and because vitamin B6 is being taken by millions of people, it is reasonable to assume that neurotoxicity at doses below 200 mg/day would have been reported by now, if it does occur at those doses. The fact that no such reports have appeared strongly suggests that vitamin B6 does not damage the nervous system when taken at doses below 200 mg/day. As the EVM did with other nutrients for which a LOAEL is known for humans, it could have divided the vitamin B6 LOAEL (200 mg/day) by 3 to obtain an SUL of 66.7 mg/day. Had the committee been allowed to evaluate both the benefits and risks of vitamin B6, it probably would have established the SUL at that level, rather than the 10 mg/day it arrived at through serial decimation of the animal data.

Manganese Guidance Level

Chronic inhalation of high concentrations of airborne manganese, as might be encountered in mines or steel mills, has been reported to cause a neuropsychiatric syndrome that resembles Parkinson's disease. In contrast, manganese is considered one of the least toxic trace minerals when ingested orally, and reports of human toxicity from oral ingestion are "essentially nonexistent."[7] The neurotoxicity that occurs in miners and industrial workers may result from a combination of high concentrations of manganese in the air and, possibly, direct entry of nasally inhaled manganese into the brain (bypassing the blood-brain barrier).

In establishing a Guidance Level for manganese, the EVM cited a study by Kondakis and others in which people exposed to high concentrations of manganese in their drinking water (1.8–2.3 mg/liter [L]) had more signs and symptoms of subtle neurological dysfunction than did a control group whose drinking water contained less manganese.[8] The committee acknowledged that another epidemiological study by Vieregge and colleagues showed no adverse effects among individuals whose drinking water contained up to 2.1 mg/L of manganese.[9] The EVM hypothesized that these studies may not really be contradictory, since the subjects in the Kondakis study were, on average, 10 years older than were those in the Vieregge study, and increasing age might theoretically render people more susceptible to manganese toxicity. Based on the results of these two studies, the EVM established a Guidance Level for supplemental manganese of 4 mg/day for the general population and 0.5 mg/day for elderly individuals.

There are serious problems with the EVM's analysis of the manganese research. First, the committee overlooked that fact that in the Kondakis

study the people in the high-manganese group were older than were those in the control group (mean age, 67.6 vs. 65.6 years). Many of the neurological symptoms that were investigated in this study are nonspecific and presumably age related, including fatigue, muscle pain, irritability, insomnia, sleepiness, decreased libido, depression, slowness in rising from a chair, and memory disturbances. The fact that the older people had more symptoms than did the younger people is not surprising, and may have been totally unrelated to the manganese content of their drinking water.

Second, the EVM broke its own rules regarding the use of uncertainty factors, presumably to avoid being faced with an embarrassingly low Guidance Level for the general population. In setting the level at 4 mg/day, the committee stated: "No uncertainty factor is required as the NOAEL [obtained from the Vieregge study] is based on a large epidemiological study." As a point of information, the Nurses' Health Study was a large epidemiological study, enrolling more than 85,000 participants. The Beaver Dam Eye Study was a medium-sized epidemiological study, enrolling more than 3,000 participants. In contrast, in the Vieregge study, there were only 41 subjects in the high-manganese group, making it a very small epidemiological study. In its evaluation of the biotin, riboflavin, and pantothenic acid research, the EVM reduced the NOAEL by an uncertainty factor of 10, in part because only small numbers of subjects had been studied. Considering that more subjects were evaluated in the pantothenic acid research[10] (94) than in the Vieregge study (41), it would seem appropriate also to use an uncertainty factor then for manganese data. Applying an uncertainty factor of 10 to the Vieregge study would have produced an absurdly low Guidance Level of 0.4 mg/day for supplemental manganese, which is well below the amount present in a typical diet (approximately 4 mg/day) and which can be obtained by drinking several sips of tea. Parenthetically, in a study of 47,351 male health professionals, drinking large amounts of tea (a major dietary source of manganese) was associated with a reduced risk of Parkinson's disease, not an increased risk.[11] In changing its methodology to avoid reaching an indefensible conclusion, the EVM revealed the arbitrary and inconsistent nature of its evaluation process.

Niacin (Vitamin B3) Guidance Level

Large doses of niacin can cause elevated liver function tests, and, rarely, other significant side effects. The EVM focused its evaluation, however, on the niacin-induced skin flush, which occurs at much lower doses. The niacin flush is a sensation of warmth on the skin, often associated with itching, burning, or irritation that occurs after the ingestion of niacin and disappears relatively quickly. It appears to be mediated in part by the release of prostaglandins. The niacin flush is not considered a toxic effect per se, and there is no evidence that it causes any harm. People who do not like the flush are free not to take niacin supplements or products that contain niacin. For those who are unaware that niacin causes a flush, an appropriate warning label on the bottle would provide adequate protection.

Granting, for the sake of argument, that the niacin flush is an adverse effect from which the public should be protected, the EVM's Guidance Level still is illogical. The committee noted that flushing is consistently observed at a dose 50 mg/day, which it established as the LOAEL. That dose was reduced by an uncertainty factor of 3, in order to extrapolate the LOAEL to a NOAEL. Thus, the Guidance Level was set at 17 mg/day, which approximates the RDA for the vitamin. The EVM also noted, however, that flushing has been reported at doses as low as 10 mg, so the true LOAEL is 10 mg/day. Applying the same uncertainty factor of 3 to the true LOAEL would have yielded a Guidance Level of a paltry 3.3 mg/day, which probably is not enough to prevent an anorexic person from developing pellagra. As with manganese, the EVM applied its methodology in an arbitrary and inconsistent manner, so as to avoid being faced with an embarrassing result.

Vitamin C Guidance Level

The EVM concluded that vitamin C does not cause significant adverse effects, although gas-trointestinal (GI) side effects may occur with high doses. The committee therefore set a Guidance Level based on a NOAEL for GI side effects. It is true that taking too much vitamin C, just like eating too many apples, may cause abdominal pain or diarrhea. The dose at which vitamin C causes GI side effects varies widely from person to person, but can easily be determined by each individual. Moreover, these side effects can be eliminated by reducing the dose. Most people who take vitamin C supplements know how much they can tolerate; for those who do not, a simple warning on bottles of vitamin C would appear to provide the public all the protection it needs. Considering the many health benefits of vitamin C, attempting to dumb down the dose to a level that will prevent the last stomachache in Europe is not a worthwhile goal. However, as mentioned previously, the EVM was instructed to ignore the benefits of vitamin C.

Granting, for the sake of argument, that there is value in setting a Guidance Level for GI side effects, the EVM did a rather poor job of setting that level. The committee established the LOAEL at 3,000 mg/day, based on a study of a small number of normal volunteers.[12] An uncertainty factor of 3 was used to extrapolate from the LOAEL to a NOAEL, resulting in a Guidance Level of 1,000 mg/day. However, anyone practicing nutritional medicine knows that some patients experience abdominal pain or diarrhea at vitamin C doses of 1,000 mg/day or less, and the EVM did acknowledge that GI side effects have been reported at doses of 1,000 mg.

It is disingenuous to set a NOAEL and then to concede that effects do occur at the no-effect level. To be consistent with the methodology it used for other nutrients, the committee should have set the LOAEL at 1,000 mg/day, and reduced it by a factor of 3 to arrive at a NOAEL of 333 mg/day. The EVM was no doubt aware of the credibility problems it would have faced, had it suggested that half the world is currently overdosing on vitamin C. To resolve its dilemma, the committee used a scientifically unjustifiable route to arrive at a seemingly politically expedient outcome.

CONCLUSION

These and other examples from the report demonstrate that the EVM applied its methodology in an arbitrary and inconsistent manner, in arriving at "safety" recommendations that are excessively and inappropriately restrictive. While the directive to evaluate only the risks, and to ignore the benefits, of nutritional supplements created a rigged game, the members of the EVM appeared to be willing participants in that game.

If the EVM report is used to relegate currently available nutritional supplements to prescription-only status, then millions of people would be harmed, and very few would benefit. It would be of little consolation that the higher doses of vitamins and minerals could still be obtained with a doctor's prescription, because most doctors know less about nutrition than do many of their patients. Moreover, the overburdened healthcare system is in no position to take on the job of gatekeeper of the vitamin cabinet; nor is there any need for it to do so.

Ironically, as flawed as the EVM report is, its recommendations may ultimately prove to be "as good as it gets" in Europe. Other European countries are recommending that maximum permitted levels be directly linked to multiples of the U.S. Recommended Dietary Allowance (RDA), which could result in limits for some nutrients being set substantially lower than those suggested in the EVM report.

While some nutritional supplements can cause adverse effects in certain clinical situations or at certain doses, appropriate warning labels on vitamin and mineral products would provide ample protection against most of those risks.

REFERENCES

1. Expert Group on Vitamins and Minerals. Safe upper levels for vitamins and minerals, 2003, p. 28. Available at: www.food.gov .uk/ multimedia/pdfs/vitmin2003.pdf.

2. Schoenen J, Jacquy J, Lenaerts M. Effectiveness of high-dose riboflavin in migraine prophylaxis: a randomized controlled trial. *Neurology* 1998;50:466–470.

3. Gaby AR: The safe use of vitamin B6. *J Nutr Med* 1990;1:153–157.

4. Schaumburg H, Kaplan J, Windebank A, et al. Sensory neuropathy from pyridoxine abuse: a new megavitamin syndrome. *N Engl J Med* 1983;309:445–448.

5. Parry GJ. Sensory neuropathy with low-dose pyridoxine. *Neurology* 1985;35:1466–1468.

6. Parry GJ. Personal communication, July 14, 1986.

7. Nielsen FH: Ultratrace minerals. In: Shils ME, Olson JA, Shike M (eds.) *Modern Nutrition in Health and Disease.* 8th ed. Philadelphia: Lea & Febiger, 1994, 276.

8. Kondakis XG, Makris N, Leotsinidis M, et al. Possible health effects of high manganese concentration in drinking water. *Arch Environ Health* 1989;44:175–178.

9. Vieregge P, Heinzow B, Korf G, et al. Long-term exposure to manganese in rural well water has no neurological effects. *Can J Neurol Sci* 1995;22:286–289.

10. Calcium pantothenate in arthritic conditions: a report from the General Practitioner Research Group. *Practitioner* 1980;224: 208–211.

11. Ascherio A, Zhang SM, Hernan MA, et al. Prospective study of caffeine consumption and risk of Parkinson's disease in men and women. *Ann Neurol* 2001;50:56–63.

12. Cameron E, Campbell A. The orthomolecular treatment of cancer. II. Clinical trial of high-dose ascorbic acid supplements in advanced human cancer. *Chem Biol Interact* 1974;9:285–315.

NEGATIVE NEWS MEDIA REPORTS ON VITAMIN SUPPLEMENTS
by Andrew W. Saul, PhD

There have been a number of widely publicized negative reports about vitamins in the news media. While trumpeting those select few, they just possibly may have missed these:

- Multivitamin supplements lower your risk of cancer by 8 percent. An 8 percent reduction in deaths means the lives of 48,000 people in the United States alone could be saved each year, just by taking an inexpensive daily vitamin pill. (Gaziano JM et al. Multivitamins in the prevention of cancer in men: the Physicians' Health Study II Randomized Controlled Trial. *JAMA* 2012;308:1871–1880.)

- **72 percent of physicians personally use dietary supplements.** The multivitamin is the most popular dietary supplement taken by doctors. (Dickinson A, et al. Physicians and nurses use and recommend dietary supplements: report of a survey. *Nutrition Journal* 2009;8:29.)

- **High serum levels of vitamin B6, methionine, and folate are associated with a 50 percent reduction in lung cancer risk.** Those with higher levels of these nutrients had a significantly lower risk of lung cancer whether they smoked or not (Johansson M, et al. Serum B vitamin levels and risk of lung cancer. *JAMA* 2010;303:2377–2385.)

- **Vitamin D reduces cancer risk.** Studies on breast and colorectal cancer found that an increase of serum 25(OH)D concentration of 10 nanograms per milliliter (ng/ml) was associated with a 15 percent reduction in colorectal cancer incidence and 11 percent reduction in breast cancer incidence (Gandini S, et al. Meta-analysis of observational studies of serum 25-hydroxyvitamin D levels and colorectal, breast and prostate cancer and colorectal adenoma *Int J Cancer* 2011;128:1414–24.)

- **Vitamin D increases breast cancer survival.** Women diagnosed with breast cancer had increased survival for those with higher serum 25(OH)D concentrations. In those with lower vitamin D concentrations, mortality increased by 8 percent. (Vrieling A, et al. Serum 25-hydroxyvitamin D and postmenopausal breast cancer survival: a prospective patient cohort study. *Breast Cancer* Res 2011;13:R74.)

- **Risk of heart failure decreases with increasing blood levels of vitamin C.** Each 20 micromole/liter (μmol/L) increase in plasma vitamin C was associated with a 9 percent reduction in death from heart failure. If everyone took high enough doses of vitamin C to reach 80 μmol/L, it would mean 216,000 fewer deaths per year. To achieve that a plasma level requires a daily dosage of about 500 milligrams (mg) of vitamin C. (Pfister R, et al. Plasma vitamin C predicts incident heart failure in men and women in European Prospective Investigation into Cancer and Nutrition-Norfolk prospective study. *Am Heart J* 2011;162:246–253.)

- **Vitamin C arrests and reverses cancer.** Oncologist Victor Marcial, MD, says: "We studied patients with advanced cancer (Stage 4). Forty patients received 40,000–75,000 mg intravenously several times a week . . . In addition, they received a diet and other supplements. The initial tumor response rate was achieved in 75 percent of patients, defined as a 50 percent reduction or more in tumor size." (Presentation at the Medical Sciences Campus, University of Puerto Rico, April 12, 2010.)

You can read about the intravenous vitamin C protocol that he used in Appendix 3, "The Riordan IVC Protocol for Adjunctive Cancer Care: Intravenous Ascorbate as a Chemotherapeutic and Biological Response Modifying Agent." Intravenous vitamin C cancer therapy for cancer is presented in detail on video, available for free access online at www.riordanclinic.org/education/symposium/s2009 (12 lectures); www.riordanclinic.org/education/symposium/s2010 (9 lectures); and www.riordanclinic.org/education/symposium/s2012 (11 lectures).

The news media have also reported claims that "vitamin E does no good at all in preventing cancer or heart disease." Here's more of what they failed to report:

- **Natural vitamin E factor yields a 75 percent decrease in prostate tumor formation.** Gamma-tocotrienol, a cofactor found in natural vitamin E preparations, kills prostate cancer stem cells. (Sze Ue Luk1, et al. Gamma-tocotrienol as an effective agent in targeting prostate cancer stem cell-like population. *Int J Cancer* 2011;128:2182–2191.)

- Gamma-tocotrienol also is effective against existing prostate tumors. (Nesaretnam K, et al. Modulation of cell growth and apoptosis response in human prostate cancer cells supplemented with tocotrienols. *Eur J Lipid Sci Technol* 2008, 110, 23-31; see also: Conte C, et al. Gamma-tocotrienol metabolism and antiproliferative effect in prostate cancer cells. *Ann NY Acad Sci* 2004;1031:391–394.)

- Vitamin E reduces mortality by 24 percent in persons 71 or older. (Hemila H, et al. *Age Ageing* 2011;40(2): 215–220.)

- 300 IU vitamin E per day reduces lung cancer by 61 percent. (Mahabir S, et al. Dietary alpha-, beta-, gamma- and delta-tocopherols in lung cancer risk. *Int J Cancer* 2008;123(5):1173–1180.)

- Vitamin E is an effective treatment for atherosclerosis. "Subjects with supplementary vitamin E intake of 100 IU per day or greater demonstrated less coronary artery lesion progression than did subjects with supplementary vitamin E intake less than 100 IU per day." (Hodis HN, et al. Serial coronary angiographic evidence that antioxidant vitamin intake reduces progression of coronary artery atherosclerosis. *JAMA* 1995;273:1849–1854.)

- 400 to 800 IU of vitamin E daily reduces risk of heart attack by 77 percent. (Stephens NG et al. Randomized controlled trial of vitamin E in patients with coronary artery disease: Cambridge Heart Antioxidant Study (CHAOS). *Lancet* 1996;347:781–786.)

Here are additional studies showing special health benefits from vitamin E:

- Increasing vitamin E with supplements prevents COPD (chronic obstructive pulmonary disease), emphysema, chronic bronchitis. (Agler AH et al. Randomized vitamin E supplementation and risk of chronic lung disease in the Women's Health Study. American Thoracic Society 2010 International Conference, May 18, 2010.)

- 800 IU vitamin E per day is a successful treatment for fatty liver disease. (Sanyal AJ, et al. Pioglitazone, vitamin E, or placebo for nonalcoholic steatohepatitis. *N Engl J Med* 2010;362:1675–1685.)

- Alzheimer's patients who take 2,000 IU of vitamin E per day live longer. (Pavlik VN, et al. Vitamin E use is associated with improved survival in an Alzheimer's disease cohort. *Dement Geriatr Cogn Disord* 2009;28 (6):536–540; see also: Grundman M. Vitamin E and Alzheimer disease: the basis for additional clinical trials. *Am J Clin Nutr* 2000;71(2):630S–636S.)

- 400 IU of Vitamin E per day reduces epileptic seizures in children by more than 60 percent. (Ogunmekan AO, et al. A randomized, double-blind, placebo-controlled, clinical trial of D-alpha-tocopheryl acetate [vitamin E], as add-on therapy, for epilepsy in children. *Epilepsia* 1989;30:84–89.)

- Vitamin E supplements help prevent amyotrophic lateral sclerosis (ALS). This important finding is the result of a 10-year-plus Harvard study of over a million persons. (Wang H, et al. Vitamin E intake and risk of amyotrophic lateral sclerosis: a pooled analysis of data from 5 prospective cohort studies. *Am J Epidemiol* 2011;173:595–602.)

- Vitamin E is more effective than a prescription drug in treating chronic liver disease. Said the authors: "The good news is that this study showed that cheap and readily available vitamin E can help many of those with this condition." (Sanyal AJ, et al. Pioglitazone, vitamin E, or placebo for nonalcoholic steatohepatitis. *N Engl J Med* 2010 May;362:1675–1685.)

Excerpted from the *Orthomolecular Medicine News Service*, November 12, 2013.

DEATH BY MEDICINE

by Gary Null, PhD, Carolyn Dean, MD, ND, Martin Feldman, MD, and Debora Rasio, MD

A close reading of medical peer-review journals and government health statistics shows that American medicine frequently causes more harm than good. The number of people having in-hospital, adverse drug reactions (ADR) to prescribed medicine is 2.2 million.[1] Richard Besser, MD, of the Centers for Disease Control and Prevention (CDC), in 1995, said the number of unnecessary antibiotics prescribed annually for viral infections was 20 million. Dr. Besser, in 2003, refers to tens of millions of unnecessary antibiotics.[2,2a] The number of unnecessary medical and surgical procedures performed annually is 7.5 million.[3] The number of people exposed to unnecessary hospitalization annually is 8.9 million.[4] The total number of iatrogenic deaths shown in the Table 1 is 783,936. It is evident that the American medical system is the leading cause of death and injury in the United States. The 2001 heart disease annual death rate is 699,697; the annual cancer death rate, 553,251.[5]

picture. Unfortunately, cause and effect go unmonitored. The figures on unnecessary events represent people ("patients") who are thrust into a dangerous healthcare system. They are helpless victims. Each one of these 16.4 million lives is being affected in a way that could have a fatal consequence (see Table 2).

TABLE 2. ANNUAL UNNECESSARY MEDICAL EVENTS STATISTICS

UNNECESSARY EVENTS	PEOPLE AFFECTED	IATROGENIC EVENTS
Hospitalization[4,15]	8.90 million	1.78 million
Procedures[3,22]	7.50 million	1.30 million
TOTAL	16.4 million	3.08 million

Simply entering a hospital could result in one of the following events:

• In 16.4 million people, 2.1 percent chance of a serious adverse drug reaction[1] (186,000).

• In 16.4 million people, 5–6 percent chance of acquiring a nosocomial infection[9] (489,500).

• In 16.4 million people, 4–36 percent chance of having an iatrogenic injury in hospital (medical error and adverse drug reactions)[15] (1.78 million).

• In 16.4 million people, 17 percent chance of a procedure error[22] (1.3 million).

Overlap of Statistics

We have added, cumulatively, figures from 13 references of annual iatrogenic deaths. However, there is invariably some degree of overlap and double counting that can occur in gathering nonfinite statistics. Death numbers don't come with names and birth dates to prevent duplication. On the other hand, there are many missing statistics.

TABLE 1. ANNUAL PHYSICAL AND ECONOMIC COST OF MEDICAL INTERVENTION

CONDITION	DEATHS	COST
Hospital ADR[1,31]	106,000	$12 billion
Medical error[6]	98,000	$2 billion
Bedsores[7,8]	115,000	$55 billion
Infection[9,10]	88,000	$5 billion
Malnutrition[11]	108,800	—
Outpatient ADR[12,38]	199,000	$77 billion
Unnecessary Procedures[3,13]	37,136	$122 billion
Surgery-Related[39]	32,000	$9 billion
TOTAL	783,936	$282 billion

The enumerating of unnecessary medical events is very important in our analysis. Any medical procedure that is invasive and not necessary must be considered as part of the larger iatrogenic

From the *J Orthomolecular Med* 2005;20(1):21–34.

As we will show, only about 5 to 20 percent of iatrogenic incidents are even recorded,[15,17,18] and, our outpatient iatrogenic statistics[12,32] only include drug-related events and not surgical cases, diagnostic errors, or therapeutic mishaps.

We have also been conservative in our inclusion of statistics that were not reported in peer review journals or by government institutions. For example, on July 23, 2002, the *Chicago Tribune* analyzed records from patient databases, court cases, 5,810 hospitals, as well as 75 federal and state agencies and found 103,000 cases of death due to hospital infections, 75 percent of which were preventable.[36] We do not include this figure but report the lower Weinstein figure of 88,000.[9]

Another figure that we withheld, for lack of proper peer review was the National Committee for Quality Assurance, September 2003 report, which found that at least 57,000 people die annually from lack of proper care for common diseases such as high blood pressure, diabetes, or heart disease.[37] Overlapping of statistics presented here may occur with the Institute of Medicine (IOM) paper that designates "medical error" as including drugs, surgery, and unnecessary procedures.[6] Since we have also included other statistics on adverse drug reactions, surgery, and, unnecessary procedures, perhaps as much as 50 percent of the IOM number could be redundant. However, even taking away half the 98,000 IOM number still leaves us with iatrogenic events as the number one killer at 734,936 annual deaths.

Even greater numbers of iatrogenic deaths will eventually come to light when all facets of healthcare delivery are measured. Most iatrogenic statistics are derived from hospital-based studies. However, health care is no longer typically relegated to hospitals. Today, health care is shared by hospitals, outpatient clinics, transitional care, long-term care, rehabilitative care, home care, and private practitioners offices. In the current climate of reducing healthcare costs, the number of hospitals and the length of patient stays are being slashed. These measures will increase the number of patients shunted into outpatient, home care, and long-term care, and the iatrogenic morbidity and mortality will also increase.

First Major Iatrogenic Study

Lucian L. Leape, MD, opened medicine's Pandora's box in his 1994 *Journal of the American Medical Association (JAMA)* paper, "Error in Medicine."[15] He began the paper by reminiscing about the famous medical maxim "First, do no harm," but he found evidence of the opposite happening in medicine. He found that Schimmel reported in 1964 that 20 percent of hospital patients suffered iatrogenic injury, with a 20 percent fatality rate. Steel in 1981 reported that 36 percent of hospitalized patients experienced iatrogenesis with a 25 percent fatality rate and adverse drug reactions were involved in 50 percent of the injuries. Bedell in 1991 reported that 64 percent of acute heart attacks in one hospital were preventable and were mostly due to adverse drug reactions. However, Leape focused on his and Brennan's "Harvard Medical Practice Study" published in 1991.[15a] They found that in 1984, in New York State, there was a 4 percent iatrogenic injury rate for patients with a 14 percent fatality rate. From the 98,609 patients injured and the 14 percent fatality rate, he estimated that in the whole of the United States 180,000 people die each year, partly as a result of iatrogenic injury. Leape compared these deaths to the equivalent of three jumbo jet crashes every two days.

Why Leape chose to use the much lower figure of 4 percent injury for his analysis remains in question. Perhaps he wanted to tread lightly. If Leape had, instead, calculated the average rate among the three studies he cites (36 percent, 20 percent, and 4 percent), he would have come up with a 20 percent medical error rate. The number of fatalities that he could have presented, using an average rate of injury and his 14 percent fatality, is an annual 1,189,576 iatrogenic deaths, or over 10 jumbo jets crashing every day.

Leape acknowledged that the literature on medical error is sparse and we are only seeing the tip of the iceberg. He said that when errors are specifically sought out, reported rates are "distressingly high." He cited several autopsy studies with rates as high as 35 to 40 percent of missed diagnoses causing death. He also commented that an intensive care unit reported an average of 1.7 errors per day per patient, and 29 percent of those errors were potentially serious or fatal. We wonder: What is the effect on someone who daily gets the wrong medication, the wrong dose, the wrong procedure? How do we measure the accumulated burden of injury? And when the patient finally succumbs after the tenth error that week, what is entered on the death certificate?

Leape calculated the rate of error in the intensive care unit. First, he found that each patient had an average of 178 "activities" (staff/procedure/medical interactions) a day, of which 1.7 were errors, which means a 1 percent failure rate. To some this may not seem like much, but putting this into perspective, Leape cited industry standards where in aviation a 0.1 percent failure rate would mean two unsafe plane landings per day at O'Hare International Airport in Chicago; in the U.S. mail, 16,000 pieces of lost mail every hour; or in banking, 32,000 bank checks deducted from the wrong bank account every hour.

Analyzing why there is so much medical error, Leape acknowledged the lack of reporting. Unlike a jumbo jet crash, which gets instant media coverage, hospital errors are spread out over the country in thousands of different locations. They are also perceived as isolated and unusual events. However, the most important reason that medical error is unrecognized and growing, according to Leape, was, and still is, that doctors and nurses are unequipped to deal with human error, due to the culture of medical training and practice. Doctors are taught that mistakes are unacceptable. Medical mistakes are therefore viewed as a failure of character and any error equals negligence. We can see how a great deal of sweeping under the rug takes place since nobody is taught what to do when medical error does occur. Leape cited McIntyre and Popper who said the "infallibility model" of medicine leads to intellectual dishonesty with a need to cover up mistakes rather than admit them. There are no grand rounds on medical errors, no sharing of failures among doctors, and no one to support them emotionally when their error harms a patient.

Leape hoped his paper would encourage medicine "to fundamentally change the way they think about errors and why they occur." It's been almost a decade since this groundbreaking work, but the mistakes continue to soar.

One year later, in 1995, a report in *JAMA* said that, "Over a million patients are injured in U.S. hospitals each year, and approximately 280,000 die annually as a result of these injuries. Therefore, the iatrogenic death rate dwarfs the annual automobile accident mortality rate of 45,000 and accounts for more deaths than all other accidents combined."[16]

At a press conference in 1997, Dr. Leape released a nationwide poll on patient iatrogenesis conducted by the National Patient Safety Foundation (NPSF), which is sponsored by the American Medical Association. The survey found that more than 100 million Americans have been impacted directly and indirectly by a medical mistake. Forty-two percent were directly affected and a total of 84 percent personally knew of someone who had experienced a medical mistake.[14] Leape is a founding member of the NPSF.

Dr. Leape at this press conference also updated his 1994 statistics saying that medical errors in inpatient hospital settings nationwide, as of 1997, could be as high as 3 million and could cost as much as $200 billion. Leape used a 14 percent fatality rate to determine a medical error death rate of 180,000 in 1994.[15] In 1997, using Leape's base number of 3 million errors, the annual deaths could be as much as 420,000 for inpatients alone. This does not include nursing home deaths, or people in the outpatient community dying of drug side effects or as the result of medical procedures.

Only a Fraction of Medical Errors Are Reported

Leape, in 1994, said that he was well aware that medical errors were not being reported.[15] According to a study in two obstetrical units in the United Kingdom, only about one-quarter of the adverse incidents on the units are ever reported for reasons of protecting staff or preserving reputations, or fear of reprisals, including lawsuits.[17] An analysis by Wald and Shojania found that only 1.5 percent of all adverse events result in an incident report, and only 6 percent of adverse drug events are identified properly.[18] The authors learned that the American

College of Surgeons gives a very broad guess that surgical incident reports routinely capture only 5 to 30 percent of adverse events. In one surgical study only 20 percent of surgical complications resulted in discussion at morbidity and mortality rounds.[18] From these studies, it appears that all the statistics gathered may be substantially underestimating the number of adverse drug and medical therapy incidents. It also underscores the fact that our mortality statistics are conservative figures.

Drug Iatrogenesis

Drugs comprise the major treatment modality of scientific medicine. With the discovery of the germ theory, medical scientists convinced the public that infectious organisms were the cause of illness. Finding the cure for these infections proved much harder than anyone imagined. From the beginning, chemical drugs promised much more than they delivered. But far beyond not working, the drugs also caused incalculable side effects. The drugs themselves, even when properly prescribed, have side effects that can be fatal. But human error can make the situation even worse.

Medication Errors

A survey of a 1992 national pharmacy database found a total of 429,827 medication errors from 1,081 hospitals. Medication errors occurred in 5.22 percent of patients admitted to these hospitals each year. The authors concluded that a minimum of 90,895 patients annually were harmed by medication errors in the country as a whole.[19] A 2002 study shows that 20 percent of hospital medications for patients had dosage mistakes. Nearly 40 percent of these errors were considered potentially harmful to the patient. In a typical 300-patient hospital the number of errors per day were 40.[20]

Problems involving patients' medications were even higher the following year. The error rate intercepted by pharmacists in this study was 24 percent, making the potential minimum number of patients harmed by prescription drugs 417,908.[21]

More Adverse Drug Reactions

More recent studies on adverse drug reactions show that the figures from 1994 may be increasing.

A 2003 study followed 400 patients after discharge from a tertiary care hospital (hospital care that requires highly specialized skills, technology, or support services). Seventy-six patients (19 percent) had adverse events. Adverse drug events were the most common at 66 percent. The next most common events were procedure-related injuries at 17 percent.[22]

In a *New England Journal of Medicine* (*NEJM*) study an alarming one in four patients suffered observable side effects from the more than 3.34 billion prescription drugs filled in 2002.[23] One of the doctors who produced the study was interviewed by Reuters News Agency and commented that, "With these 10-minute appointments, it's hard for the doctor to get into whether the symptoms are bothering the patients."[24] William Tierney, MD, who editorialized on the *NEJM* study, said ". . . given the increasing number of powerful drugs available to care for the aging population, the problem will only get worse." The drugs with the worst record of side effects were the selective serotonin reuptake inhibitors (SSRIs), the non-steroidal anti-inflammatory drugs (NSAIDs), and calcium-channel blockers. Reuters also reported that prior research has suggested that nearly 5 percent of hospital admissions—over 1 million per year—are the result of drug side effects. But most of the cases are not documented as such. The study found one of the reasons for this failure: in nearly two-thirds of the cases, doctors couldn't diagnose drug side effects or the side effects persisted because the doctor failed to heed the warning signs.

Medicating Our Feelings

We only need to look at the side effects of antidepressant drugs, which give hope to a depressed population. Patients seeking a more joyful existence and relief from worry, stress, and anxiety, fall victim to the messages blatantly displayed on TV and billboards. Often, instead of relief, they also fall victim to a myriad of iatrogenic side effects of antidepressant medication.

Also, a whole generation of antidepressant users has resulted from young people growing up on methylphenidate (Ritalin), the most commonly prescribed medication for attention-deficit hyperactivity disorder (ADHD). Medicating youth and modifying their emotions must have some impact on how they learn to deal with their feelings. They learn to equate coping with drugs and not with calling on their inner resources. As adults, these medicated youth reach for alcohol, drugs, or even street drugs, to cope. According to the *JAMA*, "Ritalin acts much like cocaine."[25] Today's marketing of mood-modifying drugs, such as fluoxetine (Prozac) or sertraline (Zoloft), makes them not only socially acceptable but almost a necessity in today's stressful world.

Television Diagnosis

In order to reach the widest audience possible, drug companies are no longer just targeting medical doctors with their message about antidepressants. By 1995 drug companies had tripled the amount of money allotted to direct advertising of prescription drugs to consumers. The majority of the money is spent on seductive television ads. From 1996 to 2000, spending rose from $791 million to nearly $2.5 billion.[26] Even though $2.5 billion may seem like a lot of money, the authors comment that it only represents 15 percent of the total pharmaceutical advertising budget. According to medical experts "there is no solid evidence on the appropriateness of prescribing that results from consumers requesting an advertised drug." However, the drug companies maintain that direct to consumer advertising is educational.

Sidney M. Wolfe, MD, of the Public Citizen Health Research Group in Washington, D.C., argues that the public is often misinformed about these ads.[27] People want what they see on television and are told to go to their doctor for a prescription. Doctors in private practice either acquiesce to their patients' demands for these drugs or spend valuable clinic time trying to talk patients out of unnecessary drugs. Dr. Wolfe remarks that one important study found that people mistakenly believe that the "FDA reviews all ads before they are released and allows only the safest and most effective drugs to be promoted directly to the public."[28]

How Do We Know Drugs Are Safe?

Another aspect of scientific medicine that the public takes for granted is the testing of new drugs. Unlike the class of people that take drugs who are ill and need medication, in general, drugs are tested on individuals who are fairly healthy and not on other medications that can interfere with findings. But when they are declared "safe" and enter the drug prescription books, they are naturally going to be used by people on a variety of other medications and who also have a lot of other health problems. Then, a new phase of drug testing called post-approval comes into play, which is the documentation of side effects once drugs hit the market. In one very telling report, the General Accounting Office (an agency of the U.S. government) "found that of the 198 drugs approved by the FDA between 1976 and 1985 . . . 102 (or 51.5 percent) had serious post-approval risks . . . the serious post-approval risks (included) heart failure, myocardial infarction, anaphylaxis, respiratory depression and arrest, seizures, kidney and liver failure, severe blood disorders, birth defects and fetal toxicity, and blindness."[29]

NBC's investigative show *Dateline* wondered if your doctor is moonlighting as a drug rep. After a year-long investigation they reported that because doctors can legally prescribe any drug to any patient for any condition, drug companies heavily promote "off-label" and frequently inappropriate and non-tested uses of these medications in spite of the fact that these drugs are only approved for specific indications they have been tested for.[30]

The leading causes of adverse drug reactions are antibiotics (17 percent), cardiovascular drugs (17 percent), chemotherapy (15 percent), and analgesics and anti-inflammatory agents (15 percent).[31]

Overmedicating Seniors

Robert Epstein, MD, chief medical officer of Medco Health Solutions (a unit of Merck & Co.), conducted a study on drug trends.[33] He found that seniors are going to multiple physicians and getting multiple prescriptions and using multiple pharmacies. Medco oversees drug benefit plans for more than 60 million Americans, including 6.3 million senior citizens who received more than 160 million prescriptions. According to the study the average senior receives 25 prescriptions annually. In those 6.3 million seniors a total of 7.9 million medication alerts were triggered: less than half that number, 3.4 million, were detected in 1999. About 2.2 million of those alerts indicated excessive dosages unsuitable for senior citizens and about 2.4 million indicated clinically inappropriate drugs for the elderly.

According to Drug Benefit Trends, the average number of prescriptions dispensed per non-Medicare HMO member per year rose 5.6 percent from 1999 to 2000—from 7.1 to 7.5 prescriptions. The average number dispensed for Medicare members increased 5.5 percent—from 18.1 to 19.1 prescriptions.[34] The number of prescriptions in 2000 was 2.98 billion, with an average per person prescription amount of 10.4 annually.[34] In a study of 818 residents of residential care facilities for the elderly, 94 percent were receiving at least one medication at the time of the interview. The average intake of medications was five per resident; the authors noted that many of these drugs were given without a documented diagnosis justifying their use.[35]

A Global Issue

A survey published in the *Journal of Health Affairs* pointed out that between 18 and 28 percent of people who were recently ill had suffered from a medical or drug error in the previous two years. The study surveyed 750 recently-ill adults in five different countries. The breakdown by country showed 18 percent of those in Britain, 25 percent in Canada, 23 percent in Australia, 23 percent in New Zealand, and the highest number was in the United States at 28 percent.[32]

What Remains to Be Uncovered

Iatrogenic morbidity, mortality, and financial loss in outpatient clinics, transitional care, long-term care, rehabilitative care, home care, private practitioners offices, as well as hospitals, is also due to the following:

• X-ray exposures (mammography, fluoroscopy, computed tomography scans)

• Overuse of antibiotics in all conditions

• Drugs that are carcinogenic (hormone replacement therapy)

• Immunosuppressive drugs, prescription drugs

• Cancer chemotherapy

• Surgery and surgical procedures

• Unnecessary surgery (cesarean section, radical mastectomy, preventive mastectomy, radical hysterectomy, prostatectomy, cholecystectomies, cosmetic surgery, arthroscopy)

• Medical procedures and therapies

• Discredited, unnecessary, and unproven medical procedures and therapies

• Doctors themselves (when doctors go on strike, it appears the mortality rate goes down)

• Missed diagnoses

■ CONCLUSION

What we have outlined in this paper are insupportable aspects of our contemporary medical system that need to be changed, beginning at its very foundations. When the number one killer in a society is the healthcare system, that system must take responsibility for its shortcomings. It's a failed system in need of immediate attention.

REFERENCES

1. Lazarou J, Pomeranz B, Corey P. Incidence of adverse drug reactions in hospitalized patients. *JAMA* 1998;279:1200–1205.

2. Rabin R. Caution about overuse of antibiotics. *Newsday* Sep 18, 2003.

2a. http://www.cdc.gov/drugresistance/community.

3. Calculations detailed in Unnecessary Surgical Procedures section, from two sources: (13) http:/ /hcup.ahrq.gov/HCUPnet.asp (see Instant Tables: 2001 prerun tables: most common procedures) and (71) U.S. Congressional House Subcommittee Oversight Investigation. Cost and Quality of Health Care: Unnecessary Surgery. Washington, DC: Government Printing Office, 1976.

4. Calculations from four sources, see Unnecessary Hospitalization section: 1) http:// hcup.ahrq.gov/HCUPnet.asp (see Instant Tables: 2001 prerun tables: most common diagnoses). 2) Siu AL, Sonnenberg FA, Manning WG, et al. Inappropriate use of hospitals in a randomized trial of health insurance plans. *NEJM* 1986;315(20):1259–1266. 3) Siu AL, WG Manning, B Benjamin. Patient, provider and hospital characteristics associated with inappropriate hospitalization. *Am J Public Health*

1990;80(10):1253–1256. 4) Eriksen BO, IS Kristiansen, E Nord, et al. The cost of inappropriate admissions: a study of health benefits and resource utilization in a department of internal medicine. *J Intern Med* 1999;246(4):379–387.

5. National Vital Statistics Reports. Vol. 51, No. 5, March 14, 2003.

6. Thomas et al., 2000; Thomas et al., 1999. Institute of Medicine.

7. Xakellis GC, Frantz R, Lewis A. Cost of pressure ulcer prevention in long-term Care. *JAGS* 43–45, May 1995.

8. Barczak CA, Barnett RI, Childs EJ, et al. Fourth National Pressure Ulcer Prevalence Survey, Advances in Wound Care 1997; Jul/Aug: 10–14.

9. Weinstein RA. Nosocomial infection update. Special issue. *Emerging Infectious Diseases* 1998 July/Sept; 4(3).

10. Fourth Decennial International Conference on Nosocomial and Healthcare-Associated Infections. *MMWR* 2000;49(7):138.

11. Greene-Burger S, Kayser-Jones J, Prince-Bell J. Malnutrition and dehydration in nursing homes: key issues in prevention and treatment. *National Citizens' Coalition for Nursing Home Reform.* 2000. Available at: www.cmwf.org/programs/elders /burger_mal_386.asp.

12. Starfield B. Is U.S. health really the best in the world? *JAMA* 2000;284(4):483–485. Starfield B. Deficiencies in U.S. medical care. *JAMA* 2000;284(17):2184–2185.

13. HCUPnet, Healthcare Cost and Utilization Project for the Agency for Healthcare Research and Quality. Available at www.ahrq.gov/data/hcup/hcupnet.htm and http://hcup.ahrq.gov/ HCUPnet.asp, http://hcup. ahrq.gov/HCUPnet.asp.

14. Leape L. National Patient Safety Foundation Press Release. Nationwide poll on patient safety Oct 9, 1997. Available at: www.npsf.org/ html/pressrel/finalgen.html.

15. Leape LL. Error in medicine. *JAMA* 1994;272(23): 1851–1857.

15a. Brennan TA, Leape LL, Laird NM, et al. Incidence of adverse events and negligence in hospitalized patients. *N Engl J Med* 1991;324:370–376.

16. Bates DW, Cullen DJ, Laird N, et al. Incidence of adverse drug events and potential adverse drug events: implications for prevention. ADE Prevention Study Group. *JAMA* 1995;274 (1):29–34.

17. Vincent C, Stanhope N, Crowley-Murphy M. Reasons for not reporting adverse incidents: an empirical study. *J Eval Clin Pract* 1999;5(1):13–21.

18. Wald H, Shojania K. Incident reporting in making health care safer: a critical analysis of patient safety practices. Agency for Healthcare Research and Quality (AHRQ), 2001.

19. Bond CA, Raehl CL, Franke T. Clinical pharmacy services, hospital pharmacy staffing, and medication errors in United States hospitals. *Pharmacotherapy* 2002;22(2):134–147.

20. Barker KN, Flynn EA, Pepper GA, et al. Medication errors observed in 36 health care facilities. *Arch Intern Med* 2002;162(16):1897–1903.

21. LaPointe NM, Jollis JG. Medication errors in hospitalized cardiovascular patients. *Arch Intern Med* 2003;163(12): 1461–1466.

22. Forster AJ, Murff HJ, Peterson JF, et al. The incidence and severity of adverse events affecting patients after discharge from the hospital. *Ann Intern Med* 2003;138(3):161–167.

23. Gandhi TK, Weingart SN, Borus J, et al. Adverse drug events in ambulatory care. *N Engl J Med* 2003;348(16):1556–1564.

24. Medication side effects strike 1-in-4. Reuters News Agency. Apr 17, 2003.

25. Vastag B. Pay attention: Ritalin acts much like cocaine. *JAMA* 2001;286(8):905–906.

26. Rosenthal MB, Berndt ER, Donohue JM, et al. Promotion of prescription drugs to consumers. *N Engl J Med* 2002;346(7): 498–505.

27. Wolfe SM. Direct-to-consumer advertising: education or emotion promotion? *N Engl J Med* 2002;346(7):524–526.

28. Ibid.

29. GAO/PEMD 90–15 FDA Drug Review: Post-approval risks, 1976–1985;3.

30. MSNBC, July 11, 2003.

31. Suh DC, Woodall BS, Shin SK, et al. Clinical and economic impact of adverse drug reactions in hospitalized patients. *Ann Pharmacother* 2000;34(12):1373–1379.

32. Five nation survey exposes flaws in the U.S. health care system. *Journal of Health Affairs.* May 14, 2002.

33. Bordon W. Study finds overmedication of U.S. seniors. *Reuters Health* May 21, 2003.

34. Average number of prescriptions by HMOs increases. *Drug Benefit Trends* 2002;14(8).

35. *Prescription Drug Trends* 2001; Kaiser Family Foundation.

36. Berens D. Unhealthy hospitals: infection epidemic carves deadly path. Poor hygiene, overwhelmed workers contribute to thousands of deaths. *Chicago Tribune* 2002. Available at: www.chicagotribune.com/news/specials/chi-0207210272jul 21.story.

37. Available at: www.imakenews.com/health-itworld/ e_article000187752.cfm.

38. Weingart SN, Wilson R, Gibberd RW, et al. Epidemiology of medical error. *West J Med* 2000;172(6):390–393.

39. Zhan C, Miller M. Excess length of stay, charges, and mortality attributable to medical injuries during hospitalization: AHRQ Study. *JAMA* 2003;290:1868–1874.

"SUPERNUTRITION" AS A STRATEGY FOR THE CONTROL OF DISEASE
by Roger J. Williams, PhD

Aside from frank starvation, there are three levels of nutrition that human beings have experienced: poor, fair, and good. "Supernutrition" (total nutrition in the most sophisticated sense) is above and beyond all these. It is concerned with the quality of nutrition, and is the opposite to calorie overnutrition (an excessive intake of fat and refined carbohydrates).

Poor nutrition in human populations brings about severe underdevelopment of the young, as well as the deficiency diseases (beriberi, scurvy, pellagra, rickets, kwashiorkor) and all the ill-defined combinations and variations of these afflictions.

Fair nutrition is good enough to prevent the well-recognized deficiency diseases but is not good enough to promote positive good health and excellent development. Certainly our present nutrition is not above suspicion when an official government report indicates that "one of every two selective service registrants called for preinduction examination is now found unqualified" (approximately, one-third of the nation[1]). Fair nutrition is unfortunately the kind that medical practitioners have generally been taught to regard as satisfactory. Many nutritionists have tended to accept the same doctrine; namely, if everyone gets the minimum daily requirements of certain specified nutrients ("recognized by the U.S. government!") and are free from overt deficiency diseases, the major aims of nutrition have been achieved.

Good nutrition is best exemplified by what we often give our cats and dogs, as well as the chickens and pigs being raised for the market. Such nutrition provides the animals not only with energy but with an abundance of protein of high quality, as well as a good assortment of minerals and vitamins far above the danger line. In accordance with extensive evidence presented in my book *Nutrition Against Disease* (1971),[2] good nutrition is probably experienced by no more than a minority of the population. For many are satisfied if their nutrition is fair and the physicians, who are typically ill-trained in this area,[3] often concur.

Supernutrition

Supernutrition exists at present only as an idea—a potential strategy for promoting health and preventing disease. It is a valid concept because there are many loopholes even in good nutrition. If all individuals had perfect digestive systems and average needs in every respect, then the loopholes would be minimal; but such individuals are probably so rare that they need not be considered.[4] If medical education had not been remiss in its attention to nutrition during the past six or eight decades, supernutrition would not by now be a strange idea, nor would seeking to attain it be an unusual goal.

The idea of supernutrition is based on two biological observations that can hardly be challenged: First, living cells in our bodies and everywhere practically never encounter perfect optimal environmental conditions. Second, living cells when furnished with wholly satisfactory environments, including the absence of pathogenic organisms, will respond with health and vigor. An ideal optimal environment for the cells in our bodies would include not only water and oxygen and a suitable ambient temperature but also an impressive team of about 40 nutrients, all blended in about the right proportions and working together. It is no wonder that cells usually have to put up with environments which fall short of ideal.

Optimal Environments

If living cells commonly lived under optimal conditions with no room for substantial improvement, then there would be no room for supernutrition. As it is, there is vast room for a serious attempt—which has never been made—to provide the cells and tissues comprising our bodies with highly favorable environmental conditions.

One of the crucial factors involved in any attempt to give our cells and tissues something

Paper presented at the National Academy of Sciences, October 1971.

like optimal environments is the teamwork that has so often been neglected.[2] If any link in the environmental chain is weak or missing, then the cells cannot remain healthy. The weak link may be a well-recognized substance like oxygen, tryptophan, thiamine (vitamin B1) or iron, or it may be something more obscure like molybdenum, folic acid, or selenium. The result is the same: an impoverished environment that leads to functional impairment.

At one time nutritionists used to speak of major and minor nutrients and of more and less important vitamins. It is true that some nutrients and some vitamins were discovered before others but once a nutrient is found to be indispensable, it can no longer be regarded as minor or less. Any nutrient that is absolutely indispensable is a link in a chain and is a major nutrient regardless of quantitative relationships.

Another factor that may be crucial in attempting to give every cell and tissue what they need is the existence of many barriers within the body. It cannot safely be assumed that the mere presence of a nutrient in our food insures its delivery to the cells and tissues that need it.

Digestion, absorption, and transportation are not automatic processes that always take place with perfection. Even if certain nutrients get into the blood, this does not mean that all cells and tissues automatically receive an adequate supply. As Dr. Linus Pauling,[5] has pointed out, the blood-brain barrier, for example, not only may protect the brain cells against unwanted metabolites, but it may also act imperfectly in the direction of excluding needed nutrients. For all we know, there may be in our bodies other barriers comparable to the blood-brain barrier.

A complicating factor, which makes it not a simple matter to provide human tissues with optimal environmental conditions, is the consistent presence of microorganisms in the intestinal tract that may help (or hinder) the attainment of this goal.

Biochemical Individuality

Another complication is the high probability that human needs are distinctive and appreciably dif-

ferent from those of other animals. The detailed needs of different species are not well-enough known to yield a definitive and adequate answer to this question.

Still another complication is the undeniable fact that each individual human being has nutritional needs that, from a quantitative standpoint, are distinctive.[6] The facts of biochemical individuality point to the possibility that computerized techniques will have to be employed before refined supernutrition can be applied to individual human beings.[7]

It becomes obvious in light of these observations that scientific expertise has not arrived at the point where we know definitely how to provide any human being (or animal) with supernutrition. This is clearly no playground for amateurs. If supernutrition is to be used to combat disease, experts must be engaged in the undertaking.

Raise the Quality of Nutrition

Despite the inherent difficulties that make attainment of this goal difficult or impossible, there are many measures that can be taken to help raise the quality of nutrition up toward the "super" level. First, we can be as sure as possible that every recognized essential nutrient is supplied in suitable amounts. This can be accomplished with a measure of success by consuming milk, eggs, and the cells and tissues of other organisms. The same building blocks—the amino acids, minerals (including trace minerals), and many of the vitamins—are universal and present in the metabolic machinery of living cells regardless of their origin. The energy storehouses (e.g., degerminated grains, fats, oils, and sugars) of plants and animals are different; they do not contain all the nutritional essentials, and if we depend largely on them for nutrition, the result will be an impoverishment of the environment of our cells and tissues.

We cannot safely assume that furnishing high-quality nutrition to an individual will inevitably provide adequate amounts of all the essential amino acids. There are numerous enzymes in our digestive juices, and strong evidence indicates that the patterns possessed by different individuals are distinctive.[2] Feeding amino acids as such would be a reasonable move in specific cases to help insure the adequacy of the amino acid environment of the cells and tissues.

Providing suitable minerals is difficult, partly because, as was shown in the investigations of Dr. Robert Shideler,[8] mineral balances are highly distinctive even for different healthy young men. As shown by the research of Dr. Henry Schroeder and others,[9–10] the trace element situation is complicated in that the amounts needed are imperfectly known and the supplies are uncertain.

Consider All Known Vitamins

One relatively easy step that may be taken to move in the direction of supernutrition is to provide generous amounts of all the vitamins, especially those which have been demonstrated to be harmless at higher than usual levels. This is relatively safe because in general vitamins that are provided in moderate excess are physiologically inactive. This is less true in the case of amino acids and minerals. Trace minerals in general cannot be tolerated at high levels. Supernutrition assuredly involves not only supplying enough of every nutrient but also avoiding excesses and imbalance.[2]

Several years ago in a different context several colleagues and I carried out an experiment[11] related to supernutrition. A group of mice already receiving a commercial stock diet that was supposedly well-supplied with all nutrients, including pantothenic acid (vitamin B5), were given an extra supply of the B vitamin in their drinking water. The result was an increased longevity of about 19 percent. If this result is achieved by strengthening only one link in the chain, one can legitimately expect the result to be even more striking if one attempted to strengthen all the links.

Every Link in the Environment Is Essential

In addition to furnishing the body with all the known nutrients, the next step in the direction toward supernutrition is that we must have concern for those nutrients which are presently unknown. That such nutrients exist is evidenced

"No orthomolecular physician ever claimed that giving 200 IU of vitamin E and 500 mg of vitamin C cured anything. Perhaps you [A.W.S.] should write a paper with tongue in cheek in which you announce, 'Antibiotics Do Not Cure Infection.' Then, report somewhere hidden in the paper that you only gave them 200 or even 20,000 IU of a drug that requires doses of 1 million or more. Such reporting is a superb example of the cynical, expensive, and sleazy research so loved by Big Pharma. This is because it delays the real introduction of good medicine, in the same way that tobacco companies denied smoking causes cancer and we supposedly needed more and more and more research to prove anything. All this allows the companies to add millions to their coffers. Their defense is delay, delay, and delay. The only objective of Big Pharma is to make money, lots and lots of it. How dare we try to prevent them from doing so!"

—ABRAM HOFFER

by the hard fact that cells in tissue culture, in general, cannot be cultivated in synthetic media. The presence of significant unknown nutrients in uncooked food has long been suspected, and researchers have partially isolated an unusual unknown nutrient for mice.[1] An attempt to supply supernutrition would involve a deep concern for all unknowns. Scientists whose work impinges on medicine need to identify these unknowns because they may constitute indispensable links in the nutritional chain. If so, their inclusion in attempts to supply supernutrition will spell the difference between success and failure. Every link in the environment is essential.

A third step in the direction of supernutrition is to supply our bodies with nutrients that ordinarily are of endogenous origin (produced within itself) but which under some circumstances are produced endogenously in suboptimal amounts. The list of such substances may be long. Certainly to be considered are inositol, glutamine, lecithin, lipoic acid, and coenzyme Q10.

What can we hope to accomplish by attempting to supply supernutrition? The results will obviously depend on how successful we are in reaching for the goal. It is equally obvious, if we assume that healthy cells and tissues spell healthy bodies, that the potentialities are vast.

Genetic Factors

Critics may immediately point out that there are genetic as well as environmental (including nutritional) factors to be thought of. This limitation becomes less severe when we realize, for example, that PKU (phenylketonuria) babies have a genetic defect, which can be corrected at least to a considerable degree by special nutritional measures. Rats can have a genetic defect, which causes severe inner ear difficulties and involves defective manganese utilization. The symptoms can be duplicated in other rats by depriving them of manganese, and can be eliminated from the afflicted rats if the animals having the genetic defect are given an abundant supply of this element.[13–15] These observations exemplify the genetotrophic concept set forth in 1950,[16] and in more detail in 1956,[17] which refers to the nutritional amelioration of genetic afflictions. The possibility that genetic defects may be involved does not cancel out the potentialities of supernutrition.

It seems unthinkable that medical science will be inclined to reject, without trial, the hypothesis that promoting the health of all body cells and tissues will result in general health, and that the total environment of these cells and tissues is of far-reaching significance in connection with maintaining their health. There may be cells and tissues that are so defective genetically that they cannot be reached by environmental (nutritional) means, but this should not be assumed to be true until serious attempts have been made to reach them by this means.

A Preventive Approach

I have presented elsewhere evidence, hitherto unassembled, which supports the conclusion that supernutrition (or something approaching it) has the capability, if expertly applied, of preventing:[2]

• The birth of defective, deformed, and mentally handicapped babies.

• The development of cardiovascular disease and premature aging.

• The high incidence of dental disease.

• Metabolic disorders, obesity, arthritis, etc.

• Mental disease with all its accompanying ramifications.

A Challenge to Medical Science

All the stresses to which we as human beings are subject can be withstood with far greater ease if all our cells and tissues, including those in the brain, are provided with excellent environments. This is a hypothesis eminently worth extensive trials. It seems probable that even "incurable" diseases, such as muscular dystrophy and multiple sclerosis, can be prevented by expert application of supernutrition, especially if it could be started with vulnerable individuals at an early age.

An Unparalleled Opportunity

This evidence offers an unparalleled opportunity to the medical profession. To the comment "it is all untried," my retort is a legitimate one: "Why hasn't it been tried?" I believe it will be and that the result will be even more impressive than that suggested by the physician Frank G. Boudreau who said in 1959: "If all we know about nutrition were applied to modern society, the result would be an enormous improvement in public health, at least equal to that which resulted when the germ theory of infectious disease was made the basis of public health and medical work."[18]

It is my considered belief that medical science has taken an extremely important and unfortunate wrong turn in its neglect of nutrition and that this wrong turn is evident in connection with the thinking about all diseases, including cancer. Cancer is very much in the public mind these days, and in the area of medical science treatments and cures are of the utmost concern. Prevention draws little attention and is thought of in a very restricted way.

Here again supernutrition merits serious consideration. There is certainly room for the hypothesis that cells will not go wild (become cancerous) if they are continuously supported by strong environmental conditions. Several studies have shown that cancer incidence in animals is decreased when their nutrition is improved in specific ways.[19-22] No one has taken the trouble to see whether attempts to strengthen every link in the nutritional chain will result in the decreased incidence or disappearance of cancer. This seems a lot to hope for, but available evidence points to the conclusion that if supernutrition can be successfully furnished, cancer initiation may be stopped. Friction, light, carcinogens, and viruses are all environmental agents that cause cells to become cancerous. It's an excellent possibility that cells provided excellent environments will increase their resistance to all these outside influences.[2]

If we spend money on cancer research wisely, we will certainly not forget about the ounce of prevention.

■ CONCLUSION

I most respectfully urge that every section of the National Research Council, which has to do with human health, join with the leaders and investigators in the National Institutes of Health and the National Cancer Institute in giving more than cursory study to "supernutrition" and its possibilities. The biological principles on which it is based are, I submit, irrefutable.

REFERENCES

1. One-third of a nation: a report on young men found unqualified for military service. Compiled by the President's Task Force on Manpower Conservation, Jan 1, 1964.

2. Williams RJ. *Nutrition Against Disease: Environmental Prevention.* New York: Pitman Publishing, 1971.

3. Williams RJ. How can the climate in medical education be changed? *Perspectives in Biology and Medicine* 1971;14:608.

4. Burton BT, ed. *The Heinz Handbook of Nutrition.* New York: McGraw-Hill, 1959, 137.

5. Pauling, L. Orthomolecular psychiatry. *Science* 1968; 160:265.

6. Williams RJ. *Biochemical Individuality.* New York: John Wiley & Sons, 1963.

7. Williams, RJ, Siegel FL. "Propetology": a new branch of medical science? *Am J Med* 1961;31:325.

8. Shideler RW. Individual differences in mineral metabolism. Doctorial dissertation. Austin, TX: University of Texas, 1956.

9. Schroeder HA. Losses of vitamins and trace minerals resulting from processing and preservation of foods. *Am J Clin Nutr* 1971;24(5):562–573.

10. Schroeder HA, Balassa JJ, Topton IH. Essential trace metals in man. Manganese: a study in homeostasis. *J Chronic Dis* 1966;19:545.

11. Pelton RB, Williams RJ. Effect of pantothenic acid on longevity of mice. *Soc Exp Biol Med* 1958;99:632.

12. Schneider HA. Ecological ectocrines in experimental epidemiology. *Science* 1967;158:597.

13. Daniels AL, Everson GP. The relation of manganese to congenital debility. *J Nutr* 1935;9:191.

14. Hurley LS, Everson GJ. Influence of timing of short-term supplementation during gestation on congenital abnormalities of manganese-deficient rats. *J Nutr* 1963;79:23.

15. Hurley LS. Studies on nutritional factors in mammalian development. *J Nutr Sup* 1967;1(91):27.

16. Williams RJ, et al. The concept of genetotrophic disease. *Lancet* 1950;1:287.

17. Williams RJ. *Biochemical Individuality.* Austin, TX: University of Texas, 1969. Also, see ref. 7.

18. Boudreau FG. *Food, Yearbook of Agriculture.* Washington, DC: USDA Publications, 1959.

19. Engel RW, et. al. Carcinogenic effects associated with diets deficient in chorine and related nutrients. *Ann NY Acad Sci* 1947;49:49.

20. Antopol W, Unna K. The effect of riboflavin on the liver changes produced in rats by p-dimethylaminoazobenzene. *Cancer Res* 1942;2:694.

21. Sugiura K. On the relation of diets to the development, prevention and treatment of cancer, with special reference to cancer of the stomach and liver. *J Nutr* 1951;44:345.

22. Kensler CJ, et al. Partial protection of rats by riboflavin with casein against liver cancer caused by p-Dimethylaminoazobenzene. *Science* 1941;93:308.

ABOUT "OBJECTIONS" TO VITAMIN C THERAPY
by Andrew W. Saul, PhD

In massive doses, vitamin C (ascorbic acid) stops a cold within hours, stops influenza in a day or two, and stops viral pneumonia (pain, fever, cough) in two or three days.[1] It is a highly effective antihistamine, antiviral, and antitoxin. It reduces inflammation and lowers fever. Administered intravenously, ascorbate kills cancer cells without harming healthy tissue. Many people therefore wonder, in the face of statements like these, why the medical professions have not embraced vitamin C therapy with open and grateful arms.

Probably the main roadblock to widespread examination and utilization of this all-too-simple technology is the equally widespread belief that there *must* be unknown dangers to tens of thousands of milligrams (mg) of ascorbic acid. Yet, since the time megascorbate therapy was introduced in the late 1940s by Frederick R. Klenner, MD,[2] there has been an especially safe and extremely effective track record to follow. Still, for some, questions remain. Here is a sample of what many people wonder about vitamin C:

Q. Is 2,000 mg per day of vitamin C a megadose?

A. No. Decades ago, Linus Pauling, PhD, and Irwin Stone, PhD, showed that most animals make at least that much (or more) per human body weight per day.[3,4]

Q. Then why has the government set the "Safe Upper Limit" for vitamin C at 2,000 mg per day?

A. Perhaps the reason is ignorance. According to nationwide data compiled by the American Association of Poison Control Centers, vitamin C (and the use of any other dietary supplement) does not kill anyone.[5]

Q. Does vitamin C damage DNA?

A. No. If vitamin C harmed DNA, why do most animals make (not eat, but *make*) between 2,000 and 10,000 mg of vitamin C per human equivalent body weight per day? Evolution would never so favor anything that harms vital genetic material. White blood cells and male reproductive fluids contain unusually high quantities of ascorbate. Living, reproducing systems love vitamin C.

Q. Does vitamin C cause low blood sugar, B12 deficiency, birth defects, or infertility?

A. Vitamin C does not cause birth defects, nor infertility, nor miscarriage. According to an article in the *Journal of the American Medical Association*, "Harmful effects have been mistakenly attributed to vitamin C, including hypoglycemia, rebound scurvy, infertility, mutagenesis, and destruction of vitamin B12. Health professionals should recognize that vitamin C does not produce these effects."[6]

Q. Does vitamin C . . .

A. A randomized, double-blind, placebo-controlled 14-day trial of 3,000 mg per day of vitamin C reported greater frequency of sexual intercourse. The vitamin C group (but not the placebo group) also experienced a quantifiable decrease in depression. This is probably due to the fact that vitamin C "modulates catecholaminergic activity; decreases stress reactivity, approach anxiety, and prolactin release; improves vascular function; and increases oxytocin release. These processes are relevant to sexual behavior and mood."[7]

Q. Does vitamin C cause kidney stones?

A. No. The myth of the vitamin C–caused kidney stone is rivaled in popularity only by the Loch Ness monster. A factoid-crazy medical media often overlooks the fact that William J. McCormick, MD, demonstrated that vitamin C actually prevents the formation of kidney stones. He did so in 1946, when he published a paper on the subject.[8] His work was confirmed by University of Alabama professor of medicine Emanuel Cheraskin, MD, DMD. Dr. Cheraskin showed that vitamin C inhibits the formation of oxalate stones.[9]

Other research reports that: "Even though a certain part of oxalate in the urine derives from metabolized ascorbic acid, the intake of high doses of vitamin C does not increase the risk of calcium oxalate kidney stones . . . In the large-scale Harvard Prospective Health Professional Follow-Up Study, those groups in the highest quintile of vitamin C intake (greater than 1,500 mg/day) had a lower risk of kidney stones than the groups in the lowest quintiles."[10]

Robert F. Cathcart, MD, said, "I started using vitamin C in massive doses in patients in 1969. By the time

I read that ascorbate should cause kidney stones, I had clinical evidence that it did not cause kidney stones, so I continued prescribing massive doses to patients. Up to 2006, I estimate that I have put 25,000 patients on massive doses of vitamin C and none have developed kidney stones. Two patients who had dropped their doses to 500 mg a day developed calcium oxalate kidney stones. I raised their doses back up to the more massive doses and added magnesium and B6 to their program and no more kidney stones. I think they developed the kidney stones because they were not taking enough vitamin C."

Q. Why did Linus Pauling die from cancer if he took all that vitamin C?

A. Dr. Pauling, a megadose-vitamin C advocate, died in 1994 from prostate cancer. Mayo Clinic cancer researcher Charles G. Moertel, MD, a critic of Pauling and vitamin C, also died in 1994, and also from cancer (lymphoma). Dr. Moertel was 66 years old. Dr. Pauling was 93 years old. One needs to make up one's own mind as to whether this does or does not indicate benefit from vitamin C.

A review of the subject indicates that "vitamin C deficiency is common in patients with advanced cancer . . . Patients with low plasma concentrations of vitamin C have a shorter survival."[11]

Q. Does vitamin C narrow arteries or cause atherosclerosis?

A. Abram Hoffer, MD, PhD, has said: "I have used vitamin C in megadoses with my patients since 1952 and have not seen any cases of heart disease develop even after decades of use. Dr. Robert Cathcart with experience on over 25,000 patients since 1969 has seen no cases of heart disease developing in patients who did not have any when first seen. He added that the thickening of the vessel walls, if true, indicates that the thinning that occurs with age is reversed . . . The fact is that vitamin C *decreases* plaque formation according to many clinical studies. Some critics ignore the knowledge that thickened arterial walls in the absence of plaque formation indicate that the walls are becoming stronger and therefore less apt to rupture . . . Gokce, Keaney, Frei and others gave patients supplemental vitamin C daily for 30 days and measured blood flow through the arteries. Blood flow *increased nearly 50*

percent after the single dose and this was sustained after the monthly treatment."[12]

Q. What about blood pressure?

A. A randomized, double-blinded, placebo-controlled study showed that hypertensive patients taking supplemental vitamin C had lower blood pressure.[13]

So why the flurry of antivitamin-C reporting in the mass media? Negative news gets attention. Positive vitamin studies do not. Is this a conspiracy? Of course not. It is nevertheless an enormous public health problem with enormous consequences.

Approximately 150 million Americans take supplemental vitamin C every day. This is as much a political issue as a scientific issue. What would happen if everybody took vitamins? Perhaps doctors, hospital administrators, and pharmaceutical salespeople would all be lining up for their unemployment checks. A skeptic might conclude that there is at least some evidence that the politicians are on the wrong side of this. After all, the U.S. Recommended Dietary Allowance for vitamin C for humans is only 10 percent of the U.S. Department of Agriculture's vitamin C standards for guinea pigs.[14] But conspiracy against nutritional medicine? Certainly not. Couldn't be.

REFERENCES

1. Cathcart RF. *Med Hypothesis* 1981;7:1359–1376.

2. Saul AW. *J Orthomolecular Med* 2007;22(1):31–38.

3. Pauling L. *How to Live Longer and Feel Better.* Corvallis, OR: Oregon State University Press, 2006.

4. Stone I. *The Healing Factor.* New York: Grosset & Dunlap, 1972.

5. Saul A. *OMNS* 2010. Available at http://orthomolecular.org/resources/omns/v06n04.shtml.

6. Levine M. *JAMA* 1999; 281(15):1419.

7. Brody S. *Biol Psychiatry* 2002;52(4):371–374.

8. McCormick WJ. *Medical Record* 1946;159(7): 410–413.

9. Cheraskin E. *The Vitamin C Connection.* York: Harper & Row, 1983. See also: Ringsdorf WM. *South Med J* 1981;74(1):41–43, 46.

10. Gerster H. *Ann Nutr Metab* 1997;41(5):269–282.

11. Mayland CR. *Palliat Med* 2005;19(1):17–20.

12. Gokce N. *Circulation* 1999;99:3234–3240.

13. Duffy SJ. *Lancet* 1999;354(9195):2048–2049.

14. Saul A. *OMNS* 2010. Available at http://orthomolecular.org/resources/omns/v06n08.shtml.

Excerpted from the *Orthomolecular Medicine News Service*, October 12, 2010.

ORTHOMOLECULAR PSYCHIATRY
by Linus Pauling, PhD

I feel that the use of substances normally present in the human body for improving the health of human beings, and especially their mental health, has been unjustifiably ignored by the medical profession for some 30 or 35 years now, and that the possibilities of improvement in the health of the American people and of other people in the world by improved nutrition are truly great. It is astounding to me that the medical profession has paid so little attention to these possibilities during the last few decades.

It is difficult for me to understand why this has come about. There was enthusiasm about vitamins and nutrition for a rather short period of time, beginning about 1910, when vitamins were first clearly recognized and when it was generally accepted that diseases such as scurvy and beriberi are not the result of the presence of a toxic substance of some sort in certain foods, which could be neutralized by other foods, but rather are the result of the absence in certain foods of vital substances: the vitamins.

Substances Vital for Physical Health

The essential amino acids also were discovered to be vital substances of this sort, required for life and health. The enthusiasm about vitamins may have been overly great for a while and the failure of vitamin therapy in some cases may have caused a disenchantment that really was not justified. My friend Albert Szent-Györgyi, who in 1928 prepared it for the first time, isolated vitamin C from natural sources, as a substance that he named hexuronic acid; later he changed the name to ascorbic acid. Dr. Szent-Györgyi has said in a letter to me that he felt that it was a great mistake for the medical profession to have concentrated on the anti-ascorbutic properties of vitamin C, the property of preventing death by scurvy. Scurvy is the final stage; he called it a "pre-mortal syndrome."

Death by scurvy can be prevented by a small amount of vitamin C. Dr. Szent-Györgyi said that we do not yet know the optimum rate of intake of this vitamin. He said that he himself has been taking 1,000 milligrams (mg) a day for many years, but that he does not know whether this is the optimum amount for him, nor does he know about other people and what their optimum requirements are. He went on to say that one thing is perfectly clear: any amount can be taken without danger.

I think that this is essentially true, not only for vitamin C, but also for the other water-soluble vitamins and for vitamin E. These substances have important physiological properties and are substances to which the human body is accustomed, because everyone requires these substances for life and good health, and there has been a weeding-out process. The process of evolution has given rise to the human race that now exists, consisting of people who can tolerate these important substances.

We do not know how much we need of these various vital substances in order to be in the best of health. There is good evidence that different people need different amounts, as has been pointed out by Professor Roger J. Williams. There is also new research by Dr. Leon Rosenberg, who has been working on the inborn errors of metabolism, and the diseases that result from the failure of an individual to manufacture a particular enzyme in the right amount or with the right activity. It is possible to cure some of these inborn errors of metabolism by the administration of amounts of vitamins, such as vitamin B6 or vitamin B12, in amounts as great as 1,000 times the amounts that seem to be essentially satisfactory for other human beings. I would like to know how to find out what the optimum rate of intake of these vital substances is.

Professor Williams has reported studies made with guinea pigs showing that for optimum growth the amounts of vitamin C required by different guinea pigs varied by as much as twentyfold. He has said that surely human beings are more heterogeneous and the range of requirements of human beings for vitamin C is greater than over a factor of twenty. I feel that we can say the same thing about

From *Schizophrenia* 1971;3(2):129–133.

vitamin B3, a very important substance which has many functions in the human body, and also vitamin B6, which is known to serve as a coenzyme in many enzyme systems. I feel sure that the needs for vitamin B3 in different human beings are different.

I have decided, on the basis of the evidence presented by Dr. Irwin Stone, that there is very strong evidence now that most human beings are suffering from hypoascorbemia, a mild sort of deficiency of ascorbic acid in the blood—perhaps it is wrong for me to call it a mild sort. The point that I call to your attention is that I believe that for all or almost all human beings the amount of vitamin C that is contained in the food is less than the optimum amount and that the state of health of almost all human beings is not so good as it would be if they were to ingest a larger amount.

The evidence that I have been able to gather so far about vitamin B3 is not so clear on this point. It suggests, rather, that for many human beings the amount of vitamin B3 that is usually recommended and that is contained in a good balanced diet, even a modern diet of processed foods of one sort or another, is not too far off from the optimum rate of intake. Nevertheless, it may be that I am wrong on that point, and that for vitamin B3 also the optimum rate of intake for almost all human beings would be considerably larger than the 17 mg per day that is recommended by the Food and Nutrition Board of the U.S. National Research Council and the National Academy of Sciences. In the course of time, we shall be able to answer this question and other related questions.

Substances as Vital for Mental Health

In the meantime, there is the evidence that many people with mental disease of one sort or another, including many children who show abnormal behavior, benefit by receiving large daily intakes of these important foods, vitamin B3 (niacin and niacinamide), vitamin C, and vitamin B6. What are we going to do about this problem in the future—the problem of finding out what the needs are of individual human beings for these important foods?

At the present time, I feel that it is essential that empirical methods be used. I feel that the evidence that exists now about the benefits to many people of an increased intake of vitamins, such as the many people who are suffering from mental disease, justifies the trial of these substances on every person who shows abnormality in behavior such as to require that he be given some sort of treatment. The situation is not the same as that with the phenothiazines—the synthetic drugs to which the human body is not accustomed, substances that are foreign to the human body and for which there might be expected possible very severe side effects of one sort or another that could produce damage.

We know the human body is accustomed to every one of the vitamin substances, that we have evolved in such a way as to be able to tolerate it. And we know by observation that for most of the vitamins, all except vitamin A and vitamin D, very large quantities may be ingested without producing symptoms of toxicity or serious side reactions. We know that these substances have physiological activity, that many of them are involved in the functioning of the brain, that they cause biochemical reactions to take place in the human body such as to change the molecular environment of the mind; and we know by observation, from the reports that have been published, that often these changes in the molecular environment of the mind are such as to lead to improved behavior.

I feel, accordingly, that it is the duty of every psychiatrist to add megavitamin therapy, orthomolecular methods, to his armamentarium and to make use of these vitamins; to try them out in proper amounts, not just doubling the Recommended Daily Allowance, but in the proper amounts as discussed by Dr. Abram Hoffer and others as having been found to be effective for many patients.

Electroshock therapy, which I do not like, seems to me to be closely analogous to a method of treatment of mental disease that I think was used traditionally by primitive man, that of hitting the patient over the head with a club, thus producing a generalized change in the structure of the brain, which had some chance of leading to a significant improvement in behavior. I hope that this crude treatment will be replaced by orthomolecular methods.

I remember looking, with my wife, at an exhibit of skulls of pre-Columbian Indians, with a piece of bone cut out from the skull. It is thought that this treatment was sometimes used for mental illness, perhaps with some success. It is evident from the skulls that some of the patients survived the operation and some of them died. For some skulls there was no sign of healing around the square where the piece of bone had been removed, but for many of them there were signs of healing. Primitive men learned so much about diet and even about medicines, the important alkaloids present in plants, that he may well have learned something about the methods of treating mental disease similar to the ones that are now used or analogous to them.

The Need for Technological Progress and Physicians with Open Minds

Professor A. B. Robinson, my associate, and our co-workers have been working on the problem of finding out what the molecular structure of a human being is, finding out how he handles vitamins, what happens to the vitamins that he ingests—does he utilize them in the same way as other human beings?

To do this, we have been trying to develop a refined method of analysis such that we can determine quantitatively the amounts of 200 or 300 hundred substances in his urine, blood, breath, or other body fluid. In the course of time, I feel that this attack will turn out to be of value. We are now trying to develop an instrument such that it does not take four hours (as it does at present) to determine quantitatively the amounts of 200 to 300 substances in a sample but will take only a few seconds.

This is a real possibility: that such an instrument can be developed on the basis of the scientific and technological developments of the last 20 or 30 years and of the technological progress that has occurred, progress in instrumentation, and in the handling of results that are obtained by these instruments by use of a computer. It is possible now to make a new attack on the whole problem of nutrition in relation to the health of human beings and especially of mental health.

We have, in our bodies, the mechanism for helping to protect the brain from the environment. This is the blood-brain barrier, which helps to keep undesirable molecules out of the brain. This barrier may also sometimes operate to keep good molecules out of the brain. I have thought that it might well be that the value of megavitamin therapy for some patients is the result of their having a blood-brain barrier that is operating too efficiently, in such a way that even though in the peripheral tissues the concentration of vitamins may be essentially optimal, there could still be a local avitaminosis in the brain itself.

It is soon going to be possible to answer this question and many similar questions. It is required only that scientists, physicians, and medical investigators have an open mind about such matters as the value of vitamins, that they not be inhibited by old and false ideas that have been handed on by the past generation of physicians and nutritionists to the present generation. Fortunately, the younger generation of physicians and of students generally is less gullible than those of earlier times—more open-minded. I think that the attitude of the young physicians and the students of today gives us hope for the future. I think that there is going to be much progress made in the field of psychiatry during the next decade.

It was very interesting to have Dr. Katz, who is chief of the clinical research branch of the National Institute of Mental Health, point out to me that he and Dr. Kubala, some 10 or 12 years ago, conducted a study of the intelligence of schoolchildren, as measured by IQ tests, in relation to the level of ascorbic acid in the blood. Their study showed, with statistical significance, an average increase of about four points in IQ for an average increase from 1.0 mg to 1.5 mg of ascorbic acid per 100 milliliter of blood plasma. This increase in performance on intelligence tests was attributed by Drs. Kubala and Katz to an increase in "alertness" and "sharpness" that presumably results from the increased level of ascorbic acid in the blood. This report seems to me to be very important.

I hope that further studies along this line, also involving other vitamins, will be made. I repeat that it is my conviction that we have for the most part neglected a very important way of improving the health of human beings—neglected it for several decades now—that way being through the ingestion of the optimal amounts of the natural foods, the essential foods, especially the vitamins, vitamin C, vitamin B3, and other vitamins. It is heartening to me to see how the interest in these possibilities is now growing.

OBSERVATIONS ON THE DOSE AND ADMINISTRATION OF ASCORBIC ACID WHEN EMPLOYED BEYOND THE RANGE OF A VITAMIN IN HUMAN PATHOLOGY

by Frederick Klenner, MD

Folklore of past civilizations report that for every disease afflicting man there is an herb or its equivalent that will effect a cure. In Puerto Rico the story has long been told that to have the health tree acerola in one's backyard would keep colds out of the front door.[1] The ascorbic acid content of this cherry-like fruit is 30 times that found in oranges. Boneset, scientifically called *Eupatorium perfoliatum*,[2] is now rarely prescribed by physicians, but was once was the most commonly used medicinal plant of eastern United States. Most farmsteads had a bundle of dried boneset in the attic or woodshed from which a most bitter tea would be meted out to the unfortunate victim of a cold or fever. Having lived in that section of the country we qualified many times for this particular drink.

The flu pandemic of 1918 stands out very forcefully in that the Klenners survived when scores about us were dying. Although bitter, it was curative and most of the time the cure was overnight. Several years ago my curiosity led me to assay this "herbal medicine" and to my surprise and delight I found that we had been taking from 10,000 to 30,000 milligrams (mg) of natural vitamin C at one time. Even then it was given by body weight. Children one cupful; adults two to three cupfuls. Cups those days held 8 ounces. Twentieth-century man forgets that his ancestors made crude drugs from various plants and roots, and that these decoctions served his purpose. Elegant pharmacy has only made the forms and shapes more acceptable.

Early Specifications, Action, and Dosages

To understand the chemical behavior of ascorbic acid in human pathology, one must go beyond its present academic status either as a factor essential for life or as a substance necessary to prevent scurvy. This knowledge is elementary. Listen to what appeared in the *Food and Life Yearbook 1939*, U.S. Department of Agriculture[3]: "In fact even when there is not a single outward symptom of

trouble, a person may be in a state of vitamin C deficiency more dangerous than scurvy itself. When such a condition is not detected, and continues uncorrected, the teeth and bones will be damaged, and what may be even more serious, the bloodstream is weakened to the point where it can no longer resist or fight infections not so easily cured as scurvy." It is true that without these infinitesimal amounts, myriad of body processes would deteriorate and even come to a fatal halt.

Ascorbic acid has many important functions. It is a powerful oxidizer and when given in massive amounts, from 50,000 to 150,000 mg, intravenously, for certain pathological conditions, and "run in" as fast as a 20-gauge needle will allow, it acts as a "flash oxidizer,"[4] often correcting the pathology within minutes. Ascorbic acid is also a powerful reducing agent. Its neutralizing action on certain toxins, exotoxins (external toxins), virus infections, endotoxins (internal toxins), and histamine is in direct proportion to the amount of the lethal factor involved *and the amount of ascorbic acid given*. At times it is necessary to use ascorbic acid intramuscularly. It should be used orally, when possible, along with the needle.

If one is to employ ascorbic acid intelligently, some index for requirements must be realized. Unfortunately, there exists today a sort of "brand" called "minimum daily requirements." This illegitimate "child" has been co-fathered by the National Academy of Sciences and the National Research Council and represents a tragic error in judgment. There are many factors that increase the demand by the body for ascorbic acid, and unless these are appreciated, there can be no real progress. It is vitally important that cognizance be taken of the demand by the body for ascorbic acid far beyond so-called scorbutic levels. Briefly these demands can be summarized by:

From the *J Orthomolecular Med* 1998;13(4):198–210.

- Age of the individual
- Body chemistry
- Body weight
- Drugs
- Habits such as smoking, alcohol use, and lifestyle
- Inadequate storage
- Kidney threshold
- Loss in the stool
- Physiological stress
- Season of the year
- Sleep, especially when induced artificially
- Trauma caused by a pathogen, work, surgery, or accident
- Variations in binders of commercial tablets
- Variations in individual absorption

With such knowledge it is no longer possible to accept a set numerical unit in terms of minimal daily requirements. This is true because of the simple fact that people are different and these same people experience different situations at various times. With ascorbic acid, today's adequate supply means little or nothing in terms of the needs for tomorrow. Let us start thinking in terms of maximum requirements. For too long a time we have under supplied our children and ourselves by accepting through negative ignorance and acquiescence so-called standards. Based on scant data on mammalian synthesis, available for the rat, a 70 kg (154 lbs) individual would produce 1.8 grams (1,800 mg)[5] to 4.0 grams (4,000 mg)[6] of ascorbic acid per day in the unstressed condition; under stress, up to 15.2 grams (15,200 mg).[7] Compare this to the 70 mg recommended for daily requirements without stress and the 200 mg for the simple stress of the obstetrical patient, and you will recognize the disparity and understand why we have been waging a one-man war against the establishment in Washington for 23 years.

Ascorbic Acid Not Synthesized by Man

Work on mammalian biosynthesis of ascorbic acid indicates that the vitamin C story, as is generally accepted, represents an oversimplification of available evidence.[6–8] This often leads to misinterpretations and false impressions. It has been proposed that the biochemical lesion that produces the human need for ascorbic acid is the absence of the active enzyme gulonolactone oxidase from the human liver.[9] A defect or loss of the gene controlling the synthesis of this enzyme in humans blocks the final phase in the series for converting glucose to ascorbic acid. Such a mutation could have happened by a virus, by radiation, or simply by chance, thus denying all progenies of this mutated animal the ability to produce ascorbic acid. Survival demanded ascorbic acid from an exogenous source. This is not remarkable. Other recognized genetic diseases in which a missing enzyme causes a pathological syndrome, in man, are phenylketonuria, galactosemia, and alkaptonuria. The inability of humans to manufacture their own ascorbic acid, due to genetic fault, has been called hypoascorbemia by Irwin Stone, PhD.[10]

Various Procedures for Testing Vitamin C Levels and Body Requirements

Various tests have been employed to determine the degree of body saturation of vitamin C, but for the most part they have been misleading. Blood and urine samples analyzed with the sodium salt 2,6-dichlorophenol-indophenol will give values roughly 7 percent less than when testing with dinitrophenol-hydrazine (a sensitive compound). The capillary fragility test is similar to the tourniquet test in results. Both can be used to estimate the quantity of vitamin C necessary to maintain capillary integrity. The intradermal test as modified by Lawrence Slobody[11] is again gaining new recruits. In principle it is the same as the lingual test of William Ringsdorf and Emanuel Cheraskin,[12] since both are based on the time required to decolorize dye. The lingual test is rapid and simple to perform but it requires a syringe with a 25-gauge needle and a stop watch. This test was helpful in gauging requirements for simple stress but not accurate enough when using needle therapy. Fifteen years ago, I helped to develop the silver nitrate–urine test.[13] This test employs 10 drops of 5 percent silver nitrate and 10 drops urine, which is placed in a test tube. When read in two minutes, it will give a color pattern showing white, beige, smoke gray, charcoal, or various combinations of any two depending upon the degree of saturation. We have found this color index test is all one will need for establishing the correct amount of ascorbic acid to use by mouth, by muscle, by vein in the handling of all types of human pathology either as the specific drug or as an adjuvant with other antibiotics or neutralizing chemicals. In severe pathological conditions the urine sample, taken every four hours, must show a fine charcoal-like precipitation.

Role of Ascorbic Acid in Intercellular Reactions, and in Neutralizing and Possibly Controlling Virus Production

In 1935, chemist Wendell Stanley isolated a crystalline protein possessing the properties of tobacco mosaic virus (the first virus to be discovered). It contained two substances: ribonucleic acid (RNA) and protein. The simple structure characteristic of tobacco mosaic virus was soon found to be a basic property of many human viruses, such as the coxsackievirus (which I believe to be the cause of multiple sclerosis), the echovirus (one of several viruses that affect the gastrointestinal tract), and the poliovirus. They all contain only RNA and protein. There exist minor variations. The adenovirus, which causes most respiratory illnesses, contains deoxyribonucleic acid (DNA) and protein. Other viruses such as those causing influenza contain added lipids and polysaccharides. DNA is used to program the large viruses like mumps; RNA is used to program the small viruses like measles. The role of the protein coat is to protect the parasitic but unstable nucleic acid as it rides the "blood highway" or "lymphatic system" to gain specific cell entry. Pure viral nucleic acid without its protein coat can be inactivated by constituents of normal blood. There are several theories as to what happens after cell entry:

• Once inside a given cell, the virus nucleic acid sheds its protein coat and proceeds to modify the host cell by either creating mutations or by directly substituting its own nucleic acid.

• The infectious nucleic acid, after entering a human cell, retains its protein coat and starts to produce its own type protein coat[14] and viral nucleic acid, so that new units can either depart to enter other cells or by destruction of the cell, thus making the infection more severe.

• The introduction of a foreign fragment of nucleic acid in the cell-virus interaction approach as postulated by virologist T. J. Starr[15] suggests that there can exist cells with partial chromosome makeup and cells with multi-nuclei. Hilary Kropowski, also a virologist, holds that these partial cells are pseudo-virons[16] and are found in some tumor-virus infections. A key factor in the Starr-Kropowski thinking is that the cell maintains its biological integrity to support virus development despite the abnormal morphology and genetic deficiency. If these invaded cells could be destroyed or the invader neutralized, the illness would suddenly terminate. Ascorbic acid has the capability of entering all cells. Under normal circumstances its presence is beneficial to the cell. However, when the cell has been invaded by a foreign substance, like virus nucleic acid, enzymatic action by ascorbic acid contributes to the breakdown of virus nucleic acid. Ascorbic acid also joins with the available virus protein, making a new macromolecule, which acts as the repressor factor. It has been demonstrated that when combined with the repressor (the operator gene) virus nucleic acid cannot react with any other substance and cannot induce activity in the structural gene, therefore inhibiting the multiplication of new virus bodies. The strength of the cell membrane is exceeded by these macromolecules with rupture and destruction.

Promptness of Massive Ascorbic Acid in Avoiding Fatal Encephalitis Related to Stubborn Head and Chest Colds

In 1953,[17] my colleagues and I presented a case history and films of a patient with viral pneumonia. This patient was unconscious with a fever of 106.8ºF when admitted to the hospital. She was given 140,000 mg of ascorbic acid intravenously over a period of 72 hours at which time she was awake, sitting up in bed, and taking fluids freely by mouth. Her temperature was normal. Since that time we have observed a more deadly syndrome associated with a virus causing head and chest colds. This is one of the adenoviruses, which strikes in the area of the upper respiratory tract with resulting fever, sore throat and watery eyes, and when in children can cause fatal pneumonia. More often death is indirect by way of incipient encephalitis (inflammation of the brain) where the child can be dead in 30 minutes. These are the babies and children found dead in bed and attributed to sudden infant death syndrome (SIDS). It is suffocation but by way of a syndrome we observed and reported in 1957,[18] which is similar to that found in cephalic tetanus-toxemia culminating in diaphragmatic spasms, with dyspnea (shortness of breath) and finally asphyxia.[19] By 1958,[20] we had collected sufficient information from our office and hospital patients to catalog this deadly syndrome into two important stages.

• **Stage 1:** There is always a history of having had the flu, which lasts 48 to 96 hours, complicated with extreme physical or mental distress, or a mild cold, similar to an allergic rhinitis, which lingers on for several weeks but does not incapacitate the individual.

• **Stage 2:** This stage, which is always sudden, presents itself in at least several forms, including convulsive seizures; extreme excitability, resembling delirium tremens if an adult and with dancing of the eyeballs if a child; severe chill; strangling in the course of eating or drinking; collapse; and stupor and hemiplegia. Other findings of this dramatic second stage are rapid pulse; respiration, two to three times normal, that in some cases is suggestive of air hunger; moderately dilated pupils; and a high white blood cell count.

The second stage of this syndrome is triggered by a breakthrough at the blood-brain barrier. The time required for neurological changes to become evident is roughly comparable to the time necessary for similar neuropathology to be demonstrated following a severe head injury. Cerebral edema (severe brain swelling) exists in both severe head injury and viral encephalitis. In my practice, I start massive

ascorbic acid therapy immediately. Physicians must recognize the inherent danger of the lingering head or chest cold and appreciate the importance of early massive vitamin C therapy. I have seen children dead in 30 minutes to two hours because their attending physician was not impressed with their illness upon hospital admission. An autopsy on one of these patients showed bilateral pneumonia (infection that affects both lungs)—all one needs to spark a deadly encephalitis.

How does the brain become involved in encephalitis? Some speculate on the pathways in which the virus gains entrance into the brain, summarized as follows:

• Through the olfactory nerves;

• Through the portals of the stomach from material swallowed, either pulmonary or upper respiratory drainage;

• Through direct extension from otitis media or from mastoid cells;

• Through the bloodstream; arriving in the brain, the virus goes through the blood cerebrospinal fluid barrier and/or the blood-brain barrier by one of three ways: electrical charge, chemical lysis of tissue, or osmosis. Louis Bakay[21] reported that the permeability of the blood-brain barrier can be changed by introducing various toxic agents into the blood circulation. Researchers R. Chambers and B. W. Zweifach[22] emphasized the importance of the intercellular cement of the capillary wall in regulating permeability of the blood vessels of the central nervous system. In this syndrome the toxic substance is an adenovirus. Ascorbic acid will repair and maintain the integrity of the capillary wall.

Burn Degrees Explained and Some Therapy Rationale

In the treatment of burns, ascorbic acid, in sufficient amounts, reflects itself as a truly miracle substance. In the early 1940s, when I was using ascorbic acid, intramuscularly, in treating bacillary dysentery (an acute infection of the intestines by shigella bacteria) with excellent results, Charles Lund and many others were using, what they called, massive doses of ascorbic acid in the treatment of burn-damaged skin. One or two grams each day, in fluids, was the recognized dose. Burns are at the beginning first degree and some remain as just an erythema (redness of the skin). Many times the first-degree burn progresses rapidly to the second-degree stage and remains as "blisters." Still others go on to a third degree, which usually is more pronounced on the third-plus post-burn day. There is a fourth stage which results from lack of knowledge in treatment. It terminates with skin grafting and plastic surgery. I believe that ascorbic acid can eliminate the third and fourth stages.

The pathologic physiology of a burn wound from the moment of the accident is in a state of dynamic change until the wound heals or the patient dies. The primary consideration is the phenomenon of intravascular agglutination or blood sludging (clotting of red blood cells) originally recognized by Melvin Knisely in 1945.[23,24] Initially, there is intravascular agglutination of red blood cells into distinctly visible, smooth, hard, rigid, basic masses. Oxygen uptake by the tissues is greatly reduced because of the sludging and subsequent reduced rate of blood flow. Research[25] in 1960 concluded that this phenomenon of sludging or agglutination results in capillary thrombosis in the area of the burn, extending proximally to involve the large arterioles (arteries) and venules (small veins), and thereby creating tissue destruction greater than that originally produced by the burn. Anoxia (a lack of oxygen in the tissues) produces added tissue destruction. Charles Lund and Stanley Levenson[26] found that after severe burns there is considerable alteration in the metabolism of ascorbic acid as shown by a low concentration of ascorbic acid in the plasma, either with the patient fasting or after saturation tests, and also low urinary excretion of vitamin C, either with the patient fasting or after the injection of test doses. The extent of the abnormality closely paralleled the severity of the burn. One study[27] reported an increase demand for ascorbic acid in burns especially when epithelization and formation of granulation tissue (connective tissue and tiny blood vessel repair) are taking place. Another study[28] also reported in 1941 a marked decrease in the plasma ascorbic acid concentration in patients with

severe burns. David Klasson,[29] although limiting the amount of ascorbic acid to a dose range of 300 mg to 2,000 mg daily, in divided doses, found that it hastened the healing of wounds by producing healthy granulation tissue and also that it reduced local edema. He rationalized that ascorbic acid used locally as a 2 percent dressing possessed astringent properties similar to hydrogen peroxide. He also reported that antibiotic therapy was rarely necessary.

Harlan Stone[30] suggested the use of the antibiotic gentamicin in major, severe burns to lower the sepsis (a severe often systemwide infection) caused by pseudomonas, a bacteria often seen in burn patients that is very resistant to antibiotics. Absorption of its exotoxin (a poisonous substance) from the infected burn wound inhibits the body's bacterial defense mechanism. Death can result either from the toxemia alone or from an associated septicemia. My colleagues and I have found that the secret in treating burns can be summarized in five steps:

1. Make a covered wagon-type cradle over the burn and keep warm with three 25-watt bulbs. The patient can control the heat by turning on and off the first bulb as needed to keep warm. No garments or dressings are allowed.

2. Spray a 3 percent ascorbic acid solution over the entire area of the burn, every two to four hours for about five days.

3. Apply a vitamin A and D ointment over the area of the burn and alternate with the 3 percent ascorbic acid solution.

4. Give massive doses of ascorbic acid intravenously and by mouth. By injection, use 500 mg per kg of body weight diluted to at least 18 cubic centimeters (cc) per gram of vitamin C using 5 percent dextrose or saline in water or Ringer's solution, repeated every eight hours for several days, then at twelve-hour intervals (include at least 1,000 mg of calcium gluconate daily). Ascorbic acid, by mouth, is given to tolerance.

5. Supportive treatment; that is, whole blood and maintaining electrolyte balance. If seen early after the burn, there will be no infections and no dead skin formations. This eliminates fluid formation,

since the dead skin traps will not exist and there will be no edema in the extremities because the venous and lymphatic systems will remain open. There will be no arterial obstruction and no nerve compression. Pseudomonas infection will not be a problem, since ascorbic acid destroys the exotoxin systemically and locally. Even if the burn is seen late when pseudomonas is a major problem, the gram-negative bacilli will be destroyed in a few days leaving a clean healthy surface. Ascorbic acid also eliminates pain so that opiates or their equivalent are not required. What has been overlooked in burns is that there are many living epithelial cells in the areas. With the use of ascorbic acid these cells are kept viable, will multiply, and soon meet with other proliferating units in the establishment of new skin.

Primary and Lasting Benefits in Pregnancy

Observations made on over 300 consecutive obstetrical cases using supplemental ascorbic acid, by mouth, convinced me that failure to use this agent in sufficient amounts in pregnancy borders on malprac-

tice. The lowest amount of ascorbic acid used was 4,000 mg and the highest amount 15,000 mg each day. Requirements were roughly 4,000 mg the first trimester, 6,000 mg the second trimester, and 10,000 mg the third trimester. Approximately, 20 percent of the pregnancies required 15,000 mg each day during the last trimester. Eighty percent of this group received a booster injection of 10,000 mg, intravenously, on admission to the hospital. Infants born under massive ascorbic acid therapy were all robust.

The simple stress of pregnancy demands supplemental vitamin C. During the pregnancy, hemoglobin levels were much easier to maintain; leg cramps were less than 3 percent; and stretch marks were seldom encountered, and when they were present they occurred due to an associated problem of too much eating and too little walking. The capacity of the skin to resist the pressure of an expanding uterus will also vary in different individuals. Labor was shorter and less painful; there were no postpartum hemorrhages; and the perineum was found to be remarkably elastic, and episiotomy was performed electively. No

NOT TAKING SUPPLEMENTS CAUSES MISCARRIAGE, BIRTHING PROBLEMS, INFANT MORTALITY
by Andrew W. Saul, PhD

It is simply incredible what people have been told about vitamins. Now the press is trying to scare women away from prenatal supplements.[1,2] Didn't see that one coming, now, did you?

Several friends who work as missionaries asked me if vitamin C supplementation would help the indigenous peoples they work with in South American rainforests. Since I think supplemental C is valuable for all humans, I said "yes." They took it from there, and for years now have been giving multi-thousand-milligram (mg) doses of ascorbic acid powder to the natives daily. The result is that miscarriage and infant mortality rates have plummeted.

Vitamin C Protects Mother and Baby

Far from being an abortifacient, vitamin C in fact helps hold a healthy pregnancy right from the start. Pediatri-

cian Lendon Smith, MD, known to TV audiences nationwide as "The Children's Doctor," had this to say: "Vitamin C is our best defense and everyone should be on this one *even before birth*. Three thousand mgs daily for the pregnant woman is a start. The baby should get 100 mg per day per month of age."

For centuries, postpartum hemorrhage was a leading cause of death in childbed. Hemorrhage very often occurs in scorbutic (vitamin-C deficient) patients.[3] Optimum dosing with vitamin C prevents hemorrhage and saves women's lives. One way it may do this is by strengthening the walls of the body's large and small blood vessels.

"Harmful effects have been mistakenly attributed to vitamin C, including hypoglycemia, rebound scurvy, infertility, mutagenesis, and destruction of vitamin B12. Health professionals should recognize that vitamin C does not produce these effects" (Levine M et al., *Journal of the American Medical Association* 1999;281:1419).

Frederick R. Klenner, MD, gave very large doses of vitamin C to over 300 pregnant women and reported virtually no complications in any of the pregnancies or deliveries.[4] Indeed, the hospital nurses around Reidsville, North Carolina, noted that the infants who were healthiest and happiest were the "vitamin C babies." Abram Hoffer, MD, has similarly reported that he has observed a complete absence of birth defects in babies born to his vitamin-C taking mothers-to-be.

Specifically, Klenner gave:

- 4,000 mg each day during the first trimester (first three months of pregnancy)

- 6,000 mg each day during the second trimester

- 8,000–10,000 mg each day during the third trimester

Some women got 15,000 mg daily during the third trimester. There were no miscarriages in this entire group of 300 women.

Klenner gave "booster" injections of vitamin C to 80 percent of the women upon admission to the hospital for childbirth. But just with oral supplemental vitamin C, the results were wonderful. First, labor was shorter and less painful. Second, stretch marks were seldom to be seen. Third, there were no postpartum hemorrhages at all. And, there were no toxic manifestations and no cardiac distress. Among Klenner's patients were the Fultz quadruplets, which at the time were the only quads in the southeastern United States to have survived.

Vitamin C even helps with conception. Vitamin C supplementation increases sperm production. More sperm, stronger sperm, and better swimming sperm all manifested within only four days, at 1,000 mg daily C doses, in a University of Texas study. And this has been known now for over 30 years; it was first reported in *Medical Tribune*, May 11, 1983.[5]

Vitamins Vital for Pregnancy

Vitamins deliver healthier babies. The first few weeks of pregnancy are especially crucial to the developing embryo. Yet many women only begin to eat right and take necessary vitamin supplements once they know they are pregnant. This is weeks or even months too late. Nutrition needs rise during pregnancy. Even the RDA's are higher. This may be obvious to you, but many women eat really poor diets in general. Then, in a vain attempt to "get all the nutrition they need from a balanced diet" while "eating for two," they tend to eat more of that same poor diet. Telling them to not take prenatal supplements is a genuine tragedy, for which the media and the medical professions cannot easily be excused.

One can only wonder why the media continually, repeatedly fails to even mention how vitamin supplementation benefits mother and baby. Here is what they missed:

- If you *really* want to avoid miscarriages and birth defects, avoid drugs of all kinds, prescription and over-the-counter. Avoid alcohol, cigarettes, and all but the most essential medications.

- Vitamins are safer, vastly safer, than any drug. A really good diet, properly supplemented with a daily multivitamin plus appropriate quantities of other vitamins, will go a very long way to protect mother and baby.

REFERENCES

1. Howarth M. Taking multivitamins can raise risk of a miscarriage. *MailOnline*. Retrieved Jan 26, 2014 from www.dailymail.co.uk.

2. Nohr A. periconceptional intake of vitamins and fetal death. *Intl J Epidemiol* 2014. Retrieved from http://ije.oxfordjournals.org/content/early/2014/01/21/ije.dyt214.abstract.

3. Saul AW. The pioneering work of William J. McCormick. *J Orthomolecular Med* 2003;18(2):93–96.

4. Klenner F. Observations on the dose and administration of vitamin C when employed beyond the range of a vitamin in human pathology. *J Appl Nutr* 1971;23(3&4). See also: Stone, I. *The Healing Factor*. Ch 28. New York: Grosset & Dunlap, 1972.

5. Gonzalez ER. Sperm swim singly after vitamin C therapy. *JAMA* 1983;249(20):2747–2751. See also: Dawson EB. Effect of ascorbic acid on male fertility. *Ann N Y Acad Sci* 1987;498:312–23 and Dawson EB. Effect of ascorbic acid supplementation on the sperm quality of smokers. *Fertil Steril* 1992 Nov;58(5):1034–9.

Excerpted from the *Orthomolecular Medicine News Service*, January 27, 2014.

patient required catheterization. No toxic manifestations were demonstrated in this group. There was no cardiac stress, even though 22 patients had rheumatic hearts.

Infants born under massive ascorbic acid therapy were all robust. Not a single case required resuscitation. No feeding problems were experienced. The Fultz quadruplets (the first identical African-American quadruplets on record) were in this group. They took milk nourishment on the second day. These babies were started on 50 mg of ascorbic acid the first day and, of course, this dosage was increased as time went on. Our only nursery equipment was one hospital bed; an old, used single-unit hot plate; and an equally old 10-quart kettle. Humidity and ascorbic acid tells this story. They are the only quadruplets to have survived in the southeastern United States. Another case of which I am justly proud is one in which we delivered 10 children to one couple. All are healthy and good looking. There were no miscarriages. All are living and well. They are frequently referred to as the "vitamin C kids."

I was able to take women who had had as many as five abortions without a successful pregnancy and carry them through two and three uneventful pregnancies with the use of supplemental vitamin C. The German literature is stacked with articles recommending high doses of vitamin C during gestation because they believe that this substance is of great benefit in influencing the health of the mother and in preventing infections. The vital contribution of ascorbic acid to the body tissues can be summed up in the formation and maintenance of normal intercellular material, especially in the connective tissue, bones, teeth, and blood vessels. Genetic errors might be prevented if prospective mothers were advised to take 10,000 mg or more of ascorbic acid daily. It is significant that we found in the simple stress of pregnancy, a normal physiological process, that equivalent requirements paralleled those found in the rat when under stress. Experiments by many researchers have shown that the need for supplemental vitamin C begins with the embryo.

Diabetes Mellitus Response to 10,000 Milligrams of Ascorbic Acid by Mouth

Over the past 17 years my coworkers and I have studied the effects of 10,000 mg of vitamin C taken by mouth in patients with diabetes (types 1 and 2). We found that every diabetic not taking supplemental vitamin C could be classified as having subclinical scurvy (long-term marginal deficiency). For this reason they find it difficult to heal wounds. Diabetes patients will use the supplemental vitamin C for better utilization of insulin. It will assist the liver in the metabolism of carbohydrates and will reinstate the body to heal wounds like a normal individual. We found that 60 percent of all diabetics could control their condition with diet and 10,000 mg of ascorbic acid daily. The other 40 percent needed much less needle insulin and less oral medication.

Observations Following Post-Surgery Cases on Blood Plasma Levels of Ascorbic Acid

Deduction is evident of the need for substantial amounts of ascorbic acid prior to surgery. Plasma levels, recorded before starting anesthesia and after cessation of such inhalants and completion of surgery, remained unchanged. We found, however, that samples of blood taken six hours after surgery showed drops of approximately one-quarter the starting amount of vitamin C, and at 12 hours the levels were down to one-half. Samples taken 24 hours later, without added ascorbic acid to fluids, showed levels three-quarters lower than the original samples. A Baylor University research team reported similar findings in 1965. Marshall Bartlett, Chester Jones,[35] and others reported that in spite of low blood levels of plasma ascorbic acid at the time of surgery, normal wound healing may be produced by adequate vitamin C therapy during the postoperative period. Thomas Lanman and Theodore Ingalls[36] showed that the strength of healing wounds is decreased at low plasma levels of vitamin C. Schumacher and colleagues[37] reported that the pre-operative use of as little as 500 mg of vitamin C given orally was remarkably successful in preventing shock and weakness following dental extractions. Many other investigators have shown in both laboratory and clinical studies, that optimal primary wound healing is dependent to a large extent upon the vitamin C content of the tissues.

In 1949, it was my privilege to assist at an abdominal exploratory laparotomy. A mass of small viscera was found glued together. The area was so friable that every attempt at separation produced a torn intestine. After repairing some 20 tears the surgeon closed the cavity as a hopeless situation. Two grams (2,000 mg) of ascorbic acid was given by syringe every two hours for 48 hours and then four times each day. In 36 hours, the patient was walking the halls and in seven days was discharged with normal elimination and no pain. She has outlived her surgeon by many years. We recommend that all patients take 10,000 mg of ascorbic acid each day. At least 30,000 mg should be given, daily, in solutions, post-operatively, until oral medication is allowed and tolerated.

In surgery, the use of ascorbic acid resolves itself into a must situation. The 24-hour frank scurvy levels should be sufficient evidence to encourage all surgeons to use vitamin C freely in their fluids. Proper employment of vitamin C by the surgeons will all but eliminate post-surgical deaths.

Could Ascorbic Acid Have Anticancer Features?

Jorgen Schlegel from Tulane University has been using 1,500 mg of ascorbic acid daily to prevent recurrences of cancer of the bladder.[38] He and other biochemists have been able to demonstrate that in the presence of ascorbic acid, carcinogenic metabolites will not develop in the urine. They suggest that spontaneous tumor formation is the result of faulty tryptophan metabolism while urine is retained in the bladder. Schlegel termed ascorbic acid "an anticancer vitamin." Research has also shown that that the depletion of mast cells (initiators of inflammation) from guinea pigs skin was due to ascorbic acid deficiency.[39] The possibilities indicated are that vitamin C is necessary either directly or indirectly for the formation of mast cells, or for their maintenance once formed or both.

Ascorbic acid will control myelocytic leukemia (a cancer that affects white blood cells) provided 25,000 to 30,000 mg are taken orally each day.

Cholesterol Is Not a Problem When Daily Intake of Ascorbic Acid Is High

Mention should be made of the role played by vitamin C as a regulator of the rate at which cholesterol is formed in the body.[40] A deficiency of the vitamin speeds the formation of this substance. In experimental work, guinea pigs fed a diet free of ascorbic acid showed a 600 percent acceleration in cholesterol formation in the adrenal glands. Take 10,000 mg or more each day and then eat all the eggs you want—that is my schedule and my cholesterol remains normal. Russia has published many articles demonstrating these same benefits.

Infectious Hepatitis Relieved

Viral hepatitis needs brief mentioning. There are two types: infectious hepatitis and needle

INTRAVENOUS APPLICATION

Ascorbate must be given by needle to bring about quick reversal of various insults to the human body. We have found that doses must range from 350 mg to 1,200 mg per kilogram (kg) body weight per day. Under 400 mg per kg of body weight the injection can be made with a syringe provided the vitamin is buffered with sodium bicarbonate with sodium bisulfite added. Above 400 mg doses per kg body weight, the vitamin must be diluted to at least 18 cc of 5 percent dextrose in water, saline in water, or Ringer's solution. Many times adenosine 5-monophosphate, 25 mg in children and 50 to 100 mg in adults, given intramuscularly, is necessary to achieve results. In debilitated individuals or when the pathology is serious, desoxycorticosterone acetate (DCA), aqueous solution, must also be added to the schedule. Usually 2.5 mg for children and 5 mg for adults is the daily intramuscular dose required. Sudden swelling of the feet indicates abnormal sensitivity and the drug must be discontinued.

hepatitis. Physical activity has always been considered to increase the severity and prolong the course of the disease.[41] Researchers in Vietnam showed that pick-and-shovel details had no effects on the 199 controls as against the 199 kept at bed rest.[42] One thing is certain: given massive intravenous ascorbic acid therapy, patients are well and back to work in from three to seven days. In these cases, the vitamin is also employed by mouth as follow-up therapy. A study at the University of Switzerland Clinic in Basel reported that just 10,000 mg daily, intravenously, proved the best treatment available.

Various Maladies

We could continue indefinitely extolling the merits of ascorbic acid . . .

• Excellent results have been reported in the healing of corneal ulcers even though the massive dose was 1,500 mg daily.[43]

• One single injection of ascorbic acid, calculated at 500 mg per kg of body weight, will reverse heat stroke.

• One to three injections of the vitamin in a dose range of 400 mg per kg of body weight will effect a dramatic cure in viral pancarditis (inflammation of the heart).

• Intravenous injections will quickly relieve pain and erythema even of second-degree burns when precautions are not taken.

• One to three injections of 400 mg per kg of body weight given every eight hours will dry up chickenpox in 24 hours; if nausea is present, it will stop the nausea.

• A 5 percent ointment using a water-soluble base will cure acute fever blisters if applied 10 or more times a day, and a 30 percent ointment can remove several small basal cell epithelioma with a 30 percent ointment.

• Very promising results have been reported in glaucoma with a dose schedule of 100 mg per kg of body weight taken after meals and at bed hour.[44]

• Oral doses of 1,000 mg every one to two hours during exposure will prevent sunburn.

• In arthritis, those taking at least 10,000 mg daily, and those taking 15,000 to 25,000 mg daily, will experience commensurate benefit. Supportive treatment must also be given. Repair of collagenous tissue is dependent on adequate ascorbic acid.

• In herpes zoster, 2,000 mg of vitamin C given intramuscularly with 50 mg of adenosine-5 monophosphoric acid, also intramuscularly, every 12 hours is beneficial.

• In massive shingles, ascorbic acid should also be given by vein and always as much by mouth as can be tolerated. Heavy metal intoxication is also resolved with adequate vitamin C therapy.

• In the common cold, 1,000 mg each hour for 48 hours and then 10,000 mg each day by mouth can help reduce the cold's symptoms and duration. Regnier[48] reported that the larger the dose of ascorbic acid, the better were the results.[48]

Note: Injections are usually given with a syringe in a dilution of 1,000 mg to 5 cc of fluid. This concentration will produce immediate thirst and can be prevented by having the patient drink a glass of juice just before giving the injection.

We have reviewed many other pathological conditions in which ascorbic acid plays an important part in recovery. To these might be added cardiovascular diseases, abnormally heavy or prolonged menstruation, peptic and duodenal ulcers, post-operative and radiation sickness, rheumatic fever, scarlet fever, polio, acute and chronic pancreatitis, tularemia (rabbit fever), whooping cough, and tuberculosis.

In one case of scarlet fever in which penicillin and the sulfa drugs were showing no improvement, 50,000 mg of ascorbic acid given intravenously resulted in a dramatic drop in the fever curve to normal. Here the action of ascorbic acid was not only direct but also as a synergist.

In one spectacular case of a black widow[52] spider bite in a three-year-old child, in coma, 1,000 mg of calcium gluconate and 4,000 mg of ascorbic acid were administered intravenously. Then 4,000 mg of ascorbic acid were given every six hours using a syringe. The child was awake and well in 24 hours. On physical examination, the child was comatose with a rigid abdomen. The area about the umbilicus was red and indurated, suggesting a strangulated hernia. With a 4x camera lens, fang marks were in evidence. Thirty hours after starting the vitamin C therapy the child expelled a large amount of dark clotted blood; there was no other residual. A review of the literature confirmed that this individual has been the only one to survive with such findings—the others were reported at autopsy.

As for other bites, 10,000 mg of vitamin C with 200 to 400 mg of vitamin B6, by mouth, daily will shield one from mosquito bites. Twenty percent of these patients will also require 100 mg of vitamin B6 intramuscularly each week.

General All-Around Benefit

Vitamin C plays a very important role in general health. A deficiency of this substance in sufficient amounts can be a factor in loss of appetite, loss of weight or failure to grow, muscular weakness, anemia, and various skin lesions. The relationship between vitamin C and the health of the gums and teeth has long been recognized. Laboratory studies on gum-teeth connective tissue have reaffirmed this relationship.[53] Our son who will be 19 in July has never developed a tooth cavity. Since age 10 he has received at least 10,000 mg of ascorbic acid, daily, by mouth. Before age 10, the amount given was on a sliding scale.[54]

In general, vitamin C is beneficial for all-around good health, and its benefits accrue with daily use. The brain will be clearer, the mind more active, the body less wearied, and the memory more retentive with a daily dosage of 1,000 to 10,000 mg of ascorbic acid per day for adults and 1,000 mg for each year of life for children under 10.

▪ CONCLUSION

The types of pathology treated with massive doses of ascorbic acid run the entire gamut of medical knowledge. Body needs are so great that so-called minimal daily requirements must be ignored. A genetic error is the probable cause for our inability to manufacture ascorbic acid, thus requiring exogenous sources of vitamin C. Simple dye or chemical test are available for checking individual needs. Ascorbic acid destroys virus bodies by taking up the protein coat so that new units cannot be made, by contributing to the breakdown of virus nucleic acid with the result of controlled purine metabolism. Its action in dealing with viral pneumonia and viral encephalitis has been outlined. The clinical use of vitamin C in pneumonia has a very sound foundation. In experimental tests, monkeys kept on a vitamin-C free diet all died of pneumonia while those with adequate diets remained healthy.[45] Many investigators have shown an increased need for ascorbic acid in this condition,[46,47] as well as for burns, cancer, high cholesterol, diabetes, pregnancy, healing from surgery, and many more conditions.

It must be remembered when using ascorbic acid that experiments on man are the only experiments that can give positive evidence of therapeutic action in man. Likewise, the use of ascorbic acid in human pathology must follow the law of mass action: in reversible reactions, the extent of chemical change is proportional to the active masses of the interacting substance. I am in full agreement with statistician Lancelot Hogben who said, "A scientific idea must live dangerously or die of inanition. Science thrives on daring generalizations. There is nothing particularly scientific about excessive caution. Cautious explorers do not cross the Atlantic of truth."

REFERENCES

1. Correspondence with colleague from Puerto Rico.

2. Jennings OE, A. Avinoff. *Wild Flowers of Western Penna. & Upper Ohio Basin.* University of Pittsburgh Press, Vol. 2, Plate 156.

3. Food and Life. 1939 Yearbook, U.S. Dept. Agriculture, US Printing Office, Washington, DC: 236.

4. Klenner FR. Correspondence with Dr. Bauer, University of Switzerland.

5. Salomon LL, et al. *NY Acad Sci* 1961;93:115.

6. Grollman AP, AL Lehninger. *Arch Biochem* 1957;69:458.

7. Chattejee IB, NC Kar, BC Guha. *NY Acad Sci* 1961;92:36.

8. Isherwood FA, LW Mapson. *NY Acad Sci* 1961;92:6.

9. Burns JJ. *Am J Med* 1959;26:740.

10. Stone I. Brief Proposal Per. *Biology & Medicine*, Autumn 1966.

11. Slobody LB. *J Lab & Clinical Med* 1944;29(5):464–472.

12. Ringsdorf WM, E Cheraskin. Sec., Oral Med., U. of Ala. Med. Center, Birmingham, Ala. ref.

13. Klenner FR. *Tri-State Med J*, Feb 1956. ref .

14. Larson C. *Ordnance*, Jan–Feb 1967:359–360.

15. Starr TJ. *Hospital Practice*, Nov 1968: 52.

16. Kropowski H. *Med. World News*, June 1970: 24

17. Klenner FR. *J Applied Nutr*, 1953.

18. Klenner FR. *Tri-State Med J*, June 1957.

19. Klenner FR. *Tri-State Med J*, Oct 1958.

20. Klenner FR. *Tri-State Med J*, Feb 1960.

21. Bakay L. *The Blood-Brain Barrier.* Springfield, IL: C. Thomas, 1956.

22. Chambers R. et al, *Physiol Rev* 1947;27:436–463.

23. Knisely MH. et al, *Archives Surgery* 1945:51–220.

24. Knisely MH. *Science* 1947;106:431.

25. Berkeley WT. Jr. *Southern Med J* 58:1182–1184.

26. Lund C, SM Levenson. *Arch Surg* 1947;55:557.

27. Bergman HC. et al, *Am Heart J* 1945;29:506–512.

28. Lam CR. *Col Rev Surg Gyn & Obst* 1941;72:390–400.

29. Klasson DH. *NY J Med* 1951;51:2388–2392.

30. Stone HH. *Med J* Aug 1970:6–10.

31. Meakins JC. *The Practice of Med.* St. Louis, MO: C.V. Mosby, 1938.

32. Kelli & Zilva. *J Biochemistry* 1935;29:1028.

33. Lambden MP. et al. *Proc Sec Exp Biol Med* 1954;85: 190–192.

34. Patterson JW. *J Biological Chemistry* 1950:81–88.

35. Bartlett MK, et al. *New Eng J Med* 1942;226: 474.

36. Lanman TH, TH Ingalls. *Am Surgery* 1937;105:616.

37. Schumacher. *Ohio State Med J* 1946;42:1248.

38. Schlegel GE, et al. *Trans Am Ass Genito-Urinary Surgery* 1989;61:ref 51.

39. Glick D, Hosoda T. *Proc Soc Exp Biology and Med* 1965:119.

40. Becker RR. et al. *J Am Chem Sec* 1953;75:2020.

41. Capps RB. *Modern Med*, Jan. 11, 1971.

42. Freeben RK, LR Repsher. *Mod World News*, Jan. 23, 1970.

43. Boyd TA, FW Campbell. *B Med J* 1950;2:1145.

44. Virno M. *Eye, Ear, Nose & Throat Monthly* 1967;46:1502.

45. Sabin J. *Exp Med* 1939;89:507–515.

46. Wright. *Ann Int Med*, Oct 1938;12(4):518–528.

47. Brody HD. *J Am Diet Assoc* 1953;29:588.

48. Regnier E. *Review of Allergy*, Oct 1968;22:948.

49. Pollock H, SL Halpern. Washington Nat Research Council Publication, 234, 1942.

50. Greenblatt RB. *Obstet & Gynec* 1953;2:530.

51. King CC, et al. *New York Times*, Nov. 2, 1952.

52. Klenner FR. *Tri-State Med J*, Dec. 1957

53. Baume LJ. *Science News Letter* 1953;64:103.

54. Klenner FR. *Tri-State Med J*, Nov 1955.

EVIDENCE-BASED MEDICINE:
NEITHER GOOD EVIDENCE NOR GOOD MEDICINE
by Steve Hickey, PhD, and Hilary Roberts, PhD

Evidence-based medicine (EBM) is the practice of treating individual patients based on the outcomes of huge medical trials. It is, currently, the self-proclaimed gold standard for medical decision-making, and yet it is increasingly unpopular with clinicians. Their reservations reflect an intuitive understanding that something is wrong with its methodology. They are right to think this, for EBM breaks the laws of so many disciplines that it should not even be considered scientific.

The assumption that EBM is good science is unsound from the start. Decision science and cybernetics (the science of communication and control) highlight the disturbing consequences. EBM fosters marginally effective treatments, based on population averages rather than individual need. Its mega-trials are incapable of finding the causes of disease, even for the most diligent medical researchers, yet they swallow up research funds. Worse, EBM cannot avoid exposing patients to health risks. It is time for medical practitioners to discard EBM's tarnished gold standard, reclaim their clinical autonomy, and provide individualized treatments to patients.

The key element in a truly scientific medicine would be a rational patient. This means that those who set a course of treatment would base their decision-making on the expected risks and benefits of treatment to the individual concerned. However, EBM statistics are not good at helping individual patients: rather, they relate to groups and populations.

What Use Are Population Statistics?

EBM relies on a few large-scale studies and statistical techniques to choose the treatment for each patient. Practitioners of EBM incorrectly call this process using the "best evidence."

Much medical research relies on early 20th-century statistical methods, developed before the advent of computers. In such studies, statistics are used to determine the probability that two groups of patients differ from each other. If a treatment group has taken a drug and a control group has not, researchers typically ask whether any benefit was caused by the drug or occurred by chance. The way they answer this question is to calculate the "statistical significance." This process results in a p-value: the lower the p-value, the less likely the result was due to chance. Thus, a p-value of 0.05 means a chance result might occur about one time in 20. Sometimes a value of less than 1 in 100 ($p < 0.01$), or even less than 1 in 1,000 ($p < 0.001$) is reported. These two p-values are referred to as "highly significant" or "very highly significant" respectively.

Some people assume that "significant" results must be "important" or "relevant." This is wrong: the level of significance reflects only the degree to which the groups are considered to be separate. Crucially, the significance level depends not only on the difference between the studied groups, but also on their size. So, as we increase the size of the groups, the results become more significant–even though the effect may be tiny and unimportant.

Consider two populations of people, with very slightly different average blood pressures. If we take 10 people from each, we will find no significant difference between the two groups because a small group varies by chance. If we take 100 people from each population, we get a low level of significance ($p < 0.05$), but if we take a thousand, we now find a very *highly significant* result. Crucially, the magnitude of the small difference in blood pressure remains the same in each case. In this case a difference can be highly significant (statistically), yet in practical terms it is extremely small and thus effectively insignificant. In a large trial, highly significant effects are often clinically irrelevant. More

Excerpted from the *Orthomolecular Medicine News Service*, December 7, 2011.

important and contrary to popular belief, the results from large studies are less important for a rational patient than those from smaller ones.

Once researchers have conducted a pilot study, they can perform a power calculation, to make sure they include enough subjects to get a high level of significance. Thus, over the last few decades, researchers have studied ever bigger groups, resulting in studies a hundred times larger than those of only a few decades ago. This implies that the effects they are seeking are minute, as larger effects (capable of offering real benefits to actual patients) could more easily be found with the smaller, old-style studies.

The Ecological Fallacy

There is a further problem with the dangerous assertion implicit in EBM that large-scale studies are the best evidence for decisions concerning individual patients. This claim is an example of the ecological fallacy, which wrongly uses group statistics to make predictions about individuals.

To explain this, suppose we measured the foot size of every person in New York and calculated the mean value (total foot size/number of people). Using this information, the government proposes to give everyone a pair of average-sized shoes. Clearly, this would be unwise—the shoes would be either too big or too small for most people. Individual responses to medical treatments vary by at least as much as their shoe sizes, yet despite this, EBM relies upon aggregated data. This is technically wrong; group statistics cannot predict an individual's response to treatment.

EBM Selects Evidence

Another problem with EBM's approach of trying to use only the "best evidence" is that it cuts down the amount of information available to doctors and patients making important treatment decisions. The evidence allowed in EBM consists of selected large-scale trials and meta-analyses that attempt to make a conclusion more significant by aggregating results from wildly different groups. This constitutes a tiny percentage of the total evidence. Meta-analysis rejects the vast majority of data available,

because it does not meet the strict criteria for EBM. This conflicts with yet another scientific principle, that of not selecting your data.

More EBM Problems

The human body is a biological system and, when something goes wrong, a medical practitioner attempts to control it. To take an example, if a person has a high temperature, the doctor could suggest a cold compress; this might work if the person was hot through overexertion or too many clothes. Alternatively, the doctor may recommend an antipyretic, such as aspirin. However, if the patient has an infection and a raging fever, physical cooling or symptomatic treatment might not work, as it would not quell the infection.

In the above case, a doctor who overlooked the possibility of infection has not applied the appropriate information to treat the condition. This illustrates a cybernetic concept known as requisite variety, first proposed by an English psychiatrist, Dr. W. Ross Ashby. In modern language, Ashby's law of requisite variety means that the solution to a problem (such as a medical diagnosis) has to contain the same amount of relevant information (variety) as the problem itself. Thus, the solution to a complex problem will require more information than the solution to a straightforward problem. Ashby's idea was so powerful that it became known as the first law of cybernetics. Ashby used the word *variety* to refer to information or, as an EBM practitioner might say, evidence.

As we have mentioned, EBM restricts variety to what it considers the "best evidence." However, if doctors were to apply the same statistically based treatment to all patients with a particular condition, they would break the laws of both cybernetics and statistics. Consequently, in many cases, the treatment would be expected to fail, as the doctors would not have enough information to make an accurate prediction. Population statistics do not capture the information needed to provide a well-fitting pair of shoes, let alone to treat a complex and particular patient. A doctor who arrives at a correct diagnosis and treatment in an efficient manner is called, in cybernetic terms, a good regulator. According to

Roger Conant and Ross Ashby, every good regulator of a system must be a model of that system. Good regulators achieve their goal in the simplest way possible. In order to achieve this, the diagnostic processes must model the systems of the body, which is why doctors undergo years of training in all aspects of medical science. In addition, each patient must be treated as an individual. EBM's group statistics are irrelevant, since large-scale clinical trials do not model an individual patient and his or her condition; they model a population, albeit somewhat crudely. They are thus not good regulators. Once again, a rational patient would reject EBM as a poor method for finding an effective treatment for an illness.

Real Science Means Verification

As we have implied, science is a process of induction and uses experiments to test ideas. From a scientific perspective, therefore, we trust but verify the findings of other researchers. The gold standard in science is called Solomonoff induction, named after Ray Solomonoff, a cybernetic researcher. The power of a scientific result is that you can easily repeat the experiment and check it. If it can't be repeated, for whatever reason (because it is untestable, too difficult, or wrong), a scientific result is weak and unreliable. Unfortunately, EBM's emphasis on large studies makes replication difficult, expensive, and time-consuming. We should be suspicious of large studies, because they are all but impossible to repeat and are therefore unreliable. EBM asks us to trust its results but, to all intents and purposes, it precludes replication. After all, how many doctors have $40 million and 5 years available to repeat a large clinical trial? Thus, EBM avoids refutation, which is a critical part of the scientific method.

EBM generates large numbers of risk factors and multivariate explanations, which makes choosing treatments difficult. The more risk factors you use, the less chance you have of getting a solution. This finding comes directly from the field of pattern recognition, where overly complex solutions are consistently found to fail. Too many risk factors mean that noise and error in the model will overwhelm the genuine information, leading to false predictions or diagnoses.

Medicine for People, Not Statisticians

Diagnosing medical conditions is challenging because we are each biochemically individual. As explained by an originator of this concept, nutritional pioneer Dr. Roger Williams: "Nutrition is for real people. Statistical humans are of little interest." Doctors must encompass enough knowledge and therapeutic variety to match the biological diversity within their population of patients. The process of classifying a particular person's symptoms requires a different kind of statistics (Bayesian), as well as pattern recognition. These have the ability to deal with individual uniqueness.

The basic approach of medicine must be to treat patients as unique individuals, with distinct problems. Personalized, ecological, and nutritional (orthomolecular) medicines are converging on a truly scientific approach. We are entering a new understanding of medical science, according to which the holistic approach is directly supported by systems science. Orthomolecular medicine, far from being marginalized as "alternative," may soon become recognized as the ultimate rational medical methodology. That is more than can be said for EBM.

EARLY EVIDENCE ABOUT VITAMIN C AND THE COMMON COLD
by Linus Pauling, PhD

For many years there has existed the popular belief that ascorbic acid has value in providing protection against the common cold and in ameliorating the manifestations of this viral disease. This belief has not, however, been generally shared by physicians, authorities on nutrition, and official bodies.

I was puzzled by the contradiction between the popular belief and the official opinion, and I made a study of published reports of controlled trials of ascorbic acid in relation to the common cold. On the basis of this study and of some general arguments about orthomolecular medicine (the preservation of good health and the treatment of disease by varying the concentrations in the human body of substances that are normally present in the body and are required for health[1]), I reached the conclusion that ascorbic acid, taken in the proper amounts, decreases the incidence of colds and related infections, and also decreases the severity of individual colds. These arguments were presented in my book *Vitamin C and the Common Cold*, which was published in November 1970.[2]

In this book I presented a discussion of the studies that had been made, including several carefully controlled double-blind studies carried out by competent medical investigators. The evidence and arguments presented in this book apparently were not convincing to some physicians, experts in nutrition, and health officials. Since 1970 several reports of new investigations have been published. All the studies of subjects given ascorbic acid (or a placebo) over a period of time and exposed to cold viruses in the usual way, by contact with other people, have given the result that the ascorbic-acid subjects had less illness than the placebo subjects. There is no doubt that ascorbic acid provides some protection against the common cold, as well as against other diseases.

In the course of the years, I have learned about some early studies other than those discussed in my 1970 book. These studies are not so reliable as the later ones, but they provide some significant evidence, and their existence raises again the question of why the nutritional and medical authorities have continued for 30 years to contend that vitamin C has no value in combating the common cold.

An account of some of the early papers is given in the following sections. [Editor's note: All statistical analyses conducted in the following studies were one-tailed unless otherwise noted.]

Korbsch, 1938

In 1938 Dr. Roger Korbsch of St. Elisabeth Hospital, Oberhausen, Germany, published an account of his observations.[3] He mentioned the fact that ascorbic acid had been reported to be effective against several diseases, including gastritis and stomach ulcers, suggested that he try it in treating acute rhinitis and colds. In 1936 he found that oral doses of up to 1,000 milligrams (mg) per day were of value against rhinorrhea (runny nose), rhinitis (common cold), and accompanying manifestations of illness, such as headache. He then found that the injection of 250 or 500 mg of ascorbic acid on the first day of a common cold almost always led to the immediate disappearance of all the signs and symptoms of the cold, with a similar injection sometimes needed on the second day. He stated that ascorbic acid is far superior to other cold medicines, such as aminopyrine (Pyramidon) and injected calcium ion, and is, moreover, without danger, in that there is no evidence that hypervitaminosis C occurs, even with large doses.

Ertel, 1941

In the spring of 1941 a trial was made of vitamin C in Germany in which 357 million daily doses of vitamin C were distributed among 3.7 million pregnant women, nursing mothers, suckling infants, and schoolchildren.[4] Dr. H. Ertel reported that the recipients of the vitamin C enjoyed better health, in several different respects, than the corresponding control populations. The only quantitative information given by him is that with one group of schoolchildren for which good statistical data were

From the *J Orthomolecular Psych* 1974;3(3):139–151.

collected the amount of illness with respiratory infections was 20 percent less than the year before.

Glazebrook and Thomson, 1942

In 1942 Drs. A. J. Glazebrook and Scott Thomson, of the Department of Clinical Medicine and Bacteriology, University of Edinburgh, reported a study carried out with about 1,500 boys, 15 to 20 years old, in a large training school in Scotland.[5] The subjects received a normal diet rather low in ascorbic acid, the daily ration being estimated to contain only 10 to 15 mg. The principal study, carried out over a period of six months, involved 1,100 control subjects and 335 ascorbic-acid subjects. The control subjects, in seven dining groups, received the ordinary diet. The ascorbic-acid subjects, in two dining groups, received the ordinary diet, but with ascorbic acid administered in the milk and cocoa that was served. The average amount of ascorbic acid administered is somewhat uncertain. The authors state that vitamin C was added to the supplies of cocoa or milk serving the tables for the appropriate divisions. In their discussion of preliminary experiments carried out to determine the daily urinary excretion of ascorbic acid, it is stated that initially 200 mg per day was given to each boy, 100 mg being placed in the morning cocoa and 100 mg in an evening glass of milk, the mixing being done in bulk in the kitchens. Analysis of the cocoa and milk showed an average of 63 mg per cup of cocoa and 98 mg per glass of milk, suggesting that about 160 mg per day was the average intake.

Because a number of preliminary studies had been carried out, and the ascorbic acid was added in the kitchens, it is likely that this investigation can be considered to have been a blind study. The authors mention that careful records had been kept of the incidence of all infections for 18 months before the observations described in their paper were begun and that in the preceding year there had been an epidemic of tonsillitis that had affected all the divisions uniformly, so that they could not be regarded as separate units within the larger population. All of the divisions had a population more or less the same as regards the duration of stay in the establishment. Records were kept of the common cold (coryza), tonsillitis (hemolytic streptococcal disease of the nose and throat, covering tonsillitis, sore throat, otitis media, pharyngitis, and cervical adenitis), and other infective conditions (conjunctivitis, boils, impetigo, etc., as well as pneumonia and acute rheumatism).

The total numbers of cases of colds during the six-month period of the study are given in Table 1 for the control group and the ascorbic-acid group. There is a decrease in incidence in all colds by 17 percent, and in colds serious enough to require hospitalization (sick quarters) by 23 percent. For other infectious diseases, a decreased incidence for the ascorbic-acid group was also reported (except for tonsillitis with inclusion of the mild cases). The reported decreases of 100 percent for pneumonia and acute rheumatism are significant.

Glazebrook and Thomson in their paper point out that the difference in incidence of pneumonia and acute rheumatism in the control group and the

TABLE 1. THE PRINCIPAL STUDY BY GLAZEBROOK AND THOMSON: INCIDENCE OF ILLNESS					
	CONTROL GROUP (N = 1,100)		ASCORBIC-ACID GROUP (N = 335)		DECREASE
Colds	286	0.260	72	0.215	17%
Colds, sick quarters	253	.230	59	.176	23%
Tonsillitis	94	.086	29	.087	−1%
Tonsillitis, sick quarters	83	.075	18	.053	28%
Pneumonia	17	.016	0	.000	100%
Acute rheumatism	16	.015	0	.000	100%

ascorbic-acid group is statistically significant, and also that the period of hospitalization for tonsillitis is statistically significant. They give the average stay in the hospital for control subjects (83) hospitalized with tonsillitis as 16.7 days, and for the vitamin-C subjects (18) as 10.05, and state that analysis shows that a difference as great as or greater than that obtained would be expected only once in 50 times in a homogeneous population. Glazebrook and Thomson give information in their paper that permits the severity of individual colds or other infectious diseases and the integrated morbidity, as measured by the number of days hospitalized, to be calculated. These values are given in Tables 2 and 3.

TABLE 2. THE PRINCIPAL STUDY BY GLAZEBROOK AND THOMSON: SEVERITY OF ILLNESS, MEASURED BY AVERAGE NUMBER OF DAYS HOSPITALIZED PER HOSPITALIZED CASE

	CONTROL GROUP	ASCORBIC-ACID GROUP	DECREASE
Common cold	1.47	1.11	24%
Tonsillitis	1.26	0.54	57%
All infective conditions*	5.0	2.5	50%

*Common cold, tonsillitis, pneumonia, acute rheumatism, conjunctivitis, boils, impetigo, etc.

TABLE 3. THE PRINCIPAL STUDY BY GLAZEBROOK AND THOMSON: INTEGRATED MORBIDITY, MEASURED BY AVERAGE NUMBER OF DAYS HOSPITALIZED PER SUBJECT*

	CONTROL GROUP	ASCORBIC-ACID GROUP	DECREASE
Common cold	0.334	0.195	41%
Tonsillitis	.095	.029	69%

*Values for all infective conditions not available because total number of hospitalized cases not reported.

The results described in Tables 1, 2, and 3 thus indicate that ascorbic acid has the effect of decreasing the incidence and severity of tonsillitis, pneumonia, and acute rheumatism, as well as the common cold, for the principal population studies by Glazebrook and Thomson.

A smaller study was also reported by Glazebrook and Thomson, with 150 recruits who entered the institution and were studied during the second half of the six-month period. The results of this trial, as reported by the authors, are given in Table 4. A decrease in the incidence of colds by 12 percent was noted, with, however, little statistical significance. The incidence of tonsillitis was 79 percent less for the ascorbic-acid group than for the control group.

An interesting aspect of the report by Glazebrook and Thomson is that they refer to the numbers in Table 1 for the incidence of colds and tonsillitis in the following words: "It is obvious, therefore, that vitamin C had no effect on the incidence either of the common cold or tonsillitis." It is hard to explain why this statement is made, when in fact the observed incidence of the common cold was 17 percent less for the ascorbic-acid subjects than for the controls, and the number of subjects was so large that the decrease is significant. The authors reported the statistical significance correctly for several of their comparisons, but apparently failed to make the calculation in this case. Some results with statistical significance were obtained also in the smaller study (Table 4). Nevertheless, in their summary the authors state that "the incidence of common cold and tonsillitis were the same in the two groups." They also say that "the average duration of illness due to the common cold was the same in the two groups," although the values that they reported in their paper (Table 2) correspond to a decrease by 24 percent for the ascorbic-acid subjects relative to the controls.

A similar failure of the investigators to describe their own results completely and correctly is found in the report by Drs. Cowan, Diehl, and Baker, discussed next. These misrepresentations by the investigators may well have delayed the general acceptance of vitamin C as a protective agent against the common cold and other diseases by the medical profession.

	CONTROL GROUP (N = 90)		ASCORBIC-ACID GROUP (N = 60)		DECREASE
	TABLE 4. **THE SMALLER STUDY BY GLAZEBROOK AND THOMSON:** **INCIDENCE OF COLDS AND TONSILLITIS**				
Common cold	29	0.322	17	0.283	12%
Tonsillitis	7	.078	1	.017	79%
Colds plus tonsillitis	36	.400	18	.300	25%

Cowan, Diehl, and Baker, 1942

The best of the early studies of ascorbic acid and the common cold was reported by Drs. D. W. Cowan, H. S. Diehl, and A. B. Baker in 1942, when all three were at the University of Minnesota.[6] The principal work on ascorbic acid was done during the winter "cold season" of 1939–1940. The subjects were all students in the University of Minnesota who volunteered to participate in this study because they were particularly susceptible to colds. Persons whose difficulties seemed to be due primarily to chronic sinusitis or allergic rhinitis, as shown by examination of the nose and throat and consideration of symptoms of allergy, were excluded from the study. The subjects were assigned alternately and without selection to an experimental group and a control group. The subjects in the control group were treated exactly like those in the experimental group, except that they received a placebo instead of the ascorbic acid. The subjects were instructed to report to the Health Service whenever a cold developed, so that special report cards could be filled in by a physician. The study was a double-blind one, with neither the subjects nor the physicians knowing which group a subject was in. Each subject was interviewed every three months in order to check the completeness of the reports.

The study was continued for 28 weeks. Of the 233 students initially in the ascorbic-acid group, 183 received 200 mg per day throughout the period of 28 weeks, and 50 received 200 mg per day for two weeks, followed by 100 mg per day except on inception of a cold, when an additional 400 mg per day for two days was administered. This group numbered 208 subjects at the completion of the study, 25 having dropped out. If the composition of the group remained unchanged, the average intake of ascorbic acid was 180 mg per day. The students in the control group initially numbered 194, of whom 155 completed the study (see Table 5).

The authors report the observed incidence of colds by giving the average and the probable error. The corresponding values of the standard deviation, as calculated from the probable error, are given below in parentheses. The average number of colds per person during the period of study was 2.2 for the control group and 1.9 for the ascorbic-acid group.

	PLACEBO GROUP (N = 155)	ASCORBIC-ACID GROUP (N = 208)	DECREASE
	TABLE 5. THE STUDY BY **COWAN, DIEHL, AND BAKER**		
Incidence of colds	2.2	1.9	14%
Severity (days of illness per cold)	0.73	0.58	21%
Integrated morbidity (days of illness per person	1.6	1.1	31%

The authors state in their paper that "the actual difference between the two groups during the year of the study amounts to one-third of a cold per person. Statistical analysis of the data reveals that a difference as large as this would arise only three or four times in a hundred through chance alone. One may therefore consider this as probably a significant difference, and vitamin C supplements to the diet may therefore be judged to give a slight advantage in reducing the number of colds experienced."

Because the authors rounded off the numbers giving the actual numbers of colds per person, the difference is not known exactly. The original records and the original calculations are no longer available. There is evidence, however, that the actual difference between the average number of colds in the two groups is 0.32. The statement by the authors that the difference would arise only three or four times in a hundred through chance alone accordingly restricts the difference to the range 0.31 to 0.33, with 0.32 as the likely value. This difference represents a decrease by 14.4 percent in the incidence of colds in the ascorbic-acid group as compared with the control group.

The observed differences are statistically significant. The average number of days lost from school per person in the placebo group was reported as 1.6, and in the ascorbic acid group as 1.1, giving a decrease of 31 percent in integrated morbidity. The average number of days lost from school per cold was 0.73 for the placebo group and 0.58 for the ascorbic-acid group, a decrease in severity of individual colds by 21 percent. Despite the fact that they had found statistically significant differences between their two groups in Table 5, Cowan, Diehl, and Baker wrote the following sentence as the entire summary of their important paper: "This controlled study yields no indication that either large doses of vitamin C alone or large doses of vitamins A, B1, B2, C, and D and nicotinic acid have any important effect on the number or severity of infections of the upper respiratory tract when administered to young adults who presum-

ably are already on a reasonably adequate diet." This statement would be completely false if it did not contain the adjective "important." Drs. Cowan, Diehl, and Baker apparently thought that a 31 percent decrease in the amount of illness, simply as the result of taking a vitamin C tablet every day, was not important. It is hard to understand this attitude, which, however, seems still to be held by some prominent physicians and nutritionists.

Franz, Sands, and Heyl, 1956

A double-blind study of ascorbic acid and the common cold was carried out by Drs. Warren Franz, Winthrop Sands, and Henry Heyl of Dartmouth Medical School during the three-month period from February to May 1956, with 89 volunteer medical students and student nurses.[7] The subjects were divided, in a random way, into four groups, three of 22 subjects and one of 23 subjects. One group received tablets containing ascorbic acid, the second ascorbic acid and a bioflavonoid (naringin), the third a placebo, and the fourth naringin only. The daily amount of ascorbic acid was 205 mg and that of the bioflavonoid was 1,000 mg. Symptoms of colds were systematically recorded. The results for the bioflavonoid groups, with or without ascorbic acid, were the same as for the corresponding groups without bioflavonoid. The authors concluded that the administration of a bioflavonoid had effect neither on the incidence or the cure of colds nor on the ascorbic-acid level of the blood. The results reported by the authors are given in Table 6. From this table we see that the incidence of colds in the two ascorbic-acid groups is nearly the same as in the other groups (4.5 percent less).

TABLE 6. THE PRINCIPAL STUDY BY FRANZ, SANDS, AND HEYL			
GROUP	NUMBER IN GROUP	TOTAL	NUMBER OF COLDS NOT CURED OR IMPROVED IN 5 DAYS
Ascorbic acid	22]44	8]14	0]1
Ascorbic acid plus bioflavonoid	22	6	1
Placebo	23]45	7]15	4]8
Bioflavonoid	22	8	4

The authors point out that the subjects receiving ascorbic acid showed more rapid improvement in their colds than those not receiving it and that this difference is statistically significant. In the placebo and bioflavonoid groups, 8 of the total of 15 colds remained uncured or unimproved in five days, whereas of the 14 colds in the two groups receiving ascorbic acid only one remained unimproved or uncured in five days, a decrease in the incidence of severe colds by 87.5 percent. This double-blind study shows with statistical significance that ascorbic acid has a greater effect than a placebo in decreasing the incidence of severe colds. A comparison with statistical information about the duration of colds leads to the conclusion that the integrated morbidity for the ascorbic-acid subjects was 40 percent less than for the placebo subjects.

Ritzel, 1961

An important study that gave results with high statistical significance was reported in 1961 by Dr. G. Ritzel, a physician with the medical service of the School District of the City of Basel, Switzerland.[8] The study was carried out in a ski resort with 279 boys during two periods of five to seven days. The conditions were such that the incidence of colds during these short periods was large enough (approximately 20 percent) to permit results with statistical significance to be obtained. The subjects were of the same age (15–17) and had similar nutrition during the period of study. The investigation was double-blind, with neither the participants nor the physicians having any knowledge about the distribution of the ascorbic-acid tablets (1,000 mg) and the placebo tablets. The tablets were distributed every morning and taken by the subjects under observation such that the possibility of interchange of tablets was eliminated. The subjects were examined daily as to symptoms of colds and other infections, as listed in the footnote of Table 7. The records were largely on the basis of subjective symptoms, partially supported by objective observations (measurement of body temperature, inspection of the respiratory organs, auscultation of the lungs, and so on). People who showed cold symptoms on the first day were excluded from the investigation.

TABLE 7. THE STUDY BY RITZEL			
	PLACEBO GROUP (N = 1,100)	ASCORBIC-ACID GROUP (N = 139)	DECREASE
Number of colds	31	17	
Incidence of colds	0.221	0.122	45%
Total days of illness	80	31	
Total individual symptoms*	119	42	
Severity of individual colds, from days of illness per cold from individual symptoms per cold	2.58	1.82	29%
Severity of individual colds, from individual symptoms per cold	3.84	2.47	36%
Integrated morbidity from days of illness per person	0.571	0.223	61%
Integrated morbidity from individual symptoms per person	0.850	0.302	64%

* Pharyngitis, laryngitis, tonsillitis, sore throat; bronchitis, coughing; fever, chills; otitis media; rhinitis; herpes labialis; other symptoms (muscle ache, headache, abdominal pain, vomiting, diarrhea, general malaise).

After the completion of the investigation a completely independent group of professional people was provided with the identification numbers for the ascorbic acid tablets and placebo tablets, and this group carried out the statistical evaluation of the observations. The principal results of the investigation are given in Table 7. The author points out that the group receiving ascorbic acid showed only 39 percent as many days of illness per person as the group receiving the placebo, and that the number of individual symptoms per person was only 35 percent as great for the ascorbic-acid group as for the placebo group, and states that the statistical evaluation of these differences by two-by-two tables gives a significant difference. The author also points out that the average number of days per cold for the ascorbic-acid group was 1.8 (more accurately 1.82), 29 percent less than the value for the placebo group, 2.6 (2.58), and that this difference is statistically significant.

In Table 2 of the paper by Ritzel (not included here), the values of the number of patients showing different symptoms (the seven classes of symptoms listed in the footnote to Table 7) are given, and the number of days of illness for each symptom. It is interesting that for each of these seven classes of symptoms the number of patients showing the symptom is less for the ascorbic-acid group than for the placebo group, and that, moreover, the number of days of illness per patient showing the symptom is also less.

Let us discuss separately the effect of ascorbic acid on the incidence of the common cold and its effect on the severity of individual colds in Table 7. The number of colds was 31 for the placebo group and 17 for the ascorbic-acid group. (The number of colds was not given explicitly in the paper. However, the number of days of illness for each of the two groups was given [80, 31], and the average number of days of illness per cold [2.6, 1.8]. The only integral values for the number of colds allowed by these numbers are 31 for the placebo group and 17 for the ascorbic-acid group.) The incidence of colds is accordingly 0.221 per person for the placebo group and 0.122 for the ascorbic acid group, a decrease by 45 percent for the ascorbic-acid group. This investigation accordingly

"Never put your trust into anything but your own intellect. The world progresses, year by year, century by century, as the members of the younger generation find out what was wrong among the things that their elders said. So you must always be skeptical— always think for yourself."—LINUS PAULING

shows that the hypothesis that ascorbic acid has only the same effect as the placebo is to be rejected.

Two values may be calculated for the effect of ascorbic acid on the severity of individual colds. In Table 7 the number of days of illness per cold for the placebo group is given as 2.58 and for the ascorbic-acid group as 1.82, 29 percent smaller. Moreover, the average number of individual symptoms recorded per cold (they were recorded daily) is given as 3.84 for the placebo group and 2.87 for the ascorbic-acid group, 36 percent smaller. Each of these differences is statistically significant, the hypothesis that the two populations are the same with respect to the number of days of illness per cold and the individual symptoms per cold is also to be rejected.

Two values are given in Table 7 for the integrated morbidity, one as measured by the number of days of illness per person and the other as measured by the number of symptoms (recorded daily) per person. These values are 61 percent and 64 percent less, respectively, for the ascorbic-acid subjects than for the placebo subjects.

This investigation seems to have been very well-planned and executed. Ritzel was aware of the problem of obtaining reliable results in the study of the common cold, and he discussed the problem in some detail. His paper is provided with an English-language summary, reading as follows: "The possibility of preventing infection by administration of vitamin C was investigated in a moderately large test population during a period of increased exposure. The trial was conducted in such a way as to exclude sources of error in assessing subjective symptoms. Statistical evaluation of the results confirmed the efficacy of vitamin C in the prevention and treatment of colds."

It is interesting that in an often-quoted review of the evidence about ascorbic acid and the common cold, which ended with the statement that "there is no conclusive evidence that ascorbic acid has any protective effect against, or any therapeutic effect on, the course of the common cold in healthy people not depleted of ascorbic acid," the work of Ritzel was covered in two sentences, stating quite erroneously that he had reported "a reduction of 39 percent in the number of days ill from upper respiratory infections and a reduction of 35 percent in the incidence of individual symptoms in the supplemented group as compared with the placebo group." (The correct values are 61 percent and 64 percent, respectively.)[9]

■ CONCLUSION

Since 1970 several careful double-blind studies of ascorbic acid in relation to the common cold have been carried out. They leave no doubt that ascorbic acid in amounts greater than the officially recommended dosage decreases the amount of illness with the common cold. The point of the present paper is that the evidence for this protective effect was already moderately strong by 1942 and was very strong by 1961.

Despite the strength of the evidence, which has been systematically misrepresented by the medical and nutritional authorities, the possible value of an increased intake of vitamin C in decreasing the amount of suffering and loss of time from work of the people has been ignored by almost all physicians. The official stand of the American Medical Association is still, in 1974, that extra vitamin C has no value in controlling the common cold or in any other way, and that an increased intake of vitamin E or other vitamins also has no value in controlling disease. [Editor's note: That negative stance has changed, but not much, in the four decades since.]

The case of vitamin C and the common cold has, I believe, a lesson for us. It is that we cannot rely on the medical and nutritional establishment to give us good advice about health and nutrition. What is the optimum daily intake of vitamin C? Can vitamin C decrease the age-specific incidence of diseases other than the common cold? There is, in fact, considerable evidence that it can, in part cited above and in the review of the more recent work.[10] What is the *optimum* daily intake of vitamin E, and of other vitamins and other nutrient factors? Very little research is being done at the present time on these important problems.

REFERENCES

1. Pauling L. Orthomolecular psychiatry. *Science* 1968;160:265.

2. Pauling L. *Vitamin C and the Common Cold.* San Francisco: W.H. Freeman & Co, 1970.

3. Korbsch R. Ober die Kupierung entzundlich-allergischer Zustande durch die L-Askorbinsaure. *Medizinische Klinik* 1938;34:1500–1501.

4. Ertel H. Der verlauf der vitamin-C-prophylaxen im Fruhjahr. *Die Emahrung* 1941;6:269–273.

5. Glazebrook AJ, Thomson S. The administration of vitamin C in a large institution and its effect on general health and resistance to infection. *J Hygiene* 1942;42:1–19.

6. Cowan DD, Diehl HS, Baker AB. Vitamins for the prevention of colds. *J Am Med Assoc* 1942;120:1267–1271.

7. Franz WL, Sands GW, Heyl HL. Blood ascorbic acid level in bioflavonoid and ascorbic acid therapy of common cold. *J Am Med Assoc* 1956;162:1224–1226.

8. Ritzel G. Kritische beurteilung des vitamins C als prophylacticum und therapeuticum der Ertaltungskrankheiten. *Helv Med Act* 1961;28:63–68.

9. Anonymous. Ascorbic acid and the common cold. *Nutr Rev* 1967;25:288.

10. Stone I. *The Healing Factor: Vitamin C Against Disease.* New York: Grosset & Dunlap, 1972.

DYNAMIC FLOW: A NEW MODEL FOR ASCORBATE

by Steve Hickey, PhD, Hilary Roberts, PhD, and Robert F. Cathcart, MD

This paper introduces the dynamic flow model, which describes the function and pharmacokinetics of vitamin C. In dynamic flow, an excess of oral ascorbate provides a steady flow of electrons (electrically charged particles essential to every cellular processes) through the body. Human physiology is restored to the condition before the evolutionary loss of the ability to synthesize ascorbate. The model supports and extends the ideas of Linus Pauling, PhD, Nobel Prize winner and founder of orthomolecular medicine. Back in the early 1970s, Pauling popularized the idea that high doses of vitamin C are essential to health.[1] The ensuing controversy about vitamin C requirements continues to this day. However, this situation is about to change, since the dynamic flow model brings together evidence from both sides of the argument, resolving the apparent contradictions.

Shortly after Pauling's death in 1994, the National Institutes of Health (NIH) published a highly acclaimed series of papers, concerning the pharmacokinetics of ascorbate.[2,3,4] These appeared to show that the claims of Pauling and others for megadose supplementation were incorrect. The NIH reported that doses of vitamin C as low as 200 mg per day saturate the body. This saturation claim was highly influential, becoming a cornerstone of the Recommended Dietary Allowance (RDA).[5-11] A purpose of this brief review is to establish definitively that the NIH papers, and hence the justification for the RDA, contain serious errors. Furthermore, when interpreted correctly, the NIH data supports the claims for high daily intakes.[12,13]

Low-Dose Hypothesis

The low-dose hypothesis, which forms the basis for the RDA, is that humans require only a few milligrams (mg) of ascorbate each day. This is in contrast to the majority of other animals, which manufacture their own vitamin C at substantially higher levels. In humans, an intake of less than 10 mg per day will prevent acute sickness and death from the deficiency disease scurvy. Researchers initially assumed that people do not need vitamin C above the scurvy-prevention level. However, objectors to this hypothesis pointed out that such a minimal intake may not be optimal; low doses could result in degenerative diseases, a compromised immune system, and a reduced ability to respond to stress.[14,15]

"Patients ask me, 'How dangerous is vitamin therapy?' I answer them, 'You are going to live a lot longer. Is that a problem for you?'"

—ABRAM HOFFER

The U.S. Institutes of Medicine (IOM), the organization responsible for setting the recommended allowances, used the NIH pharmacokinetic papers to justify their low dose RDA. Their argument was simple: if the body is saturated at an intake of 200 mg per day, there is no point considering a higher dose, as it will just be excreted. The NIH had themselves recommended an RDA, based on their studies of ascorbate pharmacokinetics in blood plasma and white blood cells. The IOM used these results, somewhat arbitrarily, to determine a recommended intake within the range 0–200 mg per day.

Megadose Hypothesis

The megadose hypothesis, popularized by Drs. Linus Pauling and Irwin Stone, suggests that people need 1,000 mg or more of ascorbate per day. The proponents based their ideas largely on evolutionary arguments. Most animals synthesize large amounts of ascorbate internally or, less commonly, obtain equivalent gram-level intakes from their diets. Animals also increase their production of vitamin C when they are diseased. Therefore, researchers proposed that higher doses provide

From the *J Orthomolecular Med* 2005;20(4):237–244.

increased resistance to many, if not all, diseases. These suggestions are consistent with known biology and evolution.

Following Pauling's death, the NIH pharmacokinetic results led to a widespread assumption that the megadose hypothesis was wrong. If body saturation occurs at a daily intake level of 200 mg, the opponents argued, higher doses are unnecessary. They added that there is no point risking the possible side effects of higher doses, if such doses offer no benefit. Perhaps surprisingly, this second objection is logically inconsistent with the first. Saturation implies that higher doses are ineffective because the doses are not absorbed. However, if a high dose offers no benefits because the body does not absorb it, then similarly it should not lead to toxic effects, because it has not been absorbed.

Dual-Phase Excretion

The ascorbate plasma levels corresponding to varying intakes of ascorbate exhibit dual-phase pharmacokinetics. The first phase occurs when blood levels are low: below 70 µM/L. In this phase, the kidney's sodium-dependent vitamin C transporters (SVCT) reabsorb ascorbate, but not its oxidized form, dehydroascorbate,[16,17] When levels are relatively low, the transporters prevent ascorbate being lost in the urine. The second phase occurs when blood levels are high; during this phase, the body excretes ascorbate rapidly, as it does other small, water-soluble, organic molecules.[18]

The plasma half-life of ascorbate is widely reported to be between 8 and 40 days.[11,19] However, this applies only to periods of deficient intake, when the kidney transporters are actively reabsorbing the vitamin to prevent acute scurvy. When intake levels are higher, rapid excretion occurs; during this phase, ascorbate has a half-life of about half an hour. The NIH pharmacokinetic data shows the rapid excretion phase clearly: we calculated this result from their initial plasma-concentration decay slope for intravenous doses. This rate of decay follows the principles of pharmacology, as applied to a molecule with the characteristics of ascorbate.

Blood Plasma Levels

The NIH performed a series of pharmacokinetic experiments purporting to show that, with oral ascorbate, blood plasma is saturated at approximately 70 micromoles per liter (µM/L). This figure, however, is inconsistent with the researchers' own data in the same and later papers. The original papers show graphs in which the plasma level, following oral administration, is much higher than 70 µM/L. Subsequent papers suggest sustained plasma levels of at least 220 µM/L, following oral administration.[20] These higher plasma levels are consistent with other reports in the literature.[49,21,22]

Bioavailability

In order to be used by the body, a dose of ascorbate must be absorbed. The NIH chose bioavailability as their measure of the absorption of oral doses, claiming this was essential to establish an RDA for vitamin C.[2,3] Bioavailability is a relative measure, which compares the oral absorption of a substance to an equal injected dose. If the oral dose results in the same plasma level as an equivalent intravenous dose, then the bioavailability is said to be complete. The NIH stated that the bioavailability of ascorbate is complete at an intake of 200 mg. This means that a dose of 200 mg or less is completely absorbed by the body, whereas a smaller proportion (although a higher absolute amount) of higher doses is absorbed. Unfortunately, the name is misleading:

IN BRIEF

This paper presents a new account of the action of ascorbate in humans: the dynamic flow model. The model is consistent with previous studies and with the known properties of vitamin C. Based on this model, we propose a mechanism by which human physiology can compensate for losing the ability to synthesize vitamin C. The dynamic flow approach links Linus Pauling's megadose suggestions with other reported effects of massive doses for the treatment of disease. The model also refutes the current low dose hypothesis and resulting recommendations for dietary intakes.

many people think bioavailability means the amount available to the tissues, which is wrong.

In considering bioavailability, the NIH ignore the short half-life of vitamin C during the rapid excretion phase. They indicate that bioavailability is complete for a single 200 mg dose then, implicitly, jump to an RDA (i.e., daily dose) of 200 mg. Since blood plasma levels above 70 µM/L have a half-life of approximately half an hour, doses taken several hours apart are independent, as is their bioavailability. Two doses taken 12 hours apart have the same absorption characteristics as each other, which means that splitting a single large dose into several smaller ones, taken a few hours apart, increases the effective bioavailability of the large dose.

The NIH's assertion, that bioavailability is complete at 200 mg, implies that this is a fixed property of ascorbate. However, Dr. Cathcart's bowel tolerance method[23] indicates that individual bioavailability can vary by a factor of at least two orders of magnitude. This widely confirmed variation depends upon the current state of health of the subject. This means that bioavailability is not a static property of ascorbate but is subject to individual differences and varies with the timing of the dose. If, as the NIH and IOM have suggested, bioavailability is fundamental to determining the RDA, then it follows that the appropriate intake will vary widely, both between individuals and also over time for the same person, depending on factors such as state of health and intake patterns. [Editor's note: To read more about Dr. Cathcart's method, see his article "The Method of Determining Proper Doses of Vitamin C for the Treatment of Disease by Titrating to Bowel Tolerance" later in Part One.]

Ascorbate Transporters

Two families of biochemical pumps, SVCT and glucose transporters (GLUT), pump vitamin C into cells. The SVCT pumps are specific to ascorbate,[24] whereas GLUT transporters normally transport glucose but, since dehydroascorbate is structurally similar to glucose, can also transport oxidized ascorbate.[25,26] Their transport rates for glucose and dehydroascorbate are similar, for equal plasma concentrations. However, glucose is normally several orders of magnitude more concentrated, so the role of GLUT transporters in pumping dehydroascorbate, as a mechanism for cellular accumulation of ascorbate, may have been overemphasized. The transporters' role may be to remove dehydroascorbate, which is relatively toxic, from the plasma, so the cells can reduce it back to ascorbate. The electrons used to reduce the dehydroascorbate come from normal metabolism.[27]

An important feature of ascorbate transporters is often overlooked. Cell types in the body have different and characteristic forms of transporters on their surfaces. Even cells with identical transporter types may differ in the quantity and rate of ascorbate accumulation. The absorption and resulting intracellular concentration depend on the quantity, or concentration, of transporter molecules on the cell surface.[13,28,29] This value can change between cells and even within a group of cells; for example, the number of GLUT4 transporters in the cell membrane increases rapidly in response to the hormone insulin.[30]

Red Blood Cells

Red blood cells could provide a model for the uptake of ascorbate by many tissue cells. They are easily sampled cells that might be used to indicate the body's ascorbate requirements for the following reasons. The concentration of ascorbate in red blood cells is similar to that of the surrounding plasma.[31–33] Under physiological conditions, transport of ascorbate across the red blood cell mem-

USING THE BOWEL TOLERANCE METHOD TO DETERMINE YOUR VITAMIN C REQUIREMENT

A person wishing to estimate his or her own requirement needs to determine their bowel tolerance level. To do this, start with a low dose and repeat it each hour until unpleasant bowel effects (gas, distensions, and loose stools) are observed. This level of intake is your bowel tolerance levels and the optimal intake is 50 to 90 percent of this maximum.

brane is relatively slow and internal concentrations (20–60 µM) correspond to plasma levels in unsupplemented individuals.[34–36] Hence, raising the mean plasma concentration will lead to high levels of ascorbate in these cells, while transient changes will have little effect. Erythrocytes (red blood cells) have a high capacity to import dehydroascorbate using GLUT1 and reduce it back to ascorbate.[37–39] Uptake of dehydroascorbate by erythrocytes is a protective mechanism that can lower its concentration in healthy plasma to levels lower than 2 µM/L.[40,41] Once inside the red blood cell, dehydroascorbate is reduced to ascorbate.[36,39,42] Thus, we can suggest uptake of dehydroascorbate by red blood cells is an antioxidant mechanism to prevent damage in many disease states.

White Blood Cells

White blood cells are highly specialized in terms of their redox metabolism,[43] ascorbate transport,[44,45] and biochemistry. White blood cells use oxidants to damage and absorb foreign bodies. Metabolism, ascorbate absorption, and cycling (discussed next) increase greatly when white blood cells are activated.[46] Transporters and related mechanisms in white blood cell membranes allow them to accumulate ascorbate, even when levels are low in the surrounding medium.

White blood cells provide a model for a limited number of cells in the body, for which ascorbate deprivation is critical. Such cells contain transport mechanisms that prevent loss when the rest of the body is deficient. Therefore, they do not provide a model for levels of ascorbate in the body as a whole. Most tissues do not accumulate ascorbate in the same way as white blood cells; if they did, such cells would contain millimolar (mM) levels, giving a total body pool at least 10 times greater than the observed value of 1,000 to 2,000 mg.

Redox Cycling and Tissue Health

Ascorbate and dehydroascorbate are involved in a redox cycle.[47] Ascorbate loses a single electron, forming the ascorbyl radical, which can lose a further electron, forming dehydroascorbate. Ascorbate can also be oxidized to dehydroascorbate in a single step by donating two electrons. Dehydroascorbate may be oxidized by the cellular metabolism or it can be lost from the tissue and excreted in the urine. The ratio of ascorbate to dehydroascorbate, and by implication that of other related antioxidants, such as the reduced glutathione-oxidized glutathione couple, provides a measure of the redox environment of a tissue. Since oxidation appears to be a factor in many disease processes, this ratio is lower in damaged tissue. Restoring the ratio, by supplying additional ascorbate, reverses the oxidized state of the tissue and decreases free radical damage.[48]

Ascorbate Synthesis

Ascorbate is abundant throughout the plant and animal kingdoms, where its main function appears to be as an electron donor. Humans and a few other animals do not synthesize ascorbate. This loss may be the largest, single, biochemical difference between these and other animal groups. It is generally stated that humans cannot manufacture ascorbate because they have lost the enzyme gulonolactone oxidase, which is used in the synthetic pathway from glucose to ascorbate. The evidence for such a strong statement is inadequate.[49] It is possible that some humans can manufacture ascorbate, at a low level. Such low-level manufacture, by specific individuals, could explain some of the variation in the incidence of scurvy under deprivation conditions.

Dynamic Flow

The dynamic flow model proposes restoring human physiology to approximate that of animals that synthesize their own vitamin C. This can be achieved by consuming excess ascorbate, over and above the amount normally absorbed. This intake is spread throughout the day, so a consistent supply is achieved. Some of the excess ascorbate is absorbed into the blood plasma, while the rest remains in the gut. As in animals that synthesize the molecule, some ascorbate is lost through the kidneys. However, there is a steady flow of antioxidant electrons through the body, with a reserve available to combat stress or free radical damage.

The absorption from the gut of a single oral dose is not instantaneous, but occurs over a period of several hours. As the ascorbate is absorbed, it is transported to other body compartments, such as lymph, and into cells. However, this transportation is limited by the short plasma half-life. A single, oral dose increases plasma levels for a maximum of two to three hours following intake, and then decays back towards baseline levels. The average plasma level, and thus the intake into erythrocytes and typical cells, remains low after single daily doses.

However, repeated doses, at an interval of less than five half-lives, produce a high, steady-state value in blood plasma. This also leads to a large increase in erythrocyte and other typical cell ascorbate levels. Ascorbate levels in white blood cells and other redox sensitive tissues is not greatly increased, because these cell types accumulate ascorbate preferentially, at low external concentrations. When dynamic flow has been achieved, the mean and minimum plasma levels are relatively high: consistent levels of 220 μM can be attained. The body pool is also increased, because of increased absorption by tissues whose levels are related to those in the surrounding microenvironment. More ascorbate is available when required and the ratio of ascorbate to dehydroascorbate is high. Hence, the tissues are maintained in a reduced state, through ascorbate's interaction with other antioxidants, such as the tocopherols, tocotrienols, and glutathione.

"New nutrition research exposes the weakness of current medical doctrine. Nature is not dumb." —ABRAM HOFFER

If the person encounters a viral infection or other free radical stress, high levels of ascorbate are immediately available, providing electrons to neutralize the free radicals and quench the disease process. Additional ascorbate for this process is recruited by absorption from the intestines, while dehydroascorbate is excreted preferentially by the kidney.

During Illness

Under normal conditions, such as mild stress, dynamic flow is predicted to maintain a reducing state in the body, reducing the incidence of disease. However, diseased tissues may generate large numbers of free radicals, in which case the maximum absorption from the gut may increase greatly. Under such conditions, dynamic flow cannot be maintained by normal intakes. The intake required to sustain plasma levels during illness may increase to 200,000 mg, or more. During illness, achieving dynamic flow corresponds to the bowel tolerance technique, described earlier. For severe illnesses, intravenous doses may be required, to maintain a reducing state in the damaged tissue.

Cancer

Cancer is an exception to the role of ascorbate as an antioxidant. Depending on the conditions, ascorbate can act as a pro-oxidant or reducing agent; this feature is common to many organic antioxidants. In normal tissues, ascorbate acts as an antioxidant. However, in the presence of free iron, ascorbate can participate in a Fenton reaction and become an oxidant, generating free radicals that lead to cellular damage. Cancer cells can absorb high levels of ascorbate, and their disturbed metabolism produces redox cycling and free radical production.[50] High levels of ascorbate kill cancer cells by apoptosis, while leaving normal cells undamaged. In cancer, and other infected or damaged cells, ascorbate's beneficial effects may involve oxidation.

Research Implications

The research implications of the dynamic flow model are profound. Many studies have used low doses of ascorbate, assuming wrongly that, because of the low-dose hypothesis or tissue saturation, the results could be extrapolated to higher intakes. Since doses many times higher than 200 mg can be absorbed and utilized by the body, such extrapolation is unjustified. Clearly, an intake of 5,000 mg per day could have quite different effects to an intake of 100 mg. To take a specific example, it is not valid to conclude that vitamin C has no effect on heart disease, based on inconclusive or even negative results with low doses.

The short half-life presents immediate and wide-ranging implications for research into this vitamin. Most studies have used single, daily doses of vitamin C or, occasionally, twice daily doses. Occasional studies have used low-dose, slow-release formulations. These studies all require urgent re-evaluation. A single dose will produce a transient increase in blood plasma levels, leaving the mean and minimum concentrations largely unchanged. Such doses will not load tissues, such as red blood cells, or increase the body pool substantially. A large, single, daily dose of ascorbate will therefore produce a minimal biological effect.

To be explicit, consider Linus Pauling's suggestion for prevention of the common cold. It is occasionally reported that this suggestion has been refuted.[51,52] However, these once or twice daily megadose supplementation studies would not be expected to show more than a minimal biological effect, when compared with dynamic flow. In light of the dynamic flow model, the available results are consistent with Pauling's proposal. Similar statements can be made for a multitude of other conditions, such as atherosclerosis and arthritis.

CONCLUSION

The dynamic flow model provides a new paradigm that is consistent with the known pharmacokinetics of ascorbate. It is also consistent with claims for the health benefits of high doses.

Current knowledge of ascorbate pharmacokinetics and tissue biology challenges the low-dose hypothesis. In particular, it is not valid to model human intakes on the specialized properties of white blood cells. Red blood cells are also specialized, but have characteristics closer to those of typical body tissues. Such body tissues gain their supply of ascorbate through the blood supply: mean and minimum blood plasma values are thus of central importance to the availability of ascorbate. Previously, the NIH data on ascorbate pharmacokinetics have been misinterpreted, resulting in inappropriate recommended intakes.

Considering that the scientific data is consistent with claims for large health benefits with higher doses, the result of adhering to the low-dose hypothesis may be unnecessarily high rates of illness and premature death.

REFERENCES

1. Pauling L. *Vitamin C and the Common Cold.* New York: W.H. Freeman & Co, 1970.

2. Levine M, Conry-Cantilena C, Wang Y, et al. Vitamin C pharmacokinetics in healthy volunteers: evidence for a recommended dietary allowance. *Proc Natl Acad Sci USA* 1996;93: 3704–3709.

3. Levine M, Wang Y, Padayatty SJ, et al. A new recommended dietary allowance of vitamin C for healthy young women. *Proc Natl Acad Sci USA* 2001;98(17): 842–9846.

4. Levine M, Rumsey SC, Daruwala R, et al. Criteria and recommendations for vitamin C intake, *JAMA*, 1999; 281: 1415–1423.

5. Expert Group on Vitamins and Minerals. UK government update paper EVM/99/21/P, 1999.

6. Expert Group on Vitamins and Minerals. Revised review of vitamin C. UK government publication, EVM/99/21; 2002.

7. Expert Group on Vitamins and Minerals. Safe upper limits for vitamins and minerals. UK government publication, 2003.

8. Expert Group on Vitamins and Minerals. Review of vitamin C, UK Government publication, 2003.

9. Committee on Medical Aspects of Food Policy. Dietary reference values for food energy and nutrients for the united kingdom: report on health and social subjects. No. 41; HMSO, London, 1991.

10. Food and Nutrition Board (RDA Committee). *Recommended Dietary Allowances* (Dietary Reference Intakes). 10th ed. Washington: National Academies Press, 1992.

11. Food and Nutrition Board (RDA Committee). *Dietary Reference Intakes for Vitamin C, Selenium and Carotenoids.* Washington: National Academies Press, 2001.

12. Hickey S, Roberts H. *Ascorbate: The Science of Vitamin C.* Raleigh, NC: Lulu Press, 2004.

13. Hickey S, Roberts H. *Ridiculous Dietary Allowance.* Raleigh, NC: Lulu Press, 2004.

14. Stone I. *The Healing Factor: Vitamin C Against Disease.* New York: Putnam, 1974.

15. Pauling L. *How to Live Longer and Feel Better.* New York: Avon Books, 1986.

16. Wang Y, Mackenzie C, Tsukaguchi H, et al. Human vitamin C (L-ascorbic acid) transporter SVCT1. *Biochem Biophys Res Commun* 2000;267(2):488–494.

17. Takanaga H, Mackenzie B, Hediger MA. Sodium-dependent ascorbic acid transporter family SLC23. *Euro J Physiol* 2004;447(5):677–682.

18. Hardman JG, Limbird LE, Gilman AG. *The Pharmacological Basis of Therapeutics.* 10th ed. New York: McGraw-Hill Professional, 2005.

19. Kallner A, Hartmann D, Hornig D. Steady-state turnover and body pool of ascorbic acid in man. *Am J Clin Nutr* 1979;32: 530–539.

20. Padayatty SJ, Sun H, Wang Y, et al. Vitamin C pharmacokinetics: implications for oral and intravenous use. *Ann Intern Med* 2004;140:533–537.

21. Benke KK. Modelling ascorbic acid level in plasma and its dependence on absorbed dose. *Journal of the Australasian Coll Nutr Environ Med* 1999;18(1):11–12.

22. Ely J. Ascorbic acid and some other modern analogs of the germ theory. *J Orthomolecular Med* 1999;14(3):143–156.

23. Cathcart RF. Vitamin C: titrating to bowel tolerance, anascoremia, and acute induced scurvy, *Med Hypoth* 1981;7:1359–1376.

24. Liang WJ, Johnson D, Jarvis SM. Vitamin C transport systems of mammalian cells. *Mol Membr Biol* 2001;18(1):87–95.

25. Mueckler M. Facilitative glucose transporters. *Eur J Biochem* 1994;219:713–725.

26. Olson AL, Pessin JE. Structure, function and regulation of the mammalian facilitative glucose transporter gene family. *Ann Rev Nutr* 1996;16:235–256.

27. Brown S, Georgatos M, Reifel C, et al. Recycling Processes of cellular ascorbate generate oxidative stress in pancreatic tissues in in vitro system. *Endocrine* 2002;18(1):91–96.

28. Rumsey SC, Daruwala R, Al-Hasani H, et al. Dehydroascorbic acid transport by GLUT4 in *Xenopus oocytes* and isolated rat adipocytes. *J Biol Chem* 2000;275:28246–28253.

29. Rumsey SC, Kwon O, Xu GW, et al. Glucose transporter isoforms GLUT1 and GLUT3 transport dehydroascorbic acid. *J Biol Chem* 1997;272:18982–18989.

30. Kodaman PH, Behrman HR. Hormone-regulated and glucose-sensitive transport of dehydroascorbic acid in immature rat granulosa cells. *Endocrinol* 1999;140:3659–3665.

31. Hornig D, Weber F, Wiss O. Uptake and release of 1-14C ascorbic acid and 1-14Cdehydroascorbic acid by erythrocytes of guinea pigs. *Clin Chim Acta* 1971;31:25–35.

32. Evans RM, Currie L, Campbell A. The distribution of ascorbic acid between various cellular components of blood, in normal individuals, and its relation to the plasma concentration. *Br J Nutr* 1982;47:473–482.

33. Mendiratta S, Qu ZC, May JM. Erythrocyte ascorbate recycling: antioxidant effects in blood. *Free Radic Biol Med* 1998;24(5):789–797.

34. Hughes RE, Maton SC. The passage of vitamin C across the erythrocyte membrane. *Brit J Haematol* 1968;14:247–53.

35. Wagner ES, White W, Jennings M, et al. The entrapment of 14C ascorbic acid in human erythrocytes. *Biochim Biophys Acta* 1987;902:133–136.

36. Okamura M. Uptake of L-ascorbic acid and L-dehydroascorbic acid by human erythrocytes and HeLa cells. *J Nutr Sci Vitaminol* 1979;25:269–279.

37. May JM. Ascorbate function and metabolism in the human erythrocyte. *Frontiers in Bioscience* 1998;3:1–10.

38. Rose RC. Transport of ascorbic acid and other water-soluble vitamins. *Biochim Biophys Acta* 1988; 947:335–366.

39. Bianchi J, Rose RC. Glucose-independent transport of dehydroascorbic acid in human erythrocytes. *Proc Soc Exp Biol Med* 1986;181:333–337.

40. Okamura M. An improved method for determination of L-ascorbic acid and L-dehydroascorbic acid in blood plasma. *Clin Chim Acta* 1980;103:259–268.

41. Dhariwal KR, Hartzell WO, Levine M. Ascorbic acid and dehydroascorbic acid measurements in human plasma and serum. *Am J Clin Nutr* 1991;54:712–716.

42. Vera JC, Rivas CI, Fischbarg J, et al. Mammalian facilitative hexose transporters mediate the transport of dehydroascorbic acid. *Nature* 1993;364:79–82.

43. Wang Y, Russo TA, Kwon O, et al. Ascorbate recycling in human neutrophils: induction by bacteria. *Proc Natl Acad Sci USA* 1997;94(25):13816–13819.

44. Washko P, Yang Y, Levine M. Ascorbic acid recycling in human neutrophils. *J Biol Chem* 1993; 268(21):15531–15535.

45. Washko P, Rotrosen D, Levine M. Ascorbic acid transport and accumulation in human neutrophils. *J Biol Chem* 1989;264(32):18996–19002.

46. Halliwell B, Gutteridge JMC. *Free Radicals in Biology and Medicine.* 3rd ed. Oxford, England: Oxford University Press, 1999.

47. Cathcart RF. A unique function for ascorbate. *Med Hypoth* 1991;35:32–37.

48. Cathcart RF. Vitamin C: the non-toxic, non-rate limited, antioxidant free-radical scavenger. *Med Hypoth* 1985;18:61–77.

49. Lewin S. *Vitamin C: Its Molecular Biology and Medical Potential.* Burlington, MA: Academic Press, 1976.

50. Gonzalez MJ, Miranda-Massari JR, Mora EM, et al. Orthomolecular oncology: a mechanistic view of intravenous ascorbate's chemotherapeutic activity. *PR Health Sci J* 2002; 21(1):39–41.

51. Hemila H. Vitamin C supplementation and the common cold: was Linus Pauling right or wrong? *Int J Vitam Nutr Res* 1997;67(5):329–335.

52. Douglas RM, Chalker EB, Treacy B. Vitamin C for preventing and treating the common cold (Cochrane Review). *CochranDatabase of Systematic Reviews* 2004;4:CD000980.

THE THREE FACES OF VITAMIN C
by Robert F. Cathcart, MD

Clinical experience prescribing doses of ascorbic acid up to 200,000 milligrams (mg) or more per 24 hours to over 20,000 patients during the past 23-year period has revealed its clinical usefulness in all diseases involving oxidation damage from free radicals. The controversy continues over the value of vitamin C mainly because inadequate doses are used for most free-radical scavenging purposes. Paradoxically, the non-controversial use of minute doses of vitamin C in the prevention and treatment of scurvy has set the minds of many against more creative uses.

Vitamin C has differing benefits in increasing dose ranges. Its usefulness is in three such distinct realms that I will describe them as the three faces of vitamin C.

• **Face 1.** Vitamin C to prevent scurvy in dosages up to 65 mg per day.

• **Face 2.** Vitamin C to prevent acute induced scurvy[1,2] and to augment vitamin C functions at 1,000 to 20,000 mg per day.

• **Face 3.** Vitamin C to provide reducing equivalents in dosages from 30,000 to 200,000 mg per day.[3]

One might criticize the wisdom of my use of these massive doses but Frederick Klenner, MD, had previously used large doses intravenously.[4,5,6,7] The works of Irwin Stone, PhD,[8,9,10] Linus Pauling, PhD,[11,12,13] and Archie Kalokerinos, MD,[14] have supported many of my observations. In all published studies yielding negative or equivocal results, inadequate doses were used. In some studies, doses barely bordering on adequate, tease the investigator with statistically significant but not very impressive beneficial results.

My early discovery was that the bowel tolerance to ascorbic acid of a person with a healthy gastrointestinal tract was somewhat proportional to the toxicity of their disease.[15] Bowel tolerance doses are the amounts of ascorbic acid tolerated orally that almost, but not quite, cause a marked loosening of stools. A patient who could tolerate orally 10,000–15,000 mg of ascorbic acid per 24 hours when well might be able to tolerate 30,000–60,000 mg per 24 hours if he had a mild cold, 100,000 mg with a severe cold, 150,000 mg with influenza, and 200,000 mg or more per 24 hours with mononucleosis or viral pneumonia.[1,2] Marked clinical benefits in these conditions occur only at the bowel tolerance or higher levels. I named the process whereby the patient determined the proper dose as titrating to bowel tolerance. These increases in bowel tolerance in the vast majority of patients normally tolerant to ascorbic acid (perhaps 80 percent of patients) are invariable. The marked clinical benefits are noted only when a threshold dose, usually close to the bowel tolerance dose, is consumed. I call this benefit the "ascorbate effect."

Most patients are started at first with hourly doses of ascorbic acid powder dissolved in small amounts of water. Later, after the patient has learned to accurately estimate the dose necessary to achieve the ascorbate effect, comparable doses of ascorbic acid tablets or capsules are also used. Where patients are intolerant to adequate amounts of ascorbic acid orally and the severity of the disease warrants it, intravenous sodium ascorbate is used. Failures are related to individual difficulties in taking the proper adequate doses. In patients who tolerate adequate doses, the results are almost invariably as described. I now have had 23 years to gather clinical experience and to reflect on this phenomenon.[16–19]

I want to emphasize the importance of this increasing bowel tolerance with increasing toxicities of diseases. The sensation of detoxification one experiences at these doses is unmistakable. The effect is so reliable and dramatic in the tolerant patient as to make obvious the fact that something very important, which has not been widely appreciated before, is going on.

From the *J Orthomolecular Med* 1993;7(4):197–200.

The First Face

Vitamin C probably always functions by being an electron donor. At the lowest dose level (up to 65 mg per day), it is necessary as a vitamin to prevent scurvy. It is essential for certain metabolic functions that are well described and mostly non-controversial.

The Second Face

At the middle dose level, vitamin C is still used as a vitamin but larger doses are necessary to maintain its basic vitamin C functions because the vitamin is destroyed rapidly in diseased or injured tissues where there is an overabundance of free radicals. When an ascorbate molecule gives up two reducing equivalents (available electrons) to neutralize free radicals, it becomes dehydroascorbate (DHA). If the DHA (a relatively unstable form of ascorbate) is not rapidly re-reduced by reducing equivalents from the mitochondria (site of energy production within the cell), the DHA is irreversibly lost. I describe the resulting state of deficiency, if the vitamin C is not replaced, as acute induced scurvy.[12] There is ample evidence of this depletion of vitamin C by stress and disease as recently reviewed in the literature.[20] Additionally, the recent extensive research on vitamin C has concerned itself with certain functions that may be augmented by higher than minimal doses of vitamin C.[20] Strangely, any usefulness of these larger than minimal doses of vitamin C remain mostly neglected by clinicians. This level is from about 1,000 to 20,000 mg a day. Benefits vary from person to person.

At this second level, as in studies reviewed by Pauling[11] and more recently by Harri Hemilä, MD, PhD,[20] there may be expected a slight decrease in the incidence of colds but a more significant reduction in the complications and the duration of colds. Personally, I am impressed by the number of patients (but certainly not all) who tell me that they have not had a cold for years since reading Pauling's book *Vitamin C and the Common Cold and the Flu* (1976) and taking vitamin C. Patients with chronic infections frequently have their infections cured for the first time. Antibiotics work synergistically with these doses. A surprising number of elderly people benefit from doses of this magnitude and may indeed have what Irwin Stone described as chronic subclinical scurvy.

The Third Face

The highest dose level is virtually undiscussed in the literature but is the most interesting. These doses range usually from 30,000 to 200,000 mg or more per 24 hours. The most important concept to understand is that while incidentally at these dose levels the vitamin C performs all its level one and two functions, yet it is mostly thrown away for the reducing equivalents it carries.[3] With these dosages, it is possible to saturate the body with reducing equivalents. Inflammations mediated by free radicals can be eliminated or markedly reduced. In many instances patients with allergies or autoimmune diseases have their humoral immunity (antibody-mediated) controlled, while their cellular immunity is augmented.[19] To the extent that free radicals are either

---

IN BRIEF

Bowel tolerance, the amount of ascorbic acid tolerated orally without producing diarrhea, increases with the toxicity of diseases. Bowel tolerance to ascorbic acid with a disease such as mononucleosis may reach 200,000 milligrams (mg) or more per 24 hours. A marked clinical amelioration or cure is achieved in many disease processes when threshold doses near bowel tolerance are given. In a very important sense, it is the reducing equivalents (available electrons) carried by free-radical scavengers that quench free radicals, not the free-radical scavengers themselves. Ascorbic acid can be dramatically useful in quenching free radicals because it is usually tolerated in amounts needed to provide the reducing equivalents necessary to quench almost all the free radicals generated by severe disease processes. Vitamin C functions are incidental at these dose levels; the benefit is from the reducing equivalents carried. To the extent that free radicals are either essential to the perpetuation of a disease or just part of the cause of symptoms, the disease will be cured or just ameliorated. These effects are even more dramatic with intravenous sodium ascorbate.

essential to the perpetuation of a disease or just part of the cause of symptoms, the disease will be cured or just ameliorated.

The list of diseases involving free radicals continues to grow. Infections, cardiovascular diseases, cancer, trauma, burns both thermal and radiation, surgeries, allergies, autoimmune diseases, and aging are now included. It is more difficult to think of a disease that does not involve free radicals. Progressive nutritionists routinely give vitamin C, vitamin E, beta-carotene, selenium, N-acetyl cysteine, and other antioxidant compounds to counter free radicals. I certainly agree with this practice. However, there is one important concept neglected that results in these nutrients not being as effective as described.

In the spirit that if you throw a bucket of water on a fire, it is the water that puts the fire out, not the bucket; it is the reducing equivalents carried by the free-radical scavengers that quench the free radicals, not the free-radical scavenger itself.

Dietary free-radical scavengers carry in on ingestion only a small percentage of the total reducing equivalents carried by those scavengers during their lifetime in the body. After their first pass neutralizing free radicals, the free-radical scavenger must be recharged with reducing equivalents made available in the mitochondria.

The problem in inflamed tissues or in patients with severe illnesses is not so much that all the free-radical scavengers have been lost (although they may be lost), but that the mitochondria cannot furnish the reducing equivalents fast enough to re-reduce adequate amounts of free-radical scavengers. The dynamic nature of this process must be emphasized. When free radicals injure cells, particularly their mitochondria, more free radicals are formed and some injure adjacent cells. An inflammatory cascade results. Without enough reducing equivalents being provided by glycolysis in the mitochondria and the continuing re-reduction of free-radical scavengers, the inflammatory cascade cannot be properly contained.

Early in this study, a 23-year-old, 98-pound librarian with severe mononucleosis claimed to have taken 2 heaping tablespoons every two hours, consuming a full pound of ascorbic in two

days without it producing diarrhea. She felt mostly well in three to four days, although she had to continue about 20,000–30,000 mg a day for about two months. Subsequently, all my young mononucleosis patients with excellent gastrointestinal tracts have responded similarly and have had equivalent increases in bowel tolerance during the acute state of the disease. What is important here is the magnitude of this increased bowel tolerance.

"No one dies from vitamins."
—ABRAM HOFFER

I believe that the loose stools caused by excessive doses of ascorbic acid orally ingested are due to a resulting hypertonicity of ascorbate in the rectum. Water is attracted into the rectum by the increased osmotic pressure and results in a loosening of the stools. With toxic illnesses, the ascorbate is destroyed rapidly in the involved tissues and this results in a rapid absorption of ascorbate from the gut. Of the ascorbate, what does not reach the rectum does not cause diarrhea. Intravenous sodium ascorbate does not cause diarrhea. With hypertonicity of the ascorbate both in the blood and in the rectum, the osmotic pressure of the ascorbate is more equal on both sides of the bowel wall so no diarrhea results. If the diarrhea was caused by other metabolic processes, diarrhea would be caused by intravenous ascorbate.

It should be noted that in some cases of pathological diarrhea, ascorbic acid *stops* the diarrhea. Presumably in these cases some of the increased destruction of ascorbate is from free radicals in the bowel. However, in most toxic systemic diseases, there is no reason to believe that the destruction of the additional ascorbate tolerated occurs directly in the bowel, so it is a safe hypothesis that this increased destruction occurs in the interior of the body. The increased tolerance to ascorbic acid orally provides an interesting and somewhat useful measure of the toxicity of a disease. Probably it is somewhat a measure of the free radicals involved in a disease.

I describe a cold that at its maximum makes it possible for a patient to just tolerate 100 grams (100,000 mg) of ascorbic acid orally per 24 hours without diarrhea, as a "100-gram cold." Patients, appearing to be well, who have a tolerance over 20–25 grams (20,000–25,000 mg) per 24 hours probably have some subclinical condition that is being hidden by their own free-radical scavenging system. Patients with chronic infections (and a normally strong stomach) can ingest enormous amounts of ascorbic acid. One of my chronic fatigue patients is functional only because of his ingestion of 65 pounds of ascorbic acid in the past 12 months. In 22 years, I, personally, have ingested approximately 361 kilos (about 797 lbs, 4.3 times my body weight) of ascorbic acid because of chronic allergies and perhaps chronic Epstein-Barr virus.

Considering the reducing equivalents carried by such amounts of ascorbic acid, one can only guess at the turnover rate of the non-enzymatic free-radical scavengers in a patient acutely ill with a 200-gram (200,000-mg) mononucleosis. However, one gains the impression that all the non-enzymatic free-radical scavengers would have to be re-reduced many times a day.

An Analogy

Suppose you owned a farm and on one end of the property there was a barn and on the other end of the property there was a water well. One day the barn catches fire and neighbors come with buckets to set up a bucket brigade between the water well and the barn and are putting out the fire when the well goes dry. My use of ascorbate is like thousands of neighbors coming from miles around, each with a bucketful of their own water, throwing their own water on your fire once, and then leaving.

■ CONCLUSION

Because of the invariable (in patients tolerant to ascorbic acid) increasing bowel tolerance to ascorbic acid in patients roughly in proportion to the toxicity of their disease, there has to be something happening to ascorbate in the sick patient other than its being used as vitamin C in the classic sense. The amelioration or sometimes cure of different diseases appears related to the importance of free radicals in the perpetuation of the particular disease.

The sudden marked benefit in many disease processes, which is achieved at dosages near to the bowel tolerance level, suggests that a reducing redox potential is forced into the affected tissues only at those dose levels. This ascorbate effect only at the high-dose levels is also suggestive that something other than classic functions of vitamin C is involved. This ascorbate effect is more compatible with principles of redox chemistry.

Only a small percentage of the total reducing equivalents donated by non-enzymatic free-radical scavengers to neutralize free radicals come into the body through the ingested nutritional free-radical scavengers. Ascorbate is unique in that the body can tolerate doses adequate to supply the necessary reducing equivalents to quench the free radicals generated by severely toxic disease processes. The vitamin C is thrown away for the reducing equivalents it carries. Only in this way can the large amounts of free radicals generated by the most toxic disease processes be rapidly quenched.

REFERENCES

1. Cathcart RF. The method of determining proper doses of vitamin C for the treatment of disease by titrating to bowel tolerance. *J Orthomolecular Psych* 1981;10:125–32.

2. Cathcart RF. Vitamin C: titrating to bowel tolerance, anascorbemia, and acute induced scurvy. *Med Hypotheses* 1981;7:1359–1376.

3. Cathcart RF. A unique function for ascorbate. *Med Hypotheses* 1991;35:32–37.

4. Klenner FR. Virus pneumonia and its treatment with vitamin C. *J South Med and Surg* 1948;110:60–63.

5. Klenner FR. The treatment of poliomyelitis and other virus diseases with vitamin C. *J South Med and Surg* 1949;111:210–214.

6. Klenner FR. Observations on the dose and administration of ascorbic acid when employed beyond the range of a vitamin in human pathology. *J App Nutr* 1971;23:61–88.

7. Klenner FR. Significance of high daily intake of ascorbic acid in preventive medicine. *J Int Acad Prev Med* 1974;1:45–49.

8. Stone I. Studies of a mammalian enzyme system for producing evolutionary evidence on man. *Am J Phys Anthro* 1965;23:83–86.

9. Stone I. Hypoascorbemia: the genetic disease causing the human requirement for exogenous ascorbic acid. *Perspect Biol Med* l966;10:133–134.

10. Stone I. *The Healing Factor: Vitamin C Against Disease.* New York: Grosset & Dunlap, 1972.

11. Pauling L. *Vitamin C and the Common Cold.* San Francisco: W.H. Freeman & Co, 1970.

12. Pauling L. *Vitamin C, the Common Cold and the Flu.* San Francisco: W.H. Freeman & Co, 1976.

13. Pauling L. *How to Live Longer and Feel Better.* New York: W.H. Freeman & Co, 1986.

14. Kalokerinos A. *Every Second Child.* New Canaan, CT: Keats Publishing,, 1981.

15. Cathcart RF. Clinical trial of vitamin C. Letter to the Editor. *Medical Tribune,* June 25, 1975.

16. Cathcart RF. Vitamin C in the treatment of acquired immune deficiency syndrome (AIDS). *Med Hypothesis* 1984;14(4):423–433.

17. Cathcart RF. Vitamin C: the non-toxic, non-rate-limited, antioxidant free-radical scavenger. *Med Hypothesis* 1985;18:61–77.

18. Cathcart RF. HIV infection and glutathione. Letter. *Lancet* 1990;335(8683):235.

19. Cathcart RF. The vitamin C treatment of allergy and the normally unprimed state of antibodies. *Med Hypothesis* 1986;21(3):307–321.

20. Hemilä H. Vitamin C and the common cold. *Br J Nutr* 1992;67:3–16.

THE "EXPENSIVE URINE" MYTH

by Andrew W. Saul, PhD

Ever heard this one before? "Your body doesn't absorb extra vitamins. All you get from taking vitamin supplements is expensive urine." Sure you have. And you still will, at websites such as www.dietitian.com and www.americanchronicle.com/articles/67769. Even the British Broadcasting Company (BBC) has reported it (http://news.bbc.co.uk/1/hi/health/109881.stm). Some people will tell you that any vitamin consumption higher than the lowly RDA is simply a "waste of money."

"Expensive urine." It is an old saw, and one terrific sound byte. Too bad it is also false.

Vitamin C Overflow

Urine is what is left over after your kidneys purify your blood. If your urine contains, say, extra vitamin C, that vitamin C was in your blood. If the vitamin was in your blood, you absorbed it just fine. It is the absence of water-soluble vitamins in urine that indicates vitamin deficiency. If your body excretes vitamins in your urine that is a sign that you are well nourished and have nutrients to spare. That is good.

Here's another way to think of it: Standing at the base of the Hoover Dam looking up, you cannot tell how much water is behind it. However, by observing the overflow spillway, you can tell. If the spillway is dry and dusty, full of tumbleweeds and foxes are making their dens, there has been a drought for some time, and the water level in the dam must be low. If water is pouring down the spillway, the dam must be full. "Waste" indicates fullness, just as an overflowing cup is unmistakably a full cup. Urine spillage of vitamins indicates nutritional adequacy. A lack of water-soluble vitamins in the urine indicates inadequacy.

"Expensive urine," writes veteran nutritional reporter Jack Challem, is "a bizarre argument because a $50 restaurant meal and a bottle of fine wine also lead to expensive urine, but no one seems to be complaining about those things. Numerous studies have shown, however, that vitamin supplements do increase people's blood levels of those nutrients."[1]

Former faculty member at the University of Auckland Michael Colgan, PhD, measured how much vitamin C is actually used with increasing daily doses. He found that "only a quarter of our subjects reached their vitamin C maximum at 1,500 milligrams (mg) a day. More than half required over 2,500 mg a day to reach a level where their bodies could use no more. Four subjects did not reach their maximum at 5,000 mg." Indeed, says one commentator, "Increasing vitamin C intake from 50 to 500 mg tends to double serum vitamin C levels. Increasing intake to 5,000 mg a day will double serum levels again."[2]

Time for a Second Opinion?

Thomas Levy, MD, JD, a board-certified cardiologist, says, "There's a popular medical view that taking vitamin C just makes expensive urine. Some of it is lost in urine, but the more you consume, the more stays in your body."[3]

William Kaufman, MD, a physician with a PhD in nutritional biochemistry as well, wrote: "Those who believe that you can get all the nourishment including vitamins and minerals you need to sustain optimal health throughout life from food alone can be very smug. They have the equivalent of an orthodox religious belief: "food is everything." They don't have to concern themselves with the fact that the nutritional value of foods their patient eats may be greatly inferior to the listed nutritional values given in food tables . . . The two-liner 'We get all the vitamins we need in our diets. Taking supplements only gives you an expensive urine' completely overlooks the benefits vitamin supplements can produce in our bodies before being excreted in our urine."[4]

Expensive Breath

We all know that we breathe in oxygen and breathe out carbon dioxide. We also breathe out oxygen, and quite a lot of it, too. Inhaled air is about 21 percent oxygen. We typically consume only about a quarter of that. So exhaled breath is approximately 15 percent oxygen.[5] Exhaled breath has enough oxygen for CPR to save lives. That also must mean that scuba divers have "expensive breath." For that matter, oxygen-tent patients from preemies to geriatric patients, and those receiving surgical anesthesia all receive far more oxygen than their bodies can actually use. We do not consider that a waste; we consider that a good idea. Abundance is not a bad thing.

Expensive "Drug Urine"

"When it comes to really expensive urine," says one editorial, "doctors fail to look at the cost of all those pharmaceuticals and chemotherapy drugs they're shoving down the throats of patients. Those drugs are excreted through the urine, too, and when you add up the cost of those, just the financial cost, not even counting the cost in devastat-ing side effects, they far outweigh the cost of eating healthy foods and taking supporting supplements."[6]

Benefits of Excess Vitamin C

Dr. Kaufmann adds: "During the early part of World War II, GIs treated with penicillin had to save all their urine so that the penicillin which had been excreted in their urine could be recovered and then used to treat other GIs with life-threatening wound infections. If one only considered the penicillin that was excreted in the urine and not the benefits that the GI had in having his infection cured by penicillin, one could sneer that penicillin's only function was to give the GI expensive urine. If one considered only the function of penicillin in the GI's body, one would have to marvel at the miracle of its curing a potentially lethal infection."[4]

Good nutrition saves lives. The therapeutic use of vitamin supplements, to both treat and prevent serious diseases, has tens of thousands of scientific references to support it.[7] Can all of those researchers and physicians be dumber than the reporter you may have just have heard intone that "vitamins just give you expensive urine"?

So many of us modern-day people are deficit eaters, attempting to obtain our vitamins from a selection of nutritionally weak foods. Foods alone cannot meet our vitamin needs for optimum health. Vitamin supplements are the solution, not the problem. Good health is not about the vitamins you excrete; it's about the vitamins you retain.

REFERENCES

1. Challem J. *The Nutrition Reporter*, 1996.

2. http://annieappleseedproject.stores.yahoo.net/expensive urine.html.

3. Levy T. *Vitamin C, Infectious Diseases & Toxins: Curing the Incurable*. Henderson, NV: Livon Books, 2002.

4. Kaufman W. *J Orthomolecular Med* 2007;22(2):83–89.

5. Measurement of gas concentration in exhaled breath. *Patent Storm*. Available at www.patentstorm.us/patents/5069220.html.

6. Adams M. *Natural News*. Available at www.naturalnews.com /021393.html.

7. Many full-text nutrition therapy papers are posted for free access at http://orthomolecular.org/library/jom; 17 extensive bibliographies of nutrition research are posted at www.doctory-ourself.com.

Excerpted from the *Orthomolecular Medicine News Service*, November 10, 2008.

THE METHOD OF DETERMINING PROPER DOSES OF VITAMIN C FOR THE TREATMENT OF DISEASE BY TITRATING TO BOWEL TOLERANCE
by Robert F. Cathcart, MD

My experience in utilizing vitamin C in large doses has extended over a nine-year period and has involved over 9,000 patients.[4–7] Much of the original work with large amounts of vitamin C was done by Fred R. Klenner of Riedsville, North Carolina.[11–14] Klenner found that viral diseases could be detoxified and subsequently cured by intravenous sodium ascorbate in amounts up to 200,000 milligrams (mg) per 24 hours. Irwin Stone pointed out the potential of vitamin C in the treatment of many diseases, the inability of humans to synthesize ascorbate and the resultant condition hypoascorbemia.[18–19] Linus Pauling reviewed the literature on vitamin C and led the crusade to make known its medical uses to the public and the medical profession.[16–17] Ewan Cameron, in association with Pauling, has shown the usefulness of ascorbic acid in the treatment of cancer.[2–3]

The purpose of this paper is to describe a method that maximizes the effectiveness of ascorbic acid (vitamin C) taken orally for various diseases and stress processes. Much of the controversy about ascorbic acid has been due to studies utilizing totally inadequate doses of vitamin C. It seems incredible to the growing number of physicians familiar with the proper doses of ascorbic acid that recent papers would describe studies utilizing only up to 4,000 mg per 24 hours. Also, the hypothesis that not only do humans suffer from chronic hypoascorbemia, but that stress and disease can induce localized and systemic aascorbemia (a type of scurvy) will be presented.

Bowel Tolerance Method

In 1970, I discovered that the sicker a patient was, the more ascorbic acid he would tolerate by mouth before diarrhea was produced. At least 80 percent of adult patients will tolerate 10,000 to 15,000 mg of ascorbic acid powder in one-half cup of water in four divided doses per 24 hours without having diarrhea. The astonishing finding was that almost all patients will absorb far greater amounts without having diarrhea when ill. This increased tolerance is somewhat proportional to the toxicity of the disease being treated. Tolerance is increased by stress (e.g., by anxiety, exercise, heat, cold, etc.). Admittedly, increasing the frequency of doses increases tolerance perhaps to half again as much; but the tolerance exceeding sometimes 200,000 mg per 24 hours was totally unexpected. Representative doses taken by patients titrating their ascorbic acid intake between the relief of most symptoms and the production of diarrhea are shown on Table 1.

The maximum relief of symptoms that can be expected with oral doses of ascorbic acid is obtained at a point just short of the amount that produces diarrhea. The amount and the timing of the doses are usually sensed by the patient. The physician should not try to regulate exactly the amount and timing of these doses because the optimally effective dose will often change from dose to dose. Patients are instructed on the general principles of determining doses and given estimates of the reasonable starting amounts and timing of these doses. I have named this process of the patient determining the optimum dose, titrating to bowel tolerance. The patient tries to titrate between that amount that begins to make him feel better and that amount that almost but not quite causes diarrhea.

Aascorbemia

The term "aascorbemia" is coined to mean complete absence of ascorbate from the blood. It accompanies acutely and chronically induced scurvy.

The object of this titration to bowel tolerance is to eliminate the toxicity of the disease and to maintain a high level of ascorbate in all tissues of the body, especially in the tissues directly involved by the disease process. Bearing in mind that almost

From the *J Orthomolecular Psych* 1981;10(2):125–132.

TABLE 1. USUAL BOWEL TOLERANCE DOSES

CONDITION	MILLIGRAMS (MG) PER 24 HOURS	NUMBER OF DOSES PER 24 HOURS
Normal, well	4,000–15,000	4–6
Mild cold	30,000–60,000	6–10
Severe cold	60,000–100,000 or more	8–15
Influenza	100,000–150,000	8–15
Echovirus, coxsackievirus	100,000–150,000	8–15
Mononucleosis	150,000–200,000 or more	12–18
Viral pneumonia	150,000–200,000 or more	12–18
Hay fever, asthma	15,000–25,000	4–8
Burn, injury, surgery	25,000–150,000	6–15
Anxiety, exercise and other mild stresses	15,000–25,000	4–6
Cancer	15,000–100,000	4–15
Ankylosing spondylitis	15,000–100,000	4–15
Rheumatoid arthritis	15,000–100,000	4–15
Bacterial infections	30,000–200,000 or more	10–18
Infectious hepatitis	30,000–100,000	6–15
Candidiasis	15,000–200,000 or more	6–25

continual sipping of ascorbic acid would be optimum (especially with the more toxic diseases), for practical purposes compromising to the number of doses listed in Table 1 often suffices. Apparently, there is an almost unbelievable and unappreciated potential draw by diseased tissues on ascorbic acid. Only by fully satisfying this need of stressed tissues can the condition of aascorbemia and localized scurvy be absolutely prevented. Fully satisfying this need probably accounts for the striking amelioration of symptoms just before bowel toler-ance is reached. This need for ascorbate is probably the reason many toxic diseases or stressful situations produce complications or even secondary diseases later on. The induced aascorbemia may predispose to pneumonia, heart attacks, phlebitis, Guillian-Barre syndrome, and perhaps rheumatoid arthritis and cancer.

It is my custom to speak of 20- to 100-gram colds, and so on. A 100-gram cold would mean that the patient is capable of ingesting 100 grams (100,000 mg) of vitamin C per 24 hours at the peak of the disease. In the case of systemic viral infections, it is often more important to properly estimate what milligram disease it is and persuade the patient to take adequate doses than to know what virus is being treated. A patient who learns to start titrating at the earliest symptoms of a disease will have the best results. Nevertheless, adequate doses will usually reduce symptoms even late in the disease.

By this method large amounts of ascorbate are spilled in the urine, but this is necessary to push adequate amounts of ascorbate into the tissues of the very seat of the disease and to maintain full vitamin C functions. One who argues that ascorbate can have no effect above renal (kidney) threshold misses the point entirely and would, I suppose, maintain that one could not become more intoxicated on ethyl alcohol above renal threshold. Also, large amounts of ascorbate in the urine will prevent many kidney and bladder infections.

In the case of the more toxic conditions, half-hourly doses may be necessary. Absorption and presumably destruction of ascorbate occur so rapidly as to require this frequency of doses for adequate amounts of ascorbic acid to keep the diseased tissues saturated without requiring too large doses that produce diarrhea. Even short delays in taking these doses may prolong the disease and reduce the effectiveness of ascorbic acid in blocking symptoms.

Infants and children tolerate ascorbic acid remarkably. I encourage the use of water rather than juice because the unsweetened taste aids in helping the patient select the proper dose. Juice is allowed only if the child refuses doses otherwise. Children who are 10 years old take adult doses; most teenagers take half again as much as adults.

Older adults often tolerate ascorbic acid less well and more frequently require intravenous (IV) ascorbate. Young children refusing to take oral ascorbic acid often will subsequently take oral doses after intramuscular (IM) injections of ascorbate. Although this method of persuasion seems cruel, it is better than the complications of serious diseases and probably hurts no more than a penicillin shot.

IV and IM Injections

Per milligram intravenous and intramuscular sodium ascorbate is more effective than oral ascorbic acid.[11,14] Solutions with 250 mg of sodium ascorbate per cubic centimeter (cc) with no preservative except for ethylenediaminetetraacetic acid (EDTA) must be used. The volume of a single IM injection can be as much as one could give as a saline shot. Usually 2 cc are used; sometimes a little more, sometimes in two sites. The object of the intramuscular injection is to avert a crisis, break the fever, or whatever the symptom. Usually a very rapid conversion to oral doses is possible.

In adults, intravenous injections can be made with the same 250 mg per cc solutions in pushes of 10 cc or very slowly up to 50 cc. Care is necessary here to make sure that the vein does not hurt as the injection is made and that the patient does not dehydrate or have tetany (muscle, spasm). IV bottles can be prepared using a salt solution called lactated Ringer's solution, or one half normal saline, or normal saline, and diluting the solution with 60,000 mg of sodium ascorbate per liter. At this concentration, sterile water can be used but care must be taken to make absolutely sure straight sterile water is never given. These solutions can be run in two to eight hours for a liter. It is my experience that sodium ascorbate intravenously in an edematous patient will usually act as a diuretic. However, one should think about the sodium and examine the patient frequently. The most frequent difficulty is dehydration or tetany from running solutions too rapidly. Oral water will prevent dehydration. A 10 cc vial of calcium gluconate (1,000 mg) should be added to one bottle per day if solutions are run more than one day. Remember that most patients will convert to oral doses of ascorbic acid rapidly. In some cases such as severe viral or bacterial pneumonias, one may want to give IV solutions of ascorbate at the same time that oral doses are being given.

Mononucleosis

Mononucleosis, an infectious viral disease, responds dramatically to ascorbic acid although the doses required can be very high. Early in this study a 23-year-old, 98-pound-female librarian with severe mononucleosis claimed to have taken two heaping tablespoons of powdered vitamin C every two hours, consuming a full pound of ascorbic acid in two days. She felt mostly well in three to four days, although she had to continue about 20,000 to 30,000 mg a day for about two months. Most cases do not require maintenance doses for more than two to three weeks. The duration of need can be sensed by the patient. Common symptoms such as swollen lymph nodes and swollen spleen return to normal rapidly.

Viral Hepatitis

Viral hepatitis (inflammation of the liver) of all types (A, B, and C), in my experience, is one of the easiest diseases for ascorbic acid to cure. A difficulty is that hepatitis often causes diarrhea; so titrating to bowel tolerance is more difficult. However, with experience one judges what milligram disease it is and gives this amount regardless of diarrhea. This amount could be from 40,000 to 100,000 mg. It soon becomes obvious whether it is the disease or the ascorbic acid causing the diarrhea. There is usually a paradoxical stopping of the diarrhea within a day or two. If too much difficulty is experienced in judging the dosages, intravenous ascorbate is extremely effective. Stools and urine return to normal color within two to three days in acute cases. Chronic cases take longer but in my experience respond rapidly. In acute cases the patient will usually feel fairly well in two to four days but it usually takes the jaundice about six days to clear. There would appear to be a staining of the skin that persists even though physical findings and laboratory results return rapidly to normal. Liver function test values so high as to be unmeasurable, rapidly fall and reflect objectively the subjective feelings of the patient.

Gastroenteritis

Gastroenteritis of viral origin (stomach flu) responds very rapidly but one must titrate boldly and anticipate paradoxical stopping of the diarrhea. If titration starts in the first hour of the disease, experienced ascorbic-acid takers may never develop the diarrhea and only suspect what they have avoided because of the disease being epidemic. These diseases may require 60,000 to 150,000 mg of ascorbic acid to almost totally block symptoms. If a patient overtitrates and develops diarrhea from the ascorbic acid, the change in character of the diarrhea to a relatively painless, less foul, more watery-like enema diarrhea, and generalized relief of malaise signals that the doses should be lowered.

Other acute self-limiting viral diseases respond similarly when the patient titrates properly. Antihistamines and decongestants should be used when appropriate.

Belfield and Stone have observed similar results in veterinary medicine with usually fatal viral diseases when intravenous ascorbate is utilized.[1]

Bacterial Infections

Ascorbic acid should be used in conjunction with the appropriate antibiotic. The effect of ascorbic acid is synergistic with antibiotics and would appear to broaden the spectrum of antibiotics considerably. The high incidence of allergic reaction to penicillin in patients saturated with ascorbate is almost zero. One must understand that ascorbate does not always effectively protect against allergic reactions until the patient has titrated up to bowel tolerance. If a patient has an allergic reaction to penicillin before bowel tolerance is reached, subsequent saturation with ascorbate in conjunction with usual medications will more rapidly than expected resolve the reaction. It is especially interesting that mononucleosis would appear to cause more rapid destruction of ascorbate than other commonly encountered viral diseases. The high incidence of allergic reaction to penicillin in patients mistakenly given penicillin when they have mononucleosis is usually prevented by saturation with ascorbic acid. It is probable that this high incidence of allergic reaction to penicillin in mononucleosis patients is due to the tremendous draw on ascorbate by the disease. It has been my experience the indications for ampicillin are markedly reduced by ascorbic acid.

Candidiasis

Candida (yeast) infections occur less frequently in patients being treated with antibiotics if bowel tolerance doses of ascorbic acid are simultaneously used. Antibiotics, which kill beneficial bacteria along with harmful ones, allow *Candida albicans* overgrowth. Ascorbic acid seems to have little effect on established Candida infections. It should be used, nevertheless, to help the patient with the stress of the disease.

Fungal Infections

Although ascorbic acid should be given in some form in some way to all sick patients to help them meet the stress of the disease, it is my experience that ascorbate has little effect on the primary fungal infection. It will probably be found certain complications can be reduced in incidence. It may be found that appropriate antifungal agents will penetrate tissues saturated in ascorbate better.

Trauma, Surgery

Swelling and pain from trauma and surgery is markedly reduced by bowel-tolerance doses of ascorbic acid. Doses should be given a minimum of six times a day. More major surgeries should require IV sodium ascorbate postoperatively. The effect of ascorbate on anesthetics should be studied. Barbiturates and many narcotics are blocked. Refer to the work of Libby and Stone.[15] The need for these substances postoperatively is greatly reduced.

Cancer

I have avoided the treatment of cancer patients for legal reasons; however, I have given nutritional consults to a number of cancer patients and have observed an increased bowel tolerance to ascorbic acid. Were I treating cancer patients, I would not limit their vitamin C ingestion to a set amount but would titrate them to bowel tolerance. Dr. Cameron's advice against giving cancer patients with widespread metastasis large amounts of ascorbate too rapidly at first should be heeded. He found that sometimes extensive necrosis, or hemorrhage of the cancer, could kill the patient if the vitamin was started too rapidly in patients with widespread metastasis. Hopefully, ascorbic acid will become the first treatment given cancer patients and not the last. The nutritional treatment of cancer should not be limited to ascorbic acid.

Stress and Disease in General

After considerable experience with patients in stressful situations and with diseases producing stress, it is my opinion that saturation with ascorbate markedly reduces the incidence of secondary complications.[7] It is difficult to prove, but it is my definite impression that the incidence of disease in the months following stress is reduced.

Allergies

Hay fever and asthma are most frequently benefited. Sometimes, pantothenic acid and/or pyridoxine (vitamin B6) are helpful in acting synergistically with ascorbic acid. Frequently, hay fever and asthma are benefited at dose levels lower and more comfortable than bowel tolerance doses. However, treatment should begin with bowel tolerance doses at least six times a day so that the response of some more difficult cases will not be missed.

Back Pain from Disc Disease

Greenwood observed that 1,000 mg a day would reduce the incidence of necessary surgery on discs.[8] At bowel tolerance levels, ascorbic acid more markedly reduces pain about 50 percent and lessens the difficulties with narcotics and muscle relaxants. It is not the total answer for back pain patients, however.

Rheumatoid Arthritis and Ankylosing Spondylitis

Bowel tolerance is increased in rheumatoid arthritis and ankylosing spondylitis (a type of arthritis that affects the base of the spine). Clinical response varies. Sometimes these diseases are put into remission; sometimes not. I would advise the patient's increased needs for ascorbate be met regardless.

Scarlet Fever

Three cases with typical sandpaper-like rash, peeling skin, and diagnostic laboratory findings of scarlet fever have responded within an hour or overnight. It is thought this immediate response is due to the neutralization of the small amount of residual streptococcus toxin causing the disease.

Herpes: Cold Sores, Genital Lesions, and Shingles

Acute herpes infections are usually ameliorated with bowel tolerance doses of ascorbic acid. However, recurrences are common especially if the disease has already become chronic. Zinc in combination with ascorbic acid is more effective for herpes infections.

Crib Deaths (Sudden Infant Death Syndrome)

I would agree with Kalokerinos and Klenner that crib deaths are caused by sudden ascorbate depletions.[10,13] The induced aascorbemia in some vital regulatory center kills the child. This induced deficiency is more likely to occur when the diet is poor in vitamin C. All the epidemiological factors predisposing to crib deaths are associated with low-vitamin C intake or high-vitamin C destruction. I have never heard of a crib death in an infant saturated with ascorbate.

Maintenance Doses

I advise patients to take bowel tolerance doses of vitamin C for about a week and observe if anything beneficial happens. Some patients clear sinuses, or get a lift from it, and so forth. In these cases, doses are reduced to a comfortable effective level. If a patient feels nothing, then the amount is lowered to about 4,000 mg a day divided in about three to four doses for a good day. During a stressful day, doses are raised to a total of perhaps 10,000 mg or more. When ascorbic acid crystals are used dissolved in a small amount of plain water, the patient usually develops a taste for the substance that tells him how much to take. At the slightest hint of a threatening viral disease, doses are increased in frequency and to bowel tolerance.

In many patients viral infections still occur despite high ascorbic acid intake, although the symptoms of the disease will be mostly ameliorated. Vitamin A in dosages from 25,000 to 50,000 international units (IU) per day should be taken if high doses of ascorbic acid are maintained for more than several months. Supplements of all essential minerals should also be taken along with long-run maintenance doses of vitamin C.

Avoidance of sugar and processed foods will prove valuable if a patient's goal is almost complete prevention of viral diseases.

Complications

It is my experience that ascorbic acid never causes kidney stones but, in fact, probably prevents them. Acute and chronic urinary tract infections are usually eliminated. One patient in a thousand will experience some discomfort while urinating. A small number will develop a light rash that usually clears with subsequent doses. Patients with hidden peptic ulcers may have pain but some are benefited. The few patients complaining of canker sores with small doses of vitamin C do not usually have problems with large bowel tolerance closes. Patients with canker sores should be given large doses of vitamin E.

Some patients complaining of acid conditions do not tolerate ascorbic acid. These cases are very few. Older patients will have more nuisance problems with ascorbic acid and have more difficulty reaching bowel tolerance.

Patients started on maintenance doses of ascorbic acid when well will have a moderately high incidence of nuisance complaints. Patients treated with bowel tolerance doses for acute diseases have

very few complaints because of the increased tolerance and the marked relief of symptoms. It is my experience that high maintenance doses of vitamin C reduce the incidence of gouty arthritis. Since that discovery, I have not had difficulties giving large amounts of ascorbic acid to patients with gout.

There has been no evidence as Herbert and Jacob suspected that ascorbic acid destroys vitamin B12.[9]

The major problem, if one wishes to call it a problem, is a certain dependency on ascorbic acid that a patient acquires over a long period of time when he takes large maintenance doses. Apparently, certain metabolic reactions are encouraged by large amounts of ascorbate and if the substance is suddenly withdrawn, certain problems result such as a cold, return of allergy, fatigue, and so forth. Mostly, these problems are a return of problems the patient had before taking the ascorbic acid. Patients have, by this time, become so adjusted to feeling better that they refuse to go without vitamin C. Patients do not seem to acquire this dependency in the short time they take doses to bowel tolerance to treat an acute disease. Maintenance doses of 4,000 mg per day do not seem to create a noticeable dependency. The majority of patients who take 10,000 to 15,000 mg of vitamin C per day probably have a certain metabolic need for ascorbate that exceeds the universal human species need.

The major problem feared by patients benefiting from these large maintenance doses of ascorbic acid is that they may be forced into a position when their body is deprived of ascorbate during a period of great stress such as emergency hospitalization. Physicians should recognize the consequences of suddenly withdrawing vitamin C under these circumstances and be prepared to meet these increased metabolic needs for it in even an unconscious patient. These consequences, which may include shock, heart attack, phlebitis, pneumonia, allergic reactions, and more, can be averted only by intravenous vitamin C. All hospitals should have supplies of large amounts of ascorbate for intravenous use to meet this need. The millions of people taking ascorbic acid make this an urgent priority. Patients should carry warning of these needs in a card prominently displayed in their wallets or should have a medic alert bracelet or necklace engraved with this warning. Physicians should, in addition, carefully ask patients' families about the patients' ascorbic acid maintenance doses. Regardless of a physician's philosophical feelings about the usefulness of vitamin C, the physician should not withhold this essential nutrient from patients who have previously adjusted their body's metabolism to their increased needs. It would be like withholding vitamin B12 from a patient with pernicious anemia just because he was hospitalized. In the case of ascorbic acid, the effect would be much more rapid however.

CONCLUSION

The method of titrating a patient's dosage of ascorbic acid between the relief of most symptoms and bowel tolerance has been described. This titration method is absolutely necessary to obtain excellent results. Studies of lesser amounts are almost useless. This method cannot by its nature be studied by double-blind methods because no placebo will mimic this bowel tolerance phenomenon. The method produces such spectacular effects in all patients capable of tolerating these doses, especially in cases of acute self-limiting viral diseases as to be undeniable. A placebo could not possibly work so reliably, nor work in infants and children, and have such a profound effect on critically ill patients. More stable patients will tolerate bowel tolerance doses of vitamin C and almost uniformly have excellent results. The more suggestible unstable patient is more likely to have difficulty with the taste.

REFERENCES

1. Belfield WO, Stone I. Megascorbic prophylaxis and megascorbic therapy: a new orthomolecular modality in veterinary medicine. *Journal of the International Academy of Preventive Medicine* 1975;2:10–26.

2. Cameron E, Pauling L. Supplemental ascorbate in the supportive treatment of cancer: prolongation of survival times in terminal human cancer. *Proc Natl Acad Sci USA* 1976;73:3685–3689.

3. Cameron E, Pauling L. The orthomolecular treatment of cancer: reevaluation of prolongation of survival times in terminal human cancer. *Proc Natl Acad Sci USA* 1978;75:4538–4542.

4. Cathcart RF. Clinical trial of vitamin C. *Medical Tribune*, June 25, 1975.

5. Cathcart RF. Clinical use of large doses of ascorbic acid. Annual Meeting of the California Orthomolecular Medical Society, San Francisco, Feb 19, 1976.

6. Cathcart RF. Vitamin C as a detoxifying agent. Annual Meeting of the Orthomolecular Medical Society, San Francisco, Jan 21, 1978.

7. Cathcart RF. Vitamin C: the missing stress hormone. Annual Meeting of the Orthomolecular Medical Society, San Francisco, Mar 3, 1979.

8. Greenwood J. Optimum vitamin C intake as a factor in the preservation of disc integrity. *Med Ann Dist Columbia* 1964;33:274–276.

9. Herbert V, Jacob E. Destruction of vitamin B12 by ascorbic acid. *JAMA* 1974;230:241–242.

10. Kalokerinos A. *Every Second Child.* New Canaan, CT: Keats Publishing, 1981.

11. Klenner FR. Virus pneumonia and its treatment with vitamin C. *J South Med and Surg* 1948;110: 60–63.

12. Klenner FR. The treatment of poliomyelitis and other virus diseases with vitamin C. *J South Med and Surg* 1949;111:210–214.

13. Klenner FR. Observations on the dose and administration of ascorbic acid when employed beyond the range of a vitamin in human pathology. *J App Nutr* 1971;23:61–88.

14. Klenner FR. Significance of high daily intake of ascorbic acid in preventive medicine. *J Int Acad Prev Med* 1974;1:45–49.

15. Libby AF, Stone I. The hypoascorbemia-kwashiorkor approach to drug addiction therapy: a pilot study. *J Ortho Psychiat* 1977;6:300–308.

16. Pauling L. *Vitamin C and the Common Cold.* San Francisco: W.H. Freeman & Co, 1970.

17. Pauling L. *Vitamin C, the Common Cold, and the Flu.* San Francisco: W.H. Freeman & Co, 1970, 1976.

18. Stone I. Studies of a mammalian enzyme system for producing evolutionary evidence on man. *Am J Phys Anthro* 1965;23:83–86.

19. Stone I. Hypoascorbemia: the genetic disease causing the human requirement for exogenous ascorbic acid. *Perspect Biol Med* 1968;10:133–134.

20. Stone I. *The Healing Factor: Vitamin C Against Disease.* New York: Grosset & Dunlap, 1972.

THE ORIGIN OF THE 42-YEAR STONEWALL OF VITAMIN C
by Robert Landwehr

In the late spring of 1949, the United States was in the grip of its worst polio epidemic ever. On June 10, a paper on ways to save the lives of bulbar polio victims was read at the Annual Session of the American Medical Association (AMA), and subsequently was printed in its journal, the *Journal of the American Medical Association* (*JAMA*), on September 3, 1949.[1] In bulbar polio, the virus attacks the brainstem and the nerve centers. Following the talk, members of the audience were invited to comment. The first speaker, a leading authority, focused on details of tracheotomy techniques caused when paralyzed breathing, swallowing, and coughing muscles of victims threatened their lives. Why the next person was recognized is puzzling. The only national recognition he had received—and it was obviously very limited—was that his picture appeared in *Ebony* magazine in 1947 for having delivered to a deaf-mute black woman, the first-known surviving, identical quadruplets in the country. Here is the abstract of his remarks as recorded in *JAMA*:

> Dr. F. R. Klenner, Reidsville, North Carolina: It might be interesting to learn how polio was treated in Reidsville, during the 1948 epidemic. In the past seven years, virus infections have been treated and cured in a period of 72 hours by the employment of massive frequent injections of ascorbic acid, or vitamin C. I believe that if vitamin C in these massive doses—6,000–20,000 milligrams (mg) in a 24-hour period—is given to these patients with poliomyelitis, none will be paralyzed and there will be no further maiming or epidemics of poliomyelitis.

The discussion period was, of course, to be devoted to hearing relevant comments of the world's leading authorities on the treatment of bulbar polio symptoms, not to airing another claim of a cure. One can imagine the silence that must have greeted this sweeping, out-of-place declaration by a small-town general practitioner. Four other speakers, three more bulbar experts, and an anesthesiologist followed. None referred to Dr. Klenner's remarks.

Data from Human Beings Not Experimental Animals

The empirical, clinical basis for Klenner's statement is found in his paper "The Treatment of Poliomyelitis and Other Virus Diseases with Vitamin C," published in the July 1949 issue of the *Journal of Southern Medicine and Surgery*.[2] He writes:

> In the polio epidemic in North Carolina in 1948, 60 cases of this disease came under our care. These patients presented all or almost all of these signs and symptoms: fever of 101°F–104.6°F, headache, pain at the back of the eyes, conjunctivitis, scarlet throat; pain between the shoulders, back of the neck, one or more extremity, the lumbar back; nausea, vomiting and constipation. In 15 of these cases, the diagnosis was confirmed by lumbar puncture; the cell count ranging from 33 to 125. Eight had been in contact with a proven case; two of this group received spinal taps. Examination of the spinal fluid was not carried out in others for the reasons: 1) Simon Flexner and Harold Amoss had warned that 'simple lumbar puncture attended with even very slight hemorrhage opens the way for the passage of the virus from the blood into the central nervous system and thus promotes infection. 2) A patient presenting all or almost all of the above signs and symptoms during an epidemic of polio must be considered infected with this virus. 3) Routine lumbar puncture would have made it obligatory to report each case as diagnosed to the health authorities. This would have deprived me of valuable clinical material and the patients of most valuable therapy, since they would have been removed to a receiving center in a nearby town.

> The treatment employed was vitamin C in massive doses. It was given like any other antibiotic every two to four hours. The initial dose was 1,000–2,000 mg, depending on age. Children up to four years received the injections

From the *J Orthomolecular Med* 1991;6(2):99–103.

intramuscularly. Since laboratory facilities for whole blood and urine determinations of the concentration of vitamin C were not available, the temperature curve was adopted as the guide for additional medication. The rectal temperature was recorded every two hours. No temperature response after the second hour was taken to indicate the second 1,000 or 2,000 mg. If there was a drop in fever after two hours, two more hours was allowed before the second dose. This schedule was followed for 24 hours. After this time the fever was consistently down, so the drug was given 1,000–2,000 mg every six hours for the next 48 hours. All patients were clinically well after 72 hours. After three patients had a relapse the drug was continued for at least 48 hours longer—1,000–2,000 mg every eight to 12 hours. Where spinal taps were performed, it was the rule to find a reversion of the fluid to normal after the second day of treatment.

For patients treated in the home the dose schedule was 2,000 mg by needle every six hours, supplemented by 1,000–2,000 mg every two hours by mouth. The tablet was crushed and dissolved in fruit juice. All of the natural 'C' in fruit juice is taken up by the body; this made us expect catalytic action from this medium. Rutin [a bioflavonoid], 20 mg, was used with vitamin C by mouth in a few cases, instead of the fruit juice. Hawley and others have shown that vitamin C taken by mouth will show its peak of excretion in the urine in from four to six hours. Intravenous administration produces this peak in from one to three hours. By this route, however, the concentration in the blood is raised so suddenly that a transitory overflow into the urine results before the tissues are saturated. Some authorities suggest that the subcutaneous method is the most conservative in terms of vitamin C loss, but this factor is overwhelmingly neutralized by the factor of pain inflicted.

Two patients in this series of 60 regurgitated fluid through the nose. This was interpreted as representing the dangerous bulbar type. For a patient in this category postural drainage, oxygen administration, in some cases tracheotomy, needs to be instituted, until the vitamin C has had sufficient time to work—in our experience

36 hours. Failure to recognize this factor might sacrifice the chance of recovery. With these precautions taken, every patient of the series recovered uneventfully within three to five days.

This paper is quoted at length to allow readers to judge for themselves whether or not Dr. Klenner made up all these details. In subsequent publications he gave details about curing life-threatening polio cases, and described his general procedures in his paper "The Vitamin and Massage Treatment for Acute Poliomyelitis," appearing in the *Journal of Southern Medicine and Surgery* in August 1952.[3]

One of the reasons why Klenner's declaration at the AMA annual session was undoubtedly met with silence was that since 1939 polio experts were quite certain that vitamin C was not effective against polio. There seemed little doubt that Albert B. Sabin, a highly respected figure in medical research even before he developed his successful vaccines, had demonstrated that vitamin C had no value in combating polio viruses. In 1939 he published a paper showing that vitamin C had no effect in preventing paralysis in rhesus monkeys experimentally infected with a strain of polio virus. He had tried to corroborate the work of Claus W. Jungeblut, another highly respected medical researcher, who had published in 1935 and 1937 papers indicating that vitamin C might be of benefit. Sabin could not reproduce Jungeblut's results even though he consulted Jungeblut during the course of the experiments. It seemed to be a fair trial, and Sabin's negative results virtually ended experiments with vitamin C and polio.

How then could a Frederick Klenner, a virtually unknown general practitioner specializing in diseases of the chest, from a town no one ever heard of, with no national credentials, no research grants, and no experimental laboratory, have the nerve to make his sweeping claim in front of that prestigious body of polio authorities?

More Data Collection

Around 1942, Klenner's wife suffered bleeding gums and her dentist recommended pulling out all her teeth. Dr. Klenner thought that solution too draconian and remembered reading about research using vitamin C to cure chimpanzees with a similar problem. He gave her several injections of the vitamin and the bleeding stopped. Soon after, this dramatic result encouraged him to try vitamin C on an obstinate man who was near death from viral pneumonia. Klenner described this seminal experience in a 1953 paper "The Use of Vitamin C as an Antibiotic"[3]:

> Our interest with vitamin C against the virus organism began 10 years ago in a modest rural home. Here a patient who was receiving symptomatic treatment for virus pneumonia had suddenly developed cyanosis. He refused hospitalization for supportive oxygen therapy. X-ray had not been considered because of its dubious value and because the nearest department equipped to give such treatment was 69 miles distant. Two grams [2,000 mg] of vitamin C were given intramuscularly with the hope that the anaerobic condition existing in the tissues would be relieved by the catalytic action of vitamin C acting as a gas transport aiding cellular respiration. This was an old idea; the important factor being that it worked. Within 30 minutes after giving the drug (which was carried in my medical bag for the treatment of diarrhea in children), the characteristic breathing and slate-like color had cleared. Returning six hours later, at eight in the evening, the patient was found sitting over the edge of his bed enjoying a late dinner. Strangely enough, his fever was three degrees less than it was at 2:00 P.M. that same afternoon. This sudden change in the condition of the patient led us to suspect that vitamin C was playing a role of far greater significance than that of a simple respiratory catalyst. A second injection of 1,000 mg of vitamin C was administered, by the same route, on this visit and then subsequently at six-hour intervals for the next three days. This patient was clinically well after 36 hours of chemotherapy. From this casual observation, we have been able to assemble sufficient clinical evidence to prove unequivocally that vitamin C is the antibiotic of choice in the handling of all types of virus diseases. Furthermore, it is a major adjuvant in the treatment of all other infectious diseases.

Again this paper is quoted at length to allow readers to judge for themselves whether or not the author made this up or deluded himself in some way. From 1943 through 1947, Dr. Klenner reported successful treatment of 41 more cases of viral pneumonia using massive doses of vitamin C. From these cases he learned what dosage and route of administration—intravenously, intramuscularly, or orally—was best for each patient. Klenner gave these details in a February 1948 paper published in the *Journal of Southern Medicine and Surgery* entitled "Virus Pneumonia and Its Treatment with Vitamin C."[4] This article was the first of Dr. Klenner's 28 scientific publications published through 1974.

Klenner realized, of course, that vitamin C's effectiveness with viral pneumonia opened up the possibility of curing other viral diseases. "With a great deal of enthusiasm," in Klenner's phrase, he tried its effectiveness with all of the childhood diseases, particularly measles. By the spring of 1948, when a measles epidemic came to Reidsville, Klenner was so confident of vitamin C's efficacy with these diseases that he devised what would ordinarily be an outrageous experiment with his two little daughters. He had them play with children known to be in the contagious phase of measles. When the usual syndrome of measles had developed and his daughters were obviously sick, vitamin C was started.

Again Dr. Klenner's words from his 1953 paper:

> In this experiment it was found that 1,000 mg every four hours, by mouth, would modify the attack. Smaller doses allowed the disease to progress. When 1,000 mg was given every 2 hours all evidence of the infection cleared in 48 hours. If the drug was then discontinued for a similar period (48 hours) the above syndrome returned. We observed this off and on picture for thirty days at which time the drug (vitamin C) was given 1,000 mg every 2 hours around the clock for four days. This time the picture cleared and did not return.

With this background of experiences—with human beings, not experimental animals—Klenner gained confidence in and control over his vitamin C treatment. One reason he turned his attention early to treating measles was that he knew that measle viruses were about as small as polio viruses and he hoped massive doses of vitamin C would be effective against the dreaded disease known as the "Crippler." By 1948 he was ready to treat polio with vitamin C, and in that year North Carolina suffered its worst epidemic ever—2,518 new cases. Dr. Klenner's hopes were realized when, as has been related above, he cured 60 patients with massive frequent injections of vitamin C. With seven years of experience behind him one can understand not only why Dr. Klenner had the nerve to speak up on June 10, 1949, but why he undoubtedly felt morally obligated to do so.

After 1949, polio epidemics continued to take their terrible toll. The peak year for the Crippler in the United States was 1952: 57,628 cases. During the 1950s, isolated doctors around the world tried Klenner's cure. Those who used vitamin C at doses below those recommended by Klenner reported no benefit; those who followed his dosages reported good results. Bauer of the University of Switzerland Clinic, Basel, in 1952 reported benefits to his polio patients with 10,000–20,000 mg of vitamin C per day. Edward Greer, using doses in Klenner's recommended range of 50,000–80,000 mg per day, recorded in 1955 good clinical results with five serious cases of polio. Abram Hoffer recalls that a controlled study, conducted in Great Britain in the late fifties with 70 young polio victims, confirmed Klenner's cure. All those given vitamin C recovered completely, while a significant number of those not given vitamin C suffered some permanent damage. (This study was not published because of the success of the polio vaccines.) Klenner himself reported that he received scores of letters from doctors in the United States and Canada corroborating his striking results. Some of the letters described how they cured their own children; others, how the doctors had cured themselves.

A Simple, Inexpensive Cure for Many Viral Diseases

What kind of reception did Dr. Klenner's discoveries receive from the medical establishment? There are two references to Klenner's 1949 paper in national, mainstream publications. The title of

that paper was included in the October 7, 1949, issue of the *Current List of Medical Literature*, published by the U.S. Army Medical Library. The paper was also included in the second edition of *A Bibliography of Infantile Paralysis—1789–1949*, published in 1951 and prepared under the direction of the National Foundation for Infantile Paralysis. Instead of abstracting the paper in the usual manner, it printed only Dr. Klenner's last paragraph, which was not a summary but an obvious rhetorical statement Klenner felt necessary to counter the skepticism he knew would greet his quick, inexpensive cures. Other than these two references, mainstream medical publications made no mention of Klenner and his work. One of *JAMA's* regular departments was *Current Medical Literature*, in which its editors abstracted papers they considered of special note. Many polio papers were abstracted in 1949, but not Klenner's.

"Let no one who has the slightest desire to live in peace and quietness be tempted, under any circumstances, to enter upon the chivalrous task of trying to correct a popular error." —WILLIAM THOMS, deputy librarian for the House of Lords, c. 1873

The National Foundation for Infantile Paralysis was founded in 1938 by polio's most famous victim, President Franklin Roosevelt, to raise money through the March of Dimes to combat the disease. Most polio research was funded by the National Foundation. There is no mention of Dr. Klenner's work or of vitamin C's possible benefits to polio victims in any of the foundation's annual reports. Not one dime was spent to prove or disprove Klenner's claim. Before 1949 a claim of a cure was promptly looked into and money spent until it was proved false. But with Klenner's claim nothing happened.

It was certainly not for lack of research funds that nothing happened. John M. Russell, in the 1960 book *The Crisis in American Medicine*, edited by Marion K. Sanders, described the glut and waste of money for medical research in the 1950s. Russell points out that the public clamor for a cure for polio was so great that in 1954 Congress appropriated $1,000,000 specifically earmarked for polio research. It turned out that there was so much polio money floating around that the recipient of this largess, the U.S. Public Health Service, classified such unlikely diseases as hepatitis as "polio-like."

Five International Polio Congresses were convened every three years from 1948 to 1960 to deal with the polio epidemics around the world. In all of the voluminous reports of these conferences, there is no reference to Klenner or to vitamin C. Only the first congress dealt briefly with the possible effect of nutrition, and this was dismissed by the statement of an expert "that no clinical evidence is known to me which justifies an increase in intake of vitamins beyond usual recommended allowances."

Thus, in 1949, the polio experts at the Annual Session of the AMA knew of Klenner's claim, as did the many readers of *JAMA's* lead article of its September 3 issue, the many researchers who used the National Foundation's bibliography, those that kept up with the titles in the *Current List of Medical Literature*, and the relatively few readers of the *Journal of Southern Medicine and Surgery*. All this exposure led to no official inquiry or follow-up of Dr. Klenner's work by U.S. government health authorities or the National Foundation. No one in authority anywhere stepped forward to insist that it be checked out. The strategy of medical leaders—conscious or unconscious, planned or unplanned—was clearly to ignore Dr. Klenner and hope his claims would be forgotten.

It worked. Klenner's cure never became well known and today has sunk almost into oblivion. A synopsis of polio infection and research by Ernest Kovacs entitled *The Biochemistry of Poliomyelitis Viruses*, published in 1964, makes no reference to Klenner. In 1985 Friedrich Koch and Gebhard Koch published *The Molecular Biology of Poliovirus*. It contains in its opening chapter a history of the disease, but it says nothing about Klenner, or even about the extensive vitamin C research done by Jungeblut and Sabin with monkeys in the 1930s. It's as though polio-vitamin C research never happened.

To this day it is mainstream medicine's position that there is no cure for polio. *The Encyclopedia American* quotes Richard W. Price of Memorial Sloan-Kettering Cancer Center of New York City: "No specific treatment is effective once neurological involvement becomes manifest." A thoroughly exasperated Klenner concluded a February 1959 paper in the *Tri-State Medical Journal* with these words:

Should the disease be present in the acute form, ascorbic acid given in proper amounts around the clock, both by mouth and needle, will bring about a rapid recovery. We believe that ascorbic acid must be given by needle in amounts from 250 mg to 400 mg per kg [kilograms] body weight every 4 to 6 hours for 48 hours and then every 8 to 12 hours. The dose by mouth is the dose that can be tolerated. To those who say that polio is without cure, I say that they lie. Polio in the acute form can be cured in 96 hours or less. I beg of someone in authority to try it.

Today, there are areas of the world where polio vaccine is still not used and where the incidence of polio is increasing. Polio remains the Crippler, and the only effort of the World Health Organization is to increase vaccination. The leading medical authorities—the editors of the leading journals, the heads of the AMA and the National Foundation, U.S. Surgeons-General, and the heads of other U.S. governmental health agencies—were, and are, responsible for stonewalling for 42 years Dr. Klenner's simple, inexpensive cure for many viral diseases, including the dreaded polio. 1949—a year in medicine that will live in infamy.

REFERENCES

1. *JAMA* September 3, 1949;(141):1:1–8.

2. Klenner F. The treatment of poliomyelitis and other virus diseases with vitamin C. *Journal of Southern Medicine and Surgery* 1949;111(7):211–212.

3. Klenner F. The vitamin and massage treatment for acute poliomyelitis. *Journal of Southern Medicine and Surgery* 1952;113(4):101–107.

4. Klenner F. Virus pneumonia and its treatment with vitamin C. *Journal of Southern Medicine and Surgery* 1948;110(2):36–38.

CHILDREN, VITAMIN C, AND MEDICAL PROGRESS
by Lendon H. Smith, MD

My dad was a pediatrician: modern, scientific, and respected by his peers. In the 1920s and '30s, it was standard medical practice to fluoroscope babies to search for an enlarged thymus, which "everyone knew" was the cause of sudden infant death syndrome (SIDS), as a large thymus would crush the windpipe. If you did not have a fluoroscope x-ray machine, you were a bad doctor. It was standard medical practice, at least that is what the fluoroscope salesman told Dad. If Dad found an enlarged thymus, he sent that patient off to the radiologist, who x-rayed it down to a more "normal" size. It was almost an emergency to get this done before the thymus suffocated the child.

Dad was always supposed to wear the lead gloves to protect himself from the radiation, but sometimes he forgot. After 20 years he got cancer of his fingers, six of them had to be amputated, and skin grafts were necessary for the rest. Some of the children so treated grew up to get cancer of the thyroid. That was science in the 1920s and '30s. One wonders what we are doing now that will be an embarrassment to the medical profession in the years to come.

A Shift in My Practice of Medicine

After I had been in the practice of pediatrics for about 20 years, I began to realize that medical school did not teach us everything we needed to know to be a reliable doctor. I shifted my practice to a more nutrition-oriented approach when I realized that conditions like bed-wetting and hyperactivity were not psychological in origin, but related to diet and nutrient deficiencies. My wife and I could not tolerate the idea that these conditions in our children were the result of poor parenting skills. What a relief to know that these things were related to nutrition and not psychogenic factors.

I found, in general, that many of these so-called psychiatric conditions were really genetic problems that became manifest when the diet was not appropriate. Sometimes bad parenting skills were to blame but often academic failure was due to bad teaching techniques, and even school phobia could be due to the big dog on the way to school.

I conducted a clinical study over 10 years involving 8,000 youngsters who had been diagnosed by their teacher as being hyperactive or academic failures. I discovered that 75 percent of them were blue-eyed blondes or green-eyed redheads. Boys outnumbered girls five to one. A few had been injured at birth enough to be a causative factor, but most had a genetic tendency that only showed up if they were eating the wrong foods or if they had a deficiency of calcium or magnesium.

Most of them were very ticklish. I could hardly touch them. The stethoscope and the otoscope were like knives to them. I found that response to my exam correlated well with being distractible in the classroom. Hair and blood tests showed me that the children, who were distractible, were also low in magnesium. Magnesium is necessary for the function of the limbic system, part of which is devoted to screening or filtering out unimportant stimuli. These children are unable to disregard unimportant stimuli. This gets them into trouble because the teacher asks them to sit down and pay attention, but they are unable to do this. There are too many distractions, just from the children in the class breathing or from cars going by outside.

The other give-away clue that the diet is faulty is that these children have mood swings or are the Jekyll-and-Hyde type of person. This is not psychiatric but is due to their blood sugar fluctuating up and down. When I gave these children calcium and magnesium, and stopped the sugar and any food to which I found them sensitive, 80 percent of them were 60 to 100 percent better, and the methylphenidate (Ritalin), which so many of them were taking, could be discontinued.

Headed in the Right Direction

Other confirmatory research helped me become more comfortable in saying that hyper kids had a

From the *J Orthomolecular Med* 1991;6(3&4):181–196.

nutrition problem. Stephen Schoenthaler, a criminal justice professor in Turlock, California, has done much research to show diet is a key in maladaptive behavior in children. He is the person who did the famous study with the New York school children. Back in 1979, he started changing the breakfasts and lunches of the 800,000 children. He first stopped the sugar, then the next year he pulled out the food colors, then the flavors and the additives. In five years he moved up the average achievement tests from a sad 39 points to a better than average 55 points. The children who were getting the worst scores in 1979 were eating the school food; at the end of the five years, the children who were getting the best grades were eating the school food. But remember, the food had gotten better. If children eat good food, their scores improve. We don't need any more studies. We have the proof. What are the school and government authorities doing about this? Who is implementing this?

But Schoenthaler went on. In a detention home for boys in Oklahoma, he conducted a double-blind, crossover, placebo-controlled study on 71 rough, surly adolescents. Before the program started, the administration had a list of complaints about these youths: fights, throwing things, non-compliance, and escape attempts. Half of these boys got a multiple vitamin and mineral capsule; the other half got a placebo. Within two weeks, the kids on the vitamins became more compliant, escape attempts and fights dropped by 75 percent, and surliness almost disappeared. There was a 5 percent change in the placebo group, but nothing significant. At six weeks the groups were switched. The placebo group got the vitamin capsule, and the incidence of antisocial behavior got better to the same 75 percent as the other group had, but the group now on the placebo began to go back to their previous nasty behavior.

This vitamin capsule would cost the state about a dollar or two per week per youngster. They decided not to use it because they have diazepam (Valium) to control behavior, and besides, they feed these kids good food, don't they? Schoenthaler even has documentation of the vitamin and mineral status of these youngsters: hyperkeratosis (overgrowth of skin tissue), white spots on the nails, cracks at the corners of their mouths, swelling of the gum tissue, and capillary dilatation on the sclera.

So research has proven that diet and behavior are related. Why doesn't it happen to everyone in the same way? Vitamin and mineral deficiencies affect different people in different ways. Some people go into crime. Some get depressed. Some will get sick or will have a headache. Some will become hyperactive; some hypoactive.

I am in touch with a former patient of mine who just got out of federal prison after 11 years serving time for bank robbery. I took care of his pediatric needs until he was an adolescent. He was surly and uncooperative. He hated school. I tried to get him to change his diet, but he craved and stole sugar. When he robbed a bank when he was 20 years old, he had not eaten breakfast. Now, if you are going to rob a bank, you would assume it will be very stressful, and being a smart person, you would load up with complex carbohydrates, some protein, and extra vitamin C and B complex. During the robbery he killed his uncle by mistake, and wounded a policeman. After they caught him, he could hardly remember the episode, he was so spacey. I believe as part of the arresting procedure, the police should ask if the accused had been drinking or eating, and if so, what.

Other Sources of Confirmation

I have learned a great deal from other researchers and also from books about nutrition. As an example, Australian physician Archie Kalokerinos wrote a book some years ago called *Every Second Child* (1981). He was referring to the deaths among aboriginal children after the government doctors gave them their immunization shots for diphtheria, pertussis, and tetanus (DPT). Every second child died. Kalokerinos knew it wasn't pneumonia or meningitis; it was the shots. He knew that the impoverished diet that these people were on could do nothing to support the immune system, so in the absence of the appropriate vitamins and minerals, the stress of the shots wiped them out.

On his own, Kalokerinos supplied each child in his district with some vitamin C. They received 1,000 milligrams (mg) per day per year of age. The two year olds got 2,000 mg a day and so on until age five, when they all got 5,000 mg per day. When the shots were administered, nobody died. Kalokerinos is still convinced that the DPT shots are the most likely cause of SIDS. (I believe that there must be at least 10 reasons for SIDS, and the DPT shots administered to a baby with a truncated immune system is but one.) When I heard this from Kalokerinos, I began to do this in my practice. I'd give a DPT shot in one of the baby's muscles, and immediately would give a shot of vitamin C (50 mg) mixed with the B complex (1 cubic centimeter total fluid) in another muscle. Infants that had trouble with irritability and fever with the previous shots had no trouble at all with this method. I am convinced I was shoring up the immune system by this method. If the vitamin-C and B-complex mixture is unavailable to parents, I have them give 1,000 mg of vitamin C, 100 mg of pyridoxine (vitamin B6), and 1,000 mg of calcium by mouth on the day before, the day of, and the day after the shots. People who are malnourished or under some stress will have trouble with shots; vitamins and minerals can be used preventively as well as therapeutically.

As time passed I became more and more enthusiastic about large doses of vitamin C and the B complex as therapy. I had to turn away from my teaching of the use of antibiotics. It was working. I billed insurance companies when I gave intravenous (IV) vitamin C, hoping they would see that this cheap, safe method was vastly superior to expensive hospital stays. What those companies were supposed to do is alert the other doctors that Smith was on to something and why doesn't everyone do this—it would save vast sums of money. Instead, they called the Board of Medical Examiners to say that Dr. Smith was doing something unproven and unsafe. The board suggested I retire.

I then realized that the only way to encourage a change in our health management was to show doctors and laypeople alike that there are other safe, effective, alternative methods of treatment. I discovered that the pressure from the pharmaceutical companies was so overwhelming and pervasive that the allopathic doctor feels compelled to

"No amount of evidence will persuade someone who is not listening."
—ABRAM HOFFER

treat everything with drugs. That is why I began to write my own books and put together the published works of the late Frederick Klenner in the *Clinical Guide to the Use of Vitamin C* (1988). Doctors tell me, "Smith, if you can get this nutrition stuff published in peer-review journals, I might believe you." So here it is. Now what are they all waiting for? Klenner began in the late 1930s to use vitamin C for almost any pathology, from viruses to germs, injuries to shock, coma to burns and snake bites. "While you are pondering the diagnosis," Klenner said, "give vitamin C."

He experimented on his own children: when one would come down with chickenpox or measles, he would give a small dose of C to help take the edge off the symptoms—maybe 200 mg two or three times per day. But his wife, Ann, upset with his experimenting, would plead, "Get them well, Fred." He would give them 1,000 mg every couple of hours and they would be well in a day or two.

Laughter with Vitamin C

I have been further encouraged by the work of the later Norman Cousins. He used to get a disease every 10 years and then write a book about it. The last illness did him in. His first book *An Anatomy of an Illness* (1979) was about his struggle with ankylosing spondylitis, a long-term type of arthritis that affects and the bones and joints at the base of the spine. This disease is very painful as it bends the victim into a pretzel-like position. He had heard about humor and vitamin C, so he talked his doctor into moving him out of the stifling hospital to a motel across the street and treat him with Groucho Marx movies and *Candid Camera* vignettes. Along with laughter therapy, he got intravenous vitamin C, at first a paltry 10,000 mg, but finally moving up to 20,000 mg at a time. He found that if he could laugh for 20 minutes, he would have two hours of

117

pain-free sleep. He could get the same blessed relief with the IV of vitamin C. They both had the same effect on pain. And his sedimentation rate (a test for inflammation in the body) would improve by about 10 percent—a meaningful change. He fully recovered from the ankylosing spondylitis, only to suffer from a devastating heart attack 10 years later. The assumption is that laughter or vitamin C will encourage the brain to produce endorphins, the brain's "feel-good" chemicals. Vitamin C is also a fighter against inflammation and helps the body make the stress hormone cortisol.

We cannot go back to the way we are meant to be in the hunting and gathering days of 2 million years ago. We have to make do with what we've got. Dr. Linus Pauling tells us that those ancestors were eating about 600 mg of vitamin C daily, and maybe far more. Food was whole and natural. A parting thought: eat food that rots, but eat it before it does rot.

CAN SUPPLEMENTS TAKE THE PLACE OF A BAD DIET?
by Andrew W. Saul, PhD

Can supplements take the place of a bad diet? They'd better. In spite of decades of intense and well-funded mass education, the great majority of adults and children in the United States do not consume even the government's very modest recommended daily quantities of fruits and vegetables. To a considerable degree, the people have spoken by their choices: they still eat terribly.

Vitamins Provide for Special Concerns

Traditional dieticians have set themselves the heroic but probably unattainable goal of getting every person to eat well every day. Even if obtained, such vitamin intake as good diet provides is inadequate to maintain optimum health for everyday people in real-life situations. Tens of millions of women have a special concern. Oral contraceptives lower serum levels of B vitamins, especially vitamin B6, plus niacin (B3), thiamine (B1), riboflavin (B2), vitamin B12, folic acid, and vitamin C.[1] It is uncommon, even rare, for a physician to instruct a woman to be sure to take supplemental vitamin C and B-complex vitamins as long as she is on the Pill.

Vitamins Fill in Nutritional Gaps

It is widely appreciated that at least 100 international units (IU) of vitamin E (and probably 400 IU or more) daily is required to prevent cardiovascular and other disease. Yet, it is literally impossible to obtain 100 IU of vitamin E from even the most perfectly planned diet. To demonstrate this, I've challenged my nutrition students to create a few days of "balanced" meals, using the food composition tables in any nutrition textbook, to achieve 100 IU of vitamin E per day. They could attempt their objective with any combination of foods and any plausible number of portions of each food. The only limitation was that they had to design meals that a person would actually be willing to eat.

As this ruled out prescribing whole grains by the pound and vegetable oils by the cup, they could not do it. Nor can the general public.

"Supplements" by definition are designed to fill nutritional gaps in a bad diet. They fill in what may be surprisingly large gaps in a good diet as well. In the case of vitamin E, doing so is likely to save millions of lives. A 1996 double-blind, placebo-controlled study of 2,002 patients with clogged arteries demonstrated a 77 percent decreased risk of heart attack in those taking 400 to 800 IU of vitamin E.[2] Again, such effective quantities of vitamin E positively cannot be obtained from diet alone.

To illustrate how extraordinarily important supplements are to people with a questionable diet, consider this: children who eat hot dogs once a week double their risk of a brain tumor. Kids eating more than twelve hot dogs a month (that's barely three hot dogs a week) have nearly ten times the risk of leukemia as children who eat none.[3] However, hot-dog-eating children taking supplemental vitamins were shown to have a reduced risk of cancer.[4] It is curious, that while theorizing many "potential" dangers of vitamins, the media often choose to ignore the very real cancer-prevention benefits of supplementation.

Vitamins Supply Nutrients Easily and Cheaply

Critics also fail to point out that supplements are economical. For low-income households, taking a three-cent vitamin C tablet and a five-cent multivitamin, readily obtainable from any discount store, is vastly cheaper than getting those vitamins by eating right. The uncomfortable truth is that it is often less expensive to supplement than to buy nutritious food, especially out-of-season fresh produce. Milligram for milligram, vitamin supplementation is vastly cheaper than trying to get vitamins from food.

Few people can afford to eat several dozen oranges a day. A single large orange costs at least 50 cents and may easily cost one dollar. It provides less than 100 milligrams (mg) of vitamin C. A bottle of 100 tablets of ascorbic acid vitamin C, 500 mg each, costs about five dollars. The supplement gives you 10,000 mg per dollar. In terms of vitamin C, the supplement is 50 to 100 times cheaper, costing about one or two cents for the amount of vitamin C in an orange. Those who wish to follow Linus Pauling's perennially wise recommendation to take daily multi-gram doses of vitamin C can do so easily and cheaply.

Vitamins Supply Nutrients Essential to Health

Since the ancient Egyptians, through the time of Hippocrates, and right up to the present, poor diet has been described and decried by physicians. Little has changed for the better, and much has changed for the worse. Though nutritionists place a nearly puritanical emphasis on food selection as our vitamin source, everyone else eats because they are hungry, because it makes them feel better, and because it gives pleasure. No one likes the "food police." Telling people what they should do is rarely an unqualified success, and with something as intensely personal as food, well, good luck. We could, of course, legislate Good Food Laws and make it against the law to make, sell, or eat junk. That is as likely to work as Prohibition.

Our somewhat less draconian choice of "noble experiment" has been to educate, to implore, and to exhort the citizenry to be "choosy chewers," to "eat a balanced diet," and to follow the food groups charts. The result? Obesity is more prevalent and cancer is no less prevalent. Cardiovascular disease is still the number one killer of men and women. "Health is the fastest growing failing business in western civilization," writes Emanuel Cheraskin, MD, in *Human Health and Homeostasis*.[5] "We can say with reasonable certainty that only about 6 percent of the adult population can qualify as 'clinically' healthy." We can try to sort out each of the many negative behavior variables (such as smoking), which certainly must be factored in. When we have done so, we are left with the completely unavoidable conclusion that our dinner tables are killing us.

Decide for Yourself

The good diet vs. supplement controversy may be reduced to four logical choices:

1) Shall we eat right and take supplements and be healthy?

2) Or, shall we eat right and take no supplements, be vitamin E and C deficient for our entire life span, and greatly increase our risk of sickness and death at any age?

3) Or, shall we eat wrong and take no supplements, and be even worse off?

4) Or, shall we eat wrong, but take daily vitamin supplements, and be a lot less sickly than if we did not take supplements?

While each of these four options constitutes a popular choice, there is one best health-promoting conclusion:

Supplements make any dietary lifestyle, whether good or bad, significantly better. Media supplement scare-stories notwithstanding, taking supplements is not the problem; it is a solution. Malnutrition is the problem. As it has been for thousands of years of human history, so malnutrition remains with us today. The biggest difference is that we are now malnourished even though overeating. Only in the last century have supplements even been available. Their continued use represents a true public health breakthrough on a par with clean drinking water and sanitary sewers, and can be expected to save as many lives.

REFERENCES

1. Wynn V. *Lancet* 1975 Mar 8;1(7906):561–564.
2. Stephens NG. *Lancet* 1996;347:781–786.
3. Peters JM. *Cancer Causes Control* 1994;5(2):195–202.
4. Sarasua S. *Cancer Causes Control* 1994;5(2):141–148.
5. Cheraskin E. *Human Health and Homeostasis*. Birmingham, AL: Natural Reader Press, 1999.

From the *J Orthomolecular Med* 2003;18(3&4):213–216.

CLINICAL PROCEDURES IN TREATING TERMINALLY ILL CANCER PATIENTS WITH VITAMIN C

by Abram Hoffer, MD, PhD

Let me tell you what I am not: I am not an oncologist, I'm not a pathologist, I'm not a general practitioner. I am a psychiatrist. Therefore, you may want to know what a psychiatrist is doing messing about with cancer. I think that's a legitimate question, so I'd like to tell you briefly how I got into this very interesting field.

In 1951, I was made director of psychiatric research for the Department of Health for the province of Saskatchewan in Canada. I didn't really know what to do. I had one major advantage, I think, over my colleagues. I didn't know any psychiatry. You may laugh but that's very important, because I didn't have anyone who could tell me what we could not do. The most important problem at that time was the schizophrenias. (Schizophrenia is a group of severe brain disorders that is characterized by delusions and hallucinations. It still takes up half the hospital beds and we still don't have an effective treatment for it.) Humphry Osmond and I began to research schizophrenia. We developed the hypothesis that those with schizophrenia were producing a toxic chemical made from adrenaline called adrenochrome. Adrenochrome is a hallucinogen that we felt was producing toxemia, in the sense that the adrenochrome worked on the brain in the same way as LSD. That was our hypothesis.

We knew that most hypotheses turn out to be wrong. We didn't think we were going to be correct, but we felt that since we didn't have much choice we ought to work with it and we also wanted to develop a treatment for our schizophrenic patients. Those were the days before tranquilizers. We didn't have any effective treatment. We had electroshock treatment, which was only temporarily helpful, and insulin coma therapy (the use of insulin to induce stupor) was going out of style.

Adrenochrome is made from adrenaline, a major stress hormone, so we thought that if we could do something to cut down the production of adrenaline and if we could also prevent the oxidation (burning) of adrenaline to adrenochrome, then we might have a therapy for our patients. And that immediately led us to look at two chemicals: one is called niacin (also known as niacinamide and vitamin B3). Vitamin B3 is known to be a methyl acceptor, which by depleting the body of its methyl groups, could cut down the conversion of noradrenaline to adrenaline and that would be helpful, we thought. The other chemical we wanted to use was vitamin C as an antioxidant. Looking back now it seems that we were 30 or 40 years ahead of antioxidant theories. We wanted to decrease the oxidation of adrenaline to adrenochrome. Vitamin C will do it but not very effectively. And that drew our attention to these two vitamins: vitamin C and niacin. I had an advantage because I had taken my PhD at the University of Minnesota on vitamins, so I knew their background. That's why we started working with these two compounds.

My Introduction to Cancer and Orthomolecular Treatment

Why did we start working with cancer? We were very curious about what these compounds would do. I recall that in 1952 when I was working as a resident in psychiatry at the General Hospital in Regina, a woman who had her breast removed for cancer was admitted to our ward. She was psychotic. This poor woman had developed a huge ulcerated lesion, she wasn't healing, and she was in a toxic delirium. Her psychiatrist decided that he would give her shock treatment. I decided I would like to give her vitamin C instead. As director of research, I had the option of going to the physicians and asking them if I could do this with their patients. A friend of mine was her doctor and he said, "Yes, you can have her." He said, "I'll withhold shock treatment for three days."

From the *J Orthomolecular Med* 1991;6(3&4):155–160.

I had thought that I would give her 3,000 milligrams (mg) per day, which was our usual dose at that time, for a period of weeks, but when he told me I could have three days only, I decided that this would not do. Therefore, I decided to give her 1,000 mg every hour. I instructed the nurses that she was to be given 1,000 mg per hour except when she was sleeping. When she awakened, she would get the vitamin C that she had missed. We started her on a Saturday morning and when her doctor came back on Monday morning to start shock treatment she was mentally normal. I wanted to know if vitamin C would have any therapeutic effect. To our amazement her lesion on her breast began to heal. She was discharged, mentally well, still having cancer and she died six months later from her cancer. This was an interesting observation that I had made at that time and that I have never forgotten.

There was another root to this interest. In 1959, we found that the majority of schizophrenic patients excreted in their urine a factor that we call the "mauve factor," which we have since identified as kryptopyrrole. I was looking for a good source of this urinary factor. We had thought that the majority of schizophrenics had it. We thought that normal people did not have it, but I was interested in determining how many people who were stressed also had the factor. Therefore, I ran a study of patients from the hospital who were on the physical wards. They had all sorts of physical conditions including cancer. I found to my amazement that half the people with lung cancer also excreted the same factor. By 1960, a very famous man of Saskatchewan, one of the professors, retired and was admitted to the psychiatric department at our hospital. He was psychotic. He had been diagnosed as having lung cancer. It had been biopsied and was visualized in the x-ray and it had also been seen in the bronchoscope. While his physicians were deciding what to do, he became psychotic so they concluded that the cancer had metastasized to his brain. Because he became psychotic, he was no longer operable and instead they gave him cobalt radiation. It didn't help the psychosis any. He was admitted to our ward where he stayed for about two months, completely psy-

chotic. He was placed on the terminal list. I discovered that he was on our ward, so I thought he might have some mauve factor in his urine. On analysis, he revealed huge quantities.

I had discovered by then that, if we gave large amounts of vitamin B3 along with vitamin C to these patients, regardless of their diagnosis, they tended to do very well. He was started on 3,000 mg per day, each of niacin and ascorbic acid, on a Friday. On Monday he was found to be normal. A few days later I said to him, "You understand that you have cancer?" He said, "Yes, I know that." He was friendly with me because I had treated his wife for alcoholism some time before. I said to him, "If you will agree to take these two vitamins as long as you live, I will provide them for you at no charge." In 1960, I was the only doctor in Canada who had access to large quantities of vitamin C and niacin. They were distributed through our hospital dispensary. He agreed. That meant he had to come to my office every month in order to pick up two bottles of vitamins. I didn't know that it might help his cancer. I was interested only in his psychological state.

However, to my amazement he didn't die. After 12 months, I was having lunch with the director of the cancer clinic, a friend of mine, and I said to him, "What do you think about this man?" And he said, "We can't understand it, we can't see the tumor anymore." I thought he'd say, "Well, isn't that great." So I asked, "Well, what's your reaction?" He responded, "We are beginning to think we made the wrong diagnosis." The patient died, 30 months after I first saw him, of a heart attack.

A Doctor Who Likes to Work with Vitamins

Here's another case that is very interesting. A couple of years later, a mother I had treated for depression came back to see me. Once more she was depressed. She said she had a daughter, age 16, who had just been diagnosed as having bone cancer of the arm. Her surgeon had recommended that the arm be amputated. She was very depressed over this and so I asked her, "Do you think you can persuade your surgeon not to amputate the arm right away?" And I told her the story about the man with the lung cancer. She brought her daughter in, and I started her on 3,000 mg of niacin per day, plus 3,000 mg of vitamin C per day. She made a complete recovery and is still well, not having had to have surgery.

When I moved to Victoria, British Columbia, another strange event happened. In 1979, a woman developed jaundice and during surgery a 6 centimeter in diameter lump in the head (first part) of the pancreas was found. The surgeons were too frightened to do a biopsy, which apparently is quite standard. They thought that the biopsy might cause the tumor to spread. The surgeon closed the incision and told the woman to write her will. They said she might have three to six months at the most. She was a very tough lady and she had read Norman Cousins's book *Anatomy of an Illness* (1979). So, she said to her doctor, "To hell with that, I'm not going to die." And she began to take vitamin C on her own, 12,000 mg per day. When her doctor discovered what she was doing, he asked her to come and see me because by that time I was identified as a doctor who likes to work with vitamins.

"Without health there is no happiness. An attention to health, then, should take the place of every other object."
—THOMAS JEFFERSON, *1787*

I started her on 40,000 mg of vitamin C per day, to which I added niacin, zinc, and a multivitamin/multimineral preparation. I had her change her diet by staying away from large amounts of protein and fat. I didn't hear from her again for about six months. One Sunday, she called me. Normally when I get a call from a patient on a Sunday, it's bad news. She immediately said, "Dr. Hoffer, good news!" I asked, "What's happened?" She said, "They have just done a computer tomography (CT) scan and they can't see the tumor." So then she said, "They couldn't believe it. They thought the machine had gone wrong; so they did it all over again. And it was also negative the sec-

ond time." She had her last CT scan in 1984, no mass, and she is still alive and well today.

By this time I had learned about Ewan Cameron's and Linus Pauling's work with vitamin C, and I began to realize that the main therapeutic factor might be vitamin C rather than vitamin B3. The reason I want to present four cases is that one might say that I have seen four spontaneous recoveries and the question is, how many spontaneous recoveries would one physician see in his lifetime? I don't know. Maybe this is not unusual, but I think it is.

The last cancer case I'm going to give details of was born in 1908. His mother died of cancer and his father had a heart attack at the age of 80. My patient had had a heart attack in 1969, and again in 1977, followed by a coronary bypass. In March 1978, he suddenly developed pain in his left groin and down the left leg. In February 1979, he developed a bulge in his left groin, and later, severe pain with movement. In surgery, a large-mass, invasive tumor was found, part of which was removed. But a mass the size of a grapefruit was left. The tumor was eroding into the pubic ramus at the front of the pelvis. In March, he had palliative radiation. The pain was gone at the end of the radiation. On May 28, he developed a severe staph infection, and in June he was very depressed because his wife was dying of cancer and also he was suffering from drainage of chronic infection. In July, he still had a purulent discharge in two areas. Now the mass was visible and palpable in the groin and lower part of the abdomen.

In January 1980, he saw me for the first time. I started him on 12,000 mg of vitamin C per day and I recommended to his referring doctor that he give him intravenous ascorbic acid, 2,500 mg, twice per week, which he agreed to. I gave him niacin, pyridoxine (vitamin B6), and zinc to balance it out. In April, the mass began to regress and the oncologist wrote, "This is interesting. It must be something else." In other words, the patient said, the vitamin C is helping and the oncologist said, no it isn't. The oncologist put a note in the file, "He's probably responding to chemotherapy." But he had never had chemotherapy. The infection was gone. In May 1980, his x-ray showed reconstruction of the left superior pubic ramus. In July, he wrote to me telling how grateful he was to be so well. In February 1988, he went back to the cancer clinic for some recurrent facial skin carcinoma. He died in the fall of 1989 of coronary disease when he was 81. This man survived 10 years after having been diagnosed with cancer.

Nutrients and Hope

My practice began to grow because the first patient felt it was her duty to tell as many people as possible that I had the cure for cancer. Now I should tell you the nature of my practice. In Canada we have a referral service. I do not take walk-ins. Every patient that comes to my office must be referred by their family doctor or by a specialist. During the early years, patients usually went to their doctor and said, "I have had all this treatment, you have told me I'm not going to do any better, will you please refer me to Dr. Hoffer." So I call these patient-generated referrals. The past four or five years, it has swung around and I am now getting a lot more doctor-generated referrals. Doctors, themselves are beginning to refer their patients to me.

I would think that 80 percent of my patients had failed to respond to any combination of treatment, including surgery, radiation, or chemotherapy. Usually, the story was that they were told by either the cancer clinic or their doctor that there was nothing more that they could do. Most of them were terminal, but not all. I see three to five new cases of cancer every week. All of them have been treated by their own doctor, their own oncologist, their own surgeon. What I do is advise them with respect to diet and the kind of nutrients they ought to take. I try to improve their general health and immune system to the point that it can cope more successfully with their tumors. Many of these patients were depressed when they came to see me. The first thing I do is to create a bit of hope. I don't think many doctors in cancer clinics realize the absolute importance of hope.

Hope is extremely important. Attitude is very important. Patients must want to live. You may be surprised to know that many people, when they are told they have cancer, are quite relieved, because they now know they don't have to live much longer. They are really quite happy to go. So you

have to test the attitude of the patient. Those who came to see me, of course, were preselected, they selected themselves. So they did have the right attitude; they did want to live. They have to be optimistic and I do think it helps if they laugh a lot. I agree with Norman Cousins, that if you combine laughter with vitamins, you do get better results.

Then I advise my patients on what kind of nutrition they ought to follow. The first thing I try to do is to cut their fat intake way down. I try to cut it down below 30 percent of calories, down to 20 or 10 percent, if possible. I find that, in our culture, the easiest way to do that is to totally eliminate all dairy products. If you eliminate all dairy products and cut out all fatty meats, it's pretty hard to get too much fat in the diet. So, I put all my patients on a dairy-free program. I reduce but I don't eliminate meat and fish, and I ask them to increase their vegetable intake, especially of raw vegetables, as much as they can. I think it's a good, reasonable diet that most people can follow without too much difficulty.

Having spent some time with them going over what they ought to eat, I begin to talk about the nutrients. The first one, of course, is vitamin C. I am convinced today that vitamin C is the most important single nutrient that one can give to any person with cancer. The dose is variable. I find that most patients can take 12,000 mg of crystalline vitamin C per day without much difficulty. They take 1 teaspoon three times a day. If they do not develop diarrhea, I ask them to increase it until this occurs and then to cut back below that level. I think in many cases it would be desirable to use intravenous vitamin C and there are doctors now in Canada doing that. The amount that one gives is limited by the skill of the physician, not by the patient.

I also add vitamin B3, either niacin or niacinamide. I prescribe from 500 mg to 1,500 mg per day. Before I did that empirically, now there is a lot of evidence that B3 does have pretty interesting anticancer properties. I also add a B-complex preparation with 50 or 100 mg of each major B vitamin. I think vitamin E is an extremely important antioxidant and I use 800 to 1,200 international units (IU) of that as well. They also get 25,000 to 75,000 IU of beta-carotene and sometimes I use preformed vitamin A. I like to use folic acid for lung cancer, and for cancer of the uterus. I use selenium (200 micrograms) three times per day. I use some zinc, especially for prostatic cancers and I do use calcium-magnesium preparations. So this is the basic nutrient program that they all follow. The cost of the supplements is relatively low.

What are this program's advantages? Well, first of all, the increase in longevity. We have increased the longevity from 5.7 months to approximately 100 months, which is very substantial, and half the patients are still alive. There has been a tremendous decrease in pain and anxiety, even among those who were dying. We do not have the final answer, but we have at least a partial answer. The use of nutrients like vitamin C and B3 increase the efficacy of chemotherapy by increasing its killing effect on the tumor and decreasing its toxicity on normal tissues. The same has been shown to be true with radiation therapy. My conclusion is that vitamin C must be a vital component of every cancer treatment program. I believe the other nutrients help, adding 20 to 30 percent to longevity.

I am not telling you that we have a treatment for cancer. I say that we have improved the results of treatment. My conclusion is that the best treatment for cancer today is a combination of the best that modern medicine can offer—surgery, radiation, chemotherapy—combined with the best of what orthomolecular physicians can offer, which is nutrition, nutrients, and hope.

PART TWO

PIONEERS OF ORTHOMOLECULAR MEDICINE

BETWEEN 1930 AND 1950 MOST of the vitamins were discovered and their chemical structures determined. This was the golden age of vitamin discovery. Some of the excitement filtered into our medical schools, but it was effectively quenched after 1950 by a number of events such as the discovery of antibiotics and the wonder drugs. Physicians lost interest in nutrition and turned it over to biochemists and non-clinical nutritionists. Medical schools happily turned to medicine, surgery, psychiatry, and the minor specialties. Away from patients, nutritionists lost the incentive that moves physicians to make discoveries—patients who do not get well. We all, patients and public, were the losers.

Then, in 1968, Linus Pauling made a statement that would challenge more medical paradigms than practically any other he'd ever made: "Orthomolecular therapy consists in the prevention and treatment of disease by varying the concentrations in the human body of substances that are normally present." Since then, the *Journal of Orthomolecular Medicine* has continuously published new research expanding our understanding of orthomolecular medicine and verifying its effectiveness. Such work has been possible only because of the foundational contributions of inquisitive and innovative clinicians in decades past. Part Two presents brief biographies of those who, through their observation, and analysis, advanced knowledge in the orthomolecular field in significant (and usually controversial) ways.

Many of these pioneering men and women are inductees into the Orthomolecular Medicine Hall of Fame. An event that was established in 2004 to honor and not forget the scientists, physicians, and biochemists who have discovered vitamins, their properties, and their clinical uses. Without their work, nutritional therapy would have remained very primitive, and orthomolecular therapy, solidified under Dr. Linus Pauling's excellent term, would not have arisen.

— ABRAM HOFFER, *Journal of Orthomolecular Psychiatry* 1984

(updated by A.W.S.)

Editor's note: Most of these individual profiles were written by Andrew W. Saul or Steven Carter. Other contributors are listed individually.

A TIME LINE OF ORTHOMOLECULAR MEDICINE

by Andrew W. Saul, PhD

1935: Claus Washington Jungeblut, MD, professor of bacteriology at Columbia University, first publishes on vitamin C as prevention and treatment for polio; in the same year, Jungeblut also shows that vitamin C inactivates diphtheria toxin.

1936: Evan Shute, MD, and Wilfrid Shute, MD, of Ontario, Canada, demonstrate that vitamin E-rich wheat germ oil cures angina.

1937: Dr. Jungeblut demonstrates that ascorbate (vitamin C) inactivated tetanus toxin.

1939: William Kaufman, MD, PhD, in Connecticut, successfully treats arthritis with niacinamide (vitamin B3).

1940: The Shute brothers publish that vitamin E prevents fibroids and endometriosis, and is curative for atherosclerosis.

1942: Ruth Flinn Harrell, PhD, at Columbia University, measures the positive effect of added thiamine (vitamin B1) on learning.

1945: Vitamin E is shown to cure hemorrhages in the skin and mucous membranes, and to decrease the diabetic's need for insulin.

1946: Vitamin E is shown to greatly improve wound healing, including skin ulcers. It is also demonstrated that vitamin E strengthens and regulates heartbeat, and is effective in cases of claudication, acute nephritis, thrombosis, cirrhosis, and phlebitis; also, William J. McCormick, MD, shows how vitamin C prevents and also cures kidney stones.

1947: Vitamin E is successfully used as therapy for gangrene, inflammation of blood vessels (Buerger's disease), retini-tis, and choroiditis; Roger J. Williams, PhD, publishes on how vitamins can be used to treat alcoholism.

1948: Frederick R. Klenner, MD, a board-certified specialist in diseases of the chest, publishes cures of 41 cases of viral pneumonia using very high doses of vitamin C.

1949: Dr. Kaufman publishes *The Common Form of Joint Dysfunction*.

1950: Vitamin E is shown to be an effective treatment for lupus erythematosus, varicose veins, and severe body burns.

1951: Vitamin D treatment is found to be effective against Hodgkin's disease (a cancer of the lymphatic system) and epithelioma.

1954: Abram Hoffer, MD, PhD, and colleagues demonstrate that niacin can cure schizophrenia; the Shutes' medical textbook *Alpha Tocopherol in Cardiovascular Disease* is published; and Dr. McCormick reports that cancer patients tested for vitamin C were seriously deficient, often by as much as 4,500 milligrams.

1955: Niacin is first shown to lower serum cholesterol.

1956: Mayo Clinic researcher William Parsons, MD, and colleagues confirm Dr. Hoffer's use of niacin to lower cholesterol and prevent cardiovascular disease; Dr. Harrell demonstrates that supplementation of the pregnant and lactating mothers' diet with vitamins increases the intelligence quotients of their offspring at three and four years of age.

1957: Dr. McCormick publishes on how vitamin C fights cardiovascular disease.

A TIME LINE . . . CONTINUED

1960: Dr. Hoffer meets Bill W., cofounder of Alcoholics Anonymous, and uses niacin to eliminate Bill's long-standing chronic depression.

1963: Vitamin D is shown to prevent breast cancer.

1964: Vitamin D is found to be effective against lymph nodal reticulosarcoma (a non-Hodgkin's lymphatic cancer).

1968: Linus Pauling, PhD, publishes the theoretical basis of high-dose nutrient therapy (orthomolecular medicine) in psychiatry in *Science*, and soon after defines orthomolecular medicine as "the treatment of disease by the provision of the optimum molecular environment, especially the optimum concentrations of substances normally present in the human body."

1969: Robert F. Cathcart, MD, uses large doses of vitamin C to treat pneumonia, hepatitis, and, years later, acquired immune deficiency syndrome (AIDS).

1970: Dr. Pauling publishes *Vitamin C and the Common Cold* and Dr. Williams publishes *Nutrition Against Disease*.

1972: Publication of *The Healing Factor: "Vitamin C" Against Disease* by Irwin Stone, PhD.

1973: Dr. Klenner publishes his vitamin supplement protocol to arrest and reverse multiple sclerosis; so does H. T. Mount, MD, reporting on 27 years of success using thiamine. Also, Ewan Cameron, MD, and Dr. Pauling publish their first joint paper on the control of cancer with vitamin C, two years after Cameron began using high-dose intravenous vitamin C.

1975: Hugh D. Riordan, MD, and colleagues successfully use large doses of intravenous vitamin C against cancer.

1976: Ewan Cameron, MD, and other physicians in Scotland show that intravenous vitamin C improved quality and length of life in terminal cancer patients.

1977: Alfred Libby, MD, and Dr. Stone present findings that the use of high doses of vitamins hastens and eases withdrawal from highly addictive drugs.

1981: Dr. Harrell and colleagues demonstrate that very high doses of nutritional supplements help overcome learning disabilities in children, and bring about highly significant improvement to those with Down syndrome.

1982: In Japan, Murata, Morishige, and Yamaguchi show that vitamin C greatly prolonged the lives of terminal cancer patients.

1984: Robert F. Cathcart, MD, publishes on the vitamin C treatment of AIDS.

1986: Publication of *How to Live Longer and Feel Better* by Linus Pauling.

1988: Dr. Lendon H. Smith publishes *Vitamin C as a Fundamental Medicine: Abstracts of Dr. Frederick R. Klenner's Published and Unpublished Work*, now known as *Clinical Guide to the Use of Vitamin C*.

1990: American doctors successfully use vitamin C to treat kidney cancer, and, in 1995 and 1996, other cancers.

A TIME LINE . . . CONTINUED

1993: Large-scale studies show that vitamin E supplementation reduces the risk of coronary heart disease in men and women.

1995: Dr. Riordan and colleagues publish their protocol for intravenous vitamin C treatment of cancer.

2002: Vitamin E shown to improve immune functions in patients with advanced colorectal cancer, by immediately increasing T-helper 1 cytokine production.

2004: Doctors in America and Puerto Rico publish more clinical cases of vitamin C successes against cancer.

2005: Research sponsored by the U.S. National Institutes of Health shows that high levels of vitamin C kill cancer cells without harming normal cells.

2006: Canadian doctors report intravenous vitamin C is successful in treating cancer.

2007: Harold D. Foster, PhD, and colleagues publish a double-blind, randomized clinical trial showing that HIV-positive patients given supplemental nutrients can delay or stop their decline into AIDS.

2008: Korean doctors report that intravenous vitamin C "plays a crucial role in the suppression of proliferation of several types of cancer," notably melanoma. And, natural vitamin E is demonstrated to substantially reduce risk of lung cancer by 61 percent.

2009, 2010, 2012: Intravenous Vitamin C and Cancer symposiums filmed and made available for free access online at:

www.riordanclinic.org/education/symposium/s2009 (12 lectures)

www.riordanclinic.org/education/symposium/s2010 (9 lectures)

and www.riordanclinic.org/education/symposium/s2012 (11 lectures)

2011: Each 20 micromole per liter (μmol/L) increase in plasma vitamin C is associated with a 9 percent reduction in death from heart failure. Also, B-complex vitamins are associated with a 7 percent decrease in mortality, and vitamin D with an 8 percent decrease in mortality.

2012: Vitamin C shown to prevent and treat radiation-damaged DNA.

2013: B-vitamin supplementation found to slow the atrophy of specific brain regions that are a key component of the Alzheimer's disease process and are associated with cognitive decline.

2014: In patients with mild to moderate Alzheimer's disease, 2,000 international units (IU) of vitamin E slows the decline compared to a placebo. Data from 561 patients showed that those taking vitamin E function significantly better in daily life, and required the least care; vitamin C greatly reduces chemotherapy side effects and improves cancer-patient survival.

From the *Orthomolecular Medicine News Service*, February 15, 2014.

HALL OF FAME PIONEERS

Ilya Metchnikov, PhD

(1845–1916) • Hall of Fame 2009

"Death begins in the colon."—ILYA METCHNIKOV

Born in 1845 in Ukraine, Ilya Metchnikov studied natural sciences at the University of Kharkov and pioneered research in immunology. In 1904, he became the deputy director at the Pasteur Institute laboratory in Paris from where he discovered the process of phagocytosis, which demonstrated how specific white blood cells can engulf and destroy harmful bacteria in the body. His theories were radical and the "sophisticated" microbe hunters in the West—Louis Pasteur, Emil von Behring, and others—scorned the Russian and his humble theory.

Nevertheless, history vindicated Metchnikov's brilliant theory and he was awarded the Nobel Prize for medicine in 1908.

Although references to the nutritional power of fermented foods date back thousands of years, Ilya (anglicized as Élie) Metchnikov is regarded as the father of modern probiotics. He made a landmark observation that the regular consumption of lactic acid bacteria in fermented dairy products, such as yogurt, was associated with enhanced health and longevity in Bulgarian peasant populations. He linked this to the "Bulgarian bacillus," which was discovered by a 27-year-old Bulgarian physician Stamen Grigorov, and he later demonstrated how healthy bacteria in yogurt helped digestion and improved the immune system. The reduction of the harmful bacteria coupled with the increase in good bacteria in the intestines appear to improve the immune system and reduce the burden on the cleansing organs such as the kidneys and liver.

The scientific rationale for the health benefit of lactic acid bacteria was provided in his book *The Prolongation of Life* published in 1907, in which he asserted that some of the bacterial organisms present in the large intestine were a source of toxic substances that contributed to illness and aging. This book also delved into the potential life-lengthening properties of lactic acid bacteria. He suggested that "the dependence of the intestinal microbes on the food makes it possible to adopt measures to modify the flora in our bodies and to replace the harmful microbes by useful microbes." He wrote two other books: *Immunity in Infectious Diseases* (1905) and *The Nature of Man* (1938).

In recognition of Metchnikov's place in the probiotic realm, the International Dairy Federation created, in 2007, the IDF Élie Metchnikov Prize to recognize outstanding scientific discoveries in the fields of microbiology, biotechnology, nutrition, and health with regard to fermented milk products.

Joseph Goldberger, MD

(1874–1929) • Hall of Fame 2008

"Goldberger is my model of a brilliant scientist."
—ABRAM HOFFER

Joseph Goldberger was born in 1874 and studied medicine at Bellevue Hospital Medical School in New York, graduating with honors in 1895. After an internship at Bellevue Hospital College, he engaged in private practice for two years and then joined the Public Health Service Corps in 1899. During routine work as a quarantine officer on Ellis Island, Goldberger rapidly acquired a reputation for outstanding investigative studies of various infectious diseases, including yellow fever, dengue fever, and typhus. Goldberger devoted the latter part of his career to studying pellagra. After quickly contradicting the contemporary general belief that pellagra was an infectious disease, he spent the last 15 years of his life trying to prove that its cause was a dietary deficiency. During the first half of the 20th century, an epidemic of pellagra produced roughly 3 million cases in the United States, about 100,000 of which were fatal (from Elmore JG, et al. "Joseph Goldberger: an unsung hero of American clinical epidemiology." *Ann Intern Med* 1994).

Abram Hoffer adds: "In the early 1940s, the U.S. government mandated the addition of niacinamide (a form of niacin or vitamin B3) to flour. This eradicated the terrible pandemic of pellagra in just two years, and ought to be recognized as the most successful public health measure for the elimination of a major disease in psychiatry: the pellagra psychoses. The reaction of contemporary physicians was predictable. Indeed, at the time, Canada rejected the idea and declared the addition of vitamins to flour to be an adulteration. The United States has long been the leading nation in nutrition research."

Knowledge comes at a cost: Goldberger had yellow fever, dengue fever, and very nearly died of typhus. The U.S. National Institutes of Health says he "stepped on Southern pride when he linked the poverty of Southern sharecroppers, tenant farmers, and mill workers to the deficient diet that caused pellagra" (http://history.nih.gov/exhibits/goldberger/index.html).

In the end, Goldberger was nominated for the Nobel Prize. Had he not died earlier in the year, he might well have shared it in 1929 with vitamin researchers Christiaan Eijkman and Frederick G. Hopkins.

Alan Kraut's prize-winning book *Goldberger's War: The Life and Work of a Public Health Crusader* (2003) is an excellent source on this outstanding pioneer.

William McCormick, MD

(1880–1968) • Hall of Fame 2004

"Vitamin C is a specific antagonist of chemical and bacterial toxins."—WILLIAM MCCORMICK

Over 50 years ago, it was Toronto physician William McCormick, who pioneered the idea that poor collagen formation, due to vitamin C deficiency, was a principal cause of diverse conditions ranging from stretch marks to cardiovascular disease and cancer. This theory would become the foundation for Linus Pauling and Ewan Cameron's decision to employ large doses of vitamin C to fight cancer.

Over 20 years before Pauling, McCormick had already reviewed the nutritional causes of heart disease and noted that four out of five coronary cases in hospitals show vitamin C deficiency. McCormick also early proposed vitamin C deficiency as the essential cause of, and effective cure for, numerous communicable illnesses, becoming an early advocate of using vitamin C as an antiviral and an antibiotic. Modern writers often pass by the fact that McCormick actually advocated vitamin C to prevent and cure the formation of some kidney stones as far back as 1946. And 50 years ago, McCormick "found, in clinical and laboratory research, that the smoking of one cigarette neutralizes in the body approximately 25 milligrams of ascorbic acid." His early use of gram-sized doses to combat what then and now are usually regarded as nondeficiency-related illnesses set the stage for today's 100,000-millgrams-a-day, antiviral/anticancer intravenous injections of vitamin C.

Max Gerson, MD

(1881–1959) • Hall of Fame 2005

"I know of one patient who turned to Gerson therapy having been told she was suffering from terminal cancer and would not survive another course of chemotherapy. Happily, seven years later, she is alive and well. So it is vital that, rather than dismissing such experiences, we should further investigate the beneficial nature of these treatments."

—H.R.H. CHARLES, Prince of Wales

In the late 1920s, Max Gerson, a German physician who had left Nazi Germany for the United States before it was too late to leave, began observing that cancer could be cured with nutrition in tandem with systemic detoxification. His daughter Charlotte Gerson writes: "Dr. Gerson found that the underlying problems of all cancer patients are toxicity and deficiency. One of the important features of his therapy was the hourly administration of fresh vegetable juices. These supply ample nutrients [especially vitamin C, potassium, and important enzymes], as well as fluids to help flush out the kidneys. When the high level of nutrients re-enter tissues, toxins accumulated over many years are forced into the bloodstream. The toxins are then filtered out by the liver. The liver is easily overburdened by the continuous release of toxins and is unable to release the load . . . Dr. Gerson found that he could provide help to the liver by the caffeine in coffee, absorbed from the colon via the hemorrhoidal vein, which carries the caffeine to the portal system and then to the liver. The caffeine stimulates the liver/bile ducts to open, releasing the poisons into the intestinal tract for excretion."

The Gerson therapy is not specifically a cancer treatment but rather a metabolic treatment, one that cleanses while strengthening the body's ability to heal itself. In addition to the administration of fresh vegetable juices and liver-detoxifying coffee enemas, the therapy emphasizes a strict fat-free, salt-free, low-protein, essentially vegetarian dietary regimen with large doses of supplements, particularly vitamin C, potassium, iodine, digestive enzymes, niacin, thyroid, liver extracts, and vitamin B12. Not surprisingly, the program is effective against a wide variety of serious illnesses. Gerson's approach has been shown, for over seven decades, to greatly improve both quality and length of life in the sickest of patients.

There is no higher compliment possible than this summation by the great Dr. Albert Schweitzer, Nobel Prize laureate: "I see in Dr. Max Gerson one of the most eminent geniuses in medical history."

Casimir Funk, PhD

(1884–1967) • Hall of Fame 2010

"I had already at that time (1912) no doubt about the importance and the future popularity of the new field."
—CASIMIR FUNK

Casimir Funk is remembered as an outstanding biochemist and early explorer in the field of nutritional science, who is best known for the first formulation of the concept of vitamins in 1912. It was Funk who coined the term "vitamine," to describe compounds that were "vital" to health and were centered around an "amine" group. He also postulated the existence of vitamins B1, B2, C, and D. In 1936, he determined the molecular structure of thiamin and was the first to isolate niacin, vitamin B3. He discovered that many human diseases are caused by a lack of particular nutrients that are readily available in certain foods. He found cures for such devastating illnesses as beriberi, pellagra, rickets, and scurvy. Funk later did extensive research on hormones.

Born in Warsaw, Poland, the son of a renowned dermatologist, Casimir Funk studied organic chemistry at Switzerland's University of Berne, from which he received his PhD in 1904. Funk worked at the Pasteur Institute in Paris until 1906, and then at London's Lister Institute of Preventative Medicine. It was at the Lister Institute that Funk's career as a scientist truly began. He was assigned to research beriberi, a common illness in the Far East that causes peripheral nerve damage and heart failure. Scientists had thought the disease was due to insufficient dietary protein, but Funk discovered that the typical Far Eastern diet of polished rice was deficient in thiamine. Adding this vitamin back into the diet cured beriberi. Later that year, he isolated a substance now known as niacin (vitamin B3). When he published his findings in 1912 and his book *The Vitamin*, in 1913, Funk immediately became well known in the scientific world.

The publication of *The Vitamin* earned him public recognition and a Beit Fellowship from the University of London. He become head of the biochemistry department at the Cancer Hospital Research Institute and later became head of research at H. A. Metz and Company, where he remained until 1921. While at Metz, Funk developed a vitamin A and D concentrate. He began a job in New York as a consulting scientist for the U.S. Vitamin Corporation, and in 1940 he became president of the Funk Foundation for Medical Research.

During his lifetime, Funk published more than 140 articles, advanced humankind's understanding of nutrition, and revolutionized the way people looked at their health. His original insight that lack of vitamins in the diet was responsible for disease helped develop effective preventive and curative measures for anemia, beriberi, rickets, and pellagra. The Polish Institute of Arts and Sciences of America annually honors Polish-American scientists with the Casimir Funk Natural Sciences Award. —STEVEN CARTER AND GREG SCHILHAB

considered him to be one of his peers in the fight for the acceptance of nutritional medicine.

Cornelis Moerman was a practicing physician for over 55 years. His work lives on today in the "Moermanvereniging," an ever-growing Dutch association of patients who advocate nutritional therapy for cancer. —GERT SCHUITEMAKER AND A.W.S.

Cornelis Moerman, MD

(1893–1988) • Hall of Fame 2005

"Dr. Moerman was a steadfast pioneer in the successful treatment of cancer with good nutrition and dietary supplements, the first Dutch orthomolecular doctor."

—GERT SCHUITEMAKER

Cornelis Moerman withstood the strongest opposition of his colleagues during his entire professional life. Even today in the Netherlands, his name remains symbolic, forever connected to nutritional therapy, especially of cancer. Prior to World War II, Dr. Moerman published his view that cancer is not a local disease, but the tumor is the end stage of the deterioration of the total body. Strengthening the immune system, he said, is the answer to this disease, and nutrition plays the central role.

Moerman, a passionate pigeon-fancier, observed that healthy birds did not develop cancer, whereas the weak and malnourished ones did. He argued, based on his own experiments with his pigeons, that cancer was a derangement of metabolism, a deficiency of iodine, citric acid, B vitamins, iron, sulfur, and the vitamins A, D, E, and later C. A strictly proper diet, supplemented with these substances, forms the basis of the Moerman therapy.

Cutting-edge nutritional science has now caught up with Dr. Moerman's viewpoint. His principles for the treatment of cancer were, at the time, revolutionary. In September 1976, Moerman was invited by Linus Pauling to the conference of the International Association of Cancer Victors and Friends in Los Angeles. As the guest of honor, Moerman received an award for his valuable work with cancer patients and for his original approach to the treatment of cancer. Meeting Moerman, Dr. Linus Pauling praised him and

Albert Szent-Györgyi, MD, PhD

(1893–1986) • Hall of Fame 2005

"Discovery consists of seeing what everybody has seen and thinking what nobody has thought."

—ALBERT SZENT-GYÖRGYI

"Dr. Szent-Györgyi depended on thought, as did Pauling, rather than on equipment," wrote Abram Hoffer. Albert Szent-Györgyi was born in Hungary and spent World War I in the Austrian army. After the war, he studied at Groningen in the Netherlands and with biochemist Frederick Hopkins at Cambridge. It was here that he became interested in a chemical agent, present in plant juices, which had the effect of delaying oxidation, such as the browning of a sliced apple exposed to the air. He suggested that this agent, which was also present in cabbages and oranges, was the mysterious vitamin. By 1933, he had isolated the substance in kilogram lots and named it "ascorbic acid," which means "the acid that prevents scurvy."

At that time, most researchers saw vitamins as substances required in miniscule amounts to prevent deficiency diseases, such as scurvy. However, writes Jack J. Challem, "Szent-Györgyi quickly began to see vitamin requirements in terms different from those of his peers. He questioned the validity of minimal daily requirements to prevent disease and asked instead the implications of the *dosis optima quotidiana*—the quantity of vitamins needed to achieve optimal health. 'I think we must call perfect health not the absense of scurvy or other disease,' he said, 'but a condition of the body in which it is capable of the highest performances, in which it shows the greatest resistance against all noxious influences, physical, chemical and biological'" (*J Orthomolecular Med* 1997;12:77).

"During World War II, Szent-Györgyi was in constant danger from the Nazis and finally took refuge in the Swedish legation in Budapest. The Gestapo raided the legation but he escaped and remained in hiding for the rest of the war. He was rescued by the Russian armies and taken to Moscow on the direct orders of Soviet Foreign Minister Vyacheslav Molotov. He went to the United States in 1947 where he settled at the Marine Biological Laboratories at Woods Hole, Massachusetts" (from *Albert Szent-Györgyi and Vitamin C* by Nigel Bunce and Jim Hunt, University of Guelph, 1987).

"Albert Szent-Gyorgyi, MD, PhD, won the 1937 Nobel Prize for his discovery of vitamin C. In fact, it was he who named the vitamin ascorbic acid and first predicted its use in cancer. When Szent-Györgyi was on his deathbed, at the age of 93, Linus Pauling flew from California to Szent-Györgyi's home at Woods Hole to say goodbye. Holding his hand, Linus said wistfully, 'You know, Albert, I always thought that someday we two would work together.' Szent-Györgyi looked up and said, humorously, 'Well, if not in this life, then maybe in the next'" (from the *Cancer Decisions Newsletter* by Ralph Moss, July 18, 2004).

Roger J. Williams, PhD

(1893–1988) • Hall of Fame 2004

"When in doubt, try nutrition first."
—ROGER J. WILLIAMS

Another pioneer in the concept of orthomolecular nutrition was Roger Williams, professor of chemistry, discoverer of pantothenic acid (vitamin B5), and founder and director of the Clayton Foundation Biochemical Institute at the University of Texas, which under the directorship of Dr. Williams, was responsible for more vitamin-related discoveries than any other laboratory in the world. He also developed the genetotrophic concept of biochemical individuality or biological diversity.

Biochemical individuality is the concept that the chemical makeup and nutritional needs of each person are unique. According to Williams, the concept formed the basis of this new approach to nutrition: "The nutritional microenvironment of our body cells is crucially important to our health, and deficiencies in this environment constitute a major cause of disease." Making sure the body has all the raw materials it needs to function properly—and that higher than usual needs for certain nutrients are met—can influence our health and our susceptibility to, and treatment of, disease.

Williams was the son of missionary parents and was born in India. At age two, his family returned to the United States, where he grew up in Kansas and California. His formal education culminated in a PhD degree from the University of Chicago. It was while he was at Chicago that he did his initial work on pantothenic acid. He taught at the University of Oregon, Oregon State University, and, beginning in 1940, at the University of Texas at Austin.

Williams became president of the American Chemical Society in 1957. His *New York Times* obituary notes, "His first book, *Introduction to Organic Chemistry*, published in 1928, was an instant success and within a year was used as a text by more than 300 colleges. Among his other books were *Nutrition and Alcoholism* (1951), *Free and Unequal* (1953), *Nutrition Against Disease* (1971) and the *Physicians' Handbook of Nutritional Science* (1975)" (*NYT*, Glenn Fowler, Feb 23, 1988).

He was nearly killed by an unexpected individual reaction to a common drug in surgery—an event that changed his life and led to study of biochemical individuality and to the writing of his most well-known book *Biochemical Individuality* (1956).

William Griffin Wilson

(1895–1971) • Hall of Fame 2006

"Bill Wilson is the greatest social architect of the 20th century." —ALDOUS HUXLEY

The man who would cofound Alcoholics Anonymous (AA) was born to a hard-drinking household in rural Vermont. When he was ten, his parents split up and Bill was raised by his maternal grandparents. He served in the Army in World War I, and, although not seeing combat, Bill had more than ample opportunities to drink. In the 1920s, Wilson achieved considerable success as an inside trader on Wall Street, but a combination of drunkenness and the stock market crash drained what was left of his fortune and his capability to enjoy life. Hard knocks, religious experience, and a growing sense that by helping other alcoholics he could best help himself led Bill to create one of the world's most famous introductions: "My name is Bill W., and I'm an alcoholic."

Even as Alcoholics Anonymous slowly grew, many of Bill's financial and personal problems endured, most notably depression. Abram Hoffer writes: "I met Bill in New York in 1960. Humphry Osmond and I introduced him to the concept of megavitamin therapy. Bill was very curious about it and began to take niacin, 3,000 milligrams daily. Within a few weeks fatigue and depression, which had plagued him for years, were gone. He gave it to 30 of his close friends in AA. Of the 30, 10 were free of anxiety, tension, and depression in one month. Another 10 were well in two months. Bill then wrote *The Vitamin B3 Therapy* (1967) and thousands of copies of this extraordinary pamphlet were distributed. Bill became unpopular with the members of the board of AA International. The medical members, who had been appointed by Bill, 'knew' vitamin B3 could not be therapeutic as Bill had found it to be. I found it very useful in treating patients who were both alcoholic and schizophrenic" (from Hoffer, A. "Vitamin B3: niacin and its amide." *Townsend Letter for Doctors* 1995;147:30–39, and two reports by Bill Wilson "The Vitamin B3 Therapy: The First Communication to AA's Physicians," 1967 [www.doctoryourself.com /BOOK1BILL_W. pdf] and "A Second Communication to AA's Physicians," 1968 [www.doctoryourself.com/ BOOK2BILL_W.pdf].

Ruth Flinn Harrell, PhD

(1900–1991) • Hall of Fame 2006

"Nobody knows anything about the area of dietary supplementation, but the National Institutes of Health knows for sure it's impossible."

—RUTH F. HARRELL

The start of World War II was breaking news when Ruth Flinn Harrell conducted her first investigations into what she called "superfeeding." Her 1942 Columbia University doctoral thesis, "Effect of Added Thiamine on Learning," was published by the university in 1943 and would be followed by "Further Effects of Added Thiamine on Learning and Other Processes" in 1947. Her research was not about enriched or fortified foods ("added" meant "provided by supplement tablets"). In a 1946 *Journal of Nutrition* article, Dr. Harrell stated that "a liberal thiamine intake improved a number of mental and physical skills of orphanage children." One reporter wrote, "An experiment was conducted by Dr. Ruth Flinn Harrell which involved 104 children from 9 to 19 years of age. Half of the children were given a vitamin B1 (thiamine) pill each day, and the other half received a placebo. The test lasted six weeks. It was found by a series of tests that the group that was given the vitamin gained one-fourth more in learning ability than did the other group." By 1956, Harrell had investigated the effect of mothers' diets on the intelligence of offspring, finding that "supplementation of the pregnant and lactating mothers' diet by vitamins increased the intelligence quotients of their offspring at three and four years of age."

Harrell recognized that thiamine and the rest of the vitamins work better as a team. She used two clinically effective but oft-criticized therapeutic nutrition techniques: simultaneous supplementation with many nutrients (the "shotgun" approach), and megadoses. Working on the reasonable assumption that learning disabled children, because of functional deficiencies, might need higher than normal levels of nutrients, she progressed from her initial emphasis on thiamine to later providing a wide variety of supplemental nutrients. Early in 1981, Harrell and colleagues published a study in the *Proceedings of the National Academy of Sciences* showing that high doses of vitamins improved intelligence and educational performance in learning disabled children, including those with Down syndrome. Dr. Harrell, who had been investigating vitamin effects on learning for 40 years, had at last succeeded in focusing much-needed public attention on the role of nutrition in learning disabilities.

Linus Pauling, PhD

(1901–1994) • Hall of Fame 2004

"Linus Pauling was right."—ASSOCIATED PRESS

Orthomolecular medicine describes the practice of preventing and treating disease by providing the body with optimal amounts of substances that are natural to the body. Two-time Nobel Prize winner and molecular biologist Dr. Linus Pauling coined the term "orthomolecular" in his 1968 article "Orthomolecular Psychiatry" in the journal *Science*. Pauling described orthomolecular psychiatry as the treatment of mental disease by the provision of the optimum molecular environment for the mind, especially the optimum concentrations of substances normally present in the body.

It was a natural progression for Pauling, who had identified sickle-cell anemia as the first molecular disease and subsequently laid the foundation for molecular biology, to then develop a theory that explained the molecular basis of vitamin therapy.

Orthomolecular is a term made up of *ortho*, which is Greek for "correct" or "right," and *molecule*, which is the simplest structure that displays the characteristics of a compound. So it literally means the "right molecule."

Pauling later broadened his definition to include orthomolecular medicine, which he defined as "the preservation of good health and the treatment of disease by varying the concentration in the human body of substances that are normally present in the body." He stressed that the adjective "orthomolecular" is used to express the idea of the right molecules in the right concentra-

tion. Pauling firmly believed that daily supplementation of vitamins in optimum amounts, in addition to following a healthy diet, was the most important step that anyone could take to live a long and healthy life, and, by following his own advice, he lived productively for 93 years.

Henry Turkel, MD

(1903–1992) • Hall of Fame 2007

"Dr. Turkel had the nerve to make his claims when everyone 'knew' that children with genetic defects could not possibly be treated successfully."

—ABRAM HOFFER

Vitamin therapy in Down syndrome began in 1940, when Henry Turkel of Detroit became interested in treating the metabolic disorders of Down syndrome with a mixture of vitamins, minerals, fatty acids, digestive enzymes, lipotropic nutrients, glutamic acid, thyroid hormone, antihistamines, nasal decongestants, and a diuretic. By the 1950s he had devoted his practice almost entirely to Down syndrome patients, on whom he kept exceptionally detailed records, including serial photographs of their progress. Conventional medicine ignored Dr. Turkel, and he eventually retired and moved to Israel. Turkel clearly demonstrated that one of the "worst" genetic defects—trisomy, leading to Down syndrome—could be modified through what is largely a nutritional program with moderately high-dose supplements. The program never corrected the basic genetic defects in Down syndrome, of course, but it did correct much of the collateral biochemical consequences, leading to improvements in cognition, physical health, and appearance. Many believe Turkel to be the first to show that nutrition can improve genetic programming, and that genetic predeterminism is limited. Turkel contributed four important articles to the *Journal of Orthomolecular Psychiatry*, including "Medical Amelioration of Down's Syndrome Incorporating the Orthomolecular Approach" (1975), and "Intellectual Improvement of a Retarded Patient Treated with the 'U' Series" (1984).

Adelle Davis, MSc

(1904–1974) • Hall of Fame 2008

"One of the pioneers of the movement toward healthier eating, Adelle Davis, raised many food safety and health issues based on her own research. Her views were not accepted by the scientific community at the time. Now the weight of medical evidence, including former Surgeon General Koops' Report on Nutrition and Health, *has vindicated her views."*

—SENATOR PATRICK LEAHY

Adelle Davis, one of America's best-known nutritionists, was born Daisie Adelle Davis and raised on a farm in Lizton, Indiana. She attended Purdue University from 1923 to 1925 and received her bachelor's degree in dietetics from the University of California, Berkeley, in 1927. Trained in hospital dietetics at Bellevue and Fordham Hospitals in New York City, Davis served as a nutritionist for the New York City public schools until 1931. After several years of private practice as a consulting nutritionist, she earned her MS in biochemistry from the University of Southern California in 1939. She continued to see patients in southern California, many thousands of which were referred to her by physicians.

The Adelle Davis Foundation (adelledavis.org) comments that "She repeatedly stated that the body does best when provided with all of the known nutrients, as well as fresh food sources for obtaining nutrients yet to be discovered by science. Knowing the amounts of nutrients that the body requires under given conditions, one can make educated decisions . . . Without knowing the research, one cannot judge what amounts are necessary to avoid vitamin deficiencies. Deficiencies in vitamins, minerals, and other nutrients can cause illness that is reversed when the nutrients are added to the diet."

Adelle Davis wrote four best-selling books, starting with *Let's Cook It Right* in 1947. *Let's Have Healthy Children* (1951), *Let's Eat Right to Keep Fit* (1954), and *Let's Get Well* (1965) would follow, each later revised and updated. She was a popular speaker and frequent guest on television, beginning in 1947 and continuing for over 25 years, including a number of appearances on *The Tonight Show* with Johnny Carson.

Linus Pauling considered Adelle Davis to be "a pioneer in the health movement. She was essentially correct in almost everything she said." In 1990, *Natural Food and Farming* magazine wrote, "Today's research shows that she was indeed ahead of her time."

Thomas L. Cleave, MD

(1906–1983) • Hall of Fame 2009

"Cleave saw that many of the diseases of civilization could be explained as the consequences of eating refined carbohydrates, pointing out the crucial fact that refined foods are an artifact of technological civilization."

—KENNETH W. HEATON, Bristol Royal Infirmary, England

Thomas Latimer Cleave was born in Exeter, England, and entered Bristol Medical School at the age of 16, finished his training at St. Mary's Hospital, and went straight into the Royal Navy. There he was a medical specialist in various hospitals at home and abroad, ending up as surgeon captain and director of medical research until he retired in 1962.

After working in obscurity for many years, in the 1970s Cleave received international acclaim as the father of the dietary fiber hypothesis. His great vision was to see that the human body was maladapted to the refined foods of civilization, primarily carbohydrates, sugar, and white flour. He reasoned that if man avoided unnatural foods he would avoid unnatural diseases that were generally absent in wild animals or primitive communities. He spent his life gathering evidence and developing arguments to support this view, which culminated in his grand hypothesis that a range of diseases—from obesity to diabetes, coronary heart disease, ulcers, dental caries, constipation, and appendicitis—were caused by maladaptation to foods containing refined carbohydrates. Since they all had a common cause, he viewed them as a single master disease that he called "the saccharine disease." His book of the same name, published in 1974, sold thousands of copies and was written in laymen's language that the public could readily grasp. In 1986, the British Medical Association finally answered Cleave's voice in the wilderness in its report *Food, Nutrition and Health,* which recommended an increase in consumption of fresh food, and vegetables and whole grains.

One of Cleave's most effective advocates was Denis Burkitt, the legendary cancer researcher, and their collaboration was a turning point in the fortunes of Cleave's hypothesis. Burkitt's connections with 150 third-world hospitals enabled him to confirm many of Cleave's epidemiological observations, and even to add to his list of Western diseases that can be attributed to refined carbohydrates. Burkitt acknowledged his debt to his friend, stating "Cleave was one of the most revolutionary and far-sighted medical thinkers of the 20th century, seeing far beyond the small vision of intricate details of individual diseases."

Carl C. Pfeiffer, MD, PhD

(1908–1988) • Hall of Fame 2004

"For every drug that benefits a patient, there is a natural substance that can achieve the same effect."

—PFEIFFER'S LAW

Carl C. Pfeiffer made his first contribution in 1974, contributing 22 papers by the time he died in 1988. He made major contributions to the understanding of trace element and mineral metabolism in the schizophrenias, made a rational division of the schizophrenias into three biochemical groups, and discussed amino acids in medicine. His contributions were of the greatest value. Dr. Pfeiffer was one of the original members of the Committee on Therapy of the American Schizophrenia Association.

"If there's a drug that can alter the brain's biochemistry, there's usually a combination of nutrients that can achieve the same thing without side effects," said Pfeiffer, founding director of the Brain Bio Center in Princeton, New Jersey. Pfeiffer

spent most of his life researching for the causes and cure of mental illness. He found that biochemical imbalances in the body were the blame for many psychological problems. His observation and treatment of more than 20,000 schizophrenic patients led him to be able to show that there were several types of schizophrenia.

Lendon Smith, a supporter of the Pfeiffer approach, wrote: "Carl C. Pfeiffer, in his book, *Nutrition and Mental Illness* (1987), listed well-known causes of schizophrenia . . . He said, 'All of these are chemically induced metabolic disorders, which suggests the strong possibility that the true schizophrenias left in the wastebasket might also be due to biochemical abnormalities'" (www.smithsez.com/hypertension.html).

Pfeiffer's other books include *Mental and Elemental Nutrients* (1975), *The Healing Nutrients* (1987), *Dr. Pfeiffer's Total Nutrition: Nutritional Science and Cookery* (1980–1985), and *Neurobiology of the Trace Metals Zinc and Copper* (1972). His contributions to orthomolecular medicine live on through his writings, the clinics he inspired, and the annual Society of Orthomolecular Medicine lecture that bears his name.

Irwin Stone, PhD

(1907–1984) • Hall of Fame 2004

"Irwin Stone was totally in love with ascorbic acid. On behalf of all humanity, I thank the stars that he was."

—ABRAM HOFFER

Irwin Stone, a biochemist and chemical engineer, born in 1907, was educated in the public schools of New York City and the College of the City of New York. He considers as part of his education his employment from 1924 to 1934 at the Pease Laboratories, a then well-known biological and chemical consulting laboratory, first as assistant bacteriologist, then as assistant to the chief chemist, and then finishing his tenure as chief chemist. In 1934, he was offered the opportunity of setting up and directing an enzyme and fermentation research laboratory for the Wallerstein Company, a large manufacturer of industrial enzymes.

He employed ascorbic acid to stabilize foodstuffs against the undesirable and deteriorating effects of exposure to air and oxidation. Three patent applications were filed in 1935 and the patents were granted in 1939 and 1940. Thus, Dr. Stone obtained the first patents on an industrial application of ascorbic acid.

By the late 1950s, Stone's research on the genetics of scurvy had progressed to a point where it could be said that scurvy was not a dietary disturbance but was a potentially fatal problem in medical genetics. Ascorbic acid thus did not behave like trace vitamin C but was a stress-responsive liver metabolite produced endogenously in large daily amounts in the livers of most mammals, but not in humans. Between 1965 and 1967 he produced four papers describing a human birth defect existing in 100 percent of the population due to a defective gene in the human gene pool, the potentially fatal genetic liver enzyme disease, which he named "hypoascorbemia," as the cause of scurvy. He had difficulty publishing his hypoascorbemia work because the ideas were so advanced and contrary to the existing theories of the etiology of scurvy.

After Irwin Stone retired from his paid employment and moved to San Jose in 1971, he devoted the rest of his life to studying and publicizing the need for multi-gram daily consumption of vitamin C by humans. Stone repeatedly stated that ignoring this fact is fatal. His classic 1972 book, *The Healing Factor: Vitamin C Against Disease*, contains over 50 pages of scientific references, making it one of the first, and still one of the best, reviews of megascorbate therapeutics. It is doubtful that many skeptics have been as thorough as Stone has in checking vitamin C literature. His book and published articles summarize the successful vitamin C treatment of infections (bacterial and viral), allergies, asthma, poisoning, ulcers, the effects of smoking, and eye diseases including glaucoma. Ascorbate's role in treating cancer, heart disease, diabetes, fractures, bladder and kidney diseases, tetanus, shock, wounds, and pregnancy complications is also discussed in the book that the National Health Federation said, "may be the most important book on health ever written" (www.vitamincfoundation.org/healing.html).

In his immensely productive 77-year lifetime, Stone, building on the work of Albert Szent-Györgyi, constructed both the theoretical and practical foundations of megascorbate therapy with such skill that it became the focus of 25 years of Linus Pauling's life. Pauling spoke of this highly influential first contact when Stone sent him "copies of some papers that he had just published, with the general title 'Hypoascorbemia: A Genetic Disease' . . . The 3,000 milligrams per day that he recommended is 50 times the RDA. My wife and I began taking this amount of the vitamin . . . [and] the severe colds that I had suffered from several times a year all of my life no longer occurred. After a few years I increased my intake of vitamin C to 100 times, then 200 times, and then 300 times the RDA (now 18,000 milligrams per day)."

"Disease is the censor pointing out the humans, animals, and plants who are imperfectly nourished."
— T. G. WRENCH, *1941*

In the book *Linus Pauling in His Own Words* (1995), Pauling wrote, "Among the several arguments Irwin Stone presented to support his thesis that the proper physiological intake of vitamin C is 50 or more times the RDA . . . is that animals manufacture very large amounts of ascorbate. The amount manufactured is approximately proportional to the body weight, and, converted to the weight of a human being, ranges from about 2,000 to 20,000 milligrams per day. Irwin Stone concluded that human beings with an average diet are accordingly all suffering from hypoascorbemia, a deficiency of ascorbate in the blood and tissues."

There could be no finer tribute to Irwin Stone than this.

Josef Issels, MD

(1907–1998) • Hall of Fame 2005

"Dr. Issels is an intelligent and profound clinician, with principles and applications of medical treatment which I admire."

—JOHN ANDERSON, King's College Hospital, London

Josef Issels' roots were in the German tradition of *naturheilverfahren* (natural practice). Because of his well-known professional skills, his kindness, and relatively high rate of survivors, many cancer patients in the terminal stage came to consult him. In 1951, one wealthy and grateful patient funded his private clinic, the Ringbergklinik in Rottach-Egern (Bavaria) with 36 beds. Dr. Issels' successful work continued until 1960, when he was arrested by the German *kriminalpolizei* on the instigation of his medical opponents. He had to close down his clinic for years, in spite of a report from an independent scientist who had concluded that, of 252 terminal cancer patients with histologically proved metastases, 42 had survived for at least five years (17 percent) with the Issels therapy. For terminal patients, such a score is disproportionately high.

Issels believed that cancer was the end stage, the ultimate symptom, of a lifetime of immune system damage that had created an environment for the tumor to grow. Issels argued that conventional therapy just looked at the tumor without recognizing this longtime preconditioning period. Just cutting out or irradiating the tumor *mit stahl und strahl* ("with scalpel and radiation") was not eradicating cancer. Instead, Issels saw the body as having great potential to heal itself. Good nutrition and a clean environment were central to his therapy. Like Dr. Max Gerson, he recognized the importance of detoxification.

In the end, Issels was proven to be right. From 1967 to 1970, Professor J. Anderson of King's College Hospital and member of the World Health Organization inspected Issels' reopened clinic. He confirmed the highly significant survival rate of Issels' terminal cancer patients. His legacy is continued by the work of his wife Ilsa and his son Christian. —GERT SCHUITEMAKER and A.W.S.

Frederick Klenner, MD

(1907–1984) • Hall of Fame 2005

"Vitamin C is the safest substance available to the physician."—FREDERICK KLENNER

Born in Pennsylvania, Frederick Klenner received his medical degree from Duke University in 1936. After three years post-graduate training to specialize in diseases of the chest, Dr. Klenner continued his general practice. "His patients were as enthusiastic as he in playing guinea pigs to study the action of ascorbic acid. The first massive doses of ascorbic acid he gave to himself. Each time something new appeared on the horizon he took the same amount of ascorbic acid to study its effects so as to come up with the answers" (*Appl Nutr* 1971).

Abram Hoffer writes: "In the early 1950s, Dr. Frederick Klenner began his work with megadoses of vitamin C. He used doses up to 100 grams per day orally or intravenously. In clinical reports he recorded the excellent response he saw when it was given in large doses. For example, polio patients given vitamin C suffered no residual defects from their polio. A controlled study in England on 70 children, half given vitamin C and half given placebo, confirmed that none of the ascorbate-treated cases developed any paralysis while up to 20 percent of the untreated group did. This study was not published because the Salk polio vaccine had just been developed and no one was interested in vitamins. Dr. Klenner's work was ignored."

Klenner was the first physician to emphasize that small amounts of ascorbate do not work. He said, "If you want results, use adequate ascorbic acid." As a result of seeing consistent cures of a great variety of viral and bacterial diseases—from pneumonia, herpes, mononucleosis, hepatitis, multiple sclerosis, childhood illnesses, fevers, encephalitis, and many other diseases—with huge doses of vitamin C, he published over 20 medical reports. Orthodox medicine's rejection of his life-saving work stands as a reminder to all medical mavericks practicing today. "Some physicians," Klenner wrote, "would stand by and see their patient die rather than use ascorbic acid because, in their finite minds, it exists only as a vitamin."

Wilfrid Shute, MD (1907–1982)
Evan Shute, MD (1905–1978)

Hall of Fame 2004

"We didn't make vitamin E so versatile. God did. Ignore its mercy at your peril."—EVAN SHUTE

In 1933, Wilfrid and Evan Shute were some of the first doctors to use large doses of vitamin E to treat heart disease. At that time, antioxidants and free radicals were rather obscure concepts in the chemistry of oxidation, far removed from issues of health and disease. Also at that time, using vitamins to treat serious diseases such as heart disease and diabetes was considered by the medical establishment as misguided at best and as outright fraud at worst. Yet thanks to the observant practitioners such as the Shutes, who were more interested in what helped their patients most, medical researchers became motivated to study it scientifically. The results would speak for themselves.

For decades, vitamin E was lampooned as a "cure in search of a disease." In 1985, Linus Pauling wrote: "The failure of the medical establishment during the last 40 years to recognize the value of vitamin E in controlling heart disease is responsible for a tremendous amount of unnecessary suffering and for many early deaths. The interesting story of the efforts to suppress the Shute discoveries about vitamin E illustrates the shocking bias of organized medicine against nutritional measures for achieving improved health." Pauling would most likely have appreciated this comment from the February 1999 *Harvard Health Letter:* "A consistent body of research indicates that vitamin E may protect people against heart disease . . . The data generally indicate that taking doses ranging from 100 to 800 international units per day may lower the risk of heart disease by 30 to 40 percent." Over half a century ago, the Shute brothers and colleagues showed that with even higher doses than those, and with an insistence on the use of natural vitamin E, the results are better still.

By the 1970s, the Shutes had published numerous mainstream books on vitamin E, including *The Heart and Vitamin E* (1972), and had successfully treated over 30,000 patients with huge doses of vitamin E. Today's growing appreciation of the role of d-alpha tocopherol in preventing and reversing cardiovascular disease is due primarily to the Shute brothers.

Allan Cott, MD

(1910–1993) • Hall of Fame 2004

"Dr. Cott was one of the trusted teachers of orthomolecular psychiatry, indeed one of the most eminent of pioneers. If any physician deserved to be honored by the medical profession at large, he was one."

—ABRAM HOFFER

Allan Cott turned from his practice of psychoanalysis to become one of the first orthomolecular psychiatrists. What persuaded him most of all were the recoveries he saw in patients who had not responded to other treatment, and how swift the recoveries often were.

Dr. Cott fasted psychiatric patients while an attending physician at Gracie Square Hospital in New York City. In so doing, Lendon Smith writes that Cott was following the work of Dr. Yuri Nikolayev of Moscow, "who has fasted more than 10,000 mentally ill patients . . . The manic phase of manic-depressive illness can be brought under control in the first week of a fast. Cott made them exercise by taking long walks. They drank two quarts of water every day as a minimum. If a patient failed to drink this amount, he terminated the fast . . . By the end of the first week, the medicines they had been on were usually discontinued." Using this treatment, which often also incorporated vitamin B6 (pyridoxine) in large doses, Cott healed enormous numbers of patients —from children to the very elderly.

In addition to two popular books on supervised fasting, Cott wrote *Dr. Cott's Help for Your Learning Disabled Child: The Orthomolecular Treatment* (1985) and was a frequent contributor to the *Journal of Orthomolecular Psychiatry*. His papers on "Controlled Fasting Treatment for Schizophrenia" and the "Orthomolecular Approach to the Treatment of Learning Disabilities" were presented at the Nutrition and Mental Health Hearing before the Select Senate Committee on Nutrition and Human Needs in 1977.

Carlton Fredericks, PhD

(1910–1987) • Hall of Fame 2008

"Carlton Fredericks repeatedly kicked the shins of public health officials because of their failure to protect the nutritional health of the public."

—MICHAEL BARBEE, *Politically Incorrect Nutrition*

Carlton Fredericks, born Harold Carlton Caplan, grew up in the Flatbush section of Brooklyn in New York. He earned his bachelor's degree at the University of Alabama in 1931 and received a master's degree in 1949 and a PhD in 1955, both in Public Health Education, and both from New York University. He wrote over 20 books, lectured widely, and was associate professor of public health at Fairleigh Dickinson University in New Jersey.

Fredericks became famous, and in some circles infamous, for his pioneering use of the media to educate people about vitamin and nutrition therapy. On the radio for nearly half a century, his most famous 30 years began in 1957 at New York City station WOR. Fredericks' call-in "Design for Living" program, broadcast six days a week and syndicated nationally, resulted in literally millions of letters to a man whom many considered to be "America's foremost nutritionist." KABC–Los Angeles presented his program "Living Should Be Fun" saying that "Dr. Fredericks presents interviews with doctors and nutritionists (and) examines the fact or superstition in certain nutrition beliefs." In one such 1978 interview, he interviewed orthomolecular niacinamide pioneer William Kaufman.

Fredericks, a colleague of Robert Atkins and Linus Pauling, was heavily criticized as a vitamin "promoter" and food "faddist." Today, he might be seen more as an orthomolecular version of famous radio broadcaster Paul Harvey. The *New York Times* described Fredericks' voice as having "crisp diction and authoritative delivery." Fredericks constantly made fun of junk foods and brought his listeners many a memorable moment. He quipped that if you lack the time to learn what you ought to know about healthy eating, just follow the average grocery store shopper and purchase only what he or she doesn't. When callers asked about white bread, he replied that it "makes a wonderful way of cleaning off your counter tops. You can dust your furniture with it." The irrepressible Fredericks appeared on the television talk program *The Merv Griffin Show,* and was a columnist for *Prevention* and *Let's Live* magazines.

William Kaufman, MD, PhD

(1910–2000) • Hall of Fame 2004

"I noted that niacinamide (alone or combined with other vitamins) in a thousand-patient years of use has caused no adverse side effects."

—WILLIAM KAUFMAN

William Kaufman was among the very first physicians to therapeutically employ megadoses of vitamin B3 (as niacin or niacinamide). He prescribed as much as 5,000 milligrams of niacinamide daily, in many divided doses, to dramatically improve and restore range of joint motion in arthritic patients. Many of his patients also found their joint paint reduced or completely eliminated. This groundbreaking work remains important to this day. In his 1949 book *The Common Form of Joint Dysfunction,* Kaufman published the details of his niacinamide arthritis treatment, which also incorporated the use of vitamins C, B1 (thiamine), and B2 (riboflavin), all in large doses. He kept meticulous patient records that repeatedly verified the safety and effectiveness of megavitamin therapy. His arthritis treatment may have been more widely embraced had it not been for the development and introduction of corticosteroid hormones for arthritis, which were considered the wonder drugs of that decade.

Over 50 years ago, Kaufman also showed

remarkable foresight half a century into the future of orthomolecular medicine, describing how the lack of just a single nutrient can cause diverse diseases, including what is now known as attention-deficit hyperactivity disorder (ADHD).

Charlotte Kaufman lovingly writes of her husband, "He was always ready to help someone else. He truly was a healer and a problem solver. He played the piano; he loved Mozart. He wrote poems, plays, essays, and subscribed to about 30 medical journals, which he read. He practiced medicine in his own way, without regard to fads or fashion. He seemed to know intuitively what the clinical answers were, but he was a thoughtful person who did not make decisions lightly. He was an independent thinker who was constantly studying and learning, not just from the printed word, but also from his patients. He really listened to his patients. His main objective was to help people live healthy lives."

Hugh MacDonald Sinclair, MD

(1910–1990) • Hall of Fame 2009

"He may prove to be one of those people whose long term influence is far greater than ever seemed likely while he was alive" —DAVID HORROBIN

Hugh MacDonald Sinclair was one of the 20th century's outstanding experts in human nutrition. He was born in Duddington House, Edinburgh, Scotland, and went to Oriel College, Oxford, to study animal physiology. He was appointed departmental demonstrator in biochemistry, before going on to study clinical medicine at University College Hospital Medical School, London. Sinclair spent most of his working life as a fellow of Magdalen College, Oxford, though he made many forays into a wider world, notably during the World War II when he was involved in planning how the British could be properly nourished and in famine relief in the Netherlands and the Rhineland.

Sinclair is most widely known for claiming that "bad fats" worsened what he called "diseases of civilization," such as coronary heart disease, cancer, diabetes, inflammation, strokes, and skin disease. He believed that diets deficient in essential fatty acids are the cause of most degenerative illnesses. Sinclair's forceful arguments on this matter preceded firm scientific evidence, however. His self-experimentation, including the infamous 100-day-seal-meat diet, dramatically demonstrated the importance of long-chain fatty acids of fish oils in decreasing the aggregation of platelets, and thus the incidence of thrombosis. Sinclair's main contributions were intellectual. He recognized the central importance of nutrition to human life and, at a time when it had become unfashionable, he constantly emphasized the importance of the right food for proper health. In a famous letter to the *Lancet* in 1956, he made a particular contribution in identifying the crucial role of essential fatty acids in health, which readers classed as either visionary or lunatic, depending on their point of view. His letter foreshadowed half a century of research on a nutritional topic, which is steadily increasing in importance.

"He who lives by rule and wholesome diet is a physician to himself."
—Concise Directions on the Nature of Our Common Food, 1790

Sinclair's greatest dream was to establish an international center for the study of human nutrition. He argued that nutrition is an important area of science in its own right, and that new insights into the relationships between food and human health should guide developments in medicine, agriculture, and food technology. Many of his ideas have relevance for us today.

Arthur M. Sackler, MD

(1913–1987) • Hall of Fame 2006

*"Arthur M. Sackler was one of the few
20th-century Renaissance figures."*

—SOLOMON H. SNYDER,

Johns Hopkins School of Medicine

Brooklyn-born Arthur Sackler was educated at New York University. He worked at Lincoln Hospital in New York City as an intern and a house physician and then completed his residency in psychiatry at Creedmoor State Hospital. His National Academies of Sciences' biography states that "there, in the 1940s, he started research that resulted in more than 150 papers in neuroendocrinology, psychiatry, and experimental medicine. He considered his scientific research into the metabolic basis of schizophrenia his most significant contribution to science, and served as editor of the *Journal of Clinical and Experimental Psychopathology* from 1950 to 1962." It was in this very journal that Dr. Sackler introduced the world to the Hoffer-Osmond high-dose niacin therapy for mental illness. In his memoirs, Abram Hoffer writes: "I wonder if our first paper on schizophrenia treatment with niacin would even have been published, had Arthur Sackler not been both my professional colleague and friend." Back in 1951, Hoffer had met the Sackler brothers, "who were doing groundbreaking research on histamine as a schizophrenia treatment. Their work would inspire some of our initial biochemical research."

Sackler would continue to publish and to inspire physicians worldwide. He started the highly respected *Medical Tribune* newspaper in 1960, which would grow to an international readership of over 1 million, with Sackler himself contributing over 500 articles on a wide variety of health issues. In 1981, Sackler ran a page-one story on Ruth Harrell's study showing that high doses of vitamins improve IQ in Down syndrome children. In one 1982 column, he personally declared his support for bowel-tolerance doses of ascorbate, including with his comments the text of "a letter we just received from Robert F. Cathcart, MD"

whom Sackler described as "brilliant." Many physicians first saw these words in the *Tribune:* "Ascorbic acid administered orally to bowel tolerance (just short of producing diarrhea) has a definite antipyretic effect (and) administered intramuscularly to small infants will usually have a dramatic effect on elevated temperatures."

Max J. Vogel, MD

(1915–2002) • Hall of Fame 2006

"Max Vogel was among the first general orthomolecular practitioners in Canada."—ABRAM HOFFER

Max Vogel was the first family physician to embrace the practice of orthomolecular medicine in 1960 and became one of its most successful physicians who continued against the usual odds facing those who practice outside the box. During World War II, Vogel became a physician in the accelerated course at Queens University, following pre-clinical years at the University of Saskatchewan, Saskatoon, 1939 to 1942. He served as captain with the Canadian armed forces in England, then volunteered for duty in the Pacific, specializing in tropical medicine at Walter Reed Hospital in Washington, DC.

In 1955, after obtaining more training in obstetrics and gynecology in New York, Vogel began a practice in Calgary, where he retired in 1997. Vogel fought tirelessly for causes in which he believed, and when he became convinced of the value of using large doses of vitamins for treatment of the schizophrenias and other diseases he became involved in trying to educate the profession, the public, and the government.

Years ago, the government of Alberta announced that patients receiving vitamins would not be covered by Medicare. With his family and friends, Vogel organized a massive effort to petition the government and, after thousands of names had been submitted, the government reversed its decision. When Vogel was on the associate staff of the Department of Psychiatry at Calgary Hospital, a new director tried to get him fired because of his controversial (orthomolecular) practices. Again,

Vogel circulated a petition that was signed by 200 staff members. At the conclusion of this debate, the director left the hospital. One of his colleagues wrote, "Apart from Max's tremendous intellectual capacity and his enthusiasm for life and challenges, I must admit I respected him as a rebel. His reputation was of a person who constantly challenged the status quo."

Vogel was a long-standing member of the board of directors of the Canadian Schizophrenia Foundation and served on the editorial review board of the *Journal of Orthomolecular Medicine*. He was presented with the Lifetime Achievement Award by the International Society of Orthomolecular Medicine in 2002.

Emanuel Cheraskin, MD, DMD

(1916–2001) • Hall of Fame 2005

"Man is a food-dependent creature. If you don't feed him, he will die. If you feed him improperly, part of him will die."—EMANUEL CHERASKIN

Emanuel Cheraskin was born in Philadelphia and received his medical degree from the University of Cincinnati College of Medicine. He was awarded his doctor of dental medicine in the first graduating class of the University of Alabama School of Dentistry, where he would stay on for several decades as chairman of the Department of Oral Medicine. Dr. Cheraskin was among the very first to recognize and demonstrate that oral health indicates total body health. He wrote over 700 scientific articles and authored or coauthored 17 textbooks, plus eight more books for the public, including the best seller *Psychodietetics: Food as the Key to Emotional Health* (1975). His last two books, *Vitamin C: Who Needs It?* (1993) and *Human Health and Homeostasis* (1999), were published when he was past 80. In addition to being a professor, physician, and prolific author, Cheraskin was a singularly popular speaker. "Health is the fastest growing failing business in western civilization," he said. "Why is it so many of us are 40 going on 70, and so few 70 going on 40?" The answer, he

said, was our neglect of the paramount value of nutrition, an educational deficiency that Cheraskin devoted a lifetime to eradicating. Longtime friend Abram Hoffer writes: "Emanuel Cheraskin was a great scientist, investigator, and physician. His papers are models of brevity, scientific clarity, and productivity."

Cheraskin's educational legacy continues through the Cheraskin archive in upstate New York, which contains the doctor's lecture slides and copies of his papers in the care of Andrew Saul.

"Cherri," a regular speaker at the annual Orthomolecular Medicine Today conferences, was always informative and entertaining. He last presented in Vancouver for the 25th conference in 1996, where he received the Orthomolecular Medicine Physician of the Year Award.

Abram Hoffer, MD, PhD

(1917–2009) • Hall of Fame 2006

"Abram Hoffer has made an important contribution to the health of human beings . . . through the study of the effects of large doses of vitamin C and other nutrients."

—LINUS PAULING

In the documentary film *Masks of Madness: Science of Healing*, Abram Hoffer says, "Mental illness is usually biochemical illness. Schizophrenia is niacin dependency." Plainspoken statements such as these have ignited a revolution in psychiatry. The person who would forever change the course of medicine was born on a Saskatchewan farm and educated in a one-room schoolhouse. In 1952, just completing his residency, he had demonstrated, with the first double-blind placebo-controlled studies in the history of psychiatry, that vitamin B3 could cure schizophrenia. But in a medical profession that "knows" vitamins do not cure "real" diseases, the young director of psychiatric research was a dissenter. For over half a century Dr. Hoffer dissented. Researcher Harold Foster, writes:

Fathering a new paradigm does not promote popularity. Fortunately, Dr. Hoffer was not just highly intelligent; he consistently proved able to stand up for the truth, regardless of personal cost.

Author Robert Sealey asks, "What made Dr. Hoffer study schizophrenia so carefully? What did he think when his patients heard voices? What could cause the human brain to hallucinate? What motivated him to research, develop, and nourish the concept of orthomolecular medicine? What intrigued him so much that, as he reached 90, he still consulted, he still researched, and he still wrote?" Hoffer's scientific memoirs, he says, share the fascinating story of his life's work and his medical adventures. In them, Hoffer's memoirs explain that, according to the Hoffer-Osmond adrenochrome hypothesis, the dysfunctional metabolism of adrenaline (a healthy brain chemical) can cause psychosis, in some people. Vulnerable patients metabolize adrenaline to hallucinogenic compounds: adrenochrome and adrenolutin. Hoffer and Osmond believed that unbalanced brain chemistry could be restored. By means of the first double-blinded clinical trials in psychiatry mentioned above, they tested two vital amines: divided doses of either niacin or niacinamide (vitamin B3, a methyl acceptor) with ascorbic acid (vitamin C, an antioxidant). This proved the efficacy of their double-barreled treatment, which, for years, has continued to work better than antipsychotic medications alone, tranquilizers, insulin comas, and metrazole therapies.

"If patients look up 'schizophrenia' in the old textbooks," says Hoffer, "they'll die of frustration and fear. That is why I wrote my first book, *How to Live with Schizophrenia* (1966). Linus Pauling was 65 and planning to retire. He chanced to see this book on a friend's coffee table. Pauling did not go to bed the first night he read this book. He decided not to retire because of it." After researching the biochemistry for himself, Pauling then championed orthomolecular medicine. Other researchers had tested specific nutrient therapies before and used them to treat nutritional deficiencies and metabolic problems: vitamin C for scurvy (Lind, 1795), foods rich in vitamin B3 for pellagra (Goldberger, 1914–1928), and insulin for diabetes (Banting and Best, 1920–1925). When these cures were first discovered, uninformed doctors disputed, discounted, and denied the

healing value of nutrients. Before long, clinicians proved the treatments so safe and so effective that biochemical supplements became the standard of care for these three illnesses, which affected millions of patients.

Hoffer had a favorite way of illustrating the powerful resistance to change and the reluctance to accept new ideas, particularly among members of the medical establishment. "Have you ever wondered why Moses spent 40 years in the desert with the Israelites after leading them out of captivity and slavery in Egypt?" Hoffer would say. "The journey could have been accomplished in a matter of months, yet Moses knew that the generation born in slavery must die out before the people could be led to claim and govern a new land for themselves. Old ideas are very difficult to dislodge, new ideas take at least 40 years to become established."

Hoffer had many clinical adventures as he determined the optimum doses of smart nutrients for his patients and encouraged ethical colleagues around the world to apply his methods. In order to share research results and educate caregivers, Hoffer cofounded the *Journal of Orthomolecular Psychiatry* (later renamed the *Journal of Orthomolecular Medicine*) and served as its editor for four decades. He wrote over 500 papers and more than two dozen books including *Niacin Therapy in Psychiatry* (1962), *Orthomolecular Medicine for Physicians* (1989), *Smart Nutrients* (1994), *Vitamin B3 & Schizophrenia: Discovery, Recovery, Controversy* (1998), *Orthomolecular Treatment for Schizophrenia* (1999), *Healing Schizophrenia: Complementary Vitamin and Drug Treatments* (2004), and *Healing Cancer* (2004, revised in 2011 with Linus Pauling). *Adventures in Psychiatry*, his scientific memoir, was published in 2005.

Through more than five decades as a practicing physician and researcher, Abram Hoffer experienced the slow shifting of attitudes regarding orthomolecular medicine. He never lost his courageous vision or his remarkable receptivity to new ideas. As he entered his 90s, Hoffer was sharper than many of his colleagues half his age. He worked four days a week at his Orthomolecular Vitamin Information Center in Victoria, British Columbia, and was busy preparing several new publications. Having treated thousands of patients, upon his retirement he wryly said that "Everyone should have a career change every 55 years." — A.W.S., ROBERT SEALEY, and STEVEN CARTER

Humphry Osmond, MD

(1917–2004) • Hall of Fame 2004

"Humphry changed my life and the life of thousands of schizophrenic patients who are today well."

—ABRAM HOFFER

In his book *Linus Pauling in His Own Words* (1995), Dr. Pauling wrote: "In 1967, I happened to read a number of papers published by two psychiatrists in Canada: Dr. Abram Hoffer and Dr. Humphry Osmond . . . They were giving very large amounts of niacin to the schizophrenic patients, as much as 17,000 milligrams per day . . . I was astonished that niacin . . . should be so lacking in toxicity that 1,000 times the effective daily intake could be taken by a person without harm. This meant that these substances were quite different from drugs, which are usually given to patients in amounts not much smaller than the lethal dosages."

Osmond's remarkable medical career included decades of distinguished psychiatric practice and a prodigious output of writing and research. He attended Guy's Hospital Medical School of the University of London. In World War II, he was a surgeon-lieutenant in the Navy, where he trained to become a ship psychiatrist. He was widely recognized as a pioneer investigator into the chemistry of consciousness. At St. George's Hospital in London, Osmond, along with colleague Dr. John Smythies, developed the theory that schizophrenics suffer due to endogenous production of an adrenaline-based hallucinogen. When the theory was not embraced by the British mental-health establishment, Osmond moved to Canada to continue the research at Saskatchewan Hospital in Weyburn, where over half the patients were schizophrenic and where he met Abram Hoffer.

Their collaborative research led to the very origin of orthomolecular psychiatry in the early 1950s. Osmond and Hoffer continued their close associa-

tion for decades, successfully treating not only schizophrenics but alcoholic patients as well. They cofounded the Canadian Schizophrenia Foundation, now the International Schizophrenia Foundation; cowrote *How to Live with Schizophrenia* (1966), as well as many other books and papers; and together created the *Journal of Orthomolecular Psychiatry*, now the *Journal of Orthomolecular Medicine*.

The popular press may today remember Humphry Osmond for coining the term "psychedelic," but countless thousands of grateful patients will remember him as the co-discoverer of niacin therapy for schizophrenia.

Lendon H. Smith, MD

(1921–2001) • Hall of Fame 2006

"ADHD is not a disease; it is a nutritional deficiency."

—LENDON H. SMITH

Lendon Smith was perhaps among the most courageous physicians of all time, as he was one of the first to unambiguously support high-dose vitamin regimens for children. Such a position did not endear Dr. Smith to every one of his fellow members of the American Academy of Pediatrics, and it is therefore further to his credit that he boldly stepped forward and, in the best traditions of Linus Pauling, took orthomolecular therapy directly to the people. In this he was particularly successful, achieving renown by way of his newsletter *The Facts*, and his many popular books, articles, videos, and primetime television appearances. He appeared on *The Tonight Show* 62 times, an exposure such as orthomolecular medicine has rarely seen. Even Pauling never won an Emmy award. Smith did.

The man who would become nationally known as "The Children's Doctor" received his medical degree in 1946 from the University of Oregon Medical School. He served as captain in the U.S. Army Medical Corps from 1947 to 1949, went on to a pediatric residency at St. Louis Children's Hospital, and completed it at Portland's Doernbecker Memorial Hospital in 1951. In 1955, Smith became clinical professor of pediatrics at the University of

Oregon Medical Hospital. He would practice pediatrics for 35 years before retiring in 1987 to lecture, write, and continue to help making "megavitamin" a household word.

And yet it was not until over 20 years of medical practice that Smith first began to use megavitamin therapy. It is a remarkable transformation. A patient "wanted me to give her a vitamin shot," he writes of an alcoholic woman from 1973. "I had never done such a useless thing in my professional life, and I was a little embarrassed to think that she considered me to be the kind of doctor who would do that sort of thing" (*Feed Yourself Right*, 1983).

"That sort of thing" consisted of an intramuscular injection of 0.5 cubic centimeters of B complex, which, Smith reported, proved successful enough such that "she walked past three bars and didn't have to go in." This was the beginning of his evolution from conventional pediatrician to orthomolecular spokesperson. As he learned about nutritional prevention and megavitamin therapy, he began to discuss it. In *Feed Your Kids Right* (1979), Smith briefly recommends up to 10,000 milligrams (mg) of vitamin C during illness. In *Foods for Healthy Kids* (1981), he recommended bowel-tolerance levels of ascorbate. But even his relatively mild statements such as "eat no sugar" and "stress increases the need for vitamin B and C, calcium, magnesium, and zinc" can be a walk on the wild side for pharmophilic physicians.

Smith couldn't have cared less about his critics. By 1979, he was a *New York Times* best-selling author, and by 1983 an advocate of four-day water fasts, 1,000-microgram injections of B12, and megavitamins for kids. There were no RDA-level vitamin recommendations to be found in a Lendon Smith book. He was an outspoken critic of junk food. Two of his trademark phrases were, "People tend to eat the food to which they are sensitive" and "If you love something, it is probably bad for you."

In 1981, in *Foods for Healthy Kids*, Smith was confidently in favor of fluoridation: "There is no doubt that it works; fluoridation is not a Communist plot." Twenty years later, writing at his website, www.smithsez.com, he appears less convinced, having written, "If we continue to eat store-bought food, we will have store-bought

teeth." What's more, he turned very cautious about routine vaccination. "The best advice I can give to parents is to forgo the shots, but make sure that the children in your care have a superior immune system. This requires a sugarless diet without processed foods [and] an intake of vitamin C of about 1,000 mg per day for each year of life up to 5,000 mg at age five."

These are long evolutionary steps for a pediatrician who, 22 years earlier, wrote of vitamin C: "Excess is a waste and will not prevent colds" (*The Children's Doctor*, 1978). Had he held to such politically safe beliefs, Smith might have avoided being compelled to stop practicing medicine in 1987, under pressure from insurance companies and his state's Board of Medical Examiners. Nonetheless, for 14 more years, he would speak out in favor of megavitamin therapy. In this, he did the job second to none.

The popularization of orthomolecular medicine by courageous physicians such as Dr. Smith has enabled the benefits of nutritional therapy to reach families with sick little kids at 3:00 A.M. Smith's exceptional visibility has done a great deal to educate and encourage fathers and mothers to use vitamins to prevent and cure illness. For this, Lendon Smith ranks as one of the most influential pediatricians of our time, and one of the true pioneers of orthomolecular medicine.

Ewan Cameron, MD

(1922–1991) • Hall of Fame 2007

"It has been known for many years that cancer patients have depressed circulating, cellular, and tissue ascorbate reserves, and ascorbate is involved in many aspects of host resistance to cancer."

—EWAN CAMERON

"Ewan Cameron was born in Glasgow, Scotland, in 1922. He received his medical degree from the University of Glasgow in 1944 and immediately joined the British Army, where he served as a medical officer in Burma for three years. A gifted surgeon, Cameron worked as a consultant surgeon at Vale of Leven Hospital in Dunbartonshire, Scotland, from 1956 to 1982, becoming the senior consultant surgeon in 1973. He received the Queen's Coronation Medal in Britain in 1977, as well as fellowships from the Royal Colleges of Surgeons in Glasgow and Edinburgh, and the Royal Faculty of Physicians and Surgeons in Glasgow. In 1966, Cameron published his first book *Hyaluronidase and Cancer*. In 1971, Cameron began corresponding with Linus Pauling and his Institute of Science and Medicine. He completed many scientific studies in conjunction with the institute, and published *Cancer and Vitamin C* with Pauling in 1979. After retirement from Vale of Leven Hospital in 1982, Cameron became the medical director and senior research professor at the Linus Pauling Institute" (excerpted Oregon State University Libraries Special Collections).

While best known today for his pioneering use of intravenous ascorbate against cancer, Cameron also made additional, remarkable discoveries. One was that high doses of vitamin C provided profound pain relief. Another was that such doses, in Cameron's own words, "enabled opiates to be withdrawn without withdrawal symptoms."

Fannie H. Kahan

(1922–1978) • Hall of Fame 2007

"Her talent lay in being able to translate the language of the researcher and clinician into laymen's language. She wrote simply and lucidly about many things normally discussed only in the obscure jargon of medicine."

—IRWIN KAHAN

Fannie Hoffer Kahan was born in 1922 on a farm in southern Saskatchewan, the youngest of Israel and Clara Hoffer's six children. A gifted writer from a young age, she graduated from the University of Minnesota with a journalism degree. Newspapers and magazines throughout North America published her articles on a variety of topics and she authored a number of books.

From the beginning of her writing career up until her death, Kahan fought passionately for bet-

ter understanding and treatment of schizophrenia. A true pioneer in recognizing and promoting a holistic orthomolecular approach to health, she was one of the first journalists to write about the early research on schizophrenia conducted by Abram Hoffer, her brother, and Humphry Osmond. She continued through the years with a large number of articles and pamphlets that provided the public with much needed information about schizophrenia and its treatment. In conjunction with Drs. Hoffer and Osmond she wrote *How to Live with Schizophrenia* (1966), using her talent for clear language to explain to laypeople the basics of schizophrenia from an orthomolecular medicine perspective. Also with Hoffer and Osmond, Kahan wrote the companion book *New Hope for Alcoholics* (1968). Another key publication was her book *Brains and Bricks* (1965), a history of the Yorkton Psychiatric Center, designed to take into account schizophrenics' experiences of different architectural features.

"Do not follow where the path may lead. Go instead where there is no path and leave a trail."— ANONYMOUS

Throughout her writing career Fannie was strongly supported by another orthomolecular pioneer, her husband Irwin Kahan, who among other activities worked tirelessly to establish the Canadian Schizophrenia Foundation. In turn, Fannie supported Irwin in his efforts to improve the quality of life for schizophrenics and their families.

In 1972, Kahan became managing editor of the *Journal of Orthomolecular Psychiatry* and editor of the *Huxley Institute for Biosocial Research/Canadian Schizophrenic Foundation* newsletter. During her last illness, with the dedication and selflessness that was so characteristic of her, she worked on the journal up until a few days before her death in 1978. She left behind an important body of work related to orthomolecular medicine. —MEKTON KAHAN

R. Glen Green, MD

(1923–2010) • Hall of Fame 2007

"When I was a sick little girl, Dr. Green changed my life. I will never forget him."—Former patient

R. Glen Green, a nutrition pioneer, received his medical degree from McGill University in 1947 after completing his BA and Certificate of Medicine at the University of Saskatchewan in 1945. He began life as a general practitioner in 1949 in Prince Albert, Saskatchewan, where he lived with his wife, Peggy.

Dr. Green served as the medical staff president of two hospitals and was a board member of the Saskatchewan College of Physicians and Surgeons. In 1968, his own poor health became the impetus for examining how doctors diagnose and treat patients. He was a voracious reader and regularly connected with luminaries such as Linus Pauling and Abram Hoffer, eager to exchange innovative ideas and new treatments.

His 1970 study of 1,200 schoolchildren lead to his discovery of subclinical pellagra, an indication that the body is lacking in vitamin B3 that, if untreated, may lead to schizophrenia. He also developed the Perceptual Dysfunction Test to diagnose more accurately subclinical pellagra. Children who fell into this category (some 17 percent) had difficulty reading and often had behavior problems. The cause was a cerebral allergy, overtaxing the digestive system. Sensory illusions stopped when orthomolecular therapy and diet were used.

Green's pursuit of help for patients who did not respond to traditional medicine lead him further into alternative medicine. In his book, *Doctors* (1988), Martin O'Malley wrote that Green was the most "radical holistic doctor in Canada," a mantel he wore with pride. Green lost his license to practice medicine in 1982 for the belief that people must alter their lifestyles and learn how to nourish their bodies to rediscover the joy of good health.

Green was one of the 24 founding members of the Academy of Orthomolecular Psychiatry established in 1976. He contributed five articles on subclinical pellagra to the *Journal of Orthomolecular Psychiatry.* —SUSAN GREEN

Archie Kalokerinos, MD

(1927–2012) • Hall of Fame 2009

"Any attempt to adequately write about Archie Kalokerinos would incorporate many such adjectives as far-sighted, intelligent, sensible, observant, honest, caring, altruistic, congenial, meticulous, brave, dogged, intrepid, and last but not least, great."

—OSCAR FALCONI, advocate of nutritional medicine

Archie Kalokerinos was born in Glenn Innes, Australia, in 1927 and received his medical degree from Sydney University in 1951. He was appointed medical superintendent of the hospital at Collarenebri, Australia, where he served until 1975. His practice is based on Linus Pauling's theory that many diseases result from excessive free radicals and can accordingly be prevented or cured by vitamin C.

Kalokerinos is well known worldwide as the doctor who spent much of his time fighting for the well-being of the aboriginal inhabitants of Australia. He became very concerned about the high death rate of aboriginal children in New South Wales and came to the conclusion that the infants had symptoms of scurvy, a deficiency of vitamin C. In his groundbreaking book, *Every Second Child* (1981), he discovered that the an acute vitamin C deficiency provoked by the vaccinations was the reason why, at a certain point, up to half of the vaccinated aboriginal infants died. Instead of being rewarded for this lifesaving observation, Kalokerinos was harassed, and his methods were disregarded by the authorities, probably because they were too simple, too cheap, and too efficacious to be accepted by the vested interests of modern medicine. And, besides, they were meant to protect a population that, in its own native county, is regarded by some as not worth taking the trouble for anyway. Kalokerinos, however, thought differently, and the Nobel Prize winner Linus Pauling (who wrote the foreword to *Every Second Child*) endorsed his views.

Kalokerinos is a life fellow of the Royal Society for the Promotion of Health, of the International Academy of Preventive Medicine, of the Australasian College of Biomedical Scientists, and of the Hong Kong Medical Technology Association; he is also a member of the New York Academy of Sciences. In 1978, he was awarded the Australian Medal of Merit for outstanding scientific research. He is an author of 28 papers listed in PubMed. He retired from full time practice in 1993 and spent most of the next two decades doing private research.

David R. Hawkins, MD, PhD

(1927–2012) • Hall of Fame 2006

"David Hawkins was among the first psychiatrists to show that both schizophrenic and alcoholic patients could be treated successfully with vitamin B3."

—ABRAM HOFFER

David Ramon Hawkins grew up in rural Wisconsin and served aboard a U.S. Navy minesweeper during the closing months of World War II. He earned his bachelor's degree from Marquette University in 1950 and his medical degree from the Medical College of Wisconsin in 1953. Dr. Hawkins interned at Columbia Hospital in 1954, was awarded a fellowship in psychiatry at Mt. Sinai Hospital in 1956, and then became supervising psychiatrist for the New York State Department of Mental Hygiene. From 1956 to 1980, he was medical director of North Nassau Mental Health Center in Manhasset, New York, one of the largest psychiatric practices in New York with 50 employees and 1,000 new patients each year. He was also director of research at Brunswick Hospital in Long Island from 1968 to 1979, and a guest on TV shows including *The MacNeal-Lehrer News Hour* and *Today*.

In 1973, along with Nobel Prize winner Linus Pauling, Hawkins co-edited *Orthomolecular Psychiatry: Treatment of Schizophrenia*, the first psychiatric textbook of its kind. Among other honors, Hawkins received the Huxley Award in 1979 and, interestingly enough, a Physicians Recognition Award from the American Medical Association in 1992. He served on the *Journal of Orthomolecular Psychiatry* editorial board and was founding president of the Academy of Orthomolecular Psychiatry. The *Journal of Orthomolecular Psychiatry* has published book reviews and seven papers by Hawkins; two of these, on the prevention and nutritional treatment of tardive dyskinesia (muscle movement disorder caused by drug therapy). During retirement, he developed an especially keen interest in spirituality and consciousness, resulting in his writing a best-selling trilogy, *Power vs. Force* (1995), *The Eye of the I* (2001), and *I: Reality and Subjectivity* (2003).

Bernard Rimland, PhD

(1928–2006) • Hall of Fame 2007

"Bernard Rimland calls drugs 'toximolecular medicines,' meaning involving toxic molecules instead of the 'correct' molecules of orthomolecular medicine. I agree with his choice of words."—LINUS PAULING

In the early 1960s, Bernard Rimland was the man who made the then revolutionary discovery that autism is a biological disorder. He outlined the evidence in his 1964 book, *Infantile Autism: The Syndrome and Its Implications for a Neural Theory of Behavior*. Based on reports from parents of autistic children, Rimland investigated high-dose vitamin B6 therapy. While other authorities in the autism field considered the idea that a vitamin could correct a brain disorder to be preposterous, to date, 22 studies (including 13 double-blind studies) show that vitamin B6, typically combined with magnesium, benefits a large percentage of autistic children.

When Dr. Rimland learned that most childhood vaccines contained thimerosal (a preservative that is nearly 50 percent mercury and a powerful neurotoxin), he realized that the escalating numbers of vaccines given to children could be the culprit behind skyrocketing rates of autism. The medical establishment, not surprisingly, expressed great antagonism toward this theory. To overcome such resistance, Rimland created the

Autism Society of America, the Autism Research Institute, and the Defeat Autism Now! (DAN) project, which grew from a small first meeting into a worldwide movement. He also served on the board of the *Journal of Orthomolecular Medicine* for many years.

Writes Dr. Woody R. McGinnis, "Any mechanistic hypothesis for autism should accommodate the successful application of high-dose vitamin B6 pioneered by Bernard Rimland" (excerpted in part from www.autismwebsite.com).

Bruce Ames, PhD

(b. 1928) • Hall of Fame 2010

"Better diet and supplementation would result in less neurodegenerative disease, less cancer, less Alzheimer's, less Parkinson's, less diabetes."—BRUCE AMES

Bruce Ames is a professor of biochemistry and molecular biology at the University of California, Berkeley, and a senior scientist at Children's Hospital Oakland Research Institute. In the 1950s, Dr. Ames began working at the National Institutes of Health, where he investigated ways of mutating the DNA of bacteria in order to learn more about gene regulation. This work led him to develop the Ames Test, one of the key diagnostic tools for detecting mutagens that is still used worldwide. With that breakthrough test, Ames and other investigators were able to show that most cancer-causing chemicals act by damaging genes—a finding that now seems obvious only because Ames helped prove it. The revolution in the Ames Test was its speed and cost: it can be done in an afternoon, whereas previously animal cancer tests cost millions of dollars and took years to complete.

Ames is a National Medal of Science winner, has published more than 450 scientific papers, and has become one of the most cited scientists alive. Ames has been interested in the free radical theory of aging for many years. Free radicals are highly reactive molecules that ravage cell machinery, bond indiscriminately with other molecules, break chromosomes, and cripple enzymes. In 1990, Ames published the first evidence that deoxyribonucleic acid (DNA) oxidation actually increases with age. This research led him to look more closely at mitochondria because they are a significant source of the body's free radicals. In order to burn fats and carbohydrates to make metabolic fuel, mitochondria take electrons from the enzyme nicotinamide adenine dinucleotide (NADH) and shuffle them among a suite of molecules in a complex chain reaction that ends in the reduction of oxygen to water. Invariably, some of the electrons escape from this "respiratory chain," creating free radicals.

His breakthrough in aging research, which came in the mid-1990s, took a closer look at a dietary supplement, acetyl-L-carnitine (ALCAR). Ames reasoned that high levels of ALCAR might also combat the problems of aging membranes and decrepit enzymes. He began feeding ALCAR to his old rats and within weeks, he noticed improvements in the animals' biochemistry and behavior. Their mitochondria were going full bore again, and they had become far more active; they were still churning out oxidants at a very high rate. Ames decided to add an agent to the rats' diet to neutralize the oxidants. He tried lipoic acid, a mitochondrial antioxidant. The results were profound. Oxidants and oxidative damage to mitochondrial components dropped dramatically. Both the structure and function of the mitochondria improved.

Three years ago, Ames set up a company called Juvenon, which sells tablets containing 200 milligrams of alpha-lipoic acid and 500 mg acetyl-L-carnitine, to be taken twice a day. Ames is also convinced that simple B-vitamin therapy could combat many diseases and has published an exhaustive review, with more than 300 references, showing that no fewer than 50 genetic diseases might be remedied with high doses of vitamins, minerals, and amino acids. Most recently, he has published on his novel "triage theory," which posits that some functions of micronutrients are restricted during shortage and that functions required for short-term survival take precedence.

—STEVEN CARTER and GREG SCHILHAB

Robert F. Cathcart III, MD

(1932–2007) • Hall of Fame 2008

"I have never seen a serious reaction to vitamin supplements. Since 1969 I have taken over 2 tons of ascorbic acid myself. I have put over 20,000 patients on bowel-tolerance doses of ascorbic acid without any serious problems, and with great benefit."

—ROBERT F. CATHCART

Robert Cathcart's observations on the clinical use of ascorbic acid drew worldwide renown, along with the respect of Linus Pauling. A native of Texas, Dr. Cathcart came to Northern California as a child and spent most of his life in the Bay Area. He earned his medical degree from the University of California in San Francisco in 1961 and then completed his internship and residency at Stanford Hospital. Cathcart was an instructor in orthopedic surgery at Stanford after his residency. The Cathcart prosthesis (used to replace the ball portion of the hip joint) has been implanted in over 100,000 hips.

Cathcart became interested in vitamin C when he read Linus Pauling's *Vitamin C and the Common Cold*, and he began using it for his own allergies and his patients' viral infections. He thought about a common side effect of high-dose ascorbate, namely diarrhea, in a new way. He observed that a person's tolerance for the vitamin increased considerably in the presence of viral illness, seemingly in proportion to the severity of the illness. A person who ordinarily develops diarrhea from, say, a 12-thousand-milligram (mg) dose of ascorbate, might be able to tolerate upwards of 100,000 mg when ill with a cold or flu. Cathcart found that titration of vitamin C dosage to bowel tolerance permitted quicker resolution of an illness.

Cathcart treated tens of thousands of patients with vitamin C megadoses. He was a popular lecturer at medical meetings, where he freely shared his findings with his colleagues. However, he was not well published. Like Linus Pauling himself, Cathcart encountered rejection and even scorn at the hands of scientific and medical journal editors. The *Journal of Orthomolecular Medicine* is proud to be one of the few platforms to have brought Cathcart's work to the attention of the world's healing professions.

Robert Cathcart received the Linus Pauling Award from the Society for Orthomolecular Health Medicine in 2002. He leaves a reminder for all who would do science: progress and success rest more on dispassionate observation and creative thinking than on all the gee-whiz technology mankind has ever come up with. —RICHARD HUEMER

Richard Kunin, MD

(b. 1932) • Hall of Fame 2008

"Richard Kunin is an authentic trailblazer who merits the name."—NATIONAL HEALTH FEDERATION

Educated at the University of Minnesota, Richard Kunin received his medical degree in 1955. Following psychiatric residency training at New York Hospital, which he completed in 1959, he served for two years in the U.S. Army Medical Corps. Dr. Kunin has been in private practice since 1963, now in San Francisco.

Inspired by Dr. Linus Pauling's work with vitamin C and antioxidants in orthomolecular medicine, his 1973 discovery of manganese as a cure for drug-induced dyskinesia (a muscle-movement disorder caused by drug therapy) was the first orthomolecular research to verify the efficacy of mineral therapy for a disease (other than simple deficiency). His 1975 studies on the effects of niacin were the first to identify prostaglandins in the niacin flush and aspirin as an antidote.

He cofounded the Orthomolecular Medical Society with Drs. Michael Lesser and Linus Pauling in 1976 and served as its president from 1980 to 1982. Kunin's clinical research led to the "Ortho-Carbohydrate Diet," the first diet plan based on individualized carbohydrate-protein-fat effects on mood, energy, and weight. The "Listen to Your Body Diet," popularized in his best-selling books *Mega-Nutrition* (1980) and *Mega-Nutrition for Women* (1983) remains one of the safest, most user-friendly and effective diet-energy plans.

In 1986, Kunin began a 12-year stint as a newspaper columnist for San Francisco's *The New Fillmore*. His column, "Putting Nutrition First," was a big hit with its readers.

He achieved the first measurement of eicosapentaenoic acid (EPA) in snake oil (a fatty acid also abundant in coldwater fish) in 1989, substantiating its anti-inflammatory benefits. Kunin demonstrated that snake oil is, oddly enough, not quackery after all!

In 1994, he founded the Society for Orthomolecular Health Medicine (OHM) in San Francisco, which brings together physicians and other health practitioners to discuss current nutritional approaches to treating disease, and organized its annual scientific meetings for 14 years. In the same year, Kunin became the first interim president of the International Society for Orthomolecular Medicine. Kunin is also director of research of Ola Loa Products, leaders in powdered nutrition supplements.

Kunin also serves on the board of governors of the National Health Federation, a not-for-profit organization advocating for freedom of choice in health care and has been on the editorial review board of the *Journal of Orthomolecular Medicine* since 1982.

Hugh Desaix Riordan, MD

(1932–2005) • Hall of Fame 2005

"Hugh Riordan was an amazing influence on my family and on all who knew him."

—JULIE HILTON, the Hilton Family Foundation

Of all the medical mavericks, Hugh Riordan was one of the most knowledgeable, both as a maverick par excellence and as a historian of mavericks. Hugh was an orthomolecular fighter, who fought hard and consistently on behalf of orthomolecular concepts. He was challenged legally when he wanted to treat his patients with high-dose vitamins in the hospital. He won. He was the first to demonstrate how large doses of vitamin C are chemotherapeutic for cancer patients. He was a pioneer in establishing the new vitamins-as-treatment paradigm.

"We worked together on the editorial board of the *Journal of Orthomolecular Medicine* (*JOM*), and on the board of the International Schizophrenia Foundation. Riordan joined the editorial board of *JOM* in 1991 and then became its associate editor in 2000. He published several books, including three volumes of *Medical Mavericks* (1988, 1989, and 2005), and about 70 clinical and research reports. His main work had to do with the schizophrenic syndrome and with the treatment of cancer using nontoxic vitamin C chemotherapy. Riordan was the leader in making available to cancer patients a treatment that is effective, safe, economical, and very tolerable. Few oncologists have ever seen these advantages unless they visited Riordan's clinic. The vitamin C intravenous chemotherapy studies established so well by Dr. Riordan are being continued at the University of Kansas and at McGill University, Montreal. In 2002, Riordan was honored by the International Society for Orthomolecular Medicine with the Orthomolecular Physician of the Year award. He worked tirelessly, founding and developing the Center for the Improvement of Human Functioning International (now called the Riordan Clinic) in Wichita, Kansas, as a superb treatment center." This year, the center celebrates its 30th anniversary. Riordan's dedicated staff of more than 70 like-minded medical mavericks continue their founder's pioneering work. —ABRAM HOFFER

Masatoshi Kaneko, PhD

(b. 1935) • Hall of Fame 2007

"Orthomolecular nutritional medicine pioneers such as Dr. Kaneko look beneath the surface, and search for answers that may remain hidden to the superficial observer."—HUGH D. RIORDAN

Masatoshi Kaneko started his career in the pharmaceutical industry, where his research involved studying the development of molecular mechanisms of carcinogenesis. Dr. Kaneko came to believe that there must be a better approach to the treatment of cancer. He recalls, "I came to realize that there was no single chemotherapeutic substance—no single magic bullet." In the early 1970s, during a fellowship in the United States, Kaneko met Dr. Rei Kitahara, from Kumamoto University Medical School in Japan, which ultimately led him to orthomolecular medicine and meeting Linus Pauling. "This," Kaneko says, "was a major turning point of my life."

With iatrogenic (doctor-caused) disease on the rise, Kaneko realized that an understanding of nutritional medicine was absent among Japan's medical establishment. Wishing to spare the public from the dangers of invasive and often unnecessary medical procedures, he began educating the people of his homeland in the art and science of managing their own health. The Kaneko School and the Know Your Body Club (KYB) were formed, and a new movement in Japan's modern health care system was born (condensed from *Medical Mavericks* by Hugh Riordan, 93–107).

Since 1984, the vision of Kaneko has nurtured the growth of the KYB Club in Japan. His goal is to provide the public with valid scientific information on the proper use of nutritional supplements and to promote a healthier nation. Affiliated with orthomolecular pioneers Linus Pauling and Abram Hoffer, the KYB Club today now represents over 30,000 professional clinicians, registered dietitians, and orthomolecular medical nutritionists all over Japan, and encompasses the Orthomolecular Nutrition Laboratory, the KYB Medical Services and Clinic, and the non-profit Orthomolecular Medical Nutrition and Associates.

Hiroyuki Abe, MD, PhD

(b. 1938) • Hall of Fame 2013

"The work of the doctor will, in the future, be ever more that of an educator, and ever less that of a man who treats ailments."

—DR. SIR THOMAS J. LORD HORDER OF ASHFORD, physician to several British monarchs

Hiroyuki Abe is a leading pioneer in orthomolecular medicine in Japan. Encouraged and inspired by Abram Hoffer, he established the Japanese Society for Orthomolecular Medicine, serving as cofounder and honorary chairman, with Tsuyoshi Kitahara as director and Abram Hoffer as honorary member. Dr. Abe has incorporated into his practice and teaching the work of many orthomolecular pioneers, including Drs. Carl Pfeiffer, Hugh Riordan, Richard Kunin, and Michael Lesser. He has attended the Orthomolecular Medicine Today conferences for the last decade and brought what he has learned to Japan.

Abe graduated from Sapporo Medical University in 1964. During his surgical training, he was appointed a clinical fellow in surgery at Philadelphia Children's Hospital and at Cleveland Clinic. After returning to Japan, he was appointed as lecturer at Juntendo University in 1975 and as associate professor of radiology at Nihon University School of Medicine in 1981, while also a visiting professor in diagnostic radiology at Stanford University School of Medicine and in cardiology at the University of California, San Francisco. Abe is widely published in leading professional journals and he is the author of many chapters on cardiac surgery for medical textbooks.

Abe opened new medical frontiers for cancer treatment, with personalized medicine based on molecular diagnostics as his underlying theme. Abe developed a dendritic cell-based cancer vaccine and uses IV therapy, onco-hyperthermia (heat treatments for tumors), immunotherapy, and other orthomolecular treatments.

Orthomolecular psychiatry is Abe's other key interest. Following Abram Hoffer, he treats many schizophrenia and autism patients.

Abe is founder, chief executive officer, and medical director of Hakushin Koseikai Medical Foundation and director of Life Science Research Institute. He is also chairman of the International Society of Personalized Medicine.

Additionally, Abe has contributed to the advancement of orthomolecular medicine as the author of *New Ways to Treat Autism* (in Japanese), and as editorial supervisor for the Japanese editions of *The Brain Chemistry Diet* (2011) by Michael Lesser, *The Puzzle of Autism* (2006) by Garry Gordon and Amy Yasko, and *What Really Causes Schizophrenia* (2006) by Harold Foster.

Chris Reading, MD

(1938–2011) • Hall of Fame 2012

"Men who achieve greatness do not work more complexly than the average man, but more simply."
— WILLIAM J. MAYO and CHARLES H. MAYO, founders of the Mayo Clinic

Reading was a dynamic force in the International Holistic Health Care community, tirelessly caring for his many thousands of patients and helping hundreds of thousands of others through his writings. He was also an original thinker, many of whose ideas were decades ahead of their time. Finally, Dr. Reading was a courageous practitioner, who fought for the beliefs and values he championed in practicing orthomolecular medicine, at its very inception, in Australia.

Christopher Michael Reading was born in his parents' farmhouse in the village of Boxted on the Essex-Suffolk border in England. In 1954, the family emigrated to Australia, where Reading gained a commonwealth scholarship to study science at the University of Sydney. There he remained for 11 years, living at St Paul's College, and taking first his bachelor's degree, then a diploma in agricultural science, and finally his medical qualifications. After his internship, he decided to study psychiatry—the field that was to become his life's passion. He became a fellow of the Royal Australian and New Zealand College of Psychiatrists, and of the Australian College of Nutritional and Environmental Medicine and was a contributor to the Support for Orthomolecular Medicine Association (SOMA) of Australia newsletter.

A regular correspondent with Abram Hoffer, Reading reported on orthomolecular activities in Australia in the *Journal of Orthomolecular Medicine* and contributed articles to the journal, most recently in 2005. Of Reading's 2002 book *Trace Your Genes to Health: Use Your Family Tree to Guide Your Diet, Enhance Your Immune System and Overcome Chronic Disease*, Hoffer wrote: "This first book on genetic sleuthing and treatment will be one of the classics of our time."

Many journal readers are aware of Reading's pioneering and dedicated work as he explored the role of diet, allergies, vitamins, and genetics across a wide range of illnesses and conditions. His memoirs, *A Doctor in Orthomolecular Medicine*, were published in 2012. Medicine was never merely an abstract idea to him: he lived to help others and to alleviate suffering. —A.W.S., DAVID RICHARDS, and MICHAEL ANDREWS-READING

David Horrobin, MD, PhD

(1939–2003) • Hall of Fame 2005

"Luckily for schizophrenic patients, David Horrobin became dissatisfied with the results of treatment that modern psychiatry provides." —ABRAM HOFFER

David Horrobin was one of the most original scientific minds of his generation. His study of human physiology lead him to investigate the role of essential fatty acids (EFAs) and their derivatives in human disease. He applied his vast knowledge of lipids to investigate their therapeutic potential in medicine. Dr. Horrobin was a scholar of Balliol College, Oxford, where he obtained a first-class honors medical degree. To this he added a clinical medical degree and a doctorate in neuroscience. He was a fellow of Magdalen College where he taught medicine alongside Dr. Hugh Sinclair, one of the pioneers in the field of essential fatty acids. After further research on EFAs at the universities of Newcastle and Montreal, he became increasingly fascinated by lipid biochemistry and its application to human disease. His research on the medical benefits of gamma-linolenic acid opened a doorway into the profound influence of lipids towards health, sparking a minor revolution of lipid studies and research around the world.

Throughout his travels in East Africa and work in Kenya, he developed the kernel of thought about fatty acids and schizophrenia, and its role in evolution. He later elaborated this idea in his 2001 book, *The Madness of Adam and Eve*, which was short-listed in 2002 for the Aventis Science Book of the Year. Abram Hoffer wrote: "This is a remarkable book. I agree with his interpretation that schizophrenia is an evolutionary advantage and that its genes are slowly moving into the general population."

Horrobin was the founder and editor of *Medical Hypotheses*, a forum for the dissemination of new ideas in medicine. He was also the founder and editor of the journal *Prostaglandins, Leukotrienes, and Essential Fatty Acids*. He was a prolific writer who authored and edited 139 books on a wide range of subjects, contributed to over 800 scientific publications, and applied for 114 patents in which he is the named inventor, bringing the grand total to 1053. From his first publication in 1964 through to his death, this is equivalent of one publication every two weeks for 39 years—a prodigious achievement. In addition, he served as medical adviser and president for the Schizophrenia Association of Great Britain. He also served on the board of the International Schizophrenia Foundation from 1998 to 2003.

Horrobin was a favorite speaker at the annual Orthomolecular Medicine Today conference, where his presentations were models of clarity and logic.

Michael Lesser, MD

(b. 1939) • Hall of Fame 2008

"Dr. Lesser is one of the pioneers in the development of orthomolecular psychiatry and medicine."

—ABRAM HOFFER

Michael Lesser received his medical degree from Cornell University in 1964 and has maintained a private practice since 1971 in Berkeley, California. He became a member of the Academy of Orthomolecular Psychiatry in 1972 and served as vice president from 1976 to 1986. During the same period he served on the Board of Trustees for the Huxley Institute for Biomedical Research. On numerous occasions since 1972, Dr. Lesser has served as an expert witness in psychiatry and orthomolecular medicine in criminal and civil cases before municipal, state, and federal courts in California and Arizona.

Along with ten other doctors, Lesser founded the Orthomolecular Medical Society in San Diego, in 1975. He served as its first president (1975–1979), with Drs. Linus Pauling, as honorary president, and Richard Kunin, as vice president.

"Life in all its fullness is Mother Nature obeyed."— WESTON PRICE

Lesser gave testimony before the California State Legislature leading to passage of Orthomolecular Medicine Bills in 1976 and 1977. He also gave testimony before the U.S. Select Senate Committee on Nutrition and Human Needs, "Diet Related to Killer Diseases, V: Nutrition and Mental Health," in Washington, DC, on June 22, 1977. An excerpt of his testimony was broadcast on CBS and NBC News that night and he appeared as a guest on ABC's *Good Morning America*, June 23, 1977.

In 1997 he founded Nutritional Medicine, a communications company that sponsors conferences on nutrition and vitamin therapy. With Dr. Kaneko of Japan, he organized the Orthomolecular Nutrition Laboratory Symposium in New York, October 1997.

Lesser's books include *Nutrition and Vitamin Therapy* (1980), which sold 350,000 copies; *Fat and the Killer Diseases* (1991); and *The Brain Chemistry Diet* (2002) in which he identifies six primary psychological types—each type evinces certain strengths when health is optimal and suffers from specific psychiatric vulnerabilities when imbalances occur. His dietary and supplement recommendations are predicated on these differences.

He has published over 50 papers and lectures on orthomolecular medicine and psychiatry and has served on the editorial review board for the *Journal of Orthomolecular Medicine*.

Erik T. Paterson, MD

(b. 1941) • Hall of Fame 2011

"I am morally compelled to remain an orthomolecular physician; indeed, I am alive because of orthomolecular medicine." —ERIK PATERSON

Erik Paterson is a fine example of the orthomolecular general practitioner working "in the trenches"—in his case in a small town in the Kootenay River valley of British Columbia, Canada, a few miles north of the Idaho border.

He was born in Cambridge, England, and graduated with a medical degree from the University of Glasgow, Scotland, where he practiced until 1970 before emigrating to Creston, British Columbia. He served his rural community until his recent retirement in January 2011.

Erik Paterson's father, T. T. Paterson, began working with Dr. Humphry Osmond on the administrative aspects of psychiatry in 1956. When he established his own private practice, Paterson was dissatisfied with the standard drug approach used by the local psychiatrist for all mentally ill patients. Believing there had to be a better way, he spent time with Abram Hoffer in Saskatoon in 1974. Combining what he learned from Hoffer with material presented by Drs. Carl Pfeiffer and Allan Cott at the 1974 meeting of the Canadian Schizophrenia Foundation, he was able to help more than three quarters of his schizophrenic patients become well.

Since those early days of discovery and success, Paterson has helped hundreds of patients through orthomolecular treatment. He also credits orthomolecular techniques for improving his condition and enhancing his survival since receiving a diagnosis of acute myeloid leukemia over fifteen years ago. In the *Journal of Orthomolecular Psychiatry* and the *Journal of Orthomolecular Medicine*, he has made dozens of contributions including many useful case reports from his general practice and he has served on the editorial board of the *Journal of Orthomolecular Medicine* since 1995. A regular presenter at the Orthomolecular Medicine Today conferences from 1981 to 2006, Paterson also participated in the 1998 documentary film *Masks of Madness: Science of Healing*.

Sister Theresa Feist

(b. 1942) • Hall of Fame 2006

"I'd like the whole world to know schizophrenia is an illness as physical as a broken leg." —SISTER THERESA FEIST

Born in northern Saskatchewan, the fifth of 12 children, Theresa attended multi-grade classrooms and St. Angela's Academy, a residential high school, where she entered the community of Ursuline Sisters and began a 17-year teaching career. In 1970 she became severely depressed and suicidal. She was later diagnosed with schizophrenia and was referred to Dr. Abram Hoffer.

On a sugar-free diet and niacin, she had a remarkable rapid recovery. *How to Live with Schizophrenia* (1966) by Drs. Hoffer and Osmond became the precious book that gave her insight into her illness. Moved to share her story with others, in 1979 Sister Theresa wrote *Schizophrenia Cured*, a valuable case history and source of hope and inspiration. Theresa also wished to establish a place to provide shelter and orthomolecular support for the mentally ill.

She shared her dream with George Morris, a Saskatchewan businessman and a director of the Canadian Schizophrenia Foundation (CSF), whom she met at a CSF conference; he financed the first Morris Center, which opened in Winnipeg, Manitoba, in 1981. Here, Theresa and another devoted woman, Mabel Fowler, carried on the ministry of teaching and accompanying all who came to learn a new lifestyle for good health. Eighteen years later, with the help of businessman Frank Flaman, the center was moved to Lebret, Saskatchewan, and renamed the Flaman-Morris Home. This residence, employing three full-time and two part-time staff, can house up to eight people seeking guidance and nutritional care. In the foreword to her book *Schizophrenia Cured*, Dr. Hoffer wrote: "All of us in the field of orthomolecular psychiatry, including doctors, patients and families, depend upon the hard work of the Sister Theresas of the world, the people who move mankind."

Harold D. Foster, PhD

(1943–2009) • Hall of Fame 2010

"What can one say about a scientist as accomplished, as brilliant, as knowledgeable as Harry Foster? His scientific writing is superb. He has a remarkable ability to examine all the data and to draw from that data, conclusions that are going to be of the greatest value to mankind. His work must be taken very seriously and followed up."—ABRAM HOFFER

Harold Foster was deeply invested in the resilience of life on the planet and in improving the quality of life for all living things. For more than 40 years, Dr. Foster worked as a geomorphologist, a professor of medical geography, a consultant to the United Nations and NATO in disaster planning, and an avid researcher, which culminated in the formation of the Harold Foster Foundation in Victoria, British Columbia.

A Canadian by choice, Foster was born in Tunstall, Yorkshire, England, and educated at the Hull Grammar School and University College London. While at university, he specialized in geology and geography, earning a bachelor of science in 1964 and a doctorate in 1968. He was a faculty member in the Department of Geography, University of Victoria, from 1967 to 2008. As a tenured professor, he authored or edited over 300 publications, the majority of which focused on reducing disaster losses or identifying the causes of chronic degenerative and infectious diseases.

His numerous books include *Disaster Planning: The Preservation of Life and Property* (1980); *Reducing Cancer Mortality: A Geographical Perspective* (1986); and *Health, Disease, and the Environment* (1992). He also wrote six books in the What Really Causes series, including those on AIDS, Alzheimer's disease, multiple sclerosis, schizophrenia, sudden infant death syndrome (SIDS), and breast cancer.

Foster became one of the giants in orthomolecular medicine, with boundless enthusiasm, a prolific gift of writing, and as a researcher who made unique contributions in our understanding of health and disease. Foster's soaring scientific mind combined his expertise in geography, epidemiology, and orthomolecular medicine to create new insights into nutritional medicine. He had a gift for synthesizing diverse, seemingly unrelated phenomena and showing us the orthomolecular whole.

A fixture at many of the Orthomolecular Medicine Today conferences, Foster's eagerly anticipated presentations were always fresh and original as he explored the complex relationships between genetic inheritance, health, and the nutritional geographies of the world. He also conducted many groundbreaking studies of selenium in AIDS therapy in Africa—a low-tech, but surprisingly effective approach that large pharmaceutical companies ignored in favor of expensive western therapies that, in the end, few Africans would be able to afford.

Foster's accomplishments as a writer, researcher, and educator are many and cover a broad range, including serving on the editorial board of the *Journal of Orthomolecular Medicine* for 15 years, and on the board of directors for the International Schizophrenia Foundation for 13 years. —STEVEN CARTER and GREG SCHILHAB

Jonathan V. Wright, MD

(b. 1945) • Hall of Fame 2012

"Dr. Wright is one of the smartest clinicians I have ever met. His remarkable insights and medical wisdom have proven miraculous for so many."—JOSEPH PIZZORNO, founding president of Bastyr University

Harvard University and University of Michigan graduate Jonathan V. Wright is a forerunner in research and application of natural treatments for healthy aging and illness. Along with Alan Gaby, MD, he has since 1976 accumulated a file of over 50,000 research papers about diet, vitamins, minerals, botanicals, and other natural substances from which he has developed non-patent medicine (non-drug) treatments for health problems. Since 1983, Drs. Wright and Gaby have regularly taught seminars about these methods to tens of thousands of physicians in the United States and overseas.

He was the first to develop and introduce the use of comprehensive patterns of bio-identical hormones (including estrogens, progesterone, DHEA, and testosterone) in 1982 and (at Meridian Valley Laboratory) directed the development of tests to ensure their safe use. He teaches use and laboratory monitoring of bio-identical hormones at several seminars each year.

He also originated successful natural treatment for the elimination of childhood asthma; popularized the use of D-mannose treatment for *E. coli* urinary tract infections; developed effective natural treatment for seborrheic dermatitis, allergic and viral conjunctivitis, and Osgood-Schlatter's disease (inflammation of the tendon below the kneecap); and discovered the effect of cobalt and iodine on estrogen and other steroid detoxification.

Wright founded the Tahoma Clinic (1973), Meridian Valley Laboratory (1976), and the Tahoma Clinic Foundation (1996); all located in Renton, Washington. Tahoma Clinic was established to approach disease by natural means and to emphasize correction of imbalances in the body that lead to disease. The infamous 1992 FDA Tahoma Clinic "raid" ("The Great B-Vitamin Bust") was a major impetus for Congressional reform of vitamin/mineral regulation. Dr. Wright continues to be an advocate for patient freedom of choice in health care.

Internationally known for his books and medical articles, Wright has authored or co-authored 11 books, selling over 1.5 million copies, with two texts achieving best-selling status: *Dr. Wright's Book of Nutritional Therapy* (1982) and *Dr. Wright's Guide to Healing with Nutrition* (1993). He authors *Nutrition and Healing*, a monthly newsletter emphasizing nutritional medicine that reaches over 118,000 in the United States, and another 15,000 or more worldwide.

Jeffrey Bland, PhD

(b. 1946) • Hall of Fame 2009

"Jeff is the most important innovator and educator in natural medicine in North America."—ABRAM HOFFER

Jeffrey Bland was born in 1946 in Illinois and grew up in Southern California, where he graduated from the University of California, Irvine, in 1967 with degrees in biology and chemistry. In 1971, he completed his doctorate degree in synthetic organic chemistry and began his career as a university professor and researcher at the University of Puget Sound with a dual appointment in chemistry and environmental sciences. In 1976, Dr. Bland was certified as a clinical laboratory director and was tenured in 1977. From 1976 to 1995, he served as a prominent educator for the natural foods and nutritional supplement industries and was involved in the founding of Bastyr University of Natural Health Sciences in Seattle, the first accredited university of naturopathic medicine in North America. In 1981, Bland was invited by Linus Pauling to become the director of nutritional supplement analysis at the Linus Pauling Institute in Palo Alto, California.

In 1984, he started HealthComm International, a company dedicated to teaching physicians and other licensed health-care providers how to successfully implement nutrition intervention into their practices. Since 1978, Bland has authored four books on nutrition and health for the general public and six books for health professionals. He is also the principal author of over 100 peer-reviewed research papers on nutritional biochemistry. He established the Institute for Functional Medicine in 1991 and published his *Textbook of Functional Medicine* in 2005.

Since 2000, Jeffrey Bland has served as the chief science officer of Metagenics and the president of MetaProteomics, a nutrigenomic research and development company employing more than 40 scientists and physicians at its research centers.

Tsuyohi (Ken) Kitahara

(b. 1948) • Hall of Fame 2011

"Do not let either the medical authorities or the politicians mislead you. Find out what the facts are, and make your own decisions about how to live a happy life and how to work for a better world."— LINUS PAULING

Tsuyoshi (Ken) Kitahara was born in Tokyo and graduated from the University of Keio, Faculty of Law. As an international businessman he has lived in the United States, Europe, Singapore, and Japan. His keen interest in integrative medicine led him to a few medical doctors in Japan who were frustrated with the current system of medicine and who wished to investigate diet and the orthomolecular approach.

In 2001, Kitahara needed psychiatric help for his son. When told that his son would never get well and would have to take drugs for the rest of his life, Kitahara decided this was not acceptable. He found one of Dr. Abram Hoffer's articles on vitamin therapies for psychiatric disorders, which provided hope for patients and families. After sending one email to Dr. Hoffer, Kitahara's whole world changed. With his son, he visited Dr. Hoffer in Victoria in 2002, where he received immediate support that he had not found in Japan. Dr. Hoffer kindly explained what the original problem was and how to advance the treatment. Kitahara decided that the benefit and the blessing received from Dr. Hoffer should be available to all people suffering from these problems in Japan.

In 2003, Kitahara established the Japanese Society for Orthomolecular Medicine (JSOM) along with Dr. Hiroyuki Abe and Dr. Osamu Mizukami. The JSOM focuses on orthomolecular treatment for psychiatric illness, autism, and various stress-related disorders. The JSOM hosts research and study meetings every year for medical doctors, as well as several orthomolecular seminars for patients and their families. In addition, a number of orthomolecular nutrition books have been published in Japanese with Ken's assistance.

It is always a great joy when patients improve; in JSOM's and Kitahara's office, five former schizo-phrenic patients are working and performing various office tasks. His next goal is to open a group home where orthomolecular therapy will be at the core of living to assist the patients and to provide meaningful work.

Today, Kitahara still feels his most important duty is to spread information on the orthomolecular approach, which has been established by our pioneers, and to maintain and lead an active movement forward for the sake of those in need.

Alan R. Gaby, MD

(b. 1950) • Hall of Fame 2012

"This physician, teacher, scientist, researcher, and writer is a modern Renaissance man."

—BILL MANAHAN, past president of the American Holistic Medical Association

Alan Gaby received his undergraduate degree from Yale University, his master of science in biochemistry from Emory University, and his medical degree from the University of Maryland. He was in private practice for 17 years, specializing in nutritional medicine.

He is past-president of the American Holistic Medical Association and gave expert testimony to the White House Commission on Complementary and Alternative Medicine on the cost-effectiveness of nutritional supplements. He is the author of *Preventing and Reversing Osteoporosis* (1994) and *The Doctor's Guide to Vitamin B6* (1984), is the co-author of *The Patient's Book of Natural Healing* (1999), and has written numerous scientific papers in the field of nutritional medicine. He has been the contributing medical editor for the *Townsend Letter for Doctors* since 1985, and contributing editor for the *Alternative Medicine Review* since 1996.

Over the past 30 years, he has developed a computerized database of tens of thousands of individually chosen medical journal articles related to the field of natural medicine. He was professor of nutrition and a member of the clinical faculty at Bastyr University in Seattle from 1995 to 2002. He is chief science editor for *Aisle 7* (formerly

Healthnotes, Inc.) and has appeared on the *CBS Evening News* and the *Donahue Show.* In 2011, Dr. Gaby published his 30-year project: a comprehensive textbook, *Nutritional Medicine,* which discusses dietary modifications, nutritional supplements, and other natural substances for the prevention and treatment of more than 400 health conditions. It has been widely acclaimed as the leading textbook in its field.

Ronald E. Hunninghake, MD

(b. 1951) • Hall of Fame 2013

"Dr. Ron exemplifies the qualities that make an exceptional orthomolecular physician. In addition to his knowledge of nutritional medicine, he understands how human relationships influence health and disease. His personal warmth enables him to connect immediately with patients."

—JACK CHALLEM, health and nutrition writer

Ron Hunninghake graduated from the University of Kansas School of Medicine in 1976. Board certified in family medicine, his early practice years reflected a conventional perspective seeking a wellness expression. All through medical school he had annoyed his professors with a burning question: "When will we learn more about health?"

His quest for a new paradigm of true health care was fulfilled in his association with Dr. Hugh Riordan, which began in 1989. Riordan's synthesis of patient as co-learner, his detective approach to identifying root causes rather than simply treating symptoms, and his own passion to find orthomolecular treatments resonated with Dr. Ron's original insight of using health as the ultimate antidote for chronic disease.

With Riordan's untimely passing in 2005, Dr. Ron was appointed chief medical officer of what is now the Riordan Clinic (formerly the Center for the Improvement of Human Functioning International). In the challenging years that followed, he advanced the scope and vision of the clinic, inspiring staff and patients as co-learners to take better care of themselves, form new and sustainable

habits of health, and assume greater responsibility for their own health care.

Serving as the face of the Riordan Clinic, Dr. Ron drew upon a vast array of its original orthomolecular research to eloquently present Riordan's message of hope to audiences in Japan, Spain, the Netherlands, Canada, and Mexico, as well as extensively in the United States. He hosted his third IV Vitamin C and Cancer Symposium in 2012, gathering doctors from all over the world to lead a new generation of orthomolecular researchers and clinicians.

The quality that makes Hunninghake a strong and effective leader can be summed up in one word: compassion. His strong commitment and devotion to leading the Riordan Clinic and his pursuit of excellence are unmatched. He is loved and respected by all who meet him.

Atsuo Yanagisawa, MD, PhD

(b. 1951) • Hall of Fame 2011

"Maintaining optimal anti-oxidative reserve by taking vitamin C is essential for cancer prevention and treatment, anti-aging, radio-protection, and optimum health."—ATSUO YANAGISAWA

Atsuo Yanagisawa graduated from the Kyorin University School of Medicine in 1976 and completed his graduate work in 1980 from the Kyorin University Graduate School of Medicine in Tokyo, Japan. Dr. Yanagisawa served as Professor in Clinical Medicine at the Kyorin University School of Health Sciences, and concurrently as professor in clinical cardiology at Kyorin University Hospital until 2008.

Yanagisawa has served as the director of the International Education Center for Integrative Medicine in Tokyo since 2008. He has introduced many well-known teachers from North America in Japan, including Drs. Burt Berkson, Michael Janson, John Hoffer, and Steve Hickey. He is a fellow of the American College for Advancement in Medicine and is board certified in chelation therapy. In 2004, he established the SPIC Salon Medical Clinic (anglicized Japanese for Lifestyle Personal Image Creator), which combines IV treatments in a spa setting. The Japanese College of Intravenous Therapy was founded in 2007, with Dr. Yanagisawa as president. The college has grown to almost 400 doctors in 200 clinics in every region of Japan. Dr. Yanagisawa presented at the 2nd IV C Symposium in Wichita, Kansas, in October 2010 and launched the International College of IV Therapy, which held their first conference, also in October 2010, bringing together experts in the field from Japan and around the world.

Dr. Yanagisawa is the author of 140 scientific papers in English and Japanese and has published several books in cardiology, chelation, nutrition, coaching, and IV vitamin C for cancer. His significant contribution as a pioneer in intravenous therapy in Japan has earned him a place in the Orthomolecular Medicine Hall of Fame.

Gert Schuitemaker, PhD

(b. 1952) • Hall of Fame 2011

"For over 30 years, Gert Schuitemaker has been an advocate for orthomolecular medicine. He organized the orthomolecular movement in the Netherlands and has long been a leader in building it internationally. He has wisdom as well as broad knowledge of nutritional medicine research."

—BO H. JONSSON, St. Goran's Hospital, Stockholm

Trained as a pharmacist, Gert Schuitemaker completed his PhD in medicine at University of Maastricht in 2004. He was introduced to orthomolecular medicine through the work of Linus Pauling, whom he first met and interviewed in Palo Alto, California, in 1985, Abram Hoffer, and others. Schuitemaker founded the Ortho Institute in 1982, the leading center for orthomolecular expertise in the Netherlands, which publishes *Orthomoleculair* (*Orthomolecular*) magazine for health professionals *Fit mit Voeding* (*Fit with Nutrition*) for the public. The Maatschappij ter Bevordering van de Orthomoleculaire Geneeskunde (Society for the Advancement of Orthomolecular

Medicine) was founded by Schuitemaker in 1987, and he served as its first president until 1997. Schuitemaker organized conferences on vitamin C with Robert Cathcart in 1986, and on nutrition and behavior with Stephen Schoentaler, which attracted much attention in 1988, the same year he began the "Around the World" column in the *Journal of Orthomolecular Medicine*. In 1994, along with his partner, Elsedien de Groot, Schuitemaker started the Ortho Company, makers of the Plantina line of supplements, for which he is product developer and formulator. Plantina products are very popular among Dutch athletes, including Nicolien Sauerbreij who won gold in snowboarding at the 2010 Olympic Games.

"Of several remedies, the physician should choose the least sensational."

—HIPPOCRATES

Schuitemaker served as president of the International Society for Orthomolecular Medicine from 1999 to 2009 and received the 2005 Orthomolecular Doctor of the Year Award, cited as a "leader in establishing orthomolecular medicine in Europe." To celebrate the 40th anniversary of Pauling's orthomolecular article in *Science*, Schuitemaker hosted a meeting in Anholt, Germany, with other leading orthomolecular scientists and practitioners in Europe. His book, *New Light on Vitamin D*, published in 2008, increased the awareness of this important nutrient in the Netherlands. A member of the advisory board of the International Schizophrenia Foundation and the editorial board of the *Journal of Orthomolecular Medicine*, Schuitemaker has published several books and more than 300 articles.

Schuitemaker's influence has led many physicians in the Netherlands to use food supplements in their daily practice and to affirm that they do "orthomolecular therapy."

Steven Carter

(b. 1954) • Hall of Fame 2012

"Whatever your hand finds to do, do it with all your heart."—ECCLESIASTES 9:10

With the exception of Abram Hoffer himself, no one person has had as much influence on the Canadian orthomolecular movement as has the current executive director, Steven Carter. Responding to the invitation of Abram Hoffer, Carter came to the Canadian Schizophrenia Foundation (CSF) in 1985 from his position as editor of *Alive Magazine* in Vancouver. He inherited an organization consisting of a small core group of like-minded orthomolecular doctors, an emerging professional journal, and a modest annual meeting. From these roots, Carter patiently nurtured and grew something greater than Abram could ever have imagined. He became the executive director of the International Schizophrenia Foundation, the managing editor of the *Journal of Orthomolecular Medicine,* and also led the International Society for Orthomolecular Medicine. In 1987 Carter took on the challenge of rebuilding the dormant CSF, envisioning a revived organization leading the way in complementary and alternative medicine (CAM). He moved the CSF office from Regina to Vancouver to be closer to the growing CAM environment. His duties included serving as director of the annual CSF meeting, and re-organizing and expanding the annual conference.

In 1988, Carter changed the conference focus towards healthcare professionals, renamed it Nutritional Medicine Today, and, in 2006, brought it to its present form: the annual international Orthomolecular Medicine Today conference. Under Carter's leadership, the conference attracts hundreds of people to Canada, including delegates, speakers, and exhibitors from 18 countries.

Serving in the multiple roles of educator, editor, publisher, planner, facilitator, and producer, Carter has worked to establish diet, nutrition, and lifestyle choices as the cornerstones of optimum health, and consistently kept professional and public attention focused on the importance of individual responsibility in health care. His commitment to orthomolecular medicine is demonstrated not only through his staying power but also in his ongoing effort to raise awareness and to educate Canadians to incorporate health-care approaches that may not be covered by the medical system. After 25 years, Carter's mission has been a great success. —GREG SCHILHAB

Andrew W. Saul, PhD

(b. 1955) • Hall of Fame 2013

"Andrew Saul is one of the best reviewers I have ever known. He is an amazing scientist and contributor."

—ABRAM HOFFER

Andrew W. Saul was born and raised in Rochester, New York. He entered university at the age of 15. After study at the Australian National University and the Canberra Hospital, he received his bachelor of science from the State University of New York, Brockport, at age 19. He then did graduate work at the University of Ghana, Legon, West Africa, and also at the Brigham and Women's Hospital in Boston. Shortly thereafter, he began lecturing on the history of nutrition research and vitamin therapy and was in private practice as a consultant for the next 35 years. He continued his education by winning three New York Empire State Teaching Fellowships, earning a master of science in 1989. Saul taught nutrition, addiction recovery, health science, and cell biology for nine years for the State University of New York, and clinical nutrition for New York Chiropractic College. He completed his non-traditional PhD in ethology (behavioral biology) in 1995. Based on his dissertation, he created www.DoctorYourself.com in 1999. This, and his writing and publishing the *Doctor Yourself Newsletter,* brought him to the attention of Dr. Abram Hoffer. Saul served as a columnist for the *Journal of Orthomolecular Medicine* beginning in 2002, as a contributing editor from 2003 to 2006, and as an assistant editor from 2006 to 2010. He remains on the editorial board of the *Journal of Orthomolecular Medicine* and of *Orthomolecular* magazine (Netherlands).

Saul testified before the Parliament of Canada in 2005 on behalf of the safety of nutrition therapy. That same year, he founded the free-access, peer-reviewed *Orthomolecular Medicine News Service* and has served as editor-in-chief for over 135 issues. In 2006, *Psychology Today* named Saul as one of seven natural health pioneers. He has won the Citizens for Health Outstanding Health Freedom Activist Award, is an honorary director of the Gerson Insti-tute and a member of the board of the Japanese College of Intravenous Therapy, and is featured in two documentaries, *Dying to Have Known: The Evidence Behind Natural Healing* (2006) and the very popular *Food Matters* (2008). He has authored or co-authored fourteen books, including four with Abram Hoffer. Saul is currently editor of Basic Health Publications' popular *Vitamin Cure* book series, with over a dozen titles in print or in progress.

OTHER NUTRIENT PIONEERS

James Caleb Jackson, MD

(1811–1895)

"In order to live free from sickness and die from old age, we need only to understand and obey the laws upon which life and health depend."—JAMES C. JACKSON

James Caleb Jackson was one of the most influential natural health practitioners of the 19th century. Jackson was a personal friend of both Frederick Douglass and Susan B. Anthony, and he was Clara Barton's personal physician. It was not by mere coincidence that the first chapter of the American Red Cross was founded in Dansville, New York. It is here that Dr. Jackson had established and operated what his grateful patients affectionately called "our home on the hillside." The 122-bed facility was the preeminent health center of the Northeast as well as "the largest hygienic institution in the world." The sanatorium even had its own rail spur.

Jackson's nutritional health contributions have been largely obscured by his much better known contemporary, Dr. John Harvey Kellogg. It was Jackson, not Kellogg, who was the true originator of the first dry breakfast cereal. Basically, twice-toasted, crumbled-up, whole-wheat graham crackers, Jackson's "granula" was neither flaked nor as successfully mass marketed. Nutritional supplements were completely unavailable a century and a half ago. Vitamins were not discovered until 1895, the year Dr. Jackson died, and not synthe-sized until the 1930s. Strict adherence to fresh, raw, or unprocessed sanatorium dining, extreme as it might superficially seem, was the only sensible orthomolecular regimen of the day.

Even Jackson's emphasis on the curative powers of water has considerable merit. Jackson had been a very sick young man and attributed his dramatic reversal to hydropathy. He was far from alone: in his century, the practice of water-cure was widespread. While the dietary doctrine that accompanies hydropathy almost certainly had a major role in the doctor's personal recovery and that of his patients, much of hydropathy has been quietly assimilated into conventional medical practice. Bathing, proper hygiene, Epsom salts soaks, sitz baths, hot and cold compresses, massage, and a keen appreciation of dietary trace minerals and the importance of proper hydration is now regarded as commonsense medicine.

President Ronald Reagan's personal physician, Ralph Bookman, has long been urging his patients with allergies to drink lots of water to relieve their symptoms. In an interview, Dr. Bookman said, "Unquestionably, the single most important element in the treatment of asthma and other bronchial allergy symptoms is hydration. Unless adequate fluids are available to the mucous glands in the bronchial tree, their secretions will be tenaciously hard to raise. In asthma, liquids are medications . . . Liquids make mucous liquid. They change it from a troublesome solid that makes breathing difficult to an easy-to-cough up liquid. I demand that my patients drink 10 full glasses of liquid every day, and I question them constantly to make sure they understand how important it is . . . Water is best, of course, but I tell them to drink what they like . . . Any fluids will work but you must make a fetish of it." Jackson would have agreed, word for word.

What made the nature-cure hospital so popular, even in a location as remote as Dansville? Perhaps it was the water, or the huge organic vegetable gardens. Perhaps in the beginning it was Jackson's personality, which by all accounts was impressive. In later generations, certainly Bernard Macfadden's charisma was an important factor (see next). But perhaps it was simply the sanatorium's success rate that brought in the crowds. Nutrition-based therapy works. It worked then and it works now.

Bernard Adolphus Macfadden

(1868–1955)

"Civilized man is manufacturing and eating many substances that slowly but surely lead to degeneration, disease, and premature death."—BERNARD MACFADDEN

Bernard "Bernarr" Adolphus Macfadden was born in 1868, orphaned by age 11, and a millionaire by age 35. He was the immensely successful publisher of long-running popular magazines including *True Detective, Photoplay,* and *Physical Culture.* The archetypal "health nut," Macfadden personally led a mass health walk every year all the way from New York City to Dansville, which is upstate near Rochester, so that is quite a hike. The 325-mile health-food-powered marathon was dubbed the "Cracked Wheat Derby."

Those who today speak only of the eccentricities of the health "faddists" like Macfadden and James Caleb Jackson (see above) marginalize their many lasting medical contributions. Too much of what the public hears today effectively distracts it from the real success nature-cure advocates have achieved. When we dwell less on the practitioners' personalities, and focus more on their actual treatments, we see an ahead-of-the-times' emphasis on physical activity and eating right. Long ago, Macfadden's "physical culture creed" specifically called for "reasonable regular use of the muscular system" and a "wholesome diet of vital foods." He and other health-food "faddists" were first to promote abstinence from tobacco, alcohol, junk food, and overeating. What the old-time "faddists" insisted on then is now universally regarded as part and parcel of good health. Macfadden, regarded by traditional vegan natural hygienists as a milk-diet revisionist, nevertheless offered menus that were nutritious, low fat, low cholesterol, low sugar, and high fiber. Though Macfadden's expansive claims for such a diet continuously got him into trouble with regulatory authorities, recently, rather strict vegetarianism has been shown by cardiologist Dean Ornish to be a highly effective way to prevent and even reverse serious cardiovascular disease. This is a therapy straight out of the past, as Dr. Ornish acknowledges. Ornish's diet prescription invites comparison with "Bernard Macfadden's culinary creed," which reads, in part:

For saving money, cutting down food costs, and building better health:

Do not discard the green outer leaves of cabbage or lettuce.

Never discard leftover vegetable pot juices; they can be used in soups or served as vegetable cocktails.

Cook carrot and beet tops with your soups; they contain valuable minerals. Fresh beet tops can be used as a green vegetable. Add parsley, mint, pimento, watercress, and lemon wherever possible to salads and dishes.

Throughout winter months, continue to use as many fresh fruits and vegetables as possible to procure; they are the protective foods.

Wash fruits and vegetables for residues of insecticide sprayings containing poisons, which frequently account for diseases of an insidious kind that are difficult to trace.

Use salt sparingly.

All raw vegetable juices are especially recommended.

Eat plenty of dandelions found in fields during many months of year. You can make teas containing valuable nutrients from grass, alfalfa, or clover leaves dried in your own kitchen.

Do not use chemically bleached white flour or sugar. Use vital foods only, those that contain all necessary vitamins and minerals. Thoroughly masticate and mix your food with saliva when eating.

The foods mentioned above are far better sources of vitamins and minerals than are highly processed factory foods, and before the advent of food fortification, they were the only sources.

Because Macfadden happened to be on a short fast when he died at the age of 87, his death has often been wrongly attributed to fasting. While Macfadden did suggest one- or two-week fasts in some of his writings, he primarily endorsed short fasts and in particular habitual undereating. In his creed he wrote, "If no appetite at meal time, wait until the next meal" and "To prolong life, do not eat to repletion. Stop when you could enjoy more, or better still, fast on water alone or fruit juices for one day each week." These are hardly reckless recommendations. Physicians, notably Allan Cott, have authored how-to books recommending therapeutic fasting for weight loss and also to promote general health and well-being.

That he completed innumerable fasts throughout his entire long and doctor-free life is generally downplayed. As a matter of fact, for decades he routinely fasted every Monday, year after year, with many additional extensive fasts. Macfadden was known to all for his long workdays and notorious for his physical stamina. This is a man who could rip a deck of cards in half, twice over, and repeatedly lift 100 pounds overhead with one hand. No wonder a young man named Angelo Siciliano became a Macfadden protegé and would later achieve his own fame as Charles Atlas.

Certainly Macfadden's charisma was an important factor in drawing flocks of people to grand health hotels to "take the cure." But his methods still largely stand up today.

Elmer McCollum, PhD

(1879–1967)

"He said he could just as well have chosen the last letter of the alphabet instead of the first, because he had no idea that there would be any more vitamins."

—A. R. PATTON

If anyone could be called the "father of nutrition science," it would be Elmer McCollum. It was he who first used rats in nutrition research. His invention of the method of biological assay turned mere feeding trials into a chemical science. He was the first to discover that there are fat-soluble and water-soluble compounds in the diet that are essential to life. He believed in telling about his discoveries in simple words so everybody could understand them, and in 1957 he wrote a popular book called *A History of Nutrition*. This helped people to believe that nutrition is based on chemistry.

His career began forty years earlier, in 1907, when the Wisconsin State Agricultural Experiment Station had tried feeding groups of dairy cows on various grains to see which was best. The cows getting wheat went blind. They decided to hire a young PhD chemist to analyze the wheat and find out what there was in it that made the cows blind. They hired Elmer McCollum, just out of Yale.

It didn't take long for McCollum to see that using cows as test animals was much too slow. What he needed was a test animal with a short life span that gave birth often, and would eat anything: he chose rats. This was the first experimental rat colony in America. McCollum knew rats grew well on milk. He decided to use a mixture of chemicals duplicating milk, leaving out one chemical at a time, and then to observe what happened. He planned a ration of lactose, butterfat, milk protein, and mineral salts. But the lead chemist wouldn't let McCollum use butterfat. Wisconsin is a dairy state, and in those days practically all the money value of milk was in the butterfat. He made McCollum use the cheaper lard instead. The rats didn't grow well. After a short time, they couldn't see in a dim light. They were going blind. McCollum remembered the blind cows.

Secretly, he replaced the lard with butterfat, which soon cured the rats. Then he did chemical work on the butterfat and got out a chemical that wasn't fat itself, but was soluble in fat. It was so potent that he could put a tiny bit in lard and keep the rats well. That was in 1913. McCollum had just discovered the first vitamin. Since it would dissolve in fat, he named it "fat-soluble A." He said he could just as well have chosen the last letter of the alphabet instead of the first because he had no idea that there would be any more vitamins.

When McCollum's boss heard that he was using butter, he said McCollum would have to cut cost somewhere else. Sucrose, ordinary table sugar, was a lot cheaper than milk sugar, so he could change to sucrose. On sucrose the rats once again began to fail in health. They lost appetite, failed to grow, became sick and nervous. McCollum put the milk sugar back, and the rats almost immediately perked up and were well again. McCollum found that the lactose contained an impurity, something soluble in water. He made an extract, which kept the rats healthy even on sucrose instead of lactose. That was in 1915. He had discovered a second vitamin. Using the next letter of the alphabet, he named it "water-soluble B." Later this turned out to have several fractions, the B complex.

In 1917 Johns Hopkins University asked McCollum to become the first professor of biochemistry in their new School of Hygiene and Public Health, and he moved to Baltimore. McCollum had wanted to study the vitamin that prevents scurvy. Using the next letter, he named it "water-soluble C." He must have remembered stories his mother had told him about how the doctor said he had scurvy when he was one year old out in Kansas, and how his mother had saved his life with apple scrapings when the doctor said he would die. (Apple peel contains a modest portion of vitamin C.) Many times, over the long years when he had been working his way through the University of Kansas, and then on to Yale for a doctorate, McCollum had remembered the apple cure. From Kansas farm boy to scientist, he lived to name the vitamin that had saved his life.

When he learned that guinea pigs need vitamin C, he used guinea pigs to prove that rats make their own vitamin C. He did this by feeding rat livers to the deficient guinea pigs. Within minutes they recovered from the typical "face ache" position, got up, and began eating.

McCollum next tackled the problem of rickets, a bone-deforming disease of children. The Scots protected their babies with bad-smelling oil from the livers of cod fish. McCollum had tried cod liver oil and knew it contained his fat-soluble A. He wondered if vitamin A would prevent rickets too. He changed his rat food so the rats would get rickets, and the cod-liver oil worked. Then he did chemical work on the oil and got out an unsaponifiable fraction, very powerful in antirachitic effect. The next letter of the alphabet was D. McCollum had discovered vitamin D. He contributed in many other areas as well.

Elmer Verner McCollum was born in 1879. He retired from Johns Hopkins in 1946 and lived 21 years more, a legend in his own time.

Claus Washington Jungeblut, MD

(1898–1976)

"Vitamin C can truthfully be designated as the antitoxic and antiviral vitamin."

—CLAUS JUNGEBLUT

Everyone today knows the names of Drs. Albert Sabin and Jonas Salk. Albert Sabin developed the live oral polio vaccine, which with time would be found to be a leading cause of the disease, and Jonas Salk, the killed injectable vaccine, which is the vaccination used to this day. By contrast, the public as well as orthodox medicine are yet to pay proper attention to the work of Dr. Claus Jungeblut.

Jungeblut received his medical degree from the University of Bern in 1921 and between 1921 and 1923 conducted research at the Robert Koch Institute in Berlin. After employment as a bacteriologist for the New York State Department of Health from 1923 until 1927, he taught at Stanford University in California and then joined the faculty at the Columbia University College of Physicians and Surgeons in New York. Jungeblut retired in 1962 and died in 1976 at the age of 78.

In his day, Jungeblut was justly regarded as an important player in polio research. While recent revisionist history of the fight against polio has generally downplayed his contribution to the crusade, it has totally sidestepped what was arguably his most important discovery: that ascorbate is prevention and cure for polio. Amazingly, Jungeblut first published this idea in 1935 shortly after vitamin C had been identified and isolated (*J Exper Med* 1935). His research on ascorbate was sweeping and profound, extending well beyond the topic of polio. By 1937 he had also shown that vitamin C inactivated tetanus toxins (*Proc Soc Exper Biol Med* 1935 and *J Immunol* 1937). Jungeblut's research went on to show that vitamin C could inactivate toxins and protect against numerous vital and bacterial toxins, including diptheria, hepatitis, herpes, and staphylococcus (http://arxiv.org/html/physics/0403023).

Unlike oral polio vaccination, vitamin C has never caused polio. Yet how many people have you met, physicians included, who know vitamin C has been known to prevent and cure polio for nearly 70 years? It was never really a secret. On September 18, 1939, *Time* magazine reported that "Last week, at the Manhattan meeting of the International Congress for Microbiology, two new clues turned up. [One is] Vitamin C." The article describes how Jungeblut, while studying statistics of the 1938 Australian polio epidemic, deduced that low vitamin C status was associated with the disease. After that, Jungeblut is rarely highlighted by the popular or professional media.

Jungeblut performed experiments that suggested high doses of vitamin C were greatly beneficial in monkeys with polio. Sabin, who was interested in producing a vaccine at that time, failed to replicate Jungeblut's results. However, Sabin effectively prevented a positive result by using larger doses of virus and smaller doses of vitamin C; he also gave the vitamin C far less frequently. Sadly, Sabin's poorly conducted experiments convinced experts that vitamin C was ineffective, clearing the way for a polio vaccine and effectively stopping Jungeblut's research. Our loss has been a 75-year period in which vitamin C's antiviral effects have been ignored.

Conrad Elvehjem, PhD (1901–1962)
Tom Spies, MD (1902–1960)

"Never does nature say one thing and wisdom another."

—JUVENAL, Roman poet

"Connie" Elvehjem was born and raised on a farm near Madison, Wisconsin. From a young age, he was very intrigued by the rapid growth of the corn plant and the reactions within the plant that allowed that to happen. In 1906, across the globe, an English chemist, Frederick G. Hopkins, fed rats a corn diet and they died. Then he isolated a substance from milk that he named tryptophane (later the "e" was dropped). He added this to the corn diet, and the rats lived. Food had always been thought of as a source of energy. Hopkins was the first to think there are tiny amounts of undetected chemicals in some natural foods, which are necessary for life. He called them "accessory food factors." He didn't know, of course, that tryptophan in the body can make niacin.

In 1923 Elvehjem began graduate work as a teaching assistant in agricultural chemistry at the University of Wisconsin, Madison, and in 1927 he received his PhD. During these years, he and his students made many discoveries, but the most unusual is the way he discovered nicotinic acid, the long-sought cure for pellagra. At one time called the P-P factor (pellagra preventive), I first knew it as vitamin G (for Joseph Goldberger), and it is now known as vitamin B3. It was Goldberger who had proved that pellagra was not an infection but due to lack of something not present in the traditional diet of "spoonbread (cornmeal), sow belly, and long sweetening."

Serendipity is an overworked word. But something prompted Elvehjem to reach up on the shelf, and take down a bottle of a simple, inexpensive chemical compound, known since 1867; namely, nicotinic acid. He mixed a tiny bit of it in the food for his dogs, and it cured their black tongue disease. Vitamin B3 is nicotinic acid. He discovered it in 1937.

Tom Spies was a young unmarried physician when I first encountered him in 1944. He was

169

spending much of his off-duty time, at his own expense, traveling among the hill folk of the South he knew so well, with a bottle of nicotinic acid in his pocket. (It was common knowledge that all this while, a rival for his girlfriend kept trying to get him drafted into the Army and out of the way.) Spies roamed the hills looking for dogs with black tongues. The first warning he would have that he was coming to a log cabin in the woods was when the hounds began to bark. This would bring a woman to the cabin door, wiping her hands on her apron, shy children clinging to her skirt.

"Ma'am," he would begin, "I see these here hound dogs of yours got black tongues; they're sick dogs. But I got here in my pocket some medicine that can fix them up real good."

"Well, tell you what. You can try it out first on my old man. If it don't kill him, then you can go ahead on the dogs."

This was what he was after. He knew that mostly the dogs got the table scraps, so if they had black tongues, chances were the people in the cabin were coming down with pellagra. Spies did great pioneer work, proving the practical power of nicotinic acid. He spread it among the hill people like Johnny Appleseed once planted trees.

Spies also made the rounds of the mental institutions. I heard him tell of many cases he helped. Here is one I recall: "I'd found this young woman, violently insane they said. They had to keep her tied down. What had happened, back home she had suddenly grabbed the axe and tried to kill her husband; would've, too, if he hadn't been too fast for her. Just to think, I've sent people like this home, well and happy, all with 15 cents worth of nicotinic acid." When added nicotinic acid was listed on bread labels, there was so much confusion with nicotine that the name was changed to niacin. The derivative nicotinamide thus became niacinamide.

I've always wondered how the Indians, including those in Mexico and Central America, where corn (maize) was first developed from teosinte, knew to soak the kernels in limewater until they were soft, before wet milling. If the Europeans who first settled the South had followed this practice, instead of dry milling, they would have got sufficient niacin to prevent pellagra, and there never would have been the 14 government hospitals full of pellagra victims, suffering and dying from lack of the "four Ds vitamin," meaning, dermatitis, diarrhea, delirium, and death. — A. R. Patton

Ed Desaulniers, MD
(1949–2000)

"For all of us who have been honored to know Ed, we are richer for the experience."
—Janet Shute

Ed Desaulniers was medical director of the Shute Medical Clinic in London, Ontario. Dr. Desaulniers was the last physician trained by world-renowned vitamin E researcher, Evan Shute. Desaulniers carried forward his mentor's legacy with integrity and commitment to the principles of orthomolecular, integrative medicine.

Born and raised in West Stockbridge, Massachusetts, Desaulniers was the oldest of 12 children. He graduated in medicine from the University of Western Ontario in 1975 and joined the Shute Medical Clinic in September 1976. Dr. Shute taught Desaulniers about the merit of supplements and nutritional medicine and Desaulniers became the medical director after Dr. Shutes's death in 1978.

Diagnosed with lung cancer in May 1999, Desaulniers continued working throughout his treatment until April 2000.

He was a man of integrity, wisdom, and courage—a beloved, compassionate, and respected physician who cared for his patients, friends, and family to the utmost of his ability. Dr. Desaulniers lived out his life in service to others. Dr. Julian Oates, who was tutored by Desaulniers, will continue the tradition established by the Shute brothers 60 years ago. —Janet Shute

PART THREE

ORTHOMOLECULAR TREATMENT

N EARLY TWO-THIRDS OF A MILLION men died in the Civil War. All other U.S. wars put together add about another two-thirds of a million soldiers killed. That means that about 1,350,000 Americans have died, totally, in all the wars in U.S. history. Yet we lose close to that number of Americans each year because of cardiovascular disease and cancer. Nearly 10 million soldiers were killed in World War I, charging machine guns and getting mowed down month after month for four terrible years. The Centers for Disease Control (CDC) and Prevention report that there are now 8 million cancer deaths worldwide in just one year. That rate is over three times as many deaths from cancer as from machine guns. A different approach is needed immediately.

Nutrient therapy, properly dosed and administered, can be the answer to many chronic medical problems. The list is far longer than the deficiency diseases. A drug in either low or high doses cannot act as a vitamin will, but a vitamin in large doses can act as a drug. Very high blood concentrations of vitamin C, for example, are selectively toxic to cancer cells. Nutritional supplementation is not the answer to every health problem, but it does not have to be. The standard is not perfection; the standard is the alternative.

Drug medicine is increasingly obsolete. The center has shifted. It is pharmacy that is the alternative if nutrition fails, and that is rarely. Roger J. Williams so well said: "When in doubt use nutrition first." Dr. Frederick R. Klenner said: "Vitamin C should be given while doctors ponder the diagnosis." And long ago, Sir William Osler, a medical doctor, said: "One of the first duties of the physician is to educate the masses not to take medicine." Dr. Abram Hoffer said: "Drugs make a well person sick. Why would they make a sick person well?"

Applying the body of knowledge accumulated by orthomolecular physicians and researchers can be done. We've all been taught that anything that is safe and inexpensive cannot possibly be really effective against "real diseases." It is time to rethink that, and especially to see what has already been accomplished. Improbable does not mean impossible. Physicians who categorically rule out nutritional therapy mimic their forbearers by overreliance on patent remedies. Much of "modern medicine" may be defined as "the experimental study of what happens when poisonous chemicals are placed into malnourished human bodies." Someday, health care without orthomolecular nutrition therapy will be seen as we today see childbirth without sanitation or surgery without anesthetic.

Here in Part Three we present the vitamin therapies and nutritional approaches pioneering physicians then and now are using to successfully treat many of our most common chronic diseases.

—A.W.S.

ALCOHOLISM

EVER SINCE I (AH) MET BILL W, the cofounder of Alcoholics Anonymous (AA), and we became close friends, I have had a personal interest in the treatment of alcoholism. Bill taught that there were three components to the treatment of alcoholism: spiritual, mental, and medical. AA provides a spiritual home for alcoholics that many cannot find anywhere else and helps them sustain abstinence. But for many AA alone is not enough; not everyone in AA has been able to achieve a comfortable sobriety. Bill recognized that the other two components of recovery were important. When he heard of our use of niacin (vitamin B3) for treating alcoholics, he became very enthusiastic about it because niacin gave these unfortunate patients immense relief from their chronic depression and other physical and mental complaints.

Niacin is the most important single treatment for alcoholism, and it is one of the most reliable treatments. And it is safe, much safer than any of the modern psychiatric drugs. Niacin does not work as well when alcoholics are still drinking, but in a few cases it has decreased the intake of alcohol until they were abstinent. This conclusion is based on the work my colleagues and I have done since 1953.

I know of many alcoholics who did not want to stop drinking but did agree to take niacin. Over the years, they gradually were able to reduce their intake until they brought it under control. Some alcoholics can even become social drinkers on a very small scale. I have not found many who could. But I think that, if started on the program very early, many more could achieve normalcy. I suspect that treatment centers using those ideas will be made available one day and will be much more successful than the standard treatment today. This all too often still consists of dumping them into hospitals and letting them dry out, with severe pain and suffering. When they are discharged, most go right back to the alcohol, the most dangerous and widely used street drug available without a prescription.

Orthomolecular treatment is the treatment of choice. This chapter on alcoholism outlines the importance of the nutritional factors that have been shown to be very successful on treating this condition. The treatment can be used alone but is best combined with dietary advice and additional nutrients.

—ABRAM HOFFER AND ANDREW W. SAUL, *The Vitamin Cure for Alcoholism,* 2009 (updated by A.W.S.) and reprinted with permission from Basic Health Publications

TERMS OF ALCOHOLISM

ALCOHOL. Alcohol is a very simple carbohydrate that is similar to sugar. It is also a slow-acting poison, and the most dangerous and widely used street drug available without a prescription.

ALCOHOL DEHYDROGENASE. An enzyme in the stomach that breaks down alcohol before it reaches the bloodstream.

ALCOHOLIC. A person whose drinking interferes with his or her psychological, social, and economic well-being.

ALCOHOLISM. A complex genetic-biochemical disorder more closely related to malnutrition—not of calories but of the nutrients that are essential to properly metabolize food—than to any behavioral or psychological disorder.

DELIRIUM TREMENS (DTS). A severe form of alcohol withdrawal that includes severe mental or nervous system changes such as body tremors, confusion, delirium, and hallucinations and that commonly occurs in people who stop drinking after a period of acute alcohol intoxication.

FUNCTIONAL HYPOGLYCEMIA. Also known as reactive hypoglycemia, or low blood sugar. A condition in which the blood sugar rises rapidly after ingestion of simple sugars, then plummets just as rapidly a short time later. Emotional and physical effects include mood swings, heart palpitations, fatigue, loss of coordination, and fainting.

LIVER. The liver processes 95 percent of alcohol ingested. It performs many essential functions related to digestion, metabolism, and the storage of nutrients in the body, and it filters out toxins and foreign substances. The liver cannot regenerate after being severely damaged by alcohol.

THE ALCOHOLIC: HOW SICK INTO TREATMENT?
HOW WELL WHEN DISCHARGED?

by Elizabeth Gentaial

I worked seven years with skid-road alcoholics, and later with some of their estranged families on welfare. We speak of skid roaders derogatorily. They are society's failures, school failures (the majority were learning-disabled), and our treatment program failures. Many, once well employed, had alcoholism treatment at expensive facilities and later, as treatment failures, skidded down the road to welfare and Salvation Army–type treatments. They included a doctor, a public health director, two lawyers, a civil engineer, and then on down to less-trained professions. They were jailed, hospitalized, stabbed and beaten, robbed, and were starving and dying without care, yet many clung tenaciously to life.

I conducted several projects with them. For a year I visited weekly the residents of a 60-room skid-road hotel with cooking facilities, housing about 90 percent alcoholics. In another project, my volunteers and I researched case-record information, including medical reports, on over 400 alcoholics. These alcoholics presented varying degrees of complications from alcoholism; no two were alike, but all were treatment failures. The average cost to the state for medical care for these alcoholics was about $25,000. I began to glimpse the thousands of dollars wasted by lack of a comprehensive approach to their problems. One suicidal alcoholic woman in her late 30s cost over $200,000 for one hospitalization and was discharged totally incapacitated into a nursing home. Being motivated by concern over the terrible financial and mental cost of alcoholism to the patient, relatives, and general public, and being of a curious mind, I have attended alcoholism conferences and classes—national and abroad—and probed at the problem off and on. Lastly, I studied nutrition to understand the disordered metabolism of alcoholism.

I have reviewed considerable research on alcoholism and have drawn together biochemical approaches. One of the best articles I have read is "Alcoholism and Malnutrition" by Robert W. Hillman.[1] The article, which appears in the book *The Biology of Alcoholism* (1974), cites about 500 articles—all of which focus not on theoretical aspects of the illness but on the its clinical aspects, and on the human research and nutritional complications of the disease. The extent of alcoholism research and types of treatment is staggering, yet if one evaluates the number of effective programs for the alcoholic, is the expenditure of the time and money involved justified?

In 1978, I attended the National Drug Abuse Conference in Seattle, Washington, where 700 speakers presented papers, including a few on the nutritional and biochemical approaches to addiction. Most of the speakers spoke "at" the problem, when what we clearly need is a practical holistic approach that speaks to the fastest, cheapest, most satisfying sobriety. A basic part of this is in the nutritional-biochemical approach to remove the depression and craving that precludes success in therapy. We need to know what are the derangements in metabolism that the alcoholic has when coming into treatment to help him or her to lasting sobriety when discharged, that is, to supply the ill body with those nutrients that lead to a feeling of wellness.

How Sick? The Biochemically Unique Alcoholic

Let's assume that the alcoholic coming to treatment has been through the detoxification process and is free of the short-range effects of alcohol. To determine how sick the person is, we need to answer: How adequate is this individual's diet? What are the correctable predisposing genetic factors he may have? What are the correctable long-range adverse effects of alcohol on this person? What other toxins besides alcohol may be disturbing the body's metabolic processes? And are stresses depleting the alcoholic of nutrients? These

From the *J Orthomolecular Psychiatry* 1979;8(4):253–264.

are interrelated factors, no one a clear-cut cause of alcoholism, but they act together, leading to the progression of the disease as the body gets depleted of nutrients. Each alcoholic has his own individual biochemical needs, which are influenced by these variables. Each one of us is unique biochemically and influenced by the same factors.

Here, I want to impress on you Dr. Roger Williams' concept of biochemical individuality, a basic principle of orthomolecular medicine. This concept says that externally, we are different and unique; internally, we are also unique. We have varying shapes and sizes of organs and glands—no two people are alike. These differences also indicate we have differing needs for the 50 or more nutrients the body utilizes in its manufacturing plant, where it chomps food to small particles and chemically separates, stores, transfers, and burns up energy substances that keep its motor going. Load a toxin such as alcohol into the body and we will have burnout in our weakest organs. Those of us with altered metabolic enzymes are genetically predisposed to quickly become alcoholic, but others will become alcoholic where dependence develops more slowly because of poor diet, increased regular drinking, and psychological stresses. According to the *Heinz Handbook of Nutrition*, about 98 percent of us are deficient in at least one of five major nutrients.[2]

Alcohol has a toxic effect on the gastrointestinal tract, pancreas, and liver,[3] which in turn causes malabsorption and malnutrition in the alcoholic. Let's follow the nutrients through the body, showing the disturbances alcohol can cause. Malabsorption is the most pronounced in alcoholics with cirrhosis of the liver.[4] The extent of the malnutrition produced depends on the diet of the person and how much alcohol was consumed and for how long.

Alcohol's Effect in the Gastrointestinal Tract

First, alcohol affects the gastrointestinal tract in conjunction with other toxic substances[4] such as salicylates from aspirin or from other insults such as an allergic response in the stomach. It can damage the intestinal lining (the mucosa), inhibiting hydrochloric acid and pepsin secretion, thus partially blocking protein digestion.[4] Further problems with protein can be caused by alcohol's irritation of the pancreas, thus decreasing secretion of the enzyme trypsin.[5] If all three secretions (hydrochloric acid, pepsin, trypsin) are blocked, the undigested protein will cause putrefaction in the bowel with attendant bowel troubles, gas, diarrhea, and reduced absorption of nutrients. A doctor can test for this lack of digestive enzymes. Supplemental hydrochloric acid and digestive enzymes can be given as needed until normal secretions are restored. Research has shown that out of 92 alcoholics tested, 43 had below-normal levels of hydrochloric acid.[6] While not technically an enzyme, hydrochloric acid interacts with digestive enzymes as they perform their essential functions.

Protein is needed to build enzymes (substances that facilitate all body processes), hormones (substances that help regulate all these body processes), and neurotransmitters (substances that help send messages between the brain and the body). One of the most important brain messengers rendered deficient in the alcoholic is serotonin,[5] a mood-elevating substance, whose precursor tryptophan is rendered deficient in the diet by alcohol. The tryptophan absorbed may not be converted to serotonin because of an alcohol-caused lack of vitamins and minerals on the conversion pathway. The reduced serotonin (the more alcohol ingested, the greater the lack) causes depression and sleep disturbances. Different neurotransmitters have effects in different areas of the brain, so a lack of serotonin triggers a computer section of the brain where external cues can bring out negative responses and depressed thinking.

Alcohol also impairs the body's digestion of fats and carbohydrates. Its disturbance of pancreatic function blocks the release of enzymes that digest fats and carbohydrates (starches and sugars), the body's other two main energy foods. Here again the alcoholic needs oral enzymes to facilitate digestion until the body rebuilds this function.

Alcohol's Effect in the Liver

Our next problem is the damaged liver. Damage to the intestinal lining by the heavy load of alcohol also makes it difficult for food to be properly absorbed into the liver.[3] The liver converts fats, carbohydrates, and proteins into energy (glucose) for immediate use or into glycogen as storage for later use. It also activates and stores vitamins, makes enzymes and hormones, and detoxifies the body from our insults. Alcohol can also damage the liver itself and causes a condition known as fatty liver (liver dysfunction). It can take the place of energy foods, which are instead changed when ingested into fat-type molecules (triglycerides) that are stored away in the muscle and liver. This accounts for the flabby appearance of the alcoholic. Remember, not much fat is digested (for lack of fat-digesting enzymes) but is eliminated via the bowel, causing steatorrhea, a frothy light-colored stool that floats in the toilet due to excess fat. As the liver becomes more damaged, other more serious problems like cirrhosis of the liver ensue (more on this later).

Another problem with increasing liver dysfunction in the alcoholic is his inability to absorb and store vitamins.[7] The water-soluble B complex of vitamins, necessary for the production of energy, and vitamin C, important in the metabolism of fats, proteins, and carbohydrates metabolism, and in neutralizing alcohol and drugs, are malabsorbed and so become deficient. There are also deficiencies in the fat-soluble vitamins (A, D, and E), which among many functions help maintain and repair the linings of the gastrointestinal tract, lungs and eyes, producing night blindness. Niacin, folic acid, and potassium are other nutrients that are often depleted.

Because the alcoholic uses more alcohol for energy, he fails to have available the building blocks for repair and proper mental functioning. One problem is that the body can no longer make enough glucose (blood sugar) from fats and protein, and also there are insufficient stores of glucose in the liver because it is damaged. This brings us to the problem of hypoglycemia or low blood sugar. Hypoglycemia can be of two types in the alcoholic: fasting hypoglycemia and functional or reactive hypoglycemia. The first type, fasting hypoglycemia, is caused by the lack of stored glucose and an inability to make glucose.[8] When the alcoholic is active, he uses up the glucose in his body. Then, with a lack of stores to supply the glucose, the brain's glucose level goes down and all the numerous confusional, emotional states of the very low-sugar hypoglycemic are exhibited. He is faint, sweats, trembles, is anxious, and depressed. He badly needs a drink to build up his energy level and, as he drinks, his sugar metabolism yo-yos up and down.

Alcohol's Effect in the Pancreas

The second type, functional or reactive hypoglycemia, is the more common. It is associated with malnourishment (rather than liver damage) and comes from insult to the pancreas from alcohol, as well as other toxins such as caffeine in coffee, large quantities of sugar and simple starches, nicotine, stimulants in chocolate and tea, and other drugs and foods. When these substances are overused, they cause an overreaction in the pancreas, which continues to secrete insulin (a blood sugar-regulating hormone),[9] which in turn causes blood sugar levels to drop to abnormally low levels.

The shut-down mechanism in the brain does not work, so that from the first to the third hour after ingestion of food, the alcoholic suffers hypoglycemic symptoms. With depleted diets the alcoholic can lack chromium, a part of the glucose tolerance factor, which makes insulin work more effectively. Dr. Louis Smith, a psychiatrist and former alcoholic, finds in the thousands of alcohol and drug abusers he has contacted, either as patients he directs or in Alcoholic Anonymous groups he attends in or out of prisons, that most of them eat poorly, are sugar freaks, and started smoking and using drugs early. Low blood sugar is often associated with violent behavior. It can be the cause of the mood swings, the addictive potential, the dry drunks (a condition of returning to old ways of thinking and behaving like an alcoholic although sober), and of binge drinking. Hypoglycemia also can be the cause of depression, the result of not having enough sugar (energy) in the brain, and violence. Barbara Reed and Alex Schauss, both directors of probation and parole offices, found that violent alcoholics, when placed on a hypoglycemic regime, calmed down and had changes of personality, sometimes within two weeks.

Special emphasis should be placed on a diet to alleviate hypoglycemia, similar to the diet researched by T. G. Kiehm and associates on diabetics,[10] who on it were able to decrease or discontinue supplemental insulin. The diet consists of eating 75 percent of one's calories from complex carbohydrates (whole grains and fresh vegetables, raw or lightly cooked), 15 percent from protein (part of this coming from complex carbohydrates), and 10 percent from fat (unsaturated) to get the essential fatty acids.

If we accepting that alcohol depletes all vitamins to some extent and that all nutrients are essential to body functions, then it only makes sense to include these in treatment of the alcoholic. Intravenous injections of vitamins may be required when there is evident depletion. By injecting the nutrients, malnourished alcoholics could get faster utilization of the substances, such as the B vitamins to get a clearer mind, and thus would be enabled to remain in treatment and benefit more from treatment. Some of the alcoholics I saw were so confused that they couldn't remember their names. Multivitamin and mineral supplements should be used after the injected ones, or in place of them.

While working with alcoholics, I read about facilities that used a multivitamin and mineral supplements successfully. I got a vitamin manufacturer to donate samples and a kind doctor to prescribe them—three a day for two weeks, and one daily after—to several of my test-case alcoholics. One of them, Tim, an ex-logging camp cook, who, when drunk, successfully passed himself off as an ex-art professor from Columbia University, was one of my first successes. Tim, when working, had tried a posh alcohol-aversion program and had been through numerous programs numerous times. He became a neat periodic drinker. When he received his welfare check, he bought about 18 bottles of wine, which he arranged near his bed, spread the floor with news-

paper, placed an oblong dishpan on this, and put about five bottles of an over-the-counter antacid medication on the dresser. He then proceeded to drink in bed. Somewhere along the way he vomited, took the antacid, and so on for about a week. With the vitamins, the first month he drank, the second he came to the door cheerfully, had bought shirts he needed, was playing cards at the firehouse nearby, visited friends in the hospital, and had gone down the street whistling, and said to himself, "Tim, you might be happy, but you aren't *that* happy!"

The next month Tim had alcohol on his breath. I asked, "What happened?" He said, "Ms. Genta-ial, look at that one bottle in the kitchen and note that it is two-thirds full. I can sit here in the chair and look at it, but don't have to drink it." He marveled because he had that compulsion for years. The vitamins worked. This happened, also, to Pearl, the ex-caseworker alcoholic, and several others. Unfortunately, I did not know enough about nutrition to guide their eating habits and, of course, got little support from other agencies. Tim has managed for four years, with only a slip or two. What is most important is that he found out he was not hopeless and in his new self-respect has contacted his family. The vitamins healed the impaired function that brought on the binge drinking. His was a simple case.

The more complicated cases are those in which the mental dysfunctions have a genetic basis.

Alcohol and Cerebral Food Allergies

The first I will discuss are the allergies. I have heard disparaging comments about allergies not causing alcoholism in the days when only a few allergy specialists were giving skin tests to determine causes for asthma, hay fever, and other common symptoms of allergic reaction. Now, much more is known about allergic responses in the brain tissue, and newer types of tests are being performed.[11] Finn and Cohen at the University of Liverpool conducted a study with six patients showing mental disturbances, along with physical symptoms, that could not be helped by any previous therapy.[12] The researchers determined these were allergic symptoms by using a nasogastric tube (through the nose to the stomach) to test reactions to foods put into the tube where the patient did not know what was given. One patient's abdominal pains and mental symptoms were due to alcohol and tea. Another researcher in the United States, Dr. Randolph, whose results were rejected or ignored, also found that alcoholics could be allergic to the protein factor of substances from which alcohol is made, such as the grains or corn. They might be allergic to one type of beverage and not another.[13] Hemmings from the University College of South Wales also reports from his laboratory studies that when protein has not been properly digested, these breakdown products pass through the gut wall and through the blood-brain barrier, where they can cause psychotic symptoms, a manifestation of a cerebral-allergic response.[14]

Dr. Coca has indicated another important effect of allergies on alcoholics, that is, the allergic response to allergens such as house dust can cause the person to crave alcohol. He found that reducing allergen exposure stopped the craving.[15] It appears that the inhalant allergen could cause a reaction in the part of the hypothalamus controlling appetite (addiction). Dr. Philpott reports that hypoglycemia (discussed earlier) can be evoked by allergic response, and that there is a close association between allergies and addictions.[16] The body craves substances to which it is allergic. As health builds up, the craving is reduced. Drs. Smith and Hawkins use megadoses of niacin for alcoholics to reduce their anxiety and depression. Interestingly, niacin releases histamine from the mast cells (the cellular response in an allergic reaction).

Drs. Newbold, Philpott, and Mandell also found that alcoholics who tested allergic to practically everything were more psychotic. This could be caused by the alcoholics' incomplete digestion of the protein factor in those foods.[17] About 20 percent of the schizophrenics display cerebral food allergies. When the allergic response is in the brain tissue, the psychosis or other reaction can be periodic, lasting from four to twenty days, or it can be seasonal depending on the allergens to which one responds.

Alcohol and Defective Enzymes

As previously mention, enzymes are catalysts that increase the rate of reaction in another tissue. They are like the match that sets the paper on fire. They are involved in converting foodstuffs to absorbable and usable forms for storage or reconverting to energy (fuel for body functioning). Some people inherit an increased probability of manufacturing defective enzymes that can't fulfill their function without help from a cofactors such as a mineral or a vitamin. In alcoholics, several enzyme defects may cause nutritional problems.

One digestive disorder caused by an enzyme defect is celiac disease. Celiacs are deficient in an enzyme normally present in the intestinal wall that is used to digest gluten, a protein most commonly found in wheat, rye, and barley. When a person with celiac disease consumes gluten, it causes a flattening out of the intestinal villi (tiny hairlike projections), which impairs the body's ability to absorb nutrients, mainly, the B vitamins, vitamins A, D, and E, as well as carbohydrates and protein. Physical symptoms of celiac disease are diarrhea with offensive, fatty light-colored stools that float in the toilet, consequent thinness, skin rash, and anemia.

Celiac disease is common in the mentally ill,[18] and it could cause part of the psychotic symptoms in alcoholics. Its presence in mild form (gluten sensitivity) could lead to a rapid addiction process; with poor absorption of energy foods, the celiac could use alcohol for his energy needs. The celiac or gluten-sensitive person has genetically inherited an increased membrane permeability and may be unusually allergic to the very grains (wheat, rye, barley) used to make alcohol. The gluten factor gliadin that causes the problem is soluble in alcohol.[19]

Interestingly, Solomons and associates also found that celiacs were highly deficient in zinc due to malabsorption and protein loss, and in other minerals for the same reason but to a lesser degree. Because gluten and milk lactose reactions (caused by a lack of the enzyme lactase) seem to act together,[18] the alcoholic with this problem should go on a milk-free, gluten-free diet. This will cause reversal of symptoms in up to six months, including reversal of psychosis.[20]

Psychotic alcoholics are the most likely treatment failures. About 15 percent of alcoholics have psychotic biochemistries (about 2 to 3 percent of the world have it) and about 15 percent are neurotics.[21] Dr. Nathan Brody found the psychotics fell into several distinct groupings: one of these is zinc and pyridoxine (vitamin B6) dependent (about 30 percent), who exhibit nervous exhaustion, depression, fear of people, flat affect, insomnia, and lack of dreams.[22] Physical complaints are abdominal pains, no appetite for breakfast, severe headache, rapid pulse, weight loss, sensitivity to cold, and white spots on the fingernails. These persons could use alcohol to mask symptoms. The test for this deficiency is a urine test for kryptopyrrole (also known as the "mauve factor").

The defective enzyme transketolase is implicated in Wernicke-Korsakoff syndrome, which causes brain deterioration and peripheral neuropathy (a gradual paralysis of the hands and feet).[23] The cofactor thiamine (vitamin B1) is needed in massive amounts to correct this defect. A dietary lack of thiamine by alcoholics who eat a poor diet increases the deterioration. Mardones has implicated low thiamine as inducing high alcohol drinking in mice.[24] Thiamine deficiency is implicated in lack of appetite, weight loss, weakness, depression, inflamed gastrointestinal tract, liver degeneration, and skin edema. Of course, other nutrient deficiencies may be involved. Alcoholics whose improvement appeared hopeless have recovered from this brain syndrome when administered thiamine. I saw several in a dumpy-appearing nursing home. When provided a good diet, they recovered lucidity in several months. The others may not have needed nursing homes if the doctor had prescribed the nutritional adjunct thiamine and probably a multivitamin.

Another disease process in alcoholics, cirrhosis of the liver (an often fatal disease), is associated with zinc deficiency[25] and may be linked with the apo-enzymes alcohol dehydrogenase and glutamic dehydrogenase.[1] The liver processes the majority of the alcohol ingested. The dehydrogenase enzymes along with zinc help break down alcohol. Depleted diets and large quantities of alcohol have been implicated in alcoholics with cirrhosis, both of which deplete zinc. Strain and associates also explain that zinc deficiency is prevalent in glaciated soils, plants, and food animals, so it could also be in man, who uses these for foods.[26] Oysters, nuts, and green leafy vegetables are rich sources of zinc and are absent from the diets of most alcoholics. One important function for zinc is for growth and healing, as the cofactor for the enzyme system involved in synthesis of proteins and nucleic acids. Zinc, as with other nutrients, may not be adequately supplied to all parts of the body if one has suffered a severe deficiency, even if one part is supplied. Zinc supplements should be taken over a long period of time and another hair sample test given to determine if the cellular level has returned to normal.

Another mineral, magnesium, in short supply in alcoholics through urinary loss, has been implicated in seizures, withdrawal symptoms, and delirium tremens.[27] All human tissue contains a small amount of magnesium, and it is essential for enzyme systems responsible for transfer of energy. In the alcoholic, low magnesium levels can be associated with low levels of calcium and potassium, so depletion of these could be associated, as could all the vitamins in withdrawal symptoms. Problems of low magnesium levels can also be compounded in people taking tranquilizers. Alcohol has been used in the depressant phase by the manic-depressive as a tranquilizer. A number of them become alcoholic after long imbibing. Interestingly, researchers Louis and Brenda Herzberg found significantly deficient magnesium in depressed patients as opposed to controls.[28] They stated it is possible that lithium, now administered to manic depressives, may interfere with the metabolism or binding of magnesium and that the cause of the illness may be a defect in magnesium metabolism. One of the functions of magnesium is the transmission of nerve impulses. Deficient magnesium causes the depression in the cycle of manic-depression.

Recent research on alcoholic hepatitis (a condition in which liver cells become inflamed and may die) by Carrol Leevy indicates that acetaldehyde, a metabolite of alcohol, is toxic to the liver of 40 percent of the alcoholics who are deficient in vitamin B6.[29] This deficiency, due to underconversion of vitamin B6, is corrected by administering pyridoxal-5-

phosphate (the activated form of vitamin B6). Another substance protective to the liver that Dr. Leevy administers is glutathione, an antioxidant involved in countless metabolic processes.

It is important to test alcoholics for low levels of these minerals, especially magnesium and zinc. A hair analysis test can be run to determine cellular levels of minerals in the body. This is an accepted medical test not yet widely used, which is more effective to determine body cellular level of minerals than that of the blood and urine. The main thing is to have adequate amounts prescribed by the doctor, and a follow-up hair test made to see that the cells are receiving adequate amounts.

More Substances and Conditions That Affect Malabsorption and Malnutrition

Other drugs and stimulants common in our diets can perpetuate the addictive state. These include caffeine in coffee, tea, and colas; theophylline in tea; theobromine in chocolate and cola drinks; and nicotine in cigarettes. Use of tranquilizing drugs to reduce the effects of alcohol, such as depression and tremors, causes reduction in body nutrients, and eventually adds to the problem, as many of these drugs are addictive. Jerry, one of my ex-alcoholics, continued to smoke and take the barbiturate phenobarbitol, which made his hypoglycemia worse. He worked for the welfare office four years before he died from cancer.

Sugar and white flour cause an insult to the pancreas and add to the hypoglycemic problem. Unfortunately, most treatment facilities and most alcoholics eat highly refined carbohydrate diets. We need to return to our forefathers' unrefined carbohydrate diets that contain the needed vitamins, minerals, and proteins in a balance for proper metabolism.

Stress causes depletion of nutrients. Under stress the brain can use up to 50 percent of the body's glucose output. Reducing stress in the life of your alcoholics is the psychotherapist's or counselor's function. Specific stresses can affect the alcoholic nutritionally: the alcoholic with surgical dissections such as gastrectomy (partial or full removal of the stomach) needs certain nutrients, as does the accidentally brain-injured, the woman on the pill (which depletes vitamin B6), and the pregnant woman needing extra supplementation of all the nutrients previously mentioned for two.

Lack of exercise induces stress, as does the alcoholic's very real craving for alcohol. Means of alleviating this craving included in this paper are niacin for hypoglycemia, a hypoglycemic diet, and reducing allergies.

The alcoholic's adaptation to a lowered nutritional state makes all thinking negative and is another type of stress to which the alcoholic is exposed. Name any subject and many an alcoholic can find something wrong with the situation. The negative alcoholic becomes hard to help unless the individual has hit bottom and has been shocked out of this mind-set. My approach to motivation to stop drinking is to encourage the alcoholic when drunk to tell me what a despicable person he is to get him to a high emotional pitch, as learning takes place under emotion. I tell the alcoholic that he can change his life, be proud of himself, be a credit to his family, that he is no different from others who stopped drinking, and so on. To do this, one needs to know the individual's concerns and interests, and to have his or her respect. I found the strong motivation to change lasted one or two months. The reason for this effect is that during intoxication, when acetaldehyde is present in the brain, it has a stronger hypnotic effect, about 35 times, that of alcohol.[30] It is as though one used hypnosis to effect the change in attitude. I've used this approach on six people so far. One woman was so drunk she was barely able to talk. I conned her into a reversal of attitude. She went to jail for her violent behavior, was released to a nursing home at my suggestion, woke up next morning, called to tell me she had a brilliant idea as to what to do to help her fellowman; it was an involved realistic plan. She did not know why the thought came to her. She said, "Maybe you think I am crazy." Another told me when drunk, "I am a no-good drunken Indian." I replied, "That's a lie; all but for one word. You are Indian." I proceeded to tell her how great she was, real things. She became a beautiful, dedicated Alcoholics Anonymous member in an Indian group. One old man, running out of nursing homes who would accept him, stayed sober several months for the first time in years. I saw him flying down the street with his cane to a grocery store that sold wine and watched as he came out with an ice cream bar and razor blades.

Treatment facilities should hire a nutritionist or someone on staff to teach proper nutrition, planning, and preparation of meals. What are you serving in your treatment facilities? Is it the type of food served in hospitals where patients die of malnutrition? The standard nursing home diet served in institutions is a depleting diet, mostly carbohydrates that do not provide the needed vitamins and minerals for rebuilding depleted bodies.

I hope I have given you cues from how sick the alcoholic is to what you can do to improve his nutrition. Starting at the mouth, see that he ingests proper foods. He needs zinc and vitamin B1 to restore his appetite. Arrange for your facility to serve a hypoglycemic diet for patients that need it. Make sure each patient is absorbing the food and has no hindrances to its utilization. Find a doctor for your patient who is concerned about nutrition to ensure this. Doctors, you owe it to all of us to treat alcoholics nutritionally. Do a hair analysis and a good blood workup. Test for allergies. Be aware of new research. Help your alcoholic toward nutritional relief of depressive thinking and alcoholic craving, and continue with your psychological and sociological support systems, so that when he comes out of treatment, he is weller than all his previous wells.

REFERENCES

1. Hillman W. Alcoholism and malnutrition. In: *The Biology of Alcoholism, Vol. 3: Clinical Pathology* edited by B. Kissin and H. Begleiter. New York: Plenum Press, 1974.

2. Burton B. *The Heinz Handbook of Nutrition.* New York: McGraw-Hill, 1976.

3. Roe D. *Drug-Induced Nutritional Deficiencies.* Westport, CT: Avi Publishing Co, 1976.

4. Leevy CM. Biochemistry of gastrointestinal and liver disease in alcoholism. In: *The Biology of Alcoholism, Vol. 1: Biochemistry* edited by B. Kissin and H. Begleiter. New York: Plenum Press, 1971.

5. Orten JM, Sardesai VM. Protein, nucleotide, and porphyrin metabolism. In: *The Biology of Alcoholism, Vol. 1: Biochemistry* edited by B. Kissin and H. Begleiter. New York: Plenum Press, 1971.

6. Janis LB. Achlorhydria in alcoholics. *Med Annuals DC* 1971;40:651.

7. Tao H, Fox H. Measurement of urinary pantothenic acid excretion of alcoholic patients. *J Nutr Sci Vitaminol* 1976;22:33–337.

8. Badawy A. A review of the effects of alcohol on carbohydrate metabolism. *British Journal on Alcohol and Alcoholism* 1977;12.

9. Moynihan, NY, Benjafield MB. Alcohol and blood sugar. New research to be published on hair analysis of alcoholics by *Practitioner* 1967;198:552–589. Miller Pharmacal Co, Inc.

10. Kiehm TG, Anderson JW, Ward K. Beneficial effects of a high carbohydrate, high fiber diet on hyperglycemic diabetic men. *Am J Clin Nutr* 1976;29:895–899.

11. Ulett G, Itil E, Perry S. Cytotoxic food testing in alcoholics. *Quart J Studies Alcoholism* 1974;35:930–942.

12. Finn R, Cohen HN. Food allergy: fact or fiction? *Lancet* 1978:426–428.

13. Mandell M. Cerebral reactions in allergic patients. In: *A Physician's Handbook on Orthomolecular Medicine* edited by R. Williams and D. Kalita. New York: Pergamon Press, 1977.

14. Hemmings WA. Food allergy. *Lancet* 1978:608.

15. Coca AF. *The Pulse Test.* New York: Lyle Stuart, Inc, 1956.

16. Philpott WH. The value of an ecologic examination as an aspect of the differential diagnosis of chronic physical and chronic emotional reactions. *International Academy of Metabology* 1974;3(1):62.

17. Newbold HL, Philpott WH, Mandell M. Psychiatric syndromes produced by allergies: ecological mental illness. *J Orthomolecular Psych* 1973;2(3):84–92.

18. Dohan FD, Grasberger JD, Lowell FM, et al. *British Journal of Psychiatry* 1969;115:595.

19. Hekkens JM. The relation of gliadin structure and its toxicity to gluten-sensitive patients. *Minerva Pediatrica* 1977;29:2191–2196.

20. Singh MM, Kay SR. Wheat gluten as a pathogenic factor in schizophrenia. *Science* 1976;191:401–402.

21. Lesser M. Lecture delivered at the Huxley Institute for Biosocial Research, New York, June 1977.

22. Brody, N. Guidelines in treating the alcoholic patient in the general hospital: orthomolecular therapy. *J Orthomolecular Psych* 1977;6(4):299–344.

23. Blass J, Gibson G. Abnormality of a thiamine-requiring enzyme in patients with Wernicke-Korsakoff Syndrome. *N Engl J Med* 1977;25:1367–1370.

24. Mardones J. Experimentally induced changes in alcohol appetite. *International Symposium: The Finnish Foundation for Alcohol Studies* 1972;20,15–27.

25. Vallee BL, Wacker W, Bartholomay SD, et al. Zinc metabolism in hepatic dysfunction. *N Engl J Med* 1987;257:1055–1065.

26. Strain W, Steadman L, Lankau C, et al. Analysis of zinc levels in hair for the diagnosis of zinc deficiency in man. *J Lab & Clin Med* 1966;68:244.

27. French SW. Acute and chronic toxicity of alcohol. In: *The Biology of Alcoholism, Vol. 1: Biochemistry* edited by B. Kissin and H. Begleiter. New York: Plenum Press, 1971.

28. Herzberg L, Herzberg B. Mood change and magnesium. *Journal of Nervous and Mental Diseases* 1977;165:423–426.

29. Leevy CM. Nutrients can ease hepatitis, research shows. *U.S. Journal of Alcohol and Drug Dependence.* Mar 6, 1978.

30. Truitt E, Walsh M. The role of acetaldehyde in the actions of ethanol. In: *The Biology of Alcoholism, Vol. 1: Biochemistry* edited by B. Kissin and H. Begleiter. New York: Plenum Press, 1971.

SUGAR: THE FIRST ADDICTION

by Abram Hoffer, MD, PhD, and Andrew W. Saul, PhD

Addictions begin during infancy. One suspicious factor starts very early: baby formulas are commonly made up of cow's milk and sugar. This may be a basis of a food addiction later in life, especially among bottle-fed infants, to one of their main foods—cow's milk. Sugar is the first major addicting substance, and many children are just as addicted to sugar as alcoholics are to alcohol. Alcohol, a very simple carbohydrate, is similar to sugar. We know of one boy, seven years old, who was seen crawling on his hands and knees to the kitchen in the middle of the night to reach the sugar bowl, and he gulped down the sugar by the handful. The sweet taste, so essential to animals in deciding which foods are ripe and safe, becomes one of the main factors in creating the addiction. Later, many of these children as teenagers are addicted to milk. In some cases, they drink huge amounts each day, as much as half of their calories. But as they grow older and have access to alcohol, many find that this makes them feel better than either sugar or milk could, and they become addicted to alcohol. At Alcoholics Anonymous meetings, members often drink coffee super-saturated with sugar.

The Sugarholic Alcoholic

And let's not forget that children commonly drink colas laced with caffeine on top of high sugar content: 12 or more teaspoons of sugar in a single can of soda. According to the Center for Science in the Public Interest, "Soda pop is Americans' single biggest source of refined sugars . . . 12- to 19-year-old boys get 44 percent of their 34 teaspoons of sugar a day from soft drinks. Girls get 40 percent of their 24 teaspoons of sugar from soda. Because some people drink little soda pop, the percentages are higher among actual drinkers."[1] The crossover between a sugarholic and an alcoholic is illustrated by this patient's letter:

"All my 45-plus years, I've fought against sugar, refined carbohydrates, and the fatigue and mood swings they bring about. However, like an alcoholic, I always seem to end up craving, and then getting back with sugar products.

"I read the following post on an Internet newsgroup: 'In order to control your addiction, follow the protocol for alcohol at www.doctor yourself.com/alcohol_protocol.html.' My daughter treated a sugar addiction nutritionally exactly as alcoholism is treated, and it works. Many people who have sugar addiction have alcoholics in the family. When alcoholics go off alcohol, they nearly always start eating lots of sugar. Unfortunately, this usually keeps the addiction going.

"I'd love to see a diet and tactics suggested to get off a sugar addiction. I am the son of alcoholics, and addicted to a terrible sugar and refined carbohydrate diet that leaves me exhausted and stressed out. Your assertion that alcoholism can be 'cured' really is heresy to my way of thinking, but maybe you might be right. I would like to find a nutritional key that might help me in my ongoing white-knuckled struggle as I hurry past the baked goods and candy."

Vital Supplements for the Sugar Junkie

Probably the most reliable and most powerful help for the sugar junkie is indeed to diligently follow the nutritional program for alcoholism developed by Roger J. Williams, PhD, author of *Alcoholism: The Nutritional Approach* (1959). Large quantities of the B-complex vitamins are a cornerstone of the treatment. We think that the cheap and easy key is to take the entire B-complex at least six times daily. Chromium, vitamin C, lecithin, the amino acid L-glutamine, and a vegetable-rich, high-fiber, complex-carbohydrate diet are also very important.

REFERENCES

1. Center for Science in the Public Interest. Liquid candy: how soft drinks are harming American's health. Available at www.cspinet.org/new/pdf/liquid_candy_final_w_new_supplement.pdf.

Excerpted from *The Vitamin Cure for Alcoholism* (2009) by Abram Hoffer and Andrew W. Saul, and reprinted with permission from Basic Health Publications.

THE REFLECTION OF HYPOGLYCEMIA AND ALCOHOLISM ON PERSONALITY: NUTRITION AS A MODE OF TREATMENT

by Elsa Colby-Morley, EdD, PhD

Early reviews on the alcoholic personality generally failed to establish any specific set of personality traits in alcoholics that would predispose a person to alcoholism.[1] It was generally held that "no satisfactory evidence has been discovered that justifies a conclusion that persons of one type are more likely to become alcoholics than persons of another type."[2] A decade later researchers had conceded that "we cannot reject the idea that personality factors play a very significant role in determining who will become an alcoholic and who will not."[3] Dr. Gordon Barnes, teacher and researcher in the area of alcohol and drug abuse, suggests that "there does appear to be a clinical alcoholic personality."[4] He explains that, no doubt, this personality pattern exists as a cumulative result of a pre-alcoholic personality and the effects of a person's drinking history on that personality pattern. In contrast, the neurotic characteristics of alcoholics seem to be more a result of the disorder than of a pre-alcoholic personality trait.[5]

In commenting on the psychiatric aspects of alcoholism, Dr. Ruth Fox, medical director at the National Council on Alcoholism, suggests that alcoholism is a chronic behavioral disturbance. Psychological characteristics found with a battery of tests on 300 consecutive private patients of Dr. Fox's showed the following character traits: "inner battle between passivity and aggression, low frustration tolerance; inability to endure anxiety or tension; feelings of isolation, devaluation of self-esteem, sometimes with overcompensation; undue sensitiveness; impulsiveness; repetitive acting out of conflicts, masochism; self-punitive behavior and extreme narcissism or exhibitionism, strong sense of guilt, hostility (either overt or covert); strong dependent needs; marked rebellion . . . "[6]

Dr. Carlton Fredericks, nutrition expert and author of *Low Blood Sugar and You* (1973) tells us that the brain and nervous system are exquisitely sensitive to disturbances of body chemistry that may not noticeably affect other organs, and that a chronic defect in the utilization of sugar in the body may not cause a single physical symptom—although it often does. According to Fredericks, low blood sugar can make you claustrophobic or a hypochondriac, fill you with obsessive and unbased fears, or prod you into alcoholism or asthma.[7]

The Effects of Alcohol and Diet on the Brain

There is a growing body of knowledge from studies with both animals and people, which suggests that dietary factors might well represent some of the most serious primary proneness factors in the development of alcoholism and the alcoholic syndrome.[8] The etiology of malnutrition in alcoholics is quite complex. Physician and psychiatrist Abram Hoffer suggests that a number of physical diseases, depression, anxiety states, alcoholism, and other addictions are the end product of ingesting excessive quantities of sucrose (table sugar).[9] Dr. Roger Williams, author of *Alcoholism: The Nutritional Approach* (1959), suggests that malnutrition may develop as a forerunner of alcoholism, and that it is only when brain cells become severely malnourished that true alcoholism appears. Williams positively asserts that "no one who follows good nutrition practices will ever become an alcoholic."[10] To this growing consortium of doctors, alcohol may, if taken in large enough quantities, actively damage the brain cells as well as deprive the brain cells of the necessary substances in the nutritional chain of life.

Williams explains that alcohol consumption, at high levels, undoubtedly acts in several ways to damage brain cells. It is thought to slow blood flow to the brain; poison the cells, and deprive them of the vitamins, minerals, and amino acids by substituting empty calories for good food. Whatever the mechanisms are, the effect is the same: brain cells

From the *J Orthomolecular Psych* 1982;11(2):132–139.

are impaired and die off with greater rapidity when alcohol levels in the blood are allowed to remain high. Williams suggests that from these facts it is reasonable to deduce that alcoholism likely results from an impairment of the cells in the appetite-regulating mechanism in the hypothalamus region of the brain. He explains that in individuals who are prone to become alcoholics, these cells are vulnerable and may become so seriously damaged that the sight of food is nauseating and only alcohol has appeal.

Dr. Fredericks suggests that "all alcoholics are hypoglycemic, for it is an inevitable result of substituting whisky for food. Some alcoholics," he explains "begin by becoming hypoglycemic, and at the point where their low blood sugar would ordinarily cause a craving for sweets, they pervert the craving into an appetite for alcohol. That group in the alcoholic population can be 'cured' of alcoholism by adopting and staying on a high protein-low carbohydrate hypoglycemic diet. The heavy consumer of sweets who becomes an alcoholic is suspect of being in this group. So is the drinker who, when drying out, eats large amounts of candy."[11]

Drs. Edwin Kepler and Frederick Moersch were among the first to describe the physical and mental manifestations of hypoglycemia (from the Greek, meaning "low sugar in the blood"). In a 1937 article appearing in the *American Journal of Psychiatry*, they described them as follows: "In attacks of any severity, the attitude and general behavior of the patient are always disturbed. Any one of the following mental states may dominate the clinical picture: apathy, irritability, restlessness, fatigue, anxiety, incorrigibility, negativism, automatic behavior, somnambulism, confusion, excitement, disorientation, 'drunken behavior,' fugue states, unconscious attacks, delirium, mania, stupor, coma; motor activity may be decreased or increased; speech is distorted; emotional instability ranges from all forms of anxiousness to querulousness and violence; thinking becomes confused and sluggish; obsessions, compulsions, and even hallucinations or delusions frequently may be present . . . and the patient may become disoriented as to time, place and persons."[12]

The behavioral disorders associated with hypoglycemia are quite varied, and it is often misdiagnosed as some neurological or emotional disorder. Hypoglycemics are often labeled as neurotics, psychotics, or hypochondriacs. Drs. Cheraskin and Ringsdorf also note that the hypoglycemic symptoms include anxiety, irritability, fatigue, mental confusion, and uncontrolled emotional outbursts.[13] A comparison of the traits commonly reported by the "sober" alcoholic and the hypoglycemic include irritability, depression, aggression, fatigue, restlessness, confusion, desire to drink, nervousness.[14]

Drs. Hoffer and Osmond give us a comprehensive look at the personality of the alcoholic who is also hypoglycemic: "Some alcoholics long noted that although dry, they remained unhappy, tense, depressed, or in many ways neurotic. Some would remain dry for awhile and then, out of sheer desperation, return to drink. It made sense that many of this group might be suffering from a biochemical malfunction instead of from ordinary varieties of neurosis, as was previously supposed."[15]

The Hypoglycemic Alcoholic

The body constantly strives to maintain a precarious balance. For example, if the concentration of sugar (glucose) in the blood is too high, the blood will draw fluid from the tissues to dehydrate the cells and dilute the blood. If untreated, diabetes will develop. On the other hand, if blood sugar is too low for a prolonged period, the cells will not receive enough food or fuel, and hypoglycemia results. This delicate balance of blood sugar is maintained by internal mechanisms. A group of cells (alpha cells) in the pancreas secrete the hormone glucagon when there is a slight drop in the blood's normal level. This spurs the liver to release stored sugar back into the blood. The pituitary gland also secretes somatotropic hormones (STH), which keep this sugar from entering muscle and fat cells and conserve it for the nervous system, which absolutely requires it.

The adrenal medulla secretes adrenaline if blood sugar drops below a critical level. The secretion of glucagon, STH, and adrenaline switches off as soon as the blood sugar level rises above normal. The liver stops issuing sugar and rapidly starts absorbing it. The entry of glucose into muscle, liver, and fat cells is promoted by a second group of cells (beta cells), which secrete the hormone insulin. The process is reversed if blood sugar becomes too low. Since hypoglycemia is low blood sugar and diabetes is high blood sugar, they would seem to be opposites. However, it is more accurate to say that hypoglycemia and diabetes are sister illnesses which, in some instances, have a common pathway of development.[16] Hypoglycemia may be a forerunner of diabetes in some cases but all hypoglycemics are not prediabetic. "Hypoglycemia," says Dr. Harold Harper, "is an early warning system for all the chronic degenerative diseases."[17]

One must dichotomize hypoglycemia into two main types: fasting hypoglycemia and functional or reactive hypoglycemia. Fasting hypoglycemia can occur as a result of abstaining from food for more than eight hours or it can be traced to some specific organic defect such as endocrine diseases, liver diseases, pancreatic islet-cell tumors, and hyperplasia. Most cases of hypoglycemia, and the kind with which we are concerned, are of the functional or reactive type. In functional hypoglycemia, blood sugar levels drop to abnormally low levels several hours after ingesting a meal. This suggests that diet may be the cause of functional hypoglycemia.

Most hypoglycemics have a ravenous appetite for sweets. Since the overactive pancreas—which spurs the desire for sweets—will be restimulated when sugar is eaten, this illustrates an aberration of the wisdom of the body. Characteristic of a group of alcoholics is this same desire for sweets; while sober, they may consume unbelievable quantities of candy, cookies, and sugar in their coffee. Alcohol is itself a sugar-like carbohydrate. The craving for sweets is a clue to low blood sugar. Meals are often made up of junk foods that are high in refined carbohydrates, fats, and salt; low in high quality protein; and devoid of fresh fruits and vegetables, and whole grains.

This type of diet can lead to blood sugar instability in susceptible individuals and, indeed, it is claimed that upwards of 95 percent of alcoholics suffer from low blood sugar.[18] In response to a rapid fall in blood sugar, hypoglycemia produces symptoms that result from the production of adrenaline. These symptoms include sweating, weakness, rapid heart beat, inner trembling, and hunger. When hypoglycemia appears in response to a slow fall of blood sugar (over a period of several hours), the symptoms include mental confusion, blurred vision, headache, double vision, incoherent speech, and sometimes convulsions. And if the hypoglycemia becomes chronic, a person may experience a variety of psychological and neurological symptoms that can include one or all of the following: personality changes, emotional instability, fatigue, suicidal intent, phobias, nervousness, depression, insomnia, antisocial behavior, mania, irritability, delirium, stupor, anxiety, "drunken behavior," and negativism.

Nutritional Treatment for Hypoglycemic Alcoholic

For the orthomolecular practitioner, nutrition is a primary consideration in the treatment of hypoglycemia; likewise, it is the primary mode of treatment for alcoholism. The orthomolecular practitioner attempts to treat the hypoglycemic and the alcoholic by providing the optimal molecular environment for the mind, especially the optimal concentration of substances normally present in the human body.

Fredericks suggests that other than reducing sugar intake to the lowest level possible, the treatment for hypoglycemia should consist of: "1) nutritional help for the liver . . . 2) relief for the pancreas (by reducing sugar intake and minimizing starches to 60 grams daily) . . . 3) an increase in protein intake from meat, fish, fowl, eggs, cheese, milk and dairy products, and in polyunsaturated (vegetable) fats . . . 4) timed meals controlled with six small, rather than three large, meals daily containing some protein . . . 5) and supplementation with multivitamin/mineral tablets, a vitamin B-complex concentrate, and special-purpose foods high in vitamins and minerals including wheat germ, brewer's yeast, and desiccated (dried) liver."[11]

The prime objective of this high protein-low carbohydrate diet is to minimize swift ascents, and consequently sudden drops in blood glucose. It is necessary for both the hypoglycemic and the alcoholic to eat six small meals a day with protein at each meal. This diet helps to regulate blood sugar. While medical men were neglecting the concept of hypoglycemia a few pioneers—Drs. Jerome Conn, Harry Salzer, H. S. Seltzer, John Tintera, Alan Nittler, and many others—entered the arena and demonstrated the devastating effect of hypoglycemia on the body and mind, and the almost miraculous recoveries that followed a high-protein diet restricted in sugar and starch.[19–22]

The alcoholic is among those individuals at high nutritional risk for developing protein-energy malnutrition and vitamin depletion. Chronic protein-energy malnutrition characterized by wasting is caused by inadequate diet, maldigestion, malabsorption, and alcoholic liver disease.[23] The vitamin requirements of alcoholics exceed those of nonalcoholics. Multiple causes of vitamin depletion may coexist in individual alcoholics, including dietary insufficiency, malabsorption, hyperexcretion, and impaired synthesis of the active or coenzyme form of some vitamins.[24] Alcohol damage to the gut reduces absorption of some vitamins, including folic acid and thiamine (vitamin B1).[25–26] Alcohol damage to precursor blood cells in the bone marrow increases the body's need for folic acid, pyridoxine (vitamin B6), and cobalamin (vitamin B12).[27] It has been shown that, if alcoholic subjects are placed on a low-folate diet, they will develop a type of anemia called megaloblastic hemopoiesis more rapidly than nonalcoholic subjects.[28] Chronic alcoholics are known to have depleted body folic acid stores. One study found that the hemopoietic response was suppressed in those patients who were deficient in folic acid and were also receiving alcohol; this effect could be reversed by eliminating alcohol.[29] Another study found a significant impairment of vitamin B1 absorption in the alcoholic.[26] The Wernicke-Korsakoff syndrome, peripheral neuritis, and pellagrous psychosis are neurological disorders associated with nutritional deficiencies in alcoholics.[24] In Wernicke-Korsakoff syndrome, the most common of these disorders, brain damage is due to vitamin B1 deficiency.[30]

The acute state of the Wernicke-Korsakoff syndrome, called Wernicke's encephalopathy, can be effectively treated with intravenous vitamin B1. In the early stages, the greatest nutritional risk is that the disease will not be recognized and the patient may develop an irreversible chronic brain syndrome characterized by memory loss and an inability to function independently.[31–32]

It is known that deficiencies of vitamins B1, B6, and B12, which help to maintain the health of the nerves, play a role in the development of certain psychotic states; for example, the deficiencies of vitamin B1 in Wernicke-Korsakoff psychosis[33] and some depressive states.[34] Alcoholics are often depleted in folic acid, ascorbic acid (vitamin C), vitamin B6, vitamin B12, magnesium, and zinc, and often quite depleted in protein.[11] Magnesium depletion and abnormally low levels of magnesium (hypomagnesemia) in the blood are common in chronic alcoholics and appear to arise through the combined effects of poor diet and rapid elimination of magnesium in the urine.[35] Magnesium deficiency is associated with neuromuscular dysfunction characterized by tetany, seizures, ataxia, muscle weakness, tremors, behavioral disturbances, and hypomagnesemia. Abnormally low magnesium levels combined with excessive alkalinity in the blood (alkalosis) are believed to be the factors that induce seizures and other symptoms of delirium tremens associated with alcohol withdrawal.[36]

Also, chronic alcoholics often experience night blindness. The night blindness can may be caused by a deficiency of vitamin A and zinc, and it responds to administration of either vitamin A, or vitamin A and zinc. Zinc stimulates synthesis of retinol-binding protein (necessary for transporting vitamin A in the blood). It is also necessary for optimal activity of alcohol dehydrogenase, an enzyme in the stomach that breaks down alcohol before it reaches the bloodstream and that converts retinol to retinal.[37]

The orthomolecular treatment for alcoholism requires the same high protein–low carbohydrate diet for hypoglycemics, along with megadoses of vitamins and minerals, especially ascorbic acid, niacin, vitamin B1, vitamin B6, vitamin E, a high-potency multivitamin and mineral, a high-potency

B complex, the amino acid L-glutamine, and sometimes vitamin B12 injections.

Dr. Williams has demonstrated that alcoholics who are treated with supernutrition may spontaneously stop drinking, and may even recover the ability to take a single drink and stop. Drs. Hoffer and Osmond recommend a diet devoid of junk foods and, in the appropriate instances, a regime of nutritional supplements. Williams has repeatedly noticed that nutritional support reduces the physiologic craving for alcohol. He recommends a high-protein diet supplemented with therapeutic amounts of the available vitamins and minerals. Williams made the following assertion: "It is our opinion that in the great majority of individual alcoholics, the practical elimination of alcoholic craving can be assured, provided the recommendations that we have made are followed. Whether they are followed is a question that must be answered separately in each individual case."

Put to the Test

At a large prestigious hospital in New York City, the author individually treated a group of physicians who had been referred by their peers because of excessive drinking. The orthomolecular approach to treatment was quite successful with these patients, who were alcoholics with hypoglycemia symptoms. I had read the papers of Drs. Hoffer, Williams, Pauling, Osmond, and others in the field of orthomolecular.[38-41] Following their lead, I treated the nutritional deficiencies of these physicians with a high protein–low carbohydrate diet and megadoses of certain vitamins and minerals. In accordance with Dr. Williams' concept of biochemical individuality, each regime was unique for that person.[42] In addition, each day they received megadoses of vitamin C-complex with bioflavonoids (8,000–12,000 milligrams [mg] in divided doses), niacin (2,000–4,000 mg in time-release capsules of 400 mg each), a vitamin B complex (100 mg, 2 to 3 times a day), a high-potency multivitamin/mineral supplement, L-glutamine (2,000–3,000 mg), tryptophan (1,500–3,000 mg at bedtime), a magnesium and calcium supplement, and vitamin Bl (500–1,500 mg).

This nutritional support reduced the craving for alcohol in every case where the recommendations were completely followed. Every patient was able to "dry out" without the devastating effects of hallucinations (the imaginary pink elephants of the alcoholic with delirium tremens). To give them support and to encourage them to stay on their regime, I saw these patients two to three times a week at first. It was very important that they have success immediately. After several weeks many of them found they had lost their craving for alcohol. Perhaps this was because they also did not substitute their craving for alcohol (at the early stages of the regime) with candy, cake, coffee, soft drinks, and other sugary foods. They substituted protein such as almonds, seeds, cheese, plain yogurt, cottage cheese, a chicken leg, or a slice of turkey instead. Eventually, this new way of eating became a habit with them. After six weeks to three months, those patients who had stayed on their regime were able to stay sober with none of the drying-out effects. Those who were still on their regime at the end of a year were sober and reported a phenomenal ability to concentrate, remember names, and relax; an ability to quit smoking; and a feeling of well-being that they had not experienced in years.

"Overdosing" with vitamins is actually beneficial for alcoholics. Usually, because of substituting alcohol for food, their bodies are depleted in most vitamins.[38-41] If within six weeks on a hypoglycemic diet, the alcoholic's blood sugar remains low, it would be advisable for him or her to have some intravenous feedings of protein. An alcoholic who is put into the hospital and is given protein intravenously with intensive vitamin therapy responds rapidly to this regime.

Dr. Williams has said that "when alcoholics, as a group, are familiar with the story of nutrition, they will be among those most anxious to learn what their own peculiar individual nutritional needs are." I found this to be true. From all the facts relating alcoholism to biological factors and nutritional deficiencies, it becomes clear that whatever measures maybe taken to prevent alcoholism, the neglect of the nutritional approach cannot be justified.

REFERENCES

1. Armstrong JD. The search for the alcoholic personality. *Ann Am Acad Polit Soc Sci* 1958;315: 40–47.

2. Sutherland EH, Schroeder HG, Tordella CL. Personality traits and alcoholism: a critique of existing studies. *Quart J Studies Alcohol* 1950;2:547–561.

3. Lisansky ES. The etiology of alcoholism: The role of psychological predisposition. *Quarterly Journal of Studies on Alcohol* 1960;21:314–341.

4. Barnes GE. The alcoholic personality: an analysis of the Literature. *J Studies Alcohol* 1979;40:7.

5. Kammeier ML, Conley JJ. Currents in alcoholism: toward a system for prediction of post treatment abstinence adaptation. *Currents Alcoholism* 1979:111–119.

6. Fox R. Psychiatric aspects of alcoholism. *Amer J Psychotherapy* 1965;19(3):408–416.

7. Fredericks C. *Low Blood Sugar and You.* New York: Constellation International, 1973.

8. Cheraskin E, Ringsdorf WM. *New Hope for Incurable Diseases.* New York: Exposition Press, 1971.

9. Hoffer A, Walker M. *Orthomolecular Nutrition.* New Canaan, CT: Keats Publishing,1978.

10. Williams RJ. *Alcoholism: The Nutritional Approach.* Austin, TX: University of Texas Press, 1959.

11. Fredericks C. *Psycho-Nutrition.* New York: Grosset & Dunlop, 1976.

12. Kepler EJ, Moersch FP. The psychiatric manifestations of hypoglycemia. *Am J Psychiatry* 1937;64:89–110.

13. Cheraskin E, Ringsdorf WM, Clark JW. *Diet and Disease.* New Canaan, CT: Keats Publishing, 1968.

14. Worden M, Rosellini G. The dry drunk syndrome: a toximolecular interpretation. *J Orthomolecular Psych* 1980;9(1):41–47.

15. Hoffer A, Osmond H. *New Hope for Alcoholics.* New York: University Books, 1968.

16. Poulos CJ, Stoddard D, Carron K. The relationship of stress to hypoglycemia and alcoholism. Huntington Beach, CA: International Institute of Natural Health Sciences, 1976.

17. Harper H. *How You Can Beat the Killer Diseases.* Westport, CT: Arlington House, 1978.

18. Meiers RL. Relative Hypoglycemia in Schizophrenia. In: *Orthomolecular Psychiatry* edited by D. Hawkins and L. Pauling. San Francisco: W.H. Freeman, 1973.

19. Conn JW, Seltzer HS. Spontaneous hypoglycemia. *Am J Med* 1955;19(3):460–478.

20. Salzer HM. Relative hypoglycemia as a cause of neuropsychiatric illness. *J Natl Med Assn* 1966;58(1):12–17.

21. Tintera JS. Endocrine aspects of schizophrenia: hypoglycemia of hypoadrenocorticism. *J Schizo* 1967;1:150–181.

22. Nittler A. *A New Breed of Doctor.* New York: Pyramid Books, 1974.

23. Blackburn GL, Bistrian BR. Curative nutrition: protein calorie management. In: *Nutritional Support of Medical Practice.* Hagerstown, MD: Harper & Row, 1977.

24. Fenerlein W. Neuropsychiatric disorders of alcoholism. Second European Nutrition Conference (Munich). *Nutr Metabol* 1977;21:163.

25. Sinclair HM. Nutritional aspects of alcohol consumption. *Proc Nutr Soc* 1972;31:117.

26. Tomasulo PA, Kater RM, Iber FL. Impairment of thiamin absorption in alcoholism. *Am J Clin Nutr* 1968;21:1340–1344.

27. Hines JD. Hematologic abnormalities involving vitamin B6 and folate metabolism in alcoholic subjects. *Ann NY Acad Sci* 1975;252:316.

28. Eichner ER, Hillman RS. Effect of alcohol on serum folate level. *J Clin Invest* 1973;52:584–591.

29. Roe A. *Drug-Induced Nutritional Deficiencies.* Westport, CT: Avi Publishing Co., 1978.

30. Cole M, et al. Extraoccular palsy and thiamin therapy in Wernicke's encephalopathy. *Am J Clin Nutr* 1969;22:41–51.

31. Victor M, Adams RD, Collins GH. The Wernicke-Korsakoff syndrome: a clinical and pathological study of 245 patients: 82 with postmortem examination. Philadelphia: F.A. Davis Co, 1971.

32. Riggs HE, Boles RS. Wernicke's disease: a clinical and pathological study of 42 cases. *Quart J Studies Alcohol* 1944:5:361.

33. Freedman AM, Kaplan HI, Sadouk BJ. *Comprehensive Textbook of Psychiatry* II. Vol 1. Baltimore, MD: Williams & Wilkins Co, 1975.

34. Dickerson JWT, Lee HA, eds. *Nutrition in the Clinical Management of Disease.* London: Edward Arnold Publishers, 1978.

35. Lim P, Jacob E. Magnesium states of alcoholic patients. *Metabolism* 1972;21:1045–1051.

Marks V, Rose FC. *Hypoglycemia.* Oxford: Blackwell, Scientific Publications, 1965.

36. Victor M. The role of hypomagnesium and respiratory alkalosis in the genesis of alcohol-withdrawal symptoms. *Ann NY Acad Sci* 1973;215:235–248.

37. Russell RM, Morrison SA, Rees-Smith F, et al. Vitamin A reversal of abnormal dark adaptation in cirrhosis. study of effect on the plasma retinol transport system. *Ann Intern Med* 1978;88:622.

38. Hoffer A, Osmond H. *The Chemical Basis of Clinical Psychiatry.* Springfield, IL: C.C. Thomas, 1960.

39. Williams RJ. *Nutrition Against Disease: Environmental Prevention.* New York: Bantam Books, 1971.

40. Pauling L. Orthomolecular psychiatry. *Science* 1968;160:265–271.

41. Pauling L. Vitamin therapy: treatment for the mentally ill. *Science* 1968;160:1181.

42. Williams RJ. *Biochemical Individuality: The Basis for the Genotropic Concept.* New York: John Wiley & Sons, 1959.

GUIDELINES IN TREATING THE ALCOHOLIC PATIENT IN THE GENERAL HOSPITAL WITH ORTHOMOLECULAR THERAPY

by Nathan Brody, MD

My interest and activity in the field of alcoholism has intensified greatly, and over the past 23 years I have evaluated and treated thousands of alcoholic patients. In my work in this field I have utilized almost every known approach at one time or another, but the successes were relatively meager until I began using a psychobiological and nutritional approach. This approach encompasses a combination of elements that based on research accumulated over the years has direct bearing on the etiology and treatment of alcoholism. Since the inception of this particular treatment regimen, the successes have increased in vast proportion, and even the so-called failures respond and do better than the therapeutic successes of the past.

Relative Hypoglycemia

One factor that I investigate in my alcoholic patients is the existence of functional or relative hypoglycemia, as either a cause or a result of the alcoholism. In many research reports, it has been stated that abnormal fluctuations in levels of blood sugar can cause neuropsychiatric difficulties (such as anxiety, tension, and depression), which could lead a patient to alcoholism.[1] It is also known that consuming large amounts of carbohydrates (of which alcohol is one), over a long period of time, can cause hypoglycemia, thus causing more disturbances.

Nutritional Deficiencies

Over the years it has been well established that alcoholics in particular suffer certain nutritional deficiencies due either to malabsorption of nutrients, an inadequate intake of nutrients, or both. The most common deficiencies found in alcoholics are those of thiamine (vitamins B1), riboflavin (vitamin B2), niacin (vitamin B3), pyridoxine (vitamin B6), and folic acid;[2] the minerals zinc, calcium, magnesium, and potassium; and proteins. In my treatment program, I test for deficiencies in all these nutrients.

I have found very few alcoholics who are not zinc deficient. Alcoholics with cirrhosis (liver damage) have the lowest zinc levels of all, and I believe that severe zinc deficiency plays a role in the development of cirrhosis. Magnesium deficiency may play an important role as a cause of confusion and "the shakes" (delirium tremens, or DTs) during the withdrawal phase of chronic alcoholism.

Psychiatric Disturbances

It is well established that psychiatric difficulties of all types can lead to, or develop as a result of, alcoholism. These can range from anxiety and depression to antisocial behavior and aggression. The determination as to whether or not psychotic symptoms exist in a patient is based on the results of the Hoffer-Osmond Diagnostic (HOD) test.[3] The HOD test, which was initially developed for use with schizophrenics, measures disturbances in a person's thought processes, perceptions, and moods. If the scores of a particular patient are found to be above normal, established cut-off scores, a psychiatric determination can be made as to the existence of psychiatric symptoms.

Based on the test results, I can usually distinguish between the toxic psychosis often found in alcoholics as a result of over-ingestion of alcohol, and other psychotic illnesses such as schizophrenia. Toxic psychoses usually respond quickly and dramatically simply to withdrawal of the toxic agent, whereas the remission of symptoms in severe psychiatric disorders is usually very slow and may even worsen during this period. An investigation of various physiological elements is accomplished in order to ascertain biochemical correlations to psychotic symptoms and thus be able to specify treatment.

A great deal of research has been devoted to the biochemical factors involved in the onset of

From the *J Orthomolecular Psych* 1977;6(4):339–344.

psychotic symptoms. The following is a short summary of some of the biochemical factors linked to psychotic illness that I routinely test my patients for, particularly those with abnormal HOD scores.

Kryptopyrroluria (Pfeiffer et al., 1974)[4]

Kryptopyrrole (also known as KP or "mauve factor") is a chemical substance found present in the urine of about 30 percent of all schizophrenic patients, which was found to lock up with zinc and vitamin B6 to cause a deficiency of these two substances. This deficiency has been found to cause certain symptoms (even psychotic symptoms) that respond to large doses of vitamin B6 and a zinc supplement. The onset of these manifestations is insidious but responds quickly to treatment. I also have found that a great many alcoholics, even those not manifesting psychoses, maintain an elevated level of kryptopyrrole. For these reasons all of my patients are evaluated and tested for this element, regardless of their HOD scores. Treatment is begun immediately if a patient's KP level is found to be above the normal range.

Hypercupremia (Pfeiffer and Iliev, 1972)[5]

Another factor in the biochemical aspects of psychotic symptoms has been found to be abnormal elevations of serum copper (hypercupremia). Copper is now known to be excitatory and a source of stimulation to brain tissue, which in and of itself can cause psychotic symptoms. Copper also is found to be antagonistic to zinc (which is tranquilizing to brain tissue). Elevated serum copper levels may be lowered, therefore, by the use of zinc supplements alone. If a patient's level of serum copper is found to be very high, then a preparation of penicillamine (Cuprimine, Depen), which binds to copper and helps remove it from the body, may be administered as well as the zinc supplement.

Histapenia and Histadelia
(Pfeiffer et al., 1973)[6]

Levels of serum histamine either higher than normal (histadelia) or lower than normal (histapenia) have been found to cause psychotic symptoms, by virtue of the nature of the chemical action of histamine on brain tissue. The determination of a patient's histamine level is of particular importance because there is a distinct and different treatment program to follow for each classification, either high or low. A patient who exhibits a low histamine level should have his or her histamine level raised, and conversely for the patient with a high-histamine level.

Because I often have great difficulty obtaining accurate histamine levels, I also check the patient's basophil count, which correlates well with histamine levels. A high basophil count correlates with high histamine level, and the low basophil count correlates with the low histamine level.

Treatment Program

My treatment protocol varies slightly depending on whether the individual is a long-term or chronic alcoholic, who presents no acute emergency and can be treated as an outpatient, or an alcoholic, who is experiencing severe, acute difficulty and must, for a time at least, be treated as a hospital inpatient.

When an alcoholic is admitted to a hospital experiencing acute difficulty, certain procedures are performed immediately—even before treatment is begun—in order to ascertain his or her true status prior to therapeutic intervention. Stats for blood alcohol and blood sugars are drawn. The blood alcohol is to ascertain the level of alcohol in the bloodstream that will later be used in confrontation tactics with the patient. The blood sugar level is to determine whether or not the patient is in a hypoglycemia state. Also, at this time, blood samples are drawn for calcium, copper, folic acid, magnesium, potassium, and zinc to determine the nutritional status of the patient.

The next step in my treatment of the acute hospitalized patient is to administer an intravenous solution of B-complex vitamins with an additional 200 milligrams (mg) of vitamin B6 added. Large doses of the B-complex vitamins are the cornerstone of the treatment. In the case of the very sick patient, I will double the above amount of vitamins. This phase of treatment serves two purposes: 1) to immediately improve the nutritional and physiochemical status of the patient; and 2) to help sedate the patient. The literature has shown that certain vitamins included in this preparation, especially niacin (vitamin B3), have a sedative effect.

This process of administering intravenous solutions of vitamins is continued once a day for at least five days, or until such time as substantial clinical improvement is achieved. Concomitantly with this phase of treatment, since approximately 70 percent of my patients experience hypoglycemia symptoms, orange juice is given every two hours when possible, and the patient is placed on a high protein–low carbohydrate hypoglycemic diet. Since the physician must not ignore the withdrawal symptoms often experienced by these patients (such as insomnia, convulsions, profuse perspiration, hallucinations), appropriate doses of an anti-anxiety medication are utilized when needed.

At the same time as the previously outlined treatment program is in process, or at such time as the patient is able, the patient is administered vitamins and minerals by mouth, three times a day, according to the following regimen: vitamin B1 (100 mg), vitamin B2 (25 mg), vitamin B3 (500 mg), vitamin B6 (100 mg), vitamin C (500 mg), vitamin E (200 IU), calcium pantothenate (100 mg), plus a zinc and manganese supplement.

This oral regimen is followed until the lab reports are returned; then, the regimen is altered suitably to fit the patient's individual needs. Additional items such as folic acid and cobalamin (vitamin B12) can be added if it is found necessary, or an already established medication can be increased or decreased if necessary.

In most cases significant improvement has been achieved within 24 hours on this program, and, as soon as this improvement is seen and the patient is deemed to be able, the HOD test is administered to determine whether or not a psychotic process is in effect.

After a two- or three-day period on the hypoglycemic diet, the patient is given a five-hour glucose test to determine the existence of relative or functional hypoglycemia. When the results for histamine level or basophil count and mauve factor return, the patient's therapeutic regimen is altered to suit his particular physiological needs according to a

protocol established by Dr. Carl C. Pfeiffer, founding director of the Brain Bio Center, in Princeton, New Jersey. The regimen administered to patients found to be low in serum histamine includes niacin, folic acid, vitamins B5 (pyridoxine) and B12, and zinc and manganese; the regimen for high-histamine patients includes calcium, methionine, zinc, manganese, and diphenylhydantoin (Dilantin).

Besides the attention given to the physiochemical, nutritional, and psychobiological needs of the patients, attention is also paid to the patient's psychosocial and physical needs. For example, an extensive program with some kind of movement, exercise, and physical therapy is instituted especially for the patients seen as suffering from depression, as evidenced by the HOD test.

The patients also are given the benefit of contact with psychiatric social workers, who perform further evaluation if necessary. They assist in ascertaining the existence and nature of various other difficulties such as intrapersonal, marital, and family problems, and social difficulties, and, if need be, they assist in job placement. The psychiatric social workers also hold group therapy sessions for these patients while they are in the hospital, and members of Alcoholics Anonymous (AA) help by holding AA meetings in the hospital setting.

All the previously mentioned facets to the program tend to lend support to the patient. Another supportive measure used for those patients who are interested is that of providing reading material, which explains the nature of hypoglycemia and gives insight and knowledge about the condition. All this tends to solidify the entire concept in the patients' minds and gives to them the reassurance they so desperately need.

One case brought to mind is that of a young man who had been hospitalized at ten different psychiatric institutions with no resultant solution to his problem. When he came to me, he was diagnosed as having hypoglycemia and was given a book *Body, Mind, and Sugar* (1951) by E. M. Abramson to read about 6 P.M. one night. The following morning, when rounds were made at 7 A.M., he was sitting up reading the book and had stayed up all night. When questioned as to why he had such an avid interest in the book, he stated with more than a little relief that it was as though he were reading his own biography. Cases such as this one give me the impetus to continue to elaborate and refine my treatment protocol and program.

Sustaining Recovery

The fully recovered patient is discharged from the hospital with all the necessary materials, medications, and information needed to sustain recovery. A return appointment for follow-up is established prior to discharge. At this time, the patient is also given all pertinent information concerning AA meetings and other support groups in the area and is strenuously urged to attend. Follow-up for these patients is done by myself in conjunction with the psychiatric social workers and members of AA. The entire program outlined here provided the medium for substantial and rapid recovery and provides the means for sustaining recovery.

My treatment for the outpatient alcoholic is basically the same as that outlined for inpatients with the exception that intravenous solutions of vitamins are not given. All the testing and medication formats previously outlined are also utilized for outpatients, in order to give them the same opportunity for sustained recovery as is given the hospitalized alcoholic.

REFERENCES

1. Salzer HM. Relative hypoglycemia as a cause of neuropsychiatric illness. *Journal of the National Medical Association* 1966;58(1):12–17.

2. Special Committee of the Diet Therapy Section, American Dietetic Association. *Guidelines for Nutrition Care of Alcoholics During Rehabilitation.* Chicago: American Dietetic Association, 1971.

3. Kelm H, Hoffer A, Osmond H. *Hoffer-Osmond Diagnostic Test Manual.* Saskatoon, Sask., 1967.

4. Pfeiffer CC, Sohler A, Jenny EM, et al. Treatment of pyroluric schizophrenia (malvaria) with large doses of pyridoxine and a dietary supplement of zinc. *J Orthomolecular Psych* 1974;3(4).

5. Pfeiffer CC, Iliev V. A study of zinc deficiency and copper excess in the schizophrenias. In: *International Review of Neurobiology* edited by C. Pfeiffer. New York: Academic Press, 1972,141–165.

6. Pfeiffer CC. *Observations on the Therapy of the Schizophrenias.* Princeton, NJ: Neuropsychiatric Institute, 1973.

B3, BILL W., AND AA
by Abram Hoffer, MD, PhD

I met Bill W. (William Griffith Wilson), cofounder of Alcoholics Anonymous (AA), at a meeting in New York in 1958. I introduced him to vitamin B3 (niacin) and suggested that he try it. He had been suffering from severe tension, fatigue, and insomnia for many years, although he did not let that deter him from his important work with AA International Headquarters. A few weeks after he started taking 1,000 milligrams (mg) of niacin after each of three meals for a total of 3,000 mg a day, his fatigue, chronic tension, insomnia, and discomfort disappeared. Bill immediately became a strong supporter of our work with niacin, but he did not leave it at that. He told his colleagues and friends about his own recovery and discussed the research we were doing in Saskatchewan. He was aware of the extraordinary properties of vitamin B3 from his discussions with me and his examination of the medical literature.

Bill was not shy about passing on this information, much to the chagrin of the International Board of AA. He had created this board and, many years before, had invited physicians to become members. They were all friends of his, but the doctors on the board were not happy with Bill and accused him of meddling with medical matters, which were none of his business. Bill did not agree—his business was to help as many alcoholics as possible get well, and, if vitamins were going to help, he was all in favor of using them. And he knew that vitamins were extraordinarily safe. But this was news to the doctors, who were not aware that vitamins in large or optimum doses had properties that they did not have when used in the very low, usual doses then being recommended.

I remember two examples that Bill told me about. One was a man with severe arthritis, who found it very difficult to continue his job as a gardener. Bill told him about niacin, and, after he was on this vitamin for a while, his arthritis vanished. This was another confirmation of Dr. William Kaufman's excellent research between 1940 and 1950. By 1949, Dr. Kaufman had published two books summarizing his studies on arthritis: *The Common Form of Niacinamide Deficiency Disease—Aniacinamidosis* and *The Common Form of Joint Dysfunction, Its Incidence and Treatment*. These were very careful, clinically controlled experiments on many hundreds of arthritics, in which he showed that most of the patients given the vitamin became normal, or so much better that they were no longer seriously handicapped.

Another example from Bill was a wealthy individual from the West Coast, who called him up very depressed. He had been suffering from manic-depressive (now called bipolar) disease for many years and had been helped somewhat by a psychoanalyst. However, his psychoanalyst died and he had become severely depressed. Bill told him that he would send him a jug of niacin (500-mg tablets) and that he should take two tablets (1,000 mg) three times daily. Within a few months, his friend was well without the need of any more psychiatric treatment.

A Great Advocate of Vitamin Therapy

The more people Bill told about niacin, and the more responses he saw, the more convinced he was of the merit in our work. Bill went even further. One evening when I was visiting him at his downtown hotel in New York, he pulled out 30 files and said, "Abram, I want to show you the results of my research." He had given niacin to 30 of his associates and friends in AA after carefully telling them about niacin and its properties, how much to take, and so on. After one month, 10 of them were well. After two months, another 10 were well. And after three months, the last 10 had not responded. I was delighted and impressed, as his response rate was very similar to what I was seeing in my practice. Bill W. was thus the first layperson to repeat our research trials and to confirm our findings.

Bill wrote three communications to AA's physicians called "The Vitamin B3 Therapy," the first distributed in 1965, the second in 1968, and the third in 1971. However, he did not think that the words niacin or nicotinic acid (niacin's original chemical name) would capture enough attention. One evening, he asked me about this, and I told him that niacin had previously been designated as vitamin B3 because it was the third water-soluble B vitamin to be identified. So, Bill began to use the designation vitamin B3, even though by then the use of letters to identify vitamins was being discontinued in the medical world. But Bill's use brought it back and it is today called vitamin B3, even in the most conservative medical literature.

Bill's Recommendations

Bill strongly promoted niacin as a nutritional treatment. He thought that AA should take the following actions:

- Fund and advocate research on niacin.

- Encourage its members to take niacin and improve their nutrition (eat whole foods and reduce intake of excessive sugars, refined carbohydrates, and caffeine).

- Advocate that all AA physicians as well as any physicians treating alcoholism should advise their patients about vitamin therapy.

Unfortunately, AA rejected these recommendations then and evidently continues to reject them. We now know that niacin decreases the mortality from delirium tremens (DTs), and niacin reduces acetaldehyde levels from the metabolism of alcohol, thus reducing oxidative stress.[2] A whole-foods diet, along with a decreased intake of sugar and refined carbohydrates, are necessary to boost long-term recovery rates. Bill's recommendations, if adopted, might have alleviated a great deal of suffering.[3] To read for yourself what he had to say, his three amazing pamphlets are available online at:

- www.doctoryourself.com/BOOK1BILL_W.pdf

- www.doctoryourself.com/BOOK2BILL_W.pdf

- www.doctoryourself.com/BOOK03BILL_%20W.pdf

Had Bill lived another ten years, the use of niacin in alcoholics would have been well established. However, his important contribution will not die. Over the years, I have seen a large number of members of AA who chose to use niacin, and it has been extraordinarily successful.

Excerpted from *The Vitamin Cure for Alcoholism* (2009) by Abram Hoffer and Andrew W. Saul, and reprinted with permission from Basic Health Publications.

A Biochemical Denominator in the Primary Prevention of Alcoholism

by Emanuel Cheraskin, MD, DMD, and William M. Ringsdorf, Jr., DMD

The primary prevention of alcoholism and/or the alcoholic syndrome, like the primary prevention of any other so-called health problem, hinges on an awareness of two fundamental ingredients: identification of the constellation of risk factors, and elimination of some if not all of these risk elements.

Risk Factors

There seems to be little or no disagreement regarding these two strategic points to accomplish primary prevention or prevention of occurrence. There is, on the other hand, considerable confusion as to what constitutes a risk factor. Serum cholesterol, to pick a popular parameter, is viewed as a risk agent in the genesis of certain types of cardiovascular disease. Serum uric acid, as a second example, is regarded as a risk variable for gout. However, the question then to be resolved is, what is it that makes for high cholesterol (hypercholesterolemia) and high uric acid (hyperuricemia)?

And so, at best, blood cholesterol and uric acid levels can be viewed as secondary risk factors. We now know that serum cholesterol and uric acid concentrations are a function of physical activity, tobacco use, coffee/tea intake, and certain dietary indiscretions, as well as other already defined and other still-to-be identified lifestyle characteristics. These lifestyle components are the true or primary risk factors. For those students of predictive medicine, no matter what the syndrome, it is possible to identify a mosaic of primary and secondary risk factors.[1] It would follow that such must be the case when one examines the alcohol-prone person.

Ecology of Health and Sickness

There is one additional point not generally considered that is critical to this discussion of primary prevention. In the final analysis, health or disease is a function of the mosaic of environmental challenges and the organism's capacity to cope, variously termed "constitution," "predisposition," or "tissue tolerance." The terms most frequently utilized are "host resistance" and "host susceptibility." For most investigators, resistance and susceptibility are simply viewed as opposites. Thus, it matters little, by this definition, whether one's resistance goes down or whether one's susceptibility goes up.

However, when viewed analytically,[2] resistance may be regarded as any agent that, when administered, tends to discourage the development of disease. When absent, however, it encourages disease. For example, thiamine (vitamin B1) may be regarded as a dietary resistance agent, for its administration tends to discourage the development of beriberi, and its absence causes it. In a sense, therefore, resistance agents—dietary and nondietary—are pluses. They should be added to our lifestyle if not already a part of it. In contrast, a susceptibility agent invites disease when present and discourages the development of disease when it is withdrawn. Thus, sugar is to be viewed as a dietary susceptibility agent because its introduction tends to encourage dental caries, and its absence exerts a preventive action. Hence, in one sense, susceptibility agents—dietary and nondietary—are minuses. They should be subtracted if they exist as part of our lifestyle.

Parenthetic mention should be made that an agent is never a resistance factor for one disease or one system or organ or site, and a susceptibility factor for another. Since vitamin C, for example, is known as a resistance agent for scurvy, it would seem that it should be a resistance agent for other syndromes. On the other hand, since sugar is viewed as a susceptibility factor in the mouth, it is likely the same for the whole body.

Proneness Profiles

Over the past few years, we have been studying primary prevention in a number of systems and have already reported an oral disease proneness profile,[3] mental illness proneness profile,[4] musculoskeletal disease proneness profile,[5] and the syndrome of sickness profile.[6] The resistance agents for each of these systems are strikingly the same. Likewise, for all systems, the susceptibility factors are identical. It would follow, if there is indeed a wisdom of the body of man, that these same resistance and susceptibility factors should prevail in the alcohol proneness profile.

A Common Denominator in Alcoholism

Apropos to alcohol consumption, it is generally agreed that different individuals drink alcohol for different reasons. Some people drink because they like the taste of alcohol. Within this group, some such persons may eventuate as alcoholics where some will not. Others will drink because of the relaxing and other tranquillizing benefits derived from alcohol. Within this second group, some may eventually turn to alcoholism but the majority will not. Third, there are those who drink because of real or supposed social pressures. Here again, some few may become alcoholic; others not. Finally, there is a group that drinks because of an urge, a chemical craving, to drink. This thirst is critical for without it alcoholism and the alcoholic syndrome do not exist.

There is no question but that alcohol is a chemical agent. As such, the desire for the first drink and, more important, the desire created by the first for the second and third one, stems from a deranged cellular metabolism. Setting aside for the moment the pathologic consequences, the wish for one and then another alcoholic drink is similar to the urge for water when the tissues are dehydrated and for food when the tissues are starved. However, under physiologic conditions, once the tissues are satisfied, the individual stops drinking water and eating food. This is not the picture in the heavy drinker following a spree. Notwithstanding the cause for the celebration, be it social pressure, or psychotrauma, or whatever else, it is well-documented that the hangover is devastating. Yet, a common "solution" is more alcohol!

The phenomenon of more and more alcohol in alcoholism is not unique. If it were unique then it might be possible to explain away alcoholism on a specific psychologic basis rather than in physiologic terms. After all, morphine, cocaine, and nicotine are also habit-forming drugs. These agents have in common with alcohol the fact that one dose produces an appetite for more and more of the same. Such cravings have never been shown to be psychologic or mental in nature. Rather, these bizarre appetites stem from a derangement in cellular metabolism induced by one or another chemical agent.

Just as elevated serum cholesterol is one, surely not the only, secondary risk factor for certain cardiovascular syndromes and just as high uric acid is one, certainly not the only, secondary risk factor for gout, it would follow that there should be biochemical repercussions of deranged metabolism in alcoholism and in the alcoholic syndrome. And, so it is. Low blood sugar appears to be one, clearly not the only, chemical parameter serving as a secondary risk factor. It is estimated that about 70 percent of alcoholics have hypoglycemia and that the blood sugar problems existed before the addiction the alcohol. The question now to be resolved is what are the primary risk factors that explain the deranged cellular metabolism?

There is a body of knowledge, admittedly not large but exciting, in both lower animals and in man, that suggests that dietary factors might well represent some of the most serious primary proneness factors in the development of alcoholism and the alcoholic syndrome.

Lower Animal Observations

Dr. Jorge Mardones at the Institute of Pharmacology and the Institute of Research on Alcoholism at the University of Chile in Santiago,[7] and subsequently Professor Roger Williams and his colleagues at the Clayton Institute of Biochemical Research at the University of Texas in Austin,[8] in brilliant monumental reviews, examined the experimentally induced changes in the free selection of alcohol in lower animals.

First and foremost, the point was emphasized that lower animals, like man, possess a "wisdom of the body." The overall conclusions drawn from many studies on the self-selection of foods was that the rat, for example, chooses the best combination of foods for physiologic growth and reproduction. Also, it is abundantly clear that food choice predictably compensates for pathologic imbalances; thus, rats will regularly and reliably increase their salt consumption after adrenalectomy and reduce carbohydrate intake after pancreatectomy.

The most relevant conclusions may be summarized in the following three statements: First, the quantity of alcohol consumed under free-choice conditions varies in different laboratory animals. Second, the deprivation of most of the water-soluble vitamins invites an increase in ethanol (alcohol) consumption. Third, when sugar solutions or a fat emulsion is offered as a third choice, ethanol intake decreases.

A second direction of investigation has looked at the possible effects of ordinary human diets upon alcohol intake in lower animals. In 1972, Drs. Register, Marsh, Thurston, Fields, and coworkers from the Departments of Nutrition and Biochemistry of the School of Health and the School of Medicine at Loma Linda University in California conducted a series of studies to ascertain whether a typical teenage-type American diet, generally held to be marginally suboptimal in certain nutrients, could provoke alcoholic behavior in rats similar to the observations obtained with the purified diets

mentioned earlier.[9] Additionally, included in these same testing schedules, an attempt was also made to examine the possible effects of other lifestyle elements such as coffee and caffeine upon drinking behavior. In one such study, the Loma Linda group provided a choice of 10 percent alcohol versus water under rigidly controlled circumstances.

Bottles of these two fluids were made equally available in the cages so that there was no technical reason for choosing one versus the other liquid. One group of rats were fed a typical teenage-type American diet, which is usually relatively high in refined-carbohydrate foodstuffs and marginally low in most of the vitamins and minerals. A second group received a control diet containing adequate concentrations of all nutrients as compared with recommended intakes for adolescents plus additional vitamins and minerals. A comparison of these two groups showed that, in a matter of a few short weeks, the subjects with the typical teenage-type diet consumed five times as much alcohol!

In an attempt to simulate further the human experience, another group of animals were supplied the very same teenage diet plus spices. A comparison of the alcohol intake in this group versus those on the teenage diet alone showed no difference. In other words, the increased consumption of alcohol with the typical American teenage diet

---

From the wife of a former alcoholic . . .

"I am the wife of an alcoholic who came out of a 30-day detox two months ago, has not been back to work for months, and was showing no promise of doing so, relapsing every three to four days . . . up until this past week.

"Your basic alcohol protocol is already working . . . and he tested it today to my initial dismay. He has been taking the vitamins you list on the site, in the dosing suggested, plus whole grain foods, vegetables, no sugar, for about a week now. Had indicated no cravings for the past four to five days, but decided to get 'a shot and a beer' this afternoon out of habit, not from craving— a whim.

"Normally this would have led to a relapse, ending

up in three to five shots and five to six beers and a lot of headache and heartache for me (and him too). Guess what?! He took the one shot, one beer . . . said it tasted disgusting, didn't give him the pleasurable physical response, and threw out the unopened second shot and beer. That's huge . . . almost unbelievable. He's not drunk and he was able to control the drinking and stopped the cycle.

"On behalf of my husband, in memory of my father (another alcoholic), and the millions of very wonderful human beings who think this 'disease' is incurable and they just have to 'manage' their symptoms, I am militant about getting the word out about this."

Source: Personal communication (AWS), 2014

was not significantly altered by virtue of the spices. In a third instance, and once again designed to duplicate if possible the typical human lifestyle, a group of rats were supplied with the same teenage diet plus the spices and the coffee equivalent of 18 cups per day. Under these circumstances, the alcohol intake was higher by 13 percent with coffee with the teenage diet than with the diet alone, and sixfold greater than the alcohol intake with the so-called good (control) diet! It would appear that the addition of coffee encourages significantly greater alcohol ingestion. Parenthetic mention should be made that this experiment resembles the experiences in limited human studies.

In order to establish what it is in coffee that contributes to the desire for alcohol, two other studies were performed. In one instance, the typical teenage diet plus spices was supplied along with caffeine (instead of coffee) and, in another experiment, the caffeine was substituted by decaffeinated coffee. In the case where caffeine was added to the teenage diet, the consumption of alcohol was very much like that observed with coffee. In other words, caffeine and coffee behaved very much alike.

In the experiment in which decaffeinated coffee was utilized, the results approached those of the teenage diet alone. Hence, within the limits of these studies, it appears that the active ingredient in coffee that makes for greater alcohol consumption is caffeine. Finally, and once again in an attempt to simulate the human experience, the teenage diet plus spices and coffee were supplemented with vitamins and minerals. Under these conditions, there was a significant reduction in alcohol intake even though the diet was not grossly deficient in any one nutrient fraction.

Human Implications

On the basis of the reports cited here and others not included in the interest of expedition, many investigators view these results as evidence of "experimental alcoholism." It should, however, be underlined that, while there are many glaring similarities, there are striking differences between the observations reported in lower animals and the experiences in man.

It is well known that the craving for alcohol observed in the human is usually overbearing and critical. The withdrawal syndrome includes insomnia, anxiety, tremor, and a host of other psychological symptoms and signs that are, to a degree, alleviated for a time by supplementation with additional alcohol. This overriding desire for alcohol is almost unique to the behavior of the human alcoholic subject. On the other hand, the desire for alcohol in laboratory animals is much less intense. This point obviously sets apart "human alcoholism" from "experimental alcoholism."

Second and generally speaking, alcoholics consume alcohol until they are intoxicated and this is demonstrated by changes in their behavior (the alcoholic syndrome). Generally speaking, laboratory animals do not display any overt signs of intoxication. Perhaps the only similarity between the lower animal and human studies is the fact that both, sooner or later, demonstrate liver damage.

A third fundamental difference between human alcoholism and experimental alcoholism is the presence of withdrawal symptoms after cessation of drinking in the human organism. Parenthetic mention should be made that the symptoms observed in the alcoholic syndrome are encountered in other so-called psychological disorders. In contra-distinction, the clinical picture of tremulousness, nausea, perspiration, insomnia, convulsions, hallucinations, and delirium are not observed in laboratory animals.

On the other hand, there are actually more similarities than differences in human versus experimental alcoholism. The urge to drink is a function of the diet and other lifestyle characteristics (Williams, 1978).[8] Individuals with suboptimal dietary regimes are more prone to become alcoholics. Persons who engage in suboptimal physical activity, who drink coffee and tea, and who use tobacco are more alcohol-prone. As a matter of fact, it is not infrequent to observe that, when individuals cease drinking alcohol, they turn to a greater consumption of refined carbohydrate foods (foods made primarily of sugar and white flour), a larger intake of coffee and caffeinated beverages (cola drink, cocoa, tea), and an increase in nicotine intake. Therefore, the mere fact that one can eliminate alcoholism (defined as the cessation of alcohol consumption) may not necessarily mean the elimination of the alcoholic syndrome since, as we have just seen, the individual simply switches his or her "fix" from alcohol to food indiscretions, coffee/tea, nicotine, and sugar. Actually, sugar is such a powerful reinforcer of behavior that it may the mother of addictions.

Controlled laboratory experiments cited by Dr. Michael B. Cantor of the Department of Psychology at Columbia University in New York City convincingly demonstrate the power of sweet taste to determine behavior. These lower animals and human studies show that the higher the concentration of sweetener, the greater the preference and the more avid the behavior in its pursuit.

Citing John Falk and his colleagues at Rutgers University, Dr. Cantor illustrates the unusual power of sweetness to control behavior and raises the question of whether it is appropriate to consider sweetness as addictive.[10] In an attempt to wean rats from ethanol, Falk found that only a sweet taste could compete with the alcohol dependence. When 5 percent ethanol was pitted against 3 percent dextrose, alcohol was preferred. When the concentration of dextrose was increased to 5 percent, it was preferred over alcohol. In choosing the sweet taste over ethanol, the animals drank so much sugared water that they suffered convulsions and faced death from malnutrition. Since Falk's animals were addicted to alcohol and this was supplanted by overindulgence in sugar, may one conclude that these animals gave up one addiction for another?

■ CONCLUSION

There is no question but that the alcohol problem, like any other problem, is multifactorial. If one surveys the literature, the overwhelming body of facts suggests that alcohol proneness is the result of psychologic, social, economic, ethnic, religious, cultural, and spiritual factors. There are only a few publications dealing with the biochemistry of alcohol-proneness.

On the other hand, if one examines the research funding process, it becomes clear that the ratio of monies is fairly proportional to the ratio of nonchemical versus chemical studies. It would be interesting in the coming years to inaugurate the following experiment. Let us, for once, shift our emphasis, meaning our time and money skills, from our present strivings to discover more nonchemical denominators in the genesis of alcoholism to a study of the risk potential of the air we breathe, the water we drink, and the food we eat. We predict, if this is done properly, we shall unearth a boundless fountain of fascinating and fruitful data in support of the chemistry of alcohol-proneness.

REFERENCES

1. Cheraskin E, Ringsdorf WM Jr. *Predictive Medicine.* New Canaan, CT: Keats Publishing, 1977.

2. Schneider HA. Nutrition and resistance-susceptibility to infection. *Amer J Trop Med* 1951;31(2):174–182.

3. Cheraskin E, Ringsdorf WM Jr, Hicks BS, et al. The prevention of oral disease. *J Intern Acad Prevent Med* 1975;2(11):22–52.

4. Cheraskin E, Ringsdorf WM Jr. The mental illness proneness profile. *Alabama J Med Sci* 1973;10(1):32–45.

5. Cheraskin E, Ringsdorf WM Jr, Medford FH, et al. The musculoskeletal disease proneness profile. *ACA J Chiropract* 1977;14 (51):41–51.

6. Cheraskin E, Ringsdorf WM Jr. Fabric of man. *J Amer Soc Prevent Dent* 1971;1(4):10–12,15–17.

7. Mardones J. Experimentally induced changes in the free selection of ethanol. *Internal Rev Neurobiol* 1960;2:41–76.

8. Williams RJ. *Alcoholism: The Nutritional Approach.* Austin: University of Texas Press, 1959, 1978.

9. Register UD, Marsh SR, Thurston CT, et al. Influence of nutrients on intake of alcohol. *J Amer Dietet Assn* 1972;61 (2):159–162.

10. Cantor M, Eichler RJ. Sweetness: a supernormal reinforcer. *Chemtech* 1977;7(4):214–216.

ALZHEIMER'S DISEASE

LZHEIMER'S DISEASE IS as prevalent as schizophrenia, probably affecting some 6 million people in Canada and the United States, and is growing rapidly. In contrast to schizophrenia, which strikes at the beginning of life's most productive period, this senile psychosis strikes at the end. I see few situations as tragic as the loss of a spouse or parent to this incipient, irresistible, overwhelming conversion of a normal, fully functional and productive human being into a shell of the same person, shuffling toward a merciful death for both victim and family.

The incidence of schizophrenia has remained constant over the past century, but the incidence of Alzheimer's is increasing. When I started in psychiatry it was extremely rare, but today it is overwhelming. We therefore need as much investigation of the facts as possible, and as much good hypothesis formation as possible, so that we can allocate funds in the right direction.

We need to spend a lot more money searching out the multiple causes of Alzheimer's disease and less money looking for new drugs. Drugs cannot restore abnormal body reactions. For this we must use molecules that are normally found in life, we have to use orthomolecular theory and practice. We must identify the toxins, remove them from the environment, discover the vulnerable part of the population so that preventive measures can be started early, and use any treatment that is shown to be effective and is not toxic.

—ABRAM HOFFER, *JOM* 2000

TERMS OF ALZHEIMER'S DISEASE

APOLIPOPROTEIN-E4. A gene that increases the risk of developing Alzheimer's.

BETA-AMYLOID. A sticky snippet of protein found in the core of plaque.

CATECHOLAMINERGIC SYSTEM. A neurotransmitter system that is essential for the regulation of general physiological changes, which prepare the body for physical activity stress and the fight-or-flight response.

CEREBRAL CORTEX. The outer layer of the cerebrum that is densely packed with nerve cells.

CEREBRUM. The two largest, most complex and most developed lobes of the brain.

CHOLINERGIC SYSTEM. A neurotransmitter system that is essential for memory and learning and that is progressively destroyed in Alzheimer's.

CYTOPROTECTIVE. Protects cells against harmful agents.

DENDRITES. Small branches from nerve cells that contain the receiving stations for signals from other neurons.

GLUTAMATERGIC SYSTEM. Central to the brain's activity, this neurotransmitter system is involved in exciting nerves between neurons so that information may be transmitted.

HIPPOCAMPUS. An area in the brain linked to the formation, organization, and storage of memories.

HOMOCYSTEINE. An amino acid that is naturally formed in the body as the result of the breakdown of another amino acid, methionine.

NEURITIC PLAQUE. Abnormal clusters of dead and dying nerve cells, other brain cells, and protein.

NEUROFIBRILLARY TANGLES. Twisted fragments of protein within nerve cells that clog up the cell.

NEURONS. Nerve cells; tangles and plaques cause neurons to lose their connection to one another and die off, and brain tissue to shrink (atrophy).

NEUROTOXIC. Poisonous to cells.

NEUROTRANSMITTERS. Messenger molecules; major neurotransmitters include acetylcholine, dopamine, glutamate, norepinephrine, and serotonin.

RECEPTORS. Molecules found on the surface of cells that receive chemical signals from outside the cell.

SENILE PLAQUES. Areas where products of dying nerve cells have accumulated around protein.

TAU. Protein that strangles neural synapses and prevents normal chemical and electrical signaling activity.

HIGH DOSES OF VITAMINS FIGHT ALZHEIMER'S DISEASE
by Andrew W. Saul, PhD

The news media reported that "huge doses of an ordinary vitamin appeared to eliminate memory problems in mice with the rodent equivalent of Alzheimer's disease." They then quickly added that "scientists aren't ready to recommend that people try the vitamin on their own outside of normal doses."[1] In other words, extra-large amounts of a vitamin are helpful, but don't take them.

Researchers at the University of California at Irvine gave the human dose equivalent of 2,000 to 3,000 milligrams (mg) of vitamin B3 to mice with Alzheimer's disease.[2] It worked. Kim Green, one of the researchers, is quoted as saying, "Cognitively, they were cured. They performed as if they'd never developed the disease."

Specifically, the study employed large amounts of nicotinamide, the vitamin B3 widely found in foods such as meat, poultry, fish, nuts, and seeds. Nicotinamide is also the form of niacin found, in far greater quantity, in dietary supplements. It is more commonly known as niacinamide. It is inexpensive and its safety is long established. The most common side effect of niacinamide in very high doses is nausea. This can be eliminated by taking less; by using regular niacin instead, which may cause a warm flush; or by choosing inositol hexaniacinate, which does not. They are all vitamin B3.

A *HealthDay* reporter mentioned how cheap the vitamin is; the study authors "bought a year's supply for $30" and noted that it "appears to be safe." Even so, one author said that "I wouldn't advocate people rush out and eat grams of this stuff each day."[1]

The British Broadcasting Company (BBC) quoted Rebecca Wood, chief executive of the United Kingdom's Alzheimer's Research Trust, who said, "Until the human research is completed, people should not start taking the supplement . . . People should be wary about changing their diet or taking supplements. In high doses vitamin B3 can be toxic."[3]

The *Irish Times* reiterated it: "People have been cautioned about rushing out to buy high dose vitamin B3 supplements in an attempt to prevent memory loss . . . The warnings came today one day on from [after] the announcement . . .Vitamins in high doses can be toxic."[4]

The Facts

Their choice of words is quaint but hardly accurate. There is no wild "rush"; half the population already takes food supplements. And as for "toxic," niacin isn't. Psychiatrist Abram Hoffer asserts that it is actually remarkably safe. "There have been no deaths from niacin supplements," Dr. Hoffer says. "The LD 50 (the dosage that would kill half of those taking it) for dogs is 5,000–6,000 mg per kilogram (kg) of body weight. That is equivalent to almost a pound of niacin per day for a human. No human takes 375,000 mg of niacin a day. They would be nauseous long before reaching a harmful dose." Dr. Hoffer conducted the first double-blind placebo-controlled clinical trials of niacin. He adds, "Niacin is not liver toxic. Niacin therapy increases liver function tests. But this elevation means that the liver is active. It does not indicate an underlying liver pathology."

The medical literature repeatedly confirms niacin's safety. Indeed, for over 50 years, orthomolecular physicians have used vitamin B3 in doses as high as tens of thousands of milligrams per day. Cardiologists frequently give patients thousands of milligrams of niacin daily to lower cholesterol. Niacin is preferred because its safety margin is so very large. The American Association of Poison Control Centers' Toxic Exposure Surveillance System annual reports indicate there is not even one death per year due to niacin in any of its forms.[5]

On the other hand, there are 140,000 deaths annually attributable to properly prescribed prescription drugs.[6] And this figure is just for one year, and just for the United States. Furthermore, when overdoses, incorrect prescriptions, and

Excerpted from the *Orthomolecular Medicine News Service*, December 9, 2008.

"If everyone started on a good nutritional program supplemented with optimum doses of vitamins and minerals before age 50, and remained on it, the incidence of Alzheimer's disease would drop precipitously."

— ABRAM HOFFER

adverse drug interactions are figured in, total drug fatalities number over a quarter of a million dead. Each year.

The BBC's curious mention that we should even be "wary about changing our diets" is especially odd. More and more scientists think our much-in-need-of-improvement diets are what contribute more than anything to developing Alzheimer's. "There appears to be a statistically significant link between a low dietary intake of niacin and a high risk of developing Alzheimer's disease. A study of the niacin intake of 6,158 Chicago residents, 65 years of age or older, established that the lower the daily intake of niacin, the greater the risk of becoming an Alzheimer's disease patient." The group with the highest daily intake of niacin had a 70 percent decrease in incidence of this disease compared to the lowest group. "The most compelling evidence to date is that early memory loss can be reversed by the ascorbate (vitamin C) minerals. Greater Alzheimer's disease risk also has been linked to low dietary intake of vitamin E and of fish."[7]

Prevention and Cure

Nutrient deficiency of long standing may create a nutrient dependency. A nutrient dependency is an exaggerated need for the missing nutrient, a need not met by dietary intakes or even by low-dose supplementation. Robert P. Heaney, MD, uses the term "long-latency deficiency diseases" to describe illnesses that fit this description. He writes: "Inadequate intakes of many nutrients are now recognized as contributing to several of the major chronic diseases that affect the populations of the industrialized nations. Often taking many years to manifest themselves, these disease outcomes should be thought of as long-latency deficiency diseases . . . Because the intakes required to prevent many of the long-latency disorders are higher than those required to prevent the respective index diseases, recommendations based solely on preventing the index diseases are no longer biologically defensible."[8] Where pathology already exists, unusually large quantities of vitamins may be needed to repair damaged tissue. Thirty-five years ago, in another paper, Hoffer wrote: "The borderline between vitamin deficiency and vitamin-dependency conditions is merely a quantitative one when one considers prevention and cure."[9]

As there is no recognized cure for Alzheimer's, prevention is vital. In their article, the *Irish Times* does admit that "Healthy mice fed the vitamins also outperformed mice on a normal diet" and quoted study coauthor Frank LaFerla saying that "This suggests that not only is it good for Alzheimer's disease, but if normal people take it, some aspects of their memory might improve."[4] And study author Green added, "If we combine this with other things already out there, we'd probably see a large effect."

The U.S. Alzheimer's Association's Dr. Ralph Nixon has said that previous research has suggested that vitamins such as vitamin E, vitamin C, and vitamin B12 may help people lower their risk of developing Alzheimer's disease. At their website (although you have to search for it), the Alzheimer's Association says, "Vitamins may be helpful. There is some indication that vitamins, such as vitamin E, or vitamins E and C together, vitamin B12, and folate may be important in lowering your risk of developing Alzheimer's . . . One large federally funded study[10] showed that vitamin E slightly delayed loss of ability to carry out daily activities and placement in residential care." But overall, at their website (www.alz.org), the Alzheimer's Association has strikingly little to say about vitamins, and they hasten to tell people that "No one should use vitamin E to treat Alzheimer's disease except under the supervision of a physician."

"They write as if these safe vitamins are dangerous drugs," comments Dr. Hoffer. "I have been using them for decades."

Niacin and Nerves Go Together

Orthomolecular physicians have found niacin and other nutrients to be an effective treatment for obsessive-compulsive disorder, anxiety, bipolar disorder, depression, psychotic behavior, and schizophrenia. New research confirms that niacinamide (the same form of B3 used in the Alzheimer's research) "profoundly prevents the degeneration of demyelinated axons and improves the behavioral deficits" in animals with an illness very similar to multiple sclerosis.[11]

A measure of journalistic caution is understandable, especially with ever-new promises for pharmaceutical products. Drugs routinely used to treat Alzheimer's disease have had a disappointing, even dismal, success rate. So when nutrition may be the better answer, foot-dragging is inexplicable, even inexcusable. Nutrients are vastly safer than drugs. Unjustified, needlessly negative opinionating is out of place. Over 5 million Americans now have Alzheimer's disease, and the number is estimated to reach 14 million by 2050. Potentially, 9 million people would benefit later from niacin now.

"Man is a food-dependent creature," wrote University of Alabama professor of medicine Emanuel Cheraskin, MD. "If you don't feed him, he will die. If you feed him improperly, part of him will die."

When that part is the brain, it is dangerous to delay the use of optimum nutrition.

REFERENCES

1. Doting R. Vitamin holds promise for Alzheimer's disease. *Health-Day*, Nov 5, 2008. Available at: www.washingtonpost.com/wpdyn/content/article/2008/11/05/AR2008110502796.html.

2. Green KN, Steffan JS, Martinez-Coria H, et al. Nicotinamide restores cognition in Alzheimer's disease transgenic mice via a mechanism involving sirtuin inhibition and selective reduction of Thr231-phosphotau. *J Neurosci* 2008;28(45):11500–11510.

3. BBC. Nov 5, 2008. Available at: http://news.bbc.co.uk/2/hi/health/7710365.stm.

4. Donnellan E. Caution urged over using vitamin B3 to treat Alzheimer's. *Irish Times*. Nov 5, 2008. Available at: www.irishtimes.com/newspaper/breaking/2008/1105/breaking91.htm.

5. Annual Reports of the American Association of Poison Control Centers' National Poisoning and Exposure Database, 1983–2006. AAPCC. Available at: www.aapcc.org/annual-reports.

6. Classen DC, Pestotnik SL, Evans RS, et al. Adverse drug events in hospitalized patients: excess length of stay, extra costs, and attributable mortality. *JAMA* 1997;277(4):301–306.

7. Hoffer A, Foster HD. *Feel Better, Live Longer with Vitamin B-3: Nutrient Deficiency and Dependency.* Kingston, ON: CCNM Press, 2007. Also: Foster HD. *What Really Causes Alzheimer's Disease.* Victoria, BC: Trafford, 2004.

8. Heaney RP. Long-latency deficiency disease: insights from calcium and vitamin D. *Am J Clin Nutr* 2003;78(5):912–919.

9. Hoffer A. Mechanism of action of nicotinic acid and nicotinamide in the treatment of schizophrenia. In: *Orthomolecular Psychiatry: Treatment of Schizophrenia* edited by D. Hawkings and L. Pauling. San Francisco: W.H. Freeman, 1973, 202–262.

10. Sano M, Ernesto C, Thomas RG, et al. A controlled trial of selegiline, alpha-tocopherol, or both as treatment for Alzheimer's disease: the Alzheimer's Disease Cooperative Study. *NEJM* 1997;336(17):1216–2122.

11. Kaneko S, Wang J, Kaneko M, et al. Protecting axonal degeneration by increasing nicotinamide adenine dinucleotide levels in experimental autoimmune encephalomyelitis models. *J Neurosci* 2006;26(38):9794–9804.

THE PREVENTION OF MEMORY LOSS AND PROGRESSION TO ALZHEIMER'S DISEASE WITH B VITAMINS, ANTIOXIDANTS, AND ESSENTIAL FATTY ACIDS: A REVIEW OF THE EVIDENCE

by Patrick Holford

Episodic memory impairment is the most common initial symptom of mild cognitive impairment (MCI).[1] Poor performance in verbal or visuospatial memory recall, processing speed, attention, and executive function tasks requiring planning or judgment and semantic fluency are common predictors of Alzheimer's risk.[2-4] The process of memory decline and brain shrinkage associated with Alzheimer's disease is thought to occur over a 30- to 40-year period, hence identifying the need for screening ideally from age 50.

High Homocysteine, and Low Folic Acid and Cobalamin Status as Markers

Both high plasma levels of homocysteine levels and low blood levels of folic and cobalamin (vitamin B12) correlate with increasing risk for Alzheimer's disease, according to a systematic review.[5] A review in 2008 concluded: "Seventy-seven cross-sectional studies on more than 34,000 subjects and 33 prospective studies on more than 12,000 subjects have shown associations between cognitive deficit or dementia, and homocysteine and/or B vitamins."[6] Homocysteine levels also predict and correlate with rate of cognitive decline,[7] as does vitamin B12 status.[8,9] There is, therefore, ample evidence to propose that lowering homocysteine by giving appropriate supplemental levels of homocysteine-lowering nutrients, including pyridoxine (vitamin B6), vitamin B12, and folic acid, would reduce risk. At what point in the process is cognitive decline reversible, and what dosage of nutrients confers maximum protection?

Clinical Trials of B Vitamins in Relation to Prevention of Memory Decline

Durga et al. provided adults, 50 years or older, without MCI but with raised homocysteine levels, supplemental folic acid (0.8 milligrams [mg]/day) or a placebo for three years.[10] The results demonstrated a highly significant improvement in memory, information processing speed, and sensorimotor speed in the treatment group.

In another study, Smith et al. investigated the effects of giving B vitamins versus a placebo in a randomized controlled trial to those with MCI by measuring brain shrinkage (atrophy) with a magnetic resonance imaging (MRI) scan as well as cognitive function.[11] In this study, a homocysteine level above 9.5 micromoles per liter (μmol/L) correlated with accelerated brain shrinkage and cognitive decline. Those given folic acid (0.8 mg/day), vitamin B12 (0.5 mg/day), and vitamin B6 (20 mg/day) had a significant reduction in the rate of brain shrinkage. Treated patients with baseline homocysteine levels greater than 13 μmol/L had rates of atrophy that were 53 percent lower than other patients in the treatment group. Greater rates of atrophy were associated with lower final cognitive test scores.

De Jager evaluated changes in cognition in patients with MCI from the previous study, who were given B vitamins or the placebo. These results indicate a greater decrease in cognitive function with higher baseline homocysteine, with effectively no significant further decline in those taking the B vitamins. In patients with a baseline of homocysteine above 11 μmol/L, the difference in cognitive decline between the placebo and supplemental group was significant.[12]

Aisen et al. gave homocysteine-lowering B vitamins to those already diagnosed as suffering from mild to moderate Alzheimer's disease.[13] Patients were not selected on the basis of homocysteine values (mean homocysteine was 9.1 μmol/L at baseline), and brain scans were not conducted. The patients received folic acid (5 mg/day), vita-

From the J Orthomolecular Med 2011;26(2):53–58.

min B6 (25 mg/day), and vitamin B12 (1 mg/day) over a period of 18 months. No overall difference occurred in the rate of cognitive decline in those on the supplements versus the placebo. However, when the patients were divided into those with high and low cognitive test scores at the start, those who had milder Alzheimer's disease did significantly respond. Those taking the B vitamins hardly got worse over 15 months, while those on the placebo showed a steady decline. Over the 18 months, homocysteine levels dropped from an average of 9.1 µmol/L to 6.8 µmol/L.

Kwok et al. studied 140 subjects with mild to moderate Alzheimer's disease or vascular dementia. Vascular dementia is the second most common form of dementia and is caused by problems in the supply of blood to the brain. Subjects were given either vitamin B12 as methylcobalamin (1 mg/day) and folic acid (5 mg/day) or a placebo for 24 months.[14] They found a significantly smaller decline in the Mattis Dementia Rating Scale (a neuropsychological test) in the supplemented subjects with a baseline homocysteine greater than 13 µmol/L.

In another study, Ford et al. gave 299 older hypertensive men without cognitive impairment either vitamin B12 (0.4 mg), folic acid (2 mg), vitamin B6 (25 mg), or a placebo over two years.[15] No change was found in the cognitive subscale of the Alzheimer's Disease Assessment Scale (another widely used assessment test). However, this test is not sufficiently sensitive to changes outside of the scope of MCI and dementia. Also, homocysteine levels were not measured.

These studies suggest that homocysteine-lowering B vitamins can, at least, arrest cognitive decline and possibly improve it in people over age 50, with or without cognitive decline but with a raised homocysteine level (> 9.5 µmol/L), and may arrest or slow down cognitive decline in those with mild Alzheimer's, but not in those with moderate to severe Alzheimer's disease. However, it is conceivable that Alzheimer's patients with raised homocysteine may respond differently. Further research is needed to determine if these improvements prevent the development of Alzheimer's disease, and what combination and intake of homocysteine-lowering nutrients have the most significant clinical effect. This is also the conclusion of a recent review.[16]

The effect of lowering homocysteine could potentially have many positive effects on brain function. Homocysteine is a toxic amino acid capable of inducing neurotoxicity through N-methyl-d-aspartate (NMDA) receptor activation and increased oxidative stress. Homocysteine also damages blood vessels potentially impairing oxygen and nutrient flow to the brain, associated with vascular dementia. Raised homocysteine also reflects faulty methylation. Methylation is required for the formation of neurotransmitters and phospholipids. Lowering homocysteine is also associated with reducing oxidative stress.

The Role of N-Acetyl Cysteine, Glutathione, and Methylcobalamin

Methylation requires the synthesis of S-adenosyl methionine (SAMe) from homocysteine, a pathway that is B12 and folic acid dependent. SAMe synthesis is impaired by oxidative stress, while vitamin B12 is also vulnerable to oxidative deactivation. Oxidative stress increases the requirement for SAMe but decreases its synthesis. In the liver, homocysteine

IN BRIEF

Memory loss and increased risk of Alzheimer's disease is strongly associated with low levels of vitamin B12 and folic acid, fish consumption and raised plasma homocysteine. Placebo controlled trials have shown protection from memory loss and/or reduced brain shrinkage in older people with raised homocysteine levels given high dose supplements of vitamin B12, folic acid, vitamin B6, or docosahexaenoic acid (DHA). In those with early stage Alzheimer's disease, there is some evidence of a reduction in cognitive decline in those given high dose B vitamins. There is inconclusive evidence regarding the combined supplementation of high dose vitamin C, together with vitamin E. The need for early screening for cognitive decline and raised homocysteine is essential given the growing body of evidence that homocysteine-lowering nutrients arrest cognitive decline and accelerated brain shrinkage.

can also be metabolized via the pathway to synthesize the antioxidant glutathione. Theoretically, by providing glutathione, or its precursor N-acetyl cysteine (NAC), together with methylcobalamin, SAMe can be spared and homocysteine lowered.

A small number of general practitioners have been implementing a B vitamin–based homocysteine management approach, including NAC, and reporting good outcomes. A series of case reports have been published.[17] Quoting the author: "Patients presenting with mild cognitive impairment frequently have raised blood homocysteine levels; I routinely measure this in all such cases. There is now good evidence for lowering elevated levels with high dose B vitamins. I also prescribe the antioxidant NAC to further lower homocysteine. In my experience, I have found significant clinical improvement from this approach."

Homocysteine can also be processed in the liver by the betaine-homocysteine methyl transferase (BHMT) pathway, requiring trimethylglycine (TMG), and zinc. The addition of NAC, TMG, and zinc to the usual combination of vitamin B12 (ideally as methylcobalamin, a more active form of cobalamin), folic acid, and vitamin B6 has yet to be tested in a clinical trial and may yield further reductions in homocysteine with associated clinical improvements.

Vitamins C and E

A cross-sectional and prospective study of 4,740 Cache County, Utah, elderly residents found the combination of vitamins C and E to be associated with reduced Alzheimer's disease prevalence of 78 percent and incidence of 63 percent. A trend toward lower Alzheimer's risk was also evident in users of vitamin E, together with multivitamins containing vitamin C, but there was no evidence of a protective effect with use of vitamin E or vitamin C supplements alone, with multivitamins alone, or with vitamin B-complex supplements. The lowest risk was reported in those supplementing with at least 1,000 mg a day of vitamin C with at least 1,000 international units (IU) a day of vitamin E.[18] In a double-blind study, subjects with MCI were randomly assigned to receive 2,000 IU a day of vitamin E, 10 mg a day of donepezil (Aricept), or a

placebo for three years. There were no significant differences in the rate of progression to Alzheimer's disease between the vitamin E and the placebo groups at any point.[19] These results suggest that there might be more therapeutic gains when treating patients that have yet to develop either MCI or Alzheimer's disease. These results also suggest that both vitamins E and C are likely to be more beneficial than using vitamin E alone.

Fish Consumption and Omega-3 Essential Fatty Acid Supplementation

Eating fish once a week reduces risk of developing Alzheimer's disease by 60 percent, according to a study by Morris et al.[20] Researchers followed 815 people, ages 65 to 94, for seven years and found that the dietary intake of fish was strongly linked to Alzheimer's disease risk. They found that the strongest link was the amount of docosahexaenoic acid (DHA) in the diet: the higher the intake of this fatty acid, the lower the risk of developing Alzheimer's disease. The lowest amount of DHA per day that offered some protection was 100 mg. Eicosahexaenoic acid (EPA) intake did not have a significant impact; however, the highest intake of EPA consumed was 30 mg a day.

In a randomized controlled trial, 900 mg of DHA was taken daily for 24 weeks with reported improvements in learning and memory function among those with age-related cognitive decline.[21] In a further trial by the same research group, 2,000 mg per day of algae-sourced DHA or a placebo given to 402 subjects with mild to moderate Alzheimer's disease for 18 months resulted in no cognitive improvement.[22]

Clinical Recommendations

Alzheimer's disease is an advanced disease process that requires many years of progression before it can be clinically diagnosed. Using nutritional supplements late in the disease process may yield limited benefits. However, the low cost and potential benefits of nutritional supplements make them attractive therapeutically. On the basis of the evidence, there is good logic to pursue specific clinical recommendations, especially among patients without any evidence of cognitive impairment. Patients 50 years or older should have their cognitive function tested. Homocysteine should also be tested in patients who exhibit signs of reduced cognitive function.

If the homocysteine result is above 9.5 µmol/L, supplement with the following homocysteine-lowering nutrients daily: folic acid (400–800 micrograms), vitamin B6 (20–40 mg), and vitamin B12 (0.5–1.0 mg, preferably as methylcobalamin).

There is good logic in using these additional daily nutrients: NAC (500–1,000 mg), omega-3 essential fatty acids (fish source containing 500–1,000 mg of DHA), TMG (1,000–2,000 mg), and zinc (10–15 mg).

While there might be some logic in supplementing with vitamin E (1,000 IU/day) and vitamin C (1,000 mg/day or more) among elderly individuals without MCI or Alzheimer's disease, further research is needed.

Dietary Guidelines

There is an increasing body of evidence linking metabolic syndrome (blood-fat/blood-sugar disorders), insulin resistance, and diabetes with risk for dementia/Alzheimer's disease. Following a low-glycemic-load (low-sugar) diet, high in oily fish, nuts, seeds, and beans, with plenty of antioxidant-rich fruits and vegetables is likely to be protective. Limit or avoid coffee, which is known to raise homocysteine levels. Whether or not coffee intake increases or reduces risk for Alzheimer's disease is currently inconclusive.

REFERENCES

1. Peterson RC. Mild cognitive impairment: prevalence, prognosis, aetiology, and treatment. *J Int Med* 2004;256:183–194.

2. deJager CA, Hogervorst E, Combrinck M, et al. Sensitivity and specificity of neuropsychological tests for mild cognitive impairment, vascular cognitive impairment and Alzheimer's disease. *Psychol Med* 2003;33:1039–1050.

3. Perry RJ, Hodges JR. Attention and executive deficits in Alzheimer's disease: a critical review. *Brain* 1999;122(Pt 3):383–404.

4. Oulhaj A, Wilcock GA, Smith AD, et al. Predicting the time of conversion to MCI in the elderly. *Neurology* 2009;73:1436–1442.

5. Van Dam F, Van Gool WA. Hyperhomocysteinemia and Alzheimer's disease: A systematic review. *Arch Gerontol Geriatr* 2009;48:425–430.

6. Smith AD. The worldwide challenge of the dementias: a role for B vitamins and Hcy? *Food Nutr Bull* 2008; 29(2 Suppl):S143–S172.

7. Oulhaj A, Refsum H, Beaumont H, et al. Hcy as a predictor of cognitive decline in Alzheimer's Disease. *Int J Geriatr Psychiat* 2010;25:82–90.

8. Smith AD, Refsum H. Vitamin B-12 and cognition in the elderly. *Am J Clin Nutr* 2009:89:707S–711S.

9. Tangney CC, Tang Y, Evans DA, et al. Biochemical indicators of vitamin B12 and folate insufficiency and cognitive decline. *Neurology* 2009;72:361–367.

10. Durga J, van Boxtel MP, Schouten EG, et al. The effect of 3-year folic acid supplementation on cognitive function in older adults in the FACIT trial: a randomized, double-blind, controlled trial. *Lancet* 2007;369:208–216.

11. Smith AD, Smith SM, de Jager CA, et al. Hcy-lowering by B vitamins slows the rate of accelerated brain atrophy in mild cognitive impairment: a randomized controlled trial. *PLoS One*, 2010;5(9):e12244.

12. de Jager CA. Cognitive and clinical outcomes of Hcy-lowering B vitamin treatment in mild cognitive impairment: a randomized controlled trial. Unpublished manuscript. 2011.

13. Aisen PS, Schneider LS, Sano M, et al. High-dose B vitamin supplementation and cognitive decline in Alzheimer disease. *JAMA* 2008;300:1774–1783.

14. Kwok TJ, Lee A, Lawb CB, et al. A randomized placebo controlled trial of Hcy lowering to reduce cognitive decline in older demented people. *Clin Nutr* 2011;30(3):297–302.

15. Ford AH, Flicker L, Alfonso H, et al. Vitamins B12, B6, and folic acid for cognition in older men. *Neurology* 2010 Oct 26;75(17):1540–1547.

16. Sachdev PS. Hcy and Alzheimer disease: an intervention study. *Nature Rev Neurology* 2011;7:9–10.

17. McCaddon A. Homocysteine and cognitive impairment; a case series in a general practice setting. *Nutr J* 2006;5:6.

18. Zandi PP, Anthony JC, Khachaturian AS, et al. Reduced risk of Alzheimer disease in users of antioxidant vitamin supplements: the Cache County Study. *Arch Neurol* 2004;61:82–98.

19. Petersen R, Thomas R, Grundman M, et al. Vitamin E and donepezil for the treatment of mild cognitive impairment. *N Engl J Med* 2005;352:2379–2388.

20. Morris MC, Evans DA, Bienias JL, et al. Consumption of fish and n-3 fatty acids and risk of incident Alzheimer disease. *Arch Neurol* 2003;60:940–946.

21. Yurko-Mauro K, McCarthy D, Rom D, et al. Beneficial effects of docosahexaenoic acid on cognition in age-related cognitive decline. *Alzheimers Dement* 2010;6:456–464.

22. Quinn JF, Raman R, Thomas RG, et al. Docosahexaenoic acid supplementation and cognitive decline in Alzheimer disease: a randomized trial. *JAMA* 2010;304:1903–1911.

HOW ALUMINUM CAUSES ALZHEIMER'S DISEASE: THE IMPLICATIONS FOR PREVENTION AND TREATMENT OF FOSTER'S MULTIPLE ANTAGONIST HYPOTHESIS

by Harold D. Foster, PhD

Aluminum has been identified as a neurotoxin for over 100 years.[1] Its toxic impacts were demonstrated most dramatically when long-term hemodialysis patients (with chronic renal failure) were treated with aluminum-containing phosphate binders, and/or a dialysate made using water with high-dissolved aluminum levels.[2] Many of these kidney patients developed dialysis dementia and other complications.

There are similarities between the brains of Alzheimer's and dialysis-dementia patients. Senile plaques have been observed in both, as have decreased levels of the enzyme choline acetyltransferase activity and concentrations of the neurotransmitter gamma-aminobutyric acid.[3–6] Such similarities have provided further support for the hypothesis that aluminum toxicity is the key to Alzheimer's disease, although many researchers reject this suggestion.[7] Opponents of this viewpoint argue that aluminum deposition in the brains of Alzheimer's patients only occurs late in the disorder because the blood-brain barrier prevents aluminum entry until it is damaged by extensive nerve cell death or by other causes, such as amyloid deposition. Secondly, they claim that even when incorporated into the brain, aluminum is relatively benign. Thirdly, they point out that pathological changes caused experimentally in animals by aluminum are not identical to those seen in the brains of Alzheimer's disease patients.[8] This article provides evidence to refute such objections.

Geographical and Epidemiological Evidence of Aluminum's Involvement in Alzheimer's Disease

Drinking water usually contains between 0.01 and 0.15 milligrams (mg) per liter of aluminum. Some potable water, however, may have as much as 0.40 mg or more per liter.[9] While this represents only a small percentage of total dietary aluminum, it is possible that because of repetitious exposure aluminum from drinking water may provide a large component of the total aluminum absorbed. Priest[10] has shown that the fraction of dietary aluminum entering the tissues may vary from as much as 0.01 for aluminum citrate to 0.0001 for insoluble forms, such as aluminum silicates and oxides. Most of this absorbed aluminum tends to be excreted if kidney action is normal, but about 5 percent is deposited in the body, mainly in the skeleton.[11] It was established by Sohler and coworkers[12] as early as 1981, however, that in 400 psychiatric outpatients in New Jersey, memory loss increased as blood aluminum levels rose.

It has been shown that in Norway,[13–14] England, Wales,[15] and Canada[16] the prevalence of Alzheimer's disease rises as the amount of aluminum in the water supply increases. Other sources of exposure to aluminum include tea, certain food additives (such as those often found in chocolate), aluminum foil, cans and cookware, antacids, enteric-coated aspirin, and some antiperspirants and deodorants.[20]

Aluminum also is always present in the air but numerous industrial workers inhale far more than the 4.4 micrograms (mcg) average daily intake from the air.[10] Inhaled aluminum appears to be neurotoxic under certain special conditions. To illustrate, the mineral silica has a well-known ability to protect against aluminum and vice versa. For this reason, between 1944 and 1979, many miners were given aluminum powder as a preventative against silicotic lung disease. An aluminum "bomb" was let off after each shift and the miners inhaled its dust in an effort to protect themselves against silica. During a study[21] conducted during 1988 and 1989, miners who had been exposed to aluminum dust in this way were found to show abnormal cognitive

From the *J Orthomolecular Med* 2000;15(1):21–51.

deficits, their neurological problems increasing with the duration of their exposure.

Probably the most significant evidence of the possible link between dementia and aluminum comes from an Ontario study involving 668 autopsy-verified Alzheimer's disease brains. These showed that the risk of developing Alzheimer's disease is about 2.5 times greater in individuals from communities drinking water containing more than 100 mcg per liter of aluminum, than it is in individuals from communities where the potable water contains less than this level of aluminum.[22]

It is not my objective here to present all the epidemiological and geographical evidence that is available to support a role for aluminum in Alzheimer's disease. Readers wanting a more comprehensive introduction to this literature are directed to Doll's "Review: Alzheimer's disease and environmental aluminum" in *Age and Ageing* (1993)[9] and to the double edition of *Environmental Geochemistry and Health* (1990), which is devoted largely to this topic.[23]

A Multiple Antagonist Hypothesis

Numerous hypotheses have attempted to explain the neurodegenerative processes that ultimately culminate in Alzheimer's disease. These focus, for example, on calcium homeostasis,[24] beta-amyloid protein, and the apolipoprotein-E4 gene.[25] None of these hypotheses, however, appear able to account for all the diverse geographical, sociological, pathological, biochemical, and clinical aspects of the disease. For this reason, I am presenting a new multiple antagonist hypothesis that appears capable of explaining more fully the etiology of Alzheimer's disease.

Antagonism among elements is widely established. To illustrate, many diseases in livestock occur because fodder, enriched in particular minerals, results in shortages of others. Cobalt deficiencies, which cause wasting in sheep and cattle, for example, can usually be linked to a high iron and manganese soil content.[26] Such relationships between minerals are commonplace and appear to occur because ions with similar electronic configurations[27–30] are antagonistic toward each other. Aluminum shows this type of antagonism toward metals, including zinc, phosphorus, calcium, and magnesium.[31–34] Aluminum's biological activity is influenced further by silicon and fluorine, some compounds of which are able to chelate (bond with) it, while others promote its solubility. Dietary levels of minerals formed from these six elements greatly affect aluminum's absorption by the digestive tract and its ability to cross the blood-brain barrier. If it reaches the brain, aluminum's negative impact again is due largely to its antagonism with calcium, magnesium, phosphorus, and zinc, since it has a strong tendency to replace them in important enzymes and proteins. The resulting novel compounds then create cascades of biochemical dysfunctions, which eventually cause neuronal degeneration, ultimately culminating in Alzheimer's disease. Evidence to support this hypothesis is presented now, together with a discussion of its implications for the prevention and treatment of this form of dementia.

Alzheimer's Disease: The Challenge

Alzheimer's disease affects at least 6 million people in the United States and Canada, and probably 30 million more worldwide, chiefly in the developed world.[25] It is most common in the elderly, but between 2 and 7 percent of cases are associated with inherited genetic mutations, which can cause the disease in people as young as 30 years old. Three rare genes have been implicated in such early-onset Alzheimer's cases, but these stand apart from the major susceptibility genes linked to Alzheimer's in the elderly. Most Alzheimer's patients, however, develop the disease after age 65, without any previous family history of this disorder.[25] Apart from genetic susceptibility and aging, other identified risk factors for the disease are malnutrition, lack of education, and head trauma.[25,35–36]

Alzheimer's disease, a normally irreversible brain disorder, is characterized by insidious onset and progressive loss of intellectual capacity. This decline in the ability of the brain to function is linked to the formation of senile plaques and neurofibrillary tangles, and to the degeneration of neurons in the cerebral cortex.[37] Other nerve cell degeneration in the subcortical area of the brain also has been recorded.[38] Such brain abnormalities were documented first by the German physician Alois Alzheimer in 1907,[39] hence the name of the disease.

Biochemically, Alzheimer's disease is known to involve malfunctions in the cholinergic and catecholaminergic systems, which are linked for example to deficiencies of the neurotransmitters acetylcholine and dopamine. Another hallmark of Alzheimer's disease is a decrease in brain glucose metabolism. Such changes in the brains of Alzheimer's patients are not typical of aging. Indeed, Byell and Coleman[40] suggest that while degenerative dendritic changes do occur in some cells as a usual consequence of aging, these seem associated with a simultaneous thickening of branches in other neurons. This suggests that in normal aging there is an attempt to compensate for neural degeneration, which does not occur in Alzheimer's brains.[41]

Typically, memory loss is the first obvious sign of the early stage of Alzheimer's disease. Then subtle personality shifts begin to appear, including signs of apathy and withdrawal. By the middle stage of the disease appearance and behavior tend to deteriorate and wandering may become more apparent. Intellectual personality disturbances increase and depression or delusions may appear, followed by delirium. As progression occurs, the patient may become mute, incontinent, and incapable of self-care. Death ultimately follows. From onset to mortality, the average course of Alzheimer's disease is usually between five to eight years.

Any hypothesis attempting to explain the cause of Alzheimer's disease must, therefore, be able to account for the disorder's known risk factors (such as its increasing frequency with age), its links to genetic aberrations, its associated neurological and biochemical abnormalities, and its clinical symptoms.[25] The rest of this article is an attempt to meet this challenge.

Aluminum's Absorption by the Intestinal Tract

While exposure to aluminum is ubiquitous, how much of it is absorbed by the intestinal tract and how easily it is excreted depends on a variety of complex interrelationships. To illustrate, there is considerable evidence to show that, when dietary calcium intake is low or when aluminum intake is very high, the latter may substitute for the former, or may use some of the same transport mechanisms to gain access to the brain.[42] This is most likely to occur in individuals drinking acidic water, which may explain why the prevalence of Alzheimer's disease increases in areas that experience acid rain.[43] Relationships between aluminum and calcium are complex, as illustrated by the impact of aluminum-containing antacids on the absorption of calcium and other minerals.[44] Even small doses of such antacids significantly increase fecal fluoride, indicating a decline in its intestinal absorption. Antacids that contain aluminum also impact phosphorus and calcium metabolism, and their primary effect is binding with intestinal phosphorus, which results in its depletion. This change in phosphorus metabolism results in a rise in urinary and fecal calcium excretion, which often is sufficient to produce a negative calcium balance. Animal experiments suggest that aluminum absorption also is greatly affected by parathyroid hormone and vitamin D levels, both of which help maintain an appropriate balance of calcium in the bloodstream and in tissues. Rats[45] fed on a diet containing elevated aluminum, for example, produced high levels of parathyroid hormone, which in turn increased gastrointestinal aluminum absorption. This element was subsequently deposited in the brain. Chickens given supplements of vitamin D also developed increased aluminum brain content.[46] In contrast, dogs with low levels of vitamin D suffered significantly more aluminum accumulation in their bones, independently of parathyroid hormone status.[47]

Such animal studies also demonstrate that diets deficient in calcium alone, or low in calcium and magnesium (with or without added aluminum), can reduce absorption of magnesium and increase that of aluminum.[48] Low calcium–high aluminum diets in rats, for example, diminish magnesium in the bones and in the central nervous system and induce a loss of calcification in the former and tissue degeneration in the latter.[49] Furthermore, aluminum has been shown to decrease zinc concentration in the bones and soft tissues of rats fed a low calcium-magnesium diet.[50] Beyond this, it has been established that in rats fed magnesium-deficient diets there is diminished kidney function,[51] which seems likely to provide greater access of aluminum to soft tissues. This decline in kidney function is associated with calcium deposition in its tubules. The antagonism between magnesium and aluminum, therefore, is clearly established,[52] but it would appear that magnesium intake also influences the bioavailability of both calcium and zinc.

Aluminum also has a strong affinity for silicon, which influences its absorption by the intestinal tract. This was demonstrated by a British clinical trial, conducted by Edwardson and coworkers,[53] in which volunteers were given an aluminum tracer[26] dissolved in orange juice. Elevated levels of this element were later detected in their blood. Six weeks later the same volunteers drank orange juice, again containing aluminum but to which sodium silicate also had been added. After this second challenge, blood aluminum levels rose to only 15 percent of that previously reached in the absence of silica. Edwardson and colleagues argued that the geographical association between Alzheimer's disease and levels of aluminum in water supplies reflects this inverse relationship between aluminum and silicates. It is believed silica promotes the formation of an aluminum-silicate complex, limiting the gastrointestinal absorption of aluminum.

Fluorine also has an affinity for aluminum and influences its absorption. Fucheng and coworkers,[54] for example, have described high incidences of osteoporosis, osteomalacia, spontaneous bone fractures, and dementia in certain villages in Guizhou Province, China. These diseases are very similar to those occurring in European dialysis patients, treated with water and gels containing aluminum.[55] Fucheng and colleagues discovered that such Chinese health problems stemmed from eating maize, which had been baked in fires of coal mixed with kaoline (formed from aluminous minerals). The latter contained 19.3 percent aluminum and 7,000 parts per million (ppm) of fluorides. In this area, fluoride levels in drinking water also were elevated. Bone aluminum and fluoride levels were found to be 25 times higher in maize-eating villagers than they were in controls. Tests with rats confirmed that in the presence of elevated fluorides, the toxic dose of aluminum in food may be reduced to 100 ppm or less. The implications of this fluoride-aluminum relationship to Alzheimer's disease are unclear but demonstrate that aluminum can be neurotoxic in individuals who do not suffer from kidney malfunction.

The solubility of aluminum (Al), and probably the ease with which it is absorbed, varies markedly with pH (acid/alkaline balance), being lowest at about pH 6.5.[56] Aluminum's solubility, therefore, is greatest in highly acid or highly alkaline waters. However, since the latter usually contain elevated calcium and/or magnesium, it tends to be the greatest health threat when dissolved in acidic water. It is also believed that fluorine binds with aluminum at acidic pH values, forming compounds such as solvated $AlF2+$ and $AlF2$. At a higher pH, the predominant form of aluminum is $Al(OH)4$. These relationships have been discussed at length by Forbes and coworkers.[19] In general, therefore, aluminum is most soluble in acidic water, especially if it contains fluorides. Tennakone and Wickramanayake[58] for example, have shown that the presence of only 1 ppm of fluoride in water adjusted with sodium bicarbonate or citric acid to pH3, and boiled in an aluminum vessel, releases nearly 200 ppm of aluminum in 10 minutes. Prolonged water boiling can elevate dissolved aluminum to 600 ppm. In contrast, if such water contains no fluoride, only 0.2 ppm aluminum levels are reached. In addition, in 10 minutes, 50 grams of acidic crushed tomatoes cooked in 200 milliliters (ml) of water containing 1 ppm of fluoride produced a paste containing 150 ppm of aluminum.

In summary, acidic food or water, especially if fluoride is present, can leach excessive aluminum from cooking vessels. Furthermore, tea brewed in soft (acidic) water or flavored with lemon juice and aluminum may be of great significance in Alzheimer's disease since, Varner and coworkers[61] have demonstrated that the chronic administration of the fluoride-aluminum complex (AlF3) to rats, in drinking water, resulted in elevated aluminum levels in brains and kidneys. These high levels of aluminum were associated with damage to rat neuronal integrity, not seen in controls drinking double-distilled deionized water.

Beyond such antagonistic and synergistic relationships with these specific elements, it is clear that certain aluminum compounds inherently are more easily absorbed than others. McLachlan and Kruck,[62] for example, have fed a wide variety of aluminum compounds to rabbits to establish variations in absorption rates. They discovered that aluminum citrate, formed when aluminum reacts with the citric acid in oranges or tomatoes, caused the absorption of aluminum to increase by a factor of 2.5. This is of particular interest because oranges and tomatoes also are known to increase calcium absorption, which needs acid for assimilation.[63] McLachlan and Kruck's rabbit experiments further established that aluminum maltolate, produced when this metal reacts with maltol (an additive that usually is found in hot chocolate, beer, and some commercially baked goods), raised aluminum uptake some 90-fold. Aluminum citrate and aluminum maltolate, therefore, seem particularly capable of entering the body.

Aluminum and the Blood-Brain Barrier

Investigators who oppose the pathogenicity of aluminum in Alzheimer's disease have claimed that the blood-brain barrier will prevent this neurotoxic metal from impacting on the brain until after serious damage already has occurred from other causes.[64–65] This argument is incorrect. Yumoto and coworkers[66] injected the radioisotope[26]Al into healthy rats and showed that a considerable amount of this aluminum isotope was incorporated into the cerebrum within five days after one injection and continued to show a gradual increase in the brain for a further 70 days. This accumulation of aluminum was accompanied by a decline in dendrites in cortical nerve cells and in attached spines. These changes implied a decrease in the amount of information that could be received. Many similar changes have been reported from Alzheimer's brains.

Aluminum's ability to cross the blood-brain barrier is influenced by the form in which it is absorbed and the levels of other compounds in the blood. To illustrate, it has been discussed previously that aluminum maltolate is absorbed easily by the intestinal tract. It appears also to be capable of quickly crossing the blood-brain barrier.[67] Furthermore, as it does, it increases the permeability of this barrier, a process with subsequent serious toxicity implication. That is, aluminum maltolate may affect the blood-brain barrier adversely, making it permeable to other damaging toxins. This may account for the variety of symptoms seen in subtypes of Alzheimer's disease and even in some other forms of dementia. Interestingly, Rao and colleagues[68] have suggested that maltolate-treated, elderly rabbits can be used as a good animal model of Alzheimer's disease because of their neurofibrillary pathology.

Aluminum maltolate is not the only substance that can enhance aluminum's ability to cross the blood-brain barrier. To illustrate, Deloncle and coworkers[69] have shown that, when there is an increase in sodium L-glutamate in blood, aluminum penetrates red blood cells. This suggests that aluminum crosses the red blood cell's membrane as a glutamate complex. Experiments with rats have demonstrated that similarly, aluminum can pass the blood-brain barrier as a glutamate complex and then be deposited in the cortex. This aluminum-L-glutamate complex is neurotoxic in vivo.[70] Nevertheless, aluminum enters neurons and alone induces possible conformational changes in the tau. Aluminum combined with glutamate or glutamate by itself do not.[71]

Aluminum and the Brain

On reaching the brain, aluminum begins to antagonistically replace calcium, magnesium, zinc, and phosphorus in various enzymes and proteins. As a consequence, it sets in motion a series of biochemical cascades involving abnormal processes, which together eventually culminate in the pathologic and clinical symptoms known as Alzheimer's disease. Several examples will now be provided, but no claim is made here that all such antagonistic relationships have been identified, or that they are necessarily limited to calcium, magnesium, zinc, and phosphorus.

Aluminum and Glucose Metabolism

Decreased glucose metabolism is a hallmark of Alzheimer's disease.[72] It appears to occur because of aluminum's binding with the phosphate enzyme, glucose-6-phosphate dehydrogenase and its interference with hexokinase (a group of enzymes that speed carbohydrate metabolism).[73] To illustrate, Cho and Toshi[74] purified two isozymes (enzymes important in cell signaling) from pig and human brains and established that they contained an enzyme-aluminum complex. They were then able to demonstrate that glucose-6-phosphate could be completely inactivated by aluminum, but that this enzyme's potency could be restored by the three aluminum chelators: citrate, sodium fluoride, and apotransferrin. Aluminum's negative impact on glucose metabolism, however, is not limited to inhibiting the glucose-6-phosphate enzyme. Lai and Blass[75] have shown that this metal also inhibits hexokinase activity in the rat brain, but that high levels of magnesium can reverse this process. Aluminum also appears to inactivate hepatic phosphofructokinase, an important control site in the glycolytic pathway in which glucose is converted to simpler compounds.[76]

Aluminum and the Cholinergic System

Cholinergic neurotransmitter deficits are characteristic of Alzheimer's disease.[25] Indeed, a deficiency of acetylcholine is the basis for a recognized diagnostic test for this disorder.[77] Such malfunctioning of the cholinergic system appears to be caused by aluminum's ability to inhibit the activities of the enzyme choline acetyltransferase,[78-80] a deficiency of which has been confirmed in Alzheimer's disease by several researchers including Perry,[81] Gottfries,[80] and Quirion and coworkers.[82] In addition, some neuritic plaques have been shown to contain acetylcholinesterase-beta amyloid protein complexes, further compromising the functioning of the cholinergic system.[83] As is described in the following discussion, the development of such plaques is also the result of aluminum's disruptive influence.

Interestingly, Gottfries and colleagues[84] have established that in the early stages of Alzheimer's disease, elevated serum homocysteine appears to be a sensitive marker for cognitive impairment.[85] Choline deficiency raises homocysteine levels by altering the metabolism of methionine[86] and would, therefore, account for both homocysteine's presence at high levels in the serum and associated cognitive impairment. Certainly, there is an extensive literature[87-91] that indicates that the malfunctions that occur in the cholinergic system in Alzheimer's disease are accompanied by selective degeneration of cholinergic neurons in the cortex, hippocampus, and base of the forebrain. This is highly significant because such acetylcholine-containing neurons play a key role in memory and affect the highest levels of cognitive functioning.

Aluminum and the Catecholaminergic System

Altman and coworkers[92] have shown that, in patients on hemodialysis, levels of the enzyme dihydropteridine reductase are inversely related to aluminum concentrations. When such patients were given the aluminum-chelating agent desferrioxamine, their dihydropteridine reductase activity doubled. This depression of dihydropteridine reductase by aluminum is extremely significant, since this enzyme is essential for the maintenance of normal brain concentrations of tetrahydrobiopterin, which is itself required for the synthesis of the neurotransmitters, dopamine, norepinephrine, and serotonin.

As might be expected, if Alzheimer's disease is caused by aluminum neurotoxicity, levels of tetrahydrobiopterin are depressed significantly in the cerebrospinal fluid of patients suffering from this disease.[93] As a consequence, the brains of Alzheimer's patients contain less dopamine, norepinephrine, and serotonin than those of controls.[94-96] Several studies have demonstrated that the subnormal production of these neurotransmitters appears to be linked to the death of dopamine receptors and noradrenergic and serotonergic neurons in the cortex and elsewhere in the Alzheimer's brain. Joyce and coworkers,[97] for example, argued that the loss of the dopamine D2 receptor-enriched modules in the brains of Alzheimer's patients contributed to disturbances in information processing that may be responsible for cognitive and non-cognitive impairments. Similarly, Palmer[98] has suggested that the absence of noradrenergic and serotonergic neurons probably contributes to the non-cognitive impairments in behavior seen in Alzheimer's patients.

It is possible that aluminum impacts more directly on the catecholaminergic system. Marinho and Manso,[99] for example, have studied the effects of different concentrations of aluminum sulfate on the non-enzymatic oxidation of dopamine, conducting these experiments to evaluate the action of aluminum on neuromelanin synthesis. Their results indicate that aluminum partially inhibits dopamine self-oxidation, decreasing the formation of such intermediate compounds as dopaminequinone and dopaminochrome. This suggests that if, as believed, neuromelanins have a cytoprotective function in the central nervous system, where they are thought to act as free scavengers of metal ions and free radicals (unstable and damaging molecules), then their reduction by aluminum could accelerate the damage of neuronal tissues by oxidative stress.

Furthermore, Singh and colleagues[100] have described the high toxicity of aluminum phosphide, which is used widely as a fumigant in India. Accidental poisoning with this aluminum compound is relatively common and its dominant clinical feature is severe hypotension related to dopamine. This appears to further confirm that aluminum has a direct impact on the catecholamine system.

Wenk and Stemmer[101] have shown that, in rats, the neurotoxic effects of ingested aluminum are dependent on the dietary intake of copper, zinc, iron, and magnesium. To illustrate, norepinephrine levels in the cortex and cerebellum are depressed in rats receiving a high aluminum–low copper diet. Similarly, suboptimal iron levels reduce norepinephrine in the cerebellum. Furthermore, diets containing aluminum but little copper or zinc decreased cortex dopamine levels. These data suggest that aluminum's impact on the catecholaminergic system is complex and depends very much on the presence, or absence, of adequate levels of these various elements in diet.

Aluminum and Parathyroid Hormone

Adenylyl cyclase is a catecholamine-sensitive enzyme[102] that plays a significant role in parathyroid hormone secretion. Parathyroid hormone, as previously mentioned, helps to maintain an appropriate balance of calcium in the bloodstream and in tissues. Calcium inhibits adenylyl cyclase activity but magnesium promotes it, so stimulating the production of parathyroid hormone.[103] Indeed, Zimmerman and colleagues[104] have suggested that the adenylyl cyclase catalytic mechanism involves two magnesium ions. Animal studies have established that aluminum can cause an irreversible activation of adenylyl cyclase that Ebstein and coworkers have suggested may be one reason for this metal's neurotoxicity.[105] Indeed, although while adenylyl cyclase activity declines in the non-demented elderly, no such reduction is seen in Alzheimer's patients, who typically show abnormally high-brain adenylyl cyclase activity.[106]

Aluminum and the Glutamatergic System

There is a profound reduction in glutamatergic neurotransmission in Alzheimer's disease that results from neuron loss and cholinergic innervation.[107] This deficit is associated with significantly depressed plasma glutamate levels and abnormally low glutamine concentrations in cerebrospinal fluid.[108] There appears to be a strong correlation between behavior and coping ability in Alzheimer's patients and cerebrospinal fluid glutamate levels, which provides clear evidence of a role for the disruption of amino acid metabolism in the disease.

Studies with rabbits that have been injected with aluminum powder have shown that this element causes significant decreases in glutamate decarboxylase activity in the cerebellum.[109] In addition, aluminum impairs the glutamate-nitric oxide-cyclic GMP pathway in neurons[110] and appears to inhibit glutamate release from the rat hippocampus.[111] Aluminum chloride also has been shown to slow the rate of accumulation of L-glutamate in the rat forebrain nerve-ending particles, in a dose-dependent fashion, so influencing neurotransmitter substance transport.[112] As has been discussed previously when reviewing aluminum's ability to cross the blood-brain barrier, aluminum can react with glutamate to form an aluminum L-glutamate complex that is neurotoxic in vivo.[69,70] This may be because aluminum, as has been shown, potentiates both glutamate-induced calcium accumulation and iron-induced oxygen free-radical formation,[113] suggesting that the aluminum-glutamate association may increase oxidative stress in neurons.

Aluminum and Neuritic Plaques

The brains of Alzheimer's patients are characterized by neuritic plaques, which are composed of abnormal proteins. The cores of such plaques consist of beta-amyloid, a sticky snippet of a larger protein, amyloid-precursor protein. It has been established that beta-amyloid, involved in such plaques, is created when the brain is deficient in acetylcholine, a shortage that causes amyloid-precursor protein to break down.[78,114] As has been discussed previously, acetylcholine deficiency is a hallmark of Alzheimer's disease because of aluminum's ability to inhibit the activities of the enzyme choline acetyltransferase,[78] so interfering with the normal operation of the cholinergic system.[83] In addition, as pointed out already, some neuritic plaques contain acetylcholinesterase–beta-amyloid protein complexes, which further disrupt the cholinergic system.[83]

Perry[115] has demonstrated that in postmortem Alzheimer's brain tissue, there is an inverse relationship among the activities of choline acetyltransferase and acetylcholinesterase and senile plaque numbers. Furthermore, plaques that contain acetylcholinesterase have a higher resistance to low pH and to anticholinesterase inhibitors and are more cytotoxic than normal plaques.[116]

Aluminum and Neurofibrillary Tangles

Neurofibrillary tangles also are a characteristic of Alzheimer's brains. Such tangles consist mainly of an abnormal form of the protein tau, which is highly and unusually phosphorylated.[117] Calcium/calmodulin kinase II acts as a cataylst in the addition of phosphate (phosphorylation) of tau,[118] a process that is stimulated by two phospholipids,[119] phosphatidylserine and phosphatidylethanolamine. However, aluminum interacts with calmodulin to form a stable Al-calmodulin complex.[117–120] Under these circumstances, calmodulin becomes less flexible, is prevented from reacting with several other proteins, and is inhibited in its regulatory functions. In addition, aluminum creates fatty acid abnormalities in the phospholipids, which normally stimulate the phosphorylation of tau.[117,121] Beyond this, Yamamoto and colleagues[122] have shown that aluminum appears to inhibit the dephosphorylation of tau in the rat brain. It seems likely, therefore, that in the presence of elevated aluminum both phosphorylation and dephosphorylation of tau are disrupted, largely by the replacement of calcium by aluminum in calmodulin.

Furthermore, hemodialysis patients exposed to elevated aluminum develop depressed phosphatase levels.[123] Abnormally low phosphatase concentrations also have been reported from Alzheimer's patients' brains.[124] Aluminum-induced abnormalities in levels of phosphatases, enzymes required to remove phosphate groups from protein, also appear to be involved in the formation of neurofibrillary tangles. It would appear that such aluminum-induced lack of phosphatase,[125] in the brains of Alzheimer' patients, occurs because of an excess of phosphates in tau that prevent this protein from performing its normal role of securing vital parts of the neuronal cytoskeleton. The cell, therefore, is harmed and hyper-phosphorylated tau is precipitated to form tangles. According to Roushi[126] animal studies suggest that such extra phosphates may cause neural damage even before tangles form, by interfering with one of tau's normal functions, assembling and stabilizing the microtubules that carry cell organelles, glycoproteins, and other vital nutrients through the neurons.

It has been demonstrated that the more phosphate groups that are attached to synthetic neurofilament fragments, the easier it is for aluminum ions to bind and cross-link neurofilaments.[125] The presence of aluminum, therefore, appears to change the paired helical filaments that make up neurofibrillary tangles so that they accumulate and are not removed, in the normal way, by protein-digesting enzymes.

Interestingly, a laser microprobe study of the elemental content of neurofibrillary tangles in Alzheimer's disease, conducted by Good and coworkers,[127] established that the only metallic elements found to be consistently present were aluminum and iron.

Aluminum and Brain Cell Membranes

In Alzheimer's patients, cellular brain membranes display abnormal viscosity that appears to disrupt the activities of various enzymes, receptors, and membrane carriers and may be linked to dendritic spine loss.[128] These abnormalities seem associated with irregularities in the biochemistry of the phospholipids that concentrate in such brain cell membranes. Corrigan and coworkers,[130] for example, have shown that in Alzheimer's disease phospholipids from the parahippocampal cortex (part of the brain important for remembering scenes or episodes), including phosphatidylcholine, phosphatidylserine, and phosphatidylinositol, contain below normal levels of the potent antioxidant alpha-linolenic acid. In addition to this depression of the level of omega-3 fatty acids, abnormalities also occur in levels of omega-6 essential fatty acids. It has further been demonstrated that, not only are the biochemical compositions of phospholipids from Alzheimer's patients abnormal, but that total concentrations of such membrane phospholipids are low[130] and that their regional distribution in the brain is irregular.[131]

It has been suggested that the biochemical abnormalities seen in phospholipids in Alzheimer's disease result from elevated oxidative stress.[121] However, aluminum also appears more directly involved. To illustrate, aluminum chloride has been shown to inhibit the incorporation of inositol into phospholipids.[132] Deleers and coworkers[133] also have demonstrated aluminum-induced lipid phase separation and fusion of phospholipid membranes. However, it seems more likely that disruption of phospholipase A2 by aluminum[134] is probably the main cause of the biochemical abnormalities seen in phospholipids in Alzheimer's disease, and the chief cause of associated brain membrane dysfunctions. Certainly, phospholipase A2 plays a key role in the metabolism of membrane phospholipids,[135] is decreased in Alzheimer's disease,[136] and is inhibited by aluminum chloride.[134]

In addition, aluminum has a direct effect on cell membranes. Dill and coworkers,[137] for example, have proved that the addition of micromolar quantities of aluminum chloride to phospholipid membranes containing VDAC (voltage-dependent anion channels) greatly inhibits the voltage dependence of the channels' permeability, encouraging them to remain open. It would appear, therefore, that both through its antagonism with phosphorus and by its own direct impact, aluminum adversely affects the functioning of cellular brain membranes in Alzheimer's disease.

Aluminum and Oxidative Stress

There is overwhelming evidence that Alzheimer's disease brain cells are subjected to elevated oxidative stress and that amyloid plaques are a focus of cellular and molecular oxidation. Much of the destruction of neurons, which characterizes Alzheimer's disease, has been linked to the oxidation of lipids (fat-like substances) in cell membranes caused by free radicals. This process seems to occur because of disturbed defense mechanisms in Alzheimer's disease that are associated with a self-propagating cascade of neurodegeneration.[138–139] It has been established, for example, that Alzheimer's patients display depressed antioxidant status associated with significantly low vitamin E levels.[140]

There is considerable evidence that aluminum itself reduces the body's defense against free-radical damage. In dialysis patients for example, levels of glutathione peroxidase, an enzyme that protects against the formation of free radicals, are significantly depressed.[141] Similarly, animal studies have demonstrated that the oral administration of aluminum sulfate, especially in the presence of citric acid, inhibits the activities of two free-radical scavenging enzymes in the brain: superoxide dismutase and catalase.[142] Interestingly, vitamin E, which is depressed in Alzheimer's patients, can protect rats against associated aluminum-induced free-radical damage.[143] Other evidence of the significance of oxidative stress includes a significant increase in superoxide dismutase and catalase activity in the blood of Alzheimer's patients[144] and a pronounced increase in superoxide dismutase in the tissues.

Exactly how aluminum is involved in the catastrophic loss of neurons from free radical damage is being established by van Rensburg and coworkers[139,146] and Fu and colleagues.[147] The former have shown, for example, that both beta-amyloid and aluminum dose-dependently increase lipid peroxidation in platelet membranes. Their research has established that beta-amyloid is toxic to biological membranes and that aluminum is even more so.[146] Beyond this, van Rensburg and colleagues have demonstrated that iron encourages lipid peroxidation, both by aluminum and by beta-amyloid protein. This is of considerable interest since the only metallic elements found in the neurofibrillary tangles of Alzheimer's disease are aluminum and iron.[127] Van Rensberg and coworkers' in-vitro model also showed that the hormone melatonin prevented lipid peroxidation by aluminum and beta-amyloid protein in the absence of hydrogen peroxide. If the latter were present, melatonin could only slow the process.[146]

Fu and coworkers[147] have begun to explain how beta-amyloid specifically damages neurons. Their cell culture research has shown that beta-amyloid interferes with calcium homeostasis and induces apoptosis (death) in neurons by oxidative stress. This latter process involves the catecholamines (nonepinephrine, epinephrine, and dopamine), which increase beta-amyloid's toxicity to cultured hippocampal neurons. Fu and coworkers[147] also have been able to show that the antioxidants vitamin E, glutathione, and propyl gallate (used in foods, cosmetics, and pharmaceuticals) can protect neurons against damage caused by beta-amyloid peptide and the catecholamines.

Aluminum also may increase free radical damage in Alzheimer's disease by inhibiting the protective superoxide dismutase. Normally, this is one of the major enzymes that provide protection against free radicals. However, Shainkin-Kesterbaum and coworkers[151] showed that in vitro, at the levels of the enzyme found in dialysis patients, aluminum severely inhibited its protective effects. This inhibition of superoxide dismutase's antioxidant activity was directly proportional to the level of aluminum.

Silicon was found also to have a similar inhibitory effect on the enzyme. The disruptive influence of aluminum on superoxide dismutase may account for the fact that, while zinc supplementation generally improves mental alertness in the elderly, in Alzheimer's patients it accelerates deterioration of cognition, encouraging amyloid-plaque formation.[152] This may be because in the latter stages of Alzheimer's disease, it cannot be used in disrupted superoxide dismutase production and so merely stimulates free-radical formation.

Aluminum and Established Risk Factors in Alzheimer's Disease

Any hypothesis seeking to explain Alzheimer's disease must be able to account for established risk factors, namely: malnutrition, susceptibility genes, head trauma, aging, and lack of education.[25] An attempt will be made now to do this for my multiple antagonist hypothesis.

Malnutrition

Throughout this article, evidence has been presented to show that diet influences aluminum's absorption, ability to cross the blood-brain barrier, and likelihood of causing brain damage. Furthermore, Grant[153] has shown that epidemiological evidence is consistent with the view that low fat–low calorie diets may lessen the risk of Alzheimer's disease. Interestingly, Mazur and coworkers[154] have established that, in the rat, low selenium diets increase apolipoprotein E levels. Similarly, Durlach and colleagues[155] have suggested that, in humans, vitamin E, selenium, magnesium, and other antioxidants can protect against the deleterious metabolic consequences of apolipoprotein E4.

Genetic Susceptibility to Alzheimer's Disease

Recent studies have shown that elderly Japanese and African-Americans living in the United States have a much greater prevalence of Alzheimer's disease than those still residing in their ethnic homelands. Environmental not genetic factors must, therefore, be the major agents responsible for Alzheimer's disease.[156–157] Nevertheless, the likelihood of any first-degree relative of a late-onset Alzheimer's patient also developing the disease is some four times greater than in the population at large.[158] There must be, therefore, at least one genetic component to Alzheimer's disease. In fact, there appear to be several such links. To date four genes have been identified as playing a role in either early- or late-onset Alzheimer's: beta-amyloid precursor protein, presenilin-1, presenilin-2, and apolipoprotein E (ApoE) genes.[159] Workers have linked most of these variants to familial early-onset Alzheimer's but the apolipoprotein E4 allele is a relatively common definite risk factor for developing late-onset Alzheimer's disease.[25]

Considerable progress has been made in interpreting the significance of such genetic variants. To illustrate, mutations in the presenilin-1 gene seem associated with increased superoxide production and greater vulnerability to beta-amyloid peptide toxicity.[160] Interestingly, mutations in the presenilin genes, which are linked to more than 40 percent of all familial Alzheimer's disease cases, enhanced production of an abnormal form of beta-amyloid precursor protein.[161] This protein is longer than normal, aggregates more rapidly, kills neurons in culture more effectively, and precipitates preferentially to form amyloid plaques. The same elongated protein is also produced as a result of mutations in the gene-encoding beta-amyloid precursor protein.

As has previously been described, aluminum interacts with L-glutamate to form a complex that can cross the blood-brain barrier.[69] This reaction appears to lead to depressed levels of glutamate and glutamine.[162] The largest familial Alzheimer's disease kindred discovered to date occurs in Antioquia, Columbia.[159] These individuals appear to develop Alzheimer's disease because of a genetic mutation that results in a glutamic acid-to-alanine substitution in presenilin-1. That is, members of the Antioquia disease kindred are short of glutamic acid. A similar deficiency might be expected to be associated with aluminum-induced depression of glutamate and glutamine.

An ApoE variant predisposes a significant section of the population to late-onset Alzheimer's disease.[25] This may occur in several ways. Pratico and coworkers[163] have shown that in ApoE-deficient mice, oxidative stress is increased, encouraging arteriosclerosis. Interestingly, oral supplementation with vitamin E suppresses this degenerative process. Naiki and colleagues[164] also have demonstrated that normal ApoE inhibits beta-amyloid fibril formation in vitro. Indeed, it would seem that in normal brains ApoE efficiently binds and sequesters beta-amyloid peptide, preventing it from forming senile plaques.[165] In Alzheimer's disease, associated with this genetic variant, there is impaired apo/beta-amyloid peptide binding, resulting in an accumulation of beta-amyloid peptide that facilitates senile plaque formation.

The literature suggests, therefore, that the gene variants that predispose to both early- and late-onset Alzheimer's disease do so because they either increase susceptibility to, or mimic, the aluminum-related degenerative processes previously described. That is, the genetic mutations involved in promoting the development of Alzheimer's disease duplicate some of aluminum's deleterious impacts on the brain and, in so doing, encourage at least one of the following: the growth of neuritic plaques or neurofibrillary tangles, excessive free-radical formation, and higher neural oxidative stress. As a consequence, unfortunate individuals carrying any one of the genetic variants are much more likely to develop Alzheimer's disease, whether or not they are exposed to the aluminum excess or vitamin and mineral deficiencies that are normally associated with its etiology.

Head Trauma

Controversy continues over whether or not traumatic brain injury increases the probability of developing Alzheimer's disease.[166] Launer and coworkers[167] sought to answer this question by performing a pooled analysis of four European population-based prospective studies of individuals, ages 65 years and older. These data included 528 incident dementia patients and 28,768 person-years of follow-up. Incident dementia occurs as a result of a physical disease or injury. Their analysis established that a history of head trauma with unconsciousness did not increase significantly the risk of subsequent Alzheimer's disease. Similarly, Nemetz and colleagues[168] followed up the medical histories of 1,283 traumatic brain injury cases that had occurred in Olmsted County, Minnesota, from 1935 to 1984. Thirty-one of these trauma patients subsequently had developed Alzheimer's disease, a number similar to that normally expected in individuals without head injuries. However, the data clearly shows that such head trauma had reduced the time-of-onset of Alzheimer's disease by about eight years, among persons at risk for developing it. That is, head trauma does not appear to increase the probability of developing Alzheimer's disease in the general population, however, those prone to it tend to suffer from it earlier than normally expected.

Why this happens is a question that appears to have been answered by Nicoll and coworkers.[169] These researchers have shown that the deposition of beta-amyloid in the brain had been promoted by head trauma, in approximately one third of individuals dying shortly afterward from severe injury. The probability of deposition of such beta-amyloid, following trauma, is greater than would be anticipated statistically in individuals with the ApoE4 allele, that is the gene that has been linked to late-onset Alzheimer's disease. In short, in individuals with this genotype, severe head trauma often appears to initiate beta-amyloid deposition. Not surprisingly, if they survive the trauma, such deposition reduces the time-of-onset of sporadic Alzheimer's disease in those genetically prone to it since, of course, beta-amyloid is the major constituent of neuritic plaques.

Aging and Increased Prevalence

In the United States, the prevalence of severe dementia, much of it Alzheimer's disease, found among those ages 65 to 74, is roughly 1 percent, compared to 25 percent for those over 84.[170] There is a disputed suggestion that the risk of developing dementia may decline after age 84 is reached,[171] but this hypothesis appears to be in conflict with results of detailed surveys.[172] Evans and coworkers,[173] for example, found that in East Boston, Massachusetts, an urban working class community of some 32,000 inhabitants, an estimated 10.3 percent of the population over 65 had probable Alzheimer's disease. The prevalence of this disorder increased steadily with aging, from 3.0 percent at age 65 to 74 years, to 18.7 percent for those aged 75 to 84. This trend continued so that 47.2 percent of those 85 years or older were diagnosed as suffering from probable Alzheimer's disease. This age-related increase in dementia was identified again in San Marino.[174] At age 67 only 1.8 percent of the population suffered from it, a figure that rose to 25.0 percent in those 87 years of age. The general situation was summarized by Jorm, Korten, and Henderson[175] who, after a survey of the international literature, concluded that dementia prevalence rates reflected the age of the sample population, doubling every 5.1 years.

If the multiple antagonist hypothesis presented here is correct, this increase in risk of developing Alzheimer's disease with aging is inevitable. As the individual ages, intestinal absorptive capacity is reduced, and as a consequence calcium absorption drops. In addition, kidney function declines and with it there is a corresponding reduction in the production of vitamin D, further decreasing calcium absorption in the intestines.[36] These changes typically lead to a loss of bone calcium and, as has been discussed previously, make aluminum absorption far more likely to occur.

Not only is the brain's aluminum burden likely to increase with aging in this way but its ability to protect itself also characteristically declines. Vitamin deficiency, for example, is common in the elderly,[176] who are all too frequently deficient in antioxidants and, therefore, more prone to oxidative stress. Beyond this, two hormones that decline with age, melatonin and estrogen, play roles in protecting the brain from aluminum. As their levels fall, damage from this element inevitably increases. The aluminum relationship to estrogen probably explains why, as Cohen[177] pointed out, Alzheimer's disease is more common in women then in men, a gender bias that cannot be explained entirely by the greater longevity of females.

Sleep disruption, nightly restlessness, and other circadian disturbances are common in Alzheimer's disease patients. This behavior often appears to be associated with abnormally low melatonin.[178] Interestingly, the levels of melatonin in such patients have been linked to genotype. It has been shown also that the normal daily variations in melatonin disappears in both older subjects and Alzheimer's patients.[179]

This decline of melatonin production in the elderly[180] has many significant implications for Alzheimer's risk. Melatonin, for example, has been shown to alter the metabolism of beta-amyloid precursor protein,[181] prevent peroxidation and associated toxicity to biological membranes, and reduce neural damage due.[182] In addition, Pappolla and colleagues[183] have demonstrated that melatonin is likely to prevent neural damage caused by glutamate and by beta-amyloid protein, both of which are implicated in the neuronal destruction characteristic of Alzheimer's disease.

The decline of estrogen production in post-menopausal women also increases their risk of developing Alzheimer's disease. Confirmation of this has come from the Italian Longitudinal Study on Aging, which provided convincing evidence that estrogen-replacement therapy reduces the prevalence of Alzheimer's disease.[184] It has been shown also that female Alzheimer's patients receiving this hormone have improved cognitive skills.[185] Why estrogen acts in this way is still the subject of extensive research. It has been proved, however, that, in rats, estrogen acts as a growth factor for cholinergic neurons.[186] Gibbs and Aggarwal[187] have hypothesized that there are similar effects in humans and that, as a result, in postmenopausal women receiving estrogen replacement therapy, this hormone delays the decline in basal forebrain cholinergic function, a part of the brain involving spatial learning and memory that is lost early in the development of Alzheimer's disease.

Lack of an Education

Beyond the possibility that less educated individuals may be more likely to eat inappropriate diets, there appear to be three hypotheses that may explain why the lack of an education might increase the risk of developing Alzheimer's disease. First, it is possible that the ApoE variant that predisposes a significant section of the population to late-onset Alzheimer's disease might, in some way, also adversely affect an individual's ability to cope with the demands of an education. There seems, however, to be no available evidence to support this hypothesis.

Second, education might stimulate the brain's development, so increasing its ability to withstand more degenerative damage before Alzheimer's symptoms become apparent. There is certainly growing evidence that stimulation affects brain development. To illustrate, Rosenzweig[188] showed that the number of neurons in rats' brains were influenced by the stimuli in the environment. Rats that grew up in an "enriched" milieu were found to have more neurons in the cerebral cortex than those that did not. In addition a rat from an "enriched" environment had a heavier cortex with thicker cortical coverings. Brain enzymes were also elevated. Globus[189] further discovered that such "enriched" environments increased the number of dendritic spines in the rat brain. Perhaps as Restak[190] muses, learning, memory, and other brain functions in humans may depend to a large degree on the quality of environmental stimulation.

A third hypothesis that may account for the apparent link between a lack of education and the risk of developing Alzheimer's disease would focus on exposure to toxic metals and inadequate dietary mineral intake. If a child were exposed to elevated aluminum while his or her calcium, magnesium, zinc, and phosphorus intakes were depressed, the child might be unable to handle the rigors of higher education. Ultimately, these imbalances might also result in the development of Alzheimer's disease. There is clearly this type of negative relationship between lead exposure and depressed childhood intelligence.[191] Furthermore, Varner and coworkers[61] have shown that the chronic administration of drinking water containing aluminum-fluoride or sodium-fluoride to rats causes significant deficits in neuronal integrity that show regional brain differences. It has been established also that elevated hair aluminum levels seem to be associated with classroom withdrawal by young children.[192] Much of this aluminum may come from cans but it should be noted that aluminum concentrations in most cow's milk-derived formulas are 10- to 20-fold greater than in human breast milk. They are also 100-fold greater in soy-based formulas.[193] Deficiencies in trace and bulk elements also appear to adversely influence school performance. To illustrate, Marlowe and Palmer[194] compared 26 hair trace elements in two sets of young Appalachian children: an economically disadvantaged group of 106 drawn from Head Start programs and a control group of 56 children from more prosperous backgrounds. Developmental disabilities, including communication and behav-

VITAMINS HELP PREVENT ALZHEIMER'S DISEASE

by Patrick Holford and Andrew W. Saul, PhD

Nutritional supplementation with antioxidants and the B-complex vitamins has been shown to help prevent dementia. Half of all cases of Alzheimer's disease, the most common form of dementia, could be attributable to known dietary and lifestyle risk factors, and at least one-fifth of current cases could be prevented right now.

Preventive Factors

But there's no money for prevention research, or sufficient political will to put prevention steps into action. To date, tens of billions of dollars have been spent on developing drugs, none of which have proven to stop or slow down the disease process. Yet already studies have shown that B vitamins have decreased the rate of brain shrinkage in the areas affected by Alzheimer's by almost nine times, as well as dramatically slowing down memory loss, in people with mild cognitive impairment, the precursor to Alzheimer's. Other promising preventive factors include getting exercise, controlling blood sugar and blood pressure, supplementing with omega-3 fish oils, and becoming involved in more social activities.

"Of the millions of pounds so far pledged for dementia research by the UK government, none has been spent on prevention," says Professor David Smith from Oxford University. Dr. Smith's research group first identified that almost half of people over 60 have insufficient vitamin B12 to stop accelerated brain shrinkage. He believes we need to wake up to the fact that Alzheimer's is unlikely to be prevented by drugs.

To Learn More

* *Preventing Alzheimer's Disease-Related Gray Matter Atrophy by B-Vitamin Treatment* by Gwenaëlle Douaud et al at: www.pnas.org/content/early/2013/05/16/ 1301816110.full.pdf+html.

* *Vitamins B12, B6 and Folic Acid Shown to Slow Alzheimer's in Study* by Carol Bradley Bursack at: www.healthcentral.com/alzheimers/c/62/160989/ vitamins-B12-shown-alzheimer.

* *Low Vitamin B12 Status in Confirmed Alzheimer's Disease* by H. Refsum at: http://jnnp.bmj.com/ content/74/7/959.full.pdf+html.

To learn more about how other vitamins can cut Alzheimer's risk:

* *Reduced Risk of Alzheimer's Disease in Users of Antioxidant Vitamins* by Peter Zandi et al. at: http://archneur. jamanetwork.com/article.aspx?articleid=785249 or www.cnn.com/2004/HEALTH/conditions/01/20/ alzheimers.vitamins.reut.

* *Niacinamide for Alzheimer's* by *Alternative Medicine Digest* at http://www.alternative-medicine-digest.com /alzheimers-treatment.html.

* *Nicotinamide Restores Cognition in Alzheimer's Disease* by Kim N. Green et al. at: www.jneurosci.org /content/28/45/11500.full.pdf+html.

Excerpted from the *Orthomolecular Medicine News Service*, December 20, 2013.

ioral disorders, were recorded in 13 members of the Head Start group but were absent from the control group. Hair analysis also established that the mean levels of calcium, magnesium, and zinc were significantly depressed in children from the economically disadvantaged group. Conversely, Benton[195] reviewed five studies that suggested that vitamin/mineral supplements improved many children's performances during intelligence tests. In summary, the evidence suggests that many children are exposed to excess aluminum, while being simultaneously mineral deficient. Such individuals appear to experience schooling difficulties early in life and may possibly develop Alzheimer's disease when older. This may be particularly true if they eat a high fat diet.[153]

The Prevention of Alzheimer's Disease

The number of elderly is undergoing an unprecedented increase, with the proportion of the very old doubling within one generation. In 1950, globally there were 214 million people 60 or older; by 2025 there will probably be 1 billion.[196] Not only are more people surviving into old age and, therefore, increasing their chances of developing Alzheimer's disease but those who do so are living longer after its onset. Gruenberg[197] termed this paradox the "failure of success," a tragedy caused largely by progress in medical care. As he and his colleagues[198] point out, "the old man's friend, pneumonia, is dead—a victim of medical progress." In consequence, the old man is still with us, but all too often he is demented.

As Khachaturian[25] states, the costs of this paradox will be enormous, ". . . if current demographic trends continue, the number of people with Alzheimer's disease will double every twenty years. As of 1997, The United States was already spending $100 billion a year on care for Alzheimer's patients: with the rising cost of health care, society will have a monster on its hands." America will not be alone. This trend is typical of the developed world.[199–200]

I believe that the preceding review has demonstrated that aluminum neurotoxicity is the cause of Alzheimer's disease.[201] At the political level, a series of highly unpalatable steps, therefore, must

be taken if the "monster" is not to have its way. These include setting much lower limits for aluminum in drinking water,[202] prohibiting the use of aluminum salts as coagulants in water treatment,[203] reversing the drive for water fluoridation, and banning the use of both aluminum cans[204] and the food additive aluminum maltolate.[62] It is obvious also that the recommended daily allowances of many minerals and vitamins, especially antioxidants, are too low and that this inadequacy is reflected in the contents of the average multivitamin pill.[205]

The chances that such changes will be made in the near future are poor. Fortunately, there are many steps that the individual can take to reduce his or her own probability of developing Alzheimer's disease. These include drinking low-aluminum potable water, avoiding hot chocolate and acidic drinks in aluminum cans, and not using aluminum-containing antacids or deodorants. Cooking utensils should be stainless steel or glass and foods should not be cooked or stored in aluminum foil. Mineral supplements should include calcium, magnesium, and zinc. Probably the best evidence that vitamin supplements also can reduce the risk of developing Alzheimer's disease comes from a prospective study of 633 people, ages 65 or older, whose vitamin intake was carefully established.[205] After a 4.3 year follow-up period, 91 of the participants met criteria for the clinical diagnosis of Alzheimer's disease. None of the 27 vitamin-E supplement users suffered from it, however, nor did any of the 23 elderly individuals taking vitamin C. Nevertheless, there was no relationship between the incidence of Alzheimer's disease and the use of multivitamins. These data suggest that high-dose vitamin E and C supplements lower the risk of Alzheimer's disease; but that multivitamin antioxidant levels are too low to do so.

Very few people ever come back from the abyss, but it has been done. The author is aware of only two well-documented cases of the "spontaneous regression" of Alzheimer's disease. Fortunately, both of these individuals have written books about their experiences.[206–207] In the belief that Siegel[208] is correct that "We should be paying more attention to the exceptional patients, those who get well unexpectedly, instead of staring bleakly at all who die in the usual pattern," their cases will now be reviewed.

Louis Blank[207] was confirmed to have Alzheimer's disease after detailed hospital testing. As his disorder progressed, he lost the ability to recognize his own family or to speak, and to dress, wash, or eat without assistance. For six months, at the peak of his illness in 1993, he sat virtually motionless. His recovery appeared to begin after his family replaced all its aluminum cooking utensils and started to avoid aluminum cans. In addition, he was fed a high magnesium diet, designed to chelate aluminum.

By May 1994, Louis Blank was again able to carry on conversations and venture outside. By January 1996, he had written and published his book *Alzheimer's Challenged and Conquered?*[209] despite the fact that one of his specialists continued to argue that since there is no cure for Alzheimer's disease, he must still have it. An interesting aspect of Blank's description of his experiences is that while most of his long-term memory remains he still has no recollections of his worst six months. This confirms that, as Alzheimer's disease progresses, the patient loses the ability to form short-term memories. Older-term memories appear to remain intact for much longer.

In his book *Beating Alzheimer's: A Step Towards Unlocking the Mysteries of Brain Diseases* (1991), Tom Warren[206] also describes his experiences with dementia. In June 1983, a computer assisted tomography (CAT) scan confirmed that Warren had Alzheimer's disease. His physicians gave him a maximum of seven years to live. Yet nearly four years later, a new scan indicated that the disease process had reversed. Warren's self-treatment had included rectifying low-hydrochloric stomach acid, the removal of all his teeth and mercury amalgam fragments from his gums, ethylene diamine tetracetic acid (EDTA) chelation therapy, and high doses of vitamins and minerals. The latter included zinc, calcium, magnesium, and vitamins B3 (niacin), B6 (pyridoxine), B12 (cobalamin), and folic acid.

In summary, both Blank and Warren attempted to reduce their exposure to metals, especially aluminum and/or mercury; they underwent chelation therapy and added minerals to their diet, espe-

cially in Blank's case, magnesium. These protocols seem consistent with the hypothesis presented here, that Alzheimer's disease is caused by aluminum and reflects its antagonistic relationships with zinc, calcium, phosphorus, and magnesium. It would seem essential that the Alzheimer's patient, in addition to avoiding contact with aluminum and other toxic metals, undergoes treatment to lower the body's existing burden of these elements. To illustrate, clinical trials have shown that the chelating agent desferrioxamine can slow the progression of the disorder.[210] This may be because, as Savory and coworkers[211] have shown in rabbits, aluminum-induced neurofibrillary degeneration can be effectively reduced in as little as two days by intramuscular injections of desferrioxamine. An excellent oral chelation therapy designed to remove metals from the body has been described by Pouls.[212]

Campell[213] has suggested that a daily supplement of 500 mg of calcium and a similar amount of magnesium can lower elevated hair aluminum back to normal in a year, while Bland[214] recommended the daily use of 600 mg of calcium and 300 mg of magnesium to reduce body aluminum burden. Durach[215–216] has argued that there are two types of magnesium deficit: magnesium deficiency and magnesium depletion. Magnesium deficiency, in his view, is due to insufficient magnesium intake and responds to simple supplementation. Magnesium depletion, in contrast, is the result of a dysregulation in the mechanisms responsible for magnesium metabolism. This second form of magnesium deficit can only be addressed by the correction of the responsible pathogenic dysregulation. However, since in Alzheimer's the dysregulation is apparently due to excess exposure to aluminum, which itself can be corrected by elevating magnesium intake, magnesium supplementation alone also may correct such dysregulation and with it the deficit. This appears to be what happened in the case of the "spontaneous regression" of Louis Blank's Alzheimer's disease when he both avoided aluminum and ate a high magnesium diet.[209]

Once exposure to aluminum and the existing body burden of this element have been reduced, the final stage of Alzheimer's disease treatment appears likely to involve attempts to buttress the patient's cholinergic, catecholaminergic, and glutamatergic systems and associated oxidative stress defense mechanisms (see Table 1). Scinto and coworkers,[77] for example, have used acetylcholine deficiency as the basis for the early detection of Alzheimer's disease, demonstrating that the pupils of patients with Alzheimer's disease dilate markedly in response to a dilute solution of the acetylcholine-blocking drug, tropicamide (Mydriacyl), while normal subjects are virtually unaffected by it. As a consequence, several attempts have been made to treat Alzheimer's disease by trying to increase brain acetylcholine levels. To illustrate, various clinical trials have been conducted to determine whether phosphatidylcholine or lecithin (which contains it) improve brain function in Alzheimer's patients.[217–218] Taken as a whole, these trials seem to suggest that phosphatidylcholine may slow the rate of progression of Alzheimer's disease. Again, in an attempt to elevate brain acetylcholine, clinical trials also have been conducted using acetyl-L-carnitine in the treatment of Alzheimer's patients.[219–221] Results have been promising, with statistically significant improvements being recorded in behavior, attention, and memory. It is not surprising that acetyl-L-carnitine may be valuable in the treatment of Alzheimer's disease because patients' brains are deficient in carnitine acetyl-transferase, which is necessary to catalyze interchange between L-carnitine and acetyl-L-carnitine.[222] Acetyl-L-carnitine may be of benefit in Alzheimer's disease for two reasons. It is a precursor of acetylcholine,[223] increasing the brain availability of this neurotransmitter. In addition, it also seems to evoke dopamine release from the dopaminergic

TABLE 1. ALZHEIMER'S DISEASE AND ALUMINUM: AN OVERVIEW		
ALUMINUM-IMPAIRED ENZYME	CONSEQUENCE	POTENTIAL TREATMENT
Glucose-6-phosphate	Glucose metabolism impaired	Calcium, magnesium
Hexokinase	Glucose metabolism impaired	Calcium, magnesium
Phosphofructokinase	Glucose metabolism impaired	Calcium, magnesium
Choline acetyltransferase	Acetylcholine deficiency; Malfunction of cholinergic neurons Formation of senile plaques	Vitamin B12, [zinc], estrogen, folic acid, calcium, magnesium, phosphatidylcholine, lecithin, acetyl-L-carnitine
Adenylyl cyclase	Elevated parathyroid activity	Magnesium
Dihydropteridine	Depressed dopamine, norepinephrine and serotonin	Desferrioxamine, magnesium, copper, reductase zinc, iron, calcium, magnesium
Glutamate decarboxylase	Reduction in glutamatergic neurotransmission	Calcium, magnesium
Calcium/Calmodulin kinase II	Loss of calmodulin flexibility, formation of neurofibrillary tangles	Desferrioxamine, calcium, magnesium
Alkaline phosphatase	Neurofibrillary tangles	Calcium, magnesium
Phospholipid A2	Abnormal brain cell membranes	Omega-3 and omega-6 essential fatty acids, calcium, magnesium, phosphatidylserine, phosphatidylcholine, phosphatidylcholine, phosphatidyl ethanolamine, phosphatidylinositol
Glutathione-peroxidase	Increased lipid peroxidation	Vitamin E, vitamin C, selenium, melatonin
Superoxide dismutase	Greater free radical damage	[Zinc], copper, ginkgo biloba

As zinc can accelerate amyloid plaque formation in later stages of Alzheimer's disease,[152] it may or may not be suitable treatment.

neurons.[224] Acetyl-L-carnitine, therefore, may be capable of helping to correct deficits in both the cholinergic and catecholaminergic systems, commonly found in Alzheimer's disease.

It is unfortunate that clinical trials to date have used acetyl-L-carnitine in isolation. The production of acetylcholine from choline involves other nutrients, including vitamin B12 and folic acid. These substances should not be assumed to be readily available in Alzheimer's patients. Indeed, a B12 deficiency seems characteristic of the disease,[225–226] as are high levels of its metabolites.[227] McCaddon and Kelly[228] have suggested that when B12 levels are depressed, a well-known biochemical process, the "methyl-folate trap" occurs. This trap diverts folic acid from the brain, preventing the manufacture of acetylcholine, even in the presence of abundant choline.

Nevertheless, there is increasing evidence for a role for acetylcholine in the treatment of Alzheimer's. Donepezil (Aricept), a acetylcholinesterase inhibitor,[229] has been used to produce an increase in central nervous system acetylcholine in mild to moderate Alzheimer's patients, with improvements in cognition. Similarly, vitamin B12 injections, which may increase brain acetylcholine levels, have been reported linked to significant improvement in various neuropsychiatric disorders, even when anemia is absent.[230] Since the production of acetylcholine from choline involves folic acid, it is not surprising that Snowdon's study of postmortem brains from the School Sister's of Notre Dame, Mankato, Minnesota, has identified that a deficiency of this vitamin also appears to occur in Alzheimer's disease.[231]

Three potential treatments for Alzheimer's disease also rest on reducing the availability of acetylcholinesterase for incorporation into plaque complexes with beta-amyloid. Tetrahydroaminoacridine (tacrine), for example, is a potent inhibitor of acetylcholinesterase, which reportedly improves memory deficits in Alzheimer's disease.[232] Similarly, in a dementia mouse model, created with aluminum chloride solution, the Chinese herbal medicine of tonifying kidney-depressed acetylcholinesterase levels in the cerebral cortex, led to an improvement in memory.[233] Bonnefont and coworkers[234] also have shown that estrogen protects neuronal cells from the cytotoxicity induced by acetylcholinesterase-amyloid complexes.

Ginkgo biloba is an herb that has been used traditionally to treat both memory loss and diabetes mellitus.[235] Its active components are ginkgolides, which have antioxidant, neuroprotective, and cholinergic properties. The value of ginkgo biloba extracts in the treatment of Alzheimer's have been demonstrated in placebo-controlled clinical trials and seems to be similar to those of donepezil or tacrine (Cognex), but without any undesirable side effects. One of the major benefits of ginkgo appears to be its ability to increase blood flow, not only to healthy parts of the brain, but also to disease-damaged areas.[235] Beta-amyloid, in its interaction with superoxide radicals, constricts and damages the lining of the small blood vessels supplying the brain. It is likely that ginkgo, acting as a circulation enhancer, helps to overcome this problem.[236–237] This, of course, may be why the blood thinner aspirin[238–239] may also be beneficial in the treatment of Alzheimer's disease. However, there seems to be more to ginkgo biloba extract than its antioxidant and circulation-enhancing properties since clinical trials also have established that it improves memory and cognitive performance in healthy young females.[240] In addition, in both young and old rats it increases neurotransmitter-receptor binding.[241]

There appear to have been few attempts to correct deficits in the catecholaminergic system in Alzheimer's disease. One exception to this generalization has been the testing of lisuride (Dopergin), a dopamine-receptor antagonist, more often used in the treatment of Parkinson's disease. Initial results suggest that this drug may reduce the rate of decline of verbal memory in Alzheimer's but results were not statistically significant.[242]

In contrast, several attempts have been made to assess the possibility of correcting the abnormal viscosity of cellular brain membranes in Alzheimer's disease. Trials have been conducted, for example, to test the value of phosphatidylserine in this role.[243–244] In Italy for example, Cenacchi[245] conducted a clinical trial involving 425 people, ages 66 to 93, in 23 institutions. All participants had experienced moderate to severe cognitive decline. Phosphatidylserine dosage was 300 mg per day and patients were assessed when the study began and three to six months later. Significant improvement in memory and learning scores was reported. Interestingly, phospholipids such as phosphatidylserine, phosphatidylcholine, phosphatidyl-ethanolamine, and phosphatidylinositol are available in health food stores and are widely used as memory aids by the general public.

The potential value of antioxidants such as melatonin, estrogen, and vitamins C and E in the treatment of Alzheimer's disease has been discussed earlier. However, there may be more to estrogen than its ability to protect against free radical damage. In addition to promoting the growth of cholinergic neurons and decreasing neuronal damage by acting as an antioxidant,[246] this hormone also has been shown to have powerful protective neuronal cell effects against the cytotoxicity of the acetylcholinesterase-amyloid beta-peptide complex found in the senile plaques that are characteristic of Alzheimer's disease.[116] It would appear that estrogen protects neurons against damage from both senile plaques and from amyloid beta-peptide fibrils. This helps to explain why Alzheimer's disease is considerably less common in women receiving estrogen replacement therapy.[184]

Little is known of the clinical impact of melatonin on Alzheimer's disease. However, Jean-Louis and coworkers[247] describe its effects on two cases. In one patient, melatonin enhanced and stabilized the circadian sleep/wake cycle, along with a reduction of daytime sleepiness and mood improvement. In the other patient, no significant changes were observed. Interestingly, Pierpaoli and Regelson[180] describe treating a patient who suffered from parkinsonism with melatonin and claim that, on a dose of 5 mg daily, her uncontrolled hand shaking disappeared and 10 years later she was still completely disease free.

It is well established also that melatonin plays a significant role in normalizing blood zinc levels in the elderly because it aids this mineral's absorption.[180] Zinc deficiency may cause depressed gluta-

mate dehydrogenase, resulting in the overproduction of glutamate,[248] which in excess is a powerful nerve-cell killer. Furthermore, zinc enzymes also are involved in the metabolism of neurotransmitters, including acetylcholine. A shortage of zinc, therefore, may partially account for the depression of this neurotransmitter in Alzheimer's disease. Supplementation with zinc aspartate appears beneficial in preliminary trials with Alzheimer's patients.[248] However, great care must be taken in the use of this mineral since, although it seems beneficial in improving mental alertness in the elderly, in a clinical trial in Australia it caused a serious deterioration of cognition in Alzheimer's patients within two days.[152]

In contrast, the available evidence suggests that the antioxidant selenium may be very beneficial in dementia, including Alzheimer's disease. In 1987, Tolonen and colleagues[249] described a double-blinded clinical trial in which the demented elderly were given high doses of sodium selenate (inorganic selenium), organic selenium, and vitamin E. These supplements resulted in statistically significant improvements in depression, self-care, anxiety, mental alertness, fatigue, and interest in the environment. While the roles of selenium and vitamin E in producing these improvements cannot be identified separately, this study suggests that high doses of both of these antioxidants may be of significant benefit to Alzheimer's patients.

CONCLUSION

It has been known for over a century that aluminum is a neurotoxin.[1] The uncomfortable truth that its widespread use is the major cause of Alzheimer's disease is now unavoidable.

REFERENCES

1. Doelken P. Naunynschmiedeberger. *Arch Exp Pathol Pharmakol* 40:58–120 cited by Crapper McLachlan DR., Lukiw WJ, Kruck TPA. Aluminum, altered transcription, and the pathogenesis of Alzheimer's disease. *Environ Geochem Health* 1990; 12(1–2):103–114.

2. Arieff AI. Aluminum and the pathogenesis of dialysis dementia. *Environ Geochem Health* 1990;12(1–2):89–93.

3. Brun A, Dictor M. Senile plaques and tangles in dialysis dementia. *Acta Path Microbiol Scand* 1981;89:193–198.

4. Francis PT, Palmer AM, Sims NR, et al. Neurochemical studies of early-onset Alzheimer's disease. *New Engl J Med* 1985; 313:7–11.

5. Friedland PR, Budinger TF, Ganz E, et al. Regional cerebral metabolic alterations in dementia of the Alzheimer's type: positron emission tomography with [18F] fluorodeoxyglucose. *J Comp Ass Tomography* 1983;7:590–598.

6. Rossner, MN, Iversen LL, Reynolds GP, et al. Neurochemical characteristics of early and late onset types of Alzheimer's disease. *Br Med J* 1984;288:961–964.

7. Munoz DG. Letter. *Can Med Assoc J* 1995;152(4):468–469.

8.Yumoto S, Kakimi S, Ogawa HN, et al. Aluminum neurotoxicity and Alzheimer's disease. In Hanin I, Yoshida M, Fisher A. (eds.) *Alzheimer's and Parkinson's Diseases: Recent Developments.* New York: Plenum Press, 1983;2:23–29.

9. Doll R. Review: Alzheimer's disease and environmental aluminum. *Age and Ageing* 1993;22:138–153.

10. Priest ND. The bioavailability and metabolism of aluminum compounds in man. *Proc Nutr Soc* 1992 cited by Doll, R. op. cit, 138.

11. Priest ND, Newton D, Talbot RJ. Metabolism of aluminum-26 and gallium-67 in a volunteer following their injection as citrates. *UKAEA Report AEA-EE-0206,* 1983. Harwell Biomedical Research, Harwell.

12. Sohler A, Pfeiffer CC, Papaionnov R. Blood aluminum levels in a psychiatric outpatient population. High aluminum levels related to memory loss. *J Orthomol Psychiat* 1981;19(1):54–60.

13. Vogt T. Water quality and health: study of a possible relation between aluminum in drinking water and dementia. Sosiale Og Økonimiske Studier, 61: Central Bureau of Statistics of Norway: Oslo. 1986. 60–63.

14. Flaten TP. Geographical association between aluminum in drinking water and death rates with dementia (including Alzheimer's disease), Parkinson's disease and amyotrophic lateral sclerosis, in Norway. *Environ Geochem Health* 1990;12 (1–2):152–167.

15. Martyn CN, Barker DJO, Osmond C, et al. Geographical relation between Alzheimer's disease and aluminum in drinking water. 1989;*Lancet* 1:59–62.

16. Forbes WF, McAiney CA. Aluminum and dementia. *Lancet* 1991;340:668–669.

17. Forbes WF, Hayward LM, Agwani N. Dementia, aluminum and fluoride. *Lancet* 1991; 338:1592–1593.

18. Still CN, Kelley P. On the incidence of primary degenerative dementia vs water fluoride content in South Carolina. *Neurotox* 1980;1:125–132.

19. Forbes WF, McAiney CA, Hayward LM, et al. Geochemical risk factors for mental functioning, based on the Ontario Longitudinal Study of Aging (LSA) ii. The role of pH. *Can J Aging* 1996;13(2):249–267.

20. House RA. Factors affecting plasma aluminum concentrations in non-exposed workers. *J Occup Med* 1992;34:1013–17.

21. Rifat SL, Eastwood MR, McLachlan DRC, et al. Effect of exposure of miners to aluminum powder. *The Lancet* 1980;336:1162–1165.

22. McLachlan DR. Aluminum and the risk of Alzheimer's disease. *Environmetrics* 1995;6:233–238.

23. Davies BE (ed). *Environ Geochem Health* 1990; 12(1–2):1–196.

24. Khachaturian ZS. Calcium hypothesis of Alzheimer's disease and brain aging. In Disterhoft JF, Gispen WH, Traber J, Khachaturian ZS (eds.) *Calcium Hypothesis of Aging and Dementia.* New York: New York Acad Sci, 1990;1–11.

25. Khachaturian ZS. Plundered memories. *The Sciences* 1997;37(4):20–25; 2013 data: www.alz.co.uk/research/World AlzheimerReport2013.pdf.

26. Bowie SHU, Thornton I (eds.). *Environmental Geochemistry and Health: Report to the Royal Society's British National Committee for Problems of the Environment.* D. Reidel Publishing Co: Dordrecht, 1985.

27. Hill CH, Matrone G. Chemical parameters in the study of in vivo and in vitro interactions of transition elements. *Fe Proc Fed Amer Soc Biol* 1977;29:1474–1481.

28. Hartman RH, Matrone G, Wise GH. Effect of dietary manganese on hemoglobin formation. *J Nutr* 1955, 55:429–439.

29. Thompson ABR, Olatumbosun D, Valberg LS. Interaction in intestinal transport system for manganese and iron. *J Lab Clin Med* 1971;78:642–655.

30. Chetty KN. Interaction of cobalt and iron in chicks. PhD thesis. North Carolina State University, 1972.

31. Tamari GM. Aluminum-toxicity and prophylaxis. *Data Medica* 1994;2.1:48–52.

32. Yasui M, Ota K. Aluminum decreases the magnesium concentrations of spinal cord and trabecular bone in rats fed a low calcium, high aluminum diet. *J Neurol Sci* 1998;157(1):37–41.

33. Neathery MW, Crowe NA, Miller WJ, et al. Effect of dietary aluminum and phosphorus on magnesium metabolism in dairy calves. *J Anim Sci* 1990;68(4):1133–1138.

34. Hussein AS, Cantor AH, Johnson TH, et al. Relationship of dietary aluminum, phosphorus, and calcium to phosphorus and calcium metabolism and growth performance of broiler chicks. *Poult Sci* 1990;69(6):966–971.

35. Hoffer A. *Orthomolecular Medicine for Physicians.* New Canaan: Keats Publishing, 1989.

36. Fujita T. *Calcium and Your Health,* Tokyo: Japan Publications, 1987.

37. Reisberg B. An overview of current concepts of Alzheimer's disease, Senile dementia, and Age-associated cognitive decline. In Reisberg B (ed) *Alzheimer's Disease: The Standard Reference.* New York: The Free Press, 1983.

38. Whitehouse PJ, Price DL, Clark AW, et al. Alzheimer's disease: evidence for selective loss of cholinergic neurons in the nucleus besalis. *Annals Neurol* 1981;10:122–126.

39. Enserink M. First Alzheimer's diagnosis confirmed. *Science* 1998;279:2037.

40. Byell SJ, Coleman PD. Dendritic growth in the aged human brain and failure of growth in senile dementia. *Science* 1979;206:854–856.

41. Brody H. Central nervous system. In Maddox GL (ed.) *The Encyclopaedia of Aging.* New York: Springer Verlag, 1987;108–112.

42. Crapper McLachlan DR, Farnell BJ. Aluminum and neuronal degeneration. In Gabay S, Harris J, Ho BT (eds.) *Metal Ions in Neurology and Psychiatry,* New York: Alan R Liss, 1985, 69–87.

43. Vogt T. Water quality and health: study of a possible relation between aluminum in drinking water and dementia. Sosiale Og Okonomiske Studier 61, *Statistisk Sentralbyra Oslo-Kongsvinger* 1986;60–63.

44. Spencer H, Kramer L, Norris C, et al. Effect of small doses of aluminum-containing antacids on calcium and phosphorus metabolism. *Am J Clin Nutr* 1982;36(1):32–40.

45. Mayor GH, Sprangue SM, Hourani MR, et al. Parathyroid hormone mediated aluminum deposition and regress in the rat. *Kidney Int* 1980;17:40–40.

46. Long JF, Nagoda LA, Kindig A, et al. Axonal swelling of the Purkinje cells in chickens associated with high intake of 1,25 (OH)2 D3 including microanalysis. *Neurotoxicol* 1980; 1(4):111–120.

47. Quarles LD, Dennis VW, Gitelman HJ, et al. Aluminum deposition at the osteoid-bone interface. An epiphenomenon of the osteomalacic state in vitamin D-deficient dogs. *J Clin Invest* 1985;75(5):1441–1447.

48. Yasui M, Yase Y, Ota K, et al. Evaluation of magnesium, calcium and aluminum metabolism in rats and monkeys maintained on calcium-deficient diets. *Neurotoxicol* 1991;12(3):603–614.

49. Yasui M, Ota K. Aluminum decreases the magnesium concentration of spinal cord and trabecular bone in rats fed a low calcium, high aluminum diet. *J Neurol Sci* 1998;157(1):37–41.

50. Yasui M, Ota K, Garruto RM. Aluminum decreases the zinc concentration of soft tissues and bones of rats fed a low calcium-magnesium diet. *Biol Trace Elem Res* 1991;31(3):293–304.

51. Kikuchi T, Matsuzaki H, Sato S, et al. Diminished kidney function and nephrocalcinosis in rats fed a magnesium-deficient diet. *J Nutr Sci Vitaminol* 1998: (Tokyo) 44(4):515–523.

52. Kiss SA, Dombov'ari J, Oncsik M. Magnesium inhibits the harmful effects on plants of some toxic elements. *Magnes Res* 1991;4(1):3–7.

53. Edwardson JA, Moore PB, Ferrier IN, et al. Effect of silicon on gastrointestinal absorption of aluminum. *Lancet* 1991; 342:211–212.

54. Fucheng L, Zhou L, Fang S, et al. Endemic aluminum-fluoride combined toxicosis by food chain. In eds. Tan J, Peterson PJ, Li R, Wang W. *Environment Life Elements and Health.* Beijing: Science Press, 1990;205–208.

55. Crapper McLachlan DR, Farnell BJ. Aluminum and neuronal degeneration. In eds. Gabay S, Harris J, Ho BT. *Metal Ions in Neurology and Psychiatry,* New York: Alan R. Liss, 1985;69–87.

56. Driscoll CT, Schecher WD. The chemistry of aluminum in the environment. *Environ Geochem Health* 1990;12(1/2):28–49.

57. Flaten TP. Geographical associations between aluminum in drinking water and death rates with dementia (including Alzheimer's disease), Parkinson's disease and amyotrophic lateral sclerosis in Norway. *Environ Geochem Health* 1990;12(1/2):152–167.

58. Tennakone K, Wickramanayake S. Aluminum leaching from cooking utensils. *Nature* 1987;325(6105):202.

59. Flaten TP, Odegard M. Tea, aluminum and Alzheimer's disease. *Chem Toxicol* 1988;26:959–960.

60. Slanina P, French W, Ekstrom LG, et al. Dietary citric acid enhances absorption of aluminum in antacids. *Clin Chem* 1986;32:539.

61. Varner JA, Jenseen KF, Horvath W, et al. Chronic administration of aluminum-fluoride or sodium-fluoride to rats in drinking water: alterartions in neuronal and cerebrovascular integrity. *Brain Res* 1998;784:284–298.

62. McLachlan and Kruck cited in Ross A, The Silent Scourge. *Equinox* 1991;60:86–100.

63. Anon. Incredible calcium: not just for bones. *Health Counsellor* 1992;4(5):19–20.

64. Wisniewski HM. Aluminum neurotoxicity and Alzheimer's disease. In eds. Hanin I, Yoshida M, Fisher A. *Alzheimer's and Parkinson's diseases: Recent Developments.* New York: Plenum Press, 1986;223–229.

65. Alfrey AC. *Neurobiology of Aging,* 1986;7:543 cited by Yumoto S et al. op. cit.

66. Yumoto S, Ogawa Y, Nagai H, et al. Aluminum neurotoxicity and Alzheimer's disease. In Hanin I, Yoshida M, Fisher A (eds). *Alzheimer's and Parkinson's diseases: Recent Developments.* New York: Plenum Press, 1986;223–229.

67. Favarato M, Zatta P, Perazzolo M, et al. Aluminum (III) influences the permeability of the blood-brain barrier to [14C] sucrose in rats. *Brain Res* 1992;569(2):330–335.

68. Rao JK, Katsetos CD, Herman MM, et al. Experimental aluminum encephalo-myelopathy. Relationship to human neurodegenerative disease. *Clin Lab Med* 1998;18(4):687–698.

69. Deloncle R, Guillard O, Clanet F, et al. Aluminum transfer as glutamate complex through blood-brain barrier. Possible implication in dialysis encephalopathy. *Biol Trace Elem Res* 1990;25(1):39–45.

70. Deloncle R, Huguet F, Babin P, et al. Chronic administration of aluminum L-glutamate in young mature rats: effects on iron levels and lipid peroxidation in selected brain areas. *Toxicol Lett* 1999;104(1–2):65–73.

71. Jones KR, Oorschot DE. Do aluminum and/or glutamate induce Alz-50 reactivity? A light microscopic immunohistochemical study. *J. Neurocytol* 1998;27(1):45–57.

72. Marcus DL, Wong S, Freedman ML. Dietary aluminum and Alzheimer's disease. *J Nutr Elder* 1992;12(2):55–61.

73. Joshi JG. Neurochemical hypothesis: participation by aluminum in approaching critical mass of colocalized errors in brain leads to neurological disease. *Comp Biochem Physiol C* 1991;100(1–2):103–105.

74. Cho SW, Joshi JG. Inactivation of glucose-6-phosphate dehydrogenase isozymes from human and pig brain by aluminum. *J Neurochem* 1989;53(2):616–621.

75. Lai JC, Blass JP. Inhibition of brain glycolysis by aluminum. *J Neurochem* 1984;42(2):438–446.

76. Xu ZX, Fox L, Melethil S, et al. 1990. Mechanism of aluminum-induced inhibition of hepatic glycolysis: inactivation of phosphofructokinase. *J Pharmacol Exp Ther* 1990;254(1): 301–305.

77. Scinto FM, Daffner KR, Dressler D, et al. A potential noninvasive neurobiological test for Alzheimer's disease. *Science* 1994;266(5187):1051–1054.

78. Cherroret G, Desor D, Hutin MF, et al. Effects of aluminum chloride on normal and uremic adult male rats. Tissue distribution, brain choline acetyl-transferase activity, and some biological variables. *Biol Trace Elem Res* 1996;54(1):43–53.

79. Inestrusa NC, Alarc'on R. Molecular interactions of acetylcholinesterase with senile plaques. *J Physiol Paris* 1998;92 (5–6):341–344.

80. Gottfries CG. Alzheimer's disease and senile dementia: biochemical characteristics and aspects of treatment. *Psychopharmacol* 1985;86(3):245–252.

81. Perry EK. The cholinergic system in old age and Alzheimer's disease. *Age Ageing* 1980;9(1):1–8.

82. Quirion R, Martel JC, Robitaille Y, et al. Neurotransmitter and receptor deficits in senile dementia of the Alzheimer type. *Can J Neurol Sci* 1986;13(4 suppl):503–510.

83. Yasuhara O, Nakamura S, Akiguchi I, et al. The distribution of senile plaques and acetylcholinesterase staining in the thalamus in dementia of the Alzheimer type. *Rinsho Shinkeigaku* 1980;31(4):377–382.

84. Gottfries CG, Lehmann W, Regland B. 1998. Early diagnosis of cognitive impairment in the elderly with a focus on Alzheimer's disease. *J Neural Transm* 105(8–9):773–786.

85. Riggs KM, Spiro A III, Tucker K, et al. Relations of vitamin B12, vitamin B6, folate, and homocysteine to cognitive performance in the Normative Aging Study. *Am J Clin Nutr* 1996;63(3):306–314.

86. Challem J, Dolby V. *Homocysteine: The New "Cholesterol."* New Canaan: Keats Publishing. 1996.

87. Whitehouse PH, Price DL, Struble RG, et al. Alzheimer's disease and senile dementia: loss of neurons in the basal forebrain. *Science* 1982;215(4537):1237–1239.

88. Frölich L, Dirr A, Götz ME, et al. Acetylcholine in human CSF: methodological considerations and levels in dementia of Alzheimer type. *J Neurol Transm* 1998;105(8–9):961–973.

89. Rylett RJ, Ball MJ, Calhoun EH. Evidence for high affinity choline transport in synaptosomes prepared from hippocampus and neocortex of patients with Alzheimer's disease. *Brain Res* 1983;289(1–2):169–175.

90. Chan-Palay V. Galanin hyperinnervates surviving neurons of the human basal nucleus of Meynert in dementias of Alzheimer's and Parkinson's disease: a hypothesis for the role of galanin in accentuating cholinergic dysfunction in dementia. *J Comp Neurol* 1988, 273(4):543–557.

91. Kasa P, Rakonczay Z, Gulya K. The cholinergic system in Alzheimer's disease. *Prog Neurobiol* 1997;52(6):511–535.

92. Altmann P, Al-Salihi F, Butter K, et al. Serum aluminum levels and erythrocyte dihydropteridine reductase activity in patients on hemodialysis. *N Engl J Med* 1987;317(2):80–84.

93. Kay AD, Milstein S, Kaufman S, et al. Cerebrospinal fluid biopterin is decreased in Alzheimer's disease. *Arch Neurol* 1986;43(10):996–999.

94. Hamon CG, Cattell RJ, Wright CE, et al. Visual evoked potentials and neopterin: biopterin ration in urine show a high correlation in Alzheimer's disease [letter]. *J Neurol Neurosurg Psychiat* 1988;51(2):314–315.

95. Reinikainen KJ, Soininen H, Riekkinen PJ. Neurotransmitter changes in Alzheimer's disease: implications for diagnostics and therapy. *J Neurosci Res* 1990;27(4):576–586.

96. Engelburghs S, DeDeyn PP. The neurochemistry of Alzheimer's disease. *Acta Neurol Belg* 1997;97(2):67–84.

97. Joyce JN, Myers AJ, Gurevich E. Dopamine D2 receptor bands in normal human temporal cortex are absent in Alzheimer's disease. *Brain Res* 1998;784(1–2):7–17.

98. Palmer AM. Neurochemical studies of Alzheimer's disease. Neurodegen 1996;5(4):381–391.

99. Marinho CR, Manso CF. Effect of aluminum on the non-enzymatic oxidation of dopamine. *Acta Med Port* 1994;7(11):611–615.

100. Singh S, Singh D, Wig N, et al. Aluminum phosphide ingestion: a clinico-pathologic study. *J Toxicol Clin Toxicol* 1996;34(6):703–706.

101. Wenk GL, Stemmer L. The influence of ingested aluminum upon norepinephrine and dopamine levels in the rat brain. *Neurotoxicol* 1981;2(2):347–353.

102. Kurokawa T, Kitamura Y, Moriuchi M, et al. Differences between magnesium and manganese ions in modification of effect of catecholamine on adenylate cyclase system in Ehrlich ascites tumour cells. *J Pharmacobiodyn* 1981;4(10):794–797.

103. Mahaffe DD, Cooper CW, Ramp WK, et al. Magnesium promotes both parathyroid hormone secretion and adenosine 3' 4'-mono-phosphate production in rat parathyroid tissues and reverses the inhibitory effects of calcium on adenylate cyclase. *Endocrinol* 1982;110(2):487–495.

104. Zimmermann G, Zhou D, Taussig R. Mutation uncovers a role for two magnesium ions in the catalytic mechanism of adenylyl cyclase. *J Biol Chem* 1998;273(31):19650–19655.

105. Ebstein RP, Oppenheim G, Ebstein BS, et al. The cyclic AMP second messenger system in man: the effects of heredity, hormones, drugs, aluminium, age and disease on signal amplification. *Prog Neuropsycho-pharmacol Bio Psychiatry* 1986;10(3–5):323–353.

106. Danielsson E, Eckernäs SA, Westlilnd-Danielsson A, et al. VIP-sensitive adenylate cyclase, guanylate cyclase, muscarinic receptors, choline acetyltransferase and acetylcholinesterase in brain tissue affected by Alzheimer's disease/senile dementia of the Alzheimer's type. *Neurobiol Aging* 1988;9(2):153–162.

107. Enz A, Francis PT. The rationale for development of cholinergic therapies in AD. In Fisher A, Hanin I, Yoshida M (eds). *Progress in Alzheimer's and Parkinson's Diseases.* New York: Plenum Press 1998;445–450.

108. Bosun H, Forssell LG, Almkvist O, et al. Amino acid concentrations in cerebrospinal fluid and plasma in Alzheimer's disease and healthy control subjects. *J Neural Transm Park Dis Dement* 1990;Sect 2(4):295–304.

109. Hofstetter JR, Vincent I, Bugiani O, et al. Aluminum-induced decrease in choline acetyltransferase, tyrosine hydroxylase, and glutamate decarboxylase in selected regions of the rabbit brain. *Neurochem Pathol* 1987;6(3):177–193.

110. Cucarella C, Montoliu C, Hermenegildo C, et al. Chronic exposure to aluminum impairs neuronal glutamate-nitric oxide-cyclic GMP pathway. *J Neurochem* 1998;70(4):1609–1614.

111. Provan SD, Yokel RA. Aluminum inhibits glutamate release from transverse rat hippocampal slices: role of G proteins, Ca channels and protein kinase C. *Neurotoxicol* 1992;13(2):413–420.

112. Wong PC, Lai JC, Lim L, et al. Selective inhibition of L-glutamate and gamma-aminobutyrate transport in nerve ending particles by aluminum, manganese and cadmium chloride. *J Inorg Biochem* 1981;14(3):253–260.

113. Mundy WR, Freudenrich TM, Kodavanti PR. Aluminum potentiates glutamate-induced calcium accumulation and iron-induced oxygen free radical formation in primary neuronal cultures. *Mol Chem Neuropathol* 1997;32(1–3):41–57.

114. Wurtman R. Choline metabolism as a basis for the selective vulnerability of cholinergic neurons. *Trends Neurosci* 1992;15(4):117–122.

115. Perry EK. The cholinergic system in old age and Alzheimer's disease. *Age Ageing* 1980;9(1):1–8.

116. Bonnefont AB, Muñoz FJ, Inestrosa NC. Estrogen protects neuronal cells from the cyto-toxicity induced by acetyl-cholinesterase-amyloid complexes. *FEBS Lett* 1998;441(2):220–224.

117. Levi R, Wolf T, Fleminger G, et al. Immunodetection of aluminium and aluminium induced conformational changes in calmodulin-implications in Alzheimer's disease. *Mol Cell Biochem* 1998;189;(1–2):41–46.

118. Xiao J, Perry G, Troncoso J, et al. Alpha-calcium-calmodulin-dependent kinase II is associated with paired helical filaments of Alzheimer's disease. *J Neuropathol Exp Neurol* 1996;55(9):954–963.

119. Baudier J, Cole RD. Phosphorylation of tau protein to a state like that in Alzheimer's brain is catalysed by a calcium/calmodulin-dependent kinase and modulated by phospholipids. *J Biol Chem* 1987;262(36):17577–17583.

120. Savazzi GM, Allergi L, Bocchi B, et al. The physiopathologic bases of the neurotoxicity of phosphorus chelating agents containing soluble aluminum salts in patients with renal insufficiency. *Recenti Prog Med* 1989;80(4):227–232.

121. Corrigan FM, Horrobin DF, Skinner ER, et al. Abnormal content of n-6 and n-3 long-chain unsaturated fatty acids in the phosphoglycerides and cholesterol esters of parahippocampal cortex from Alzheimer's disease patients and its relationship to acetyl Coa content. *Inst J Biochem Cell Biol* 1998;30(2):197–207.

122. Yamamoto H, Saitoh Y, Yasugawa S, et al. Dephosphorylation of tau factor by protein phosphatase 2A in synaptosomal cytosol fraction, and inhibition by aluminum. *J Neurochem* 1990;55(2):683–690.

123. Chan MK, Varghese Z, Li MK, et al. Newcastle bone disease in Hong Kong: a study of aluminum associated osteomalacia. *Int J Artif Organs* 1990;13(3):162–168.

124. Pei JJ, Gong CX, Iqbal K, et al. Subcellular distribution of protein phosphates and abnormally phosphorylated tau in the temporal cortex from Alzheimer's disease and control brains. *J Neural Transm* 1998;105(1):69–83.

125. Yamamoto H, Saitoh Y, Yasugawa S, et al. Dephosphorylation of tau factor by protein phosphatase 2A in synaptosomal cytosol fractions, and inhibition by aluminum. *J Neurochen* 1990;55(2):683–690.

126. Roushi W. Protein studies try to puzzle out Alzheimer's tangles. *Science* 1995;267(5199):793–794.

127. Good PF, Perl DP, Bierer LM, et al. Selective accumulation of aluminum and iron in the neurofibrillary tangles of Alzheimer's disease: a laser microprobe (LAMMA) study. *Ann Neurol* 1992;31(3):286–292.

128. The SMID Group 1987. Phosphatidylserine in the treatment of clinically diagnosed Alzheimer's disease. *J Neural Transm Suppl* 1987;24:287–292.

129. Corrigan FM, Horrobin DF, Skinner ER, et al. Abnormal content of n-6 and n-3 long-chain unsaturated fatty acids in the phosphoglycerides and cholesterol esters of parahippocampal cortex from Alzheimer's disease patients and its relationship to acetyl Coa content. *Inst J Biochem Cell Biol* 1998;30(2):197–207.

130. Gottfries CG, Karlsson I, Svennerholm L. Membrane components separate early-onset Alzheimer's disease from senile dementia of the Alzheimer's type. *Int Psychogeriatr* 1996;8(3):365–372.

131. Prasad MR, Lovell MA, Yatin M, et al. Regional membrane phospholipid alterations in Alzheimer's disease. *Neurochem Res* 1998;23(1):81–88.

132. Johnson GV, Jope RS. Aluminum impairs glucose utilization and cholinergic activity in rat brain in vitro. *Toxicology* 1986;40(1):93–102.

133. Deleers M, Servais JP, Wülfert E. Aluminum-induced lipid phase separation and membrane fusion does not require the presence of negatively charged phospholipids. *Biochem Int* 1987;14(6):1033–1034.

134. Jones DL, Kochian LV. Aluminum interaction with plasma membrane lipids and enzyme metal binding sites and its potential role in A1 cytotoxicity. *FEBS Lett* 1997 400(1):51–57.

135. Gattaz WF, Cairns NJ, Levy R, et al. Decreased phospholipase A2 activity in the brain and platelets of patients with Alzheimer's disease. *Eur Arch Psychiatry Clin Neurosci* 1996;246(3):129–131.

136. Gottfries CG, Karlsson I, Svennerholm L. Membrane components separate early-onset Alzheimer's disease from senile dementia of the Alzheimer's type. *Int Psychogeriatr* 1996;8(3):365–372.

137. Dill ET, Holden MJ, Colombini M. Voltage gating in VDAC is markedly inhibited by micromolar quantities of aluminum. *J Membr Biol* 1987;99(3):187–196.

138. Retz W, Gsell W, Münch G, et al. Free radicals in Alzheimer's disease. *J Neural Transm Suppl* 1998;54:221–236.

139. Van Rensburg SJ, Daniels WM, Potocnik FC, et al. A new model for the pathophysiology of Alzheimer's disease. Aluminum toxicity is exacerbated by hydrogen peroxide and attenuated by an amyloid protein fragment and melatonin. *S Afr Med J* 1997;87(9):1111–1115.

140. Sinclair AJ, Bayer AJ, Johnson J, et al. Altered plasma antioxidant status in subjects with Alzheimer's disease and vascular dementia. *Int J Geriatr Psychiat* 1998;13(12):840–845.

141. Turan B, Delilba, Si E, et al. Serum selenium and glutathione-peroxidase activities and their interaction with toxic metals in dialysis and renal transplantation patients. *Biol Trace Elem Res* 1992;33:95–102.

142. Swain C, Chainy GB. Effects of aluminum sulphate and citric acid ingestion on lipid peroxidation and on activities of superoxide dismutase and catalase in cerebral hemisphere and liver of developing chicks. *Mol Cell Biochem* 1998;187(1–2):163–172.

143. Abd el-Fattah AA, al-Yousef HM, al-Bekairi AM, et al. Vitamin E protects the brain against oxidative injury stimulated by excessive aluminum. *Biochem Mol Biol Int* 1998;46(6):1175–1180.

144. Perrin R, Brian C S, Jeandeal C, et al. Blood activity of Cu/Zn superoxide dismutase, glutatione peroxidase and catalase in Alzheimer's disease: a case-control study. *Gerontology* 1990;36(5–6):306–313.

145. Kulkarni-Narla A, Getchell TV, Schmitt FA, et al. 1996. Manganese and copper-zinc superoxide dismutase in the human olfactory mucosa: increased immunoreactivity in Alzheimer's disease. *Exp Neurol* 1996;140(2):115–125.

146. Daniels WM, van Rensburg SJ, van Zyl JM, et al. Melatonin prevents beta-amyloid-induced lipid peroxidation. *J Pineal Res* 1998;24(2):78–82.

147. Fu W, Luo H, Parthasarathy S, et al. Catecholamines potentiate amyloid beta-peptide neurotoxicity: involvement of oxidative stress, metochondrial dysfunction, and perturbed calcium homeostatis. *Neurobiol Dis* 1998;5(4):229–243.

148. Hoffer A, Osmond H. Malvaria: a new psychiatric disease. *Acta Psychiatrica Scand* 1963, 39:335–366.

149. Hoffer A, Osmond H, Smythies J. Schizophrenia: a new approach. II. Results of a year's research. *J Ment Sci* 1954;100:29.

150. Hoffer A. *Vitamin B3 Schizophrenia: Discovery, Recovery, Controversy.* Kingston, Quarry Press, 1998.

151. Shainkin-Kesterbaum R, Adler AJ, Berlyne GM, et al. Effect of aluminum on superoxide dismutase. *Clin Sci* 1989;77(5):463–466.

152. Kaiser K. Alzheimer's: could there be a zinc link? *Science* 1994;265 (5177):1365.

153. Grant W. Dietary links to Alzheimer's disease. *Alzheimer's Dis Rev* 1997;2:42–55.

154. Mazur A, Nassir F, Gueux E, et al. Diets deficient in selenium and vitamin E affect plasma lipoprotein and apolipoprotein concentrations in the rat. *Br J Nutr* 1996;76(6):899–907.

155. Durlach J, Durlach A, Durlach V. Antioxidant dietary status and genetic cardiovascular risk, or how an adequate intake of a-tocopherol, selenium, taurine, magnesium and various other natural antioxidants may overcome the deleterious metabolic consequences related to the E4–4 type of apolipoprotein E (editorial). *Magnes Res* 1996;9(2):139–141.

156. Graves AB, Larson EB, Edland SD, et al. Prevalence of dementia and its subtypes in the Japanese American population of King County, Washington State. *Am J Epidemiol* 1996; 144:760–771.

157. Hendrie HC, Osuntokun BO, Hall KS. Prevalence of Alzheimer's Disease and dementia in two communities: Nigerian Africans and African Americans. *Am J Psychiatry* 1997;152: 1485–1492.

158. Cohen GD. Alzheimer's disease. In Maddox GL (ed.) *The Encyclopaedia of Aging.* New York: Springer Verlag, 1987, 27–30.

159. Velez-Pardo C, Jimenez Del Rio M, Lopera E. Familial Alzheimer's disease: oxidative stress, beta-amyloid, presenilins, and cell death. *Gen Pharmacol* 1998;31(5):675–681.

160. Guo Q, Sebastian L, Sopher BL, et al. Increased vulnerability of hippocampal neurons from presenilin-1 mutant knock-in mice to amyloid beta-peptide toxicity: central roles of superoxide production and caspase activation. *J Neurochem* 1999;72 (3):1019–1029.

161. Haass C, Baumeister R. What do we learn from a few familial Alzheimer's disease cases? *J Neural Transm Suppl* 1998;54:137–145.

162. Basun H, Forssell LG, Almkvist O, et al. Amino acid concentrations in cerebrospinal fluid and plasma in Alzheimer's disease and healthy control subjects. *J Neural Trans Park Dis Dement Sect* 1990;2(4):295–304.

163. Pratico D, Tangirala RK, Rader DJ, et al. Vitamin E suppresses isoprostane generation in vivo and reduces atherosclerosis in apo E-deficient mice. *Nat Med* 1998;4(10):1189–1192.

164. Naiki H, Hasegawa K, Yamaguchi I, et al. Apolipoprotein E and antioxidants have different mechanisms of inhibiting Alzheimer's beta-amyloid fibril formation in vitro. *Biochemistry* 1998;37(51):17882–17889.

165. Russo C, Angelini G, Dapino D, et al. Opposite roles of apolipoprotein E in normal brains and in Alzheimer's disease. *Proc Natl Acad Sci* 1998;95(26):15598–15602.

166. Salib E, Hillier V. Head injury and the risk of Alzheimer's disease: a case control study. *Int J Geriatr Psychiat* 1997;12 (3):363–368.

167. Launer LJ, Anderson K, Dewey ME, et al. Rates and risk factors for dementia and Alzheimer's disease: results from EURODEM pooled analyses. EURODEM Incidence Research Group and Work Groups European Studies of Dementia. *Neurology* 1999;52(1):78–84.

168. Nemetz PN, Leibson C, Naessens JM, et al. Traumatic brain injury and time of onset of Alzheimer's disease: a population-based study. *Am J Epidemiol* 149(1):32–40.

169. Nicoll JA, Roberts GW, Graham DI. Amyloid beta-protein, APOE genotype and head injury. *Ann NY Acad Sci* 1996;777:271–275.

170. Cross PD, Gurland BJ. The Epidemiology of Dementing Disorders. *Contract report prepared for the Office of Technology Assessment,* US Congress.1986.

171. Mortimer JA, Hutton JT. Epidemiology and Etiology of Alzheimer's disease. In eds. Hutton JT, Kenny AD *Senile Dementia of the Alzheimer's Type.* New York: AR Liss. 1985.

172. Sayetta RB. Rates of senile dementia in Alzheimer's type in the Baltimore Longitudinal Study. *J Chronic Diseases* 1986;39:271–286.

173. Evans DA, Funkenstein HH, Albert MS, et al. Prevalence of Alzheimer's disease in a community population of older persons higher than previously reported. *J Am Med Assoc* 1989;262(18):2551–2556.

174. D'Alessandro R, Gallassi R, Benassi G, et al. Dementia in subjects over 65 years of age in the Republic of San Marino. Brit *J Psych* 1988;153:182–186.

175. Jorm AF, Korten AE, Henderson AS. The prevalence of dementia: a quantitative integration of the literature. *Acta Psychiatrica Scand* 1987;75(5):465–479.

176. Baker H. Hypovitaminosis in the elderly. *Geriatric Medicine Today* 1983;2(10):61–66.

177. Cohen GD. Alzheimer's disease. In Maddox GL (ed). *The Encyclopaedia of Aging,* New York: Springer Verlag 1987;27–30.

178. Liu RY, Zhou JN, Van Heerikhuize J, et al. Decreased melatonin levels in postmortem cerbrospinal fluid in relation to aging, Alzheimer's disease and apolipoprotein Eepsilon 4/4 genotype. *J Clin Endocrinol Metab* 1999;84(1):323–327.

179. Skene DJ, Vivien-Roels B, Sparks DL, et al. Daily variation in the concentration of melatonin and 5-methoxytryptophol in the human pineal gland: effect of age and Alzheimer's disease. *Brain Res* 1990;528(1):170–174.

180. Pierpaoli W, Regelson W, Colman C. *The Melatonin Miracle,* New York: Simon and Schuster, 1995.

181. Song W, Lahiri DK. Melatonin alters the metabolism of the beta-amyloid precursor protein in the neuroendocrine cell line PC12. *J Mol Neurosci* 1997;9(2):75–92.

182. Reiter RJ. Oxidative damage in the central nervous system: protection by melatonin. *Prog Neurobiol* 1998;56(3):359–384.

183. Pappolla MA, Sos M, Omar RA, et al. Melatonin prevents death of neuroblastoma cells exposed to Alzheimer's amyloid peptide. *J Neurosci* 1997;17(5):1683–1690.

184. Baldereschi M, Di Carlo A, Lepore V, et al. Estrogen replacement therapy and Alzheimer's disease in the Italian Longitudinal Study on Aging. *Neurology* 1998;50(4):996–1002.

185. Henderson VW, Watt L, Buckwalter JG. 1996. Cognitive skills associated with estrogen replacement in women with Alzheimer's disease. *Psychoneuroendocrinol* 1996;21(4):421–430.

186. Honjo H, Tamura T, Matsumoto Y, et al. Estrogen as a growth factor to central nervous cells. Estrogen treatment promotes development of acetylcholinesterase-positive basal forebrain neurons transplanted in the anterior eye chamber. *J Steroid Biochem Mol Biol* 1992;41(3–8):633–635.

187. Gibbs RB, Aggarwal P. Estrogen and basal forebrain cholinergic neurons: implications for brain aging and Alzheimer's disease-related cognitive decline. *Horm Behav* 1998;34(2): 98–111.

188. Rosenzweig MR. Bennet, EL, Diamond MC. Brain changes in response to experience. *Scientific American* 1972;226 (2):22–29.

189. Globus cited by Restak RM. *The Brain: the Last Frontier.* Garden City, New York: Doubleday. 1979.

190. Restak RM. *The Brain: The Last Frontier.* Garden City, New York: Doubleday, 1979.

191. Tuthill RW. Hair lead levels related to children's classroom attention-deficit behaviour. *Arch Env Health* 1996;51 (3):214–220.

192. Marlowe M, Bliss LB. Hair element concentrations and young children's classroom and home behaviour. *J Orthomolecular Med* 1993;8(2):79–88.

193. Bishop N, McGraw M, Ward N. Aluminum in infant formulas. *Lancet* 1989;8636:490.

194. Marlowe M, Palmer L. Hair trace element status of Appalachian Head Start children. *J Orthomolecular Med* 1996; 11(1):15–22.

195. Benton D. Vitamin/mineral supplementation and the intelligence of children: a review. *J Orthomolecular Med* 1992;7 (1):31–38.

196. Henderson AS. The epidemiology of Alzheimer's disease. *Brit Med Bull* 1986;42(i):3–10.

197. Gruenberg EM, The failure of success. *Millbank Mem Fund Quart* 1977;3–24.

198. Gruenberg EM, Hagnell O, Ojesjo L, et al. The rising prevalence of chronic brain syndrome in the elderly. 1976. Paper presented at the Symposium on Society, Stress and Disease: *Aging and Old Age* cited by Henderson AS. 1986. op cit, 3.

199. Dementia rates poised to soar, StatsCan says. *Times Colonist,* Canada. August 5, 1997, D3.

200. Hoffman A. Prevalence, incidence, prognosis and risk factors of dementia. *Revue D'Epidemiologie et De Sante Publique* 1987;35(3–4):287–291.

201. Hill AB. The environment and disease: association or causation? *Proc Roy Soc Med* 1965;58:295–300.

202. Crapper McLachlan DR, Kruck TP, Lukiw WJ, et al. Would decreased aluminum ingestion reduce the incidence of Alzheimer's disease? *Can Med Assoc J* 1991;145:793–804.

203. Safe Drinking Water Committee, National Research Council. Drinking Water and Health, Washington, DC: *National Acad Sci,* 1977.

204. Duggan JM, Dickeson JE, Tynan PF, et al. Aluminum beverage cans as a source of aluminum. *Med J Aust* 1992; 156(9):604–605.

205. Morris MC, Beckett LA, Scherr PA, et al. Vitamin E and vitamin C supplement use and risk of incident Alzheimer's disease. *Alzheimer Dis Assoc Disord* 1998;12(3):121–126.

206. Warren T. *Beating Alzheimer's: A Step Towards Unlocking the Mysteries of Brain Disease,* Avery: Garden City Park, New York, 1991.

207. Blank L. Medical world stunned by my miracle recovery. *The Weekly News,* Jan 20, 1996, 7.

208. Siegel BS. *Love, Medicine and Miracles.* Harper and Row: New York, 1986.

209. Blank L. *Alzheimer's Challenged and Conquered?* Foulsham: London. 1995.

210. Crapper McLachlan DR, Dalton AJ, Kruck TR, et al. Intramuscular desferrioxamine in patients with Alzheimer's disease. *Lancet* 1991;337(8753):1304–1308.

211. Savory J, Huang Y, Wills MR, et al. Reverse by desferrioxamine of tau protein aggregates following two days of treatment in aluminum-induced neurofibrillary degeneration in rabbit: implications for clinical trials in Alzheimer's disease. *Neurotoxicity* 1988;19(2):209–214.

212. Pouls M. Oral chelation and nutritional replacement therapy for chemical and heavy metal toxicity and cardiovascular disease. *Townsend Lett Doctors and Patients* 1999;192:82–91.

213. Campbell J. *Personal communication,* March 1, 1991.

214. Bland J. *Biochemical Aspects of Mental Illness.* Seattle: Schizophrenia Association of Seattle, 1979.

215. Durlach J. Magnesium depletion and pathogenesis of Alzheimer's disease. *Magnes Res.* 1990;3(3):217–218.

216. Durlach J, Bac P. Mechanisms of action in the nervous system of magnesium deficiency and dementia. In Yasui M, Strong MJ, Ota K, Verity MA (eds). *Mineral and Metal Neurotoxicology* 1997, CRC Press: Boca Raton.

217. Dysken M. A review of recent clinical trials in the treatment of Alzheimer's dementia. *Psychiatric Annals* 1987;17(3):178.

218. Duffy FH, McAnulty G, Albert M, et al. Lecithin: absence of neurophysiologic effect in Alzheimer's disease EEG topography. *Neurology,* 37(6):1015–1019.

219. Passeri M, Cucinotta D, Bonati PA, et al. Acetyl-L-carnitine in the treatment of mildly demented elderly patients. *Int J Clin Pharmacol Res* 1990;10(1–2):75–79.

220. Spagnoli A, Lucca U, Menasce G, et al. Long-term acetyl-L-carnitine treatment in Alzheimer's disease. *Neurology* 1991;41:1726–1732.

221. Rai G, Wright G, Scott L, et al. Double-blind, placebo controlled study of acetyl-L-carnitine in patients with Alzheimer's dementia. *Curr Med Res Opin* 1990;11(10):638–647.

222. Kalaria RN, Harik S. Carnitine acetyl-trans-ferase activity in the human brain and its microvessels is decreased in Alzheimer's disease. *Ann Neurol* 1992;32(4):583–586.

223. White HL, Scates PW. Acetyl-L-carnitine as a precursor of acetylcholine. *Neurochem Res* 1990;15(6):597–601.

224. Harsing LG Jr, Sershen H, Toth E, et al. Acetyl-L-carnitine releases dopamine in rat corpus striatum: as in vivo microdialysis study. *Eur J Pharmacol* 1992;218(1):117–121.

225. Levitt AJ, Karlinsky H. Folate, vitamin B12 and cognitive impairment in patients with Alzheimer's disease. *Acta Psychiatr Scand* 1992;86(4):301–305.

226. Ikeda T, Furukawa Y, Mashimoto S, et al. Vitamin B12 levels in serum and cerebrospinal fluid of people with Alzheimer's disease. *Acta Psychiatr Scand* 1990;82(4):327–329.

227. Joosten E, Lesaffre E, Riezler R, et al. Is metabolic evidence for vitamin B12 and folate deficiency more frequent in elderly patients with Alzheimer's disease? *J Gerontol A Biol Sci Med Aci* 1997;52(2):M76–79.

228. McCaddon A, Kelly CL. Alzheimer's disease: a "cobalamin-ergic" hypothesis. *Med Hypoth* 1992;37(3):161–165.

229. Rogers SL. Perspectives in the management of Alzheimer's disease: clinical profile of donepezil. *Dement Geriatr Cogn Disord.* 1998;9 Suppl 3:29–42.

230. Lindenbaum J, Healton EB, Savage DG, et al. Neuropsychiatric disorders caused by cobalamin deficiency in the absence of anaemia or macrocytosis. *N Engl J Med* 1988;318(26):1720–1728.

231. Thompson D. Our daily folate. *Time* 153(20):38–39. 1999.

232. Marquis JK. Pharmacological significance of acetyl-cholinesterase inhibition by tetrahydroaminoacridine. *Biochem Pharmacol* 1990;40(5):1071–1076.

233. Mo Q, Ma J, Gong B. Effect of Chinese herbal medicine of tonifying kidney on M-cholinergic receptor and acetyl-cholinesterase activity in dementia mimetic mice. *Chung Kuo Chung Hsi I Chieh Ho Tsa Chih* 1996;16(2):99–101.

234. Bonnefont AB, Muñoz FJ, Inestrosa NC. Estrogen protects neuronal cells from the cytotoxicity induced by acetyl-cholinesterase-amyloid complexes. *FEBS Lett* 1998;441(2):220–224.

235. Perry EK, Pickering AT, Wang WW, et al. Medicinal plants and Alzheimer's disease: Integrating ethnobotanical and contemporary scientific evidence. *J Altern Complement Med* 1998;4 (4):419–428.

236. Krieglstein J, Beck T, Seibert A. Influence of an extract of Ginkgo biloba on cerebral blood flow and metabolism. *Life Sci* 1986;39(24) 2327–2334.

237. Jung F, Mrowietz C, Kiesewetter H, et al. Effect of Ginkgo biloba and fluidity of blood and peripheral microcirculation in volunteers. *Arzneimittelforschung* 1990;40(5):589–593.

238. Beard CM, Waring SC, O'Brien PC, et al. Nonsteroidal antiinflammatory drug use and Alzheimer's disease: a case-control study in Rochester, Minnesota, 1980 through 1984. *Mayo Clin Proc* 1998;73(10):951–955.

239. Stewart WF, Kawas C, Corrada M, et al. Risk of Alzheimer's disease and duration of NSAID [nonsteroidal anti-inflammatory drugs] *Neurology* 1997;48(3):626–632.

240. Lacomblez L. Comparative effects of Ginkgo biloba extracts on psychomotor performances and memory in healthy subjects. *Therapie* 1991;46(1):33–36.

241. Taylor JE. The effects of chronic, oral Ginkgo biloba extract administration on neurotransmitter receptor binding in young and aged Fisher 344 rats. *Effects of Gingko biloba extract on organic cerebral impairment.* John Libbey Eurotext Ltd. 1985.

242. Claus JJ, de Kong I, van Harskamp F, et al A. Lusuride treatment of Alzheimer's disease. A preliminary placebo-controlled clinical trial of safety and therapeutic efficiency. *Clin Neuropharmacol* 1998;21(3):190–195.

243. Amaducci L. Phosphatidylserine in the treatment of Alzheimer's disease: results of a multicentre study. *Psychopharmacol Bull,* 24(1):130–134.

244. Amaducci L, Crook TH, Lippi A, et al. Use of phosphatidylserine in Alzheimer's disease. *Ann NY Acad Sci* 1991; 640:245–249.

245. Anon. PS. I love you, Brain. Alive: *Can J Health Nutr* 1999; 200:16–17.

246. Inestrosa NC, Marzolo MP, Bonnefont AB. 1998. Cellular and molecular basis of estrogen's neuroprotection. Potential relevance for Alzheimer's disease. *Mol Neurobiol* 17(1–3):73–86.

247. Jean-Louis G, Zizi F, von Gizycki H, et al. Effects of melatonin in two individuals with Alzheimer's disease. *Percept Mot Skills* 1998;87(1):331–339.

248. Constantinidis J. Alzheimer's dementia and zinc. *Schweiz Arch Neurol Psychiatr* 1990;141(6):523–556.

249. Tolonen M, Hulme M and Sarna S. Vitamin E and selenium supplementation in geriatric patients: a double-blind clinical trial. 1987. In Combs Jr. GF, Levander PA, Spallholz JE, Oldfield JE (eds.) *Selenium in Biology and Medicine* Part B. Proceedings of the Third International Symposium, May 27–June 1, 1984. New York: Van Nostrand Reinhold.

CANCER

ANCER MAY BE HUMANITY'S MOST feared disease, and with reason. Much of that fear can be displaced with well-researched, clinically-tested, practical nutrition. Physician reports of vitamin-taking patients who achieved significantly longer life, and vastly improved quality of life, should not be dismissed. Not everyone agrees with this. Certain politically powerful medical authorities have openly discouraged cancer patients from taking large doses of vitamin C and other nutrients. It is unethical for any doctor to deny therapy that might be of value to her patient. Still, the number of cancer patients who have ever had their doctor recommend a therapeutic trial of large quantities of vitamin C orally and/or intravenously remains small. There may eventually be a class-action lawsuit brought against orthodox medicine by patients who were wrongly kept from supportive high-dose vitamin therapy.

The grounds for disparagement usually center on three inaccurate claims: 1) vitamins are ineffective against cancer; 2) vitamins interfere with conventional cancer therapies; and 3) vitamins are themselves harmful to the cancer patient. These are common but fallacious views.

Take vitamin C for example. There are many controlled studies that demonstrate that vitamin C is indeed effective against cancer. A number of nutrients reduce the side-effects of chemotherapy, surgery, and radiation therapy. Patients on a strong nutritional program have far less nausea, far less fatigue, and often experience little or no hair loss during chemo (Carr, *NZ Med J* 2014). They experience reduced pain and swelling following radiation. They have faster, uncomplicated healing after surgery. Such vitamin-mediated benefits mean that oncologists can give vitamin-taking patients the full dose of chemotherapy, rather than having to cut the dose to keep the patient from giving up entirely. Obviously, full-strength chemo is more likely to be effective against cancer than reduced-strength chemo. A similar benefit is at work with radiation therapy: the full intensity of treatment is far better tolerated by an optimally nourished, nutritionally fortified patient. With surgery, the risk reduction aspects of supplemental vitamins, both pre- and post-op, are well established. Therefore, vitamin C and other nutrients, far from being detrimental, make a most positive contribution to the conventional treatment of cancer. Even at very high doses, vitamin C is an unusually safe substance; countless studies have verified this. As an antioxidant, collagen-building co-enzyme, and reinforcer of the immune system, vitamin C is vital to a cancer patient. Yet the blood work of cancer patients will invariably show that they have abnormally low levels of the vitamin. What is dangerous is vitamin deficiency.

Fortunately, there are physicians who still look to the patient, and not the test tube, for their answers. A patient's therapeutic response is the highest of all guiding principles in medicine. If it works, do it. If it seems to work, do it. If it does no harm, do it. If there were a sure cure for cancer, you would have heard about it. There isn't. But this just makes it all the more important for patients to demand adjunctive vitamin therapy from their physicians. The number of conventionally educated physicians, including oncologists, that now support vitamin therapy is growing. This section will provide considerable basis for their doing so.

—A.W.S.

TERMS OF CANCER

ADENOCARCINOMA. A type of cancer that forms in the mucous-secreting glands throughout the body.

APOPTOSIS. Cell-induced cell death.

ASCORBIC ACID. Ascorbic acid is a weak acid, far weaker than stomach hydrochloric acid. For oral administration, orthomolecular physicians tend to specify ascorbic acid rather than the nonacidic vitamin C salts (calcium ascorbate, magnesium ascorbate, sodium ascorbate) because ascorbic acid seems to get better clinical results than do the salts do. Intravenous administration of vitamin C requires either sodium ascorbate or carefully buffered ascorbic acid.

BOWEL TOLERANCE. Loose stools when a person exceeds their requirements, or limits, for oral vitamin C. It varies with the state of health increasing by up to 100 times when a person is ill.

CARCINOMA. A malignant tumor that begins in the epithelial tissues (the cells that line the entire surface of the body); approximately 80 percent of all cancers are carcinomas.

CYTOKINE. Immunoregulatory (cell-signalling) proteins.

CYTOTOXIC. Cell-killing, toxic to cells.

DYNAMIC FLOW. Taking large and frequent doses of vitamin C (ascorbic acid), at least 500–1,000 milligrams four to six times a day. Intake is adjusted for the individual concerned and should total 70–80 percent of the bowel tolerance.

GRADE. A grade for cancer that indicates how aggressive it is; the lower the grade, the less aggressive the cancer and the greater the chance for cure.

LEUKEMIA. A cancer involving the blood and blood-forming organs (bone marrow, lymphatic system, and spleen).

LYMPHOMA. A cancer involving the lymphatic system.

REDOX. A term that refers to an oxidation-reduction reaction; the loss (oxidation) or gain (reduction) of electrons.

STAGING. A way to categorize or classify patients according to how extensive the disease is at the time of diagnosis. Stage I indicates the earliest cancers. Stages II, III, and IV indicate more extensive disease. Letters may be used along with the numerals (Stage IIB, for example) to subclassify cancers based on specific tumor characteristics.

SARCOMA. A malignant tumor that grows from connective tissue such as cartilage, fat, muscle, or bone.

VITAMINS AND CANCER
by Abram Hoffer, MD, PhD

New ideas that eventually become part of medical practice do not spring forth fully formed from someone's mind. They usually begin with simple observations by one person and later by several, until someone crystallizes these ideas and observations into a coherent hypothesis.

This is the case with vitamin C and cancer. The first observations were made by many clinicians who were using vitamin C to treat a number of conditions that were not part of scurvy. During the golden age of vitamin discovery, between 1930 and 1940, physicians used these vitamins as soon as they became available, encouraged by the companies that synthesized them. Several clinicians observed or thought they had observed that their patients with cancer lived longer when they were given vitamin C in quantities substantially larger than those needed to prevent scurvy. These observations were summarized by Irwin Stone in his book, *The Healing Factor: Vitamin C Against Disease* (1974).

I am very proud of this book because Dr. Stone published it after I had been urging him for two years to summarize his vast collection of vitamin C papers so that the medical world would know something about these early clinical studies. But his book was not taken seriously by the medical establishment, which adhered to the vitamins-as-prevention paradigm. This was the paradigm that looked upon vitamins as having value only in the prevention of the classical vitamin deficiency diseases such as scurvy (severe vitamin C deficiency) or pellagra (severe vitamin B3 deficiency). In this paradigm using large doses and/or using them for treating conditions not accepted as vitamin deficiency conditions was contraindicated. One of my medical colleagues lost his medical license because he gave large doses of vitamin C intravenously.

The Great Divide

Dr. Stone's book suggested two major possible roles for vitamin C. The first was its use in preventing cancer and the second as a possible treatment.

The first possibility was accepted much more readily and has been studied for several decades. There is little doubt that a diet rich in vitamin C does tend to have preventive properties. This idea was not an anathema to the current paradigm. The second possibility was rejected except by a slowly growing school of physicians who were interested in the optimum use of vitamins, in small or large dosages, for conditions not known to be deficiency diseases such as hypercholesterolemia, schizophrenia, or arthritis. This school represented the new paradigm, the vitamin-as-treatment paradigm, which originated in 1954 with the discovery in which I participated that niacin (vitamin B3) lowered cholesterol levels. At that time Dr. William Kaufman was using megadoses of vitamin B3 for arthritis, Drs. Wilfrid and Evan Shute were treating large numbers of heart patients with vitamin E, and Dr. Fred Klenner was treating enormous numbers of patients with serious infections and cancer with very large doses of vitamin C.

Dr. Stone's review of vitamin C used in large doses excited Dr. Linus Pauling's interest. But Dr. Pauling was spurred to action only after a meeting he addressed where he suggested that vitamin C in large doses might be useful in the treatment of cancer. He was attacked by hematologist Victor Herbert who challenged him to provide some evidence. Pauling thought Herbert was right and that he should present some evidence . . . and this led to Pauling's enduring interest in the use of vitamin C. He encouraged Dr. Ewan Cameron in Scotland to investigate what were then enormous doses with 10 grams intravenously in a series of failed cancer patients. The results were very encouraging and led to a large number of reports in the medical literature and in their book *Cancer and Vitamin C* (1979). This is one of the most important books, in my opinion, published in the field of cancer treatment.

From the *J Orthomolecular Med* 2000;15(4):171–172, 193–200.

The discourse between the two vitamin paradigms has been very strained. Orthomolecular physicians continued to use optimum doses of vitamins for a variety of conditions, including cancer, and the vast body of current medicine continued to consider that this paradigm was of no value, even dangerous. The medical journals would not carry the reports prepared by the second paradigm, nor invite them to their meetings, and the second paradigm found it could only publish in their own specialty journals, usually not reviewed nor abstracted by the standard medical journals. Physicians supporting the modern vitamins-as-treatment paradigm emerged from the vitamins-as-prevention paradigm, that is, they are familiar with both. I do not know of any who moved in the reverse direction.

How a Psychiatrist Began to Treat Cancer

I am a psychiatrist who was involved with Dr. Pauling in establishing orthomolecular psychiatry and medicine. I had been routinely using several nutrients in my treatment protocols, which included vitamin B3 (as niacin or niacinamide), vitamin C, vitamin B6 (pyridoxine), B-complex preparations, vitamin E, and zinc.

I used doses of 3,000 milligrams (mg) per day and more for my schizophrenic patients. In 1952, I gave 1,000 mg each hour for 48 hours to a woman who had become psychotic after a mastectomy and had been admitted on a Thursday for electroconvulsive treatment (ECT or shock therapy), the only treatment then that had any effectiveness. Monday morning after that vitamin-C weekend, she was mentally normal and did not need the ECT. At the same time her ulcerated, infected mastectomy lesion had begun to heal. She died six months later from her cancer but she was mentally normal. This showed that huge doses of vitamin C were tolerable and potentially valuable in treating psychotic patients.

In 1960, a 75-year-old psychotic retired professor was admitted to our psychiatric ward. He had terminal, inoperable lung cancer identified by x-ray and biopsy, but he also excreted large amounts of a substance in his urine we had found present in most of our schizophrenic patients. These patients responded well to treatment with vitamin B3. I

therefore started him on niacin, 1,000 mg three times daily, and the same amount of vitamin C. A few days later he was mentally normal. Every three months his lesion was smaller on x-ray examination and after one year it was gone. He died 30 months after I first saw him.

A year or two later, a 16-year-old female with Ewing's sarcoma (a bone cancer) was slated for surgery to amputate her arm. I started her on niacinamide, 1,000 mg three times daily, and ascorbic acid (vitamin C), 1,000 mg three times daily, and suggested to the surgeon he postpone surgery. Her cancer disappeared.

In 1977, a female with jaundice was found to have a large mass in the head of the pancreas. It was inoperable and was not biopsied because of the danger of spreading the disease. She was advised she might survive six months. She began to take 10,000 mg of vitamin C each day and later was referred to me. I increased it to 40,000 mg and added several other vitamins. She is alive today.

What are the odds that the first four terminal cases of cancer I saw would all respond to simple vitamin therapy? If the woman last referred to had died, as it was expected she would, I may not have developed this part of my practice, for she told so many people about her recovery that within a few years many patients were routinely referred to me. This experience with a few patients who had responded so well preconditioned me to look upon the Cameron/Pauling studies (mentioned earlier) very seriously. I advised all my cancer patients to improve the quality of their diet and to take 12,000 mg of vitamin C daily and to increase it to bowel tolerance levels whenever possible. I also added vitamin B3, beta-carotene, and zinc.

After I had seen about 50 patients I did a follow-up on each of them. I found to my surprise and pleasure that the patients who had stuck with the program at least two months lived much longer than the smaller group who had not followed the program.[1] This was not a randomized study and I had not planned it to be. It was the use of orthomolecular treatment for a group of desperate patients, most of them with terminal and untreatable forms of cancer.

I am familiar with the double-blind methodology since under my direction in Saskatchewan we conducted the first six prospective, randomized, double-blind, therapeutic trials in psychiatry beginning in 1952, but in private practice I was not able to conduct this type of study. By the end of 1998 I had treated over 1,000 cancer patients. Arising from this large cohort, I published various reports outlining my conclusions from data I had been collecting.[2-8]

My Cohort

I hoped that every patient seen would follow the regimen but in fact they did not and it would have been very surprising if they had. Clinical research is messy. It is not the clean-cut affair many theorists would have us think it is. I decided originally to use as my control every patient who did not follow the regimen for at least two months, including many who died within two months after they first saw me. They were still on standard treatment or had already received it and I considered that this group would constitute my control. I played no role in determining who would not follow the program. The decisions were made by fate, by referring physicians, by oncologists, and by family members or by the belief the cost involved in taking nutrients was not justified. I excluded every patient who died within two months after first seeing me. This removes the argument that I had thrown the most hopeless group into the control group. Every patient who followed this program for at least two months was included in the treatment group and every patient who did not was included in the control group. It is not a randomized control group, nor would this have been possible in this series. I think it was fair to split the groups this way because, based on my experience, it takes about two months for the program to begin to take effect.

Clinical Matters

Fewer than 10 percent of the cancer patients were early-onset cases. The rest were all late-stage, or inoperable, or untreatable, or had failed to yield to treatment, or had relapsed after having had treatment. The early cases were not motivated to come

to see me and physicians did not tell the patients that vitamin treatment was an option. The desperate nature of the disease forced them all to consult with me when they had lost all hope of receiving any additional help.

I used only hard data. This was the length of time these patients lived after they had first seen me. I did not and could not use size of tumor and other clinical criteria used by oncologists for evaluating the treatment.

During the first interview I told the patients that I was not treating the tumor, that this was the

---

VITAMIN C AND OTHER ANTIOXIDANTS DO NOT INTERFERE WITH CHEMOTHERAPY

Sweeping recommendations warning cancer patients to not take supplemental vitamin C is irresponsible. Vitamin C is not just an antioxidant. Inside cancer tumors, it also acts as a pro-oxidant killing malignant cells.

Unfortunately, just over 2 percent of all cancers respond to chemotherapy. Specifically, one scientific review concluded, "The overall contribution of curative and adjuvant cytotoxic chemotherapy to 5-year survival in adults was estimated to be 2.3 percent in Australia and 2.1 percent in the United States . . . chemotherapy only makes a minor contribution to cancer survival. To justify the continued funding and availability of drugs used in cytotoxic chemotherapy, a rigorous evaluation of the cost-effectiveness and impact on quality of life is urgently required."[1]

REFERENCES

1. Morgan G. *Clin Oncol* 2004;16(8):549–560.

ADDITIONAL READING

Block KI. *Cancer Treat Rev* 2007;33(5):407–418.
Block KI. *Int J Cancer* 2008;123(6):1227–1239.
Hoffer A. *Townsend Lett.* Available at www.tldp.com/issue/11_00/hoffer.htm.
Lamson DW. *Altern Med* Rev 1999;4(5):304–329.
Prasad KN. *J Am Coll Nutr* 1999;18:13–25.
Prasad KN. *Z Onkol/J of Oncol* 1999;31:1201–1078.
Simone CB. *Altern Ther Health Med* 2007;13(1):22–28.

responsibility of their oncologists, that I was offering them a nutritional program that I hoped would increase the probability of their survival. I pointed out that this was not an alternative treatment, that it was complementary. I added that the use of nutrients was compatible with any other treatment including surgery, chemotherapy, and radiation. For many years I had to counteract the advice given these patients by the nutritionists at the cancer clinic and by their oncologist who insisted on telling them that the vitamins would interfere with the therapy. This is based upon their theoretical view that the antioxidants would decrease the effectiveness of the treatment in killing tumor cells. This is contradicted by the literature. In fact, vitamins increase the effectiveness of the treatment and decrease the toxic effect on the patient.[9]

I would see the patient again in one or two months to deal with any problems unless they were depressed or very anxious, in which case I would treat them as primary psychiatric patients.

Each year after they were first seen I would obtain a report of whether they were alive and how they were doing. I would call either the patient, their family, their physicians, or the cancer clinic and I would check the obituaries in the local paper. Since over 90 percent of my patients came from southern Vancouver Island, almost all deaths were reported in the local daily paper.

Results

A comparison between the patients who followed the program and those who did not is given in Table 1. Out of the original 134 patients, 3 were lost to follow up. Nine died within the first two months and were excluded.

At the end of year one, only 28 percent of the controls were alive compared to 77 percent of the vitamin-treated group. At year three, only 16 percent of the control group was alive compared to 56 percent of the vitamin-treated group. By year five, only 5 percent of the control group and 46 percent of the vitamin-treated group were alive, while at years seven and nine there were no survivors in the control group, but 39 percent and 34 percent, respectively, in the vitamin-treated group.

I examined further the first cohort of 134 patients as of December 1998. Thirty-three were still alive from the vitamin-treated group, all having survived at least ten years. None survived from the control group. Half the six deaths in 1992 were caused by other physical disease and were not directly from cancer.

TABLE 1. SURVIVAL TRENDS FOR FIRST CANCER PATIENTS FOLLOWED FROM 1976 TO 1988		
GROUP	ORTHOMOLECULAR TREATMENT	STANDARD TREATMENT
Number*	97	18
Alive at 1 year	77%	28%
Alive at 3 years	56%	16%
Alive at 5 years	46%	5%
Alive at 7 years	39%	0%
Alive at 9 years	34%	0%

* Editor's note: These numbers, the basis for the percentages surviving, include 3 lost and 9 that died. More exclusions could have further reduced the total from 134 to 115 after several years.

The survival trends that appeared in the first Hoffer and Pauling paper[2] and reappeared in our second[3] and in my third presentation are confirmed in this report. A comparison between the patients seen until the end of 1993, who followed the program and those who did not, is given in Table 2.

TABLE 2. SURVIVAL TRENDS FOR CANCER PATIENTS SEEN BEFORE THE END OF 1993		
GROUP	ORTHOMOLECULAR TREATMENT	STANDARD TREATMENT
Number	441	54
Alive at 1 year	73%	28%
Alive at 2 years	56%	15%
Alive at 3 years	48%	15%
Alive at 4 years	44%	13%
Alive at 5 years	39%	11%

A comparison between the patients seen until the end of 1997, who followed the program and those who did not, is given in Table 3.

TABLE 3. SURVIVAL TRENDS FOR CANCER PATIENTS SEEN BEFORE THE END OF 1997

GROUP	ORTHOMOLECULAR TREATMENT	STANDARD TREATMENT
Number	769	75
Alive at 1 year	72%	24%
Alive at 2 years	48%	12%
Alive at 3 years	37%	12%
Alive at 4 years	30%	8%
Alive at 5 years	23%	8%

Six Special Cases

The types of cancers in these cohorts were varied. They included among others cancers of the abdomen, breast, cervix, colon, intestines, kidney, lymph nodes, pancreas, prostate, spinal cord, throat, thyroid, and uterus. Following are several case histories of particularly difficult-to-treat cancers.

Case 1. A 63-Year-Old Woman with Poorly Differentiated Squamous Cell Carcinoma of the Lung

In November 1983, the patient presented with constitutional symptoms and collapse of the upper lobe of the right lung. Bronchoscopy and mediastinoscopy were negative, but, at thoracotomy in December 1983, she was found to have a poorly differentiated squamous cell carcinoma occluding the right upper lobe bronchus and extending to the lateral chest wall. She was deemed inoperable and was given a course of 20 sessions of cobalt irradiation to her right chest (January/February 1984). In April 1984, she began a vitamin regimen that included vitamin C, (12,000 mg), niacinamide (1,500 mg), and other vitamins. Chest x-rays in 1984 and 1985 showed extensive pleural thickening at the right lung base and fibrotic scarring extending into the right apex. The patient continued to take 12,000 mg of vitamin C per day until 1987, after which she reduced the dose to 8,000 mg

per day. She was discharged from the Victoria Cancer Clinic in 1988 as not requiring further follow-up. She had a mild stroke in January 1993, and a more severe one in December of that year. She died in January 1994, without evidence of cancer 10 years after diagnosis.

Case 22. A 14-Year-Old Girl with Ewing's Sarcoma of the Left Humerus

This patient presented to the hospital in October 1979, with a painful left upper arm. There was obvious bony swelling of the upper half of the humerus (arm). The x-ray was highly suggestive of Ewing's sarcoma, a diagnosis confirmed on surgical biopsy. There was no evidence of tumor spread and she underwent radiation and multiple courses of chemotherapy, which included cyclophosphamide, vincristine, actinomycin D, and doxorubicin, over a period of two years. During the period of therapy she developed a displaced fracture at the site of the cancer and in 1981 consideration was given to the possibility of a residual tumor. In July 1981, she was started on vitamin C (12,000 mg), niacinamide (3,000 mg), and pyridoxine (250 mg). In 1982, there was evidence of spontaneous healing at the fracture site and no evidence of recurrent malignant disease and she remains disease free. She stayed on a megavitamin regimen from 1981 to 1983, with her vitamin C intake ranging from 4,000–16,000 mg a day. She may be considered cancer free after a 20-year period without disease.

Case 23. A 39-Year-Old Woman with Carcinoma of the Ovary

The patient presented to the hospital in 1981 with ascites (fluid build-up) and a 10 by 12 centimeter (cm, 3.9 by 4.7 inch [in]) pelvic tumor was found on operation to be a Stage IIC non-mucin secreting adenocarcinoma involving a fallopian tube. Removal of the uterus and ovaries and an omentectomy were carried out. Over the year she received chemotherapy with cisplatin and doxorubicin, followed by radiation to the anterior abdomen and pelvis in October 1981, after which she was disease free. In May 1982 she was begun on a vitamin regimen that included vitamin C (12,000 mg), niacinamide (1,500 mg), pyridoxine (250 mg), zinc sulfate (220 mg), and vitamin A. She followed the program for about one year, after which she took the vitamins only intermittently. In 1995, she underwent a craniotomy (brain surgery) to remove a tumor in the left cerebellum. This was found to be a papillary (slow-growing) adenocarcinoma. The patient then received radiation to the brain. She resumed vitamin therapy and was well in 1998.

Case 74. A 35-Year-Old Man with Widespread Multiply Recurrent Lymphoma

In 1983, this patient was found to have a poorly differentiated, small non-cleaved cell lymphoma involving his retroperitoneum (a layer of specialized cells lining the area that contains the kidneys, pancreas, and other organs), diagnosed at abdominal surgery. A computed tomography (CT) scan revealed a pancreatic mass 12 cm (4.7 in) in diameter extending into the connective tissue (mesentery) attaching it to the abdominal wall. Over the next two years, he received several courses of chemotherapy (including doxorubicin, cyclosphosphamide, vincristine, and prednisone) and several courses of radiation for the original tumor and its multiple recurrences. In March 1984, a recurrence in the left back chest wall was treated with radiation. In May 1984, a recurrence in the left thoracic spine was treated with radiation and chemotherapy. A large right pelvic mass detected in January 1985 was treated with radiation. Progress notes in the medical record between 1983 and 1984 consistently note his dismal prognosis. Concurrent with the chemotherapy and radiation this patient received up to 40,000 mg a day of ascorbic acid, either orally or intravenously, as well as up to 12,000 mg of niacin, 1,000 micrograms (mcg) of selenium, and other vitamins and minerals. The patient stated that after his cancer had been treated for one year and he was in remission, he took himself off all the supplements. After two to three months the tumor recurred, so he resumed taking the vitamins (12,000 mg of vitamin C, 3,000 mg of niacin, and other vitamins and minerals). Since 1985 there was no further recurrence of his lymphoma despite no additional conventional anticancer therapy. He remains well.

Case 324. A 61-Year-Old Woman with Squamous Cell Carcinoma of the Lung

This patient was found to have a 9 by 10 cm mass (3.5 by 3.9 in) in the lower lobe of her right lung, with CT scan evidence of subcarinal adenopathy (an increase in lymph node size). Squamous cell carcinoma was diagnosed by transthoracic needle biopsy. In October 1990, the oncologist concluded that the cancer was Stage T2 N2 MO (a cancer that had spread far). He arranged for a 29-day course of radiation but doubted a prolonged survival because of the large size of the primary lesion. In December, the lung mass was slightly smaller. In April 1991, it was concluded that the lung mass was about the same size as before radiation. In June 1991, it was concluded that there might be improvement in the lung mass. In July 1991, she began taking vitamin C (12,000 mg), niacinamide (1,500 mg), B-complex vitamins, vitamin E (1,200 international units [IU]), and other vitamins and minerals, remaining on this program thereafter. In April 1996, a chest x-ray and CT scan examination was reported as showing no sign of tumor. In 1998, she was well.

Case 384. A 46-Year-Old Woman with Ovarian Cancer

This woman was found to have a Stage IIIB papillary serous cystoadenocarcinoma of the ovary on exploratory laparotomy for a painful abdominal mass. She was deemed to fall into the high-risk treatment category and was given 6 cycles of cisplatin chemotherapy completed in July 1991. She achieved a sustained complete clinical remission but, because of the complication of peripheral neuropathy, was started on a daily regimen of ascorbic acid (12,000 mg), niacinamide (1,500 mg), B complex, folic acid, and other vitamins and minerals. She remains in clinical remission.

■ CONCLUSION

I treated the first few patients with orthomolecular therapy because there was no other treatment available, because I was curious what the vitamin regimen might do, and because I knew that my patients could not be harmed by giving them vitamins. As my experience with the use of vitamins increased, I became more confident that there was some value in this treatment by increasing longevity and improving the quality of life, but I did not conclude that I had fully established the validity of the program. I hoped that one day this volume of data might arouse the interest of research physicians in the field, who could then conduct definitive experiments that would answer the questions: 1) Is the addition of megavitamin therapy, especially vitamin C, of value in the treatment of cancer? 2) What is the relative value of each of the nutrients and is the value of some so small that it need not be included? 3) What additional antioxidants and nutrients would improve these therapeutic results? and 4) We cannot stop the search, for the results of treatment are simply not good enough with or without megavitamin therapy. We cannot stop our search until each case of cancer can be treated as easily as most infections are today and, even more important, until we have isolated those factors that are responsible for the major increase in the incidence and prevalence of cancer.

REFERENCES

1. Hoffer A. *Orthomolecular Medicine for Physicians.* New Canaan, CT: Keats Publishing, 1989.

2. Hoffer A, Pauling L. Hardin Jones biostatistical analysis of mortality data for cohorts of cancer patients with a large fraction surviving at the termination of the study and a comparison of survival times of cancer patients receiving large regular oral doses of vitamin C and other nutrients with similar patients not receiving those doses. *J Orthomolecular Med* 1990;5:143–154. Reprinted in *Cancer and Vitamin C* by E. Cameron E and L. Pauling. Philadelphia, PA: Camino Books, 1993.

3. Hoffer A, Pauling L. Hardin Jones biostatistical analysis of mortality data for a second set of cohorts of cancer patients with a large fraction surviving at the termination of the study and a comparison of survival times of cancer patients receiving large regular oral doses of vitamin C and other nutrients with similar patients not receiving these doses. *J Orthomolecular Med* 1993; 8: 154–167.

4. Hoffer A. Orthomolecular oncology. In: *Adjuvant Nutrition in Cancer Treatment, 1992 Symposium Proceedings*, sponsored by Cancer Treatment Research Foundation and American College of Nutrition. Arlington Heights, IL: Cancer Treatment Research Foundation, 1994, 331–362.

5. Hoffer A. Orthomolecular Treatment of Cancer. In eds. *Nutrients in Cancer Prevention and Treatment* edited by K. Prasad, L. Santamaria, RM Williams. Totowa, NJ: Humana Press, 1995: 373–391.

6. One patient's recovery from lymphoma. *Townsend Lett* 1996;160:50–51.

7. Hoffer A: How to live longer even with cancer. *J Orthomolecular Med* 1996;11:147–167.

8. Simone CB, Simone NL, Simone, CB: Nutrients and cancer treatment. *Int J Integr Med* 1998; 1: 22–27.

VITAMIN C: A CASE HISTORY OF AN ALTERNATIVE CANCER THERAPY
by John Hoffer, MD, PhD

Any consideration of high-dose vitamin C in cancer therapy must include a careful analysis of its use, some 30 years ago, by the Scottish oncologic surgeon Ewan Cameron in the treatment of patients with advanced untreatable cancer at Vale of Leven Hospital in Scotland. Dr. Cameron's treatment program, which typically involved about 10,000 milligrams (mg) of ascorbic acid (vitamin C) given first by intravenous injection, followed by oral administration, was carried out in collaboration with the renowned American chemist, Linus Pauling. It became clear early in this clinical experience that while vitamin C had no important effect on the disease course of most patients, important and sometimes astounding benefits occurred for a substantial minority of them.

Patients experienced an increase in subjective well-being that was accompanied by such objective clinical evidence of retardation of tumor progression, reduced pain from bone metastases, reduced rate of accumulation of malignant effusions (fluid in the lung linings), reduced obstructive jaundice, or improved respiratory function. There were a few cases of clinical remissions, and others in which there was objective evidence of acute tumor hemorrhage (bleeding) and necrosis. This last dramatic effect did not benefit patients, for it hastened their demise. (Cameron would later find that the vitamin was working but working too fast in a very sick patient.) But these dramatic events, bolstered in many cases by the results of autopsy examinations, represent potent evidence of an important biologic effect of high-dose ascorbic acid in some situations.

Cameron and Pauling also noted that, on average, vitamin C-treated patients lived substantially longer than other patients not admitted under Cameron's service, and hence not given ascorbic acid, but otherwise similar with regard to sex, age, tumor diagnosis, and clinical stage, and treated by the same physicians in the same hospital using the same norms of clinical care. The clinical results of treatment of the first 50 patients appeared in

1974[1,2] in *Chemico-Biological Interactions*. One case control study was published in the *Proceedings of the National Academy of Sciences (PNAS)* in 1976. A second study, using different case-control matching criteria, and with the same conclusion, was published in the same journal in 1978.[3,4] In 1979, Cameron and Pauling published their book *Cancer and Vitamin C*, which describes the results of their clinical experience in detail.[5]

Subsequently, two randomized double-blind controlled trials comparing the effects of oral vitamin C and a placebo were carried out at the Mayo Clinic in Rochester, Minnesota, under the direction of Charles G. Moertel, an expert in cytotoxic chemotherapy trials.[6,7] Dr. Moertel concluded that vitamin C is of no benefit whatsoever in cancer therapy. In light of the current understanding of the mode of action of biologic response modifiers (substances that boost the body's immune system to fight against cancer) as well as other considerations pointed out at the time of the studies, these Mayo Clinic studies seem naive in conception and seriously flawed in their design and execution. The question as to the value of ascorbic acid therapy in cancer therapy thus remains unresolved nearly 30 years after the initial Vale of Leven experience.

This review provides a historical overview and interpretive analysis of the Cameron-Pauling experience and a critique of the Mayo Clinic trials. In it I endeavor to frame the issues that drove the controversy and to draw attention to the lessons that may be learned from it in a modern consideration of vitamin C as a cancer therapy. In preparing this review I drew upon the initial clinical reports, which are invaluable and irreplaceable. I previously reported on these.[8] I also drew on the revised (1993) edition of Cameron and Pauling's *Cancer and Vitamin C*,[9] and on a valuable analysis by Eveleen Richards in *Vitamin C and Cancer: Medicine or Politics?*[10]

From the *J Orthomolecular Med* 2000;15(4):181–188.

LEARNING FROM THE PAST: PRESENT-DAY PROTOCOL

Acute tumor hemorrhage and necrosis in patients with advanced cancer within a few days of starting high-dose intravenous vitamin C therapy is rare. Ewan Cameron observed this reaction in his early clinical experience in the 1970s. Campbell and Jack (*Scot Med J* 1979) reported that one patient died due to massive tumor necrosis and hemorrhaging following an initial dose of intravenous ascorbate. Since then physicians experienced with high-dose vitamin C supplementation have learned more about why these reactions may have occurred and now take precautions to prevent it. Writes Dr. Robert Cathcart: "Ewan Cameron's advice against giving cancer patients with widespread metastasis large amounts of ascorbate too rapidly at first should be heeded. He found that sometimes extensive necrosis or hemorrhage in the cancer could kill a patient with widespread metastasis if the vitamin was started too rapidly" (*Med Hypothesis* 1981). High-dose intravenous vitamin C protocol developed by the late Dr. Hugh Riordan (see Appendix 3: Riordan Clinic Protocol) recommends that treatment start at a low dose and be carried out using slow "drip" infusion. It is also now known that fatal hemolysis can occur if a patient has an inherited deficiency of the enzyme glucose-6-phosphate dehydrogenase deficiency (G6PD). It is thus recommended that G6PD levels be assessed prior to the onset of therapy. The treatment is also contraindicated in situations where increased fluids, sodium, or chelating may cause serious problems. These situations include congestive heart failure, edema, ascites, chronic hemodialysis, unusual iron overload, and inadequate hydration or urine void volume (Rivers, *Ann NY Acad Sci* 1987).

The Vale of Leven Trial

Ewan Cameron began his Phase III vitamin C trial at the Vale of Leven Hospital in November 1971, treating patients with a variety of advanced, untreatable malignancies. He was prompted to conduct this trial by theoretical considerations that vitamin C might increase host resistance to tumor spread, and by his review of some earlier, smaller reports published by others indicating that vitamin C had beneficial effects in human cancer.[1]

The treatment regimen varied somewhat, but as a rule it included the continuous intravenous (IV) infusion of ascorbic acid (10,000 mg) per day. Higher doses (up to 45,000 mg per day) were occasionally administered. After up to 10 days of intravenous vitamin C, treatment was transferred to the oral route, at a usual dose of 10,000 mg per day. Patient responses were recorded in five categories: no response, minimal response, growth retardation, cytostasis (cessation of tumor progression), tumor regression, and tumor hemorrhage and necrosis.[2] It is important to note that no more than about 4 percent of these patients had received prior chemotherapy at the time they were declared untreatable.[9]

The 1974 paper in *Chemico-Biological Interactions* describes the experience with 50 consecutive advanced cancer patients.[2] No response, or only minimal response, was observed in 27 patients. Cytostasis occurred in three patients. These included patients who were preterminal with progressive disease but became clinically well and remained normal with continuing vitamin C therapy for follow-up periods of over a year despite the continuous presence of their malignancy. Tumor regression occurred in five patients. In these cases, symptoms and clinical evidence of tumor mass disappeared (clearance of intestinal obstruction, disappearance of palpable mass, relief of obstructive jaundice, disappearance of x-ray evidence of bone metastases). Most striking of all, however, was the occurrence of tumor hemorrhage and necrosis in four patients. Cameron and his colleague Allan Campbell's descriptions of these occurrences bear an uncanny resemblance to the first description of tumor hemorrhage and necrosis (cells and tissue that have died) induced with tumor necrosis factor (a substance that can cause tumor cells to die), which coincidentally appeared in the *PNAS* one year later.[11]

In one case, a 66-year-old man with locally widespread bronchogenic cancer (lung cancer) and a large palpable subcutaneous metastasis over the right shoulder developed acute tumor necrosis and hemorrhage of the right shoulder metastasis on the sixth day of vitamin C administration. This was followed by confusion, coma, and death.

In a second case, a 42-year-old man with testicular cancer, cannonball metastases in both lungs, and a large secondary tumor mass in the left upper jaw experienced acute hemorrhage from the oral tumor, hemoptysis (coughing up blood), confusion, and death on the third day of vitamin C administration.

In a third case, a 63-year-old man with chondrosarcoma of the ilium (hip bone cancer) and a large, fixed pelvic tumor mass developed severe right hip and abdominal pain on the third day of vitamin C administration. This was followed by fever, confusion, pulmonary edema, and death. At autopsy, both the primary tumor and all the numerous metastases in the aortic region and elsewhere showed extensive hemorrhage and necrosis.

Also striking was the report, in a subsequent paper by Cameron, Campbell, and Jack of two vitamin C-induced complete remissions in the same patient of a stage IVB non-Hodgkin's lymphoma.[12] The patient was a 42-year-old truck driver who developed fever and constitutional symptoms in 1973 and was found to have a right pulmonary infiltrate (cancer that had spread to the lung). Two months later the infiltrate was worse, and a pleural effusion (water on the lungs) was present. The clinical diagnosis of lung cancer was made and no treatment offered. However, when the patient then developed an enlarged liver and spleen and enlarged lymph nodes, which is usually associated with disease, a lymph node biopsy was carried out and the diagnosis of non-Hodgkin's lymphoma was made. The accuracy of this diagnosis was later confirmed by expert pathologists.[5,10] Although the plan at that time was for radiation and chemotherapy, an administrative delay in obtaining the patient's transfer to a referral center and his poor clinical condition motivated his physicians to administer intravenous vitamin C. The response was so strikingly favorable that all indications for standard lymphoma therapy promptly disappeared. Within a few days the patient experienced a return of well-being associated with complete regression of his enlarged

lymph nodes, liver, and spleen. The water on the lungs resolved and the chest x-ray became normal. After three months, vitamin C therapy was tapered and stopped. Four weeks after stopping vitamin C, the patient's constitutional symptoms returned and a repeat chest x-ray again showed water on the lungs and right hilar enlargement (area where breathing tubes and blood vessels converge). The patient was started on oral ascorbic acid, but it was ineffective in preventing further clinical deterioration, so he was admitted to hospital for an intravenous ascorbic acid infusion (20,000 mg a day for 14 days) followed by oral ascorbic acid. A slow but sustained clinical improvement resulted. As of 1979, the patient, still on vitamin C, remained in complete remission.[5]

Another striking early case is described in the 1993 book.[9] A 68-year-old woman was admitted with severe malignant ascites (fluid buildup in the abdomen) due to a proven ovarian cancer. She had failed to respond to one prior course of chemotherapy. On this admission following palliative drainage of some of the peritoneal fluid, permitting easy palpation of a large tumor mass, she was begun on intravenous ascorbic acid as her sole treatment. There was a prompt clinical improvement, including return of appetite. In the absence of any other therapy, the tumor masses shrank and became impalpable. Then, about four weeks after starting ascorbic acid, the patient developed clinical shock and died within a few hours. At autopsy she was found to have an intestinal obstruction related to the adhesions. The great bulk of the tumor was gone, leaving only residual tumor nodules.

In summary, the Vale of Leven experience showed that intravenous, followed by oral, vitamin C exerted a favorable effect, sometimes astonishingly favorable, in a significant minority of advanced cancer patients who had not received prior chemotherapy. Indeed, the effect reported by Cameron, an experienced and well-regarded oncologist, was similar to that reported for the biologic response modifier, interleukin-2 (IL-2), in later National Cancer Institute (NCI)-funded Phase II trials that attracted wide interest in the scientific medical community.[13,14] Most important from the biologic perspective were the cases in which vitamin C induced catastrophic tumor hemorrhage and necrosis. Although IL-2 occasionally produces rapid remissions, it has never had an effect as dramatic as this.

The response of the scientific medical community to the Vale of Leven trial was silence. Part of this can be ascribed to its publication in *Chemico-Biological Interactions*, a non-medical journal, after rejection by a leading cancer journal on the grounds that it "was not of sufficiently high priority to warrant publication space."[10]

But there were more important reasons. When Pauling presented details of the Vale of Leven treatment responses to experts at the NCI, he was told his clinical data failed to prove vitamin C was effective against cancer, and therefore no clinical research on vitamin C and cancer was warranted. Cameron and Pauling then carried out retrospective examinations of the survival times of vitamin C-treated and case-control patients, published in 1976 and 1978 in the *PNAS*, demonstrating a significant prolongation of the life span of vitamin C-treated cancer patients over that of matched contemporaneous patients not treated with vitamin C.[3,4] The *PNAS* took the unprecedented step of adjoining an editorial to the second *PNAS* paper, criticizing Pauling for not using "well-established rules of clinical investigation." The editorial, by medical researcher Julius H. Comroe, called for a well-designed, double-blind randomized prospective study to confirm or refute vitamin C's anti-cancer activity. The editorial also recommended histologic (cell and tissue) matching of cancer patients randomized to vitamin C and no treatment, and that a system be established to ensure that patients randomized to a vitamin C group take their vitamin C and ones randomized to placebo take their placebo.[15]

The Mayo Clinic Trials

The results of such a Phase III study, carried out in patients with various advanced cancers at the Mayo Clinic in Rochester, Minnesota, were published the following year in the *New England Journal of Medicine*, and they were negative.[6] There ensued a vigorous exchange between Linus Pauling and the principal investigator of the Mayo Clinic trial, Charles Moertel, which brought out the fact that almost none of the Vale of Leven patients but almost all the Mayo Clinic patients had received extensive prior chemotherapy. This might have affected their responsiveness to an immune-modulating substance. As well, Pauling subsequently alluded to data that many of the patients in the placebo group were actually taking vitamin C.[9]

Another Phase III trial of vitamin C in cancer was carried out, this time only involving colon cancer patients who had not previously received cancer chemotherapy. The results of this study, published in the *New England Journal of Medicine* in 1985, were also negative.[7] Even though this trial involved only colon cancer patients, Moertel concluded that it proved vitamin C has no effect in any type of cancer. For his part, Pauling criticized the study because of several problems related to its design and conduct. There was a failure to confirm in any meaningful way the compliance of treated patients, or to assure that control patients did not supplement their diets with vitamin C; indeed, such monitoring as was carried out by measuring urinary vitamin C levels suggested that a substantial fraction of control patients were medicating themselves with vitamin C. Also, Pauling pointed out that it was incorrect to terminate vitamin C treatment as soon as evidence of tumor progression was obtained, as was done in this trial, if the aim was to learn the effect of the treatment on life span. Thus, patients started on oral ascorbic acid (no intravenous ascorbate was used as in the Cameron and Pauling trial) were instructed to take it (or a placebo) for only 75 days on average, during which time only one patient in either group died.[9] This vitiated any comparison with the Vale of Leven study and indeed, risked shortening the lives of vitamin C-treated patients, since Pauling had previously pointed out that stopping vitamin C was associated with an adverse "rebound" effect of accelerated tumor progression.

Pauling re-analyzed such data as he could obtain from the trial (the Mayo Clinic researchers refused to make their raw data public) and demonstrated an increased death rate among patients whose vitamin C was abruptly terminated. This analysis was submitted to the *New England Journal of Medicine,* but, after a two-year editorial review, was rejected for publication.[10] Because the Mayo

Clinic researchers refused to allow external scrutiny of their data, the possibility that some patients assigned to placebo were actually taking ascorbic acid, and that some patients assigned to ascorbic acid were not taking the amounts prescribed, remains unaddressed.

What Happened in Vale of Leven, Scotland, That Didn't Happen in Rochester, Minnesota?

Even though the physiologic mechanism by which vitamin C exerted its anticancer effect is quite unclear (and might bear no relation to the reasons it was given), the clinical responses recorded in the Vale of Leven patients point to an impelling biological rationale for investigating vitamin C's efficacy in at least some human cancers. Whatever its ultimate place in cancer therapy, it is impossible, in my view, to discard the clinical evidence of a vitamin C effect for at least some patients.

The *New England Journal of Medicine* published its Special Report of a Phase II NCI-sponsored IL-2 trial in advanced cancer in 1985, the same year it published the second Mayo Clinic Phase III vitamin C trial.[16] The report on IL-2 stimulated great interest both within and without the scientific community, with the result that large-scale funding of Phase II IL-2 trials continues up to this date. The clinical response to IL-2 in the NCI trial, and the detail provided in the *New England Journal of Medicine* publication, were equivalent to the experience with vitamin C at Vale of Leven Hospital; the objective documentation was certainly no better. Yet even as they rejected vitamin C based on a narrowly conceived Phase III trial, NCI researchers were vigorously promoting further in-house Phase II IL-2 research, perhaps appreciating that if they used Phase III protocols like Moertel's at this stage of investigation, they would run a high risk of coming up with a negative result.

How could they reason this way? To reach these opposite evaluations of similar data, the NCI experts had to have concluded either that the Vale of Leven results—relief of metastatic bone pain, tumor stasis or regression, tumor necrosis, and repeated remissions in one case of stage IVB non-Hodgkin's lymphoma—were, if not fabricated, grossly misinterpreted by Cameron. Perhaps they believed vitamin C therapy to be so inherently implausible that any alternative explanation for these clinical responses, no matter how far-fetched, must be true. Yet Cameron was a well-respected oncologic surgeon. One of the memorable features of Richards' account in *Vitamin C and Cancer: Medicine or Politics?* is the indelible impression it leaves of Ewan Cameron as a physician of exceptional dignity, humility, intelligence, and integrity.[10] Linus Pauling, who sponsored the examination of the data, was one of the most respected scientific figures of the century. Unlike purveyors of useless nostrums, neither Pauling nor Cameron had anything to gain and much to lose from promulgating false, unpopular data, and they knew it.

Looking back on this history, it is difficult to comprehend the cynical disrespect for Cameron and Pauling implicit in the NCI's rejection of their data. The NCI had only to agree that "something happened" at Vale of Leven to be scientifically required, from any perspective, to acknowledge the need for further investigation. Yet they refused to do this until prodded into it, and, when they finally did proceed, the studies were carried out and interpreted with a hostile bias that stacked the odds against a comprehensive, fair evaluation.

The history of the two Phase III Mayo Clinic trials is important. Whatever their deficiencies, one has to assume they were undertaken in good faith, albeit with an intellectually stifling negative bias and from a naive and ignorant perspective. While the first trial may have been appropriate, its negative findings should have prompted a reevaluation of the situation and the adoption of procedures appropriate for evaluating biologic response modifiers, namely, the conduct of sequential, intelligent, immunologically-monitored Phase II trials in patient groups with a reasonable likelihood of mounting a biologic response, such as those with hematological (blood) malignancies, renal (kidney) cancers, or melanoma (skin cancers). (Phase II IL-2 and TNF trials clearly indicate that colon cancer, the tumor type chosen for study in the second Mayo Clinic trial, is one that is least likely to respond to biologic response modifiers.)

The possibility that prior chemotherapy might obviate the anticancer effect of vitamin C is a valid one that often comes up when other biologicals are evaluated. It was apparently recognized as relevant to vitamin C's effects only after the first Mayo Clinic trial was completed. This issue remains a matter of uncertainty and conjecture but is critically important. There is evidence that prior cytotoxic therapy might even, in some situations, increase rather than decrease the immunologic response to biologic response modifier therapy.[17] More important than prior chemotherapy may have been the patients' overall debility, malnutrition, or yet other factors still unrecognized. Data indicate evidence of an important beneficial response to vitamin C is indeed possible in patients with far less advanced cancers despite and during cytotoxic therapy.

It is difficult to read Richards' account of the Mayo Clinic's second Phase III trial without sharing Cameron's concern that many patients in the active treatment group failed to take all 20 of their vitamin C tablets every day, as well as his suspicion that many in the placebo group ingested vitamin C on their own, vitiating a meaningful comparison of survival times. Any experienced clinical trial investigator will acknowledge the numbing effect on a patient's motivation of being presented with 20 tablets per day, especially when he or she has incurable cancer and when the study personnel harbor a hostile bias that might have been impossible to conceal, even if good faith efforts are made to do so. More fundamentally, by 1985, when Phase II trials of other biologic response modifiers were actively under way, NCI officials must have been aware of the error implicit in designing Phase III trials of the kind used to evaluate cytotoxics for a biologic response modifier like vitamin C if their intention was to evaluate it in good faith, and not merely to efficiently discredit what they perceived as a useless and troublesome quack remedy.

The dramatic episodes of tumor hemorrhage and necrosis at Vale of Leven Hospital suggest to me a vitamin C-triggered immunologic response, if not spearheaded by tumor necrosis factor and/or other cytokines. What unleashed this incredible effect, and why were no such dramatic cases observed in the Mayo Clinic trials? The most likely possibility is that tumor hemorrhage and necrosis is an infrequent response at best, and one which is liable to occur only when vitamin C is administered intravenously in large doses. Another possibility is suggested by the different dietary habits in the United States and Scotland. Vitamin C intakes are higher in America than Europe. Clients of the Mayo Clinic presumably had the cultural attitudes and financial means to purchase and consume orange juice, whereas the vitamin C intake of terminal cancer patients admitted to the wards of a district general hospital in Scotland would be not be expected to be comparably high.[18–20] Are responses of cancer-bearing patients to vitamin C greater when there has been a prior period of deficient intake? Is it possible that vitamin C-susceptible tumor clones develop in a chronically low vitamin-C environment?

Whatever the biologic explanation for vitamin C's effect on cancer, it is one that merits investigation. Does it represent a nonspecific immune stimulation? If so, then unlike the heavy-handed procedure of injecting large amounts of IL-2 and lymphokine-activated lymphocytes, vitamin C might stimulate cytokine release (or upregulate receptor-cell sensitivity, or both) in a coordinated fashion that increases the efficiency of the host response with far less toxicity. The episodes of tumor hemorrhage and necrosis suggest that vitamin C acts high up in the cascade of events that mobilizes an effective antitumor host response. This may be understood by analogy to the human blood coagulation system. A treatment that activates the coagulation cascade physiologically will be far more efficient than one that simply involves infusing large amounts of a single factor whose effects are exerted lower down in the cascade. On the other hand, basic investigations in recent years provide ample evidence that ascorbic acid may exert biochemical effects separate from any effects to enhance immune responsiveness.

One may conclude that apart from any immediate clinical benefit to cancer patients conferred by vitamin C, the evidence that it modulates nonspecific immunity in cancer patients suggests the value of using it to study fundamental mechanisms governing antitumor immunity. An obvious clinical trial possibility is to combine vitamin C (and other nutrients) with non-nutrient biologic response modifiers in Phase II trials. A recent report that IL-2 therapy induces a precipitous and profound reduction of circulating vitamin C levels in cancer patients has obvious implications.[21]

What Has Changed Between 1985 and Now?

In the 1993 edition of *Cancer and Vitamin C*, Cameron and Pauling present 25 cases of dramatic apparent cancer remissions that were reported to the Linus Pauling Institute of Science and Medicine. These cases are dramatic and, taken together with the Vale of Leven experience, indicate that vitamin C therapy has by far the strongest biochemical and clinical support of all alternative cancer therapies. Nevertheless, oncologists are aware of the wide variability in the natural history of cancer even when patients with the same type and stage of disease receive the same therapy. There is understandable skepticism about the meaning of highly selected "best cases" that may well merely represent extremes in the natural history of a cancer rather than a specific response to an unconventional therapy.

But unremitting narrow skepticism carries with it the risk of missing new discoveries. It is no longer appropriate for skeptics to require dramatic, "unexplainable" responses to a specific unconventional therapy before taking it seriously. Rather, it ought to suffice to observe a statistically (and clinically) significantly greater proportion of patients treated with unconventional therapies who have outcomes outside the usual range of response. Perhaps those diseases with the greatest unpredictability in natural history could be the very ones most amenable to unconventional therapy. Failing that, it ought be possible to postulate appropriate biomarkers that predict which patients respond to vitamin C therapy and to monitor that response. In this way the population of patients to be studied can be narrowed to those who are most likely to respond.

What has changed since the second Mayo Clinic trial rang the "death knell" for vitamin C

therapy in cancer? First, in the ensuing years there has been an important increase in understanding of the biology of vitamin C. Understanding of biologic response modifiers has increased, and there is more sophistication in the use of appropriate methods for evaluating them. Moreover, there are data that vitamin C has effects on the immune system that might mediate anticancer effects. Third, the idea that large doses of vitamins can affect human health is no longer considered "crackpot," as it was in 1985. Public interest in alternative therapies of all kinds is at an all-time high, and the resulting infusion of research funds for studying alternative cancer therapies (of which this one is, by orders of magnitude, the most credible of the biological therapies) seems to have a stimulant effect on academics who previously discounted it. Fourth, there is continuing clinical experience, attesting to the safety of high-dose vitamin C when used under proper surveillance, and its clinical efficacy in treating patients who have received or are receiving conventional anticancer therapy.

REFERENCES

1. Cameron E, Pauling L. The orthomolecular treatment of cancer, I. The role of ascorbic acid in host resistance. *Chem Biol Interact* 1974;9:273–283.

2. Cameron E, Pauling L. The orthomolecular treatment of cancer. II. Clinical trial of high-dose ascorbic acid supplements in advanced human cancer. *Chem Biol Interact* 1974;9:285–315.

3. Cameron E, Pauling L. Supplemental ascorbate in the supportive treatment of cancer: prolongation of survival times in terminal human cancer. *Proc Natl Acad Sci, USA* 1976;73:3685–3689.

4. Cameron E, Pauling L. Supplemental ascorbate in the supportive treatment of cancer: reevaluation of prolongation of survival times in terminal human cancer. *Proc Natl Acad Sci, USA* 1978;75:4538–4542.

5. Cameron E, Pauling L. *Cancer and Vitamin C.* Menlo Park, CA: Linus Pauling Institute of Science and Medicine, 1979.

6. Creagan ET, Moertel CG, O'Fallon JR, et al. Failure of high-dose vitamin C (ascorbic acid) therapy to benefit patients with advanced cancer. *N Engl J Med* 1979;301:687–690.

7. Moertel CG, Fleming TR, Creagan ET, et al. High-dose vitamin C versus placebo in the treatment of patients with advanced cancer who have had no prior chemotherapy. *N Engl J Med* 1985;312:137–141.

8. Hoffer LJ. Nutrients as biologic response modifiers. In: *Adjuvant Nutrition in Cancer Treatment* edited by P. Quillan, R. Williams. Arlington Heights, IL: Cancer Treatment Research Foundation, 1993, 55–79.

9. Cameron E, Pauling L. *Cancer and Vitamin C.* 2nd ed. Philadelphia, PA: Camino Books, 1993.

10. Richards E. *Vitamin C and Cancer: Medicine or Politics?* London: MacMillan, 1991.

11. Carswell EA, Old LJ, Kassel RL, et al. An endotoxin-induced serum factor that causes necrosis of tumors. *Proc Natl Acad Sci, USA* 1975;72:3666–3670.

12. Cameron E, Campbell A, Jack T. The orthomolecular treatment of cancer. III. Reticulum cell sarcoma: double complete regression induced by high-dose ascorbic acid therapy. *Chem Biol Interact* 1975;11:387–393.

13. Rosenberg SA, Lotze MT, Muul LM, et al. Progress report on the treatment of 157 patients with advanced cancer using lymphokine-activated killer cells and interleukin-2 or high-dose interleukin-2 alone. *N Engl J Med* 1987;316:889–897.

14. Durant JR. Immunotherapy of cancer: the end of the beginning? *N Engl J Med* 1987;316:939–941.

15. Comroe JH. Experimental studies designed to evaluate the management of patients with incurable cancer. *Proc Natl Acad Sci, USA* 1978;75:4543.

16. Rosenberg SA, Lotze Yt, Muul LM, et al. Special report: observations on the systemic administration of autologous lymphokine-activated killer cells and recombinant interleukin-2 to patients with metastatic cancer. *N Engl J Med* 1985;313:1485–1492.

17. Weisenthal LM, Dill PL, Pearson FC. Effect of prior chemotherapy on human tumor-specific cytotoxicity in vitro in response to immuno-potentiating biologic response modifiers. *J Natl Cancer Inst* 1991;37–42.

18. Krasner N, Dymock IW. Ascorbic acid deficiency in malignant diseases: a clinical and biochemical study. *Br J Cancer* 1974;30:142–145.

19. Dickerson JWT, Basu TK. Specific vitamin deficiencies and their significance in patients with cancer and receiving chemotherapy. *Curr Concepts Nutr* 1977;6:95–104.

20. Fain O, Mathieu E, Thomas M. Scurvy in patients with cancer. *BMJ* 1998;316:1661–1662.

21. Marcus SL, Petrylak DP, Dutcher JP, et al. Hypo-vitaminosis C in patients treated with high-dose interleukin 2 and lymphokine-activated killer cells. *Am J Clin Nutr* 1991;54:1292S–1297S.

PHYSICIAN'S REPORT:
INTRAVENOUS VITAMIN C IN A TERMINAL CANCER PATIENT
by Neil Riordan, PhD, James A. Jackson, PhD, and Hugh D. Riordan, MD

In October 1995, the author (NR) was completing a clinical rotation with a physician in a rural community as part of his Physician Assistant training. A week into the training, a home health-care agency nurse visited the clinic and asked if the medical student or the author knew of a treatment that could help a "terminal" breast cancer patient with pain control. She said the patient had cancer for several years and the latest bone scan showed that the cancer had metastasized to "nearly every bone in her skeleton." She was particularly worried about pain from a metastatic lesion in the patient's left upper arm. The patient was taking intravenous (IV) morphine for pain and needed sublingual morphine to cope with pain associated with getting up and going to the bathroom.

The medical student (who planned on a career in pain management and anesthesia), enthusiastically described a nerve block procedure that would relieve the pain but, "unfortunately," loss of function of the arm, as well. Information about the experiences at the Riordan Clinic with the control of metastatic bone pain using high doses of IV vitamin C was given to the nurse. She was also furnished with references describing the usefulness

of Vitamin C in helping cancer patients. One article, from the present authors, (NR, JAJ, HDR) described the preferential toxicity of vitamin C toward tumor cells, and presented evidence listing the plasma concentrations of vitamin C that would be beneficial as a preferential cytotoxic agent in humans.

The nurse's reaction was less than enthusiastic. She said she would ask the patient if she was interested and would also ask the physician if he would be willing to try something like vitamin C. Since the doses suggested in the article were in excess of 100,000 milligrams (mg) IV per day, and the RDA for vitamin C is 60 mg per day, a positive reply was not expected. Some physicians and health-care workers believe (wrongly) that any dose over 2,000 mg intravenously will either kill you or make you very ill by inducing an acidotic state. As fate would have it, this patient visited the clinic the next day complaining of a painful, swollen, left arm. A Doppler venogram revealed both subclavian veins to be blocked by blood clots. She was admitted to the hospital and started on anticoagulant therapy. Many staff did not think she would leave the hospital alive.

254

Treatment

During clinical rounds, the patient said that she had read the paper on vitamin C and was anxious to try the IV C therapy because it offered her some hope. Also, the home health nurse said that she and the physician had read the article and were willing to try the IV vitamin C treatments. The physician later said he was enthusiastic to try something that could actually have a positive effect on the pain and disease processes. He also said that he wanted to clear the blood clots before starting the vitamin C treatment. He was concerned that, if an embolism occurred and the patient died, it would be blamed on the IV vitamin C treatment (obviously an enlightened physician). He did start the patient on oral vitamin C, 250 mg per day, to prevent scurvy, a common occurrence in disseminated metastatic disease. The patient was treated one time with Activase R to clear the clots. An arterial blood sample was drawn from the patient's wrist shortly after the anticoagulant therapy. This resulted in extensive subcutaneous bleeding with bruising of the entire arm, and the site subsequently became infected, swollen, and hot to the touch. She continued to receive small doses of IV and oral anticoagulant therapy, antibiotic therapy, and oral vitamin C. The infection had not cleared within a week, probably due to poor circulation in the arm and depressed immune system of the patient. The next week, the patient's physician visited and spoke to Dr. Riordan at the clinic. Riordan furnished him with vitamin C to use in the IV treatment.

After two weeks, the patient was strong enough to take high doses of IV vitamin C. Her physician ordered 30,000 mg of vitamin C given IV in Ringer's lactate solution. One of the nurses said that she had never heard of such a high dose and she would not administer it "because it would kill the patient." She was assured by the author (NR) that patients at the clinic and other clinical sites had been given 100,000 mg and more of IV C without any ill effects, and that he had personally taken 60,000 mg IV with no side effects. The nurse was still not convinced. To prove the safety of the IV C, the author started an IV infusion of 30,000 mg of vitamin C in Ringer's lactate on himself. He was seated next to the nurse with the IV pole between them. The infusion lasted an hour and all the time the nurse was saying "you are going to die" and wanted witnesses to the fact that she would not be held responsible. As expected, there were no side effects and after further observation for ill effects by the head nurse for several hours, she finally agreed to give the IV vitamin C to the patient.

The patient received 30,000 mg IV vitamin C on the first day, 40,000 mg the next day and 50,000 mg the following day. After the third dose her right arm was completely without swelling and the swelling in her left arm was greatly decreased. Most notably, the infection in her left hand began to resolve, and she did not need to take sublingual morphine for pain. All, including the physician, nurses, and patient, were very impressed. The physician ordered additional shipments of vitamin C to continue the infusions. Infusions of vitamin C were increased to 100,000 mg per day, administered over five hours.

Results

Within one week of starting the increased vitamin C infusions, the patient was walking around the halls of the hospital, looking like a new person. As the clinical rotation came to an end, the patient invited everyone connected with the vitamin C treatment to her room for a pizza party. The patient had her hair done and makeup on, something she had not done in the recent past. It was a wonderful pizza party, especially for a terminally ill cancer patient, once bedridden with intractable pain due to disseminated bone metastasis who previously was given a few weeks to live. After leaving the hospital, telephone calls were made to the physician to follow up on this patient. He said that she was discharged from the hospital one week after the vitamin C treatments were begun. She continued to take high dose IV C treatments three times a week at home. Three months after she began the IV C treatments she was surviving with resolution of metastasis to the skull as shown by bone scan.

REFERENCES

1. Riordan NH. *Med Hypothesis* 1994;9;2:207–213.
2. Jackson JA. *J Orthomolecular Med* 1990;5:1:57.

From the *J Orthomolecular Med* 1996;11(2):80–82

THE REAL STORY OF VITAMIN C AND CANCER
by Steve Hickey, PhD, and Hilary Roberts, PhD

Vitamin C and cancer has become a hot news topic. For people who have followed this matter, the media's sudden interest comes as something of a surprise: the evidence that vitamin C is a selective anticancer agent has been known for decades. This story is important, as it illustrates how the head-in-the-sand conventional view (that nutritional supplements are useless) can lead to restrictive legislation, reduced health, and limited approaches to the treatment of disease. The recent news story arose from a study by researchers at the U.S. National Institutes of Health (NIH).[1] The NIH experiment showed that, when injected into mice, vitamin C could slow the growth of tumors. The NIH paper presents its findings as new, ignoring the long history of research into vitamin C and cancer. Far from being novel, many of the findings reported in this paper have been recognized for decades. What is strange, however, is that the media suddenly decided to report a story they had ignored for so long.

A History

One strand of this story begins with the work of an old friend, Dr. Reginald Holman. In 1957, Holman published a paper in *Nature* about how hydrogen peroxide (the chemical Marilyn Monroe reportedly used on her hair) destroyed or slowed the growth of tumors in mice.[2] Holman met with some hostility from the medical profession, which slowed his research and clinical work over the following half century. Nevertheless, scientists have known that hydrogen peroxide kills cancer cells for over 50 years. In 1969, when man first walked on the moon, researchers found that vitamin C would selectively kill cancer cells without harming normal cells.[3] That finding meant that vitamin C was like an antibiotic for cancer: potentially a near perfect anticancer drug. Before 1970, it was known that vitamin C was an example of a new class of anticancer substances. However, the medical research establishment largely ignored these scientific results.

In the 1970s, some members of the public and pioneering doctors experimented with high doses of vitamin C to treat cancer. By 1976, double Nobel Prize winner Linus Pauling and Scottish surgeon Ewan Cameron reported clinical trials, showing an unparalleled increase in survival times in terminal cancer patients treated with vitamin C.[4] However, by this time Pauling was considered a quack, having claimed that vitamin C could prevent or cure the common cold, so these apparently amazing findings made little impact.

Cameron and Pauling published a second report in 1978.[5] The Mayo Clinic responded with a study that suggested vitamin C had no effect, which the medical profession readily accepted, perhaps because it confirmed existing prejudices. However, despite the Mayo Clinic study being "considered definitive,"[1] it was highly criticized from the start. In particular, it used relatively low oral doses for short periods, rather than the lifetime combination of high oral and intravenous (IV) doses in the Pauling and Cameron study. The Mayo Clinic refused to provide Pauling with their data so he could check it. When we emailed the Mayo Clinic with a similar request, we received no reply.

If Cameron and Pauling's work, back in the 1970s, had been just a single study, it would have been interesting and suggestive. Such a large increase in survival time demands a proper scientific follow-up and, indeed, other studies soon backed up the findings. Japanese researchers found similar survival times,[6] apparently confirming Pauling's early results. Subsequently, Dr. Abram Hoffer, working in Canada, provided more evidence that vitamin C could enable cancer patients to live much longer. We have analyzed these results and found them to be statistically valid. They are not explicable by placebo effect or by a simple biased selection of long-lived patients. Moreover, over the last three decades, a large number of clinical and anecdotal patient reports support the claims.

From the *J Orthomolecular Med* 2008;23(3):133–138.

A long time before the NIH's mouse experiment, Pauling also studied the effects of vitamin C on cancer in mice. He worked with Dr. Art Robinson but, unfortunately, the two researchers fell out over their interpretations of the results. Robinson left the Linus Pauling Institute (which he had helped establish) and completed the experiment alone. It was eventually published in 1994.[7] The results were outstanding: mice with cancer that were given high-dose vitamin C in the diet, or fed a diet of raw vegetables, lived up to 20 times longer than controls. Translated into human terms, this might mean that a person with 1 year to live might get an extra 20. Importantly, Robinson and Pauling had been inspired to do this experiment by claims from cancer sufferers in the popular literature.

Drs. Hugh Riordan, Ron Hunninghake, James Jackson, Jorge Miranda-Massari, Michael Gonzalez, and others at the Riordan Clinic Health Center did the core research on vitamin C and cancer. They repeated and extended the early work, which had showed vitamin C would selectively kill cancer cells. They have years of experience of treating cancer patients with high-dose vitamin C. Their work is consistent with results from independent researchers and doctors worldwide.[8]

We recently reviewed the literature on vitamin C and cancer, in our book *Cancer: Nutrition and Survival* (2005).[8] We found solid evidence that vitamin C, in high enough doses, acts as a selective anticancer drug. In healthy tissues, vitamin C is an antioxidant, while in cancer it acts as an oxidant generating free radicals and killing the abnormal cells. Furthermore, an understanding of its action provides insight into the cancer development process. Oxidants, such as hydrogen peroxide, are able to make cells grow and divide erroneously. So, as the cells divide, they form a population of varying cells that compete with each other for survival. It was immediately clear that oxidation could explain how cancer starts; following which Darwin's theory of evolution takes over. Given enough time, cells divide and the "fittest" are selected. In this context, the fittest to survive are those cells that grow rapidly to form an invasive cancer. Cancer is not a mysterious disease but is a result of straightforward biological processes.

This microevolutionary model for cancer makes highly specific predictions. One is that high-dose vitamin C should prevent cancer and even higher doses should kill cancer cells. The model also predicts that there could be thousands of selective anticancer drugs. Animals, and especially plants, will contain these substances, because they evolved in the presence of cancer and had to develop ways to control it. If such predictions are correct, we should find a multitude of safe anticancer agents in food. Checking against medical databases, we immediately found numerous examples such as curcumin (from turmeric), alpha-lipoic acid, and vitamin D3. Everywhere we looked, we found substances with the predicted properties. Unfortunately, many are the very supplements the Alliance for Natural Health (ANH) is trying to protect from being banned!

To conclude our history, the NIH paper was essentially a repeat of previous animal experiments. Despite this, the NIH authors appear not to have referenced many of the scientists who did the original work on vitamin C and hydrogen peroxide in cancer. Instead, they present their work as standing alone, in an informational vacuum. With the exception of the Cameron and Pauling clinical trial, the original scientists' work is not mentioned in the NIH text. Wrongly, a reader might gain the impression that the NIH's work was fundamentally original, rather than repeating the work of others. This might mislead the media into ascribing credit for the work on vitamin C and cancer to the NIH, which would be unfair to the real pioneers of this subject.

Intravenous or Oral?

Lead researcher of the NIH study Dr. Mark Levine claims that "When you eat foods containing more than 200 milligrams (mg) of vitamin C a day—for example, two oranges and a serving of broccoli—your body prevents blood levels of ascorbate from exceeding a narrow range."[9] This statement is demonstrably false (the NIH's own data refutes it) and is an artifact of the way the NIH group interpret their experiments.

In their mouse paper, the NIH used intravenous vitamin C, rather than oral. To be more accurate, the NIH used intravenous ascorbate. Sodium ascorbate is normally used for injection, as vitamin C (ascorbic acid) can cause local inflammation at the injection site. The results they obtained are suggestive of a response but do not show the same large effects reported by Dr. Robinson. Robinson fed his mice dietary vitamin C, in very high doses. Thus, the NIH's suggestion that only intravenous vitamin C is useful as an anticancer agent does not appear to fit the animal data. Likewise, the idea that only intravenous vitamin C is effective against cancer does not fit the clinical data. Abram Hoffer, for example, used oral doses and obtained essentially the same results as Cameron and Pauling.

The NIH's insistence that the body has "tight controls," which prevent oral vitamin C from functioning as an anticancer agent, is wrong. In our book *Ascorbate: The Science of Vitamin C* (2004), we have shown that the NIH claims for blood "saturation" at a low level (70 micromoles per liter [μM/L]) are incorrect.[10] The NIH authors never admitted this error, despite a long email correspondence between Hickey and Levine. However, they have changed the wording they use, from "saturated" to "tight controls," and increased the level by about three times (to 200 μM/L). It would appear that they are holding onto an outdated idea about how vitamin C acts in the body. As an alternative, we have proposed a dynamic flow model, in which, at high doses, vitamin C flows through the body, providing antioxidant support, potentially preventing cancer growth and killing cancer cells.[11]

Dynamic Flow

Dr. Levine claims: "Clinical and pharmacokinetic studies conducted in the past 12 years showed that oral ascorbate levels in plasma and tissue are tightly controlled. In the case series, ascorbate was given orally and intravenously, but in the trials ascorbate was just given orally. It was not realized at the time that only injected ascorbate might deliver the concentrations needed to see an antitumor effect."[9] As we have explained, there is no evidence for such tight control. The suggestion that the legendary scientist, Dr. Linus Pauling, or consultant surgeon, Ewan Cameron, did not know the

difference between oral and intravenous administration[12] is bizarre and, again, demonstrably incorrect.[8] The difference between oral and intravenous vitamin C is, however, more complex than suggested by the NIH. Contrary to their conclusions, it is not clear that intravenous vitamin C necessarily provides an advantage over oral supplements in the treatment of cancer. There is a fair case for suggesting that high-dose oral administration could be more effective.

At low intakes, the body prevents vitamin C from being lost through the urine; if this were not the case, we would all be at risk of acute scurvy. The body tries to retain a minimum of about 70 μM/L of vitamin C in blood plasma. This level can be maintained with an intake as low as 200 mg a day. At higher doses, the body can afford to let some vitamin C escape in urine. This saves energy, which the kidneys would otherwise use to keep pumping the vitamin C molecules back into the blood. If dietary vitamin C is in plentiful supply, there is no need for our bodies to retain it all. So, at high doses, vitamin C flows through the body, being taken in from the gut and excreted in the urine. With such high intakes, the body has a reserve that it can call upon in times of need.

A single 5,000-mg dose of vitamin C can generate blood levels of about 250 μM/L; this is above the NIH paper's claimed maximum of 200 μM/L. Moreover, repeated large doses can sustain these levels. We have achieved vitamin C plasma levels above 400 μM/L, following a single dose of oral liposomal (oil-soluble) vitamin C.[13] It seems that the claimed "tight control" concept will need revising again soon.

People vary in their responses to vitamin C. In some people, a single 2,000-mg oral dose of vitamin C may have a laxative effect. Our collaborator, Dr. Robert Cathcart, described this as the bowel tolerance level. Strangely, bowel tolerance has been observed to increase dramatically when a person is ill, say with the flu. A person with a laxative effect at, say, 2,000 mg, may be able to tolerate 100 times more if they become ill. This increased bowel tolerance also occurs in cancer sufferers. It suggests that at times of stress or illness, the body absorbs extra vitamin C. When promoting intravenous vitamin C, the NIH authors have not considered the possibility of such increased bowel tolerance to oral doses.

To achieve the maximum blood plasma levels possible with oral vitamin C, a typical healthy person may need a total intake of about 20,000 mg, spread throughout the day (say 3,000 or 4,000 mg every four hours). However, cancer patients may require far more. Such massive intakes result in consistently high blood levels, which tumor tissues absorb, and which then generate the hydrogen peroxide that kills the cancer cells.

Other possible mechanisms for how vitamin C kills cancer cells[14] are not covered by the NIH study. The NIH based their work on laboratory studies of mice, in which vitamin C kills cancer cells over the course of, perhaps, a couple of hours. Lower levels of vitamin C may simply take longer to kill the cells, which is a standard dose-response relationship. Sustained oral doses can increase plasma vitamin C consistently, over periods measured in months or years: this may, in the end, be more effective that the short, sharp shock of intravenous therapy. Sustained levels also reduce the likelihood of tumors developing resistance to the therapy (analogous to bacterial resistance to antibiotics).

Redox Synergy

When combined with alpha-lipoic acid, selenium, vitamin K3, or a range of other supplements, vitamin C is a far more powerful anticancer agent than when used alone. Experimental data from Riordan and others shows that the cancer-destroying effect of such combinations is much higher. We have described some of these combinations in a recent book *The Cancer Breakthrough* (2007).[15] Strong scientific reasons suggest that such combinations, given orally, could provide cancer sufferers with a large increase in life span and increased quality of life. Just as your doctor advises you to take a whole course of antibiotics continuously, until all infection is gone, vitamin C-based redox therapy needs to be continuous. Like bacterial infections, cancers can rapidly become resistant to intermittent treatments. Typically, intravenous ascorbate is given at intervals, whereas oral ascorbate can maintain blood levels continuously and indefinitely. This is a valid medical reason to prefer an oral regime. Also, patients prefer the oral route, as they have greater control, lower cost, and are more involved in their treatment.

People often ask us what we would do, if we developed the disease. In the event that one of us developed a malignancy, we would opt for a vitamin C-based redox therapy as our primary approach to treatment. This would be based on oral intakes: we would consider intravenous ascorbate only as an adjunct. We might use liposomal vitamin C to sustain blood levels at 400–500 µM/L, together with alpha-lipoic acid, selenium, and other synergistic nutrients.[15] While we realize malignant cancer would place us at high risk of death, we would expect to live a greatly extended life. While the assessment of increased longevity could be inaccurate (the data is not definitive), the risks are small and the potential benefits substantial.

◼ CONCLUSION

Levine claims that the "NIH's unique translational environment, where researchers can pursue intellectual high-risk, out-of-the-box thinking with high potential payoff, enabled us to pursue this work."[9] However, the NIH study, while interesting, adds little to the studies it replicates. More interesting is the lack of historical perspective, which may detract from the people, such as Hugh Riordan, Abram Hoffer, or Linus Pauling, who deserve the credit for carrying out original research, despite conventional medicine actively suppressing their work. The groundbreaking work of doctors such as those in the British Society for Ecological Medicine, who have risked their careers to provide vitamin C-based treatments for cancer and other conditions should be recognized. These pioneering doctors are often well aware of the scientific evidence and should not be described as "complementary" or "alternative." Perhaps, one day, the media will realize the true story of vitamin C and cancer, and patients will have the opportunity to benefit.

The Alliance for Natural Health is defending our right to supplements. Over the last century, we have benefited from a large increase in life expectancy and freedom from many diseases. Much of that benefit has arisen directly from nutrition.[16] We need access to supplements, which provide the possibility of disease prevention without significant risk. If this basic right is removed by Codex Alimentarius, or similar legislation—for example, the draconian regulatory measures the natural health sector is facing in Europe—even pioneering doctors will find it difficult to progress the nutritional treatment of disease. The health of most of us will suffer. We will get more illnesses, more often, and options for medical treatment of major killers, such as cancer, heart disease, and stroke, will decline.

REFERENCES

1. Chen Q, Espey MG, Sun AY, et al. Pharmacologic doses of ascorbate act as a pro-oxidant and decrease growth of aggressive tumor xenografts on mice. *PNAS* 2008;105(32): 11105–11109.

2. Holman RA. A method of destroying a malignant rat tumour in vivo. *Nature* 1957;179:1033.

3. Benade L, Howard T, Burk D. Synergistic killing of ehrlich ascites carcinoma cells by ascorbate and 3-amino-1, 2, 4, -triazole. *Oncology* 1969;23:33–43.

4. Cameron E, Pauling L. Supplemental ascorbate in the supportive treatment of cancer: prolongation of survival times in terminal human cancer. *Proc Natl Acad Sci USA* 1976;73:3685–3689.

5. Cameron E, Pauling L. Supplemental ascorbate in the supportive treatment of cancer: reevaluation of prolongation of survival times in terminal human cancer. *Proc Natl Acad Sci USA* 1978;75:4538–4542.

6. Murata A, Morishige F, Yamaguchi H. Prolongation of survival times of terminal cancer patients by administration of large doses of ascorbate. *Int J Vit Nutr Res, Suppl* 1982;23:101–113.

7. Robinson AR, Hunsberger A, Westall FC. Suppression of squamous cell carcinoma in hairless mice by dietary nutrient variation. *Mech Aging Devel* 1994; 76: 201–214.

8. Hickey S, Roberts H. *Cancer: Nutrition and Survival.* Raleigh, NC: Lulu Press, 2005.

9. NIH. Vitamin C injections slow tumor growth in mice. *NIH News.* Aug 4, 2008.

10. Hickey S, Roberts H. *Ascorbate: The Science of Vitamin C.* Raleigh, NC: Lulu Press, 2004.

11. Hickey S, Roberts H, Cathcart RF. Dynamic flow. *J Orthomol Med* 2005;20(4):237–244.

12. Padayatty SJ, Levine M. Reevaluation of ascorbate in cancer treatment: emerging evidence, open minds and serendipity. *J Am Coll Nutr* 2000;19(4):423–425.

13. Hickey S, Roberts H, Miller NJ. Pharmacokinetics of oral ascorbate liposomes, *JNEM* 2008;17(3):169–177.

14. Toohey J. Dehydroascorbic acid as an anticancer agent. *Canc Lett* 2008;263:164–169.

15. Hickey S, Roberts HJ. *The Cancer Breakthrough.* Raleigh, NC: Lulu Press, 2007.

16. Wootton D. *Bad Medicine.* New York: Oxford University Press, 2007.

PHYSICIAN'S REPORT:

CASE STUDY: HIGH-DOSE INTRAVENOUS VITAMIN C IN THE TREATMENT OF A PATIENT WITH ADENOCARCINOMA OF THE KIDNEY

by Hugh D. Riordan, MD, James A. Jackson, PhD, and Mavis Schultz, ARNP

In late 1985, a 70-year-old, white male complained of pain in his right side. A urinalysis showed gross hematuria. He was referred to a urologist who, through x-rays and computed tomography (CT) scans, diagnosed the patient as having a small stone in the right kidney, and a large, solid, space occupying mass in the lower pole of the right kidney. Adenocarcinoma was suspected and in December 1985, a radical nephrectomy was performed on the right kidney and adenocarcinoma was confirmed by pathological studies. His left kidney was completely functional. He was followed by an oncologist at another clinic. About three months after surgery, the patient's X-rays and CT scan studies showed "multiple pulmonary lesions and lesions in several areas of his liver which were abnormal and periaortic lymphadenopathy." None of the lesions were biopsied.

Treatment

The patient decided not to undergo chemotherapy, hormone therapy, or cytotoxic treatment of any kind. He requested and was started on vitamin C intravenous (IV) treatment. He was started 30,000 milligrams (mg) of vitamin C in 250 mL in a salt solution given by intravenous injection (60 drops per minute) twice a week for seven months. The treatments were then reduced to one per week and 1 milliliter (mL) of magnesium was added to the vitamin C and salt solution. This treatment lasted for eight months, then for six months he received 15,000 mg of vitamin C weekly in 250 mL of salt solution with 1.0 mL of magnesium.

Results

In April 1986, about six weeks after the x-ray and CT scan studies, the oncologist's report showed "the patient returns feeling well. His exam is totally normal. His chest x-ray shows a dramatic improvement in pulmonary nodules compared to six weeks ago. The periaortic lymphadenopathy is completely resolved."

In June 1986, the oncologist reported the patient "has been receiving vitamin C shots now twice weekly, feeling well and playing golf. On exam day, his weight is up a couple of pounds and he looks well. He has absolutely no evidence of progressive cancer." The oncologist's report in July 1986 stated "the patient has been feeling well with no symptoms of cancer . . . Chest x-ray today is totally normal. The pulmonary nodules are completely gone. There is no evidence of lung metastasis, liver metastasis or lymph node metastasis today, whatsoever."

The report of September 1986 stated, "On exam today, there is absolutely no evidence of recurrent cancer and we have opted to continue our observation. I suggest he continue with you the vitamin C shots . . . "

In March 1987, fifteen months after surgery, the report stated, "the patient is feeling well, and on exam today there is absolutely no evidence of recurrent cancer. He wishes to continue his vitamin C shot once weekly as well, which seems reasonable to me."

To date, after three and a half years the patient remains cancer free. He returns at irregular intervals for a 30,000-mg vitamin C IV treatment.

During and after the treatments, the patient showed no toxic, or unusual side effects from the high-dosage IV vitamin C therapy. Periodic blood chemistry profiles and urine studies were normal.

Comments

Various theories have been presented on how vitamin C controls or inhibits the growth of malignant tumors. The antioxidant properties of vitamin C may prevent free radical damage to all tissues.[1] Vitamin C is also thought to increase host resistance against cancer by enhancing lymphocyte functions, by increasing resistance of the intercellular ground substance to hydrolysis produced by tumor cells, and by protecting the pituitary-adrenal axis from the effects of stress.[2] In 1974, Drs. Campbell and Cameron treated 50 advanced cancer patients with 10,000 mg of oral vitamin C daily and reported that 5 had objective tumor reactions.[3] Drs. Cameron and Pauling later reported on 100 cancer patients treated with oral vitamin C from the date when the patient's disease became untreatable. When compared to 1,000 "historical controls," the survival of the patients taking vitamin C was increased to a mean of 293 days or more compared to the control group of 30 days.[4] Dr. Noto and others showed that vitamin C and vitamin K3 had a growth-inhibiting action at high concentrations on in vitro cultured human neoplastic cell lines MCF-7 (breast carcinoma), KB (oral epidermoid carcinoma), and AN3-CA (endometrial adenocarcinoma) when given separately. When combined, the inhibition of cell growth occurred at 10 to 50 times lower concentrations.[5]

The case study presented here differs from other studies in that the amount of vitamin C administered was higher (30,000 mg versus 10,000 mg) and the route of administration was different (IV versus oral).

REFERENCES

1. Watson RR. *Am Diet Assoc* 1986;86:505–510.

2. Cameron E. *Chem Biol Interact* 1974;9:285–315.

3. *Ibid.*

4. Cameron E. Proc Natl Acad Sci 1978;75:4538–42, 1978.

5. Noto V. *Cancer* 1989;63:901–906.

SCHEDULE DEPENDENCE IN CANCER THERAPY: WHAT IS THE TRUE SCENARIO FOR VITAMIN C?

by Jorge Duconge, PhD, Jorge R. Miranda-Massari, PharmD,

Michael J. Gonzalez, PhD, and Neil H. Riordan, PhD

Many agents in cancer chemotherapy are highly schedule-dependent. The axiom underlying this pattern is: "Response is *not* proportional to cumulative drug dose or area under the disposition curve, instead response is proportional to cumulative drug effect" (meaning, same total dose size but different response depending on dosing schedule). For instance, fewer administrations of larger doses of cisplatin (Platinol) and etoposide (Etopophos), both widely used chemotherapeutic agents, were generally less satisfactory than multiple but smaller treatments. The most effective sequence was an alternating regimen, by which the cytoreductive effects (reduction in number of cancer cells) of cisplatin resulted in recruitment of quiescent (non-dividing) cells into active proliferation, enhancing in turn the efficiency of subsequent etoposide schedules: 30 milligrams (mg), 50 mg, and 15 mg (four times) every 10 hours by bolus injection to few cancer patients.[2] (Bolus injection is a method that increases the concentration of a drug in the bloodstream so the drug can start working quickly.)

Comparing the 15-mg and 30-mg doses there was no significant increase in early drug levels but a marked increase in terminal half-life (time required to divide the concentration by two). At doses higher than 30 mg, however, there was a steep increase in early drug levels too. However, in this dose range a steep dose-dependent rise in early drug levels is to be expected. As early high-serum levels correlate with congestive heart failure, administration schedules reaching effective concentration without high-peak levels, such as continuous infusion or consecutive administration of low doses, seem to be necessary.[2]

In another study the authors aimed at determining possible schedule-dependent pharmacokinetic and pharmacodynamic interactions between 800 mg of gemcitabine (Gemzar, given as 30-minute infusion) and 50 mg of cisplatin (given as one-hour infusion) in 33 patients with advanced-stage solid tumors in a Phase I trial. Sixteen patients had a four-hour interval between gemcitabine (days 1, 8, 15) and cisplatin (days 1 and 8), followed by the reverse schedule and 17 patients had a 24-hour interval between gemcitabine (days 1, 8, 15) and cisplatin (days 2 and 9), followed by the reverse schedule. Of all schedules, the treatment of patients with cisplatin, 24 hours before gemcitabine, led to the highest gemcitabine–triphosphate accumulation and levels in plasma. These characteristics formed the basis for further investigation of this schedule in a Phase II clinical study.[3]

In some circumstances, continuous infusion does not seem to be the optimal schedule because this type of administration could down-regulate (reduce or suppress) the target expression, which might constitute a mechanism of resistance to the drug. Then, repeated administration over a longer critical period should be favored.

Discussion

In a recent work, we conducted a pharmacokinetic characterization of six different intravenous vitamin C infusion dosage scheme given at high doses, following dose-escalation protocols (15,000–65,000 mg, five cycles), in a 75-year-old prostate cancer patient. The results for this pilot pharmacokinetic study of vitamin C at high-dose infusions, in a cancer patient, suggest a dual-phase kinetic behavior of ascorbate such as earlier reported in vitro.[4] This disposition pattern depends on the actual infusion-generated plasma ascorbate concentrations with respect to the saturation cut-off level (about 70 micromoles or 0.123 mg per deciliter [μM/dL]).

As Hickey and coworkers have pointed out, the short half-life of vitamin C during the rapid excretion phase is sometimes ignored, particularly

From the *J Orthomolecular Med* 2007;22(1):21–26.

262

by the National Institute of Health's dose and frequency of intake recommendations.[5] Plasma levels above 70 µM have a half-life of approximately 30 minutes, so large doses taken several hours apart should be considered independent, as should be their bioavailability.[5] This cumulative pattern means that splitting a single large dose into several smaller ones, taken a few hours apart, increases the effective bioavailability of the large dose.

In another report from a colleague in Vermont, the following results were observed for a 60-year-old, 105-pound, breast cancer patient taking 10,000 mg of oral vitamin C in divided doses each day. The plasma ascorbate levels after infusion of 75,000 mg over 75 minutes were 521 mg/dL. Strikingly, the same patient one month later was infused with 50,000 mg in 30 minutes, and then continued with another 25,000 mg over the next 90 minutes, the resulted plasma ascorbate concentration at steady-state was 423 mg/dL. According to Dr. William Warnock, the results suggest that once blood levels of ascorbate are established it is possible to maintain them over a period of time with a much lower amount. The infusion rate over the first 30 minutes was about 1,600 mg per minute and over the next 90 minutes was about 300 mg per minute. Previously, this patient had been receiving 75,000 mg of vitamin C three times a week for about two months but she did not seem to be making significant progress with her cancer (personal communication, Warnock; 2006).

Notably, in a recent survey using another dosing schedule, Dr. Warnock infused first 50,000 mg over 30 minutes (i.e., initial dosage in the same breast cancer patient) but this time he continued dosing 50,000 additional milligrams of vitamin C intravenously within the next three hours. Reportedly, the ascorbate level at the end of the 3.5 hours was 355 mg/dL. Accordingly, Dr. Warnock concluded that by using a higher infusion rate (i.e., 25,000 mg per hour for a total dose of 75,000 mg over 3 hours) he will be able to stay over 400 mg/dL indefinitely, and finally speculated about keeping a constant infusion going over 24, 48, or even 72 hours. In fact, the same schedule has been postulated by Drs. Miranda-Massari and Gonzalez for intravenous vitamin C administration based on his own experience.

All these observations together are suggesting a schedule-dependence phenomenon in vitamin C pharmacokinetic-pharmacodynamic relationship. Fractionating overall dose size and increasing the period of administration (exposure time) appear to offer a therapeutic advantage in terms of both efficacy and toxicity. It is assumed that the time during which the drug concentrations are maintained close to the "target concentration" seems to be critical for anti-tumor activity and highest efficacy.

Interestingly, Dr. Hugh Riordan and coworkers earlier reported that some cancer patients had complete remissions after high-intravenous infusion doses of vitamin C, even though the concentrations of vitamin C that kill most tumor cells in vitro (200–400 mg/dL) were not achieved (immediately) after the infusion of 30,000 mg of vitamin C.[6] Consequently, they argued that remissions in patients treated with this schedule are likely to have occurred as a result of vitamin C–induced biological response modification effect rather than direct cytotoxic effects.[6] But, what if we look at the cumulative (net) vitamin C effect instead of the cumulative vitamin C concentrations? Again, we speculate about the schedule-dependence in pharmacokinetics of vitamin C to account for such a discrepancy. The saturable kinetic for ascorbate distribution into cells call for slower intravenous infusion of high vitamin C doses.

IN BRIEF

Schedule-dependence is a very common phenomenon that is observed with drugs used for cancer therapy. Large intermittent doses are often more toxic and less effective than smaller repeated doses. The state of the art in schedule-dependence and its potential role for designing the optimal vitamin-C dosing regimen is discussed in the light of some literature reports and preliminary results from a pilot study we conducted at high-vitamin C dosage. Accordingly, we recommend that any further clinical protocol for pharmacokinetic assessment of vitamin C in cancer patients should be conducted based upon the schedule-dependence approach.

CONCLUSION

In consideration of the presented evidence, we recommend that any further clinical protocol for assessing the kinetic response of vitamin C in cancer patients should be conducted based upon the schedule-dependence approach, as necessary corroboration with experimental data is mandatory. In addition, the use of turnover concept and indirect response modeling for vitamin C pharmacometric analysis also needs further discussion.

REFERENCES

1. Durand RE, Vanderbyl SL. Schedule dependence for cisplatin and etoposide multifraction treatments of spheroids. *J Natl Cancer Inst* 1990;82(23):1841–1845.

2. Erttmann R, Erb N, Steinhoff A, et al. Pharmacokinetics of doxorubicin in man: dose and schedule dependence. *J Cancer Research and Clinical Oncology* 1988;114(5):509–513.

3. Van Moorsel CJA, Kroep JR, Pinedo HM, et al. Pharmacokinetic schedule finding study of the combination of gemcitabine and cisplatin in patients with solid tumors. *Annals Oncol* 1999;10 (4):441–448.

4. Casciari JJ, Riordan HD, Miranda-Massari JR, et al. Effects of high dose ascorbate administration on I-10 tumour growth in guinea pigs. *PRHSJ* 2005;24(2):145–150.

5. Hickey DS, Roberts HJ, Cathcart RF. Dynamic flow: a new model for ascorbate. *J Orthomolecular Med* 2005;20(4): 237–244.

6. Riordan NH, Riordan HD, Casciari JP. Clinical and experimental experiences with intravenous vitamin C. *J Orthomolecular Med* 2000;15(4):201–213.

INTRAVENOUS VITAMIN C AS CANCER THERAPY: FREE ACCESS TO 32 EXPERT VIDEO LECTURES ONLINE

There is extensive published research demonstrating vitamin C's anticancer properties.[1] In the 1970s, Hugh D. Riordan, MD, and colleagues began studying the underlying causes of cancer and ways to treat cancer in a non-toxic fashion. From this research came the Riordan Intravenous Vitamin C Protocol for Cancer (see Appendix 3). This protocol is widely recognized in the integrative and orthomolecular medicine community and is commonly used as an effective adjunct to conventional oncologic therapy.

Oncologist Victor Marcial, MD, has experience using it. He says: "We studied patients with advanced cancer (stage 4). Forty patients received 40,000–75,000 mg intravenously several times a week . . . In addition, they received a diet and other supplements. The initial tumor response rate was achieved in 75 percent of patients, defined as a 50 percent reduction or more in tumor size . . . As a radiation oncologist, I also give radiation therapy. Vitamin C has two effects. It increases the beneficial effects of radiation and chemotherapy and decreases the adverse effects. But this is not a subtle effect, is not 15–20 percent, it's a dramatic effect. Once you start using IV vitamin C, the effect is so dramatic that it is difficult to go back to not using it."[2]

In 2009, 2010, and 2011, Riordan IV-C and Cancer Symposiums brought together medical professionals, researchers and IV-C practitioners from the United States and abroad. The latest advancements in intravenous vitamin C cancer therapy were presented in detail, recorded on video, and are now available for free access at:

- **For 2009:** www.riordanclinic.org/education/symposium /s2009 (12 lectures)

- **For 2010:** www.riordanclinic.org/education/symposium /s2010 (9 lectures)

- **For 2011:** www.riordanclinic.org/education/symposium /s2012 (11 lectures)

Readers are urged to watch, and have their physicians (especially oncologists) watch, these important presentations.

REFERENCES

1. Free access to full text papers at www.riordanclinic.org /research/journal-articles.shtml and also http://orthomolecular .org/library/jom.

2. Presentation at the Medical Sciences Campus, University of Puerto Rico, April 12, 2010.

Excerpted from the *Orthomolecular Medicine News Service*, October 14, 2011.

TEN QUESTIONS FOR DOCTORS:
A CANCER PATIENT'S QUEST FOR ASCORBIC ACID THERAPY
by Graham Carey with Andrew W. Saul, PhD

These questions arise out of my experience of my local United Kingdom (UK) National Health Service (NHS) refusing to allow moderate cost intravenous ascorbic acid infusions, which could be carried out in my local doctor's office, on the grounds that this treatment has not undergone a proper scientific trial. Ascorbic acid, about which some 48,000 medical papers have been written, is one of the most used, most safe and most advocated of substances. I challenge orthodox NHS oncologists to show how the testing of substances by double-blind placebo-controlled trials is almost exclusively the way to medical excellence, and to answer the following questions.

QUESTION #1. Do you believe that there is only one valid medical tradition for health improvement—the one which currently permeates the NHS?

QUESTION #2. Was orthodox health care ineffective before double-blind placebo-controlled studies became common? Richard Horton, editor of the *Lancet* (August 2006), made a complementary point, in connection with the treatment of HIV/AIDS: "Why does our definition of science still seem to include only the laboratory experiment and the clinical trial?"

QUESTION #3. With regard to drug safety, how do you account for the tens of thousands, perhaps hundreds of thousands, of iatrogenic deaths and harms that occur in the UK, many of them relating to drugs, while as far as I can establish no one anywhere has ever died from a high oral or intravenous dose of vitamin C? We all have friends and relations who rely on and are grateful for medicines with high-risk factors attached to them. Warfarin (Coumadin) is a commonly dispensed orthodox substance that is also used to kill rats and, if it is not carefully monitored, can cause bald patches, purple toes, hepatic (liver) dysfunction, nausea, vomiting, hemorrhaging, jaundice, and diarrhea. Oral vitamin-C takers risk only diarrhea. Kidney stones, as a much touted side-effect of

megadose vitamin C, can be regarded only as a scare story used by people who have not read the literature. Drs. Hickey and Roberts (2004) write that the margin of safety for high-dose vitamin C is much greater than for aspirin, antihistamines, antibiotics, all pain medications, muscle relaxants, tranquilizers, sedatives, and diuretics.

QUESTION #4. My experience of the insistence by doctors on random control trials suggests that this requirement laid down by the NHS has become routine, almost a dogma, in the NHS. Do you think that this should always come before informed patient choice, especially when cost is not the main factor? Also, is the practice of running random control trials on seriously ill patients ethical?

QUESTION #5. How would you justify the almost total ignoring by orthodoxy of the major successes with ascorbic acid, and the prosecution of good doctors who treat with ascorbic acid? Drs. Klenner, Pauling, Cameron, Stone, Levine, Levy, Cathcart, and others must feature importantly and positively in 21st-century medical practice. Their good science resulted in the saving of life and correction of the lamentable distortion of the early expectations for, and results of, vitamin C. This is the time to press home the reiterated refrain of its advocates, "dosage, dosage, dosage," in order to attain sufficiently high blood plasma levels for it to be effective. Hickey and Roberts (2004) cite the consistently positive clinical results that Dr. Robert Cathcart has had over two decades with thousands of patients with "massive" vitamin C doses, ranging from 15,000 to over 200,000 milligrams (mg), up to the bowel tolerance limit and administered in up to 20 to 25 doses a day.

QUESTION #6. Random control trials frequently do not take into account the interactions of patients' other drugs and substances. Is it not true that when

From the *J Orthomolecular Med* 2008;23(1):3–5.

a patient is taking a second drug the trial becomes unscientific? What about the massive onslaught on the human body of both widely dispersed and localized industrial pollution of water and air, workplace stress, and multiple new sources of radiation? How can medical epidemiology, valuable as it is, deal scientifically with such complexities?

QUESTION #7. If the practice of orthodox western medicine is an unfolding and dynamic one, how does this observation square with the static dogma of random control trials as presently constituted? Hickey and Roberts write, "To object that a study is not double-blind and that treatment should be delayed for several years until such tests had been performed would be ridiculous." When a new treatment has a high safety margin and low cost, it could be made available to patients even before the results of follow-up studies were known, without medical, scientific, or ethical objections. The development of penicillin proceeded in just this way.

QUESTION #8. What ethical stand does a doctor take with regard to the "need" for high profit levels in the pharmaceutical industry, and all the injustices that spring from this? One wonders why there is such readiness to accept expensive and frequently ever more unsafe drug treatments. In my own case, an NHS nurse practitioner is able to carry out this work only 300 yards from my house, at a cost of only a few hundred pounds [in 2013, about $300–$400] depending on the protocol adopted. A typical course of cancer chemotherapy costs between £4,000 and £5,000 [about $6,000–$7,500]. There is little or nothing to lose in allowing a treatment, which is having widespread success, as a second line of defense to orthodox treatment, which is eventually liable, even likely, to fail. It would seem sensible to combine the apparent but limited success of a hormone therapy such as goserelin (Zoladex, my own present treatment) with intravenous ascorbic acid megadosing. This is what I am seeking for myself.

QUESTION #9. How am I to proceed with my health care when few if any are prepared to read the new and optimistic unorthodox work, and many happy to dismiss and debunk it? I have been receiving high-quality orthodox medical

attention from my local general practitioners for many years, as well as from hospital doctors, and I consider myself fortunate in the care that I receive. In my recent serious medical condition, however, I have discovered a resolute inability on the part of doctors who treat me to have a proper awareness of the achievements of other doctors and scientists who work outside the NHS. Perhaps this is due to high work loads or burnout. I recognize that many doctors, especially in inner urban practices, have an impossibly large health-care task. Yet even my hospital has written to say that it cannot find the time to read the clinical documents that I sent through the post. My general practitioner investigates some studies of mutual interest, but there is of course a limit to this. He has written to me that I would be "hard pushed to get any sensible doctor to prescribe" the treatment that I legitimately seek.

QUESTION #10. On what basis do doctors still insist on toxicity testing for vitamin C? Practitioner and researcher Dr. Brian A. Richards states: "There is no need for toxicity testing: ascorbate is one of the least toxic substances known. Similarly, double-blind testing is not required. We are assessing a gross effect, using large doses. DBT is not required any more than it was, at the time, to test say either anesthesia or surgical asepsis. The dramatic responses require no such subtleties of assessment."

Why We Are Still Waiting?

Figures released from the Department of Health, and a King's Fund report, "Future Trends and Challenges for Cancer Services," show that one in three will soon be contracting cancer and one in four dying from it. "Thousands of new treatments are in development but many are high-cost and currently of marginal benefit . . . We need a public debate with informed media coverage," says the report. There might be a case for making decisions "at a local level, with public involvement in policy-making and developing local criteria for clinical eligibility." Don't we have in the case of ascorbic acid just the kind of treatment, alone or with other substances, and moderate cost at that, which this report might be calling for?

Ascorbic acid is a crucial biological substance in the human body: we all once made it. Almost all other animals make it but a genetic fault somewhere down our ancestry caused us to stop doing so. If a great scientist like Pauling thinks vitamin C is thus the most important substance in the medical world, cannot we "give it a go"?

[Editor's note: The NHS refused to try the therapy Graham Carey asked for. Mr. Carey died two years after this article was first published.]

LITERATURE CITED

Steven H, Hilary R. *Ascorbate: The Science of Vitamin C.* Raleigh, NC: Lulu Press, 2004.

Thomas E. Levy. *Vitamin C, Infectious Diseases and Toxins: Curing the Incurable.* Bloomington, IL: Xlibris, 2002.

Rosy Daniel. *The Cancer Directory.* Hammersmith, UK: Harper Thorsons, 2005.

Padayatty et al. Intravenously administered vitamin c as cancer therapy: three cases. *Can Med Assoc J* 2006;174(7):937–942.

VITAMINS DECREASE LUNG CANCER RISK BY 50 PERCENT

by Robert G. Smith, PhD

A recent study[1] of the effect of B vitamins on a large group of participants reported an inverse relationship between blood serum levels of vitamin B6, methionine, and folate and the risk of lung cancer. High serum levels of vitamin B6, methionine, and folate were associated with a 50 percent or greater reduction in lung cancer risk. This exciting finding has not been widely reported in the media, but it confirms a growing body of evidence gathered over the last 40 years that B vitamins are important for preventing diseases such as cancer.

The study gathered information about the lifestyle and diet of 385,000 people in several European countries. The average age was 64 years, and most had a history of drinking alcohol daily. Blood samples were then taken from these participants, and some of those (889) that developed lung cancer were analyzed for the level of several B vitamins and related biochemicals such as methionine, an essential amino acid. These nutrients were studied because they are known to be important in the metabolism of single carbon compounds, which is necessary for the synthesis and repair of DNA in the body's tissues.[2] Thus, B vitamins are helpful in preventing defects in DNA that can cause cancer.[2–4]

Specifically, a high level of either vitamin B6, or methionine, or folate reduced the risk for lung cancer. High levels of all these nutrients together produced an even lower risk. The effects were large, so the results are highly significant.

The study divided the participants into three categories, depending on whether they currently smoked, had previously smoked, or had never smoked. While smoking is the most important lifestyle factor in the risk for lung cancer, interestingly, the effects of vitamin B6, methionine, and folate were fairly constant among the three categories. That is, those with higher levels of these B vitamins had a significantly lower risk of lung cancer no matter whether they smoked or not. The report emphasizes that this result strongly suggests that the effect of these essential nutrients in lowering the risk for cancer is real and not purely a statistical correlation. And, the report reiterates that smoking is dangerous, greatly increasing the risk for lung cancer in older people after decades of insult to the lungs.

The question begged by the report is, what role did vitamin supplements play in the blood levels reported for these essential nutrients? Taking a multivitamin that includes B-complex vitamins will obviously increase the blood levels of these essential nutrients. However, the value of supplements was not emphasized in the report.

So we will emphasize it here. Vitamins dramatically lower lung cancer risk. Supplements provide these nutrients in abundance. Modern diets do not.

REFERENCES

1. Johansson M. *JAMA* 2010 Jun 16; 303(23): 2377–2385.
2. Xu X. *J Genet Genomics* 2009; 36: 203–214.
3. Larsson SC. *JAMA* 2010;303:1077–1083.
4. Ames BN. *J Nucleic Acids* 2010;pii:725071.

Excerpted from the *Orthomolecular Medicine News Service*, November 18, 2011.

VITAMIN C AND CHEMOTHERAPY
by Steve Hickey, PhD, and Hilary Roberts, PhD

A paper in *Cancer Research* by Dr. Mark Heaney claims that vitamin C antagonizes the cytotoxic (cell-killing) effects of chemotherapeutic drugs.[1] On closer examination, the evidence presented does not support the claim. Contrary to Dr. Heaney's suggestions, vitamin C is an effective anticancer agent, capable of killing cancer cells at concentrations achievable by oral supplementation.[2] Other researchers argue that vitamin C enhances the effectiveness of chemotherapy and curbs its side effects.[3] To understand these apparent contradictions, we need to appreciate the differing roles of vitamin C in the body and in tumors.

Ascorbate and dehydroascorbate vitamin C is a simple chemical called ascorbate or ascorbic acid. Ascorbate is an antioxidant: each molecule can donate two electrons, helping to prevent free radical damage in the body. When ascorbate (vitamin C) donates its two electrons, it is oxidized to a different molecule called dehydroascorbate.

In their experiments, Heaney and others used dehydroascorbate or oxidized vitamin C, rather than ascorbate. Dehydroascorbate is an oxidant: it tends to gain electrons. Inside cells, dehydroascorbate molecules can be reduced back to ascorbate, by gaining electrons, produced using the cells' metabolic energy. In tissues, this expenditure of cellular energy may add to the stress on sick cells, which typically exist in an oxidizing environment, under free radical attack.[4,5] Vitamin C (ascorbate, antioxidant) has low toxicity, whereas dehydroascorbate (oxidized ascorbate, oxidant) is more toxic. Importantly, these two molecules can influence cancer cells in contrasting ways.

Ascorbate and Cancer

Vitamin C can act as an anticancer agent, killing cancer cells by generating hydrogen peroxide and other oxidants. In tumors, vitamin C acts as an oxidant, rather than as an antioxidant. Together with free (unbound) iron or copper, the vitamin C causes a redox cycling Fenton reaction (named after Henry Fenton, who first described it at the end of the 19th century, which releases a cytotoxic oxidant, hydrogen peroxide. Many other substances, such as alpha-lipoic acid, vitamin K3, or the chemotherapeutic drug motexafin gadolinium, work similarly with vitamin C to generate oxidation and kill cancer cells.

Dehydroascorbate and Cancer

In healthy individuals, the body maintains low dehydroascorbate levels to minimize toxicity. When dehydroascorbate is formed, cells take it up and reduce it back to ascorbate. Thus, in healthy individuals, the level of dehydroascorbate in cells is low, relative to the amount of ascorbate.[6] People taking vitamin C supplements consume ascorbate, not dehydroascorbate. Researchers have suggested dehydroascorbate for use as an anticancer agent. To quote a recent paper, the results of studies on the effects of dehydroascorbate as an anticancer agent are "truly remarkable."[8]

Dehydroascorbate is selectively toxic to cancer cells.[7,8] Its effectiveness has been demonstrated both in vitro[9] and in animal studies. In standard survival studies (using mice with a cell line of leukemia known as P388, and Ehrlich carcinoma), 50 control mice received saline injections and had an average life expectancy of 11 days. Fifty experimental mice received 2 milligrams (mg) of dehydroascorbate (80 mg/kg) and lived for a minimum of 31 days; half of these had no detectable tumor cells and went on to survive long term.[10]

These dehydroascorbate results, like those on vitamin C itself,[11,12] put chemotherapy to shame. In such experiments, even with aggressive conventional chemotherapy, an increase in life expectancy of about two days would be considered significant[13]; long-term survival is rare.[8]

In another study, researchers investigated the effects of dehydroascorbate on the growth of solid

From the *J Orthomolecular Med* 2008;23(4):183–186.

tumors (Krebs 2 sarcoma and Ehrlich carcinoma). Control mice with Ehrlich carcinoma had an average tumor size of more than 2 cm (just under 1 inch)[2], whereas the subject mice, treated with injections of dehydroascorbic acid (2 mg per day about 80 mg/kg), developed no obvious tumors. In the control group, the Krebs sarcoma tumors were on average larger than 1.6 cm[2] (just over .5 inches) yet of those in the dehydroascorbate-treated group, only two of 25 mice developed detectable (small) tumors.[14,15]

Animal studies have shown dehydroascorbate to be an effective anticancer agent, at doses lower than those for vitamin C.[16] These results were considered so unusual by an establishment accustomed to the failure of standard chemotherapy that they were considered suspect and ignored. However, continuing research into ascorbate and dehydroascorbate as anticancer agents confirms their potential.

Dehydroascorbate Is Not Vitamin C

In the study by Heaney et al.,[1] the authors assume that giving an injection of dehydroascorbate is equivalent to giving vitamin C; this is incorrect. In healthy tissues, high levels of dehydroascorbate are toxic and generate oxidative stress, whereas ascorbate's antioxidant action prevents such stress.

Within cancer tissues, the action of the two molecules is also different. Dehydroascorbate is absorbed rapidly by the cancer cells, where it may be reduced to ascorbate through use of metabolic energy. By contrast, ascorbate often remains in the extracellular space, where it takes part in a redox cycle, generating dehydroascorbate, hydrogen peroxide, and hydroxyl radicals. This results in oxidative damage to the cancer cells, which is cytotoxic.[12] In addition, the resultant dehydroascorbate may be taken up by the cancer cells and reduced, placing additional oxidative stress on the tumor.

Poor Experimental Methods

In the Heaney et al. paper, the researchers gave high doses of dehydroascorbate to cancer cells in vitro. The cancer cells absorbed the dehydroascorbate and reduced it internally, thus accumulating high levels of intracellular ascorbate (vitamin C). Our microevolutionary model[17] predicts that such levels of ascorbate could protect cancer cells from further stresses, such as chemotherapy. The intracellular ascorbate would lessen the occurrence of apoptosis (cell destruction) and might potentially aid cancer growth. However, these findings have no relevance to the use of ascorbate as an anticancer agent, nor do they suggest, as Heaney et al. argue, that high intakes of vitamin C are contraindicated during conventional chemotherapy.

Normally, the body maintains relatively high levels of ascorbate, compared to dehydroascorbate. In tumors, ascorbate is converted to dehydroascorbate, in a mechanism that generates hydrogen peroxide and hydroxyl radicals. This produces severe oxidation, which destroys cancer cells by apoptosis and other mechanisms. Thus, high levels of ascorbate lead to an environment that is toxic to cancer cells. Once this poisonous environment exists, cancer cells may absorb the dehydroascorbate. However, reducing it back to vitamin C adds a second oxidative stress, taking energy from the cellular metabolism.

Thus, high levels of ascorbate do not act as antioxidants in tumors, but as oxidants, in a process that adds an additional selective stress to the tumor as it undergoes chemotherapy. Rather than acting as an antioxidant against the chemotherapy, as suggested, high levels of ascorbate should be synergistic with it. This action has been demonstrated in previous studies.[18–23] In their study, Heaney et al. circumvented the cytotoxic vitamin C–Fenton reaction process, by using dehydroascorbate rather than ascorbate. Their study therefore has little relevance to the use of ascorbate as an anticancer agent.

Inconsistent Results

In their mouse experiments, Heaney and others report no appreciable anticancer effects with dehydroascorbate at a dose of 250 mg/kg. However, reports in the literature have demonstrated that, in mice, 300 mg/kg doses have a "truly remarkable" antitumor effect.[8] In some animal studies, dehydroascorbate appears to outperform standard chemotherapeutic approaches. The paper by Heaney et al. is inconsistent with these earlier animal studies, which are not cited in the paper.

Conventional Chemotherapy Is Rarely Effective

Conventional chemotherapy has had some success in Hodgkin's disease, acute lymphocytic leukemia, testicular cancer, and in cancers that can occur during pregnancy such as choriocarcinoma, or in childhood such as retinoblastoma and Wilms' tumor. However, these rare forms account for less than 5 percent of cancers in the United States. In the majority of cancers, there is little evidence that chemotherapy extends life substantially.[24] The contribution of chemotherapy to survival is approximately a 2 percent increase (treated versus untreated patients).[25] The cost of this is high, both financially and in terms of reducing the quality of remaining life. Given such poor therapeutic results, oncologists should ask themselves why they continue to encourage patients to accept chemotherapy and yet ignore the potential benefits of vitamin C–based redox therapy.

REFERENCES

1. Heaney ML, Gardner JR, Karasavvas N, et al. Vitamin C antagonizes the cytotoxic effects of antineoplastic drugs. *Cancer Res* 2008;68(19):8031–8038.

2. Hickey S, Roberts HJ, Miller NJ. Pharmacokinetics of oral vitamin C. *JNEM* 2008; 31 July.

3. Stoute JO. The use of vitamin C with chemotherapy in cancer treatment: an annotated bibliography. *J Orthomolecular Med* 2004;19(4):198–245.

4. Hickey S, Roberts H. *Ascorbate: The Science of Vitamin C.* Raleigh, NC: Lulu Press, 2004.

5. Hickey S, Roberts HJ, Cathcart RF. Dynamic flow: a new model for ascorbate. *J Orthomolecular Med* 2005;20(4):237–244.

6. Stone I. *The Healing Factor: Vitamin C Against Disease.* New York: Putnam, 1974.

7. Poydock ME, Fardon JC, Gallinia D, et al. Inhibiting effect of vitamins c and B12 on the mitotic activity of ascites tumors. *Exp Cell Biol* 1979;47:210–217.

8. Toohey JI. Dehydroascorbic acid as an anticancer agent. *Canc Lett* 2008;263:164–169.

9. Poydock ME, Reikert D, Rice J, et al. Inhibiting effect of dehydroascorbic acid on cell division in ascites tumors in mice. *Exp. Cell Biol* 1982;50:34–38.

10. Poydock ME, Reikert D, Rice J. Influence of vitamins C and B12 on the survival rate of mice bearing ascites tumor. *Exp Cell Biol* 1982;50:88–91.

11. Gonzalez MJ, Miranda Massari JR, et al. Orthomolecular oncology: a mechanistic view of intravenous ascorbate's chemotherapeutic activity. *PR Health Sci J* 2002;21(1):39–41.

12. Hickey S, Roberts H. *Cancer: Nutrition and Survival.* Raleigh, NC: Lulu Press, 2005.

13. Stone S, Miller I. Statistical properties of the L1210 mouse leukaemia tumor system in primary screening. *Cancer Chemother Rep* 1975;5:5–13.

14. Poydock ME, Phillips L, Schmitt P. Growth-inhibiting effect of hydroxycobalamin and ascorbic acid on two solid tumors in mice. *IRCS J Med Sci* 1984;12:813.

15. Poydock ME: Effect of combined ascorbic acid and B12 on survival of mice with implanted ehrlich carcinoma and L1210 leukemia. *Am J Clin Nutr* 1991;54,1261S–1265S.

16. Poydock ME, Harguindey S, Hart T, et al. Mitogenic inhibition and effect on survival of mice bearing L1210 leukemia using a combination of dehydroascorbic acid and hydroxycobalamin. *Am J Clin Oncol* 1985;8:266–269.

17. Hickey S, Roberts H. Selfish cells: cancer as microevolution. *J Orthomolecular Med* 2006; 23(3):137–146.

18. Taper HS, De Gerlache J, Lans M, et al. Nontoxic potentiation of cancer chemotherapy by combined C and K3 vitamin pretreatment. *Int'l J Canc* 1987;40:575–579.

19. Skimpo K, Nagatsu T, Yamada K, et al. Ascorbic acid and adriamycin toxicity. *Am J Nutr* 1991;54:1298S-1301S.

20. De Loecker W, Janssens J, Bonte J, et al. Effects of sodium ascorbate (vitamin c) and 2methyl1,4naphthoquinone (vitamin K3) treatment on human tumor cell growth in vitro: synergism with combined chemotherapy action. *Anticanc Res* 1993;13:103–106.

21. Sarna S, Bhola RK. Chemoimmunotherapeutical Studies on Dalton's lymphoma in mice using cisplatin and ascorbic acid: synergistic antitumor effect in vivo and in vitro. *Archivum Immunol et Thera Exper* 1993;41:327–333.

22. Prasad KN, Hernandez C, Edwards Prasad J, et al. Modification of the effect of tamoxifen, cisplatin, DTIC, and interferon 2b on human melanoma cells in culture by a mixture of vitamins. *Nutr Canc* 1994; 22/3: 233–245.

23. Chiang CD, Song E, Yang VC, et al. Ascorbic Acid increases drug accumulation and reverses vincristine resistance of human non-small cell lung cancer cells. *Biochem J* 1994;301:759–764.

24. Abel U. Chemotherapy of advanced epithelial cancer: a critical review. *Biomed Pharmacother* 1992;46(10):439–452.

25. Morgan G, Ward R, Barton M. The contribution of cytotoxic chemotherapy to 5-year survival in adult malignancies. *Clin Oncol (R Coll Radiol)* 2004;16(8):549–560.

SIXTEEN-YEAR HISTORY WITH HIGH-DOSE INTRAVENOUS VITAMIN C TREATMENT FOR VARIOUS TYPES OF CANCER AND OTHER DISEASES

by James A. Jackson, PhD, Hugh D. Riordan, MD, Nancy L. Bramhall, RN, and Sharon Neathery

We have reported on the use of high-dose intravenous vitamin C in the treatment of patients with various types of cancer.[1-4] Research conducted at the Riordan Clinic Health Center has also been published to help explain the scientific basis for the dynamics of intravenous vitamin C.[5-7] Many health-care workers are wary of giving high-dose vitamin C to patients due to the warning that "one could develop kidney stones with high-dose vitamin C." The possibility of kidney stones does exist, theoretically, because vitamin C (ascorbic acid) is water soluble and is excreted by the kidneys as oxalic acid. Since most kidney stones consist of some form of oxalate, it would seem to follow, to some people, that high doses of vitamin C cause kidney stones. In reality, this never happens. Were this the case, then why are there thousands of people with kidney stones who *do not* take large doses of vitamin C?

Humans cannot make ascorbic acid. They must get their vitamin C from the diet or with supplements. Millions of years ago, our ancestors lost the enzyme gulonolactone oxidase, which is key in the conversion of glucose to vitamin C. If the above theory about vitamin C causing kidney stones is correct, why is it that animals are not suffering an epidemic of kidney stones? Based on body weight, the smallest to the biggest animal can manufacture a daily amount of vitamin C that can vary from 1,000 milligrams (mg) to over 20,000 mg (about 12.5 to 250 times the Recommended Dietary Allowance for humans)! In addition, one of us (JAJ) has been taking 6,000 mg of vitamin C daily for over ten years. His kidneys are fine, but, according to the kidney stone theory, his kidneys should be concrete!

Our Data

At the center, infusing patients with high doses of intravenous (IV) vitamin C is not taken lightly. Any time an intravenous injection is given, there is always a danger to the patient. We always measure the level of the enzyme glucose-6-phosphate dehydrogenase (G6PD) in a patient before IV vitamin C is given. A deficiency of G6PD in the red blood cells of an affected individual may result in a hemolytic crisis (destruction of red blood cells) when vitamin C, or other types of substances are given. We also measure the electrolytes (minerals that conduct electricity), especially sodium, and osmolality (total salt concentration) of the patient's blood to make sure that the sodium from the sodium ascorbate (vitamin C) causes no adverse osmotic or electrolyte problem. In the 16-year history of this treatment, no patient has been troubled with a kidney stone, hemolytic, or osmolality problem.

Our data shows that we treated 153 patients (66 men, 87 women) with a diagnosis of the following types of cancer: breast (40), prostate (23), lung (11), pancreas (11), lymphoma (11), renal (10), colon (9), ovary (6), non-Hodgkin's lymphoma (5), myeloma (4), liver (3), sarcoma (3), leukemia (3), melanoma (2), bone (1), brain (1), cervix (1), thyroid (1), and

---

I have treated over 1,600 cancer patients, most of whom were given 12,000 milligrams per day or more of ascorbic acid, in combination with other nutrients. The results have been good and at least 40 percent of the 1,600 reached ten-year cure rates. A small number of patients who were on every attending physician's terminal and untreatable list were cured. Linus Pauling and I had examined the follow-up data and found that the significant prolongation of these patients' lives favors the use of the vitamins. We published this in our book Healing Cancer: Complementary Vitamin & Drug Treatments *(2004).* —ABRAM HOFFER

From the *J Orthomolecular Med* 2002;17(2):117–119.

271

colorectal (1). The total number of IV vitamin Cs given was 3,239. The lowest total dose of IV vitamin C given to one patient was 15,000 mg; the highest total dose given to one patient was 190,075 mg.[5] Total amount of IV vitamin C given to all patients was 104,432,000 mg or about 230 pounds.

Patients with diseases other than cancer were also treated with IV vitamin C. Data from 120 patients (32 men, 88 women) are shown to have fatigue (38), upper respiratory infection/influenza (25), arthritis (9), virus infections (5), and other miscellaneous conditions (43). The total number of IV vitamin Cs given was 4,708. The lowest dose given to one patient was 15,000 mg; the highest dose given was 110,947 mg. The total amount of IV vitamin C given to all patients was 890,622 mg or 197 pounds. The most IV vitamin C given at one time to a patient was 115,000 mg.

This data together represents 194,054,000 mg, or 427 pounds, of IV vitamin C administered to 275 patients with no sign of serious kidney disease, or any other significant side effects over a 16-year period. Our center is not unique in using high doses of vitamin C to treat various diseases. Dr. Abram Hoffer has been using high-dose vitamin C for years to treat patients with cancer and various other diseases.[9] There are many other pioneers in the long-term use of high-dose vitamin C. Among these are Drs. Ewan Cameron, Robert F. Cathcart, Emanuel Cheraskin, Linus Pauling, Irwin Stone, and Neil H. Riordan, just to name a few.

There is another argument used by some health-care workers against the use of vitamin C or other nutrients for the treatment of diseases. This is "the lack of double-blind, placebo-controlled studies" that the Food and Drug Administration (FDA) insists on as one means of granting approval for use of medicines in patients. Dr. Hoffer commented on double-blind controlled experiments in an editorial in 1993 that is worth reading.[10] In addition, these numerous studies that one has to do to prove the safety of medicines is not foolproof by any means, as exemplified by the recent recall of the cholesterol lowering statin drug, Tmor.[11] This drug passed all the experiments required by the FDA but still caused 100 deaths from unexpected side effects before it was recalled. It is also interesting to note

that this recall received little notice in the popular press, or the various medical "experts" on television. Also, remember the article published in 1998 in the Journal of the American Medical Association. Data calculated from 1994 showed there were 106,000 deaths in hospitals from adverse drug reactions and that the number of deaths per year remained stable over the last 30 years![11] However, when a vitamin or nutrient study has any type of negative slant to it, it is page one news and all over the television news shows!

■ CONCLUSION

Our experience over the past 16 years has shown vitamin C to be a safe and effective treatment for many diseases. We continue to use it today and will continue to do so in the future.

REFERENCES

1. Jackson JA, Riordan, HD, Schultz M. High-dose intravenous vitamin C in the treatment of a patient with adenocarcinoma of the kidneys: a case study. *J Orthomolecular Med* 1990;5–1:5–7.

2. Jackson JA, Riordan HD, Hunninghake R, et al. High-dose intravenous vitamin C and long time survival of a patient with cancer of the head of the pancreas. *J Orthomolecular Med* 1995;10–2:87–88.

3. Riordan NH, Jackson JA, Riordan HD. Intravenous vitamin C in a terminal cancer patient. *J Orthomolecular Med* 1996; 11–2:80–82.

4. Riordan HD, Jackson JA, Riordan NH, et al. High-dose intravenous vitamin C in the treatment of a patient with renal cell carcinoma of the kidney. *J Orthomolecular Med* 1998;13–2:72–73.

5. Riordan NH, Riordan HD, Jackson JA. Intravenous ascorbate as a tumor cytotoxic chemo-therapeutic agent. *Med Hypothesis* 1994; 44–3: 7–213.

6. Casciari JP, Riordan NH, Jackson, JA, et al. Cytotoxicity of ascorbate, lipoic acid and other antioxidants in hollow fibre in vitro tumors. *Brit J Canc* 2001;84–11:1544–1550.

7. Goodwin JS, Tangum MR. Battling quackery. *Arch Intern Med* 1998;158(20):2187–2191.

8. Riordan NH, Riordan HD, Casciari JP, et al. Clinical and experimental experiences with intravenous vitamin C. *J Orthomolecular Med* 2000;15:201–203.

9. Hoffer A: How to live longer and feel better—even with cancer. *J Orthomolecular Med* 1996;11–3:147–167.

10. Hoffer A. What goes around comes around: Alaskan Bears and double-blind controlled experiments. *J Orthomolecular Med* 1993;8-4:195–197.

11. Lazarou J, Pomeranz BH, Corey PN. Incidence of adverse drug reactions in hospitalized patients: a meta-analysis of prospective studies. *JAMA* 1998;279:10–15.

INTRAVENOUS ASCORBATE TREATMENT OF BREAST CANCER: A CASE REPORT

by Bernhard G. Welker, MD

A 73-year-old woman underwent diagnostic procedures in January 2010. Clinically, a solid mass of 4 centimeters (cm) in diameter (about 1.5 inches) was found between the outer upper and outer lower quadrant of her right breast with inflammation of the skin and a lymph node of 2 cm (1.2 in) in diameter in the right armpit. A biopsy revealed an inflammatory ductal carcinoma. This type of breast cancer tends to have a higher chance of spreading and a worse outlook (prognosis) than typical invasive ductal cancer.

Further diagnoses were irregular heartbeat, insufficiency of the tricuspid and mitral valves, mitral valve stenosis, hypertension, arteriosclerosis, elevated liver enzymes, and type 2 diabetes. Since 2006 she was treated with daily heart medications that included verapamil (240 milligrams [mg]), olmesartanmedoxomil (30 mg), hydrochlorothiazide (25 mg), furosemide (60 mg), pantoprazol (20 mg), iodine (100 mcg), metoprolol succinate (95 mg), and phenprocoumone (a systemic anticoagulant drug).

Patient Compliance

After all diagnostic procedures were finished, the patient refused any therapy for her breast cancer. Ten months later, in November 2010, she was seen for the first time at my office. She was also taking the estrogen modifier tamoxifen at a dose of 20 mg per day, but neither chemotherapy nor radiation was performed.

Despite not taking all of her medications daily, she assured us that she was compliant with the phenprocoumone. Her international normalization ratio (INR; indicative of clotting tendency of the blood) result was in the therapeutic range. Symptoms observed were edema of the legs, nausea, vertigo, and epistaxis (nose bleeding). The tumor in her breast, which was accompanied with inflammation of her skin that measured 4 cm in diameter, had serous secretion out of its center where the biopsy was taken.

She requested intravenous ascorbate (IVA) therapy and continued not to pursue chemotherapy or surgical treatment for her breast cancer. Abram Hoffer s daily diet (whole unprocess foods and no sugar) and supplement regimen for cancer was offered[1] but she was unwilling to follow it because she was on so many medications. She was also unwilling to abstain from sugar intake. IVA therapy was initiated and was the only treatment she agreed to. She was administered two infusions of IVA per week, and would have only one or no infusions during holidays. Each IVA treatment contained 15,000 milligrams (mg) of ascorbate and lasted approximately one hour. This dosage corresponded to 190 mg of ascorbate per kilogram (2.2 pounds) of body weight. No side effects were observed and INR monitoring remained stable. Her previously elevated liver enzymes decreased slightly and her blood pressures remained unchanged.

After three months the metastatic lymph node was not palpable anymore and could not be visualized by ultrasound. The inflammation of the skin measured 3.0 by 2.5 cm (1.2 by .8 in) and the rims of the tumor in the breast were not sharp-edged anymore.

Six months after the beginning of IVA treatment the inflammation of the skin almost disappeared. The tumor was 2.5 cm in diameter as measured by mammography. No enlarged regional lymph nodes were found. The patient always felt well. No other metastases were identified by x-ray and ultrasound.

The serum level of the tumor marker was normal in June 2011; it had not been measured earlier. Over the course of IVA therapy, her international normalized ratio (INR) values (clotting tendency of blood) ranged from 1.7 to 2.6, systolic blood pressures ranged from 130 to 170 mmHg, and diastolic blood pressures ranged from 80 to 110 mmHg. Testing of her lipids, ferritin, iron, selenium, and zinc were normal.

Unexpectedly, the patient died in July 2011 of a gastrointestinal hemorrhage. No autopsy was performed.

From the *J Orthomolecular Med* 2011;26(4):175–178.

Discussion

This report suggests resolution of a lymph node metastasis and regression of primary breast cancer from infusions of 15,000 mg of IVA therapy over the course of eight months. No other specific therapy or dietary interventions were used during this period of time. No side effects were observed and the patient did not suffer.

IVA therapy did not significantly alter the patient's daily dose of phenprocoumone (or her INR), suggesting that it might be safe to apply both simultaneously. Theoretically, kidney stone formation could occur. However, when attempting to combat cancer it might be reasonable to accept the risk of kidney stones if IVA therapy helps. Patients with histories of renal insufficiency, renal failure, systemic iron overload, glucose-6-phosphate dehydrogenase deficiency (an enzyme that helps break down oxidizing substances such as vitamin C), or who are actively undergoing dialysis should be excluded from receiving this therapy.

Spontaneous regression is often touted by individuals to dismiss the putative merits of IVA therapy. Spontaneous regression means "the partial or complete disappearance of a malignant tumor in the absence of all treatment, or in the presence of therapy that is considered inadequate to exert significant influence on neoplastic disease."[2] This assumption cannot be applied to the present case.

It is evident that the results obtained with ascorbate[3–6] in cancer treatment over the past decades are reproducible, even when the protocol is not well established, and even if chemotherapy shortly before or simultaneously with IVA might influence the efficacy of ascorbate.[7] In cases where chemotherapy has not been shown to benefit a specific cancer or when a patient refuses such treatment, it might make sense to use IVA therapy.

Riordan and others[8] elucidated that ascorbate selectively destroys cancer, but not normal cells by generating hydrogen peroxide. Chen and others[9] confirmed that tumor cell destruction is mediated by extracellular ascorbate at pharmacologic concentrations achievable through intravenous administration. It was concluded that ascorbate may serve as a prodrug (forerunner) for hydrogen peroxide delivery. There is even speculation that special preparations of oral ascorbate might achieve concentrations sufficient enough for it to function as a prodrug.[10]

More reports have been published on IVA therapy for advanced cancers than for early-stage cancers. Hopefully, this report contributes to an emerging body of literature supporting IVA therapy for early-stage diseases, as there was a definitive diagnosis of cancer, documentation of disease response, absence of confounders, and documentation of treatment history.

In summary, IVA therapy of breast cancer should be studied further, as it might be an effective primary treatment. Also, it could be considered as a strategy to prevent both metastases and cancer recurrences following primary cancer treatment.

REFERENCES

1. Hoffer A, Pauling L. *Vitamin C and Cancer: Discovery, Recovery, Controversy.* Kingston, ON: Quarry Press, 1999; republished as *Healing Cancer: Complementary Vitamin and Drug Treatments* in 2004 by CCNM Press, Toronto, Ontario.

2. Cole WH, Everson TC. *Spontaneous Regression of Cancer.* Philadelphia, PA: W.B. Saunders, 1966.

3. Cameron E, Campbell A. The orthomolecular treatment of cancer. ii. clinical trial of high-dose ascorbic acid supplements in advanced human cancer. *Chem Biol Interact* 1974;9:285–315.

4. Riordan HD, Jackson JA, Riordan NH, et al. High-dose intravenous vitamin c in the treatment of a patient with renal cell carcinoma of the kidney. *J Orthomolecular Med* 1998;13:72–73.

5. Padayatty SJ, Riordan HD, Hewitt SM, et al. Intravenously administered vitamin c as cancer therapy: three cases. *CMAJ* 2006;174:937–942.

6. Ichim TE, Minev B, Braciak T, et al. Intravenous ascorbic acid to prevent and treat cancer-associated sepsis? *J Transl Med* 2011;9:25–38.

IN BRIEF

Intravenous ascorbate (IVA) therapy was applied to a patient with breast cancer in November 2010. Continuous tumor regression was observed over the course of eight months. Neither surgery nor chemotherapy was performed. For this patient, IVA therapy was successful, safe, and without side effects. Unexpectedly, the patient died in July 2011 of gastrointestinal hemorrhage. No autopsy was performed. IVA therapy of breast cancer should be studied further, as it might be an effective treatment.

7. Hoffer LJ, Levine M, Assouline S, et al. Phase I clinical trial of IV ascorbic acid in advanced malignancy. *Ann Oncol* 2008;19:1969–1974.

8. Riordan NH, Riordan HD, Meng X, et al. Intravenous ascorbate as a tumor cytotoxic chemotherapeutic agent. *Med Hypotheses* 1995; 44: 207–213.

9. Chen Q, Espey MG, Krishna MC, et al. Pharmacologic ascorbic acid concentrations selectively kill cancer cells: action as a pro-drug to deliver hydrogen peroxide to tissues. *Proc Natl Acad Sci* 2005;102:13604–13609.

10. Hickey S, Roberts HJ, Miller NJ. Pharmacokinetics of oral vitamin C. *J Nutr Environ Med* 2008;17:169–177.

DAILY MULTIVITAMIN REDUCES CANCER RISK

by Robert G. Smith, PhD

A major new health study found that everyday multivitamin supplements lower your risk of cancer by 8 percent.[1] This is terrific news for everyone. Cancer deaths in the United States in recent years have hovered near 600,000 per year (190 per 100,000) and are increasing.[2] If taking a daily multivitamin will prevent 8 percent of these deaths, then the lives of 48,000 people in the United States could be saved each year, just by taking an inexpensive daily vitamin pill.

The study was performed on approximately 15,000 older men, half assigned randomly to take a multivitamin tablet and the other half to take a placebo. The men included in the study were medical doctors older than 50, including some older than 70, averaging about 64, and being doctors, most were in good health, exercised regularly, ate generous amounts of fruits and vegetables, and did not smoke.[1] Overall the risk of cancer was low, about 2 percent per person per year. After about 11 years, the cases of cancer in the 15,000 participants were tabulated. Those who took the multivitamin tablet were diagnosed with 89 fewer (1,379 vs. 1,290) cases of cancer, which represents a reduction of 8 percent.[1] This result, although modest, is significant because the reduction in risk was greater than would be expected by chance.

The multivitamin tablet used in the study contained doses of low-quality vitamins and minerals, some in an inaccessible form, such as magnesium oxide. The doses were similar to the recommended daily amounts published by the Institute of Medicine of the National Academies.[3] Such low doses, because they represent only an average minimum dose for health, should not be taken as the most appropriate dose for anyone. Many, perhaps most, of us require much higher levels of essential nutrients because of poor diet, stressful lifestyle, and differences in their genetic background.

Most vitamin and mineral supplements when taken at appropriate doses are extremely safe. Many nutritionists recommend doses of vitamins B1, B2, B5, and B6 in the range of 50– 100 mg/day; vitamin B3 (niacin) in the range 200–1,000 mg/day in divided doses; vitamin C in the range of 3,000–6,000 mg/day in divided doses; vitamin D in the range of 1,500–2,000 IU/day or up to 5,000– 10,000 IU/day for large or obese adults; and vitamin E in the range of 400–1200 IU. Most of us have a deficiency in magnesium, which has been implicated in an elevated risk for cancer, and a dose of 200–500 mg/day of magnesium or more, taken in the proper form to recover from deficiency, will help to prevent cancer.[4] Higher supplemental doses of vitamins and minerals, along with an excellent diet, do the best job helping the body to fight cancer and other chronic diseases.[5,6]

REFERENCES

1. Gaziano JM, et al. Multivitamins in the prevention of cancer in men: the Physicians' Health Study II Randomized Controlled Trial. *JAMA* 2012:1–10.

2. NCI. Report to the nation finds continuing declines in cancer death rates since the 1990s. Press release. Mar 28, 2012, at www.cancer.gov/newscenter/newsfromnci/2012/ReportNation Release2012

3. IOM. List of RDA for vitamins and minerals. Sept 12, 2011, at www.iom.edu/Activities/Nutrition/SummaryDRIs/DRI Tables.aspx.

4. Dean C. *The Magnesium Miracle*. New York: Ballantine Books, 2006.

5. Ames BN. Prevention of mutation, cancer, and other age-associated diseases by optimizing micronutrient intake. *J Nucleic Acids* 2010; article ID. 725071.

6. McCann JC, et al. Adaptive dysfunction of selenoproteins from the perspective of the triage theory: why modest selenium deficiency may increase risk of diseases of aging. *FASEB J* 2011; 25:1793–1814.

Excerpted from the *Orthomolecular Medicine News Service*, October 26, 2012.

CLINICAL AND EXPERIMENTAL EXPERIENCES WITH INTRAVENOUS VITAMIN C

Neil H. Riordan, PhD, Hugh D. Riordan, MD, and Joseph P. Casciari, PhD

Vitamin C has potential as a chemotherapeutic agent. Rather than possessing adverse side effects as most chemotherapeutic drugs do, vitamin C has side benefits such as increasing collagen production and enhancing immune function.

We began to study the effects of vitamin C on cultured tumor cells in 1991. We found that vitamin C was preferentially toxic to tumor cells: it killed tumor cells before killing normal cells. This phenomenon first came to our attention through the work of Benade and others in 1969.[1] They theorized that the preferential toxicity was due to the relative deficiency of catalase in tumor cells. (Less of the enzyme catalase increases the likelihood of higher hydrogen peroxide levels that kill cancer cells.) This theory has since been validated by others.[2] Our early findings on preferential vitamin C toxicity were published in 1994.[3] In that paper we also described a so-called serum effect; vitamin C's toxicity was reduced by the presence of human serum. Serum's inhibitory effects led us to the conclusion that the concentrations of vitamin C that were toxic to tumor cells in our early studies—5 to 50 milligrams per deciliter (mg/dL)—would not necessarily be toxic in vivo.

We, therefore, began a series of experiments in which we tried more closely to mimic the in vivo tumor environment. In particular, we began testing for toxicity of vitamin C toward cultured tumor cell lines using dense monolayers and hollow fiber tumor models to mimic the three dimensionality of tumors. We used human sera as culture media to include the serum inhibitory activity seen in previous assays. Using these new culture conditions we found that the cytotoxic concentration of vitamin C for most human tumor cell lines was indeed much higher than previously described.

For the purposes of this paper reference to ascorbic acid or vitamin C refers to sodium ascorbate. All in vitro studies described herein used sodium ascorbate. All intravenous vitamin C references herein refer to the use of ascorbic acid buffered to a pH range of 5.5–7.0 by sodium hydroxide and/or sodium bicarbonate.

Human Vitamin C Pharmacokinetics

Given the information that higher concentrations of vitamin C were required to become cytotoxic to tumor cells, we needed to learn more about the pharmacokinetics of vitamin C. There were no data on the concentrations of vitamin C that were achievable in human beings after high-dose intravenous vitamin C. We therefore began a series of experiments to yield data for modeling pharmacokinetics of high doses of vitamin C.

We gave a series of vitamin C infusions to a 72-year-old male who was in excellent physical condition except for slowly progressing, non-metastatic carcinoma of the prostate. Before the infusions, and at intervals thereafter, blood was drawn and the plasma analyzed for plasma vitamin C concentration. From this experiment we observed that a 30,000 mg-infusion was not adequate to raise plasma levels of vitamin C to a level that was toxic to tumor cells (>200 mg/dL for dense monolayers and >400 mg/dL for hollow fiber models). Infusion of 60,000 mg resulted in a brief (30 minute) elevation of plasma levels of vitamin C above 400 mg/dL, while 60,000 mg infused over 60 minutes immediately followed by 20,000 mg infused over the next 60 minutes resulted in a 240-minute period in which the vitamin C plasma concentration was near or above 400 mg/dL.

Potentiation of Preferential Toxicity of Vitamin C

Because plasma concentrations of vitamin C of greater than 200 mg/dL are problematic to maintain, we began looking for ways to increase the

From the *J Orthomolecular Med* 2000;15(4):201–213.

sensitivity of tumor cells to vitamin C. During experimentation we found that alpha-lipoic acid (a water- and lipid-soluble antioxidant that recycles vitamin C) can enhance the tumor toxic effects of vitamin C. Alpha-lipoic acid decreased the dose of vitamin C required to kill 50 percent of the tumor cells from 700 mg/dL to 120 mg/dL.

Effects of High-Dose Vitamin C on Tumor-Cell Collagen Production

It is well known that vitamin C is required for the hydroxylation of proline, and that low levels of vitamin C can be a limiting factor in the production of collagen. Because many tumor cells produce collagenase and other proteolytic enzymes, we wanted to determine if vitamin C supplementation would increase collagen production by tumor cells, thereby having a balancing effect on collagenase. In an experiment, we supplemented cultured tumor cells with vitamin C concentrations that are achievable with oral supplementation (2 and 4 mg/dL) and measured the collagen produced using a well-known method.[5] We found that indeed, these concentrations of vitamin C greatly increased the production of collagen.

Clinical Experiences

We have not observed toxic reactions to high-dose intravenous vitamin C. All patients are pre-screened for the genetic disorder glucose-5-phosphate dehydrogenase deficiency (G6PD).

Patients with Renal Cell Carcinoma Treated with Intravenous Vitamin C

One of us (HDR) reported positive effects of vitamin C therapy in a patient with adenocarcinoma of the kidney in 1990.[4] This report described a 70-year-old white male diagnosed with adenocarcinoma of his right kidney. Shortly after right nephrectomy, he developed metastatic lesions in the liver and lung. The patient elected not to proceed with standard methods of treatment. Upon his request, he began intravenous vitamin C treatment, starting at 30,000 mg twice per week. Six weeks after initiation of therapy, reports indicated that the patient was feeling well, his exam was nor-

mal, and his metastases were shrinking. Fifteen months after initial therapy, the patient's oncologist reported the patient was feeling well with absolutely no signs of progressive cancer. The patient remained cancer-free for 14 years. He died of congestive heart failure at the age of 84.

A second case study, published in 1998,[5] described another complete remission in a patient with metastatic renal cell carcinoma. The patient was a 52-year-old white female from Wisconsin diagnosed with non-metastatic disease in September 1995. In October 1996, eight metastatic lung lesions were found: seven in the right lung and one in the left, measuring between 1 and 3 centimeters (about 0.4 to 1.2 inches). The patient chose not to undergo chemotherapy or radiation treatments. The patient was started on intravenous vitamin C and specific oral nutrient supplements to correct diagnosed deficiencies and a broad-spectrum oral nutritional supplement in October 1996. The initial dose of intravenous vitamin C was 15,000 mg, subsequently increased to 65,000 mg after two weeks. The patient was given two infusions per week. Intravenous vitamin C treatments were continued until June 6, 1997. An x-ray taken at that time revealed resolution of all but one lung metastases. The patient discontinued intravenous vitamin C infusions at that time and continued taking the broad-spectrum oral nutritional supplement. A radiology report on a chest x-ray taken January 15, 1998, stated that no significant infiltrate was evident, and there was resolution of the left upper lobe lung metastasis. In February 1999 a chest x-ray showed no lung masses, and the patient reported being well at that time.

Combined Intravenous Vitamin C and Chemotherapy in a Patient with Stage IV Colorectal Carcinoma

In April 1997, a 51-year-old white male from Wichita, Kansas, was first seen at our center. A workup demonstrated the presence of a distal colon lesion. On December 31, 1997, he underwent an anterior colon resection and appendectomy at a local hospital. The colon tumor penetrated through the bowel wall and into the surrounding adipose tissue. Two large hepatic (liver) metastases were discovered at

277

the time of surgery; one was biopsied. Pathology revealed that the colon lesion was a moderately differentiated adenocarcinoma, and the liver biopsy was metastatic adenocarcinoma. Following surgery he received chemotherapy with weekly fluorouracil (5-FU) and leucovorin (which increases its anticancer effect) for twelve cycles. The patient and his wife, who is a registered nurse, asked the chemotherapist about getting intravenous vitamin C along with the chemotherapy. The oncologist informed them that vitamin C would not be of any value.

The patient was then seen at Pittsburg University Hospital on May 13, 1997, where he underwent liver resection to segments three and five. The pathology report showed metastatic carcinoma and segments three and five both contained multiple nodules. The Pittsburg University oncologist informed him his prognosis was very poor and that he should go home and begin chemotherapy again. He and his wife asked this oncologist if he should use intravenous vitamin C. He responded, "I know of no studies which showed that this [vitamin C] would eradicate or delay progression of cancer."

In spite of the two no-confidence recommendations for the use of intravenous vitamin C, the patient returned to our center for infusions after recovering from surgery in June 1997. He also began receiving weekly 5-FU (1,100 mg) and leucovorin (1,300 mg) treatments administered by his local oncologist. His first vitamin C infusion was 15,000 mg over one hour. The dose was gradually increased during biweekly infusions. On September 9, 1997, a post-intravenous vitamin C (100,000 mg over two hours) plasma concentration of vitamin C was 355 mg/dL. He was then started on intravenous vitamin C, (100,000 mg) twice weekly. His wife gave most of these infusions at home. In addition to the vitamin C, he was given recommendations for oral vitamin and mineral supplementation to increase levels of nutrients that he was found to be low in.

He kept up his vitamin C infusions until February 1998, when he traveled to Florida for a vacation. While on vacation he continued the 5-FU/leucovorin injections. After a two-week hiatus from the vitamin C infusions, he began to experience nausea, diarrhea, stomach pain, and stomatitis (mouth sores)—common side effects of 5-FU. The side effects stopped when he restarted intravenous vitamin C. He continued on chemotherapy and 100,000 mg biweekly intravenous vitamin C until April 1, 1998. Other than the brief period of side effects mentioned above, he had no other side effects during the year of chemotherapy. He never experienced anemia, leucopenia (low white blood cell count indicative of poor immune defense), or thrombocytopenia (low platelet count that increases the risk of internal bleeding).

During April 1998, we began to taper his intravenous vitamin C. The doses were 75,000 mg, one time per week for two months; then 75,000 mg, one time every other week for two months; then 75,000 mg, on time every month for two months; and then 50,000 mg, one time per month for six months. The patient's carcinoembryonic antigen (CEA, a tumor marker) dropped into the normal range on July 31, 1997, and has remained normal (<3.0 ng/mL) to this writing (March 20, 1999). A computed tomography (CT) scan in October 1998 showed no evidence of metastatic disease. During an interview last week, he described himself as "perfectly healthy."

This report demonstrates four things about intravenous vitamin C in this patient's case: 1) intravenous vitamin C was not encouraged by his oncologists, 2) the patient did not take the advice of his oncologists on the issue of intravenous vitamin C usage, 3) his only side effects of chemotherapy occurred during a hiatus from intravenous vitamin C therapy and disappeared upon reinstatement of vitamin C infusions, and 4) for this patient intravenous vitamin C did not work against the chemotherapy, as demonstrated by his complete remission.

Combined Intravenous Vitamin C and Chemotherapy in a Patient with Carcinoma of the Pancreas

In October 1997, a 70-year-old white male from southeastern Kansas was first seen at our center. After exploratory surgery in December 1997, he had been diagnosed with a low-grade carcinoma of the pancreas. During surgery there was found to be widely metastatic disease affecting all intra-abdominal organs. In January 1997, he was started on gemcitabine (Gemzar). He had an allergic reaction to Gemzar and was placed on weekly 5-FU for nine weeks. He was placed back on Gemzar in June 1997 along with dexamethasone (Decadron) to counteract his allergy. In spite of chemotherapy his CA-19–9 (a tumor marker) continued to elevate until he was seen at our center. His first vitamin C infusion was 15,000 mg over one hour. His plasma concentration of vitamin C was 34 mg/dL immediately following that infusion. We expect the plasma level of a healthy person to reach between 120 and 200 mg/dL. On his first visit he was also placed on a broad-spectrum nutritional program. The dose of intravenous vitamin C was increased to 75,000-mg infusions biweekly until he received the results of a CT scan of the abdomen/pelvis, which showed no change compared to a CT in January. He related that he felt he was wasting his money at that time, and stopped his biweekly intravenous vitamin C.

The evidence in this case suggests that the intravenous vitamin C was acting as a cytostatic (cell reproduction-inhibiting) and not a cytotoxic (cell-killing) agent. When the patient went off the protocol, the tumors became active again. The evidence also suggests that intravenous vitamin C was working independently of the chemotherapy, given his CA-19–9 level continued to decrease after chemotherapy was discontinued. This patient died at home on July 4, 1998.

Resolution of Non-Hodgkin's Lymphoma with Intravenous Vitamin C: Two Cases

A 66-year-old white female was diagnosed with a large perispinal (L4–5) malignant, non-Hodgkin's lymphoma in January 1995. Her oncologist recommended localized radiation therapy and doxorubicin- (Adriamycin-) based chemotherapy. She began the radiation therapy five days per week for five weeks on January 17, 1995, but refused the chemotherapy. Four days earlier, she was started on intravenous vitamin C, 15,000 mg two times per week, which she continued after completing the radiation therapy. She also began taking several oral supplements to replace those found to be deficient by laboratory testing, and coenzyme Q10 (200 mg) two times per day. She was also successfully treated at that time for an intestinal parasite. On May 6, 1995, she returned to her oncologist with swelling and painful supraclavicular (just above the

collarbone) lymph nodes. One lymph node was removed and found to contain malignant lymphoma cells. In spite of recommendations for chemotherapy and more radiation, she refused and continued with her intravenous vitamin C and oral regimen. Within six weeks, the supraclavicular nodes were barely noticeable. She continued intravenous vitamin C infusions until December 24, 1996. She has been followed with regular physical exams and has had no recurrence. During a telephone follow-up on March 23, 1999, she was well without recurrence.

Comment: This case is rare. The patient refused chemotherapy, which in all likelihood would have been curative. She also had a so-called recurrence of her lymphoma during intravenous vitamin C therapy months after her radiation therapy had ended. The possibility exists that the lymphoma cells in her lymph nodes were there at the initial diagnosis and the adenopathy occurred during immune recognition of those cells. Also of note is the fact that this patient received only 15,000 mg of vitamin C per infusion. According to our model, this is not a high-enough dose to achieve cytotoxic concentrations of vitamin C in the blood. Therefore, any effect of vitamin C could only be attributed to its biological response modification characteristics.

In the fall of 1994, a 73-year-old white male farmer from western Kansas was diagnosed with widespread non-Hodgkin's lymphoma. Biopsies and CT scan revealed bilateral tumor involvement in his anterior and posterior cervical, inguinal, axillary, and mediastinal lymph nodes. A bone marrow aspirate was negative for malignant cells. The patient was treated with chemotherapy for eight months that resulted in remission. In July 1997, he began losing weight (30 pounds). He returned to his oncologist and a CT scan at that time showed recurrence. He was placed on chemotherapy in September 1997. In December 1997, he developed leukopenia and then extensive left-sided herpes zoster. As a result the chemotherapy was stopped. In March 1998, he became a patient at our center and began receiving intravenous vitamin C and oral nutrient supplements, including alpha-lipoic acid. His vitamin C dose was escalated until he was receiving 50,000 mg two times per week. He continued on that dose for 11 months. Three months after beginning vitamin C therapy a CT scan showed no evidence to malignancy. Another CT scan, in February 1999, was also clear and he was declared to be in complete remission by his oncologist. Also of note is that this patient was addicted to sleeping pills when first seen at our center. After three months of intravenous vitamin C therapy, he replaced the sleeping pills with kava tea.

Intravenous Vitamin C in a Patient with End-Stage Metastatic Breast Carcinoma

In 1995, a hospitalized 68-year-old women with widely metastatic end-stage breast cancer was seen.[6] Her latest bone scan showed metastases to "nearly every bone in her skeleton." She was experiencing bone pain that was not controlled with narcotics. At the time of her first consultation she had blood clots in both subclavian veins and shortly thereafter contracted cellulitis (a skin infection) in her left arm and hand due to an errant arterial blood draw. After the blood clots were treated with alteplase (Activase), she was placed on intravenous vitamin C, 30,000 mg per day initially, increasing to 100,000 mg per day over five hours. Within one week, the once bed-bound patient began walking the halls of the hospital. Several hospital staff reported that she looked like a new person. Her cellulitis cleared, and she was discharged from the hospital. At home she received 100,000 mg of intravenous vitamin C three times per week. Three months after starting the vitamin C therapy a bone scan revealed resolution of several skull metastases. Six months after starting the vitamin C, she fell while shopping at a mall and subsequently died of complications from pathological fractures.

■ CONCLUSION

We have presented evidence that vitamin C may be useful in the treatment of cancer. In particular, we have produced the following evidence: vitamin C is toxic to tumor cells. Concentrations of vitamin C that kill tumor cells can be achieved in humans using intravenous vitamin C infusions. Oral vitamin C followed by slow intravenous infusion can result in sustained concentrations of vitamin C in human plasma. Alpha-lipoic acid enhances vitamin C induced tumor cell toxicity. Vitamin C in blood concentrations achievable through oral supplementation is capable of increasing collagen production by tumor cells. Vitamin C in doses up to 50,000 mg per day, infused slowly, are not toxic to cancer patients. Some cancer patients have had complete remissions after high-dose intravenous vitamin C infusions. Concentrations of vitamin C that kill most tumor cells are not achieved after infusion of 30,000 mg of vitamin C. Therefore, remissions in patients treated with this dose of vitamin C are likely to have occurred as a result of vitamin C–induced biological response modification effects rather than its cytotoxic effects.

REFERENCES

1. Benade L, Howard T, Burk D. Synergistic killing of Ehrlich ascites carcinoma cells by ascorbate and 3-amino-1, 2, 4-triazole. *Oncology* 1969;23:33–43.

2. Maramag C, Menon M, Balaji KC, et al. Effect of vitamin C on prostate cancer cells in vitro: effect on cell number, viability, and DNA synthesis. *Prostate* 1997;32:188–195.

3. Riordan NH, et al. Intravenous ascorbate as a tumor cytotoxic chemotherapeutic agent. *Med Hypothesis* 1994;9:207–213.

4. Riordan HD, Jackson JA, Schultz M. Case study: high-dose intravenous vitamin C in the treatment of a patient with adenocarcinoma of the kidney. *J Orthomolecular Med* 1990;5:5–7.

5. Riordan HD, Jackson JA, Riordan NH, et al. High-dose intravenous vitamin C in the treatment of a patient with renal cell carcinoma of the kidney. *J Orthomolecular Med* 1998;13:72–73.

6. Riordan N, Jackson JA, Riordan HD. Intravenous vitamin C in a terminal cancer patient. *J Orthomolecular Med* 1996;11:80–82.

SCHEDULE DEPENDENCE IN CANCER THERAPY: INTRAVENOUS VITAMIN C AND THE SYSTEMIC SATURATION HYPOTHESIS

by Michael J. Gonzalez, DSc, PhD, Jorge R. Miranda-Massari, PharmD, Jorge Duconge, PhD, Neil H. Riordan, PhD, and Thomas Ichim, PhD

The pharmacokinetics and pharmacodynamics of intravenous (IV) vitamin C (ascorbic acid, ascorbate) has been partially described by various groups.[1-7] Nevertheless, the issues of schedule dependence and dosage in relation to cancer therapy have not been thoroughly discussed.

The use of large doses of vitamin C has been utilized for the treatment of cancer by various groups.[8-10] The inhibitory action on cancer cells by ascorbic acid has been described since 1952.[11] High concentrations of ascorbic acid may induce apoptotic cell death in tumor cell lines, possibly via its pro-oxidant action.[12] Moreover, high doses of ascorbic acid in the presence of oxygen favor the formation of hydrogen peroxide, providing an additional mechanism of anticarcinogenic action.[12] Another anticarcinogenic action induced by high doses of ascorbic acid is angiogenesis (new blood supply) inhibition.[13]

Discussion: IV Vitamin C

The concentrations of vitamin C toxic to cancer cells in vitro can be achieved clinically by intravenous administration. Currently, IV vitamin C is used extensively by alternative medicine practitioners in the United States (11,233 patients treated in 2006; 8,876 patients in 2008).[14] Clinical studies evaluating ascorbic acid in cancer outcome have been done.[15-17] As much as a 70-fold difference in plasma concentrations is expected between oral and IV administration, depending on dose. As a matter of fact, the pharmacokinetics of orally administered ascorbic acid has been early postulated to be dose-dependent, as the fraction absorbed decreased with increasing dose.[5]

In addition, the systemic clearance of vitamin C seems to be increased with accumulative exposure, a process that has been well-described by Hickey and others in the dynamic flow model.[4] Briefly, under physiological conditions, ascorbic acid is normally removed through filtration by kidneys (and then excreted), but a fraction of this filtered amount is returned into the body and reabsorbed by the blood. Thus, this concentration-dependent tubular reabsorption of ascorbic acid by the kidneys is saturated at supra-physiological levels of ascorbate. Therefore, a shorter terminal vitamin C elimination half-life is observed in individuals who receive excessively high amounts of ascorbic acid by continuous IV infusion. We think an IV schedule affording very high doses (>100,000 milligrams [mg]) or continuous infusions will overload the body stores for vitamin C, as well as block its dynamic flow processes. In this context, it is necessary to take control of the dosing schedule for vitamin C delivery into the body so that the required systemic levels are obtained (i.e., those necessary to have in vivo anticarcinogenic activity, but not too high that they can saturate the non-linear recycling process in kidneys, and hence increase clearance of vitamin C from the body).

We have hypothesized that giving vitamin C intravenously by following a fractioned schedule over a longer period (i.e., by multiple days, intermittent short-term IV infusions of high doses instead of using the conventional long-term continuous IV infusion administration) will provide the optimal levels for anticarcinogenic activity. Such a schedule is expected to minimize the saturation of renal vitamin C reabsorption while providing a continuous dynamic flow of ascorbic acid in the body for optimal systemic exposure and effect.

We firmly believe that a good understanding of all these mechanisms and their further implementation in clinical practice will yield better therapeutic outcomes. Accordingly, a concentration-function approach to vitamin C provides new insights into its physiology and pharmacology. With IV administration, ascorbate is turned from vitamin to

From the J Orthomolecular Med 2012;27:9–12.

drug, as pharmacologic concentrations are produced that are as much as 100-fold greater than maximal oral dosing.[2]

In some circumstances continuous infusion of IV vitamin C does not seem to be the optimal therapeutic schedule for cancer and repeated administration over a longer time period should be favored. We believe this particular pharmacokinetic-pharmacodynamic behavior of high-dose IV vitamin C can be explained by the systemic saturation hypothesis.

Systemic Saturation Concept in Relation to Intravenous Vitamin C

Systemic saturation results when the concentration of ascorbic acid in plasma and tissues in the body are high enough to produce an adverse effect in the biochemical parameters or metabolism. In this way, ascorbic acid's conversion to schedule dependence in cancer therapy[11] dehydroascorbate (oxidized ascorbic acid) is reversed back to ascorbic acid. Once this takes place, the pro-oxidant action is decreased, thus ascorbic acid's anticarcinogenic and/or carcinostatic action (the slowing or stopping of the growth) is reduced. This physiological phenomenon may occur when high IV doses of ascorbic acid (100,000 mg or more) are given in a continuous schedule. When high doses of IV ascorbic acid are

ASCORBIC ACIDITY

Ascorbic acid is a weak acid. It is more alkaline than the stomach contents, which contains hydrochloric acid, a strong acid. For oral administration, orthomolecular physicians tend to specify ascorbic acid rather than the nonacidic vitamin C salts (calcium ascorbate; magnesium ascorbate; sodium ascorbate) because ascorbic acid seems to get better clinical results than do the salts do. Intravenous administration of vitamin C requires sodium ascorbate.

given continuously, it overwhelms the cellular biochemical pathways favoring the reversion of DHA to ascorbic acid. This particular action dismisses ascorbic acid's anticarcinogenic and/or carcinostatic activity. This concept may in part explain the contradictory results reported previously in clinical studies despite in vitro evidence that high concentrations kill cancer cells. The continuous high-dose ascorbic acid may pose a physiological stress to the body that may cancel or overcome the same physiological mechanisms we are trying to modify.

A pilot pharmacokinetic study of vitamin C at high dose infusions in a cancer patient suggested a dual-phase kinetic behavior of ascorbate in vitro.[18] This disposition pattern depends on the

IN BRIEF

Despite the significant number of in vitro and in vivo studies to assess vitamin C effects on cancer following the application of large doses and its extensive use by alternative medicine practitioners in the United States, the precise schedule for successful cancer therapy is still unknown. Based on interpretation of the available data, we postulate that the relationship between vitamin C doses and plasma concentration over time, the capability of tissue stores upon distribution, and the saturable mechanism of urinary excretion are all important determinants to understand the physiology of high-intravenous vitamin-C dose administration and its effect on cancer. Practitioners should pay more attention to the cumulative vitamin C effect instead of the vitamin C concentrations to account for observed discrepancy in antitumor response. We suggest that multiple, intermittent, short-term intravenous (IV) infusions of vitamin C over a longer time period will correlate with greater antitumor effects than do single continuous IV doses of the same total exposure. This approach would be expected to minimize saturation of renal reabsorption, providing a continuous dynamic flow of vitamin C in the body for optimal systemic exposure and clinical outcomes. This prevents the "systemic saturation" phenomena, which may recycle vitamin C and render it less effective as an anticancer agent. Nonetheless, more pharmacokinetic and pharmacodynamic studies are needed to fully understand this schedule-dependence phenomenon.

actual infusion-generated plasma ascorbate concentrations with respect to the saturation cut-off level (about 70 micromoles = 0.123 mg per deciliter).[4,7] All these parameters are relevant to understand the physiology of high-dose IV ascorbic acid.

■ CONCLUSION

While vitamin C alone may not be enough of an intervention in the treatment of most active cancers, it seems to improve quality of life[17] and extend survival time.[19–27] It should be considered as part of the treatment protocol for all cancer patients.

Despite multiple in vitro and in vivo studies using different schedules of vitamin C for cancer therapy, the exact administration schedule that maximizes antitumor response remains unknown. Researchers should pay more attention to the cumulative (net) vitamin C effect instead of the vitamin C concentrations. Again, we speculate that the schedule-dependence in the pharmacokinetics of ascorbic acid accounts for such a discrepancy. The relationship between ascorbate dose, steady state plasma concentration, tissue store, or cell compartments concentration/distribution, and urinary excretion is important to understand its physiological effect or more related to this discussion, its effect on cancer. In this regard, we suggest that prolonged schedules of intravenous vitamin C would yield greater antitumor effects than would single continuous IV doses of the same total exposure. As such, administration schedules reaching effective antitumor concentrations are more likely to result from intermittent IV infusion delivered on multiple days. Nonetheless, more pharmacokinetic and pharmacodynamic studies are needed to fully understand this phenomenon.

REFERENCES

1. Levine M, Conry-Cantilena C, Wang Y, et al. Vitamin C pharmacokinetics in healthy volunteers: evidence for a recommended dietary allowance. *PNAS* 1996;93:3704–3709.

2. Riordan NH, Riordan HD, Casciari JP. Clinical and experimental experiences with vitamin C. *J Orthomolecular Med* 2000; 15:201–213.

3. Padayatty SJ, Sun H, Wang Y, et al. Vitamin C pharmacokinetics: implications for oral and intravenous use. *Ann Intern Med* 2004;140:533–537.

4. Hickey DS, Roberts HJ, Cathcart RF. Dynamic flow: a new model for ascorbate. *J Orthomolecular Med*, 2005;20:237–244.

5. Duconge J, Miranda-Massari JR, Gonzalez MJ, et al. Schedule dependence in cancer therapy: what is the true scenario for vitamin C? *J Orthomolecular Med* 2007;22:21–26.

6. Duconge J, Miranda-Massari JR, González MJ, et al. Vitamin C pharmacokinetics after continuous infusion in a patient with prostate cancer. *Ann Pharmacother* 2007;41:1082–1083.

7. Duconge J, Miranda-Massari JR, Gonzalez MJ, et al. Pharmacokinetics of Vitamin C: insights into the oral and intravenous administration of ascorbate. *PR Health Sci J* 2008;27:7–19.

8. Murata A, Morishige F, Yamaguchi H. Prolongation of survival times of terminal cancer patients by administration of large doses of ascorbate. *Int J Vitam Nutr Res Suppl* 1982;23:103–113.

9. Riordan HD, Riordan NH, Jackson JA, et al. Intravenous vitamin C as a chemotherapy agent: a report on clinical cases. *PR Health Sci J* 2004;23:115–118.

10. Verrax J, Calderon PB. Pharmacologic concentrations of ascorbate are achieved by parenteral administration and exhibit antitumoral effects. *Free Radic Biol Med* 2009;47:32–40.

11. McCormick WJ. Ascorbic acid as a therapeutic agent. *Arch Pediat* 1952;69:151–155.

12. Chen Q, Espey MG, Krishna MC, et al. Pharmacologic ascorbic acid concentrations selectively kill cancer cells: action as a pro-drug to deliver hydrogen peroxide to tissues. *Proc Natl Acad Sci USA*, 2005;102:13604–13609.

13. Mikirova NA, Casciari JJ, Riordan NH. Ascorbate inhibition of angiogenesis in aortic rings ex-vivo and subcutaneous matrigel plugs in vivo. *J Angiogenes Res* 2010;18:2.

14. Padayatty SJ, Sun AY, Chen Q, et al. Vitamin C: intravenous use by complementary and alternative medicine practitioners and adverse effects. *PLoS One*, 2010;5(7):e11414.

15. Riordan HD, Casciari JJ, González MJ, et al. A pilot clinical study of continuous intravenous ascorbate in terminal cancer patients. *PR Health Sci* 2005;24:269–276.

16. Hoffer LJ, Levine M, Assouline S, et al. Phase I clinical trial of I.V. ascorbic acid in advanced malignancy. *Ann Oncol* 2008; 19:1969–1974.

17. Vollbracht C, Schneider B, Leendert V, et al: Intravenous vitamin C administration improves quality of life in breast cancer patients during chemo-/radiotherapy and aftercare: results of a retrospective, multicentre, epidemiological cohort study in Germany. *In Vivo* 2011;25:983–990.

18. González MJ, Mora EM, Miranda-Massari JR, et al. Inhibition of human breast carcinoma cell proliferation by ascorbate and copper. *PR Health Sci J* 2002;21:21–23.

19. Cameron E, Pauling L. Supplemental ascorbate in the supportive treatment of cancer: prolongation of survival times in terminal human cancer. *Proc Natl Acad Sci USA* 1976;73: 3685–3689.

20. Cameron E, Pauling L. Supplemental ascorbate in the supportive treatment of cancer: reevaluation of prolongation of survival times on terminal human cancer. *Proc Natl Acad Sci USA* 1978;75:4538–4542.

21. Morishige F, Murata A. Prolongation of survival times in terminal human cancer by administration of supplemental ascorbate. *J Int Acad Prev Med* 1979;5:47–52.

22. Murata A, Morishige F, Yamaguchi H. Prolongation of survival times of terminal cancer patients by administration of large doses of ascorbate. *Int J Vitam Nutr Res Suppl* 1982;23:101–113.

23. Hoffer A, Pauling L: Hardin Jones biostatistical analysis of mortality data for cohorts of cancer patients with a large fraction surviving at the termination of the study and a comparison of survival times of cancer patients receiving large regular oral doses of vitamin C and other nutrients with similar patients not receiving those doses. *J Orthomolecular Med* 1990;5:143–154.

24. Hoffer A, Pauling L. Hardin Jones biostatistical analysis of mortality data for a second set of cohorts of cancer patients with a large fraction surviving at the termination of the study and a comparison of survival times of cancer patients receiving large regular oral doses of vitamin C and other nutrients with similar patients not receiving these doses. *J Orthomolecular Med* 1993;8:157–167.

25. Gonzalez NJ, Isaacs LL. Evaluation of Pancreatic Proteolytic Enzyme Treatment of Adenocarcinoma of the Pancreas, with Nutrition and Detoxification Support. *Nutr Cancer* 1999;33:117–124.

26. Riordan HD, Riordan NH, Jackson JA, et al. Intravenous vitamin C as a chemotherapy agent: a report on clinical cases. *PR Health Sci J* 2004;23:115–118.

27. Padayatty SJ, Riordan HD, Hewitt SM, et al. Intravenously administered vitamin C as cancer therapy: three cases. *Can Med Assoc J* 2006;174:937–942.

PHYSICIAN'S REPORT:

HIGH-DOSE INTRAVENOUS VITAMIN C AND LONG-TIME SURVIVAL OF A PATIENT WITH CANCER OF HEAD OF THE PANCREAS

by James A. Jackson, PhD, Hugh D. Riordan, MD, Ronald E. Hunninghake, MD, and Neil H. Riordan, PhD

A 68-year-old white male was a self-referral to the Riordan Clinic Health Center in December 1993. Two months previous he was seen at another medical facility for painless jaundice, darkening of the urine, pain in the stomach, and a rapid weight loss of 21 pounds—symptoms that are common in pancreatic cancer. A computed tomography (CT) scan and abdominal angiogram suggested a blocked bile duct and a pancreatic mass. An operation was performed and because of it's location, all of the tumor could not be removed. An area of the tumor, 4 cm x 2 cm x 4 cm

(1.5 in x .8 in x 1.5 in), was removed. The gallbladder, head of the pancreas (near the right side of the abdomen), and parts of the stomach and small intestine were also removed, and a complete Whipple procedure was performed. The pathology report showed a grade I cancer of the pancreas with metastasis to one of seven regional lymph nodes.

Pancreatic cancer surgery is complex and one of the hardest for a patient to have because of the problems of the long recovery time and problems that can result. A month after the operation the patient developed hyperglycemia (high blood glucose). He was placed on the American Diabetes Association's high-protein, low-carbohydrate diet with blood glucose monitoring twice a day. After a short period, his blood glucose returned and remained at normal. Three months prior to the Whipple procedure, he had a transurethral resection for an enlarged prostate, which proved to be benign.

Patient Profile

After discussing treatment options with an oncologist, the patient decided not to take conventional chemotherapy and radiation. At our center, a complete physical, psychological, and biochemical examination was done on the patient. He was an alert, pleasant, five foot eight, 140-pound male. Significant laboratory data included blood dehydroepiandrosterone (DHEA), 39.7 nanograms per deciliter (ng/dL) (normal, 200–335); beta-carotene, 2.4 micrograms (mcg) per dL (normal, 10–85); and vitamins A, C, and E in the non-supplementing normal range. Urine vitamin C was 10 milligrams (mg) per dL (our normal is 20–40), and the red blood cell (RBC) essential fatty acid profile showed low levels of gamma-linolenic acid and palmitoleic acid, and a low stearic/oleic ratio. His fructosamine level was 313 micromoles (umol) per liter (L) (normal, 175–272), and his blood glucose was 326 mg/dL. Hair tissue analysis showed calcium, magnesium, and sodium to be low.

A blood analysis for glucose-6-phosphate dehydrogenase (G6PD), and a blood urea nitrogen (BUN), creatinine, and urinalysis was done before intravenous (IV) vitamin C was started. All were normal. Appropriate supplements were started for those identified as low or suboptimal by the laboratory results.

Treatment

The patient initially received a small dose of vitamin C in a saline solution during a one-hour infusion to screen for toxic reactions. The next infusion of 115,000 mg was given in 1,000 milliliters (mL) of the saline solution over a eight-hour period. One hour into the infusion, the patient's plasma C level was 3.7 mg/dL, and at five hours it was 19 mg/dL. During the fourth eight-hour infusion (eight days later), the one-hour plasma C level was 158 mg/dL, and at five hours the level was 185 mg/dL. Both values are well above the concentration required to kill 100 percent of human pancreatic tumor cells as found in our research laboratory.[1]

Results

The low plasma levels of C in this patient during the first infusion compared to the fourth infusion show the value of measuring the plasma level to see that adequate levels are achieved during therapy. The patient received 39 of the eight-hour infusions in doses, ranging from 57,500 mg to 115,000 mg over a 13-week period, the length of the treatment protocol with high-dose IV vitamin C. A CT scan of the abdomen six months after the surgery failed to detect any progression of the tumor. A recurrence of the tumor occurred after the amount and frequency of IV vitamin C was significantly reduced so the patient could travel in his motor home to family reunions and other functions. The patient lived for 12 months after the initial diagnosis of cancer of the head of the pancreas. He received no chemotherapy or radiation treatment and enjoyed a good quality of life until the time of his death.

Comments

Altogether, six patients have been infused intravenously with similar doses of vitamin C over eight-hour periods with no reported side effects. In all cases, the patients had either been given no further therapeutic options by their oncologists, had refused conventional treatment, or had requested IV vitamin C in conjunction with standard chemotherapy.

REFERENCES

1. Riordan NH, et al. *Med Hypotheses* 1995;44:207–213.

From the *J Orthomolecular Med* 1995;10(2):87–88.

A Nutritious Cocktail for the Treatment of Melanoma: A Case Report

by Joao Libanio G. de Oliveira, MD

The patient is a 51-year-old white engineer who has suffered from melanoma in his cervical (neck) area for three years. Although melanoma, the most serious type of skin cancer, develops in the cells that produces melanin, the pigment that gives skin its color can sometimes form elsewhere, as in this case the neck. The patient underwent surgery but the melanoma returned. He was operated on once more, and the lymphatic nodes in the neck area were taken out. He then began taking synthetic interferon in order to avoid new metastases. However, a new nodule appeared in his left lung six months later. Tissue sampling and analysis confirmed melanoma nodule metastasis. His oncologist told him to stop taking synthetic interferon, to go back home and wait for any resolution, saying to him that there was nothing to be done. He was very ill, very thin, desperate, and frustrated when he told his son to make an appointment with our office.

Case Report

We began his treatment in 1997, and he quickly improved in regard to his physical performance, sleeping, appetite, and weight. He took all nutrients methodically (50 capsules daily) and took care of his eating habits, staying away from fried food, fat, sugar, meat, and processed food, and increasing his consumption of natural seeds, vegetables, fruit juices, extra virgin olive oil, and a lot of fish and, occasionally, chicken.

He came to the office daily to have his intravenous nutrients for five weeks. He developed more vitality, but he was worried about the nodule in his left lung and requested a new x-ray after a month. At this time we found that his nodule had disappeared and he was very surprised with such a fast evolution and recovery. He visited his oncologist who was surprised with his clinical condition as well. However, the oncologist insisted that

the nodule was still present concluding: "If your doctors used x-rays techniques like we do they would also see the nodule." Although I had less experience in this regard, I was sure that there was nothing more in that lung area, compared to the x-ray prior to our treatment. But I was cautious to affirm exactly what I thought, until I could get a more specific exam and a specialist to confirm my point of view. So we decided to wait and to go on with the treatment.

Over the next 11 months we worked together. He had two more x-rays showing the same results. The patient's first hair analysis detected a great deficiency of nutrients, especially magnesium, calcium, zinc, selenium, germanium, cobalt, and copper. Some intoxication by lead, aluminum, and mercury was also detected. His blood analysis indicated a small number of leukocytes (white blood cells), probably because of the previous use of synthetic interferon or as a result of his own low immunity.

Slowly, yet progressively, however, his leukocytes increased in number. Before the beginning of orthomolecular treatment, his leukocyte count was 2,500 and now it was 4,200. The last hair analysis showed the levels of cobalt, zinc, copper, germanium, and selenium had increased and he was free from mercury and lead intoxication. However, the deficiency of magnesium and calcium persisted despite his large intake of these supplements, which suggested a greatly increased metabolic consumption of these minerals.

Today, the patient's health is improved. Now he is very happy; he has gained 10 kilograms (22 pounds), presents with no fatigue, is eating well, and has an excellent appearance. All blood analyses, liver proofs, full abdominal ultrasonography are normal too. At last, we submitted him to a new modern thorax tomography, conducted by a qualified expert, and, instead of the nodule, only a little fibrous tissue scar was evident.

Treatment Regimen and Results

To recap the results:

• June 6, 1997: X-ray shows a nodule in the left lung measuring 0.6 centimeters.

• August 11, 1997: Tomography with dirigible nodule puncture, with tissue sample, confirms a melanoma nodule metastasis after hystological analysis.

• August 20–September 10, 1997: Patient begins having his nutrients orally and intravenously (for 20 days only).

• September 10, 1997: A-ray shows the nodule absent.

• June 18, 1998: Follow-up tomography shows only a little fibrous tissue scar.

We used the following nutrients in his daily treatment:

NUTRITIONAL COMBINATIONS USED IN MELANOMA TREATMENT REGIMEN			
Vitamin A (palmitate)	10,000 IU	Molybdenum	5 mcg
Beta-carotene (pro-vitamin A)	15,000 IU	Potassium citrate	50 mg
Vitamin B2 (riboflavin)	70 mg	Selenium	100 mcg
Vitamin B3	20 mg as niacin 50 mg as niacinamide	Zinc citrate	30 mg
Pantothenic acid	70 mg	Coenzyme Q10 (CoQ10)	400 mg
Vitamin B6 (pyridoxine)	250 mg	DL-methionine	100 mg
Vitamin B12 (cobalamin)	3,000 mcg	L-citrulline	600 mg
Biotin	300 mcg	L-cysteine	120 mg
Folic acid	400 mcg	L-glutathione	50 mg
Para-aminobenzoic acid	150 mg	L-lysine	50 mg
Inositol	70 mg	L-ornithine aspartate	2,400 mg
Vitamin C	25,000 mg	L-arginine cloridrate	9,000 mg
Rutin	25 mg	Catalase	20,000 IU
Vitamin E	2,000 IU	Glutathione peroxidase	5,000 IU
Calcium dibasic phosphate	300 mg	Superoxide dismutase	5,000 IU
Calcium gluconate	40 mg	Dimethyl sulfoxide (DMSO)	
Chromium chelate	20 mg	Ethylenediaminetetracetic Acid (EDTA)	
Copper gluconate	0.5 mg	Eicosapentanoic acid (EPA)	1,800 mg
Germanium	100 mg	Docosahexaenoic acid (DHA)	1,200 mg
Magnesium aspartate	500 mg	Docosahexaenoic acid (DHA	1,200 mg
Magnesium citrate	150 mg	Manganese gluconate	2 mg

Note: milligrams (mg), micrograms (mcg), international units (IU).

■ CONCLUSION

As mentioned before, the patient submitted to a program of synthetic interferon three times a week for six months, which unfortunately was not beneficial to him and worsened his clinical condition (i.e., decreased the number of leukocytes and in the end a nodule appeared in his lung). When the patient started orthomolecular treatment in our office, he took intravenous nutrients that contained large amounts of vitamin C (a natural interferon stimulator) at a rate of 50,000 mg daily five days a week, during the first month. These intravenous treatments also contained high doses of other nutrients such as selenium, magnesium, and calcium, and in lower quantities pyridoxine, pantothenic acid, zinc, copper, manganese, and chromium. The anti-inflammatory solvent dimethyl sulfoxide (DMSO) was also added to his intravenous cocktail three times a week. Ethylenediaminetetraacetic acid (EDTA) was also used to reduce the previously detected lead and mercury levels.

Since the very beginning the patient took 400 mg of coenzyme Q10 (CoQ10) daily. My idea of using CoQ10 emerged from reading a publication by Professor Debasis Bagchi in the *Journal of Orthomolecular Medicine*,[1] who reported the successful treatment of lung metastasis of breast cancer in some cases using CoQ10 for four or five years.

The use of the anti-inflammatory DMSO in the patients "nutrient cocktail" was rather intuitive. Once I had a patient who had a metastatic nodule from the bladder diminished after taking DMSO for a period of time. I also had read some old publications about DMSO that mentioned its property to inhibit some kinds of tumors in experiments on rats. The good result obtained in this treatment made me wonder about its actual potential in treating cancer. At present, the patient goes on taking his intravenous cocktail two times a week, and also takes 400 mg of CoQ10 along with other nutrients. I think the certainty of a full recovery we need to have will come only with time and that is why we will keep the same treatment and the best nutrition.

During the treatment the patient followed all my instructions. He accepted the treatment and he trusted me, maintaining the changes in his eating habits as I prescribed. I believe this was an important factor in his recovery.

We all know that it is very difficult to believe in nutrients defeating cancer. However, non-traditional medical thinking about cancer has made great progress in numbers of cases all over the world.

This is a report about a small melanoma metastasis nodule measuring only 0.6 centimeters (1/4 inch) but containing millions of powerful cancer cells that were destined to kill its living host. We beat it with nutrients and maybe with the help of the anti-inflammatory DMSO. Putting it all together with their antioxidant action we obtained this result. That's the new orthomolecular nutrition.

REFERENCES

1. Bagchi D. Coenzyme Q10: a novel cardiac antioxidant. *J Orthomolecular Med* 1997;12:4–10.

ACUTE MYELOID LEUKEMIA: AN ORTHOMOLECULAR CASE STUDY

by Michael Friedman, ND, and Erik T. Paterson, MD

Within the memory of many physicians now living, the diagnosis of acute myeloid leukemia (AML) was an automatic death sentence for the patient.[1] AML is one of many types of leukemia, a cancer of the blood or blood-forming tissues (bone marrow, lymphatic system, and spleen). People with leukemia often have a very high number of white blood cells (leukocytes), which normally help defend the body against infections but in leukemia do not function as they should. Hope for the management of all the leukemias dawned in the 1960s when chemotherapy began to bring about complete remission for most, but not all, patients with acute lymphatic leukemia (ALL). Chronic lymphocytic leukemia (CLL) remains almost resistant to chemotherapy, although it has the best prognosis of the leukemias with some patients surviving from time of diagnosis as much as 25 years or more. Chronic myeloid leukemia (CML), with a much poorer prognosis than CLL, is starting to yield to chemotherapy, the most favorable form being the cytokines, interferon in particular. With chemotherapy or bone marrow transplants, new hope has come for patients with AML.

Diagnosis

AML is not an uncommon illness. In fact, its incidence in the population has been rising in recent decades. The age distribution tends to be from the early 20s to old age. While generally its cause remains unknown, there is a strong statistical relationship between AML and exposure to radiation—an almost linear relationship between the risk of AML and the total exposure to x-rays, for example. Another strong relationship exists between AML and previous chemotherapy for other cancers, Hodgkin's lymphoma in particular. The role of pollutants is strongly suspected but unproven (the absence of proof never meaning proof of absence).

There are two currently accepted lines of management of AML: bone marrow transplants and chemotherapy. Of the two treatments, bone marrow transplant has received the most publicity because of its promise of "cure." In a conventional allogeneic bone marrow transplant, a donor of tissue type close to that of the patient provides bone marrow. The bone marrow of the patient is, hopefully, destroyed either by radiation or aggressive chemotherapy. The donated marrow is transplanted and the almost inevitable rejection reactions are suppressed by cyclosporin. In an autologous bone marrow transplant, still an experimental procedure, the patient receives chemotherapy to kill the cancer cells. When the marrow recovers, it is removed from the patient and then harvested and grown in the laboratory, hopefully without the blast cells that are the origin of the leukemia. The patient then receives the same aggressive chemotherapy to destroy his or her marrow, and the harvested marrow is reimplanted by injection.

The other accepted line of management is chemotherapy. This consists of giving high doses of cytosine arabinoside (Ara-C), or less commonly idoxuridine, in combination with other agents such as mitoxantrone and etoposide to kill the cancer cells. Formerly, this was performed as two rounds of chemotherapy followed by maintenance oral chemotherapy. More recently, the recommended regimen consists of three rounds of chemotherapy without the oral medication afterward.

Recent results suggest that chemotherapy is marginally superior in outcome to bone marrow transplantation. In either case, the mortality rate is about 50 percent by six months after the date of diagnosis. In one center, if the patient shows no recurrence by two years following the date of diagnosis, the survival curve becomes flat at approximately 30 percent (although there are trends suggesting 45 percent survival). This, of course, means that 55 to 70 percent of patients are dead within two years.

From the *J Orthomolecular Med* 1999;14(3):161–168.

The operative word in the above account is "accepted" since most major leukemia treatment centers do not recognize additional nutritional support as an aid to enhancing the effectiveness of therapy either during the chemotherapy or after. The following case report illustrates one attempt by a patient to ensure his survival using orthomolecular means.

At the time of diagnosis the patient was a 55-year-old family physician in practice in a western Canadian rural community. He was a non-smoker and his use of alcohol was slight. Other health problems included asthma, hay fever, and a minor degree of temporal lobe (partial complex) seizures. He had no known drug sensitivities except for gastric intolerance of niacin. In the course of practice he had been exposed to x-rays and, as a patient with other health problems, had been subject to barium studies of the gastrointestinal tract. For nineteen years he had been a practicing anesthetist exposed to unvented anesthetic gases but had given this up five years before becoming ill with AML.

The first symptom suggestive of the onset of AML was unusual bleeding of his gums after brushing his teeth. About five to seven days later, he developed nausea of sudden onset followed less than one hour later by a rapidly rising temperature accompanied by mild right-sided chest discomfort. In the emergency department of the local community hospital, his family physician discovered that his white blood cell count was 41,000 (the upper level of normal being 11), more than a simple infection. Intravenous antibiotics began to be administered. The following morning, at a regional hospital, the diagnosis of AML was established, and transfer to the bone marrow transplant/leukemia unit of a tertiary care hospital was arranged.

Chemotherapy: Round One

Following a bone marrow biopsy to establish the diagnosis and subtype of the AML for prognostic purposes, a first injection of Ara-C was administered at 6,750 mg over two hours. The subtype of AML was French-American-British type M4, or acute myelomonocytic leukemia, which carries a better prognosis than some other types but not the best. The patient's white blood cell count then being 36.6. Near midnight, over 48 hours after the acute illness began, a Hickman line (a triple lumen, long-term catheter) was established into the patient's superior vena cava or right atrium. Over a period of about 72 hours, further Ara-C (3,380 mg) and mitoxantrone (27 mg) per day were administered, followed for a further 17 hours by etoposide (1,800 mg). Steroid eye drops were administered every four hours. This being completed, the patient's white blood cell count had fallen to 3.0. His platelet levels were 10.

With persistence of the patient's fever, four antibiotics (vancomycin, tobramycin, ceftazidime, and metronidazole) were continuously administered intravenously. The cytoprotective agent allopurinol was given orally to prevent kidney failure due to high uric acid levels (hyperuricemia), a common feature of early therapy for AML. The antiviral drug acyclovir was also administered to prevent super infections. Seventeen transfusions of packed cells were administered. Even more frequently, 112 platelet infusions were administered; he also received 19 units of albumin, a protein in blood. All the blood products were irradiated to prevent the transmission of infectious diseases, such as cytomegalovirus.

IN BRIEF

A case is presented of a 55-year-old male who developed acute myeloid leukemia of sudden onset. There being insufficient time for orthomolecular therapy to be effective, he was obliged to risk chemotherapy, which he survived despite numerous expected and unexpected complications. In between the three rounds of chemotherapy he tried to use orthomolecular means to improve his condition and enhance his survival. He is now in complete remission and feeling well, using such techniques. The issue requiring resolution is the advisability of using chemotherapy with orthomolecular techniques concurrently to improve survival of patients with acute myeloid leukemia.

The following complications of treatment occurred during this first round of chemotherapy:

• Vomiting, anorexia, diarrhea, and hair loss as is almost routine with aggressive chemotherapy.

• Rhabdomyolysis (breakdown of skeletal muscle) accompanied by fever, which was reported to the patient's wife as being 47°C (116°F); vigorous cooling of the patient by his family restored survivable temperatures. No action was taken by either the medical or nursing staff.

• Widespread, blistering eruption of the skin, which was initially presumed to be due to a virus in the blood but was later shown to be caused by a severe reaction to the allopurinol; by the time this drug was stopped, the hyperuricemic threat was over.

• Marked edema caused by fluid overload, which resulted in a mild form of adult respiratory distress syndrome (ARDS), a serious lung condition that causes shortness of breath (dyspena); this was managed by appropriate diuresis (increasing production of urine by the kidneys) and more careful control of fluid balance.

• Dyspnea accompanied by mild pain in the lower third of the left soleus muscle; this was presumed to be a sign of pulmonary thromboembolism, which was investigated excessively with no such state being found. It was, in fact, due to the combination of the ARDS and the patient's asthma.

• Atrial fibrillation (abnormal heartbeat) that resolved spontaneously with more careful management of his fluid balance.

• Stomatitis (mouth sores), which required intravenous morphine until it resolved spontaneously.

About four weeks after the onset of the illness, the patient's white blood cells had recovered enough that the feverishness had settled. The antibiotics could be stopped.

Six days later, a repeat bone marrow biopsy showed the number of blast cells as being less than 5 percent of the total, defined as a "complete remission."

In all this time, the patient was not permitted to receive any more than 500 mg of ascorbic acid per day, even though his usual pre-treatment dose had been 10,000 mg per day, along with vitamins A, D, E, B1 (thiamine), B6 (pyridoxine), a potent multivitamin preparation, and the minerals calcium and magnesium.

He was discharged to the care of his family in a small rental apartment near the hospital and was followed in the bone marrow transplant day-care unit. He was advised that the second round (first "consolidation" round) of chemotherapy would begin after two weeks.

Chemotherapy: Round Two

Four weeks later, at the time of the second admission, the patient's condition had spectacularly improved. During this interval he had undertaken increasing exercise and consumed increasing doses of vitamin C. Nevertheless, the vomiting still occurred at times provoked by the slightest digestive misstep. This last problem was investigated endoscopically in another tertiary care hospital and infection by Helicobacter pylori was suggested but unproven. The patient elected to delay therapy for this until it was clear that he was able to survive the subsequent rounds of chemotherapy.

The patient also experienced episodes of depression but the oncological psychiatrist felt that it was best to leave these untreated, a conclusion with which the patient agreed. The drug regimen of the second round of chemotherapy was exactly the same as the first. The antibiotics used this time were ceftazidime, tobramycin, and vancomycin. None of the above noted complications occurred except for the vomiting, diarrhea, and hair loss. However, an acute case of stomatitis, involving the cheek cavity, tongue, and pharynx occurred; this was managed by total parenteral nutrition and intravenous morphine for a period of about eleven days. Blood transfusions of 10 and 30 units of platelet infusions were administered as before. After 37 days the patient was again discharged.

The initial recovery period was marked by an infection of the Hickman line, which had to be removed because antibiotics had failed to control the infection. It is not on record what dose of vitamin C the patient reached during this seven-week interval, but continued gastrointestinal delicacy did not permit a rapid increase in dosage.

Chemotherapy: Round Three

At the start of the final round of chemotherapy, the patient showed a marked decrease in the white blood cells with a count of 2.3, which necessitated another bone marrow biopsy that turned out to show no abnormality. A fresh Hickman line was established and treatment with the Ara-C and mitoxantrone only was given as chemotherapy, the same doses as before. Again intravenous antibiotics (with the addition of acyclovir and amphotericin-B as prophylaxis for viral and fungal infections), blood transfusions (eight units), and platelet infusions (34 units) were administered. The problems in this round included a more prolonged recovery time for the bone marrow and elevated creatinine (indicative of impaired kidney function), along with low potassium and magnesium levels. These were almost certainly due to renal tubular trauma (kidney damage caused by the antifungal agent amphotericin-B), and a problem that has persisted to the time of this writing and that is unlikely to resolve.

The other significant problem was the development of a low-grade allergic reaction to the platelets, which was treated prophylactically with the antihistamine Benadryl, at the cost of considerable sedation to the patient each time it was administered.

Eight days after discharge, the Hickman line was removed by the oncologist in charge of the final round of chemotherapy, who advised the patient that there was nothing further to offer by way of aftercare except routine blood tests. Only in the event of a recurrence of the AML would any other active therapy be considered. This the patient was not prepared to accept.

Orthomolecular Therapy

At home, convalescent, the patient began a program of increasing doses of nutrients, as well as maintaining the necessary replacement of potassium (600 mg) three times per day, and magnesium (1,000 mg) per day in combination with calcium and vitamin D. Depending on his gastric tolerance, he began to take vitamin E (1,000 IU) per day; a multivitamin and mineral capsule daily; thiamine and pyridoxine (500 mg) each daily; halibut liver oil (as a source of vitamins A and D), one capsule daily; evening primrose oil (800-mg capsules) three times daily; coenzyme Q10 (150 mg) daily; and DHEA (333 mg) daily.

The dosage of vitamin C is of particular interest. At first the patient's tolerance of this was governed by his gastric tolerance. As this improved he was able, in over less than two months, to build up his total daily intake to 60,000 mg in divided doses. For the lower doses he used 1,000-mg tablets. As the amounts built up, he switched to calcium ascorbate powder dissolved in unsweetened juice (a level teaspoonful being equivalent roughly to 4,000 mg, or a level commercial coffee scoop being equivalent to 10,000 mg). The top dosage was determined by bowel tolerance, any higher dose than 60,000 mg per day caused diarrhea.

As the patient's convalescence proceeded and his condition improved, the diarrhea recurred forcing progressive reductions in dosage down from 50,000 mg, gradually through to 10,000 mg, and recently to 8,000 mg daily.

Less than 13 months after diagnosis of the AML, with persistently normal blood tests, the patient returned to full-time medical practice.

Discussion

A more detailed but non-technical account of the events described above has been published elsewhere.[2–16] One fact omitted from the case report is that the patient had considered for 20 years prior to the onset of the AML the possibility that he might at some time develop one of the leukemias. Being a practicing orthomolecular physician he had decided that, in that eventuality, he would not accept standard chemotherapy. Equally, he knew that for orthomolecular therapy to work, time in the order of several months would be needed before the benefits of such therapy would become apparent.

At the onset of his illness he was forced to reconsider the above decision because of the acuteness of the AML. He had only days to live before he would succumb to kidney failure from the hyperuricemia, a death experienced by the sister of a close friend, or infection. He was not an accept-

292

able candidate for kidney dialysis. Survival for the time necessary for orthomolecular therapy to work was highly unlikely.

When he arrived at the blood marrow transplant unit he was faced with further difficult decisions. There was a 10 percent chance that the chemotherapy would not work at all, and he would die as a result. There was another 10 percent chance that the complications of the chemotherapy would be lethal for him (and, indeed, at one stage it was presumed by the staff of the unit that he was dying of such complications). Two analogies were presented to him: The first was to imagine a garden overgrown with weeds; the garden was sprayed with gasoline and a lighted match was tossed in. The hope would be that something useful would survive the holocaust. The second was to imagine being poisoned to death and then there being an attempt to rescue him. The patient was too old for consideration for a bone marrow transplant. In any event the only likely donor, his sister, had breast cancer only a few years before and was, hence, not acceptable.

Having made the decision to proceed with the chemotherapy the patient was disturbed that no consideration was taken of his previous intake of vitamins. Indeed, it was with considerable reluctance by the medical staff of the transplant unit that he was given as little as the 500 mg of vitamin C. As far as he could, he tried to make up for this in the intervals between the rounds of chemotherapy when he was out of hospital, the limiting factor being his gastric tolerance. Having completed the chemotherapy, he could proceed to be more aggressive with his use of nutrients. What was the rationale for this, and what so far has been the outcome?

That there may be a role for ascorbate in cancer therapy has been known for more than 20 years.[17] Even more specifically it has also been known that in vitro growth of the cell cultures of AML are suppressed by ascorbate as shown by Park et al.[18] That most forms of cancer might respond favorably in a clinical setting to ascorbate and other nutrients has been shown by Hoffer and Pauling[19,20] in terms of survival times.[21,22] Whether vitamin C is given orally or intravenously, the dose tolerated is a reflection of the current condition of the patient (deteriorating or improving as the case may be) as determined by titrating to bowel tolerance as defined by Cathcart.[23]

None of the nutrients mentioned are known to have any adverse influence on the effectiveness of the chemotherapy or upon the measures taken to rescue patients from the complications of chemotherapy. As far as ascorbate is concerned Hoffer[24] has cited a meeting in 1990, cosponsored by the National Cancer Institute, at which ascorbate was shown to decrease the toxic effects of both radiation and chemotherapy against normal tissue, while sensitizing malignant cells against the same forms of therapy. Prasad and Rama[25] showed that pre-treatment with ascorbate yielded improved outcomes after radiation. Since the effect of chemotherapy on individual cells is the same as that of radiation, similar efficacy of ascorbate as a protective agent for normal tissues and as a sensitizing agent of cancerous tissues is to be predicted until proven otherwise. Vitamin B3 (niacin) has been shown in numerous animal studies to enhance the effectiveness of both chemotherapy and radiation while being protective of normal tissues. Over 50 years ago it was shown[26,27] that niacin improved outcomes in cancer patients, along with other nutrients. And Canner et al.[28] showed that this same vitamin reduced the death rate from all causes including cancer. Vitamin E may have a protective effect against cancer. Studies of its role as protective of normal tissues against the toxic effects of chemotherapy are woeful by their absence. CoQ10, a central coenzyme in oxidative phosphorylation such as reduction/oxidation or redox reactions, has been shown to prolong life in cancer patients.[29] Minerals, selenium in particular, have a cancer-fighting effect when given in deficiency states.[30]

These results consider nutrients given alone and should warrant more serious consideration by the oncological community. But what if they are given in combination? Is there evidence to suggest a synergistic effect? Rueff,[31] Kallistratos, and others,[32] and Winn and Levin[33] found that there was indeed such an effect.

Since all the nutrients mentioned here are safe in much higher doses than those of the Recommended Dietary Allowances (RDAs), can be administered safely (orally and in the event of gastric disturbance intravenously), and are effective both in the prevention of the adverse effects of chemotherapy and radiation yet while enhancing their efficacy, it seems strange that this patient was not offered their benefits during all three rounds of chemotherapy for his AML.

As of the time this is being written, the patient is at the third anniversary of the diagnosis of his AML and remains well. Does this mean that recurrence of the AML will not happen? After all he has not passed the fifth anniversary, let alone the tenth, the usually accepted criterion for cure of cancer. Time will tell.

By now it will be apparent that the patient described is the writer, myself. How do I feel about my situation? I am reminded of a conversation between myself and a very good friend of mine, who is also a clinical psychologist. I was between the first and second rounds of the chemotherapy and expressing my despondency about my future. He asked me what my response would have been if he had asked me how long I was likely to live before I knew I was ill with the AML. I muttered and stuttered. Then he asked, "What has changed?" Of course, nothing has changed. I still cannot say how long I am likely to live.

But I am determined to bias my chances by continuing the fight against a recurrence of the AML using orthomolecular techniques.

Postscript

Today, I take 10,000 mg of vitamin C per day, now over 16.5 years since the diagnosis of the AML. There is no sign of recurrence.

So, am I done with cancer? No. My father died of prostate cancer. I know that if any man lived long enough he would develop prostate cancer, and I could not be excluded. I began regular tests of my prostate specific antigen (PSA), a measure of the total bulk of prostate tissue, not a test for cancer except indirectly. For years my results were highish but stable. Suddenly, in 2010, there was a 50 percent jump in the PSA result. This was ominous. A prostate biopsy showed cancer with a Gleason score of 9, a strong hint of invasiveness.

Following hormone suppression I received 57 radiation treatments in the fall of 2011. The treatments themselves caused me very little problem, as expected with orthomolecular therapy.

With time I was not unscathed. By July 2012, I started having substantial bowel bleeds. I watched a colonoscopy and saw that the problem was radiation proctitis (a complication of radiation therapy). We tried local corticosteroids, which had no benefit. In fact, I developed such severe anemia that I had to have several blood transfusions. Then, I had two ablation treatments for prevention of recurrent bleeding, which appears—as this is being written—to have stopped the bleeding.

But, most important, what about the cancer? Repeated measures of my PSA have shown virtually undetectable levels. I remain alive because of orthomolecular therapy.

REFERENCES

1. Owens AH, Abelhoff MD. *Illustrative Neoplastic Diseases: The Principles and Practice of Medicine.* 21st ed. Norwalk, CT: Appleton-Century-Crofts, 1984.

2. Paterson ET. An encounter with leukemia, part 1: the discovery. *Med Post* 1996;19:9.

3. Paterson ET. An encounter with leukemia, part 2: the gathering of the clan. *Med Post* Nov 26, 1996:32.

4. Paterson ET. An encounter with leukemia, part 3: the "poisoning." *Med Post* Dec 3, 1996:32.

5. Paterson ET. An encounter with leukemia, part 4: the "difficult" patient. *Med Post* Dec 17, 1996:34.

6. Paterson ET. An encounter with leukemia, part 5: complications, consultations, and isolation. *Med Post* Jan 7, 1997:44–45.

7. Paterson ET. An encounter with leukemia, part 6: the waiting game. *Med Post* Jan 14, 1997:45.

8. Paterson ET. An encounter with leukemia, part 7: prisoner of pain. *Med Post* Jan 28, 1997:32.

9. Paterson ET. An encounter with leukemia, part 8: home again. *Med Post* Feb 4, 1997:36.

10. Paterson ET. An encounter with leukemia, part 9: I find my "survive" switch. *Med Post* Feb. 11, 1997:55.

11. Paterson ET. An encounter with leukemia, part 10: back to Vancouver. *Med Post* Apr 1, 1997:32.

12. Paterson ET. An encounter with leukemia, part 11: down I go again *Med Post* Apr 8, 1997:48–49.

13. Paterson ET. An encounter with leukemia, part 12: the road back. *Med Post* Apr 15, 1997: 50–51.

14. Paterson ET. An encounter with leukemia, part 13: struggling to get home. *Med Post* Apr 22, 1997:37.

15. Paterson ET. An encounter with leukemia, part 14: finding out who your friends are. *Med Post* May 6, 1997:9.

16. Paterson ET. Postscript of my encounter with leukemia: the return to work. *Med Post* Apr 7, 1999:24.

17. Cameron E, Pauling L. *Cancer and Vitamin C.* Menlo Park, CA: Linus Pauling Institute of Science and Medicine, 1979.

18. Park CH, et al. Growth suppression of human leukemic cells in vitro by L-ascorbic acid. *Cancer Res* 1980;40:1062–1065.

19. Hoffer A, Pauling L. Hardin Jones biostatistical analysis of mortality data for cohorts of cancer patients with a large fraction surviving at the termination of the study and a comparison of survival times of cancer patients receiving larger regular doses of vitamin C and other nutrients with similar patients not receiving those doses. *J Orthomolecular Med* 1990;5:143–154.

20. Hoffer A, Pauling L. Hardin Jones biostatistical analysis of mortality data for a second set of cohorts of cancer patients with a large fraction surviving at the termination of the study and a comparison of survival times of cancer patients receiving larger regular doses of vitamin C and other nutrients with similar patients not receiving those doses. *J Orthomolecular Med* 1993; 8:157–167.

21. Jackson JA, et al. Case from the Center: High dose intravenous vitamin C and long-term survival of a patient with cancer of the head of the pancreas. *J Orthomolecular Med* 1995; 10:87–88.

22. Riordan N, et al. Case from the center: intravenous vitamin C in a terminal cancer patient. *New Eng J Med* 1996;11:80–82.

23. Moertel CG, et al. High dose vitamin C versus placebo in the treatment of patients with advanced cancer who have had no prior chemotherapy. *New Eng J Med* 1985;312:137–141.

24. Hill AB. Medical ethics and controlled trials. *BMJ* 1963;1: 1043–1049.

25. Rothman KJ, Michels KB. The continuing unethical use of placebo controls. *New Eng J Med* 1994;331:394–398.

26. Cathcart RF. The third face of Vitamin C. *J Orthomolecular Med* 1992;7:197–200.

27. Hoffer A. Personal communication, 1996.

28. Prasad KN, Rama BN. Nutrition and cancer. In: *Yearbook of Nutritional Medicine* edited by J Bland. New Canaan, CT: Keats Publishing, 1985.

29. Gerson M. Dietary considerations in malignant neoplastic disease: a preliminary report. *Rev Gastroenterol* 1945;12: 419–425.

30. Ibid. Effects of a combined dietary regime on patients with malignant tumours. *Exper Med Surg* 1949;7:299–317.

31. Canner, PL et al. Fifteen-year mortality coronary drug project: patients long term benefit with niacin. *Am Coll Cardiol* 1986; 8:1245–1255.

32. Folkers K, et al. Survival of cancer patient on therapy with coenzyme Q10. *Biochem Biophys Res Comm* 1993; 192:241–245.

33. Toma S et al. Selenium therapy in patients with precancerous and malignant oral cavity lesions: preliminary results. *Cancer Detect Prev* 1991;15:491–494.

34. Rueff D. Clinical experience with antioxidant supplementation in oncological treatments: therapeutic potential of biological antioxidants. Tiburon, CA: Linus Pauling Institute of Science and Medicine, 1994.

35. Kallistratos GI, et al. Prolongation of the survival time of tumour bearing wistar rats through a simultaneous oral administration of vitamins c and e and selenium with glutathione. *Nutrition, Growth and Cancer.* New York: Alan L. Liss, 377–389.

36. Winn, RJ, Levin B. Chemoprevention of colon cancer. *Hematol/Oncol Clin North Amer* 1989;3:65–75.

ANTIOXIDANT VITAMINS REDUCE THE RISK FOR CANCER
by Michael J. Glade, PhD

The published scientific evidence that increased consumption of the antioxidant vitamins C and E reduces the risk of cancer has been growing over the last several decades. This review assesses the evidence that was reviewed previously by the Food and Drug Administration (FDA) along with the evidence that has appeared since that review was completed. The conclusions that are drawn are based on the totality of publicly available scientific evidence, with emphasis on well-designed studies, which were conducted in a manner that is consistent with generally recognized scientific procedures and principles and which provide credible scientific evidence. These conclusions are drawn with the recognition that an apparent finding of "no effect" is not equivalent to a finding of a "negative effect," and that studies that demonstrate neither beneficial nor harmful effects do not "oppose" studies that do observe a beneficial effect.

This scientific evidence reveals that vitamin C and vitamin E reduce the risk for cancer in general. Individually, they each reduce the risk of several site-specific cancers, including cancer of the colon, esophagus, stomach, larynx, lung, oral cavity, pancreas, throat, kidney, salivary glands, bladder, brain, cervix, and rectum.

Part 1: Vitamin C Reduces Cancer Risk

The scientific evidence indicates that increased consumption of vitamin C reduces the risk for cancer. In the 24-year prospective Western Electric Company Study conducted in Chicago, the risk of death from cancer was reduced significantly by greater daily intakes of vitamin C—113 to 393 milligrams (mg) vs 21– 82 mg— (adjusted for age, systolic blood pressure, body mass index [BMI], serum total cholesterol concentration, smoking status, family history of cardiovascular disease, alcohol consumption, and dietary intakes of energy, cholesterol, iron, saturated fatty acids and polyunsaturated fatty acids).[1] This protective effect of vitamin C was more pronounced among smokers. In another, 17-year prospective study of 2,974 men

in Basel, Switzerland, mean serum vitamin C concentrations were significantly lower in men who died from cancer than they were in men who remained cancer free.[2,3]

Consistent with these reports, when men and women who had participated in the National Health and Nutritional Examination Survey II between 1976 and 1980 were contacted again, 12 to 16 years later, the adjusted risk of dying from any cancer was found to be increased significantly in men with serum ascorbate concentrations less than (<) 28.4 micromoles (μM), compared to the risk in men with serum ascorbate concentrations greater than (>) 73.8 μM, in 1976 to 1980 (adjusted for age, race, education, cigarette smoking, alcohol consumption, history of diabetes, serum total cholesterol concentration, systolic blood pressure, and BMI).[4] Women were not similarly affected. However, the results of observing a cohort of 11,580 initially cancer-free residents of a retirement community for eight years indicated that the risk of developing cancer in women (but not in men) was inversely correlated with the daily consumption of vitamin C.[5] In addition, in a case-control study, people with cancer affecting different sites (breast, head and neck, genitourinary, lung, gastrointestinal, and others) exhibited significantly lower mean serum vitamin C concentrations.[6]

On the other hand, the results of a 13.8-year prospective observational study of 2,112 Welsh men indicated that differences in vitamin C intakes did not affect mortality from cancers of the respiratory tract or from cancers of the digestive tract (adjusted for age, smoking status, social class, BMI, daily intakes of total energy, and fat and alcohol consumption).[7] In the eight-year prospective Nurses' Health Study of 89,494 women in the United States, the risk of developing cancer was not affected by differences in vitamin C intakes.[8] Consistent with these reports, in a prospective observational study

From the *J Orthomolecular Med.* Part 1. 2009;24(1):15–30; Part 2. 2009; 24(2):65–87.

of 605 men and women with coronary heart disease, there were no differences in the average vitamin C intakes between those subjects who developed cancer during the study and those who did not.[9] Similarly, in a 28-year prospective observational study in Washington County, Maryland, differences in vitamin C intake had no effect on hazard ratios for all-cause mortality or death from cancer but 50 percent of subjects consumed less than the RDA for vitamin C.[10] These data suggest that among vitamin-C deficient adults, the degree of deficiency has no effect on all-cause mortality or death from cancer but increased risk for premature death is a feature of chronic vitamin C deficiency.

The scientific evidence indicates that increased consumption of vitamin C reduces the risk for cancer. The evidence documented by a prospective observational study[5] and a retrospective observational study[6] supports this conclusion and there is no evidence that increased consumption of vitamin C may increase the risk for cancer. In addition, the scientific evidence indicates that increased consumption of vitamin C reduces the risk for death from cancer. The evidence documented by four prospective observational studies[1-4] supports this conclusion and there is no evidence that increased consumption of vitamin C may increase the risk for death from cancer.

Bladder Cancer

The scientific evidence indicates that increased consumption of vitamin C reduces the risk for bladder cancer. The results of several retrospective observational studies are consistent with this conclusion. In a case-control study conducted in Los Angeles, consumption of less than 62 mg per day of vitamin C compared to the consumption of more than 168 mg per day of vitamin C reduced significantly the multivariate-adjusted odds of developing bladder cancer (adjusted for education, number of cigarettes smoked per day, number of years smoking, current smoking status, lifetime use of nonsteroidal anti-inflammatory drugs, and number of years employed as a hairdresser or barber).[11] In a similar case-control study of middle-aged men and women conducted in Washington State, individuals consuming the most dietary vita-

min C intake (>156 mg/day vs <78 mg/day) experienced significantly less risk for bladder cancer (adjusted for age, sex, county, smoking, and daily energy intake).[12] Similarly, individuals who consumed the most vitamin C from dietary supplements (>502 mg/day vs none) experienced significantly less risk for bladder cancer (adjusted for age, sex, county, smoking, and daily energy intake), and individuals who consumed the most total vitamin C from foods and dietary supplements (>335 mg/day vs <95 mg/day) experienced significantly less risk for bladder cancer (adjusted for age, sex, county, smoking, and daily energy intake).[12] Consistent with the results of these studies conducted within the United States, investigators reported that men and women in Turkey with grade 1, 2, or 3 transitional cell carcinoma of the bladder (the most common type of bladder cancer) had significantly lower serum concentrations of vitamin C than cancer-free men and women.[13]

In contrast, an epidemiologic analysis of the data obtained during the prospective, double-blind, randomized, placebo-controlled Alpha-Tocopherol, Beta-Carotene Cancer Prevention Study of 29,133 middle-aged male cigarette smokers in Finland who supplemented their diets with 50 mg of vitamin E, 20 mg of beta-carotene, or a placebo for five to eight years, indicated that the risk of developing bladder cancer was not affected by differences in the dietary vitamin C intakes of smokers.[14] However, the results of this epidemiologic analysis are relevant only to populations that match the parent experiment's subjects—middle-aged, lifelong cigarette smoking males—and despite the design of the parent experiment, carry no more "weight" than any other epidemiologic findings.

Several other prospective observational studies have failed to document a chemopreventive effect of vitamin C against bladder cancer. The results of the 12-year prospective observational Health Professionals Follow-Up Study of 51,529 initially cancer-free men, ages 40 to 75, indicated that the risk for bladder cancer was not affected by differences in vitamin C intakes (adjusted for cigarette smoking, region of the United States, total daily fluid intake, and total daily consumption of cruciferous vegetables).[15] Similarly, in the 20-year prospective Nurses' Health Study of 88,796 women in the United States, differences in daily vitamin C intakes from foods or supplements did not affect the multivariate-adjusted risk of developing bladder cancer (adjusted for age, pack-years of cigarette smoking, current smoking status, and total daily energy intake).[16] In the largest of such studies, the 16-year prospective observational American Cancer Society Cancer Prevention Study II of 991,522 men and women in the United States, the regular consumption of any amount of supplemental vitamin C for any length of time had no effect on the risk of dying from bladder cancer.[17] A lack of effect of vitamin C consumption on the prevention of bladder cancer also has been observed outside of the United States; for example, the results of a 6.3-year Dutch prospective observational study (the Netherlands Cohort Study) of 58,279 men and 62,573 women, ages 55 to 69, indicated that the age- and sex-adjusted risk of developing bladder cancer was not affected by differences in vitamin C intakes.[18]

The scientific evidence indicates that increased consumption of vitamin C reduces the risk for bladder cancer. The evidence documented by three retrospective observational studies[11–13] supports this conclusion, and there is no evidence that increased consumption of vitamin C may increase the risk for bladder cancer.

Breast Cancer

The scientific evidence indicates that increased consumption of vitamin C reduces the risk for breast cancer. In an eight-year prospective observational study of 59,036 women, ages 40 to 76, in Sweden (the Swedish Mammography Cohort), among women with a BMI >25, consuming more than the RDA for vitamin C reduced significantly the risk of developing breast cancer (adjusted for age, family history of breast cancer, BMI, education, parity, age at first birth, total daily energy intake, alcohol consumption and daily intakes of dietary fiber, monounsaturated fatty acids, and polyunsaturated fatty acids).[19]

The results of several retrospective observational studies also support the conclusion that increased consumption of vitamin C reduces the risk for breast

cancer.[20–32] In a case-control study conducted in western New York State, the multivariate-adjusted odds of developing breast cancer were reduced significantly among premenopausal women by daily vitamin C intakes >223 mg compared to daily vitamin C intakes <132 mg (adjusted for age, education, age at first birth, age at menarche, history of first-degree relatives with breast cancer, personal history of benign breast disease, BMI, and total daily energy intake).[20] This significant reduction in risk was independent of the intakes of other dietary antioxidants and did not require but was not attenuated by dietary supplementation with vitamin C, although the protection afforded by supplemental vitamin C became slightly less important with increasing consumption of vegetables. In this study, the multivariate-adjusted odds of developing breast cancer were reduced significantly in both premenopausal and postmenopausal women without a family history of breast cancer and who consumed the most vitamin C (premenopausal and postmenopausal women with daily vitamin C intakes >232 mg vs <132 mg; both adjusted for age, education, age at menarche, age at first pregnancy, and BMI).[21] These protective effects were not enjoyed by similar premenopausal women who had a positive family history of breast cancer, suggesting that these adequate but relatively modest intakes of vitamin C were insufficient to override other predisposing factors.[21]

In a case-control study conducted in Germany, the odds of developing breast cancer were halved by vitamin C intakes greater than the RDA (vitamin C intake >134.4 mg/day vs <58.5; adjusted for age, total daily energy intake, age at menarche, age at first birth, age at menopause, family history of breast cancer, current smoking status, personal history of benign breast disease, BMI, daily alcohol consumption, and current or recent use of hormone replacement therapy).[22] In a case-control study conducted in Seoul, Korea, the odds of developing breast cancer were reduced significantly by daily vitamin C intakes >210 mg compared to daily vitamin C intakes <100 mg (adjusted for age at menarche, total number of menstrual periods, parity, total number of full-term live births, total months of breastfeeding, family history of breast cancer, and BMI).[23]

In a case-control study conducted in Moscow, Russia, the odds of developing breast cancer in postmenopausal women were reduced significantly by vitamin C intake (greatest vitamin C intake vs lowest).[24] In another case-control study conducted in Navarra, Spain, the odds of developing breast cancer were reduced significantly by the consumption of vitamin C (greatest vitamin C intake vs lowest).[25] In another case-control study of women conducted in western India, the odds of developing breast cancer were significantly lower among women who consumed the most vitamin C, compared to the odds among women who consumed the least.[26] In another case-control study conducted in Uruguay, the odds of developing breast cancer were reduced significantly by moderately increased daily vitamin C intakes (3rd quartile of vitamin C intake vs 1st quartile; adjusted for age, residence, urban or rural status, family history of breast cancer in a first-degree relative, BMI, age at menarche, parity, menopausal status, and total energy intake).[27]

In another more recent case-control study conducted in Uruguay, the likelihood of breast cancer in premenopausal women was inversely correlated with vitamin C intake.[28] The data collected from a cross-sectional ecological survey in 65 rural Chinese counties indicated that breast cancer mortality was inversely correlated with serum ascorbate concentrations.[29] In other case-control studies conducted in Shanghai, China,[30] Tianjin, China,[30] Italy,[31] and Switzerland,[32] the odds of developing breast cancer were significantly inversely correlated with daily vitamin C intake. In addition, in a case-control study of women conducted in western India, the odds of developing breast cancer were significantly lower among women with the highest plasma ascorbate concentrations, compared to the odds among women with the lowest.[26] (Circulating concentrations of vitamin C can be used as biomarkers of exposure to dietary vitamin C; even small changes in vitamin C intake are reflected in changes in plasma ascorbate concentration.[33])

The results of a meta-analysis of retrospective case-control studies indicated that there was a statistically significant inverse association between vitamin C intake and risk for breast cancer.[34] In addition, other investigators performing a meta-analysis of published data on the relationship between breast cancer and the intake of vitamin C also concluded that the risk of developing breast cancer was reduced significantly by vitamin C consumption ("high" daily consumption of vitamin C vs "low").[35]

In contrast to this large body of evidence demonstrating that increased consumption of vitamin C reduces the risk for breast cancer, the prospective observational data collected from women during the Nurses' Health Study and Nurses' Health Study II in the United States failed to reveal a relationship between vitamin C consumption and the incidence of breast cancer.[36–38] After the first six years of the prospective Nurses' Health Study II of 58,628 women, differences in total vitamin C intakes from foods and supplements had no effects on the adjusted risks of developing nonproliferative benign breast disease, proliferative benign breast disease without atypia, or benign breast disease with atypical hyperplasia (adjusted for age, time period, total daily energy intake, supplement use, family history of breast cancer, oral contraceptive use, and BMI).[36] After eight years, the results of the prospective observational Nurses' Health Study II of 90,655 premenopausal women, ages 26 to 46, found the multivariate-adjusted risk of developing breast cancer from these non-cancerous breast disorders was not affected by differences in the daily intakes of vitamin C from foods or from foods plus supplements (adjusted for age, smoking status, height, parity, age at first full-term birth, BMI, age at menarche, family history of breast cancer, personal history of benign breast disease, oral contraceptive use, menopausal status, alcohol consumption, daily energy intake, and daily intake of animal fat).[37] Similarly, in the 14-year prospective Nurses' Health Study of 83,234 women, the multivariate-adjusted risk of developing breast cancer was not affected by differences in daily intakes of vitamin C from foods alone or from foods and dietary supplements (adjusted for age, length of follow-up, daily energy intake, parity, age at first birth, age at menarche, history of breast cancer in a mother or sister, history of benign breast disease, alcohol consumption, BMI at age 18 years, change in body weight since age 18 years, height, age at menopause, and post-menopausal hormone therapy).[38]

Three other prospective observational studies also failed to reveal a relationship between vitamin C consumption and the incidence of breast cancer.[39-41] In a prospective observational study of 34,387 postmenopausal women in the state of Iowa (the Iowa Women's Health Study), the multivariate-adjusted risk of developing breast cancer was not affected by differences in vitamin C intakes (adjusted for age, daily energy intake, age at menarche, age at menopause, age at first live birth, parity, BMI at entry into study, BMI at age 18 years, family history of breast cancer, personal history of benign breast disease, alcohol consumption, and education).[39] In addition, data obtained from 4,697 women, initially cancer free and ages 15 or older, after 25 years of observation failed to reveal a significant relationship between differences in daily vitamin C intakes and the occurrence of breast cancer,[40] and, after the first 4.3 years of a prospective observational study of 62,573 women, ages 55 to 69 (the Netherlands Cohort Study), the risk of developing breast cancer was not affected by differences in vitamin C intakes.[41]

The results of several retrospective observational studies[42-52] also failed to demonstrate the protective effect of increased vitamin C consumption against breast cancer. In a case-control study of women conducted in North Carolina, the multivariate-adjusted odds of developing breast cancer were not affected by dietary supplementation with any amount of vitamin C (adjusted for age, age at menarche, age at first full-term pregnancy, menopausal status, lactation history, family history, BMI, waist-to-hip circumference ratio, education, alcohol consumption, smoking history, and daily intakes of fruits and vegetables).[42] Similarly, the odds of developing breast cancer were not affected by differences in vitamin C intakes in upstate New York.[43]

Investigators performing a case-control study nested within the Canadian National Breast Screening Study of 56,837 women also reported that the multivariate-adjusted odds of developing breast cancer were not affected by differences in the daily intakes of vitamin C from either foods or dietary supplements (adjusted for age, daily energy intake, age at menarche, surgical menopause, age at first live birth, education, family history of breast cancer, and personal history of benign breast disease).[44]

In a set of case-control studies conducted in China (the Shanghai Nutrition and Breast Disease Study[45] and the Shanghai Breast Cancer Study[46-48]), differences in vitamin C intakes had no effects on the odds of developing nonproliferative benign breast disease, proliferative benign breast disease without atypia, or proliferative benign breast disease with atypical hypertrophy. In case-control studies conducted in Italy, the energy-adjusted odds of developing breast cancer were not affected by differences in vitamin C consumption.[49,50] In case-control studies conducted in Greece, the odds of developing breast cancer were not affected by differences in vitamin C intakes.[51,52]

In a case-control study nested within the Danish Diet, Cancer, and Health Study of post-menopausal women, the odds of developing breast cancer were reported to increase significantly with increased intake of vitamin C, an anomalous finding that the investigators could not explain and considered artifactual.[53]

The scientific evidence indicates that increased consumption of vitamin C reduces the risk for breast cancer. The evidence documented by a prospective observational study,[19] 13 retrospective observational studies,[20-32] and two meta-analyses[34,35] supports this conclusion, and there is no evidence that increased consumption of vitamin C may increase the risk for breast cancer.

Cervical Cancer

The scientific evidence indicates that increased consumption of vitamin C reduces the risk for cervical cancer. The results of several retrospective observational studies support the conclusion that increased consumption of vitamin C reduces the risk for cervical cancer.[54-56] Most important, in a case-control study conducted in Seattle, Washington, the odds of developing cervical cancer were halved by increased daily intakes of vitamin C.[54] In addition, the results of a case-control study conducted in four Latin American countries indicated that the odds of developing cervical cancer were inversely correlated with vitamin C intakes.[55] In a case-control study conducted in India, the odds of developing cervical cancer and the severity of cervical cancer were both inversely correlated with serum ascorbate concentrations.[56] In contrast, the results of a two-year, double-blind, placebo-controlled, randomized, factorial study in which women with colposcopically (follow-up test for an abnormal pap smear) and histologically confirmed minor squamous atypia or cervical intra-epithelial neoplasia (an established precursor lesion to cervical cancer) supplemented their diets with either a placebo, 30 mg of beta-carotene, 500 mg of vitamin C, or 30 mg of beta-carotene plus 500 mg vitamin C suggested that the rate of lesion regression was not accelerated by supplementation with this amount of vitamin C.[57] The results of several retrospective observational studies are consistent with this conclusion.[58–60] In a case-control study conducted in the state of Hawaii, the multivariate-adjusted odds of developing cervical dysplasia (a precursor to cervical cancer) were not affected by differences in plasma ascorbate concentrations (adjusted for age, ethnicity, smoking status, alcohol consumption, and presence or absence of human papillomavirus).[58] In a case-control study conducted in the state of Alabama, the multivariate-adjusted odds of developing cervical dysplasia were not affected by differences in vitamin C intakes (adjusted for age, race, age at first intercourse, number of sexual partners, parity, smoking status, use of oral contraceptives, and presence of human papillomavirus infection).[59] In a case-control study conducted in Portland, Oregon, the age-adjusted odds of developing precancerous cytological abnormalities of the cervix were not affected by differences in daily vitamin C intakes.[60]

The scientific evidence indicates that increased consumption of vitamin C reduces the risk for cervical cancer. The evidence documented by three retrospective observational studies[54–56] supports this conclusion, and there is no evidence that increased consumption of vitamin C may increase the risk for cervical cancer.

Colon Cancer

The scientific evidence indicates that increased consumption of vitamin C reduces the risk for colon cancer. In a prospective study that compared patients with adenomatous colonic polyps (an accepted risk factor for colon cancer) to subjects without polyps, one month of dietary supplementation with vitamin C (750 mg/day) produced a significantly greater decrease in cell proliferation within crypts (dimple-like indents) in normal-appearing colon lining in subjects with polyps than was produced by a placebo consumption, while there was no change in subjects without polyps—suggesting that vitamin C does not interfere with normal cell cycling but does slow abnormally accelerated proliferation in the colon's lining.[61] Consistent with this evidence of a protective effect of supplemental vitamin C, in a prospective observational study of 35,215 women, ages 50 to 69, in Iowa (the Iowa Women's Health Study), the age-adjusted risk of developing colon cancer was reduced 33 percent in women who consumed more than 60 mg of supplemental vitamin C daily, compared to the risk in women who did not consume vitamin C supplements.[62]

The results of several retrospective observational studies also support the conclusion that increased consumption of vitamin C reduces the risk for colon cancer.[63–65] In the case-control North Carolina Colon Cancer Study, a group of men and women with "high" vitamin C intakes (median: 644 mg/day) experienced half the risk for colon cancer than was experienced by another otherwise similar group of men and women with "low" vitamin C intakes (median: 59 mg/day).[63] The responses of Caucasian and African Americans to vitamin C intake were not different.[63] On average, individuals with colon cancer consumed significantly less vitamin C, although vitamin intakes appeared to have no effect on the relative incidence of microsatellite instability (a biomarker for risk for colon cancer).[64] Similarly, in a case-control study conducted in Seattle, Washington, the age- and sex-adjusted odds of developing colon cancer were reduced significantly in men and women who supplemented their diets with vitamin C (daily supplemental vitamin C intake >500 mg vs none).[65]

In a case-control study conducted in Shanghai, China, the odds of men developing colon cancer also were reduced significantly by greater daily intake of vitamin C (vitamin C intake >30 mg/day vs <30 mg/day), although the odds of women developing colon cancer were not affected by differences in vitamin C intakes.[66] However, in a 17-year prospective study of 2,974 men in Basel, Switzerland, in which dietary and lifestyle patterns were assumed to remain static, differences in pre-study serum vitamin C concentrations had no effect on the risk of developing colon cancer, a result that may reflect changing dietary and lifestyle patterns during the last quarter of the 20th century more than inherent relationships between vitamin C and the colon epithelium.[2,3]

In a case-control study conducted in Denmark, the odds of adenomatous polyp recurrence were inversely correlated with daily intakes of vitamin C.[67] In contrast, in other case-control studies, the odds of adenomatous polyp occurrence[68] or recurrence[69] were not affected by differences in daily vitamin C intakes.

The scientific evidence indicates that increased consumption of vitamin C reduces the risk for colon cancer. The evidence documented by a prospective clinical trial of vitamin C supplementation,[61] a prospective observational study,[62] and five retrospective observational studies[63–67] supports this conclusion and there is no evidence that increased consumption of vitamin C may increase the risk for colon cancer.

Colorectal Cancer

The scientific evidence indicates that increased consumption of vitamin C reduces the risk for colorectal cancer. The results of the 14-year prospective observational American Cancer Society Cancer Prevention Study II of 711,891 men and women who were initially cancer free indicated that the age- and sex-adjusted risk of developing colorectal cancer was reduced significantly by 10 or more years of dietary supplementation with any amount of vitamin C.[70] In addition, the results of several retrospective observational studies support the conclusion that increased consumption of vitamin C reduces the risk for colorectal cancer.[71–76]

In a case-control study conducted in France, the multivariate-adjusted odds of developing colorectal polyps (a risk factor for colorectal cancer) were reduced significantly by the consumption of greater amounts of vitamin C (men and women, daily vitamin C consumption >114 mg vs <61 mg; both adjusted for age, sex, BMI, tobacco use, daily energy intake and alcohol consumption).[71] In a case-control study conducted in Italy, the multivariate-adjusted odds of developing colorectal cancer were reduced significantly by increased vitamin C intakes (vitamin C intake >188 mg/day vs <189 mg/day; adjusted for age, study center, sex, education, level of physical activity, and daily intakes of energy and dietary fiber).[72] In a case-control study conducted in the Canton of Vaud, Switzerland, the multivariate-adjusted odds of developing colorectal cancer were reduced significantly by "intermediate" intakes of vitamin C (median: 112 mg/day) compared to "low" intakes (median: 65 mg/day) (adjusted for age, sex, education, smoking status, alcohol consumption, BMI, level of physical activity, and daily intakes of energy and dietary fiber).[73] Consistent with these findings, the results of a case-control study conducted in northern Italy indicated that the odds of developing colorectal cancer were reduced significantly by vitamin C consumption (5th quintile of daily vitamin C intake vs 1st quintile)[74] and, in a case-control study conducted in western New York State, the odds of developing colorectal cancer were inversely correlated with vitamin C intakes.[75] In addition, men in Turkey with colorectal tumors had significantly lower mean plasma vitamin C concentration than healthy men.[76]

In contrast, the results of a double-blind, randomized, placebo-controlled clinical trial in which men and women supplemented their diets with either a placebo, beta-carotene (25 mg/day), vitamin C (1,000 mg/day) plus vitamin E (400 mg/day), or all three antioxidants for four years indicated that combined dietary supplementation with this amount of vitamin C did not affect the incidence of colorectal polyps (adjusted for age, sex, number of prior polyps, actual length of time between clinical evaluations and study center).[77] Consistent with this finding, in a two-year double-blind, randomized, placebo-controlled clinical trial in which patients who were thought to be free of colorectal polyps after polyp removal added either a placebo or a supplement containing 400 mg of vitamin C and 400 mg of vitamin E to their diets, the multivariate-adjusted risk of developing new polyps was not affected by the combined supplement (adjusted for age and the usual frequency of consumption of meats and fish).[78]

Also consistent with these findings, the results of a secondary end-point analysis of the data obtained during the prospective, double-blind, randomized, placebo-controlled Alpha-Tocopherol, Beta-Carotene Cancer Prevention study of 29,133 middle-aged male cigarette smokers in Finland who supplemented their diets with 50 mg of vitamin E, 20 mg of beta-carotene, or a placebo for five to eight years indicated that the risk of developing colorectal cancer was not affected by the intake of vitamin C, although more than 50 percent of these subjects consumed less than the RDA for vitamin C.[79] However, the placebo-controlled trials were of inadequate duration to measure accurately the incidence of new polyps or tumors; even in patients who have undergone polypectomy (removal of polyps), the minimum time before re-examination recommended by the 2006 Consensus Update on Guidelines for Colonoscopy after Polypectomy of the U.S. Multi-Society Task Force on Colorectal Cancer and the American Cancer Society is five years.[80]

The results of two retrospective observational studies failed to support the conclusion that increased consumption of vitamin C reduces the risk for colorectal cancer.[81,82] In a case-control study conducted in Los Angeles, the multivariate-adjusted odds of developing colorectal adenoma or colorectal adenomatous polyps were not affected by differences in vitamin C intakes from foods or from supplements (adjusted for daily intakes of calories, saturated fat, folate and fiber, alcohol consumption, current smoking status, BMI, race, level of daily physical activity, and use of nonsteroidal anti-inflammatory drugs).[81] In another case-control study conducted in North Carolina, the multivariate-adjusted odds of developing colorectal adenoma were not affected by differences in vitamin C intakes in men or women (adjusted for age, BMI, daily energy intake, smoking status, use of dietary supplements, family history of colon cancer and daily intakes of fat, dietary fiber, and alcohol).[82]

The scientific evidence indicates that increased consumption of vitamin C reduces the risk for colorectal cancer. The evidence documented by a prospective observational study[70] and six retrospective observational studies[71–76] supports this conclusion and there is no evidence that increased consumption of vitamin C may increase the risk for colorectal cancer.

Endometrial Cancer

The scientific evidence indicates that increased consumption of vitamin C reduces the risk for endometrial (uterine) cancer. The results of three retrospective observational studies[83–85] support the conclusion that the consumption of increased amounts of vitamin C reduces the risk for endometrial cancer. In a case-control study nested within the Western New York Diet Study, the multivariate-adjusted odds of developing endometrial cancer were reduced significantly in women who consumed amounts of vitamin C greater than the median (daily vitamin C intake >172 mg vs <129 mg; adjusted for age, education, BMI, diabetes, hypertension, pack-years of cigarette smoking, age at menarche, parity, use of oral contraceptives, menopausal status, postmenopausal use of estrogen, and daily energy intake).[83] Similarly, the results of a case-control study conducted in Shanghai, China, indicated that the multivariate-adjusted odds of developing endometrial cancer were reduced significantly among women with greater daily vitamin C intakes (daily vitamin C intake >42 mg/1,000 kcal vs <30 mg/1,000 kcal; adjusted for age, education, menopausal status, diagnosis of diabetes, alcohol consumption, BMI, level of physical activity, and dietary intakes of animal products, fruits and vegetables, and energy).[84] In another case-control study, conducted in the Swiss Canton of Vaud and in Northern Italy, the energy-adjusted odds of developing endometrial carcinoma were reduced significantly by increased intake of vitamin C (5th quintile of daily vitamin C intake vs 1st quintile).[85]

In contrast, the data obtained from the 10-year

prospective Canadian National Breast Screening Study of 56,837 women indicated that the risk for endometrial cancer was not associated with differences in daily intakes of vitamin C.[86] Similarly, in a case-control study conducted in the state of Hawaii, the multivariate-adjusted odds of developing endometrial cancer were not affected by differences in the intake of vitamin C from foods (adjusted for parity, use of oral contraceptives, use of unopposed estrogen, history of diabetes, and BMI).[87]

The scientific evidence indicates that increased consumption of vitamin C reduces the risk for endometrial cancer. The evidence documented by three retrospective observational studies[83–85] supports this conclusion, and there is no evidence that increased consumption of vitamin C may increase the risk for endometrial cancer.

Esophageal Cancer

The scientific evidence indicates that increased consumption of vitamin C reduces the risk for adenocarcinoma of the esophagus (esophageal cancer). The results of two retrospective observational studies[88,89] support the conclusion that the consumption of increased amounts of vitamin C reduces the risk for adenocarcinoma of the esophagus. In a case-control study conducted in the United States, compared to men and women with daily vitamin C intakes less than the 25th percentile, men and women with daily vitamin C intakes greater than the 75th percentile exhibited significantly reduced odds of developing esophageal cancer (adjusted for sex, state of residence, age, race, income bracket, education, BMI, cigarette smoking, alcoholic beverage consumption, and total daily energy intake).[88] In a similar case-control study conducted in Germany, the multivariate-adjusted odds of developing adenocarcinoma of the esophagus were reduced significantly in men who consumed >100 mg of vitamin C daily compared to those who consumed <100 mg (adjusted for unspecified "known risk factors").[89]

On the other hand, in a case-control study conducted in New York State, the odds of developing adenocarcinoma of the esophagus were not affected by differences in vitamin C intakes.[90] In

another case-control study conducted in northeast China, the multivariate-adjusted odds of developing any esophageal cancer were not affected by differences in daily vitamin C intakes (adjusted for alcohol consumption, smoking status, income, and occupation).[91] In a case-control study of the impact of vitamin C deficiency on adenocarcinoma of the esophagus conducted in Sweden, the multivariate-adjusted odds of developing squamous cell carcinoma of the esophagus (see next) were not affected by differences in vitamin C intakes in a vitamin C–deficient population (adjusted for age, sex, BMI, and smoking status).[92]

The scientific evidence indicates that increased consumption of vitamin C reduces the risk for adenocarcinoma of the esophagus. The evidence documented by two retrospective observational studies[88,89] supports this conclusion, and there is no evidence that increased consumption of vitamin C may increase the risk for adenocarcinoma of the esophagus.

Squamous Cell Cancer of the Esophagus

The scientific evidence indicates that increased consumption of vitamin C reduces the risk for squamous cell carcinoma of the esophagus. This type of cancer begins in the squamous cells lining the surface of the esophagus, in contrast to adenocarcinoma of the esophagus, which begins in the cells mucus-secreting glands in the esophagus. The results of several retrospective observational studies[88,89,93–96] support the conclusion that the consumption of increased amounts of vitamin C reduces the risk for squamous cell carcinoma of the esophagus. Among men participating in a case-control study conducted in the United States, Caucasian men who consumed the most vitamin C from vegetables or who consumed dietary supplements containing vitamin C cut their risk of developing squamous cell carcinoma of the esophagus in half (adjusted for age, residence, smoking, and alcohol consumption).[93] Similarly, in the same study, African-American men who consumed the most vitamin C from fruit also cut their risk of developing squamous cell carcinoma of the esophagus in half (adjusted for age, residence, smoking, and alcohol consumption).[93] In another case-control study conducted in the United States, compared to men and women with daily vitamin C intakes less than the 25th percentile, men and women with daily vitamin C intakes greater than the 75th percentile exhibited significantly reduced odds of developing squamous cell carcinoma of the esophagus (adjusted for sex, state of residence, age, race, income bracket, education, BMI, cigarette smoking, alcoholic beverage consumption, and total daily energy intake).[88] In a case-control study conducted in Uruguay, the multivariate-adjusted odds of developing squamous cell carcinoma of the esophagus also were reduced significantly by increased intakes of vitamin C (2nd quartile of vitamin C intake vs 1st quartile; adjusted for age, sex, residence, urban or rural status, birthplace, education, BMI, smoking status, years since quit smoking, number of cigarettes smoked per day by current smokers, alcohol consumption, mate tea consumption, and total daily energy intake).[94] In a case-control study conducted in France, the multivariate-adjusted odds of developing squamous cell cancer of the esophagus were reduced significantly by intakes of vitamin C greater than the RDA (daily vitamin C intake >90 mg vs <60 mg; adjusted for interviewer age, smoking status, and daily consumption of beer, aniseed aperitives, hot Calvados, whiskey, total alcohol, and total energy).[95] In a case-control study conducted in Germany, the multivariate-adjusted odds of developing squamous cell carcinoma of the esophagus were reduced significantly in men who consumed >100 mg of vitamin C daily compared to men who consumed <100 mg (adjusted for unspecified known risk factors).[89] In another case-control study conducted in Uruguay, the multivariate-adjusted odds of developing any esophageal cancer were reduced significantly by daily vitamin C intakes greater than the lowest quartile of intake (adjusted for age, gender, residence, urban or rural status, education, BMI, smoking status, alcohol consumption, total energy intake, and daily intakes of alpha-carotene, beta-carotene, lutein, lycopene, beta-cryptoxanthin, vitamin E, glutathione, quercetin, kaempferol, total flavonoids, beta-sitosterol, campesterol, and stigmasterol).[96]

On the other hand, in one case-control study conducted in northeast China, the multivariate-adjusted odds of developing any esophageal cancer were not affected by differences in daily vitamin C intakes (adjusted for alcohol consumption, smoking status, income, and occupation).[91] In another case-control study of the impact of vitamin C deficiency on squamous cell carcinoma of the esophagus conducted in Sweden, the multivariate-adjusted odds of developing squamous cell carcinoma of the esophagus were not affected by differences in vitamin C intakes in a vitamin C–deficient population (adjusted for age, sex, BMI, and smoking status).[92]

The scientific evidence indicates that increased consumption of vitamin C reduces the risk for squamous cell carcinoma of the esophagus. The evidence documented by six retrospective observational studies[88,89,93–96] supports this conclusion, and there is no evidence that increased consumption of vitamin C may increase the risk for squamous cell carcinoma of the esophagus. In addition, the evidence documented by a retrospective observational study[92] demonstrates that squamous cell carcinoma of the esophagus is not prevented by vitamin C deficiency.

Part 2: Vitamin E Reduces Cancer Risk

Vitamin E, like vitamin C, is a powerful antioxidant. It is fat soluble, which makes it particularly effective at preventing the oxidation of fats in cell membranes. Many of the same studies discussed in Part 1 on vitamin C also investigated the role of vitamin E against cancer. [Editor's note: The amounts of vitamin E used in the following studies are often reported in milligrams (mg) rather than international units (IU), the more familiar value. A mg of vitamin E (a weight measure) is approximately 1 to 1.5 IU of vitamin E (an activity measure). The natural form is more active per mg.]

Breast Cancer

The scientific evidence indicates that increased consumption of vitamin E reduces the risk for breast cancer. The results of several retrospective observational studies support the conclusion that increased consumption of vitamin E reduces the risk for breast cancer.[10,11,16–18,21,37–39,43,98] In a case-control study conducted in New York State, the multivariate-adjusted odds of developing breast cancer were reduced significantly among premenopausal women by any daily intakes of alpha-tocopherol (the form most widely used in supplements) equal to or greater than two-thirds of the RDA (daily vitamin E intakes >10 mg vs <7 mg; adjusted for age, education, age at first birth, age at menarche, history of first-degree relatives with breast cancer, personal history of benign breast disease, BMI, and total daily energy intake).[10] This significant reduction in risk was independent of the intakes of other dietary antioxidants and did not require but was not attenuated by dietary supplementation with vitamin E, although it became less important with increasing consumption of vegetables. In a case-control study of women conducted in western New York State, the multivariate-adjusted odds of developing breast cancer were reduced significantly in both premenopausal and postmenopausal women without a family history of breast cancer and who consumed the most alpha-tocopherol, despite the almost universal prevalence of vitamin E deficiency among these women (premenopausal and postmenopausal women with daily alpha-tocopherol intake >10.4 mg vs <6.4 mg; both adjusted for age, education, age at menarche, age at first pregnancy, and BMI).[11] These protective effects were not enjoyed by similar premenopausal women who had a positive family history of breast cancer, indicating that chronic vitamin E deficiency cannot overcome factors that predispose a woman of any age to breast cancer.[11]

In a case-control study conducted in China (the Shanghai Breast Cancer Study), the odds of women developing breast cancer were reduced significantly among women who consumed more than the RDA for vitamin E, compared to vitamin-E deficient women (vitamin E intake >19.9 mg/day vs <9.4 mg/day).[37] In an extension of this study, the multivariate-adjusted odds of developing breast cancer were reduced significantly among women with diets deficient in vitamin E and who consumed dietary supplements of vitamin E (vitamin-E deficient diet plus vitamin E supplement vs vitamin-E deficient diet alone; adjusted for age, education, age at menarche, parity, BMI, menopausal status,

level of recreational exercise, history of fibroadenoma, history of breast cancer in first-degree relatives, and phase of study).[38] In addition, in a case-control study nested within the Danish Diet, Cancer, and Health Study of postmenopausal women, the odds of developing breast cancer were reduced significantly by the daily consumption of at least 25 mg of vitamin E, compared to the odds associated with the daily consumption of 10 to 15 mg (adjusted for vitamin C intake, vitamin A intake, number of childbirths, age at first childbirth, history of surgery for benign breast disease, education, years of hormone replacement therapy, alcohol consumption, and BMI).[43]

From the data obtained in a case-control study conducted in Italy, it was determined that 8.6 percent of the risk of developing breast cancer is attributable to daily vitamin E intake less than 8.5 mg.[98] The impact of poor vitamin E nutrition on risk for breast cancer was confirmed further by the results of another case-control study conducted in Italy, in which the energy-adjusted odds of developing breast cancer were reduced significantly by increased vitamin E consumption (5th quintile of daily vitamin E intake vs 1st quintile)[39] and in another, the odds of developing breast cancer were inversely correlated with daily intakes of vitamin E.[21] Furthermore, in a case-control study conducted in Uruguay, the multivariate-adjusted odds of developing breast cancer were reduced significantly by even moderately increased daily vitamin E intakes (2nd quartile of vitamin E intake vs 1st quartile; adjusted for adjusted for age, residence, urban or rural status, family history of breast cancer in a first-degree relative, BMI, age at menarche, parity, menopausal status, and total energy intake)[17] and, in a more recent case-control study conducted in Uruguay, the likelihood of breast cancer in premenopausal women was inversely correlated with vitamin E intake.[18] In addition, in a case-control study of women conducted in western India, the odds of developing breast cancer were significantly lower among women with the highest plasma alpha-tocopherol concentrations, compared to the odds among women with the lowest.[16] (Circulating concentrations of vitamin E can be used as biomarkers of exposure to dietary vita-

VITAMIN E PREVENTS LUNG CANCER YET NEWS MEDIA VIRTUALLY SILENT ON POSITIVE VITAMIN RESEARCH

by Andrew W. Saul, PhD

Researchers at the University of Texas Anderson Cancer Center have found that taking more vitamin E substantially reduces lung cancer. Their new study shows that people consuming the highest amounts of vitamin E had the greatest benefit. When they compared persons taking the most vitamin E with those taking the least, there was a 61 percent reduction in lung cancer risk.[1]

Lung cancer is the most prevalent form of cancer on earth; over 1.3 million people are diagnosed with it each year. With medical treatment, survival rates are "consistently poor," says Cancer Research UK. Lung cancer kills nearly 1.2 million per year. It accounts for 12 percent of all cancers, but results in 18 percent of all cancer deaths.[2] Anything that can reduce these dismal facts is important news . . . very important. Yet the mainstream media have virtually ignored vitamin E's important role as a cancer fighter.

A 61 percent reduction in lung cancer with vitamin E? How could the news media have missed this one?

Good News

The news media probably did not miss it: they simply did not report it. They are biased. You can see for yourself what bias there is. Try a Google search for any of the major newspapers or broadcast media, using the name of the news organization along with the phrase "vitamin E lung cancer." When you do, you will find that it will quickly bring up previous items alleging that vitamin E might (somehow) increase cancer risk. You will find little or nothing at all on how vitamin E prevents cancer.

And why not? Might the answer possibly have anything to do with money? One cannot watch television or read a magazine or newspaper without it being obvious that drug company cash is one of the media's very largest sources of revenue. Given where their advertising income comes from, it is hardly a big surprise that media reporting on vitamins is biased. Well-publicized vitamin scares feed the pharmaceutical industry. Successful reports of safe, inexpensive vitamin therapy do not. This is an enormous public health problem with enormous consequences.

Bad News

The good news about how important high quantities of vitamin E are in combating cancer is not arising out of nowhere. A U.S. National Library of Medicine Medline search will bring up over 3,000 studies on the subject, some dating back to 1946. By the early 1950s, research clearly supported the use of vitamin E against cancer.[3] Before 1960, vitamin E was shown to reduce the side effects of radiation cancer treatment.[4] In reviewing vitamin E research, one notes that the high-dose studies got the best results.

Vitamin E is not the sure cure for cancer. It is not certain prevention, either. Stopping cigarette smoking is essential. But vitamin E is part of the solution, and we need more of it. An independent panel of physicians and researchers[5] has recently called for increasing the daily recommended intake for vitamin E to 200 IU. The present U.S. RDA/DRI is less than 23 IU a day.

It is time to raise it. A lot.

REFERENCES

1. Mahabir S. *Int J Cancer* 2008;123(5):1173–1180.

2. Cancer Research UK. http://info.cancerresearchuk.org/cancerstats/geographic/world/commoncancers.

3. Telford IR. *Tex Rep Biol Med* 1955;13(3):515–521. Also: Swick RW. *Cancer Res* 1951;11(12):948–953.

4. Fischer W. *Munch Med Wochenschr* 1959;101:1487–1488. Also: Sabatini C. *Riforma Med* 1955;69(18): Suppl,1–4. Also: Graham JB. *Surg Forum* 1953; (38th Congress):332–338.

5. Doctors say, raise the RDAs now. *Orthomolecular Medicine News Service*, Oct 30, 2007.

Excerpted from the *Orthomolecular Medicine News Service*, October 29, 2008.

min E; for example, for every doubling of alpha-tocopherol intake, plasma alpha-tocopherol concentration increases 10 percent).[23,99]

In contrast to this large body of evidence demonstrating that increased consumption of vitamin E reduces the risk for breast cancer, the prospective observational data collected during the eight-year prospective observational Nurses' Health Study II of 90,655 premenopausal women, ages 26 to 46, indicated that the multivariate-adjusted risk of developing breast cancer was not affected by differences in the daily intakes of vitamin E from foods or from foods plus supplements (adjusted for age, smoking status, height, parity, age at first full-term birth, BMI, age at menarche, family history of breast cancer, personal history of benign breast disease, oral contraceptive use, menopausal status, alcohol consumption, daily energy intake, and daily intake of animal fat).[27] Similarly, in the 14-year prospective Nurses' Health Study of 83,234 women, the multivariate-adjusted risk of developing breast cancer was not affected by differences in daily intakes of vitamin E from foods alone or from foods and dietary supplements (adjusted for age, length of follow-up, daily energy intake, parity, age at first birth, age at menarche, history of breast cancer in a mother or sister, history of benign breast disease, alcohol consumption, BMI at age 18, change in body weight since age 18, height, age at menopause, and postmenopausal hormone therapy).[28] The results of a prospective observational study of 34,387 postmenopausal women in the state of Iowa (the Iowa Women's Health Study) also indicated that the multivariate-adjusted risk of developing breast cancer was not affected by differences in vitamin E intakes (adjusted for age, daily energy intake, age at menarche, age at menopause, age at first live birth, parity, BMI at entry into study, BMI at age 18 years, family history of breast cancer, personal history of benign breast disease, alcohol consumption, and education).[29]

Three other prospective observational studies also failed to reveal a relationship between vitamin E consumption and the incidence of breast cancer.[9,30,31] For example, data obtained from 4,697 women, initially cancer free and ages 15 or older,

after 25 years of observation failed to reveal a significant relationship between differences in daily vitamin E intakes and the occurrence of breast cancer.[30] After the first 4.3 years of the prospective observational study of 62,573 women, ages 55 to 69 (the Netherlands Cohort Study), the risk of developing breast cancer was not affected by differences in vitamin E intakes.[31] Interestingly, the results of an eight-year prospective observational study of 59,036 women, ages 40 to 76, in Sweden (the Swedish Mammography Cohort), among women with a BMI >25, differences in vitamin E intakes were unable to overcome the established procarcinogenic influence of excess body weight on the risk of developing breast cancer.[9]

The results of retrospective observational studies conducted in the United States[32,33,100–103] also failed to demonstrate the protective effect of increased vitamin E consumption against breast cancer. In a case-control study conducted in western New York state, the odds of developing breast cancer were not affected by differences in vitamin E intakes[33] and in a more recent case-control study of women conducted in North Carolina, the multivariate-adjusted odds of developing breast cancer were not affected by dietary supplementation with any amount of vitamin E (adjusted for age, age at menarche, age at first full-term pregnancy, menopausal status, lactation history, family history, BMI, waist-to-hip circumference ratio, education, alcohol consumption, smoking history, and daily intakes of fruits and vegetables).[32] In case-control studies nested within prospective studies conducted in Missouri,[100] Washington County, Maryland,[101,102] and within the prospective Nurses' Health Study in the United States,[103] the odds of developing breast cancer were not affected by differences in serum alpha-tocopherol concentrations.

Similarly, in a case-control study nested within the Canadian National Breast Screening Study of 56,837 women, the multivariate-adjusted odds of developing breast cancer were not affected by differences in the daily intakes of vitamin E or alpha-tocopherol from either foods or dietary supplements (adjusted for adjusted for age, daily energy intake, age at menarche, surgical menopause, age at first live birth, education, family history of breast cancer, and personal history of benign breast disease).[34] In case-control studies conducted in China (the Shanghai Nutrition and Breast Disease Study,[35] the Shanghai Breast Cancer Study,[36] and studies conducted in Shanghai and Tianjin[20]), differences in vitamin E intakes had no effects on the age-adjusted odds of developing nonproliferative benign breast disease, proliferative benign breast disease without atypia, or proliferative benign breast disease with atypical hypertrophy. In several European case-control studies conducted in Sweden,[104] Italy,[40] Greece,[41] and the UK[105] and in a similar study conducted in western India,[16] the odds of developing breast cancer were not affected by differences in daily intakes of vitamin E.

In case-control studies conducted in Germany[12] and Seoul, Korea,[13] the odds of developing breast cancer were not affected by differences in vitamin E intakes; however, over 80 percent of the subjects in these studies were chronically vitamin E deficient.

One double-blind, randomized, placebo-controlled clinical trial directly addressed the effects of dietary supplementation with vitamin E in the prevention of breast cancer. In the 10-year Women's Health Study, in which 39,876 apparently healthy women over 45 years old consumed either a placebo or 600 IU of vitamin E every other day, this amount and pattern of vitamin E supplementation did not affect the age-adjusted risk for breast cancer.[106] However, the extent to which separating episodes of vitamin E consumption by 48 hours prevents the establishment of an elevated steady-state of circulating alpha-tocopherol concentration is not known (alpha-tocopherol concentrations were not measured during this study).

The scientific evidence indicates that increased consumption of vitamin E reduces the risk for breast cancer. The evidence documented by 11 retrospective observational studies[10,11,16–18,21,37–39,43,98] supports this conclusion, and there is no evidence that increased consumption of vitamin E may increase the risk for breast cancer. In addition, the results of two studies[12,13] confirm that vitamin E deficiency does not protect against breast cancer.

Colon Cancer

The scientific evidence indicates that increased consumption of vitamin E reduces the risk for colon cancer. The results of a prospective observational study of 35,215 women, ages 50 to 69, in Iowa (the Iowa Women's Health Study), largely as a result of the protective effect of supplemental vitamin E intakes greater than 30 mg per day (supplemental vitamin E intake >30 mg/day vs none), women consuming the most vitamin E experienced significantly less risk for colon cancer (total vitamin E intake >35 mg/day vs <6 mg/day).[107] These protective effects remained significant after further adjustment of the calculated risk ratios for age, daily total energy intake, height, parity, vitamin A supplementation, and daily intakes of seafood and skinless chicken (supplemental vitamin E intake >30 mg/day vs none; total vitamin E intake >35 mg/day vs <6 mg/day).[107]

In addition, the results of retrospective observational studies support the conclusion that increased consumption of vitamin E reduces the risk for colon cancer.[99,108–113] In the case-control North Carolina Colon Cancer Study, a group of African-American men and women with "high" vitamin E intakes (median: 140 mg/day) experienced significantly less risk for colon cancer than was experienced by another otherwise similar group of African-American men and women with "low" vitamin E intakes (median: 6 mg/day).[108] In contrast, the odds of developing colon cancer were not affected by differences in vitamin E intakes among Caucasian men and women, over half of whom were vitamin E deficient.[108] On average, individuals with colon cancer consumed significantly less vitamin E but vitamin intakes appeared to have no effect on the relative incidence of microsatellite instability (a biomarker for risk for colon cancer).[109]

In a case-control study conducted in the Seattle, Washington area, the age- and sex-adjusted odds of developing colon cancer were reduced significantly in men and women who supplemented their diets with vitamin E (daily supplemental vitamin E intake >15 mg vs none)[110] and, in a case-control study conducted in Montreal, Quebec,

Canada, the multivariate-adjusted odds of developing colon carcinoma were reduced significantly by increased consumption of vitamin E (2nd quartile of vitamin E intake vs 1st quartile; adjusted for sex, age, marital status, history of colon carcinoma in first-degree relatives, and total daily energy intake).[111] In a case-control study conducted in Shanghai, China, the odds of men developing colon cancer were reduced significantly by greater daily intake of vitamin E (vitamin E intake >32 mg/day vs <26 mg/day), although the odds of women developing colon cancer were not affected by differences in vitamin E intakes.[99]

In a case-control study conducted in New York City, the odds of adenomatous polyp recurrence were reduced significantly among patients who supplemented their diets with vitamin E (vitamin E supplementation vs none).[112] Similarly, in Denmark, the odds of adenomatous polyp recurrence were inversely correlated with daily intakes of vitamin E.[113]

In contrast to these reports, when the data from 87,998 women in the prospective Nurses' Health Study were combined with the data from 47,344 men in the prospective Health Professionals Follow-Up Study, the risk for developing colon cancer was found to be unaffected by differences in vitamin E consumption.[114] In addition, in a case-control study conducted in Salt Lake City, Utah, the odds of developing colon cancer did not reflect differences in daily intakes of alpha-tocopherol.[115] In a 17-year prospective study of 2,974 men in Basel, Switzerland,[86,87] and in a case-control study nested within a prospective study in Washington County, Maryland,[101] differences in serum vitamin E concentrations had no effect on the risks of developing colon cancer.

One double-blind, randomized, placebo-controlled clinical trial directly addressed the effects of dietary supplementation with vitamin E in the prevention of colon cancer. In the 10-year Women's Health Study, in which 39,876 apparently healthy women over 45 years old consumed either placebo or 600 IU of vitamin E every other day, this amount and pattern of vitamin E supplementation did not affect the age-adjusted risk for colon cancer.[106] However, the extent to which separating

episodes of vitamin E consumption by 48 hours prevents the establishment of an elevated steady-state of circulating alpha-tocopherol concentration is not known (alpha-tocopherol concentrations were not measured during this study).

The scientific evidence indicates that increased consumption of vitamin E reduces the risk for colon cancer. The evidence documented by a prospective observational study[107] and seven retrospective observational studies[99,108–113] supports this conclusion and there is no evidence that increased consumption of vitamin E may increase the risk for colon cancer.

Colorectal Cancer

The scientific evidence indicates that increased consumption of vitamin E reduces the risk for colorectal cancer. The results of several retrospective observational studies support the conclusion that increased consumption of vitamin E reduces the risk for colorectal cancer.[53,55,63] In a case-control study conducted in North Carolina, the multivariate-adjusted odds of developing colorectal adenoma (polyps) were reduced significantly in men by intakes of vitamin E greater than the RDA (vitamin E intake >15.3 mg vs <0.3 mg; adjusted for age, BMI, daily energy intake, smoking status, use of dietary supplements, family history of colon cancer, and daily intakes of fat, dietary fiber, and alcohol).[63] In a case-control study conducted in Italy, the multivariate-adjusted odds of developing colorectal cancer were reduced significantly by increased vitamin E intakes (vitamin E intake >12.3 mg/day vs <12.3 mg/day; adjusted for age, study center, sex, education, level of physical activity, and daily intakes of energy and dietary fiber).[53] In another case-control study conducted in northern Italy, the odds of developing colorectal cancer were reduced significantly by vitamin E consumption (5th quintile of daily vitamin E intake vs 1st quintile).[55] In contrast, the results of several other retrospective observational studies failed to reveal a relationship between increased consumption of vitamin E and reduced risk for colorectal cancer.[52,63,116] In a case-control study conducted in North Carolina, the multivariate-adjusted odds of developing colorectal polyps were not affected by differences in vitamin E intakes in women (adjusted for age, BMI, daily energy intake, smoking status, use of dietary supplements, family history of colon cancer, and daily intakes of fat, dietary fiber, and alcohol).[63] In a case-control cross-sectional observational study of men and women in California, differences in vitamin E intakes, with or without supplements, had no effect on the odds of developing colorectal adenomatous polyps.[116] In a case-control study conducted in France, the multivariate-adjusted odds of developing colorectal adenoma were not affected by differences in the consumption of vitamin E.[52]

In a case-control study conducted in Los Angeles, the multivariate-adjusted odds of developing colorectal adenoma were not affected by differences in vitamin E intakes from foods or from supplements among a study population that was almost entirely vitamin E deficient, even with vitamin E supplementation (adjusted for daily intakes of calories, saturated fat, folate and fiber, alcohol consumption, current smoking status, BMI, race, level of daily physical activity, and use of nonsteroidal anti-inflammatory drugs).[62] In this study, varying the degree of vitamin E deficiency did not reduce the risk for colorectal polyps. Similarly, in a case-control study conducted in the Canton of Vaud, Switzerland, the multivariate-adjusted odds of developing colorectal cancer were not affected by differences in daily intakes of vitamin E in another population that was largely vitamin E deficient (adjusted for age, sex, education, smoking status, alcohol consumption, BMI, level of physical activity, and daily intakes of energy and dietary fiber).[54]

In a case-control study conducted in Los Angeles, the multivariate-adjusted odds of developing colorectal polyps were not affected by differences in plasma alpha-tocopherol concentration (adjusted for location, sex, age, date examined, ethnicity, serum total cholesterol concentration, serum triglyceride concentration, BMI, exercise, smoking, alcohol consumption, daily caloric intake, daily intakes of saturated fat, fruits, vegetables, folate and calcium, use of nonsteroidal anti-inflammatory drugs, and plasma ferritin concentration).[117] Similarly, in three case-control studies conducted in Japan, no relationship was observed between colorectal adenoma or cancer and circulating vitamin E concentrations.[118–120]

The results of a double-blind, randomized, placebo-controlled clinical trial in which men and women supplemented their diets with either a placebo, beta-carotene (25 mg/day), vitamin C (1,000 mg/day) plus vitamin E (400 mg/day), or all three antioxidants for four years indicated that combined dietary supplementation with this amount of vitamin E did not affect the incidence of colorectal adenoma (adjusted for age, sex, number of prior adenomas, actual length of time between clinical evaluations and study center).[58] This finding was confirmed in another two-year double-blind, randomized, placebo-controlled human clinical trial in which patients, who were thought to be free of colorectal polyps after polyp removal and who added either a placebo or a supplement containing 400 mg of vitamin C and 400 mg of vitamin E to their diets, exhibited no difference in the multivariate-adjusted risk of developing new polyps (adjusted for age and the usual frequency of consumption of meats and fish).[59] However, the placebo-controlled trials were of inadequate duration to measure accurately the incidence of new polyps or tumors; even in patients who have undergone polypectomy (removal of polyps), the minimum time before reexamination recommended by the 2006 Consensus Update on Guidelines for Colonoscopy after Polypectomy of the U.S. Multi-Society Task Force on Colorectal Cancer and the American Cancer Society is five years.[61]

The results of secondary end-point analyses of the data obtained during the prospective, double-blind, randomized, placebo-controlled Alpha-Tocopherol, Beta-Carotene Cancer Prevention study of 29,133 middle-aged male cigarette smokers in Finland who supplemented their diets with 50 mg of vitamin E, 20 mg of beta-carotene, or a placebo for five to eight years indicated that supplementation with 50 mg of vitamin E was associated with a significant increase in the incidence of colorectal polyps,[121] although the incidence of colorectal cancer was not affected.[60,122] This report is hardly credible; the incidence of new colorectal adenoma reported in the subjects who did not receive supplemental vitamin E was over 10 times the projected incidence of such cancers among the general U.S. male population in 2008[123] and an additional two- to ten-fold increase would be expected to dominate the findings of every clinical trial that employed at least 50 mg of vitamin E. This has not happened.[3,106,124–127]

The scientific evidence indicates that increased consumption of vitamin E reduces the risk for colorectal cancer. The evidence documented by three retrospective observational studies[53,55,63] supports this conclusion, and there is no evidence that increased consumption of vitamin E may increase the risk for colorectal cancer.

Esophageal Cancer

The scientific evidence indicates that increased consumption of vitamin E reduces the risk for cancer of the esophagus. The results of several retrospective observational studies[70,128,129] support the conclusion that the consumption of increased amounts of vitamin E reduces the risk for cancer of the esophagus.

In a case-control study conducted in Germany, the multivariate-adjusted odds of developing adenocarcinoma of the esophagus were reduced significantly in men who consumed more than 13 mg of vitamin E daily (daily vitamin E intake >13 mg vs <13 mg; adjusted for unspecified "known risk factors").[70] In a case-control study in Uruguay, the multivariate-adjusted odds of developing esophageal cancer were reduced significantly by daily vitamin E intakes greater than the lowest quartile of intake (adjusted for age, gender, residence, urban or rural status, education, BMI, smoking status, alcohol consumption, total energy intake, and daily intakes of beta-carotene, lutein, lycopene, beta-cryptoxanthin, vitamin E, glutathione, quercetin, kaempferol, total flavonoids, beta-sitosterol, campesterol, and stigmasterol).[128] In a case-control study conducted in China (the General Population Trial in Linxian), although the mean serum concentration of alpha-tocopherol did not differ between men and women with esophageal cancer and cancer-free men and women, for every 25 percent increase in serum alpha-tocopherol concentration above the mean, the risk for esophageal cancer decreased significantly by 10 percent.[129]

On the other hand, a secondary end-point analysis of the data obtained during the prospective, double-blind, randomized, placebo-controlled Alpha-Tocopherol, Beta-Carotene Cancer Prevention study of 29,133 middle-aged male cigarette smokers in Finland who supplemented their diets with 50 mg of vitamin E, 20 mg of beta-carotene, or a placebo for five to eight years determined that five to eight years of daily supplementation with 50 mg of vitamin E was unable to overcome the procarcinogenic effects of lifelong cigarette smoking on the incidence of esophageal cancer.[130] However, the results of this epidemiologic analysis are relevant only to populations that match the parent experiment's subjects—middle-aged, male, lifelong cigarette smokers.

The results of three retrospective observational studies[71,73,131] failed to reveal a protective effect of increased vitamin E intakes against adenocarcinoma of the esophagus. In a case-control study conducted in New York State, the odds of developing cancer of the esophagus were not affected by differences in vitamin E intakes.[71] In a case-control study of the impact of vitamin E deficiency on esophageal cancer conducted in Sweden, the multivariate-adjusted odds of developing squamous cell carcinoma of the esophagus (see next) were not affected by differences in vitamin E intakes in a vitamin E–deficient population (adjusted for age, sex, BMI, and smoking status).[73] In a case-control study conducted in the state of Hawaii, mean serum alpha-tocopherol concentrations of subjects with and without esophageal cancer were not different.[131]

The scientific evidence indicates that increased consumption of vitamin E reduces the risk for adenocarcinoma of the esophagus. The evidence documented by three retrospective observational studies[70,128,129] supports this conclusion, and there is no evidence that increased consumption of vitamin E may increase the risk for adenocarcinoma of the esophagus.

Squamous Cell Carcinoma of the Esophagus

The scientific evidence indicates that increased consumption of vitamin E reduces the risk for squamous cell carcinoma of the esophagus. The results of several retrospective observational studies[69,70,128,129,132] support the conclusion that the consumption of increased amounts of vitamin E reduces the risk for squamous cell carcinoma of the esophagus. In a case-control study conducted in the United States, compared to men and women with daily vitamin E intakes less than the 25th percentile, men and women with daily vitamin E intakes greater than the 75th percentile exhibited significantly reduced odds of developing esophageal squamous cell carcinoma (adjusted for sex, state of residence, age, race, income bracket, education, BMI, cigarette smoking, alcoholic beverage consumption, and total daily energy intake).[69] Similarly, in a case-control study conducted in France, the multivariate-adjusted odds of developing squamous cell carcinoma of the esophagus were reduced significantly by less-deficient intakes of vitamin E (daily vitamin E intake >7 mg vs <7 mg; adjusted for interviewer, age smoking status and daily consumption of beer aniseed aperitives, hot Calvados, whiskey, total alcohol, and total energy).[132] This protection was strongest among the heaviest consumers of alcoholic beverages. In a case-control study conducted in Germany, the multivariate-adjusted odds of developing this type of cancer were reduced significantly in men who consumed more than 13 mg of vitamin E daily (daily vitamin E intake >13 mg vs <13 mg; adjusted for unspecified "known risk factors").[70]

In a case-control study in Uruguay, the multivariate-adjusted odds of developing esophageal cancer were reduced significantly by daily vitamin E intakes greater than the lowest quartile of intake (adjusted for age, gender, residence, urban or rural status, education, BMI, smoking status, alcohol consumption, total energy intake and daily intakes of beta-carotene , lutein, lycopene, beta-cryptoxanthin, vitamin E, glutathione, quercetin, kaempferol, total flavonoids, beta-sitosterol, campesterol, and stigmasterol).[128] In a case-control study conducted in China (the General Population Trial in Linxian), although the mean serum concentration of alpha-tocopherol did not differ between men and women with esophageal cancer and cancer-free men and women, for every 25 percent increase in serum alpha-tocopherol concentration above the mean, the risk for esophageal cancer decreased significantly by 10 percent.[129]

In contrast, a secondary end-point analysis of the data obtained during the prospective, double-blind, randomized, placebo-controlled Alpha-Tocopherol, Beta-Carotene Cancer Prevention study of 29,133 middle-aged male cigarette smokers in Finland who supplemented their diets with 50 mg of vitamin E, 20 mg of beta-carotene, or a placebo for five to eight years, determined that five to eight years of daily supplementation with 50 mg of vitamin E was unable to overcome the procarcinogenic effects of lifelong cigarette smoking on the incidence of esophageal cancer.[130] However, the results of this epidemiologic analysis is relevant only to populations that match the parent experiment's subjects—middle-aged male lifelong cigarette smokers.

Data obtained during four retrospective observational studies[73,82,131,133] failed to reveal a protective effect of increased vitamin E intakes against squamous cell carcinoma of the esophagus. In two case-control studies conducted in Uruguay, the multivariate-adjusted odds of developing squamous cell carcinoma of the esophagus were not affected by differences in vitamin E intakes (adjusted for age, sex, residence, urban or rural status, birthplace, education, BMI, smoking status, years since quit smoking, number of cigarettes smoked per day, alcohol consumption, mate tea consumption, and total daily energy intake;[133] adjusted for age, residence, urban or rural status, education, family history of prostate cancer, BMI, and total daily energy intake).[82] In a case-control study of the impact of vitamin E deficiency on squamous cell carcinoma of the esophagus conducted in Sweden, the multivariate-adjusted odds of developing squamous cell carcinoma of the esophagus were not affected by differences in vitamin E intakes in a vitamin-E deficient population (adjusted for age, sex, BMI, and smoking status).[73] In a case-control study conducted in the state of Hawaii, mean serum alpha-tocopherol concentrations of subjects with and without esophageal cancer were not different.[131]

The scientific evidence indicates that increased consumption of vitamin E reduces the risk for squamous cell carcinoma of the esophagus. The evidence documented by five retrospective observational studies[69,70,128,129,132] supports this conclusion, and there is no evidence that increased consumption of vitamin E may increase the risk for squamous cell carcinoma of the esophagus. In addition, the evidence documented by a retrospective observational study[73] demonstrates that squamous cell carcinoma of the esophagus is not prevented by vitamin E deficiency.

Laryngeal Cancer

The scientific evidence suggests that increased consumption of vitamin E may reduce the risk for laryngeal cancer (cancer of the larynx, commonly called the voice box). The results of a retrospective observational study[134] support the conclusion that the consumption of increased amounts of vitamin E reduces the risk for laryngeal cancer. In a case-control study conducted in Uruguay, the multivariate-adjusted odds of developing laryngeal cancer were inversely correlated with vitamin E intake (adjusted for age, sex, residence, urban or rural status, education, BMI, smoking status, years since quit smoking, number of cigarettes smoked per day by current smokers, age at start of smoking, and total daily energy intake).[134] Increased vitamin E intake was most effective in the prevention of cancer of the supraglottis and less effective in the prevention of cancer of the glottis. The supraglottis is the part of the larynx above the glottis (where the vocal cords are located). Risk reduction was weakened by continuation of cigarette smoking.

On the other hand, the results of two retrospective observational studies[131,135] failed to reveal a protective effect of increased vitamin E intakes against laryngeal cancer. In a case-control study conducted in Japan, the multivariate-adjusted odds of developing laryngeal cancer were not affected by differences in vitamin E intakes (adjusted for age, sex, smoking status, alcohol consumption, use of multivitamin supplements, total daily energy intake, dental hygiene, and year of first hospital visit)[135] and, in a case-control study conducted in the state of Hawaii, mean serum alpha-tocopherol concentrations of subjects with and without laryngeal cancer were not different.[131]

The scientific evidence suggests that increased consumption of vitamin E may reduce the risk for laryngeal cancer. The evidence documented by a retrospective observational study[134] supports this conclusion, and there is no evidence that increased consumption of vitamin E may increase the risk for laryngeal cancer.

Melanoma

The scientific evidence indicates that increased consumption of vitamin E reduces the risk for melanoma. The results of a case-control study conducted in Washington County, Maryland, indicated that the odds of developing malignant melanoma were inversely correlated with age, education, and energy intake-adjusted vitamin E intakes.[136] Although the odds of men in the United States developing malignant melanoma were not affected by differences in the intakes of vitamin E from foods and supplements, the odds of women developing malignant melanoma were halved when daily total vitamin E intakes from foods and supplements exceeded the RDA.[137] Consistent with these reports, the results of observing the 39,268 male and female participants in the Finnish Social Insurance Institution's Mobile Clinic Health Survey, ages 15 to 99 and initially free from cancer, prospectively for eight years indicated that serum alpha-tocopherol concentrations were inversely correlated with the risk of developing melanoma.[138]

In contrast, the results of combining the data obtained from 73,525 female participants in the prospective observational Nurses' Health Study and from 88,553 female participants in the prospective observational Nurses' Health Study II indicated that the multivariate-adjusted risk of developing melanoma was not affected by differences in vitamin E intakes from foods or dietary supplements (adjusted for age, skin reaction after two hours of sun exposure during childhood, number of sunburns over lifetime, number of sunburns during adolescence, number of moles on left arm, number of moles on lower legs, hair color, family history of melanoma, state of residence, menopausal status, use of oral contraceptives, use of postmenopausal hormone therapies, parity, height, and BMI).[139] In a case-control study conducted in Boston, the multivariate-adjusted odds of developing malignant melanoma were not affected by differences in plasma alpha-tocopherol concentrations or vitamin E intakes (adjusted for age, sex, plasma lipid concentrations, hair color, and the ability to suntan).[140] In a series of case-control studies nested within a prospective study in Washington County, Maryland, prediagnostic serum vitamin E concentrations were not associated with the odds of developing melanoma.[101,141]

The scientific evidence indicates that increased consumption of vitamin E reduces the risk for melanoma. The evidence documented by a prospective observational study[138] and 2 retrospective observational studies[136,137] supports this conclusion, and there is no evidence that increased consumption of vitamin E may increase the risk for melanoma.

Oral Cavity Cancer

The scientific evidence indicates that increased consumption of vitamin E reduces the risk for cancer of the oral cavity (mouth). The results of four retrospective observational studies[135,142–144] support the conclusion that increased consumption of vitamin E reduces the risk for cancer of the oral cavity. In a case-control study conducted in New York City, the odds of developing cancer of the oral cavity were inversely correlated with dietary supplementation with vitamin E.[142] In another case-control study conducted in the United States, the odds of developing cancer of the oral cavity were inversely correlated with vitamin E supplementation (supplementation vs none).[143] In a case-control study conducted in Japan, the multivariate-adjusted odds of developing cancer of the oral cavity were reduced significantly in men and women by greater intakes of vitamin E (daily vitamin E intake >7.7 mg vs <4.0 mg; adjusted for age, sex, smoking status, alcohol consumption, use of multivitamin supplements, total daily energy intake, dental hygiene, and year of first hospital visit).[135] In a case-control study conducted in Italy and Switzerland, the multivariate-adjusted odds of developing either pharyngeal (throat) cancer or cancer of the oral cavity were reduced significantly by increased intake of vitamin E (adjusted for age, sex, center, education, occupation, body mass index, smoking and drinking habits, and non-alcohol energy intake).[144]

However, the results of four retrospective observational studies[131,145–147] failed to document a relationship between vitamin E and cancer of the oral cavity. For example, in a case-control study conducted in Melbourne, Australia, the odds of developing squamous cell cancer of the oral cavity were not affected by differences in dietary vitamin E intakes.[145] In a case-control study conducted in Japan, the odds of developing oral leukoplakia (white patches on the tongue or inside the cheeks that may be a precursor of cancer of the oral cavity) were not affected by differences in serum alpha-tocopherol concentrations.[146] In a case-control study conducted in the state of Hawaii, mean serum alpha-tocopherol concentrations of subjects with and without any upper aerodigestive tract cancer (i.e., cancer of the oral cavity, pharynx, esophagus, or larynx) were not different.[131] In a case-control study conducted in Washington County, Maryland, the odds of developing cancer of the oral cavity were not affected by prediagnostic serum alpha-tocopherol concentration.[147]

In addition, in the prospective, double-blind, randomized, placebo-controlled Alpha-Tocopherol, Beta-Carotene Cancer Prevention study of 29,133 middle-aged male cigarette smokers in Finland who supplemented their diets with 50 mg of vitamin E, 20 mg of beta-carotene, or a placebo for five to eight years, supplementation with 50 mg of vitamin E daily did not appear to affect the prevalence of either oral leukoplakia or dysplastic lesions of the buccal epithelium (inner lining of the cheeks) or the incidence of upper aerodigestive tract cancers.[130,148]

The scientific evidence indicates that increased consumption of vitamin E reduces the risk for cancer of the oral cavity. The evidence documented by four retrospective observational studies[135,142–144] supports this conclusion, and there is no evidence that increased consumption of vitamin E may increase the risk for cancer of the oral cavity.

Ovarian Cancer

The scientific evidence indicates that increased consumption of vitamin E reduces the risk for ovarian cancer. The results of retrospective observational studies support the conclusion that increased consumption of vitamin E reduces the risk for ovarian cancer.[74,79,149] In a case-control study of women conducted in North Carolina, total daily intakes of vitamin E in excess of 75 mg reduced significantly the odds of developing epithelial ovarian cancer (the most common type of ovarian cancer), and dietary supplementation with any amount of vitamin E also reduced significantly the odds of developing epithelial ovarian cancer.[74] Consistent with this report, in a case-control study conducted in Canada, any amount of supplementation with vitamin E for more than 10 years halved the adjusted odds of developing ovarian cancer (adjusted for age, residence, education, alcohol consumption, cigarette smoking, BMI, daily energy intake, recreational physical activity, parity, years of menstruation, and menopausal status).[79] In a case-control study conducted in Italy, the risk of developing epithelial ovarian cancer was reduced significantly among women who regularly consumed more than the median amount of vitamin E daily, compared to the risk of women who regularly consumed less than the median amount of vitamin E daily (adjusted for age, study center, year of entry into study, BMI, parity, use of oral contraceptives, occupational physical activity, and daily energy intake).[149]

In contrast, the results in two prospective[75,77] and three retrospective observational studies[78,80,150] failed to discern a relationship between vitamin E and ovarian cancer. Among 97,275 initially cancer-free women participating in the eight-year prospective California Teachers Study of women,[77] and among 80,326 initially cancer-free women participating in the 16-year prospective Nurses' Health Study,[75] the risks of developing ovarian cancer were not affected by differences in vitamin E intakes. In a case-control study conducted in Hawaii and Los Angeles, differences in vitamin E intakes did not affect the odds of premenopausal or postmenopausal women developing ovarian cancer.[78] In a case-control study nested within a prospective study conducted in Washington County, Maryland, the odds of developing ovarian cancer were not affected by differences in cholesterol-adjusted serum alpha-tocopherol concentrations.[150] In a case-control study conducted in New Hampshire and eastern Massachusetts, differences in daily intakes of vitamin

E had no effect on the odds of premenopausal or postmenopausal women developing ovarian cancer.[80]

The scientific evidence indicates that increased consumption of vitamin E reduces the risk for ovarian cancer. The evidence documented by three retrospective observational studies[74,79,149] supports this conclusion, and there is no evidence that increased consumption of vitamin E may increase the risk for ovarian cancer.

Pancreatic Cancer

The scientific evidence indicates that increased consumption of vitamin E reduces the risk for cancer of the pancreas. The results of retrospective observational studies conducted in Shanghai, China, support the conclusion that increased consumption of vitamin E reduces the risk for pancreatic cancer.[151,152] In one study, the multivariate-adjusted odds of developing pancreatic cancer were reduced significantly in men (but not women) consuming "high" amounts of vitamin E (daily vitamin E consumption >41 mg vs <26 mg; adjusted for age, income, smoking, green tea drinking, and daily caloric intake).[151] In the other, the multivariate-adjusted odds of developing pancreatic cancer were reduced significantly in both men and women consuming "high" amounts of vitamin E (men, 4th quartile of daily vitamin E consumption vs 1st quartile; women, 4th quartile of daily vitamin E consumption vs 1st quartile: both adjusted for age, income, smoking, green tea drinking, and daily caloric intake).[152]

However, in a case-control study nested within a prospective study in Washington County, Maryland, prediagnostic serum vitamin E concentrations were not associated with the odds of developing pancreatic cancer.[101] In addition, the results of a secondary end-point analysis of the data obtained in the prospective, double-blind, randomized, placebo-controlled Alpha-Tocopherol, Beta-Carotene Cancer Prevention study of 29,133 middle-aged male cigarette smokers in Finland who supplemented their diets with 50 mg of vitamin E, 20 mg of beta-carotene, or a placebo for five to eight years indicated that supplementation with 50 mg of vitamin E daily had no effect on the incidence of pancreatic carcinoma.[153] In addition, an epidemiologic analysis of that data indicated that the risk of developing pancreatic cancer was not affected by differences in the intake of vitamin E.[154]

Similarly, the results of observing a cohort of 13,979 initially cancer-free residents of a retirement community for nine years indicated that the risk of developing pancreatic cancer was not affected by differences in the daily consumption of vitamin E.[155]

The scientific evidence indicates that increased consumption of vitamin E reduces the risk for pancreatic cancer. The evidence documented by two retrospective observational studies[151,152] supports this conclusion and there is no evidence that increased consumption of vitamin E may increase the risk for pancreatic cancer.

Prostate Cancer

The scientific evidence suggests that the consumption of increased amounts of vitamin E reduces the risk for prostate cancer. In a secondary end-point analysis of the data obtained during the prospective, double-blind, randomized, and placebo-controlled Alpha-Tocopherol, Beta-Carotene Cancer Prevention study of 29,133 middle-aged male cigarette smokers in Finland who supplemented their diets with 50 mg of vitamin E, 20 mg of beta-carotene, or a placebo, it was determined that five to eight years of daily dietary supplementation with 50 mg of vitamin E produced a significant decrease in the incidence of new prostate cancer (adjusted for age, presence of benign prostatic hyperplasia, living in an urban area, presence or absence of concurrent dietary supplementation with beta-carotene, and serum total cholesterol concentration).[122,156,158] Consistent with this result, two groups of analysts performing systematic reviews of human clinical trials concluded that daily supplementation with 50 mg of vitamin E significantly reduces the risk for developing prostate cancer.[159,160]

In addition, an analysis of the effects of pre-study serum alpha-tocopherol concentrations on the development of prostate cancer 19 years later in participants in the prospective, double-blind, randomized, placebo-controlled Alpha-Tocopherol, Beta-Carotene Cancer Prevention study of 29,133 middle-aged male cigarette smokers in Finland who supplemented their diets with 50 mg of vita-min E, 20 mg of beta-carotene, or a placebo for five to eight years found that even though differences in serum alpha-tocopherol concentrations had no effect on the odds of developing prostate cancer during the study,[161] the risks for any prostate cancer and for advanced prostate cancer were inversely correlated with pre-study serum alpha-tocopherol concentrations (risk estimates were adjusted for age at blood sample collection, trial intervention arm, serum total cholesterol concentration, body weight, urban residence, and education).[162] These findings are even more remarkable given the continued cigarette smoking by the subjects during and after the study and the data from a 20-year prospective observational study (the Lutheran Brotherhood Cohort Study) of 17,633 Caucasian males, ages 35 years and older, that confirm that the use of tobacco products increases the risk of developing prostate cancer.[163]

The results of prospective observational studies also support the conclusion that increased consumption of vitamin E reduces the risk for prostate cancer.[86–88,164,165] For example, although the results of an 8-year prospective observational study (the Prostate, Lung, Colorectal and Ovarian Cancer Screening Trial) suggest that among all men, differences in vitamin E or alpha-tocopherol intakes from foods or dietary supplements do not affect the multivariate-adjusted risk of developing prostate cancer (adjusted for age, daily energy intake, race, study center, family history of prostate cancer, BMI, smoking status, physical activity, daily consumption of fats and red meats, history of diabetes, and aspirin use) among current smokers and nonsmokers who had quit smoking within 10 years, daily dietary supplementation with more than 400 IU of vitamin E reduces significantly the risk of developing advanced prostate cancer (daily dietary supplementation with >400 IU of vitamin E vs none; adjusted for age, daily energy intake, race, study center, family history of prostate cancer, BMI, smoking status, physical activity, daily consumption of fats and red meats, history of diabetes, and aspirin use).[88] Similarly, among current smokers and nonsmokers who had quit smoking within 10 years and who had consumed any amount of supplemental vitamin E for at least 10 years, daily dietary supplementation with vitamin E reduced significantly the risk of developing advanced prostate cancer (supplementation with any amount of vitamin E for at least 10 years vs none; adjusted for age, daily energy intake, race, study center, family history of prostate cancer, BMI, smoking status, physical activity, daily consumption of fats and red meats, history of diabetes, and aspirin use).

Consistent with this report, in a 17-year prospective study of 2,974 men in Basel, Switzerland, serum vitamin E concentrations <30.02 micromoles (uM) increased significantly the risk of developing prostate cancer among cigarette smokers.[86,87] On the other hand, the results of the double-blind, randomized, placebo-controlled Prevention Research Veteran Affairs E-Vitamin Nutrition Trial indicated that daily supplementation with 400 IU of vitamin E produced a significant increase in mean serum alpha-tocopherol concentration without affecting mean serum prostate specific antigen concentration[164] and the results of a 10-year prospective observational study of 35,242 men conducted in Washington State indicated that the risk for advanced (regionally invasive or distant metastatic) prostate cancer was reduced significantly by daily supplementation with at least 400 IU of vitamin E (adjusted for age, family history of prostate cancer, history of benign prostatic hyperplasia, income, use of multivitamins, and serum prostate specific antigen concentration).[165]

The results of retrospective observational studies also support the conclusion that increased consumption of vitamin E reduces the risk for prostate cancer.[95,166–168]

In a case-control study conducted in Serbia, the odds of developing prostate cancer were reduced significantly by greater daily intakes of alpha-tocopherol[95] and, in a case-control study conducted in Athens, Greece, the odds of developing prostate cancer were inversely correlated with vitamin E intakes.[166]

In a case-control study nested within a prospective study conducted in Washington County, Maryland, the multivariate-adjusted odds of developing prostate cancer were reduced significantly when serum alpha-tocopherol concentration was >1.31 mg per deciliter (dL),

serum gamma-tocopherol (another member of the vitamin E family) concentration (another member of the vitamin E family) was >0.28 mg/dL, and serum selenium concentrations were either <0.79 parts per million (ppm) (adjusted for age, education, and hours since last meal when blood was obtained) or >0.79 ppm (adjusted for age, education, and hours since last meal when blood was obtained).[167] Consistent with this report, in a case-control study conducted in India, mean erythrocyte ascorbic acid content and mean plasma vitamin E concentration were significantly lower among patients with prostate cancer.[168]

In contrast to this body of supportive evidence, the results of prospective[85,89,169,170] and retrospective[91,94,96,97,101,171–174] observational studies did not provide support for the conclusion that increased consumption of vitamin E reduces the risk for prostate cancer. After 10 years of observation, those among the 47,780 men participating in the prospective U.S. Health Professionals Follow-Up Study who consumed dietary supplements containing vitamin E exhibited no change in their multivariate-adjusted risk of developing prostate cancer (adjusted for period of study, age, family history of prostate cancer, vasectomy status, smoking status, current BMI, BMI at age 21, physical activity level at entry into study, daily energy intake, and daily intakes of calcium, lycopene, fructose, and total fat).[169] Similarly, among the 72,704 men of the American Cancer Society Cancer Prevention Study II Nutrition Cohort, the risk of developing prostate cancer was not affected by the intakes of vitamin E from either foods or supplements,[170] among the 475,726 men participating in the 18-year prospective observational American Cancer Society Cancer Prevention Study II, daily dietary supplementation with vitamin E did not affect the multivariate-adjusted rate of death from prostate cancer (adjusted for age, race, education, smoking status, family history or prostate cancer, exercise, BMI, alcohol consumption, vegetable consumption, and dietary supplementation with multivitamins, vitamin A, and vitamin C),[85] and the results of a 6.3-year prospective observational study (the Netherlands Cohort Study) of 58,279 men, ages 55 to 69, indicated that the age- and sex-adjusted risk of developing prostate cancer was not affected by differences in vitamin E intakes in that study population.[89]

In case-control studies conducted in Sweden[94] and Montreal, Quebec, Canada,[96] the odds of developing either any form of prostate cancer or advanced prostate cancer were not affected by differences in daily intakes of vitamin E (adjusted for age and daily energy intake). In a case-control study conducted in the state of Washington, the multivariate-adjusted odds of developing prostate cancer were not affected by the use of any dietary supplements of vitamin E (adjusted for dietary intakes of fat and total energy, race, age, family history of prostate cancer, BMI, serum prostate specific antigen concentration, and education).[91]

In a case-control study nested within the prospective Beta-Carotene and Retinol Efficacy Trial (CARET) of dietary supplementation of 18,314 high-risk subjects (heavy smokers and workers exposed to asbestos) with a placebo, beta-carotene, or retinyl palmitate (a form of vitamin A), the multivariate-adjusted odds of developing prostate cancer were not affected by differences in prestudy serum alpha-tocopherol concentrations (adjusted for study center, asbestos exposure, age, sex, smoking status during study, year of entry into study, and cigarette smoking history prior to the study).[171] Similarly, in a case-control study nested within the eight-country European Prospective Investigation into Cancer and Nutrition (EPIC), the multivariate-adjusted odds of developing prostate cancer were not affected by differences in prestudy plasma alpha-tocopherol concentrations (adjusted for BMI, smoking status, alcohol consumption, level of physical activity, marital status, and education).[172] In individual case-control studies nested within a prospective study in Washington County, Maryland, prediagnostic serum vitamin E concentrations were not associated with the odds of developing prostate cancer[101,173] and, when the data from two case-control studies conducted in Washington County were combined, the odds of developing prostate cancer were found to be unaffected by differences in serum concentrations of alpha-tocopherol.[97] In a case-control study conducted in Hawaii, the multivariate-adjusted odds of developing prostate

cancer were not affected by differences in serum alpha-tocopherol concentrations.[174]

The scientific evidence indicates that increased consumption of vitamin E reduces the risk for prostate cancer. The evidence documented by a secondary end-point analysis of the data obtained during a prospective trial,[122,156–158] the results of two systematic reviews,[159,160] six prospective observational studies[86–88,163,165,166] and four retrospective observational studies[95,166–168] support this conclusion, and there is no evidence that increased consumption of vitamin E increases the risk for prostate cancer.

Throat Cancer

The scientific evidence indicates that increased consumption of vitamin E reduces the risk for throat (pharyngeal) cancer. The results of a case-control study conducted in Italy and Switzerland indicated that the multivariate-adjusted odds of developing either cancer of the oral cavity or pharyngeal cancer were reduced significantly by increased intake of vitamin E (adjusted for age, sex, center, education, occupation, body mass index, smoking and drinking habits, and non-alcohol energy intake).[144]

However, in the prospective, double-blind, randomized, placebo-controlled Alpha-Tocopherol, Beta-Carotene Cancer Prevention study of 29,133 middle-aged male cigarette smokers in Finland who supplemented their diets with 50 mg of vitamin E, 20 mg of beta-carotene, or placebo for five to eight years, supplementation with 50 mg of vitamin E daily had no effect on the incidence of upper aerodigestive tract cancers (cancers of the oral cavity, pharynx, esophagus, or larynx).[130] Consistent with this report, in a case-control study conducted in Japan, the multivariate-adjusted odds of developing pharyngeal cancer were not affected by differences in vitamin E intakes (adjusted for age, sex, smoking status, alcohol consumption, use of multivitamin supplements, total daily energy intake, dental hygiene, and year of first hospital visit).[135] Similarly, in a case-control study conducted in Melbourne, Australia, the odds of developing either squamous cell cancer of the oral cavity or pharyngeal cancer were not affected by differences in dietary vitamin E intakes.[145] In addition, the results of a case-control study conducted in the state of Hawaii indicated that the mean serum alpha-tocopherol concentrations of subjects with and without upper aerodigestive tract cancer were not different.[131]

The scientific evidence indicates that increased consumption of vitamin E reduces the risk for pharyngeal cancer. The evidence documented by a retrospective observational study[144] supports this conclusion, and there is no evidence that increased consumption of vitamin E may increase the risk for pharyngeal cancer.

■ CONCLUSION

The foregoing credible scientific evidence establishes that adequate intakes of vitamin C and vitamin E safely reduce the risk for cancer in general. Individually, vitamin C reduces the risk for cancer of the bladder, breast, cervix, colon, colorectum, esophagus and squamous cell carcinoma of the esophagus, kidney, lung, oral cavity, ovary, pancreas, pharynx, prostate, salivary glands, stomach, and uterus. Vitamin C also may reduce the risk of laryngeal cancer. Individually, vitamin E reduces the risk for cancers of the breast, cervix, colon cancer, colorectum, esophagus and squamous cell carcinoma of the esophagus, melanoma, oral cavity, ovary, pancreas, throat, and prostate. Vitamin E also may reduce the risk of laryngeal cancer.

REFERENCES FOR PART 1

1. Pandey DK, Shekelle R, Selwyn BJ, et al. Dietary vitamin C and beta-carotene and risk of death in middle-aged men: the Western Electric study. *Am J Epidemiol* 1995;142:1269–1278.

2. Eichholzer M, Stähelin HB, Gey KF, et al. Prediction of male cancer mortality by plasma levels of interacting vitamins: 17-year follow-up of the prospective Basel study. *Int J Cancer* 1996; 66:145–150.

3. Eichholzer M, Stähelin HB, Lüdin E, et al. Smoking, plasma vitamins C, E, retinol, and carotene, and fatal prostate cancer: seventeen-year follow-up of the prospective Basel study. *Prostate* 1999;38:189–198.

4. Loria CM, Klag MJ, Caulfield LE, et al. Vitamin C status and mortality in US adults. *Am J Clin Nutr* 2000;72:139–145.

5. Shibata A, Paganini-Hill A, Ross RK, et al. Intake of vegetables, fruits, beta-carotene, vitamin C and vitamin supplements and cancer incidence among the elderly: a prospective study. *Br J Cancer* 1992;66:673–679.

6. Torun M, Yardim S, Gönenç A, et al. Serum beta-carotene, vitamin E, vitamin C and malondialdehyde levels in several types of cancer. *J Clin Pharm Ther* 1995;20:259–263.

7. Hertog MG, Bueno-de-Mesquita HB, Fehily AM, et al. Fruit and vegetable consumption and cancer mortality in the Caerphilly study. *Cancer Epidemiol Biomarkers Prev* 1996;5:673–677.

8. Hunter DJ, Manson JE, Colditz GA, et al. A Prospective study of the intake of vitamins C, E, and A and the risk of breast cancer. *N Engl J Med* 1993;329:234–240.

9. de Lorgeril M, Salen P, Martin JL, et al. Mediterranean dietary pattern in a randomized trial: prolonged survival and possible reduced cancer rate. *Arch Intern Med* 1998;158:1181–1187.

10. Genkinger JM, Platz EA, Hoffman SC, et al. Fruit, vegetable, and antioxidant intake and all-cause, cancer, and cardiovascular disease mortality in a community-dwelling population in Washington county, Maryland. *Am J Epidemiol* 2004;160:1223–1233.

11. Castelao JE, Yuan JM, Gago-Dominguez M, et al. Carotenoids/vitamin C and smoking-related bladder cancer. *Int J Cancer* 2004;110:417–423.

12. Bruemmer B, White E, Vaughan TL, et al. Nutrient intake in relation to bladder cancer among middle-aged men and women. *Am J Epidemiol* 1996;144:485–495.

13. Yalcin O, Karatas, F, Erulas, FA, et al. The levels of glutathione peroxidase, vitamin A, E, C and lipid peroxidation in patients with transitional cell carcinoma of the bladder. *BJU Int* 2004; 93:863–866.

14. Michaud DS, Pietinen P, Taylor PR, et al. Intakes of fruits and vegetables, carotenoids and vitamins A, E, C in relation to the risk of bladder cancer in the ATBC cohort study. *Br J Cancer* 2002;87:960–965.

15. Michaud DS, Spiegelman D, Clinton SK, et al. Prospective study of dietary supplements, macronutrients, micronutrients, and risk of bladder cancer in US men. *Am J Epidemiol* 2000;152:1145–1153.

16. Holick CN, De Vivo I, Feskanich D, et al. Intake of fruits and vegetables, carotenoids, folate, and vitamins A, C, E and risk of bladder cancer among women (United States). *Cancer Causes Control* 2005;16:1135–1145.

17. Jacobs EJ, Henion AK, Briggs PJ, et al. Vitamin C and vitamin E supplement use and bladder cancer mortality in a large cohort of US men and women. *Am J Epidemiol* 2002b;156: 1002–1010.

18. Zeegers MP, Goldbohm RA, van den Brandt PA. Are retinol, vitamin C, vitamin E, folate and carotenoids intake associated with bladder cancer risk? results from the Netherlands cohort study. *Br J Cancer* 2001;85:977–983.

19. Michels KB, Holmberg L, Bergkvist L, et al. Dietary antioxidant vitamins, retinol, and breast cancer incidence in a cohort of Swedish women. *Int J Cancer* 2001;91:563–567.

20. Freudenheim JL, Marshall JR, Vena JE, et al. Premenopausal breast cancer risk and intake of vegetables, fruits, and related nutrients. *J Natl Cancer Inst* 1996;88:340–348.

21. Ambrosone CB, Marshall JR, Vena JE, et al. Interaction of family history of breast cancer and dietary antioxidants with breast cancer risk (New York, United States). *Cancer Causes Control* 1995;6:407–415.

22. Adzersen KH, Jess P, Freivogel KW, et al. Raw and cooked vegetables, fruits, selected micronutrients, and breast cancer risk: a case-control study in Germany. *Nutr Cancer* 2003; 46:131–137.

23. Do MH, Lee SS, Jung PJ, Lee MH. Intake of dietary fat and vitamin in relation to breast cancer risk in Korean women: a case-control study. *J Korean Med Sci* 2003;18:534–540.

24. Zaridze D, Lifanova Y, Maximovitch D, et al. Diet, alcohol consumption and reproductive factors in a case-control study of breast cancer in Moscow. *Int J Cancer* 1991;48:493–501.

25. Landa MC, Frago N, Tres A. Diet and the risk of breast cancer in Spain. *Eur J Cancer Prev* 1994;3:313–320.

26. Bala DV, Patel DD, Duffy SW, et al. Role of dietary intake and biomarkers in risk of breast cancer: a case control study. *Asian Pac J Cancer Prev* 2001;2:123–130.

27. Ronco A, De Stefani E, Boffetta P, et al. Vegetables, fruits, and related nutrients and risk of breast cancer: a case-control study in Uruguay. *Nutr Cancer* 1999;35:111–119.

28. Ronco AL, De Stefani E, Boffetta P, et al. Food patterns and risk of breast cancer: a factor analysis study in Uruguay. *Int J Cancer* 2006;119:1672–1678.

29. Guo WD, Chow WH, Zheng W, et al. Diet, serum markers and breast cancer mortality in China. *Jpn J Cancer Res* 1994;85:572–577.

30. Yuan JM, Wang QS, Ross RK, et al. Diet and breast cancer in Shanghai and Tianjin, China. *Br J Cancer* 1995;71:1353–1358.

31. Favero A, Parpinel M, Franceschi S. Diet and risk of breast cancer: major findings from an Italian case-control study. *Biomed Pharmacother* 1998;52:109–115.

32. Levi F, Pasche C, Lucchini F, et al. Dietary intake of selected micronutrients and breast-cancer risk. *Int J Cancer* 2001; 91:260–263.

33. Mayne ST. Antioxidant nutrients and chronic disease: use of biomarkers of exposure and oxidative stress status in epidemiologic research. *J Nutr* 2003;133 (Suppl 3):933S–940S.

34. Howe GR, Jain M, Miller AB. Dietary factors and risk of pancreatic cancer: results of a Canadian population-based case-control study. *Int J Cancer* 1990;45:604–608.

35. Gandini S, Merzenich H, Robertson C, et al. Meta-analysis of studies on breast cancer risk and diet: the role of fruit and vegetable consumption and the intake of associated micronutrients. *Eur J Cancer* 2000;36:636–646.

36. Webb PM, Byrne C, Schnitt SJ, et al. A prospective study of diet and benign breast disease. *Cancer Epidemiol Biomarkers Prev* 2004;13:1106–1113.

37. Cho E, Spiegelman D, Hunter DJ, et al. Premenopausal intakes of vitamins A, C, and E, folate, and carotenoids, and risk of breast cancer. *Cancer Epidemiol Biomarkers Prev* 2003;12:713–720.

38. Zhang S, Hunter DJ, Forman MR, et al. Dietary carotenoids and vitamins A, C, and E and risk of breast cancer. *J Natl Cancer Inst* 1999;91:547–556.

39. Kushi LH, Fee RM, Sellers TA, et al. Intake of vitamins A, C, and E and postmenopausal breast cancer: The Iowa Women's Health Study. *Am J Epidemiol* 1996;144:165–174.

40. Järvinen R, Knekt P, Seppänen R, et al. Diet and breast cancer risk in a cohort of Finnish women. *Cancer Lett* 1997; 114:251–253.

41. Verhoeven DT, Assen N, Goldbohm RA, et al. Vitamins C and E, retinol, beta-carotene and dietary fibre in relation to breast cancer risk: a prospective cohort study. *Br J Cancer* 1997; 75:149–155.

42. Moorman PG, Ricciuti MF, Millikan RC, et al. Vitamin supplement use and breast cancer in a North Carolina population. *Public Health Nutr* 2001;4:821–827.

43. Graham S, Hellmann R, Marshall J, et al. Nutritional epidemiology of postmenopausal breast cancer in western New York. *Am J Epidemiol* 1991;134:552–566.

44. Rohan TE, Howe GR, Friedenreich CM, et al. Dietary fiber, vitamins A, C, and E, and risk of breast cancer: a cohort study. *Cancer Causes Control* 1993;4:29–37.

45. Wu C, Ray RM, Lin MG, et al. A case-control study of risk factors for fibrocystic breast conditions: Shanghai Nutrition and Breast Disease Study, China, 1995–2000. *Am J Epidemiol* 2004;160:945–960.

46. Cai Q, Shu XO, Wen W, et al. Genetic polymorphism in the manganese superoxide dismutase gene, antioxidant intake, and breast cancer risk: results from the Shanghai Breast Cancer Study. *Breast Cancer Res* 2004;6:R647–R655.

47. Malin AS, Qi D, Shu XO, et al. Intake of fruits, vegetables and selected micronutrients in relation to the risk of breast cancer. *Int J Cancer* 2003;105:413–418.

48. Dorjgochoo T, Shrubsole MJ, Shu XO, et al. Vitamin supplement use and risk for breast cancer: the Shanghai Breast Cancer Study. *Breast Cancer Res Treat* 2007 (DOI 10.1007/s 10549-007-9772-8).

49. Negri E, La Vecchia C, Franceschi S, et al. Intake of selected micronutrients and the risk of breast cancer. *Int J Cancer* 1996b;65:140–144.

50. Braga C, La Vecchia C, Negri E, et al. Intake of selected foods and nutrients and breast cancer risk: an age- and menopause-specific analysis. *Nutr Cancer* 1997;28:258–263.

51. Bohlke K, Spiegelman D, Trichopoulou A, et al. Vitamins A, C and E and the risk of breast cancer: results from a case-control study in Greece. *Br J Cancer* 1999;79:23–29.

52. Katsouyanni K, Willett W, Trichopoulos D, et al. Risk of breast cancer among Greek women in relation to nutrient intake. *Cancer* 1988;61:181–185.

53. Nissen SB, Tjønneland A, Stripp C, et al. Intake of vitamins A, C, and E from diet and supplements and breast cancer in postmenopausal women. *Cancer Causes Control* 2003;14: 695–704.

54. Verreault R, Chu J, Mandelson M, Shy K. A case-control study of diet and invasive cervical cancer. *Int J Cancer* 1989;43: 1050–1054.

55. Herrero R, Potischman N, Brinton LA, et al. A case-control study of nutrient status and invasive cervical cancer. i. dietary indicators. *Am J Epidemiol* 1991;134:1335–1346.

56. Ramaswamy G, Krishnamoorthy L. Serum carotene, vitamin A, and vitamin C levels in breast cancer and cancer of the uterine cervix. *Nutr Cancer* 1996;25:173–177.

57. Mackerras D, Irwig L, Simpson JM, et al. Randomized double-blind trial of beta-carotene and vitamin C in women with minor cervical abnormalities. *Br J Cancer* 1999;79:1448–1453.

58. Goodman MT, Kiviat N, McDuffie K, et al. The association of plasma micronutrients with the risk of cervical dysplasia in Hawaii. *Cancer Epidemiol Biomarkers Prev* 1998;7:537–544.

59. Liu T, Soong SJ, Wilson NP, et al. A case-control study of nutritional factors and cervical dysplasia. *Cancer Epidemiol Biomarkers Prev* 1993;2:525–530.

60. Wideroff L, Potischman N, Glass AG, et al. A nested case-control study of dietary factors and the risk of incident cytological abnormalities of the cervix. *Nutr Cancer* 1998;30:130–136.

61. Cahill RJ, O'Sullivan KR, Mathias PM, et al. Effects of vitamin antioxidant supplementation on cell kinetics of patients with adenomatous polyps. *Gut* 1993;34:963–967.

62. Bostick RM, Potter JD, McKenzie DR, et al. Reduced risk of colon cancer with high intake of vitamin E: The Iowa Women's Health Study. *Cancer Res* 1993;53:4230–4237.

63. Satia-Abouta J, Galanko JA, Martin CF, et al. Associations of micronutrients with colon cancer risk in African Americans and whites: results from the North Carolina Colon Cancer Study. *Cancer Epidemiol Biomarkers Prev* 2003;12:747–754.

64. Satia-Abouta J, Keku T, Galanko JA, et al. Diet, lifestyle, and genomic instability in the North Carolina Colon Cancer Study. *Cancer Epidemiol Biomarkers Prev* 2005;14:429–436.

65. White E, Shannon JS, Patterson RE. Relationship between vitamin and calcium supplement use and colon cancer. *Cancer Epidemiol Biomarkers Prev* 1997;6:769–774.

66. Chiu BC, Ji BT, Dai Q, et al. Dietary factors and risk of colon cancer in Shanghai, China. *Cancer Epidemiol Biomarkers Prev* 2003;12:201–208.

67. Olsen J, Kronborg O, Lynggaard J, Ewertz M. Dietary risk factors for cancer and adenomas of the large intestine. A case-control study within a screening trial in Denmark. *Eur J Cancer* 1994;30A:53–60.

68. Lysy J, Ackerman Z, Dabbah K, et al. Vitamin C status and colonic neoplasia. *Dis Colon Rectum* 1996;39:1235–1237.

69. Whelan RL, Horvath KD, Gleason NR, et al. Vitamin and calcium supplement use is associated with decreased adenoma recurrence in patients with a previous history of neoplasia. *Dis Colon Rectum* 1999;42:212–217.

70. Jacobs EJ, Connell CJ, Patel AV, et al. Vitamin C and vitamin E supplement use and colorectal cancer mortality in a large American Cancer Society Cohort. *Cancer Epidemiol Biomarkers Prev* 2001;10:17–23.

71. Senesse P, Touvier M, Kesse E, et al. Tobacco use and associations of beta-carotene and vitamin intakes with colorectal adenoma risk. *J Nutr* 2005;135:2468–2472.

72. La Vecchia C, Braga C, Negri E, et al. Intake of selected micronutrients and risk of colorectal cancer. *Int J Cancer* 1997;73:525–530.

73. Levi F, Pasche C, Lucchini F, et al. Selected micronutrients and colorectal cancer: A case-control study from the Canton of Vaud, Switzerland. *Eur J Cancer* 2000;36:2115–2119.

74. Ferraroni M, La Vecchia C, D'Avanzo B, et al. Selected micronutrient intake and the risk of colorectal cancer. *Br J Cancer* 1994;70:1150–1155.

75. Freudenheim JL, Graham S, Marshall JR, et al. A case-control study of diet and rectal cancer in western New York. *Am J Epidemiol* 1990;131:612–624.

76. Saygili EI, Konukoglu D, Papila C, et al. Levels of plasma vitamin E, vitamin C, tbars, and cholesterol in male patients with colorectal tumors. *Biochemistry* 2003;68:325–328.

77. Greenberg ER, Baron JA, Tosteson TD, et al. A clinical trial of antioxidant vitamins to prevent colorectal adenoma: Polyp Prevention Study Group. *N Engl J Med* 1994;331:141–147.

78. McKeown-Eyssen G, Holloway C, Jazmaji V, et al. A randomized trial of vitamins C and E in the prevention of recurrence of colorectal polyps. *Cancer Res* 1988;48:4701–4705.

79. Malila N, Virtamo J, Virtanen M, et al. Dietary and serum alpha-tocopherol, beta-carotene and retinol, and risk for colorectal cancer in male smokers. *Eur J Clin Nutr* 2002a;56:615–621.

80. Winawer SJ, Zauber AG, Fletcher RH, et al. Guidelines for colonoscopy surveillance after polypectomy: a consensus update by the US Multi-Society Task Force on Colorectal Cancer and the American Cancer Society. *Cancer J Clin* 2006;56:143–159.

81. Enger SM, Longnecker MP, Chen MJ, et al. Dietary intake of specific carotenoids and vitamins A, C, and E, and prevalence of colorectal adenomas. *Cancer Epidemiol Biomarkers Prev* 1996;5:147–153.

82. Tseng M, Murray SC, Kupper LL, et al. Micronutrients and the risk of colorectal adenomas. *Am J Epidemiol* 1996;144:1005–1014.

83. McCann SE, Freudenheim JL, Marshall JR, et al. Diet in the epidemiology of endometrial cancer in western New York (United States). *Cancer Causes Control* 2000;11:965–974.

84. Xu WH, Dai Q, Xiang YB, et al. Nutritional factors in relation to endometrial cancer: a report from a population-based case-control study in Shanghai, China. *Int J Cancer* 2007; 120:1776–1781.

85. Negri E, La Vecchia C, Franceschi S, et al. Intake of selected micronutrients and the risk of endometrial carcinoma. *Cancer* 1996a;77:917–923.

86. Jain MG, Rohan TE, Howe GR, et al. A cohort study of nutritional factors and endometrial cancer. *Eur J Epidemiol* 2000;16:899–905.

87. Goodman MT, Hankin JH, Wilkens LR, et al. Diet, body size, physical activity, and the risk of endometrial cancer. *Cancer Res* 1997;57:5077–5085.

88. Mayne ST, Risch HA, Dubrow R, et al. Nutrient intake and risk of subtypes of esophageal and gastric cancer. *Cancer Epidemiol Biomarkers Prev* 2001;10:1055–1062.

89. Bollschweiler E, Wolfgarten E, Nowroth T, et al. Vitamin intake and risk of subtypes of esophageal cancer in Germany. *J Cancer Res Clin Oncol* 2002;128:575–580.

90. Zhang ZF, Kurtz RC, Yu GP, et al. Adenocarcinomas of the esophagus and gastric cardia: the role of diet. *Nutr Cancer* 1997;27:298–309.

91. Hu J, Nyrén O, Wolk A, et al. Risk factors for oesophageal cancer in northeast China. *Int J Cancer* 1994;57:38–46.

92. Terry P, Lagergren J, Ye W, et al. Antioxidants and cancers of the esophagus and gastric cardia. *Int J Cancer* 2000; 87:750–754.

93. Brown LM, Swanson CA, Gridley G, et al. Dietary factors and the risk of squamous cell esophageal cancer among black and white men in the United States. *Cancer Causes Control* 1998;9:467–474.

94. De Stefani E, Ronco AL, Boffetta P, et al. Nutrient intake and risk of squamous cell carcinoma of the esophagus: a case-control study in Uruguay. *Nutr Cancer* 2006;56:149–157.

95. Launoy G, Milan C, Day NE, et al. Diet and squamous-cell cancer of the oesophagus: a french multicentre case-control study. *Int J Cancer* 1998;76:7–12.

96. De Stefani E, Brennan P, Boffetta P, et al. Vegetables, fruits, related dietary antioxidants, and risk of squamous cell carcinoma of the esophagus: a case-control study in Uruguay. *Nutr Cancer* 2000;38:23–29.

REFERENCES FOR PART 2

1. Castelao JE, Yuan JM, Gago-Dominguez M, et al. Carotenoids/vitamin C and smoking-related bladder cancer. *Int J Cancer* 2004;110:417–423.

2. Bruemmer B, White E, Vaughan TL, et al. Nutrient intake in relation to bladder cancer among middle-aged men and women. *Am J Epidemiol* 1996;144:485–495.

3. Yalcin O, Karata F, Erula FA, et al. The levels of glutathione peroxidase, vitamin A, E, C and lipid peroxidation in patients with transitional cell carcinoma of the bladder. *BJU Int* 2004;93:863–866.

4. Michaud DS, Pietinen P, Taylor PR, et al. Intakes of fruits and vegetables, carotenoids and vitamins A, E, C in relation to the risk of bladder cancer in the ATBC Cohort Study. *Br J Cancer* 2002;87:960–965.

5. Michaud DS, Spiegelman D, Clinton SK, et al. Prospective study of dietary supplements, macronutrients, micronutrients, and risk of bladder cancer in US men. *Am J Epidemiol* 2000;152:1145–1153.

6. Holick CN, De Vivo I, Feskanich D, et al. Intake of fruits and vegetables, carotenoids, folate, and vitamins A, C, E and risk of bladder cancer among women (United States). *Cancer Causes Control* 2005;16:1135–1145.

7. Jacobs EJ, Henion AK, Briggs PJ, et al. Vitamin C and vitamin E supplement use and bladder cancer mortality in a large cohort of US men and women. *Am J Epidemiol* 2002b;156:1002–1010.

8. Zeegers MP, Goldbohm RA, van den Brandt PA. Are retinol, vitamin C, vitamin E, folate and carotenoids intake associated with bladder cancer risk? Results from the Netherlands Cohort Study. *Br J Cancer* 2001;85:977–983.

9. Michels KB, Holmberg L, Bergkvist L, et al. Dietary antioxidant vitamins, retinol, and breast cancer incidence in a cohort of swedish Women. *Int J Cancer* 2001;91:563–567.

10. Freudenheim JL, Marshall JR, Vena JE, et al. Premenopausal breast cancer risk and intake of vegetables, fruits, and related nutrients. *J Natl Cancer Inst* 1996;88:340–348.

11. Ambrosone CB, Marshall JR, Vena JE, et al. Interaction of family history of breast cancer and dietary antioxidants with breast cancer risk (New York, United States). *Cancer Causes Control* 1995;6:407–415.

12. Adzersen KH, Jess P, Freivogel KW, et al. Raw and cooked vegetables, fruits, selected micronutrients, and breast cancer risk: a case-control study in Germany. *Nutr Cancer* 2003;46:131–137.

13. Do MH, Lee SS, Jung PJ, et al. Intake of dietary fat and vitamin in relation to breast cancer risk in Korean women: a case-control study. *J Korean Med Sci* 2003;18:534–540.

14. Zaridze D, Lifanova Y, Maximovitch D, et al. Diet, alcohol consumption and reproductive factors in a case-control study of breast cancer in Moscow. *Int J Cancer* 1991;48:493–501.

15. Landa MC, Frago N, Tres A. Diet and the risk of breast cancer in Spain. *Eur J Cancer Prev* 1994;3:313–320.

16. Bala DV, Patel DD, Duffy SW, et al. Role of dietary intake and biomarkers in risk of breast cancer: a case control study. *Asian Pac J Cancer Prev* 2001;2:123–130.

17. Ronco A, De Stefani E, Boffetta P, et al. Vegetables, fruits, and related nutrients and risk of breast cancer: a case-control study in Uruguay. *Nutr Cancer* 1999;35:111–119.

18. Ronco AL, De Stefani E, Boffetta P, et al. Food patterns and risk of breast cancer: a factor analysis study in Uruguay. *Int J Cancer* 2006;119:1672–1678.

19. Guo WD, Chow WH, Zheng W, et al. Diet, serum markers and breast cancer mortality in China. *Jpn J Cancer Res* 1994;85:572–577.

20. Yuan JM, Wang QS, Ross RK, et al. Diet and breast cancer in Shanghai and Tianjin, China. *Br J Cancer* 1995;71:1353–1358.

21. Favero A, Parpinel M, Franceschi S. Diet and risk of breast cancer: major findings from an Italian case-control study. *Biomed Pharmacother* 1998;52:109–115.

22. Levi F, Pasche C, Lucchini F, et al. Dietary intake of selected micronutrients and breast-cancer risk. *Int J Cancer* 2001;91: 260263.

23. Mayne ST. Antioxidant nutrients and chronic disease: use of biomarkers of exposure and oxidative stress status in epidemiologic research. *J Nutr* 2003;133 (Suppl 3):933S–940S.

24. Howe GR, Jain M, Miller AB. Dietary factors and risk of pancreatic cancer: results of a Canadian population-based case-control study. *Int J Cancer* 1990;45:604–608.

25. Gandini S, Merzenich H, Robertson C, et al. Meta-analysis of studies on breast cancer risk and diet: the role of fruit and vegetable consumption and the intake of associated micronutrients. *Eur J Cancer* 2000;36:636–646.

26. Webb PM, Byrne C, Schnitt SJ, et al. A prospective study of diet and benign breast disease. *Cancer Epidemiol Biomarkers Prev* 2004;13:1106–1113.

27. Cho E, Spiegelman D, Hunter DJ, et al. Premenopausal intakes of Vitamins A, C, and E, folate, and carotenoids, and risk of breast cancer. *Cancer Epidemiol Biomarkers Prev* 2003;12:713–720.

28. Zhang S, Hunter DJ, Forman MR, et al. Dietary carotenoids and vitamins A, C, and E and risk of breast cancer. *J Natl Cancer Inst* 1999;91:547–556.

29. Kushi LH, Fee RM, Sellers TA, et al. Intake of vitamins A, C, and E and post-menopausal breast cancer: The Iowa Women's Health Study. *Am J Epidemiol* 1996;144:165–174.

30. Järvinen R, Knekt P, Seppänen R, et al. Diet and breast cancer risk in a cohort of Finnish women. *Cancer Lett* 1997;114:251–253.

31. Verhoeven DT, Assen N, Goldbohm RA, et al. Vitamins C and E, retinol, beta-carotene and dietary fibre in relation to breast cancer risk: a prospective cohort study. *Br J Cancer* 1997;75:149–155.

32. Moorman PG, Ricciuti MF, Millikan RC, et al. Vitamin supplement use and breast cancer in a North Carolina population. *Public Health Nutr* 2001;4:821–827.

33. Graham S, Hellmann R, Marshall J, et al. Nutritional epidemiology of postmenopausal breast cancer in western New York. *Am J Epidemiol* 1991;134:552–566.

34. Rohan TE, Howe GR, Friedenreich CM, et al. Dietary fiber, vitamins A, C, and E, and risk of breast cancer: a cohort study. *Cancer Causes Control* 1993;4:29–37.

35. Wu C, Ray RM, Lin MG, et al. A case-control study of risk factors for fibrocystic breast conditions: Shanghai Nutrition and Breast Disease Study, China, 1995–2000. *Am J Epidemiol* 2004;160:945–960.

36. Cai Q, Shu XO, Wen W, et al. Genetic polymorphism in the manganese superoxide dismutase gene, antioxidant intake, and breast cancer risk: Results from the Shanghai Breast Cancer Study. *Breast Cancer Res* 2004;6:R647–R655.

37. Malin AS, Qi D, Shu XO, et al. Intake of fruits, vegetables and selected micronutrients in relation to the risk of breast cancer. *Int J Cancer* 2003;105:413–418.

38. Dorjgochoo T, Shrubsole MJ, Shu XO, et al. Vitamin supplement use and risk for breast cancer: the Shanghai Breast Cancer Study. *Breast Cancer Res Treat* 2007 (DOI 10.1007/s 10549007–9772–8).

39. Negri E, La Vecchia C, Franceschi S, et al. Intake of selected micronutrients and the risk of breast cancer. *Int J Cancer* 1996b; 65:140–144.

40. Braga C, La Vecchia C, Negri E, Franceschi S, Parpinel M. Intake of selected foods and nutrients and breast cancer risk: an age- and menopause-specific analysis. *Nutr Cancer* 1997;28: 258–263.

41. Bohlke K, Spiegelman D, Trichopoulou A, et al. Vitamins A, C and E and the risk of breast cancer: results from a case-control study in Greece. *Br J Cancer* 1999;79:23–29.

42. Katsouyanni K, Willett W, Trichopoulos D, et al. Risk of breast cancer among Greek women in relation to nutrient intake. *Cancer* 1988;61:181–185.

43. Nissen SB, Tjønneland A, Stripp C, et al. Intake of vitamins A, C, and E from diet and supplements and breast cancer in postmenopausal women. *Cancer Causes Control* 2003;14: 695–704.

44. Verreault R, Chu J, Mandelson M, et al. A case-control study of diet and invasive cervical cancer. *Int J Cancer* 1989;43: 1050–1054.

45. Herrero R, Potischman N, Brinton LA, et al. A case-control study of nutrient status and invasive cervical cancer. I. Dietary Indicators. *Am J Epidemiol* 1991;134:1335–1346.

46. Ramaswamy G, Krishnamoorthy L. Serum carotene, vitamin A, and vitamin C levels in breast cancer and cancer of the uterine cervix. *Nutr Cancer* 1996;25:173–177.

47. Mackerras D, Irwig L, Simpson JM, et al. Randomized double-blind trial of beta-carotene and vitamin C in women with minor cervical abnormalities. *Br J Cancer* 1999;79:1448–1453.

48. Goodman MT, Kiviat N, McDuffie K, et al. The association of plasma micronutrients with the risk of cervical dysplasia in Hawaii. *Cancer Epidemiol Biomarkers Prev* 1998;7:537–544.

49. Liu T, Soong SJ, Wilson NP, et al. A case-control study of nutritional factors and cervical dysplasia. *Cancer Epidemiol Biomarkers Prev* 1993;2:525–530.

50. Wideroff L, Potischman N, Glass AG, et al. A nested case-control study of dietary factors and the risk of incident cytological abnormalities of the cervix. *Nutr Cancer* 1998;30:130–136.

51. Jacobs EJ, Connell CJ, Patel AV, et al. Vitamin C and vitamin E supplement use and colorectal cancer mortality in a large American Cancer Society cohort. *Cancer Epidemiol Biomarkers Prev* 2001;10:17–23.

52. Senesse P, Touvier M, Kesse E, et al. Tobacco use and associations of beta-carotene and vitamin intakes with colorectal adenoma risk. *J Nutr* 2005;135:2468–2472.

53. La Vecchia C, Braga C, Negri E, et al. Intake of selected micronutrients and risk of colorectal cancer. *Int J Cancer* 1997;73:525–530.

54. Levi F, Pasche C, Lucchini F, et al. Selected micronutrients and colorectal cancer: a case-control study from the Canton of Vaud, Switzerland. *Eur J Cancer* 2000;36:2115–2119.

55. Ferraroni M, La Vecchia C, D'Avanzo B, et al. Selected micronutrient intake and the risk of colorectal cancer. *Br J Cancer* 1994;70:1150–1155.

56. Freudenheim JL, Graham S, Marshall JR, et al. A case-control study of diet and rectal cancer in Western New York. *Am J Epidemiol* 1990;131:612–624.

57. Saygili EI, Konukoglu D, Papila C, et al. Levels of plasma vitamin E, vitamin C, Tbars, and cholesterol in male patients with colorectal tumors. *Biochemistry* 2003;68:325–328.

58. Greenberg ER, Baron JA, Tosteson TD, et al. A clinical trial of antioxidant vitamins to prevent colorectal adenoma: Polyp Prevention Study Group. *N Engl J Med* 1994;331:141–147.

59. McKeown-Eyssen G, Holloway C, Jazmaji V, et al. A randomized trial of vitamins C and E in the prevention of recurrence of colorectal polyps. *Cancer Res* 1988;48:4701–4705.

60. Malila N, Virtamo J, Virtanen M, et al. Dietary and serum alpha-tocopherol, beta-carotene and retinol, and risk for colorectal cancer in male smokers. *Eur J Clin Nutr* 2002a;56:615–621.

61. Winawer SJ, Zauber AG, Fletcher RH, et al. Guidelines for colonoscopy surveillance after polypectomy: a consensus update by the US Multi-Society Task Force on Colorectal Cancer and the American Cancer Society. *CA Cancer J Clin* 2006;56:143–159.

62. Enger SM, Longnecker MP, Chen MJ, et al. Dietary intake of specific carotenoids and vitamins A, C, and E, and prevalence of colorectal adenomas. *Cancer Epidemiol Biomarkers Prev* 1996;5: 147–153.

63. Tseng M, Murray SC, Kupper LL, et al. Micronutrients and the risk of colorectal adenomas. *Am J Epidemiol* 1996;144: 1005–1014.

64. McCann SE, Freudenheim JL, Marshall JR, et al. Diet in the epidemiology of endometrial cancer in western New York (United States). *Cancer Causes Control* 2000;11:965–974.

65. Xu WH, Dai Q, Xiang YB, et al. Nutritional factors in relation to endometrial cancer: a report from a population-based case-control study in Shanghai, China. *Int J Cancer* 2007; 120:1776–1781.

66. Negri E, La Vecchia C, Franceschi S, et al. Intake of selected micronutrients and the risk of endometrial carcinoma. *Cancer* 1996a;77:917–923.

67. Jain MG, Rohan TE, Howe GR, et al. A cohort study of nutritional factors and endometrial cancer. *Eur J Epidemiol* 2000;16: 899–905.

68. Goodman MT, Hankin JH, Wilkens LR, et al. Diet, body size, physical activity, and the risk of endometrial cancer. *Cancer Res* 1997;57:5077–5085.

69. Mayne ST, Risch HA, Dubrow R, et al. Nutrient intake and risk of subtypes of esophageal and gastric cancer. *Cancer Epidemiol Biomarkers Prev* 2001;10:1055–1062.

70. Bollschweiler E, Wolfgarten E, Nowroth T, et al. Vitamin intake and risk of subtypes of esophageal cancer in Germany. *J Cancer Res Clin Oncol* 2002;128:575–580.

71. Zhang ZF, Kurtz RC, Yu GP, et al. Adenocarcinomas of the esophagus and gastric cardia: the role of diet. *Nutr Cancer* 1997;27:298–309.

72. Hu J, Nyrén O, Wolk A, et al. Risk factors for oesophageal cancer in northeast China. *Int J Cancer* 1994;57:38–46.

73. Terry P, Lagergren J, Ye W, et al. Antioxidants and cancers of the esophagus and gastric cardia. *Int J Cancer* 2000;87: 750–754.

74. Fleischauer AT, Olson SH, Mignone L, et al. Dietary antioxidants, supplements, and risk of epithelial ovarian cancer. *Nutr Cancer* 2001;40:92–98.

75. Fairfield KM, Hankinson SE, Rosner BA, et al. Risk of ovarian carcinoma and consumption of vitamins A, C, and E and specific carotenoids: a prospective analysis. *Cancer* 2001;92: 2318–2326.

76. Navarro Silvera SA, Jain M, Howe GR, et al. Carotenoid, vitamin A, vitamin C, and vitamin E intake and risk of ovarian cancer: a prospective cohort study. *Cancer Epidemiol Biomarkers Prev* 2006;15:395–397.

77. Chang ET, Lee VS, Canchola AJ, et al. Diet and risk of ovarian cancer in the California Teachers Study Cohort. *Am J Epidemiol* 2007;165:802–813.

78. Tung KH, Wilkens LR, Wu AH, et al. Association of dietary vitamin A, carotenoids, and other antioxidants with the risk of ovarian cancer. *Cancer Epidemiol Biomarkers Prev* 2005;14: 669–676.

79. Pan SY, Ugnat AM, Mao Y, et al. Canadian cancer registries epidemiology research group: a case-control study of diet and the risk of ovarian cancer. *Cancer Epidemiol Biomarkers Prev* 2004;13:1521–1527.

80. Cramer DW, Kuper H, Harlow BL, et al. Carotenoids, antioxidants and ovarian cancer risk in pre- and postmenopausal women. *Int J Cancer* 2001;94:128–134.

81. Sichieri R, Everhart JE, Mendonça GA. Diet and mortality from common cancers in Brazil: an ecological study. *Cad Saude Publica* 1996;12:53–59.

82. Deneo-Pellegrini H, De Stefani E, Ronco A, et al. Foods, nutrients and prostate cancer: a case-control study in Uruguay. *Br J Cancer* 1999;80:591–597.

83. Berndt SI, Carter HB, Landis PK, et al. Prediagnostic plasma vitamin C levels and the subsequent risk of prostate cancer. *Nutrition* 2005;21:686–690.

84. Daviglus ML, Dyer AR, Persky V, et al. Dietary beta-carotene, vitamin C, and risk of prostate cancer: results from the Western Electric Study. *Epidemiology* 1996;7:472–477.

85. Stevens VL, McCullough ML, Diver WR, et al. Use of multivitamins and prostate cancer mortality in a large cohort of US men. *Cancer Causes Control* 2005;16:643–650.

86. Eichholzer M, Stähelin HB, Gey KF, et al. Prediction of male cancer mortality by plasma levels of interacting vitamins: 17-year follow-up of the prospective Basel study. *Int J Cancer* 1996;66:145–150.

87. Eichholzer M, Stähelin HB, Lüdin E, et al. Smoking, plasma vitamins C, E, retinol, and carotene, and fatal prostate cancer: seventeen-year follow-up of the prospective Basel study. *Prostate* 1999;38:189–198.

88. Kirsh VA, Hayes RB, Mayne ST, et al. PLCO Trial: Supplemental and dietary vitamin E, beta-carotene, and vitamin C intakes and prostate cancer risk. *J Natl Cancer Inst* 2006; 98:245–254.

89. Schuurman AG, Goldbohm RA, Brants HA, et al. A prospective cohort study on intake of retinol, vitamins C and E, and carotenoids and prostate cancer risk (Netherlands). *Cancer Causes Control* 2002;13:573–582.

90. Kolonel LN, Yoshizawa CN, Hankin JH. Diet and prostatic cancer: a case-control study in Hawaii. *Am J Epidemiol* 1988;127:999–1012.

91. Kristal AR, Stanford JL, Cohen JH, et al. Vitamin and mineral supplement use is associated with reduced risk of prostate cancer. *Cancer Epidemiol Biomarkers Prev* 1999;8:887–892.

92. West DW, Slattery ML, Robison LM, et al. Adult dietary intake and prostate cancer risk in Utah: a case-control study with special emphasis on aggressive tumors. *Cancer Causes Control* 1991;2:85–94.

93. Ohno Y, Yoshida O, Oishi K, et al. Dietary beta-carotene and cancer of the prostate: a case-control study in Kyoto, Japan. *Cancer Res* 1988;48:1331–1336.

94. Andersson SO, Wolk A, Bergström R, et al. Energy, nutrient intake and prostate cancer risk: a population-based case-control study in Sweden. *Int J Cancer* 1996;68:716–722.

95. Vlajinac HD, Marinkovic JM, Ilic MD, et al. Diet and prostate cancer: a case-control study. *Eur J Cancer* 1997;33:101–107.

96. Ghadirian P, Lacroix A, Maisonneuve P, et al. Nutritional factors and prostate cancer: a case-control study of French Canadians in Montreal, Canada. *Cancer Causes Control* 1996; 7:428–436.

97. Huang HY, Alberg AJ, Norkus EP, et al. Prospective study of antioxidant micronutrients in the blood and the risk of developing prostate cancer. *Am J Epidemiol* 2003;157:335–344.

98. Mezzetti M, La Vecchia C, Decarli A, et al. Population attributable risk for breast cancer: diet, nutrition, and physical exercise. *J Natl Cancer Inst* 1998;90:389–394.

99. Chiu BC, Ji BT, Dai Q, et al. Dietary factors and risk of colon cancer in Shanghai, China. *Cancer Epidemiol Biomarkers Prev* 2003;12:201–208.

100. Dorgan JF, Sowell A, Swanson CA, et al. Relationships of serum carotenoids, retinol, alpha-tocopherol, and selenium with breast cancer risk: results from a prospective study in Columbia, Missouri (United States). *Cancer Causes Control* 1998;9: 89–97.

101. Comstock GW, Helzlsouer KJ, Bush TL. Prediagnostic serum levels of carotenoids and vitamin E as related to subsequent cancer in Washington county, Maryland. *Am J Clin Nutr* 1991;53:260S–264S.

102. Sato R, Helzlsouer KJ, Alberg AJ, et al. Prospective study of carotenoids, tocopherols, and retinoid concentrations and the risk of breast cancer. *Cancer Epidemiol Biomarkers Prev* 2002;11:451–457.

103. Tamimi RM, Hankinson SE, Campos H, et al. Plasma carotenoids, retinol, and tocopherols and risk of breast cancer. *Am J Epidemiol* 2005;161:153–160.

104. Hultén K, Van Kappel AL, Winkvist A, et al. Carotenoids, alpha-tocopherols, and retinol in plasma and breast cancer risk in northern Sweden. *Cancer Causes Control* 2001;12:529–537.

105. Russell MJ, Thomas BS, Bulbrook RD. A prospective study of the relationship between serum vitamins A and E and risk of breast cancer. *Br J Cancer* 1988;57:213–215.

106. Lee IM, Cook NR, Gaziano JM, et al. Vitamin E in the primary prevention of cardiovascular disease and cancer: the Women's Health Study–a randomized controlled trial. *JAMA* 2005;294:56–65.

107. Bostick RM, Potter JD, McKenzie DR, et al. Reduced risk of colon cancer with high intake of vitamin E: the Iowa Women's Health Study. *Cancer Res* 1993;53:4230–4237.

108. Satia-Abouta J, Galanko JA, Martin CF, et al. Associations of micronutrients with colon cancer risk in African Americans and whites: results from the North Carolina Colon Cancer Study. *Cancer Epidemiol Biomarkers Prev* 2003;12:747–754.

109. Satia-Abouta J, Keku T, Galanko JA, et al. Diet, lifestyle, and genomic instability in the North Carolina Colon Cancer Study. *Cancer Epidemiol Biomarkers Prev* 2005;14:429–436.

110. White E, Shannon JS, Patterson RE. Relationship between vitamin and calcium supplement use and colon cancer. *Cancer Epidemiol Biomarkers Prev* 1997;6:769–774.

111. Ghadirian P, Lacroix A, Maisonneuve P, et al. Nutritional factors and colon carcinoma: a case-control study involving French Canadians in Montréal, Quebec, Canada. *Cancer* 1997;80: 858–864.

112. Whelan RL, Horvath KD, Gleason NR, et al. Vitamin and calcium supplement use is associated with decreased adenoma recurrence in patients with a previous history of neoplasia. *Dis Colon Rectum* 1999;42:212–217.

113. Olsen J, Kronborg O, Lynggaard J, et al. Dietary risk factors for cancer and adenomas of the large intestine: a case-control study within a screening trial in Denmark. *Eur J Cancer* 1994;30A:53–60.

114. Wu K, Willett WC, Chan JM, et al. A prospective study on supplemental vitamin E intake and risk of colon cancer in women and men. *Cancer Epidemiol Biomarkers Prev* 2002;11: 1298–1304.

115. Slattery ML, Edwards SL, Anderson K, et al. Vitamin E and colon cancer: is there an association? *Nutr Cancer* 1998;30:201–206.

116. Enger SM, Longnecker MP, Chen MJ, et al. Dietary intake of specific carotenoids and vitamins A, C, and E, and prevalence of colorectal adenomas. *Cancer Epidemiol Biomarkers Prev* 1996;5:147–153.

117. Ingles SA, Bird CL, Shikany JM, et al. Plasma tocopherol and prevalence of colorectal adenomas in a multiethnic population. *Cancer Res* 1998;58:661–666.

118. Ito Y, Kurata M, Hioki R, et al. Cancer mortality and serum levels of carotenoids, retinol, and tocopherol: a population-based follow-up study of inhabitants of a rural area of Japan. *Asian Pac J Cancer Prev* 2005a;6:10–15.

119. Wakai K, Suzuki K, Ito Y, et al. Japan Collaborative Cohort Study Group: serum carotenoids, retinol, and tocopherols, and colorectal cancer risk in a japanese cohort–effect modification by sex for carotenoids. *Nutr Cancer* 2005;51:13–24.

120. Jiang J, Suzuki S, Xiang J, et al. Plasma carotenoid, alpha-tocopherol and retinol concentrations and risk of colorectal adenomas: a case-control study in Japan. *Cancer Lett* 2005;226:133–141.

121. Malila N, Virtamo J, Virtanen M, et al. The effect of alpha-tocopherol and beta-carotene supplementation on colorectal adenomas in middle-aged male smokers. *Cancer Epidemiol Biomarkers Prev* 1999;8:489–493.

122. Alpha-Tocopherol Beta-Carotene Cancer Prevention Study Group: the effect of vitamin E and beta-carotene on the incidence of lung cancer and other cancers in male smokers. *N Engl J Med* 1994;330:1029–1035.

123. Jemal A, Siegel R, Ward E, et al. Cancer Statistics, 2008. *CA Cancer J Clin* 2008;58:71–96.

124. Wright ME, Lawson KA, Weinstein SJ, et al. Higher baseline serum concentrations of vitamin E are associated with lower total and cause-specific mortality in the Alpha-Tocopherol, Beta-Carotene Cancer Prevention Study. *Am J Clin Nutr* 2006;84:1200–1207.

125. Lonn E, Bosch J, Yusuf S, Sheridan P, et al. HOPE and HOPE-TOO trial investigators. effects of long-term vitamin E supplementation on cardiovascular events and cancer: a randomized controlled trial. *JAMA* 2005;293:1338–1347.

126. Miller ER III, Pastor-Barriuso R, Dalal D, et al. Meta-analysis: high-dosage vitamin E supplementation may increase all-cause mortality. *Ann Intern Med* 2005;142:37–46.

127. Bjelakovic G, Nagorni A, Nikolova D, et al. Meta-analysis: antioxidant supplements for primary and secondary prevention of colorectal adenoma. *Aliment Pharmacol Ther* 2006;24: 281–291.

128. De Stefani E, Brennan P, Boffetta P, et al. Vegetables, fruits, related dietary antioxidants, and risk of squamous cell carcinoma of the esophagus: a case-control study in Uruguay. *Nutr Cancer* 2000;38:23–29.

129. Taylor PR, Qiao YL, Abnet CC, et al. Prospective study of serum vitamin E levels and esophageal and gastric cancers. *J Natl Cancer Inst* 2003;95:1414–1416.

130. Wright ME, Virtamo J, Hartman AM, et al. Effects of alpha-tocopherol and beta-carotene supplementation on upper aerodigestive tract cancers in a large, randomized controlled trial. *Cancer* 2007b;109:891–898.

131. Nomura AM, Ziegler RG, Stemmermann GN, et al. Serum micronutrients and upper aerodigestive tract cancer. *Cancer Epidemiol Biomarkers Prev* 1997b;6:407–412.

132. Launoy G, Milan C, Day NE, et al. Diet and squamous-cell cancer of the oesophagus: a French multicentre case-control study. *Int J Cancer* 1998;76:7–12.

133. De Stefani E, Ronco AL, Boffetta P, et al. Nutrient intake and risk of squamous cell carcinoma of the esophagus: a case-control study in Uruguay. *Nutr Cancer* 2006;56:149–157.

134. De Stefani E, Boffetta P, Ronco AL, et al. Dietary patterns and risk of laryngeal cancer: an exploratory factor analysis in Uruguayan men. *Int J Cancer* 2007;121:1086–1091.

135. Suzuki T, Wakai K, Matsuo K, et al. Effect of dietary antioxidants and risk of oral, pharyngeal and laryngeal squamous cell carcinoma according to smoking and drinking habits. *Cancer Sci* 2006;97:760–767.

136. Kirkpatrick CS, White E, Lee JA. Case-control study of malignant melanoma in Washington State II: diet, alcohol, and obesity. *Am J Epidemiol* 1994;139:869–880.

137. Millen AE, Tucker MA, Hartge P, et al. Diet and melanoma in a case-control study. *Cancer Epidemiol Biomarkers Prev* 2004;13:1042–1051.

138. Knekt P, Aromaa A, Maatela J, et al. Serum micronutrients and risk of cancers of low incidence in Finland. *Am J Epidemiol* 1991b;134:356–361.

139. Feskanich D, Willett WC, Hunter DJ, et al. Dietary intakes of vitamins A, C, and E and risk of melanoma in two cohorts of women. *Br J Cancer* 2003;88:1381–1387.

140. Stryker WS, Stampfer MJ, Stein EA, et al. Diet, plasma levels of beta-carotene and alpha-tocopherol, and risk of malignant melanoma. *Am J Epidemiol* 1990;131:597–611.

141. Breslow RA, Alberg AJ, Helzlsouer KJ, et al. Serological precursors of cancer: malignant melanoma, basal and squamous cell skin cancer, and prediagnostic levels of retinol, beta-carotene, lycopene, alpha-tocopherol, and selenium. *Cancer Epidemiol Biomarkers Prev* 1995;4:837–842.

142. Barone J, Taioli E, Hebert JR, et al. Vitamin supplement use and risk for oral and esophageal cancer. *Nutr Cancer* 1992;18:31–41.

143. Gridley G, McLaughlin JK, Block G, et al. Vitamin supplement use and reduced risk of oral and pharyngeal cancer. *Am J Epidemiol* 1992;135:1083–1092.

144. Negri E, Franceschi S, Bosetti C, Levi F, et al. Selected Micronutrients and Oral and Pharyngeal Cancer. *Int J Cancer* 2000;86:122–127.

145. Kune GA, Kune S, Field B, et al. Oral and pharyngeal cancer, diet, smoking, alcohol, and serum vitamin A and beta-carotene levels: a case-control study in men. *Nutr Cancer* 1993;20:61–70.

146. Nagao T, Ikeda N, Warnakulasuriya S, et al. Serum antioxidant micronutrients and the risk of oral leukoplakia among Japanese. *Oral Oncol* 2000;36:466–470.

147. Zheng W, Blot WJ, Diamond EL, et al. Serum Micronutrients and the Subsequent Risk of Oral and Pharyngeal Cancer. *Cancer Res* 1993;53:795–798.

148. Liede K, Hietanen J, Saxen L, et al. Long-term supplementation with alpha-tocopherol and beta-carotene and prevalence of oral mucosal lesions in smokers. *Oral Dis* 1998;4:78–83.

149. Bidoli E, La Vecchia C, Talamini R, et al. Micronutrients and ovarian cancer: a case-control study in Italy. *Ann Oncol* 2001;12:1589–1593.

150. Helzlsouer KJ, Alberg AJ, Norkus EP, et al. Prospective study of serum micronutrients and ovarian cancer. *J Natl Cancer Inst* 1996;88:32–37.

151. Ji BT, Chow WH, Gridley G, et al. Dietary factors and the risk of pancreatic cancer: a case-control study in Shanghai China. *Cancer Epidemiol Biomarkers Prev* 1995;4:885–893.

152. Ji BT, Chow WH, Yang G, et al. Dietary habits and stomach cancer in Shanghai, China. *Int J Cancer* 1998;76:659–664.

153. Rautalahti MT, Virtamo JR, Taylor PR, et al. The effects of supplementation with alpha-tocopherol and beta-carotene on the incidence and mortality of carcinoma of the pancreas in a randomized, controlled trial. *Cancer* 1999;86:37–42.

154. Stolzenberg-Solomon RZ, Pietinen P, Taylor PR, et al. Prospective study of diet and pancreatic cancer in male smokers. *Am J Epidemiol* 2002;155:783–792.

155. Shibata A, Mack TM, Paganini-Hill A, et al. A prospective study of pancreatic cancer in the elderly. *Int J Cancer* 1994;58:46–49.

156. Albanes D, Heinonen OP, Huttunen JK, et al. Effects of alpha-tocopherol and beta-carotene supplements on cancer incidence in the Alpha-Tocopherol Beta-Carotene Cancer Prevention Study. *Am J Clin Nutr* 1995;62(Suppl.):1427S–1430S.

157. Heinonen OP, Albanes D, Virtamo J, et al. Prostate cancer and supplementation with alpha-tocopherol and beta-carotene: incidence and mortality in a controlled trial. *J Natl Cancer Inst* 1998;90:440–446.

158. Hartman TJ, Albanes D, Pietinen P, et al. The association between baseline vitamin E, selenium, and prostate cancer in the Alpha-Tocopherol, Beta-Carotene Cancer Prevention Study. *Cancer Epidemiol Biomarkers Prev* 1998;7:335–340.

159. Shekelle P, Hardy ML, Coulter I, et al. Effect of the supplemental use of antioxidants vitamin C, vitamin E, and coenzyme Q10 for the prevention and treatment of cancer. *Evid Rep Technol Assess* (Summ) 2003 Oct;(75):1–3.

160. Coulter ID, Hardy ML, Morton SC, et al. Antioxidants vitamin C and vitamin E for the prevention and treatment of cancer. *J Gen Intern Med* 2006;21:735–744.

161. Weinstein SJ, Wright ME, Pietinen P, et al. Serum alpha-tocopherol and gamma-tocopherol in relation to prostate cancer risk in a prospective study. *J Natl Cancer Inst* 2005;97:396–399.

162. Weinstein SJ, Wright ME, Lawson KA, et al. Serum and dietary vitamin E in relation to prostate cancer risk. *Cancer Epidemiol Biomarkers Prev* 2007;16:1253–1259.

163. Hsing AW, McLaughlin JK, Schuman LM, et al: Diet, tobacco use, and fatal prostate cancer: results from the Lutheran Brotherhood Cohort Study. *Cancer Res* 1990a;50:6836–6840.

164. Hernáandez J, Syed S, Weiss G, et al. The modulation of prostate cancer risk with alpha-tocopherol: a pilot randomized, controlled clinical trial. *J Urol* 2005;174:519–522.

165. Peters U, Littman AJ, Kristal AR, et al. Vitamin E and selenium supplementation and risk of prostate cancer in the Vitamins and Lifestyle (Vital) Study Cohort. *Cancer Causes Control* 2008;19:75–87.

166. Tzonou A, Signorello LB, Lagiou P, et al. Diet and cancer of the prostate: a case-control study in Greece. *Int J Cancer* 1999;80:704–708.

167. Helzlsouer KJ, Huang HY, Alberg AJ, et al. Association between alpha-tocopherol, gamma-tocopherol, selenium, and subsequent prostate cancer. *J Natl Cancer Inst* 2000;92:2018–2023.

168. Surapaneni KM, Ramana V. Erythrocyte ascorbic acid and plasma vitamin E status in patients with carcinoma of prostate. *Ind J Physiol Pharmacol* 2007;51:199–202.

169. Chan JM, Stampfer MJ, Ma J, et al. Supplemental vitamin E intake and prostate cancer risk in a large cohort of men in the United States. *Cancer Epidemiol Biomarkers Prev* 1999;8:893–899.

170. Rodriguez C, Jacobs EJ, Mondul AM, et al. Vitamin E supplements and risk of prostate cancer in US Men. *Cancer Epidemiol Biomarkers Prev* 2004;13:378–382.

171. Goodman GE, Schaffer S, Omenn GS, et al. The association between lung and prostate cancer risk, and serum micronutrients: results and lessons learned from Beta-Carotene and Retinol Efficacy Trial. *Cancer Epidemiol Biomarkers Prev* 2003;12:518–526.

172. Key TJ, Appleby PN, Allen NE, et al. Plasma carotenoids, retinol, and tocopherols and the risk of prostate cancer in the European Prospective Investigation into Cancer and Nutrition Study. *Am J Clin Nutr* 2007;86:672–681.

173. Hsing AW, Comstock GW, Abbey H, et al. Serologic precursors of cancer. retinol, carotenoids, and tocopherol and risk of prostate cancer. *J Natl Cancer Inst* 1990b;82:941–946.

174. Nomura AM, Stemmermann GN, Lee J, et al. Serum micronutrients and prostate cancer in Japanese Americans in Hawaii. *Cancer Epidemiol Biomarkers Prev* 1997;6:487–491.

VITAMIN C AND CANCER: IS THERE A USE FOR ORAL VITAMIN C?

by Steve Hickey, PhD, and Hilary Roberts, PhD

Methods and technologies designed for drug therapies do not always apply to orthomolecular medicine. One current debate is the use of cytotoxic chemotherapy as a model for the use of vitamin C in cancer. Some claim that intravenous (IV) ascorbate is required to produce cytotoxic levels in the body. Here we show that restricting delivery to the IV route is inconsistent with available clinical,[1] animal,[2] and experimental data.[3] Furthermore, there are strong indications that, as a treatment for cancer, oral vitamin C is potentially more effective than IV administration.

The use of intravenous vitamin C in clinical trials has not delivered the promising results of early studies.[4] Recent studies have assumed that, in the early clinical trials, IV administration resulted in successful life extension. By contrast, Hickey and others have suggested that the use of IV ascorbate may generate resistance to treatment, rather than the expected benefits.[5,6] This contrasting idea has also been challenged.[7,8] We point out the main differences between oral and IV administration of ascorbate and explain why oral intakes are likely to be more effective for the treatment of cancer.

Cancer Biology

Cancer is often misunderstood as a disease based on genetic mutation. Thus, modern cancer research often attempts to find the gene, or genes, that lead to the illness. In some cases, there are correlations between cancer and either oncogenes (which are activated or increased) or tumor suppressor genes (which are deactivated or lowered). However, the genetic differences between healthy cells—or, indeed, benign cancer cells—and malignant cells are enormous.

Malignant cells are aneuploid[9,10] and, even in a single tumor, they can have vastly different numbers of chromosomes from the standard 23 matched pairs of healthy cells (ranging, say, from only 10 chromosomes to 100 or more). This change can be explained parsimoniously as a failure of the cancer cells' mechanisms for control of chromosome copying and cell division.

Biology is normally considered within the framework of evolution. Similarly, cancer can be viewed in terms of cellular microevolution, toward what we might refer to as "selfish" cells."[11] The implication for carcinogenesis is that anything that causes error-prone cell proliferation will, in the long-term, result in cancer. For example, local oxidation drives cell proliferation via redox signaling and free radical damage. When this happens, a lack of antioxidants—whether through dietary deficiency or because cells lack the energy to produce them—will drive carcinogenesis and increase the risk of cancer. This explains the widespread finding that dietary antioxidants prevent cancer.

The changes that occur during a cell's transition from healthy to malignant include varying responses to antioxidants and oxidants. Typically, malignant cells rely on oxidation to drive growth; however, they must strike a balance, as too much oxidation can kill the cells.[12] To a first approximation, both chemotherapy and radiotherapy work by increasing local oxidation and causing free radical damage, with the aim of either killing cancer cells directly, or stimulating apoptosis (cell suicide).

Antioxidants function in the opposite way: they decrease oxidation and may thus protect malignant cells from the oxidative effects of conventional treatments. For this reason, the use of standard dose antioxidant supplements in treating cancer is highly suspect, despite them being one of the main ways a person can avoid getting the disease in the first place.

Fortunately, within tumors, vitamin C and certain other dietary "antioxidants" act as oxidants, rather than antioxidants. Moreover, the same substances act as antioxidants within healthy cells. This means they can destroy cancer cells, while simultaneously improving the health of the rest of the body. This consequence of the redox chemistry of vitamin C and related substances is crucial to

From the *J Orthomolecular Med* 2013;28(1):33–44.

how they should be used for the prevention and treatment of cancer.

Microevolution provides a parsimonious explanation for the development of cancer.[11] One common consequence of carcinogenic microevolution is that tumors have a different metabolism than healthy cells. According to the microevolutionary model, the development of anaerobic metabolism is not surprising because, in its early stages, a tumor's growth is restricted by its lack of blood vessels.[13] Cells that are relatively far from blood vessels become short of oxygen and other metabolites. Thus, selection pressure favors anaerobic cells, which use glycolysis (sugar breakdown) for energy, avoiding the need for oxygen. Until the tumor learns (i.e., evolves) to stimulate local blood vessel growth, it remains small and its growth is limited. However, given time and a diversity of cell types, cancer cells that can stimulate the growth of local blood vessels will probably occur and will have a selective advantage over those that cannot.

Cells that divide with errors are likely to diverge from the normal, healthy form.[11] Slightly abnormal cells become subject to selection pressures, as the body responds with immune and other mechanisms to help prevent cancer. In abnormal and varying cells, such pressure favors those cells that have increased fitness. In this context, "increased fitness" means they behave like malignant cells, reproducing, spreading into their local environment, and setting up distant colonies (metastases).

The biochemistry of human cells includes essential core mechanisms that we share with microorganisms; over an evolutionary timescale, these have become stable. By contrast, the signaling and other cooperative mechanisms, needed in the tissues of multicellular organisms, are more recent and less robust. Damaged human cells thus have a tendency to revert to the precursor forms that helped microorganisms to become so successful. When cells from a multicellular animal, such as a human, regress to such single-celled behavior, we call the cells cancerous.

Adaptation

The large variation in chromosome numbers found in some tumors is an indication of biological diversity. A malignant tumor is not a clonal multiplication of a single cell type, but a diverse ecosystem. Malignant cells compete, cooperate, and communicate between themselves and with nearby healthy cells. Even among inanimate agents, populations with these characteristics often display an emergent property, sometimes called swarm intelligence.[14] Classic examples of flocking behavior include the behavior of flocks of birds or shoals of fish. Such populations often exhibit adaptation to threats, and this is also apparent in the way cancer cells develop resistance to treatment.

Resistance is perhaps the single most important issue in the treatment of cancer. Its eradication would be less demanding without its rapid development of tolerance to treatment. By definition, an anticancer drug is toxic to the population of cancer cells. However, some cells may get a lower than average dose: perhaps they have a relatively poor blood supply or are otherwise shielded from the drug. Alternatively, the duration of treatment may be insufficient for the drug to penetrate the whole tumor, allowing certain cells to survive the treatment. Furthermore, because of biological variation, some cancer cells are naturally more resistant to toxicity. Chemotherapy and radiotherapy kill the most susceptible cancer cells, while sparing the resistant cells. These resistant cells are now free

IN BRIEF

For several decades, the role of vitamin C in the treatment of cancer has been a subject of clinical research and controversy. It has been established that ascorbate is potentially a safe and elective anticancer agent, able to kill cancer cells while leaving healthy cells unharmed. However, its role has been viewed in the context of existing cytotoxic chemotherapy models of medicine. Consequently, many doctors and patients have come to believe that only intravenous vitamin C administration is an elective treatment for cancer. We suggest that this view is misguided and oral intakes are preferable.

from competition from cells that were easy to kill or damage and can thus grow more rapidly. In such cases, a tumor may be seen to shrink temporarily but then to grow back, as the aggressive cancer cells assert their dominance. Such adaptation is usually described as resistance to treatment, but it is an example of natural selection, occurring in a population of cells. Since the days of Wallace and Darwin, this selective process has been one of the well-studied phenomena in biology.

The primary problem in treating cancer is to deal with the cancer's natural variability and its resultant capacity to adapt to toxicity. It is well known that a cancer may respond to any single drug or other treatment, by avoiding its mechanisms of action. If the drug blocks an oncogene, for example, a cell using a different oncogene may proliferate. Alternatively, a cell with a disabled tumor suppressor gene may thrive, as competition is reduced. Generally, toxicity is not absolute and resistance can evolve rapidly.

Once again, nutrients need particular consideration. By definition, a nutrient is used for cellular health and growth. Providing nutrients to strengthen patients, or their immune systems, can equally deliver growth promoters (e.g., folic acid or iron) to a tumor. However, the cancer needs nutrients to grow and may be sensitive to the depletion of specific molecules. Relative deprivation of required nutrients will slow or reverse cancer growth, but the specific nutrients need to be identified and may vary with the individual and condition. One nutritional approach that a cancer cannot avoid is if it is starved of usable energy. Physically, the cancer needs energy to grow or even to continue to survive. "Starving" the cancer is a potential treatment[2] and is part of the reason patients should avoid carbohydrates and sugars.

A standard way of dealing with the issue of adaptation was developed as a result of experience with antibiotics. Bacteria have been found to adapt to antibiotic drugs, which are therefore given continuously, in order to apply a constant selection pressure on the infectious microorganism. In tuberculosis and some other chronic infections, multiple antibiotics may be given together. Bacterial adaptation to the treatment would then require a response that simultaneously overcomes multiple antibiotic mechanisms of action; this is far less likely to occur.

A critical point in preventing antibiotic resistance is to avoid starting and stopping the treatment, thus patients are warned to complete the whole course. This is because each break in treatment provides respite to the microorganisms and makes it more likely that they will develop an adaptive response. In principle, the mechanisms of resistance of bacteria to antibiotics are similar to those of cancer cells to chemotoxic therapies. By analogy, therefore, cancer treatment should be given continuously. Unfortunately, most conventional therapies are too toxic to be given long-term.

The Chemotherapy Model

Conventional chemotherapy exploits a difference in the susceptibility of cancer cells and healthy cells to toxic treatments. Cancer cells are slightly more susceptible to ionizing radiation and to some poisons, particularly those that involve free radical damage. However, the difference in response is small: a dose of a drug that is high enough to kill cancer cells will

ENSURING A STEADY STREAM OF VITAMIN C IN SICKNESS AND IN HEALTH

Dynamic flow occurs when taking large and frequent doses of ascorbic acid. Intakes of at least 500–1,000 mg are taken four to six times a day. The intake is adjusted for the individual concerned and should total 70–80 percent of the bowel tolerance (loose stools when a person exceeds their requirements, or limits, for oral vitamin C). Dynamic flow provides an excess of antioxidant into the system to help stay healthy and avoid disease. A person's bowel tolerance will vary with the state of his or her health increasing by up to 100 times when the individual is ill. In other words, a person who can tolerate only 2,000 mg a day when healthy might consume 200,000 mg without issues when ill with the flu. This is an evolutionary adaptation that provides the body with increased vitamin C when needed.

typically be toxic to the host's other cells as well. The side effects of radiation and chemotherapy are well known and form part of the media image of a cancer patient. In giving such treatment, oncologists aim to give the maximum effective dose, while minimizing harm to the patient.

For some rare cancers, such as childhood leukemia and testicular cancer, conventional chemotherapy is beneficial. However, chemotherapy is a hotly debated topic.[15] For the vast majority of adult solid tumors, it offers little, if any, life extension and the side effects may dominate any potential benefit. Importantly, the more precisely targeted the therapy, the greater is the chance that diverse cancer cells can adapt. Chemotherapy generally cannot be given in high enough doses to kill the tumor outright, without also killing the patient. Moreover, it cannot be continued at a lower level for a prolonged period, since a heuristic in pharmacology is that the toxicity is proportional to the total dose.

Natural Redox Agents

The development of cancer cells is a consequence of microevolutionary processes. Another consequence of evolution is that some natural substances have powerful anticancer properties. Cells in multicellular organisms, including plants, have evolved the ability to cooperate and to suppress the development of cancer. The list of natural anticancer substances is long and includes curcumin (turmeric), green tea extract, selenium, alpha-lipoic acid, and many other supplements. Every so often, a research group claims a breakthrough in finding a safe anticancer molecule,[16,17] without realizing that such substances are ubiquitous. We are particularly interested in vitamin C, which acts safely as an antioxidant in healthy tissues and as an oxidant in tumors. In other words, it is the archetype for anticancer treatments.[3]

A range of redox active molecules have the property of killing cancer cells, while helping healthy cells. Vitamin C may be considered unique in the respect it can be given in massive doses, with a high degree of safety. Although it is theoretically possible to give a toxic dose of vitamin C, it is less likely than an overdose of water, which

occasionally results in death. Oral doses of vitamin C have a single established but minor side effect: loose stools (diarrhea). Obviously, clinicians giving large intravenous doses need to realize the potential for toxic reactions, particularly with cancer patients, as tumor necrosis can occur.

Bowel Tolerance and Dynamic Flow

The late Dr. Robert Cathcart described how tolerance to oral doses varies with the individual's state of health.[18] In healthy people, as the dose of vitamin C is increased, progressively less is absorbed. The concentration of vitamin C builds up in the intestines, attracting water. At some point, usually after consuming several thousand milligrams (mg) in a single dose, the unabsorbed vitamin C causes diarrhea. Cathcart noticed, however, that sick or stressed individuals could take exceptionally large doses, without reaching their bowel tolerance level. This bowel tolerance effect is large and obvious. So, for example, a person might tolerate well over 100,000 mg per day when acutely ill but have a bowel tolerance of 3,000 mg per day when healthy. The magnitude and easy reproducibility of this effect suggests that it is important to the mechanism of action with oral intakes.

Cathcart's bowel tolerance observations imply that, during illness, the body responds by absorbing as much vitamin C as possible from the gut. A healthy person will absorb only a fraction of a single 1,000-mg dose, whereas a sick person seemingly absorbs almost all of a 10,000-mg dose. This increased absorption does not necessarily produce an abundance of vitamin C in the blood. During illness, the use of vitamin C by the tissues appears to increase dramatically, producing a relative deficit in the blood plasma. Together with Cathcart, we explained these findings in relation to high oral doses of vitamin C, in terms of a dynamic flow through the body.[19]

Dynamic flow occurs when "excess" vitamin C is available in the diet and gut. In good health, a proportion is absorbed and the rest is excreted. During illness, the body absorbs more from the gut, in an attempt to match the increased tissue requirements for antioxidants (or, to be more precise, for redox reactions). The result is a flow of vitamin C through the body; absorbed into the blood, it acts as an antioxidant (or oxidant) in the tissues, following which spent ascorbate is excreted in the urine. According to this model, the oft-cited "expensive urine" argument[20] against high doses of vitamin C is reinterpreted, as an essential and beneficial aspect of its biological function.

Blood Plasma Levels

When given by injection, the initial ascorbate level is determined by the mass of the vitamin dose and the volume of plasma. Even a small, milligram-level dose can produce immediate plasma levels in the millimole range.[21] However, the plasma level drops rapidly, with a half-life of 0.5 hours.[19] The baseline for this rapid excretion is a plasma level of about 60–70 micromoles per liter ($\mu M/L$). Below this level, the vitamin is conserved and excretion is slow, with a half-life measured in days to weeks, in healthy individuals. This conservation of ascorbate protects against acute scurvy and, thus, the baseline maintenance level may be taken as the minimum level for short-term health. In a healthy adult, 200 mg per day can preserve this baseline. However, such an intake assumes an unrealistic absence of illness or stress, which can rapidly deplete plasma levels.

When healthy people take high doses of vitamin C orally, absorption is incomplete and gradual, reflecting a balance between excretion and absorption. The plasma levels increase over an hour or two, to a level of about 250 $\mu M/L$, then gradually decay, returning to baseline after, perhaps, six hours. It is sometimes claimed that the plasma levels are saturated, or tightly controlled, at <100 $\mu M/L$, with a 200 mg per day oral intake,[21] but this is a misunderstanding. Firstly, the data for dynamic flow using repeated oral doses indicates that an intake of 20,000 mg per day (in divided doses) can maintain plasma levels at approximately 250 $\mu M/L$.[22] Moreover, the massively increased Cathcart bowel tolerance in sick people, who can sometimes consume up to 200,000–300,000 mg per day, reflects a greater absorptive capacity.

The availability of liposomal (oil-soluble) vitamin C has increased the plasma levels attainable with oral doses. These formulations greatly increase absorption in healthy individuals, to perhaps 90 percent of an oral dose. Our preliminary results indicated that a large single oral dose of liposomes could increase plasma levels of free ascorbate to a maximum of at least 400 $\mu M/L$.[22] We point out that this is free ascorbate, so does not include the amount that remains in intact liposomes, or that might be expected to have been absorbed into the tissues, given the form of administration.[23] Initial measurements suggest that liposomes and standard oral ascorbic acid are absorbed by independent mechanisms and that a combination of both can yield free molecule plasma levels at >800 $\mu M/L$. Importantly, such plasma levels can be sustained indefinitely using oral doses.

Clinical Trials

Cameron and Pauling performed a preliminary clinical trial, on the use of vitamin C in 100 terminal cancer patients.[24] Their results were remarkable, with vitamin C increasing the mean survival time more than 4.2 times, from 50 days (controls) to more than 200 days (treated). They reported that most treated patients had a lower risk of death and improved quality of life, while about 10 percent (13 patients) had survival times around 20 times longer than those of the control patients.

Cameron treated 100 patients, who he compared with 1,000 matched controls. The lack of randomization of the groups was later criticized as a limitation of the study.[25] However, this objection does not explain the observed difference in survival rates, as any selection bias would have needed to be unusually large to produce such results, and is inconsistent with the experiment as described. We have estimated that in order to select 100 patients with the observed characteristics, the experimenters would have needed about 7,000 patient records and the process would have taken nearly four person-years, assuming one hour per patient. Given the selection described for the study, it is implausible that patients were selected in this way.

The protocol included an initial 10-day course of IV ascorbate, at a relatively low daily dose of 10,000 mg per day, followed by continuous oral intakes of 10,000–30,000 mg per day, in divided doses. Notably, Cameron emphasized multiple oral dosing, to maintain plasma levels.[26] He warned against intermittent injections, which would give sawtooth plasma levels and might produce a rebound effect. In 1982, Murata and Morishige also reported extended survival times from the use of vitamin C in cancer.[27] These Japanese researchers used oral doses of up to 30,000 mg per day, supplemented with relatively low-dose 10,000–20,000-mg IV infusions. Their reported survival times were 43 days for 44 low-ascorbate patients, compared to 246 days for 55 high-ascorbate patients (5.7 times longer). In another Japanese hospital, the researchers reported survival times of 48 days for 19 control patients, compared to 115 days for six treated patients. Furthermore, at the time of publication, some treated patients were still alive. In 1982 Murata and Morishige had replicated the Cameron and Pauling trial with similar encouraging results.

Results have not all been so positive. In 1985, Creagan and Moertel of the Mayo Clinic published the results of clinical trials, claiming to replicate Cameron and Pauling's study. They compared 60 patients, who received 10,000 mg per day vitamin C orally, to 63 controls.[28] In a further study, they randomized 100 patients with colorectal cancer into two groups: the treatment group received 10,000 mg of vitamin C per day and control patients were given a placebo.[29] Creagan and Moertel failed to demonstrate a benefit. We would be keen to take a closer look at their findings, as was the late Linus Pauling, but these researchers have declined to release their raw data for independent analysis.

Since the Mayo Clinic studies, some researchers have attempted to explain away the negative findings by suggesting that the positive studies used IV ascorbate, whereas the negative studies used oral intakes.[30,31] The implication of this is that oral intakes cannot reach the levels needed to kill cancer cells, whereas injected ascorbate can reach the necessary cytotoxic levels. This interpretation is an error, which seems to have arisen through analogy with chemotherapy.

Although there were technical problems with the control selection in the Cameron and Pauling study, these were not sufficient to invalidate the results. By contrast, the Creagan and Moertel trials demonstrate a lack of understanding of the basic science, particularly the pharmacokinetics and short half-life of vitamin C. Perhaps Mayo Clinic researchers have begun to appreciate the difficulties with these negative studies, since the Mayo Clinic website currently states "more well-designed studies [on vitamin C and cancer] are needed before a firm recommendation can be made."[32] We agree and would place the emphasis on "well-designed."

Unfortunately, the Mayo Clinic studies did not take into account the short half-life of high-dose vitamin C, so their studies were flawed in terms of the basic science.[19] Ironically, proponents of vitamin C as chemotherapy suggest that the early positive trial results were just serendipity.[30,31] They claim that Pauling, arguably one of the greatest scientists in history, "may not have fully appreciated the critical difference between intravenous and oral administration."[31] This odd suggestion is easily refuted from Pauling's writings and those of his colleague Cameron.[1]

With some irony, we must point out that the suggestion that oral doses are ineffective is a fallacy. Firstly, however, we restate that Cameron and Pauling, and Murata and Morishige, used predominantly oral doses, with the stated aim of maintaining plasma levels. Furthermore, Hoffer also replicated the early trials, using oral vitamin C in cancer patients, and obtained similar positive results.[33]

The mean survival time for his 31 controls was 5.7 months. He treated approximately 100 hundred patients, of whom he classified 20 percent as "poor responders," even though they lived for approximately twice as long as controls (10 months). The remaining 80 percent of patients he classed as "good responders." Of these,[32] patients, with cancers of the breast, ovary, cervix, or uterus, had a mean survival time of 122 months, and 47 patients, with other cancers, had a mean survival time of 72 months. The assertion that oral doses of vitamin C are ineffective is not consistent with the data from these trials.

Selective Cytotoxicity

An understanding of the short-term toxicity of ascorbate to cancer cells is relevant to the chemotherapy model of vitamin C treatment. In such experiments, either a cancer cell line or healthy cells are treated with vitamin C for about an hour, and its toxicity is estimated. As an example, in a study by Chen and others,[34] the results showed the selective toxicity of vitamin C to tumor cells and healthy white blood cells (monocytes). The results show that Burkitt's lymphoma tumor cells start to die at relatively low levels of ascorbate, and with an hour's exposure at a concentration of 1,000 µM/L, cell death is approximately complete. The majority of cell death occurs in the range of blood plasma values achievable using oral ascorbic acid and liposomal vitamin C (250–800 µM/L). Similar results have been demonstrated with other cancer cell lines, although experimental cell lines differ in their sensitivity.[35,36]

The "vitamin C as chemotherapy" model assumes delivery of a relatively short, high burst of ascorbate. However, this does not apply to oral doses, which can be used to produce long-term, sustained plasma levels. The question arises, what happens when the treatment with ascorbate is maintained over a prolonged time period? Data calculated from Takemura and others, using mesothelioma cell lines,[37] show a large increase in cancer toxicity when the experimental exposure time was increased from 1 hour to 24 hours. In some cases, a prolonged exposure to vitamin C at a concentration of 100 µM/L, a level easily sustained with oral supplementation, was found to be more effective than a short exposure at the much higher level of 1,000 µM/L.

Despite this, it is important to remember that vitamin C on its own is a relatively weak anticancer agent. Crucially, however, it can be used as a driver, to supply electrons to synergistic redox agents. Often, such substances combine in a Fenton-style reaction, generating hydrogen peroxide, which kills cancer cells. Numerous other mechanisms may also be involved, such as inhibition by the combination of vitamin C and alpha-lipoic acid of NF-kappaB, which is involved in the control of DNA copying during cell replication.[38] When combined with vitamin K3, the concentration of vitamin C needed to kill cells is massively reduced (by a factor of 10–50).[39] Similarly, alpha-lipoic acid,[40] copper,[41] selenium, and other redox-active supplements greatly increase the selective cytotoxicity of ascorbate.[12]

■ CONCLUSION

Establishing the role of vitamin C in cancer is a challenging research endeavor. The pharmacokinetics of vitamin C is more complicated than that of a typical drug. It has dual-phase pharmacokinetics, with a short half-life for high doses and a long half-life for lower intakes. Importantly, the mechanisms underlying Cathcart's bowel tolerance effect during illness and stress do not yet have a scientific explanation. Although the effect is easily reproduced, it has been ignored by medical and nutritional research. With hindsight, it is clear that the simplistic "vitamin C as chemotherapy" research paradigm was likely to be misleading. We need to reconsider the available data, using orthomolecular concepts.

The rather startling clinical results of Cameron, Pauling, Murata, and Hoffer were not a result of the use of intravenous administration. Hoffer used oral doses exclusively, yet obtained results consistent with those of Cameron and Pauling. Cameron used some intravenous administration, but the majority of vitamin C in his studies was given orally. Indeed, he urged that levels should be sustained and warned against fluctuations, which are inevitable with intermittent intravenous infusions. Some have assumed that Murata and Morishiga's study used intravenous administration of ascorbate,[42] but the paper states that supplemental (500–1,000 mg), oral (6,000–30,000 mg), and intravenous routes (10,000–20,000 mg) were employed.[27]

Clinical results using intravenous ascorbate as chemotherapy have not lived up to the promise of the early trials.[4] One reason for this is that IV administration produces high but short-lived blood plasma levels. The assumption that a short sharp pulse of vitamin C will be more effective than a lower level prolonged exposure is not supported by the experimental data. As we have described, extending the exposure time more than compensates for a reduction in concentration. Indeed, longer exposures can be orders of magnitude more effective than short ones. The concentrations required to be cytotoxic over longer periods are much lower. Oral intakes, particularly with combined use of ascorbic acid and liposomal vitamin C, can easily achieve and maintain adequate levels for selective cytotoxicity.

Finally, the use of vitamin C as a sole anti-cancer agent is not recommended, as its anticancer actions are known to be greatly enhanced through use of synergistic supplements, such as alpha-lipoic acid. In clinical trials, it might be appropriate to study vitamin C in isolation, if the medical problem were to determine the details of its mechanism of action. However, such mechanisms can be determined using animal and experimental studies. We therefore see little reason to deprive patients of a more optimal therapy, purely in an attempt to determine the action of vitamin C in isolation. There is a more pressing and practical issue: the real medical problem is to keep cancer patients alive and healthy, for as long as possible.

REFERENCES

1. Cameron E. Pauling L. *Cancer and Vitamin C: A Discussion of the Nature, Causes, Prevention and Treatment of Cancer with Special Reference to the Value of Vitamin C.* Philadelphia, PA: Camino Books, 1993.

2. Robinson AB, Hunsberger A, Westall FC. Suppression of squamous cell carcinoma in hairless mice by dietary nutrient variation. *Mech Ageing Dev* 1994;76:201–214.

3. Benade L, Howard T, Burk D. Synergistic killing of Ehrlich ascites carcinoma cells by ascorbate and 3-amino-1, 2, 4, -triazole. *Oncology* 1969;23:3343.

4. Hoffer LJ, Levine M, Assouline S, et al. Phase I clinical trial of I.V. ascorbic acid in advanced malignancy. *Ann Oncol* 2008;19:1969–1974.

5. Hickey S, Roberts H. Results of study in line with predictions. E-Letter. *Ann Oncol* 2008 (June 18). Retrieved from: http://annonc.oxfordjournals.org/content/19/11/1969.abstract/reply#annonc_el_176.

6. Noriega LA, Hickey S, Roberts H. Re: Results of study in line with predictions. E-Letter. *Ann Oncol* 2008 (Nov 20). Retrieved from: http://annonc.oxfordjournals.org/content/19/11/1969.abstract/reply#annonc_el_176.

7. Hoffer LJ. Re: Results of study in line with predictions. E-Letter. *Ann Oncol* 2008 (Jul 30). Retrieved from: http://annonc.oxford journals.org/content/19/11/1969.abstract/reply#annonc_el_176].

8. Padayatti SJ. Re: Results of study in line with predictions. E-Letter. *Ann Oncol* 2008 (Sept 18). Retrieved from http://annonc.oxfordjournals.org/content/19/11/1969.abstract/reply#annonc_el_176.

9. Gordon DJ, Resio B, Pellman D. Causes and consequences of aneuploidy in cancer. *Nat Rev Genet* 2012;13:189–203.

10. Rajagopalan H, Lengauer C. Progress aneuploidy and cancer. *Nature* 2007;432:338–341.

11. Hickey DS, Roberts HJ. Selfish Cells: Cancer as microevolution. *J Orthomolecular Med* 2007;22:137–146.

12. Hickey S. Roberts H. *Cancer: Nutrition and Survival.* Raleigh, NC: Lulu Press, 2005.

13. Gonzalez MJ, Miranda Massari JR, Duconge J, et al. The bio-energetic theory of carcinogenesis. *Med Hypotheses* 2012;79:433–439.

14. Dorigo M, Birattari M. Swarm Intelligence. *Scholarpedia* 2007;2(9):1462.

15. Moss RW. *Questioning Chemotherapy.* Sheffield, UK: Equinox Press, 1996.

16. Michelakis ED, Webster IL, Mackey JR. Dichloroacetate (DCA) as a potential metabolic-targeting therapy for cancer. *Br J Cancer* 2008;99:989–994.

17. Coglan A. Cheap, "safe" drug kills most cancers. *New Scientist.* Originally published January 17, 2007. Updated May 16, 2011. Retrieved from: www.newscientist.com/article/dn10971 cheapsafe-drug-kills-most-cancers.html.

18. Cathcart RF. Vitamin C, Titrating to bowel tolerance, anascorbemia, and acute induced scurvy. *Med Hypotheses* 1981;7:1359–1376.

19. Hickey DS, Roberts HJ, Cathcart RF. Dynamic flow: a new model for ascorbate. *J Orthomolecular Med* 2005;20:237–244.

20. Cheraskin E. Are there merits in sustained-release preparations? *J Orthomolecular Med* 2001;16:49–51.

21. Padayatty SJ, Sun H, Wang Y, et al. Vitamin C pharmacokinetics: implications for oral and intravenous use. *Ann Intern Med* 2004;140:533–537.

22. Hickey S, Roberts HJ, Miller NJ. Pharmacokinetics of oral vitamin C. *J Nutr Env Med* 2008;17:169–177.

23. Gregoriadis G. *Liposome Technology, Vol III: Interactions of Liposomes with the Biological Milieu.* 3rd ed. New York: Informa Healthcare USA, 2006.

24. Cameron E, Pauling L. Supplemental ascorbate in the supportive treatment of cancer: prolongation of survival times in terminal human cancer. *Proc Natl Acad Sci USA* 1976;73:3685–3689.

25. DeWys WD. How to evaluate a new treatment for cancer. *Your Patient and Cancer* 1982;2(5):3136.

26. Cameron E. Protocol for the use of vitamin C in the treatment of cancer. *Med Hypotheses* 1991;36:190–194.

27. Murata A, Morishige F, Yamaguchi H. Prolongation of survival times of terminal cancer patients by administration of large doses of ascorbate. *Int J Vitam Nutr Res Suppl* 1982;23:103–113.

28. Creagan ET, Moertel CG, O'Fallon JR, et al. Failure of high-dose vitamin C (ascorbic acid) therapy to benefit patients with advanced cancer: A Controlled Trial. *N Engl J Med* 1979;301:687–690.

29. Moertel CG, Fleming TR, Creagan ET, et al. High-dose vitamin C versus placebo in the treatment of patients with advanced cancer who have had no prior chemotherapy: a randomized double-blind comparison. *N Engl J Med* 1985;312:137–141.

30. Ohno S, Ohno Y, Suzuki N, et al. High-dose vitamin C (ascorbic acid) therapy in the treatment of patients with advanced cancer. *Anticancer Res* 2009;29:809–815.

31. Padayatty SJ, Levine M. Reevaluation of ascorbate in cancer treatment: emerging evidence, open minds and serendipity. *J Am Coll Nutr* 2000;19:423–425.

32. Mayo Clinic. Vitamin C (ascorbic acid). Retrieved from: www.mayoclinic.com/health/vitamin-c/NS_patient vitaminc/DSECTION=evidence.

33. Hoffer A, Pauling L. Hardin Jones biostatistical analysis of mortality data for cohorts of cancer patients with a large fraction surviving at the termination of the study and a comparison of survival times of cancer patients receiving large regular oral doses of vitamin C and other nutrients with similar patients not receiving those doses. *J Orthomol Med* 1990;5:143–154.

34. Chen Q, Espey MG, Krishna MC, et al. Pharmacologic ascorbic acid concentrations selectively kill cancer cells: action as a pro-drug to deliver hydrogen peroxide to tissues. *Proc Natl Acad Sci USA* 2005;102:13604–13609.

35. Helgestad J, Pettersen R, Storm-Mathisen I, et al. Characterization of a new malignant human T-cell line (pfi-285) sensitive to ascorbic acid. *Eur J Haematol* 1990;44:9–17.

36. Park S, Han SS, Park CH, et al. L-ascorbic acid induces apoptosis in acute myeloid leukemia cells via hydrogen peroxide-mediated mechanisms. *Int J Biochem Cell Biol* 2004;36:2180–2195.

37. Takemura Y, Satoh M, Satoh K, et al. High-dose of ascorbic acid induces cell death in mesothelioma cells. *Biochem Biophys Res Commun* 2010;394:249–253.

38. Flohé L, Brigelius-Flohé R, Saliou C, et al. Redox regulation of NF-kappa B activation. *Free Radic Biol Med* 1997;22:1115–1126.

39. Noto V, Taper HS, Jiang YH, et al. Effects of sodium ascorbate (vitamin C) and 2-methyl-1,4naphthoquinone (Vitamin K3) treatment on human tumor cell growth in vitro. I. synergism of combined vitamin C and K3 action. *Cancer* 1989;63:901–906.

40. Casciari JJ, Riordan NH, Schmidt TL, et al. Cytotoxicity of Ascorbate, Lipoic Acid, and Other Antioxidants in Hollow Fibre In Vitro Tumors. *Br J Cancer* 2001;84:11, 1544–1550.

41. Bram S, Froussard P, Guichard M, et al. Vitamin C preferential toxicity for malignant melanoma cells. *Nature* 1980;284:629–631.

42. Ichim TE, Minev B, Braciak T, et al. Intravenous ascorbic acid to prevent and treat cancer-associated sepsis? *J Transl Med* 2011;9:25.

PHYSICIAN'S REPORT:
HIGH-DOSE INTRAVENOUS VITAMIN C IN THE TREATMENT OF A PATIENT WITH RENAL CELL CARCINOMA OF THE KIDNEYS

Hugh D. Riordan, MD, James A. Jackson, PhD, Neil H. Riordan, PhD, and Mavis Schultz

The authors published a similar case study in 1990 concerning a patient with cancer of the kidney and metastasis to the lung and liver, who was treated with intravenous (IV) vitamin C.[1] The patient recently died of congestive heart failure (cancer-free) 12 years after his original diagnosis of kidney cancer. We now present another patient.

Patient Profile

A 52-year-old retired white female from Wisconsin was seen in August 1995, presenting complaints of painless hematuria (blood in the urine). Because of the history of hematuria, a computed tomography (CT) scan was performed. The results of the scan revealed an enlarged left kidney with a homogenous attenuation without evidence of hydronephrosis (kidney swelling) or cysts. The image also showed a mass measuring up to 9 centimeters (cm), or 3.9 inches (in), in diameter involving the midportion of the kidney. The impression was a massive enlargement of the left kidney highly suspicious of a neoplasm (cancer tissue). A preoperative CT scan and chest x-ray showed the lung fields clear, no destructive bone lesions, and a normal liver and spleen. Removal of the left kidney was performed; histology examination confirmed renal cell carcinoma with no evidence of metastases. In March 1996, metastases to the lungs were found on a chest x-ray film. A chest x-ray in September showed interval development of a 3-cm (1.2-in) oval soft-tissue density in the left upper lobe. In addition, there were two 1-cm (.4-in) nodular densities at the right mid- and lower-lung field. In October 1996, there were eight 1–3 cm (.4–1.2 in) masses in her lungs: seven in the right lung, one in the left lung. She elected not to receive radiation or chemotherapy and did not have any new medical or surgical therapies performed prior to her first visit.

She was first seen by us in October 1996, where an extensive physical, history, psychological, and laboratory profile were performed. Her cholesterol and triglycerides were slightly elevated, and her liver enzymes were elevated to less than five times normal. Her lung capacity was decreased. The rest of the results were normal or unremarkable. Her glucose-6-phosphate dehydrogenase (G6PD) enzyme test was normal. We always check for G6PD deficiency before high-dose intravenous C to prevent intravascular hemolysis.

Treatment

She was started on treatments consisting of high-dose intravenous vitamin C in a salt solution. The initial dose was 15,000 milligrams (mg), which increased to 65,000 mg after two weeks, or two infusions per week. She was also started on N-acetyl cysteine (500 mg) by mouth one time daily; beta-1,3-glycan (a macrophage stimulator) three times daily; vitamin C (9,000 mg) orally every day; beta-carotene (25,000 international units [IU]) two times a day; fish oil to balance fatty acids, orally (three times daily); and a no-refined sugar diet. After returning home, she requested a physician to place a "port" into a vein to make the IV treatments more convenient. The physician refused to perform the procedure because the port was going to be used to administer IV vitamin C. He would install the port if it was to be used for chemotherapy! Fortunately, one of us (HDR) is licensed to practice medicine in Wisconsin and made arrangements to have the procedure done. She continued treatments until June 6, 1997, when another x-ray of the chest was done. The radiologist reported when compared to the x-ray of November 26, 1996, "the nodular infiltrate seen previously in the right lung and overlying the heart are no longer evident, and the nodular infiltrate seen in the left upper lung field has shown marked interval decrease in size and only vague suggestions of the approximately 1.0 cm [.4 in] density." No pleural fluid or pneumothorax (buildup of air that impedes breathing) is evident.

Results

Another chest x-ray was taken on January 15, 1998. The same radiologist compared the results with the x-ray of June 1997 and reported "since previous examination there has been clearing of the left upper lobe nodular infiltrate. The right upper lobe and base are clear. No significant infiltrate or significant pleural fluid is evident. Impression: interval resolution of left upper lobe nodular infiltrate."

The patient discontinued IV treatments in June 1997. She has continued on an oral nutritional support program since that time. As of January 15, 1998, she is well with no evidence of disease progression. During and after the treatments, the patient showed no toxic or unusual side effects from the high-dosage IV vitamin C therapy. Periodic blood chemistry profiles and urine studies were normal.

Comments

Some people might attribute these results to spontaneous remission, which does happen in some cases of cancer. It seems ironic that when patients with the same disease are treated with chemotherapy and/or radiation with successful results, they are "cured." When a patient is treated for cancer with an alternative method, they have a "spontaneous remission." In any case, we continue to follow this patient, who states that she is thrilled with her results. Of course, since she did not undergo the rigors of chemotherapy, her quality of life remained very high. The authors have previously commented on the various theories on how vitamin C controls or inhibits the growth of malignant tumors.[1]

REFERENCES

1. Riordan HD et al. *J Orthomolecular Med* 1990;5(1):5–7.

From the *J Orthomolecular Med* 1998;13(2):72–73.

INTEGRATIVE ONCOLOGY FOR CLINICIANS AND CANCER PATIENTS
by Michael B. Schachter, MD

According to the U.S. Centers for Disease Control and Prevention, the age-adjusted mortality rates in the United States for cardiovascular disease and cerebrovascular diseases dropped dramatically between 1950 and 2005, while those for cancer dropped only slightly. In 55 years, the annual death rate from cardiovascular and cerebrovascular conditions dropped from 586,000 to 211,000 (roughly 60 percent), while deaths from cancer dropped from 193,900 to 183,000 (about 10 percent). This implies that the conventional treatment methods for cancer have not been very effective during this time. Worldwide, conventional cancer treatment methods include surgery, radiation, chemotherapy, hormonal manipulation for certain cancers, and the newer monoclonal antibody targeted therapies. The goal of cancer treatment appears to be to destroy cancer cells at all cost without much attention being paid to the health of the host—the patient. There is little emphasis on helping patients to make lifestyle changes or to improve their nutrition. As for nutritional supplements, oncologists often tell patients to avoid them, as they might interfere with conventional treatment, since radiation and chemotherapy are largely pro-oxidant treatments and many nutritional supplements have antioxidant properties. Oncologists often tell patients that it doesn't matter what they eat, as long as they consume enough calories to keep their weight up while they are undergoing conventional treatments that often cause a loss of appetite.

However, as the mortality rates show, conventional cancer treatment alone is not really working very well. The purpose of this paper is to give a different perspective for treating cancer patients. Rather than just focusing on killing cancer cells, the treating physician should be able to considerably improve survival and the quality of life of cancer patients by taking a much broader view of the healing process. By utilizing a more integrative approach that involves educating and encouraging cancer patients to improve their nutrition, sleep routines, exercise habits, exposure to sunlight (to encourage vitamin D formation, but not sunburn), and ability to deal with stress, therapeutic results should be improved in terms of improved quality of life, prevention of recurrences, and improved survival time in advanced cases.

Evidence for the Role of Diet in Helping to Prevent Cancer

A number of studies suggest that dietary factors can either prevent or encourage the development of cancer. In his book *The China Study* (2006),[1] T. Colin Campbell, PhD, outlines the findings of the most comprehensive study of nutrition ever conducted. Other research[2-5] supports the work of Dr. Campbell who asserts that a whole-food, plant-based diet helps to prevent and treat cancer and other degenerative conditions. The elimination or marked reduction in animal-based foods will drastically cut cancer rates and improve results of cancer treatment. The elimination of refined plant-based foods containing sugar, white flour, and various additives is also important. He further presents evidence that an optimal diet drastically reduces the negative effects of carcinogens and inhibits cancer promotion. Campbell is critical of the notion of "reductionism" research in nutrition (e.g., focus on fats or proteins or carbohydrates), rather than looking at the effects of the diet as a whole. He claims that with reductionism research, you don't see the forest through the trees. He is also critical of the fact that health-care education to the public and to professionals is largely controlled by dairy, meat, and processed food and drug companies. A diet that is based largely on a whole-food, plant-based diet with a variety of colors is healthful and protective against cancer. Various organizations such as the American Institute for

Permission has been granted to publish an abbreviated version of this article that originally appeared in *International Journal of Integrative Medicine* 2010;2(1):52–92.

Cancer Research, the American Cancer Society, and the National Cancer Institute support the notion that cancer is largely preventable with an optimal, predominantly plant-based diet.

Expanding on the idea of a whole-food, plant-based diet, Gabriel Cousens, MD, in his book *There Is a Cure for Diabetes* (2008),[6] suggests that when such a diet is mostly raw, the therapeutic benefits for preventing and reversing degenerative diseases such as cancer are enhanced. He points out that the therapeutic benefits of phytonutrients (plant nutrients) that are not damaged by heat are greater because they may combine with transcription factors in the cell to upregulate (promote) expression of desirable anticancer, anti-inflammatory, and antidiabetic genes, while down-regulating (inhibiting) expression of transcription factors that have the opposite effect. Phytonutrients can function as a master switch to turn many genes on or off. The tiny amounts of phytonutrients in food can have a large effect on how the genes a person inherits get expressed.

A highly refined processed-food diet that emphasizes animal-based foods has the opposite effect. There is no question that anyone adopting a healthy whole-food, plant-based diet will drastically reduce his or her risk of developing cancer. We see that the Japanese people, when following a traditional Japanese diet, have a relatively low incidence of some of the most common cancers such as breast, prostate, and colon cancer. However, when they migrate to the United States and adopt the standard American diet, the incidence of these cancers goes up dramatically.

Another excellent book written by a nutritionally oriented oncologist and radiotherapist Charles B. Simone, MD, titled *Cancer & Nutrition* (2004),[7] outlines an extensive program to help prevent cancer. This program involves a largely whole-food, plant-based diet, exercise, dietary supplements, and stress management. It contains hundreds of references to the scientific literature that supports his program.

Not everyone agrees that a completely plant-based diet is best for everyone. Famed dentist and researcher Weston A. Price spent many years in the 1930s researching the relationship between diet and the development of degenerative disease by interviewing and examining people in many cultures throughout the world. He noted the health of the people, including careful examinations of their teeth and mouths while they ate their traditional diets and then again after Western, so-called civilized diets of refined processed foods were introduced. His observations were striking. People who ate a wide variety of whole-food diets (both animal- and plant-based) were extremely healthy, but once refined foods were introduced their health

IN BRIEF

Worldwide medical literature supports the notion that environmental and nutritional factors play a role in the development of cancer. Nutritional recommendations to the public to help prevent cancer are available from the United State's National Cancer Institute, the American Cancer Society, and other organizations. However, when it comes to treating patients who have been diagnosed with cancer, the vast majority of oncologists fail to deal with nutritional and lifestyle factors to help their patients manage their cancers. Evidence continues to mount that some of the same recommendations designed to prevent cancer should also be applied to patients who already have cancer. Implementing such a program of lifestyle modifications, improvement in diet, exercise, stress management, optimal exposure to sunlight, improving energy flow, and nutritional supplements should improve cancer patients' survival statistics and the quality of life of these patients, including significantly reducing the side effects of conventional treatments. This article focuses on dietary changes and nutrition to help clinicians educate cancer patients, so that they may better deal with their illness. Highlighted are principles involving an optimal diet, avoidance of harmful chemicals, and use of nutritional supplements. Some of the controversies surrounding nutritional supplements are reviewed. Specific topics covered include a broad range supplement program, vitamin C, amygdalin, iodine, and fermented wheat germ extract. Finally, there is a discussion about paradigms in health care and the effects of politics and economics on how health care is practiced today.

deteriorated and all kinds of chronic degenerative diseases, including cancer evolved.[8] Like Drs. Campbell, Cousens, and Simone, the Price-Pottenger Nutrition Foundation (www.ppnf.org) advocates eating whole foods and avoiding processed foods. However, it does advocate the use of certain types of animal foods such as raw dairy products and beef from grass-fed animals. It also emphasizes using organic foods and foods that do not contain chemicals.

Another extremely valuable book entitled *Beating Cancer with Nutrition* (2007)[9] by Patrick Quillin, PhD, offers very practical information to prevent cancer with nutrition, including nutritional supplements. Dr. Quillin is also not an advocate of extreme vegan (meat- and dairy-free) diets. This book should be read and implemented by any clinician who is treating cancer patients.

Although many physicians would acknowledge that nutritional factors are important in preventing cancer, when it comes to treating patients who have been diagnosed with cancer, the vast majority of oncologists fail to discuss nutritional and lifestyle factors to help their patients manage their cancers. They often give patients dietary advice that is exactly opposite to the advice contained in cancer-preventive diets. Patients are frequently told to eat high-calorie, high-fat, high-protein diets that also contain lots of sugar and other refined processed foods. They are sometimes told that it doesn't matter what they eat as long as they consume enough calories to sustain their weight during their conventional treatment.

Nutritional Recommendations for Cancer Patients

There is considerable direct and indirect evidence that some of the same recommendations designed to prevent cancer should also be applied to patients who already have cancer. Implementing such a program should improve cancer patient survival statistics and the quality of life of these patients, including significantly reducing the side effects of conventional treatments. Both Drs. Simone and Quillin in their books cited previously have chapters showing the benefits of excellent

nutrition for patients undergoing conventional cancer treatment with references to support their recommendations.

Common sense tells us that a patient's clinical outcome will be related to his nutritional intake. Food supplies the building blocks for all cellular structures in the body (cell membranes, DNA, proteins, etc.). It supplies the calories or fuel, which when combined with oxygen in the body, provides the energy for all biochemical reactions. Finally, food supplies information to the genes of the body to help regulate all biological processes. This epigenetic information can help the genes to repair and heal the body or can cause a deterioration of the healing process, depending upon what information from food is supplied.

One important area of concern for cancer patients (and for people in general) has to do with exposure to toxins and how well the body is able to rid itself of these toxins. Toxins may be carcinogenic or toxic in other ways. We are what we eat, drink, breathe, touch, absorb, and can't eliminate. We have many systems in our bodies to help protect us from toxins and to help our bodies eliminate them. First, we have the barrier function of our skin and our mucous membranes. We eliminate many toxins through bowel movements, and it is important for all us to move our bowels at least once daily. Also, one of the liver's main functions is to eliminate toxins. This is generally done in two phases with toxic organic molecules being converted to a more water-soluble form in Phase 1, and conjugated to another organic molecule in Phase 2 for easier elimination either through urine or feces via the bile. Many phytonutrients in fruits, vegetables, and herbs are capable of influencing various detoxification pathways to help the body eliminate toxins. For example, sulforaphane derived from broccoli sprouts, up-regulates Phase 2 of liver detoxification and shows many anti-cancer properties.[10,11]

It is difficult to find controlled studies comparing a group of cancer patients receiving only conventional treatment with another group that receives conventional treatment along with a dietary program, which includes many of the principles of nutrition that I discuss in this article. One such study recorded the survival time from diagnosis of pancreatic cancer patients who ingested a macrobiotic diet, which consists primarily of whole plant-based foods. In the first major scientific study of the macrobiotic approach to cancer, researchers at Tulane University reported that the one-year survival rate among patients with pancreatic cancer was significantly higher among those who modified their diet than among those who did not (17 months vs 6 months). The one-year survival rate was 54.2 percent in the macrobiotic patients versus 10.0 percent in the controls. All comparisons were statistically significant.[12]

Also, reported in this paper was a study in which prostate cancer patients were prescribed a macrobiotic diet. For patients with metastatic prostate cancer, a case-control study demonstrated that those who ate macrobiotically lived longer (177 months vs 91 months) and enjoyed an improved quality of life. The researchers concluded that the macrobiotic approach may be an effective adjunctive treatment to conventional treatment or in primary management of cancers with a nutritional association. "This exploratory analysis suggests that a strict macrobiotic diet is more likely to be effective in the long-term management of cancer than are diets that provide a variety of other foods," the study concluded.

In spite of the limited number of published studies on this subject, many nutritionally oriented clinicians are convinced that an optimal nutritional program is essential for improving the results of cancer treatment and that such a program should be recommended for cancer patients and not reserved only for those without cancer who are looking to prevent it. It should also be used by patients who have undergone successful conventional treatment and are searching for ways to help prevent a recurrence. Following are the dietary recommendations I give to my cancer patients.

Dietary Items to Avoid

Cancer patients should avoid sugar and white-flour products; foods containing bromine (a bleaching agent), hydrogenated fats, and trans fatty acids; foods containing preservatives and additives such as artificial sweeteners like aspartame (Nutrasweet or Equal) and sucralose (Splenda), and artificial colorings and flavorings; fish contaminated with mercury; and genetically modified food. Many people are sensitive to gluten (a protein found in wheat, rye, and barley) and should stay away from these foods. Other food allergens should also be avoided. I also advise patients to avoid alcohol, caffeine, and fluoridated and chlorinated water.

Non-dietary items to avoid include tobacco and drugs like marijuana and cocaine, mercury amalgam dental fillings, synthetic hair dyes, aluminum-containing antiperspirants, electromagnetic frequencies such as from cell phones (as much as possible) and microwave ovens, exposure to nuclear power plants, and even tight-fitting clothing such as wired bras that cut off lymphatic circulation from the breasts.

Dietary Items to Emphasize

My suggestions as to what to eat emphasize some of the points that have been previously made. I suggest that patients eat primarily whole foods, mostly plant-based, largely raw, and preferably organic. I tell them to shop in the outer aisles of the supermarket where most whole foods are kept, and to avoid the inner aisles where packaged, processed foods are largely to be found. A wide variety of vegetables, fruits, nuts and seeds, and legumes should be eaten, and an attempt should be made for the foods in the diet to be of many colors (a rainbow array), as this helps to ensure that a wide variety of phytonutrients are obtained in the diet. Fresh, raw vegetable juices with a smaller amount of fruit are excellent. Animal foods, though somewhat limited, should generally be unprocessed and without chemical additives. Meat should be from grass-fed animals, and organic when possible. Dairy should be certified raw if it is available. Eggs should be from free-range chickens, and organic when possible. For most people, I do not recommend total elimination of animal products, as advocated by Drs. Campbell and Cousens.

Additional Suggestions

Eat slowly and chew your food well to improve digestion and prevent gastric upset. Don't skip breakfast because studies have shown that people who eat breakfast generally have a lower intake of total calories for the day and better insulin sensitivity. Don't skip meals because doing so causes an increase in insulin resistance. Avoid frying, broiling, and roasting food as harsh cooking methods produce carcinogenic heterocyclic amines, oxidized cholesterol, lipid peroxides, and advanced glycation end products—all of which are carcinogenic. Boiling, poaching, and stewing foods is best. Avoid the microwave, which tends to destroy nutrients and change blood chemistries.[13]

If physicians caring for cancer patients helped them to improve their diets, several positive effects could be expected. These include: 1) Avoidance of malnutrition—many patients die from malnutrition rather than the cancer process itself, 2) minimization of adverse effects from conventional treatment, 3) optimization of cytotoxic effects on cancer cells, 4) protection of healthy tissue, 5) proliferation of healthy cells, 6) immune enhancement to help protect the patient against infections, and 7) beneficial hormone changes.

Lifestyle Recommendations for Cancer Patients

Although this paper will not stress all aspects of lifestyle that are important for cancer patients, the following items need to be addressed.

Hope, Attitude, and Stress Management

First and foremost, a patient needs to be given hope that the disease can be overcome or at least controlled. Unfortunately, under the guise of not giving patients false hope, oncologists frequently predict how long a patient will live. So, a patient may be told: "You have six months to live." Many people are extremely suggestible and, when given this dictum, they somehow fulfill the prophecy. It is absolutely reasonable for a physician to tell a patient that he doesn't know how long the patient will live. The physician can give a general prognosis for those with a similar situation who have received similar conventional treatments, but emphasize that this patient's response, especially with some of the integrative treatments, might be much better. The attitude of the patient is important in this equation

and helping the patient believe that he can respond to treatment will be important for his prognosis. Numerous books have been written about psychological aspects of dealing with cancer. Bernie Siegel's book *Love, Medicine and Miracles: Lessons Learned about Self-Healing from a Surgeon's Experience with Exceptional Patients,* written many years ago in 1986, is still quite applicable.[14] Lawrence LeShan's book *Cancer as a Turning Point: A Handbook for People with Cancer, Their Families, and Health Professionals* (1994) is also worthwhile.[15] Other inspirational books by people who have overcome cancer using various nutritional and other lifestyle changes are highly recommended.[16,17]

Deep Breathing and Energy Flow

The importance of learning how to breathe deeply (deep abdominal yoga-type breaths) to manage stress and improve oxygenation is key to cancer patients and should be emphasized. Cancer cells generally are anaerobic and they don't like oxygen. So, improving oxygenation should help the patient's own defenses overcome inflammation and slow down the cancer process. Improving energy flow is compatible with this notion and helping patients learn yoga, tai chi, Qigong, or other energy disciplines are almost always helpful. Acupuncture, acupressure, and massage can also be quite useful.

Exercise

Patients should be encouraged to move and exercise as tolerated. They must learn to listen to their bodies. If a person vigorously exercises and is out of commission for the next few days, he or she has done too much. But it is extremely important to begin to some form of exercise, such as walking outside or on a treadmill, or riding a stationary bike. This tones up the body and improves circulation and the defenses of the body. Stretching and limited strength training are also helpful types of exercise to include.

Sunlight and Vitamin D

Another factor that has been totally underestimated as important for healing is exposure to sunlight. John Ott, a pioneer in the therapeutic use of light, introduced the concept in the 1970s, but, like many other important insights, it has been ignored largely because of lack of financial incentives. In his book *Health and Light* (1976), Ott describes a study involving cancer patients at New York University, in which very ill cancer patients were exposed to sunlight a few hours a day. This resulted in a marked improvement in their prognoses.[18] Optometrist Jacob Liberman wrote a book in 1990 emphasizing the role of light in health and predicting its importance in the future of medicine, but the concept has not trickled down to conventional oncology.[19]

The importance of light has become somewhat more fashionable lately with the recent tremendous emphasis on the role of vitamin D in health and disease. Michael Holick has helped to fuel interest with his book *The UV Advantage* (2004).[20] In this book, he attempts to counter the nonsense promulgated by the dermatology industry that the sun is bad for you, that you should avoid it at all costs, and that, when exposed to it, you must cover yourself with sunscreen to avoid the damage. This advice, according to dermatologists, prevents damage to the skin and prevents skin cancer. But Holick points out that the risk of the most dangerous skin cancer, malignant melanoma, is increased with severely restricted sun exposure and vitamin D deficiency. The best way to get vitamin D is to have some exposure to the sun on bare skin not covered with sunscreen. It is important to avoid burning the skin, but some limited exposure to sun is generally good for you. According to Ott, it is not just vitamin D, but other aspects of exposure to full-spectrum sunlight that are therapeutic. I recommend that my patients try to expose themselves to as much sunlight as possible without allowing sunburn to occur.

Quality Sleep

Good quality sleep is essential for any type of healing program and must be addressed and tailored to the patient. Unfortunately, conventional medicine usually addresses sleep problems with prescription drugs like benzodiazepines (Valium, Dalmane), selective serotonin reuptake inhibitors (Paxil), atypical antipsychotic agents (Seroquel, Zyprexa), or various sleep medications (Ambien).

These usually wind up making the patient dependent upon the medication and do not really offer sustained deep sleep that encourages the repair process of the body. Frequently, as a result of stresses of all sorts, the patient has a hyperactive hypothalamus-pituitary-adrenal axis (the body system that helps manage stress hormones), elevated cortisol levels, and/or epinephrine surges that contribute to problems falling asleep or staying asleep. Often conventional medications contribute to the dysregulation of the hypothalamus and other areas of the brain associated with sleep. Stress management techniques such as deep breathing and regular exercise (both discussed above), the tapering of various psychotropic medications, and other strategies discussed in this paper can be extremely beneficial in helping a patient to regain healthy sleep patterns. An excellent recent book by James Harper, *How to Get Off Psychiatric Drugs Safely* (2010),[21] and the website www.theroadback.org are excellent resources to help patients taper off psychiatric drugs safely.

Healthy Relationships

Finally, it is important for cancer patients to enjoy healthy relationships. A patient's prognosis is affected by the quality of his or her relationships and desire to live. Frequently, brief or intermittent psychotherapy with an active psychotherapist, who works on the person's strengths rather than dwelling on weaknesses or problems, can do wonders. A practitioner needs to evaluate the social support system of the patient and attempt to build on positive relationships. An active support group may be helpful in this situation. However, many cancer support groups are in hospitals and are dominated by pure conventional oncology concepts, including ridiculing or criticizing integrative cancer approaches. It is important for cancer patients to avoid such groups and to find groups that will generally support what they are doing.

Use of Nutritional Supplements for Cancer Patients

One of the most controversial areas surrounding the care of cancer patients relates to whether they should receive nutritional supplements while undergoing radiation and/or chemotherapy. Many oncologists advise cancer patients not to take any nutritional supplements because they contain antioxidants, and, since radiation and chemotherapy are pro-oxidant, the nutritional supplements will interfere with the activity of these pro-oxidant treatments. So, the important question is whether taking nutritional supplements while undergoing these treatments will help the treatment results, interfere with treatment results, or have no effect on the treatment.

Before trying to answer the question as to the value of nutritional supplements while undergoing conventional cancer treatment, it might be helpful to discuss the similarities and differences between conventional treatment and nutritional supplements. An ideal chemotherapeutic agent would be one that is highly selective in its action by promoting the destruction of cancer cells, while not harming or even nurturing normal cells. Unfortunately, conventional therapy does not do this. Radiation, chemotherapy, antihormonal treatments, and even the targeted monoclonal antibody therapies generally are harmful to normal cells; hence, the adverse side effects observed during their administration.

Effect on Cancer Processes

Nutritional supplements, on the other hand, may be harmful overall to cancer cells while nurturing normal cells. In other words, nutritional supplements generally have different effects on cancer cells than on normal cells. In his excellent, well-documented book *Natural Compounds in Cancer Therapy: Promising Nontoxic Antitumor Agents from Plants & Other Natural Sources* (2001),[22] John Boik outlines a series of pro-cancer events that occur during the development of cancer and shows how natural substances can interfere with these processes without harming normal cells. These events are 1) gene mutations and genetic instability, 2) gene expression (switching genes on and off), 3) abnormal cell signal transduction; 4) abnormal cell-to-cell communication, 5) new blood vessel formation (angiogenesis), 6) invasion into tissues, 7) metastasis to other organs, and 8) immune suppression and other forms of immune evasion.

With multiple references and citations, Boik explains how various natural substances found in nutritional supplements can affect these processes. Many of these substances can affect several steps of the process. For example, curcumin, a compound found in the Indian curry spice turmeric, inhibits synthesis of protein tyrosine kinase (PTK), protein kinase C (PKC), nuclear factor kB (NFkB), and prostaglandin E2 (PGE2)—all of which play a role in inflammation and cancer; curcumin also inhibits invasive enzymes and stimulates or supports the immune system. Eicosapentaenoic acid (EPA), an omega-3 fatty acid from fish oil, inhibits PKC and PGE2 synthesis, stimulates and supports the immune system, and inhibits invasive enzymes. The active form of vitamin D (1,25 dihydroxycholecalciferol) is involved with nine possible anticancer effects; vitamin A, with thirteen; and melatonin and boswellic acid, with fifteen each.

Boik suggests that natural compounds are mild relative to chemotherapy drugs, being 30 times less potent in vitro, but about 21 times less toxic than most chemotherapy drugs. Each substance acts at several steps of the cancer process. They act synergistically and are used most effectively in combination. Boik's book contains hundreds of pages reviewing the studies that show these relationships, making it a very valuable resource for any clinician adding nutritional supplements to his cancer patient's regimen.

Another book that summarizes many of the studies that have been done on the effects of nutritional supplements on the management of cancer patients is the previously mentioned book by Patrick Quillin called *Beating Cancer with Nutrition*.[9] This is a good place to start for clinicians who wish to incorporate nutritional recommendations, nutritional supplements, and other integrative methods while working with cancer patients. They act synergistically and are used most effectively in combination.

Effect on Conventional Cancer Treatment

Two recent review papers have looked at the question of whether nutritional supplements are beneficial for cancer patients. Keith Block, MD, and others reviewed 845 peer-reviewed articles that discussed the use of nutritional supplements for patients undergoing conventional treatment. They identified 19 clinical trials, which met strict inclusion criteria. Most of the study participants had advanced or recurrent cancer and received various supplements. The conclusion was that "None of the trials reported evidence of significant decreases in efficacy from antioxidant supplementation during chemotherapy." Many studies showed that antioxidant supplementation was associated with "increased survival times, increased tumor responses, or both, as well as fewer toxicities than controls."[23]

Dr. Charles Simone, the oncologist and radiotherapist who authored a book previously mentioned,[7] reviewed 280 peer-reviewed in vitro and in vivo studies that had been published since 1970. He said that 50 of these studies were human studies involving 8,521 patients, 5,081 of whom were given nutrients. These studies consistently showed that non-prescription antioxidants and other nutrients do not interfere with therapeutic modalities for cancer and actually enhance the killing of conventional cancer therapies and decreased their side effects, protecting normal tissue. In 15 human studies, 3,738 patients who took non-prescription antioxidants and other nutrients actually had increased survival.[24]

Studies Suggesting Efficacy of Nutritional Cancer Supplementation

There aren't many studies evaluating the efficacy of nutritional supplements in part because there just isn't the economic motivation to do these studies since supplements are not patentable, and the vast majority of clinical research is carried out by pharmaceutical companies on patentable drugs. Nevertheless, there are a few suggestive studies (discussed next), but most physicians aren't aware of them. Even fewer studies have been done on a combination of a variety of supplements.

Small Cell Lung Cancer Study by Kaarlo Jaakkola

One non-randomized study carried out in Finland and published in 1992 involved 18 patients with small cell lung cancer, an aggressive cancer that usually spreads to others parts of the body. The

patients received a number of vitamins and minerals (several in relatively high doses), along with conventional treatment.[25]

- Vitamin A (retinol palmitate) 15,000–40,000 IU
- Beta-carotene 10,000–20,000 IU
- Vitamin B1 (thiamin hydrochloride)150–750 mg
- Vitamin B3 (nicotinamide) 150–400 mg
- Vitamin B5 (calcium pantothenate) 50–300 mg
- Vitamin B6 (pyridoxine HCl) 200–1,140 mg
- Vitamin B12 (cyanocobalamin) 30–1,600 mcg
- Biotin 300–1000 mcg
- Vitamin D 400–1,000 IU
- Vitamin C (ascorbic acid) 2,000–5,000 mg
- Vitamin E (alpha-tocopherol acetate) 300–800 IU
- Essential fatty acids 5,000–65,000 mg

The minerals used in the study included chromium, copper, magnesium, manganese, selenium, vanadium, and zinc.

The end point for the study was a simple one; namely, patient survival times from the time of diagnosis compared to the survival statistics of the United States' National Cancer Institute's Surveillance, Epidemiology, and End Results (SEER) Program for a similar group of patients. From the time of diagnosis, at six months, the survival of the SEER group was 50 percent and the nutrient group was almost 95 percent; at one year, 20 percent of the SEER group and 85 percent of the nutrient group were still alive; at two years, survival for the SEER group was only 10 percent, while 55 percent of the nutrient group was still alive; at two and a half years, only about 1 percent of the SEER group was alive while 40 percent of the nutrient group were still living; and finally at six years, all of the SEER group had passed on, while 44 percent (8 of 18 patients) of the nutrient group were alive and well.

The Jaakola study indicates that: 1) antioxidants and other nutrients given to small-cell lung cancer patients along with conventional treatment drastically improved long-term survival; 2) there were no side effects observed from the antioxidants and other nutrients; 3) surviving patients

346

started antioxidant treatment earlier than those who succumbed; and 4) antioxidant treatment should start as early as possible in combination with chemotherapy and/or radiation. Granted this was a very small study, but the statistics are truly amazing. An unbiased observer would expect that this study would have at least provoked some interest and an attempt would have been made to replicate it, but I could find no evidence of this in the medical literature.

Studies by Ewan Cameron, Linus Pauling, and Abram Hoffer with Advanced Cancer Patients

Two-time Nobel Prize winner Linus Pauling, PhD, was first introduced to the concept of high-dose vitamin C by biochemist Irwin Stone, PhD, in 1966. Being convinced of its worth and championing its use for the common cold, Dr. Pauling began to collaborate with Scottish cancer surgeon Ewan Cameron, MD, in 1971, on the use of intravenous (IV) and oral vitamin C as cancer therapy for terminal cancer patients. The reasoning was that cancer patients were generally depleted of ascorbate and ascorbate had numerous anticancer activities. They conducted a study involving 100 terminal cancer patients in a Scottish Hospital. After 10 days of IV vitamin C therapy, each patient was given 10,000 mg of vitamin C orally each day indefinitely. Their progress was compared to that of 1,000 similar patients treated identically, but who received no supplemental ascorbate. The mean survival time for the ascorbate group was 4.2 times more than the control subjects (more than 210 days compared to 50 days for the controls). An analysis of the survival time curves indicated that deaths occurred for about 90 percent of the ascorbate-treated patients at one-third the rate for the controls, and that the other 10 percent had a much greater survival time, averaging more than 20 times the controls.[26,27] Cameron and Pauling concluded that high doses of vitamin C should be given to all cancer patients.

The medical establishment rejected the conclusions of Cameron and Pauling after a series of papers from two Mayo Clinic studies failed to confirm their findings.[28,29] Pauling bitterly criticized these studies and claimed that they did not replicate his studies.[30] After completion of the Mayo Clinic studies, conventional medicine concluded that vitamin C was useless for cancer patients, and, despite letters from Pauling and Cameron criticizing the experimental design and the conclusions, vitamin C was relegated to use only by alternative practitioners. [Editor's note: For an in-depth account of the Mayo Clinic studies, see "Vitamin C: A Case History of an Alternative Cancer Therapy" by John Hoffer, MD, PhD.]

In the early 1980s, Abram Hoffer, MD, PhD, considered by many to be the father of orthomolecular psychiatry, evaluated a schizophrenic patient for treatment with high doses of niacin and vitamin C. This woman also had a lymphoma. Not only did the patient recover from schizophrenia, but, much to the surprise of Dr. Hoffer, her lymphoma also went into remission. The word got out and soon Hoffer was bombarded with requests from cancer patients to be put on a nutritional regimen. At the urging of Pauling, Hoffer began to keep track of all of the cancer patients that he put on this nutritional program and reported on the survival time of these patients in a series of articles.

The patients followed by Hoffer had received conventional treatments and 90 percent of them had cancer that was considered to be advanced. The end point of the study for each patient was either death or survival time at the time of the inquiry. Time was measured from the first visit with Hoffer. The control group consisted of patients who approached Hoffer but did not remain on the program for at least two months. Excluded were all patients who died during the first two months, whether they planned to continue the program or had decided not to do so.[36]

The protocol given to the treated patients included the elimination of so-called junk foods (refined, processed foods containing sugar, white flour, and additives), low in fat and void of allergic foods, in addition to the following vitamin regimen. Most nutrients were given in divided dosages two to three times daily.

- Vitamin C (oral) 10,000–40,000 mg
- Vitamin B3 (niacin or niacinamide) 300–3,000 mg

- Vitamin B6 (pyridoxine) 200–300 mg
- Folic acid 1–30 mg
- Vitamin E succinate 400–1,200 IU
- Coenzyme Q10 300–600 mg
- Selenium 200–1,000 mcg daily
- Zinc (with some copper) 25–100 mg
- Calcium and magnesium supplement (in a 2:1 ratio)
- Mixed carotenoids (as carrot juice)
- Multivitamin and mineral

The survival statistics for Hoffer's first 131 patients treated between 1976 and 1988 were as follows: At the end of one year, only 28 percent of the controls were alive compared to 77 percent of the treated group. At three years, only 16 percent of the control group was alive compared to 56 percent of the treated group. By five years, only 5 percent of the control group and 46 percent of the treated group were alive, while at seven and nine years, there were no survivors in the control group, but 39 percent and 34 percent respectively in the treated group. Survival statistics for 769 patients through 1997 also showed a marked difference in survival each year up until five years.

The Hoffer studies indicate that: 1) patients with a wide variety of advanced cancers have significantly improved survival when a nutritional program is added to their conventional treatment; and 2) the nutritional program consisted of dietary suggestions and relatively high doses of vitamins, minerals, and other nutritional supplements.

Studies That Awakened Some Interest

One recent study has outlined the possible proposed mechanisms for ascorbic acid activity in the prevention and treatment of cancer.[31] The mechanisms include enhancement of the immune system by increased lymphocyte production and activity; stimulation of collagen formation, necessary for "walling off " tumors; inhibition of hyaluronidase by keeping the ground substance around the tumor intact and preventing metastasis; inhibition of oncogenic viruses; correction of ascorbate deficiency commonly seen in cancer patients; expedi-

tion of wound healing after cancer surgery; enhancement of the anti-carcinogenic effect of certain chemotherapy drugs; reduction of the toxicity of chemotherapeutic agents; prevention of cellular free radical damage; production of hydrogen peroxide; and neutralization of carcinogenic substances. Previously, Cameron and/or Pauling had published several papers, outlining some of these mechanisms.[32–34]

More recent 2005 studies published from the National Institutes of Health (NIH) suggest that high doses of vitamin C, which can be achieved with IV doses of ascorbate, are capable of inducing cancer cell death, without harming normal cells. While this has awakened some interest in vitamin C for cancer patients,[35] most cancer specialists today still regard vitamin C as either having no effect or being harmful to cancer patients.

Intravenous (IV) Vitamin C for Cancer Patients

The first recommendations for IV vitamin C for cancer patients appeared in 1971.[37] In their book *Cancer and Vitamin C*, Drs. Cameron and Pauling summarized their work with vitamin C for cancer patients, including its intravenous use.[38] In one study, IV vitamin C at 10,000 mg was administered daily for 10 days. In 1990, the late Hugh Riordan, MD, and his group in Wichita, Kansas, reported a rather amazing case study of a patient with kidney cancer who had a long-term remission with IV treatments of vitamin C in the range of about 15,000–30,000 mg, a few times a week.[39] A paper in *Medical Hypothesis* in 1995 by Riordan's group described IV ascorbate as a tumor cytotoxic chemotherapeutic agent.[40] They reported that ascorbic acid and its salts are preferentially toxic to tumor cells in vitro and in vivo, and that "given in high enough doses to maintain plasma concentrations above levels that have been shown to be toxic to tumor cells in vitro, ascorbic acid has the potential to selectively kill cancer cells in a manner similar to other tumor cytotoxic agents." A major point here is that at these concentrations, ascorbic acid is *not* toxic to normal cells.

In 2000, Mark Levine, MD, at the NIH wrote a

commentary in the *Journal of the American College of Nutrition* pointing out that concentrations in the bloodstream of IV vitamin C were capable of killing cancer cells and not normal cells and that "ascorbate treatment of cancer should be reexamined by rigorous scientific scrutiny in the light of new evidence."[41] Levine and his group at the NIH published an extremely important paper in 2005, showing that high concentrations of ascorbate (achievable by IV infusions but not by oral doses) were capable of killing a wide range of cancer cells without harming normal cells. Furthermore, he described the mechanism by which this occurs. Ascorbate in these high concentrations acted as a pro-drug, forming hydrogen peroxide in the extracellular spaces. It is the hydrogen peroxide that is capable of killing many cancer cells and not normal cells at these concentrations.[26] The reason for the discrepancy in ascorbate's ability to kill cancer cells and not normal cells may be that cancer cells have between 10 and 100 times less catalase than normal cells.[30,42] Catalase is the enzyme that breaks down hydrogen peroxide in the body, and, with less catalase, cancer cells might be expected to be more easily killed by hydrogen peroxide.

More case studies were published in 2006.[43] In this paper, Dr. Riordan and others describe "three well-documented cases of advanced cancers, confirmed by histopathologic review, where patients had unexpectedly long survival times after receiving high-dose intravenous vitamin C therapy." They suggested that "the role of high-dose intravenous vitamin C therapy in cancer treatment should be reassessed. A good review of ascorbic acid for cancer over the previous 25 years appeared in 2005.[44]

In 2009, John Hoffer, MD, son of the late Abram Hoffer, an internist and professor at McGill University, Montreal, reported at the annual Orthomolecular Medicine Today Conference that a clinical trial that he had run on advanced cancer patients using high-dose IV ascorbate over a six-month period, failed to show any objective changes in the size of the tumor. The conclusion was that the IV ascorbate alone was not effective for the treatment of advanced cancers. However, Dr. Hoffer used the same methods that are used to evaluate toxic chemotherapeutic drugs and that are similar to the methods in the Mayo Clinic studies previously cited. Measuring the size of a tumor does not necessarily correlate well with either survival time or quality of life. So, it is possible that a longer term study that looks at the issues of survival time and various lifestyle parameters might show a different story. It is not clear at this time if clinical trials of this sort using IV vitamin C along with chemotherapy will show vitamin C to be of benefit, but I suspect if parameters such as survival and quality of life are measured, we should expect positive results. In my clinical experience, patients undergoing chemotherapy with another physician but receiving high-dose IV ascorbate at our office in between their chemotherapy treatments, invariably report that they appear to be doing better than other patients at the oncologist's office who are not receiving high-dose vitamin C.

In our practice at the Schachter Center for Complementary Medicine in Suffern, New York, we have been using high-dose IV ascorbate (10,000–120,000-mg) infusions in cancer patients for more than 30 years. Each patient receives a comprehensive program involving dietary suggestions, a variety of nutritional supplements, an exercise program, a stress management program, and other lifestyle-enhancing suggestions. Our patients appear to do very well and we believe that the infusions play an important role in their treatment. We usually give about 60,000 mg of vitamin C, 10 cubic centimeters (cc) of calcium gluconate, and 4 cc of magnesium chloride in sterile water and administer this over about two hours.

Additional Nutritional Supports for Cancer Patients

In addition to the recommendations and suggestions discussed, there are many other nutritional supports that we believe have value for our cancer patients and are among those we use to support cancer patients.

Amygdalin

Amygdalin (also known as laetrile or vitamin B17) has been one of the most controversial cancer treatments for the past 50 years. In the United States during the 1970s and '80s, a great debate waged on amygdalin. As many as 20 states passed legislation that decriminalized it, while some doctors who used it lost their medical licenses and some even wound up in prison. My first exposure to this alternative cancer therapy was a narrated film strip and book titled *World Without Cancer: The Story of Vitamin B17* (1976) by Edward Griffin.[45] His basic thesis, based on the theory of Ernest Krebs, Jr., discoverer of vitamin B17, is that cancer is largely a nutritional deficiency disease much like pellagra (vitamin B3 deficiency), scurvy (vitamin C deficiency), or beriberi (vitamin B1 deficiency), and that modern civilization ingests very little of this vitamin, which is contained in nitriloside-rich foods. A monograph with references on amygdalin is available at www.worldwithoutcancer.org.uk.

Amygdalin is one of many nitriloside compounds, which are natural cyanide-containing substances, found in many foods, including all of the seeds of the prunasin family (apricots, peaches, apples, pears, and others), millet, buckwheat, cassava melons, and many others. The compound is made up of two glucose molecules bound to a benzaldehyde, which in turn is bound to a cyanide radical (the benzaldehyde-cyanide radical is called mandelonitrile). Both benzaldehyde and the cyanide radical are potentially damaging to cells but are quite harmless when bound to the two glucose molecules.

In the body, the two glucose molecules are split off by the enzyme beta-glucosidase (probably by bacteria in the colon) and are replaced by a glucuronic acid molecule to form a compound consisting of glucuronic acid bound to mandelonitrile (the benzaldehyde-cyanide radical). This is actually the true laetrile, according to Dr. Krebs, and it differs from the original amygdalin, which has two glucose molecules instead of the glucuronic acid. Another enzyme known as beta-glucuronidase, which is found in high concentration in cancer cells (but is very scarce in normal cells), splits off the glucuronic acid, leaving benzaldehyde bound to cyanide (mandelonitrile). Once the glucuronic acid is split off, the remaining benzaldehyde-cyanide radical spontaneously splits off the cyanide, which is toxic to the cancer cell. Cancer cells do not have sufficient quantities of any enzyme capable of breaking down or converting the cyanide to a less toxic compound whereas normal cells do; hence, there is a selective toxicity to cancer cells.[46] Benzaldehyde, like formaldehyde, can also be toxic to cancer cells. So, both benzaldehyde and cyanide are released at the site of the cancer cells and can damage them.

An additional reason for amygdalin's selective toxicity to cancer cells—but not normal cells—involves the protective action of enzymes present in normal cells but lacking in cancer cells. An enzyme present in high concentration in normal cells but very low in cancer cells is the enzyme rhodanese or sulfur transferase. This enzyme transfers a sulfur atom onto the cyanide radical to create the relatively non-toxic thiocyanate. Cancer cells have trouble doing this because they lack this enzyme. So, the cancer cells get the toxic effects of cyanide, while the small amount of cyanide released around normal cells is converted to thiocyanate. Blood thiocyanate levels may be used to help monitor the proper dose of amygdalin, helping to make sure that toxic levels of cyanide are not reached but that therapeutic levels are present.

Many epidemiological studies, animal studies, and some clinical reports show evidence of amygdalin's efficacy. However, it is generally regarded by conventional medicine as the height of quackery. Most of the negative views of amygdalin emanate from a Mayo Clinic study that was was published in the *New England Journal of Medicine* in 1982.[47] A number of criticisms of this study have been published.

The adult oral dosage of amygdalin is approximately 500 mg three times daily, but the dosage can be increased or decreased depending upon the patient's clinical response and the results of serum thiocyanate levels (used to ensure that therapeutic levels are present). For most adults, the IV dosage that we use is 9,000 mg, dissolved in 100 milliliters (mL) of sterile saline. It is dripped over 10 to 20 minutes. At our center, we usually administer an IV vitamin C drip and follow it with an IV drip of amygdalin.

Two cautions should be kept in mind when using amygdalin. First, it is necessary for patients using amygdalin to have a sufficient source of sulfur in the diet, so that any excessive cyanide formed near normal cells can be converted to thiocyanate. A relatively inexpensive supplement source of sulfur is methylsulfonylmethane (MSM). Second, because thiocyanate tends to be suppressive to the thyroid gland, it is essential to have sufficient iodine (see next) to overcome any suppression of the thyroid gland by thiocyanate.

Iodine

Iodine supplementation should be considered in all cancer patients. Max Gerson, MD, successfully treated many cancer patients with a variety of unconventional techniques including more than 10 glasses a day of raw vegetable juice; coffee enemas; a vegan diet; flaxseed oil; cod liver oil; thyroid hormone; and Lugol's solution, which contains relatively high concentrations of iodine.[48]

Today, the commonly accepted medical opinion is that iodine's only role in the body is to help make thyroid hormones. Although this is an extremely important function, Guy Abraham, MD, a former professor of obstetrics, gynecology, and endocrinology at the University of California, Los Angeles, School of Medicine and author of "The Iodine Project," a series of papers that have drastically changed my thinking about this trace mineral, demonstrates that the role of iodine in the body goes far beyond its function of making thyroid hormones. Its other functions include helping to regulate moods, blood pressure, and blood sugar (useful for preventing and treating diabetes), preventing abnormal cardiac rhythms and cancer (especially in breasts, ovaries, uterus, prostate, and thyroid gland), and preventing and treating fibrocystic breast disease (a risk facor for breast cancer). For example, J. W. Finley reported that fibrocystic breast disease could be reversed with 5 mg (5,000 mcg) or more of iodine daily.[49] William Ghent, MD, using 5 mg of iodine daily for a year was able to reverse fibrocystic breast disease in more than 90 percent of the women in the study.[57] Jorge Flechas, MD, states that he is able to clear fibrocystic breast disease in women within three months of using 50 mg (50,000 mcg) of iodine daily.[51] In many areas of Japan, Japanese women (who have one of the lowest breast cancer rates in the world) ingest more than 13 mg of iodine daily

from seaweed without suffering any adverse consequences and iodine may be an important factor in this low rate of breast cancer.

Abraham started the Iodine Project around 1998 when he became aware of the many benefits of treating patients with iodine using doses far beyond the 2 mg (2,000 mcg) a day that most clinicians consider to be potentially toxic. He noted that starting in the 1820s, the French physician Jean Lugol used these higher doses to treat a wide variety of conditions. Lugol combined elemental iodine (5 percent) and potassium iodide (10 percent) with 85 percent water. He found that combining the two resulted in elemental iodine being much more soluble than when it was used alone. Prior to World War II, many American and European physicians used Lugol's solution to treat thyroid conditions, using doses higher than 2 mg daily without apparent significant adverse effects.

Abraham notes that research has shown that the thyroid gland prefers to utilize the iodide form of iodine, while other organs, such as the breast and ovaries, prefer the elemental form of iodine.[52] Both of these forms are present in Lugol's solution. Abraham points out in his preface to Dr. David Brownstein's book *Iodine: Why You Need It, Why You Can't Live Without It* (2009) that "Of all the elements known so far to be essential for human health, iodine is the most misunderstood and the most feared. Yet, iodine is the safest of all the essential trace elements, being the only one that can be administered safely for long periods of time to large numbers of patients in daily amounts as high as 100,000 times the RDA. However, this safety record only applies to inorganic nonradioactive forms of iodine . . . Some organic iodine-containing drugs are extremely toxic and prescribed by physicians. The severe side effects of these drugs are blamed on inorganic iodine although studies have clearly demonstrated that it is the whole molecule that is toxic, not the iodine released from it."[53]

In his excellent short book on iodine, Brownstein summarizes his own clinical experience with hundreds of patients for whom he has prescribed iodine. To determine whether a patient is iodine sufficient, he uses the iodine-loading test that Abraham used to determine if a person had an optimal amount of iodine in his or her body. Iodine is readily absorbed when ingested orally and readily excreted in the urine. The assumption was that if a person ingests a given amount of iodine and is iodine sufficient, most of the iodine should be found in the urine over a 24-hour period. On the other hand, if the person does not have an optimal amount of iodine in his body, when he ingests the iodine, his body will tend to hold onto it and a smaller amount will be found in the urine during the 24-hour collection period.[46]

Brownstein has found in using this test that more than 90 percent of his patients are iodine insufficient. Once a person is iodine sufficient, the maintenance dose for an adult is about 12.5 mg of iodine/iodide daily. The treatment dose when a person is iodine insufficient is generally between 12.5 mg and 50 mg daily. Preliminary research indicates that if a person is iodine insufficient, it takes about three months to become iodine sufficient while ingesting a dosage of 50 mg of iodine, and a year to become iodine sufficient while ingesting a dosage of 12.5 mg of iodine daily. However, the patient needs to be monitored closely with awareness of possible side effects and detoxification reactions. Cancer patients taking 50–100 mg of iodine daily may take more than a year to achieve iodine sufficiency as defined by this test. The dosage of about 12.5 mg of iodine daily can be obtained with two drops of Lugol's solution or from an identical over-the-counter solution.

Iodine's role in helping to prevent and treat cancer needs much more exploration and research but there is suggestive evidence that it plays a role in preventing and/or treating cancer (especially involving the thyroid gland, breasts, prostate, ovaries, and uterus). Dr. Gerson, whose previously mentioned successful alternative therapy involved using fresh vegetable juices and intensive detoxification, recommended Lugol's solution for all of his cancer patients. Numerous rat studies by Dr. Bernard Eskin show a direct relationship between iodine deficiency and breast abnormalities including cystic mastopathy (a painful breast disorder) and breast cancer.[54–56]

Iodine deficiency predisposes to breast cancer and a high-fat diet predisposes to iodine deficiency.[57] Japan and Iceland have high-iodine intake and low-goiter and breast cancer rates; just the reverse occurs in Mexico and Thailand.[58] Iodine protects against estrogenic effects in breast cancer.[54,56] Thyroid hormone replacement therapy increased the incidence of breast cancer in iodine-deficient women.[59] Female rats require 20 to 40 times the amount of iodine needed to control breast cancer and fibrocystic disease than to prevent goiter.[50,52] When iodine was used in dough during the 1960s, one slice of bread a day contained the RDA of 150 mcg. The average iodine intake was greater than 700 mcg daily and the breast cancer risk was 1:20. With the replacement of iodine in bread dough by the goitrogen bromine in the early 1980s, the average iodine intake was reduced below the RDA of 150 mcg and the rate of breast cancer increased to 1:8 (absorption of iodine from bread is much better than from iodized salt). This seems to me to be a totally unrecognized correlation that may be causal in nature. It wouldn't be the first time that a disastrous public health decision was made. As a result of exposure to goitrogens, including the addition of bromine to all baked goods, the amount of iodine needed to counteract the effects of these goitrogens has drastically increased. This is one of the main reasons that the average person needs so much iodine for optimal functioning. One researcher commented that to overcome the effects of goitrogens in the food chain such as bromine in dough, daily amounts of iodine ingested in Japan would be necessary (referring to the 13 mg daily in Japan).[60]

Brownstein, in his previously mentioned book, describes three cases of breast cancer that did remarkably well with an intake of iodine in the 50 mg range. A 60-year-old English teacher, diagnosed with breast cancer in 1989, refused conventional therapy and went on a nutritional program that included 2 mg daily of iodine. She did well over the next 10 years and continued to teach. She developed breast metastases in 2005. Under medical supervision, she increased her iodine from 50 to 62.5 mg daily and improved. Six weeks after starting the higher dose of iodine, a PET scan showed all of the existing tumors to be disintegrating. A 73-year-old, diagnosed in 2003, declined conventional treatment and took 50 mg of Iodoral (a supplement form of Lugol's solution) daily. An ultrasound of the breast 18 months later showed reduction in size of the tumor. Two years later, there was no evidence of cancer. A 52-year-old woman with breast cancer and no conventional treatment was given 50 mg per day of iodine. Three years later, mammograms and ultrasound exams showed decreasing size of the tumor with no progression.

At higher doses of iodine in the range of 50 mg daily, iodine combines with lipids to form iodinated lipids such as delta-iodolactone that causes apoptosis in cancer cells. RDA levels of iodine do not do this. Recent work shows strong anticancer activity in breast cancer cells.[61] Research in this area is beginning to pick up worldwide. A website with more information about the relationship between insufficient iodine and breast cancer is www.breastcancerchoices.org.

Given all of this information about breast cancer and some epidemiologic evidence relating to higher incidence of prostate and thyroid cancer in iodine insufficient areas, it seems reasonable to consider that suboptimal iodine levels may play a role in many, if not all cancers, and that Gerson was correct in giving all of his cancer patients iodine.

Fermented Wheat-Germ Extract

A nutritional supplement that has been well researched for cancer patients is a fermented wheat-germ extract developed by Hungarian chemist Máté Hidvégi, based on research initiated many years ago by Albert Szent-Györgyi, MD, PhD, a recipient of the Nobel Prize in Medicine. Dr. Szent-Györgyi theorized that naturally occurring compounds called quinones would suppress anaerobic metabolism in cancer cells and enhance oxidative metabolism in normal cells. This is what fermented wheat-germ does. However, it also appears to have several other mechanisms of action to help control the cancer process that include immune modulation, apoptosis induction, anti-angiogenesis activity, antimetastatic activity, and inhibition of cancerous DNA synthesis.

The supplement is produced by a patented process involving a fermented wheat-germ extract that yields a uniform, consistent, all-natural

dietary supplement. More than 100 reports have been written for presentation or publication describing research conducted in the United States, Hungary, Russia, Austria, Israel, and Italy. Its value has been validated by the publication of more than 18 peer-reviewed studies accessible on Medline. Clinical studies have shown that, when fermented wheat germ is added to a program of conventional treatment for at least a year, long-term follow-up shows reduced progression of cancer, reduction of metastases, and improved survival in a variety of cancers, including primary colorectal cancer,[62] malignant melanoma,[63] and head and neck cancers.[64] It also significantly reduces side effects from conventional treatment and improves the quality of life of patients using it. It appears to be very safe and there are no reported significant side effects in any of the studies.

Enzymes, Curcumin, Resveratrol, and More

This paper has barely scratched the surface on the use of nutritional supplements to support cancer patients. I have chosen to emphasize certain supplements that have either been very controversial (most of the ones I discussed), not widely known among clinicians, and ones that I thought could be implemented immediately to help patients. This is not to say that there aren't many other nutritional supplements for which there is a great deal of evidence for benefits. Among the areas that really deserve much more attention are the systemic use of proteolytic enzymes (as utilized by the late Donald William Kelly, DDS, and Nicholas Gonzalez, MD), high doses of vitamin D3 to produce optimal serum levels, vitamin K to help with the utilization of vitamin D, various phytonutrients such as sulforaphane (from broccoli), resveratrol (from grape skins, wine, grape juice), and curcumin (from turmeric), various prebiotics and probiotics, and many others. The trick is to try to put all of this together in a comprehensive manageable program for the cancer patient.

Old vs New Paradigms in Health Care

Finally, it is necessary to touch on the difficulties of trying to practice integrative oncology and/or integrative medicine in general in the current international environment. Julian Whitaker, MD, an integrative physician with his own newsletter and a great following, tries to explain the resistance to new ideas in healthcare, and his explanation was an eye-opener to me since my own thoughts were that the problem is entirely related to economics. However, this does not explain it all. Dr. Whitaker points out that it is very hard to change a paradigm and the paradigm for health care is very rigid.

He uses as an example the case of Ignaz Semmelweis, MD, a Hungarian physician described as the "savior of mothers," who discovered by 1847 that the incidence of puerperal fever could be drastically cut by the use of hand disinfection (by means of handwashing with chlorinated lime solution) in obstetrical clinics. Puerperal fever, which was discovered later to be due to a bacterial infection caused by physicians moving from pathology laboratories where bodies were dissected to obstetric wards, killed many women and their offspring (mortality estimated at between 10 and 35 percent). Rather than greeting him with awards, colleagues of Semmelweis belittled him and failed to follow his advice, which resulted in continued deaths. It was not until Pasteur explained Semmelweis' recommendations in terms of the germ theory that Semmelweis' recommendations were implemented many years after his death. Semmelweis died a pauper in a hospital from a psychiatric or neurological disease at the age of 47 in 1865, 18 years after first offering his theory and recommendations. Whitaker points out that in Semmelweis' situation there was no money at stake, but only the difficulty changing the medical paradigm.

Today, the conventional medical paradigm involves a doctor, collecting signs and symptoms from a patient, possibly ordering some tests, coming up with a diagnosis, and prescribing an approved patentable drug or recommending surgery or some other invasive procedure. Activity outside this paradigm is often ignored, ridiculed, or attacked. There is not much emphasis on finding underlying causes such as environmental toxins, suboptimal diets, poor lifestyle, and similar factors in interaction with the genotype of the person. Epigenetics is largely ignored.

Unlike the issue in the Semmelweis case more

that 100 years ago, money is a major factor. The entire health-care industry is supported by the pharmaceutical industry and virtually all medical school education and postgraduate training is supported by the wealthy pharmaceutical industry. Its many lobbyists have profound effects on legislation in the United States and control much of the media. In spite of all of this, the public is becoming wiser. More and more people are taking charge of their health and making their own decisions, rather than just relying on their doctors or the industry-supported media. It is essential that forward-thinking physicians begin to understand the new paradigm relating to health care and begin to incorporate this new knowledge into their care of patients in order for us to make progress in the treatment of cancer and other chronic disease.

REFERENCES

1. Campbell TC, Campbell TM 2nd. *The China Study: The Most Comprehensive Study of Nutrition Ever Conducted and the Startling Implications for Diet, Weight Loss and Long-Term Health.* Dallas, TX: BenBella Books, 2006.

2. Campbell TC. Influence of nutrition on metabolism of carcinogens (Martha Maso Honor's Thesis). *Adv Nutr Res* 1979;2: 29–55.

3. Doll R, Peto R. The causes of cancer: quantitative estimates of avoidable risks of cancer in the United States today. *J Natl Cancer Inst* 1981;66:1192–1265.

4. Wynder EL, Gori GB. Contribution of the environment to cancer Incidence: an epidemiologic exercise. *J Nat Cancer Inst* 1977;58:825–832.

5. Bruce WR, Wolever TMS, Giacca A. Mechanisms linking diet and colorectal cancer: the possible role of insulin resistance. *Nutr Cancer* 2000;37:19–26.

6. Cousens G. *There Is a Cure for Diabetes.* Berkeley, CA: North Atlantic Books, 2008.

7. Simone, CB. *Cancer & Nutrition.* Princeton, NJ: Princeton Institute, 2004.

8. Price WA. *Nutrition and Physical Degeneration.* 6th ed. La Mesa, CA: Price-Pottenger Nutrition Foundation, 2000.

9. Quillin P. *Beating Cancer with Nutrition.* Rev. ed. Tulsa, OK: Nutrition Times Press, 2007.

10. Tanito M, Masutani H, Kim YC, et al. Sulforaphane induces thioredoxin through the antioxidant-responsive element and attenuates retinal light damage in mice. *Invest Ophthalmol Vis Sci* 2005;46:979–987.

11. Kensler TW, Chen JG, Egner PA, et al. Effects of glucosinolate-rich broccoli sprouts on urinary levels of aflatoxin-DNA adducts and phenanthrene tetraols in a randomized clinical trial in He Zuo township, Qidong, People's Republic of China. *Cancer Epidemiol Biomarkers Prev* 2005;14(11 Pt 1):2605–2613.

12. Carter JP, Saxe GP, Newbold V, et al. Hypothesis:dietary management may improve survival from nutritionally linked cancers based on analysis of representative cases. *J Am Coll Nutr* 1993;12:209–226.

13. Cousens G. *There is a Cure for Diabetes.* Berkeley, CA: North Atlantic Books, 2008, 303–305.

14. Siegel BS. *Love, Medicine and Miracles.* New York: Harper & Row Publishers,1986.

15. LeShan L. *Cancer as a Turning Point: A Handbook for People with Cancer, Their Families, and Health Professionals.* Rev. ed. New York: Penguin Book, 1994.

16. Kraus P. *Surviving Mesothelioma and Other Cancers: A Patient's Guide.* Raleigh, NC: Cancer Monthly LLC, 2005.

17. Thomson PAJ. *After Shock: From Cancer Diagnosis to Healing.* New Paltz, NY: Roots & Wings Publishing, 2007.

18. Ott J. *Health and Light.* New York: Simon & Schuster, 1976.

19. Liberman J. *Light: Medicine of the Future.* Santa Fe, NM: Bear & Co, 1990.

20. Holick MF, Jenkins M. *The UV Advantage.* New York: Ibooks, 2004.

21. Harper J. *How to Get Off Psychiatric Drugs Safely.* Texas: The Road Back, 2010.

22. Boik J. *Natural Compounds in Cancer Therapy.* Princeton, MN: Oregon Medical Press, 2001.

23. Block KI, Koch AC, Mead MN, et al. Impact of antioxidant supplementation on chemotherapeutic efficacy: A systematic review of the evidence from randomized controlled trials. *Cancer Treat Rev* 2007;33:407–418.

24. Simone CB 2nd, Simone NL, Simone V, et al. Antioxidants and other nutrients do not interfere with chemotherapy or radiation therapy and can increase kill and increase survival, Part 1. *Altern Ther Health Med* 2007;13:22–28; Simone SB 2nd, Simone NL, Simone CB, et al. Antioxidants and other nutrients do not interfere with chemotherapy or radiation therapy and can increase kill and increase survival, Part 2. *Altern Ther Health Med* 2007;13:40–47.

25. Jaakkola K, Lähteenmäki P, Laakso J, et al. Treatment with antioxidant and other nutrients in combination with chemotherapy and irradiation in patients with small-cell lung cancer. *Anticancer Res* 1992;12:599–606.

26. Cameron E, Pauling L. Supplemental ascorbate in the supportive treatment of cancer: Prolongation of survival times in terminal human cancer. *Proc Natl Acad Sci* 1976;73:3685–3689.

27. Cameron E, Pauling L. Supplemental ascorbate in the supportive treatment of cancer: reevaluation of prolongation of survival times in terminal human cancer. *Proc Natl Acad Sci* 1978;75:4538–4542.

28. Creagan ET, Moertel CG, O'Fallon Jr, et al. Failure of high-dose vitamin C (ascorbic acid) therapy to benefit patients with advanced cancer: Aa controlled trial. *N Engl J Med* 1979;301:687–690.

29. Moertel CG, Fleming TR, Creagan ET, et al. High-dose vitamin C versus placebo in the treatment of patients with advanced cancer who have had no prior chemotherapy: a randomized double-blind comparison. *N Engl J Med* 1985;312:137–141.

30. Pauling L. Vitamin C therapy and advanced cancer (letter). N Engl J Med, 1980;302:694.

31. Gonzalez MJ, Rosario-Perez G, Guzman AM, et al. Mitochondria, energy and cancer: The relationship with ascorbic acid. *J Orthomolecular Med* 2010;25:29–38.

32. Cameron E, Pauling L. The orthomolecular treatment of cancer. Part I. The role of ascorbate in host resistance. *Chem Biol Interact* 1974;9:273–283.

33. Cameron E., Campbell A. The orthomolecular treatment of cancer. II. Clinical trial of high dose ascorbic acid supplements in advanced human cancer. *Chem Biol Interact* 1974;9:285–315.

34. Cameron E, Campbell A, Jack T. The orthomolecular treatment of cancer. III. Reticulum cell sarcoma: double complete regression induced by high dose ascorbic acid therapy. *Chem Biol Interact* 1975;11:387–393.

35. Chen Q, Espey MG, Krishna MC, et al. Pharmacologic ascorbic acid concentrations selectively kill cancer cells: Action as a pro-drug to deliver hydrogen peroxide to tissues. *Proc Natl Acad Sci USA* 2005;102:13604–13609.

36. Hoffer A. Antioxidant nutrients and cancer. *J Orthomolecular Med* 2000;15:193–200.

37. Klenner F R. Observations on the dose and administration of ascorbic acid when employed beyond the range of a vitamin in human pathology. *J Appl Nutr* 1971;23:61–88.

38. Cameron E, Pauling L. Cancer and Vitamin C. Philadelphia, PA. Camino Books, Inc. 1993.

39. Riordan H, Jackson J, Schultz M. Case study:high-dose intravenous vitamin C in the treatment of a patient with adenocarcinoma of the kidney. *J Orthomolecular Med* 1990;5:5–7.

40. Riordan NH, Riordan HD, Meng X, et al. Intravenous ascorbate as a tumor cytotoxic chemotherapeutic agent. *Med Hypotheses* 1995;44:207–213.

41. Levine M. Commentary: reevaluation of ascorbate in cancer treatment: emerging evidence, open minds and serendipity. *J Amer Coll Nutr* 2000;19:423–425.

42. Benade L, Howard T, Burk D. Synergistic killing of Ehrlich ascites carcinoma cells by ascorbate and 3-amino-1,2,4-triazole. *Oncology* 1969;23:33–43.

43. Paayatt SJ, Riordan HD, Hewitt SM, et al. Intravenously administered vitamin C as cancer therapy: three cases. *CMAJ* 2006;174:937–942.

44. Gonzalez MJ, Miranda-Massari JR, Mora EM, et al. Orthomolecular oncology review: ascorbic acid and cancer 25 years later. *Integr Cancer Ther* 2005;4:32–44.

45. Griffin GE. World Without Cancer: The Story of Vitamin B17. Rev. ed. Westlake Village, CA: American Media, 1997; video available at (www.youtube.com/watch?v=QeYMduufa-E&feature =gv).

46. Bradford RW, Culbert ML. *The Metabolic Management of Cancer: A Physician's Protocol and Reference Book.* Los Altos, CA: Robert W. Bradford Foundation. 1979.

47. Moertel C, Fleming T, Rubin J, et al. A clinical trial of amygdalin (laetrile) in the treatment of human cancer. *N Engl J Med* 1982;306:201–206.

48. Gerson MA. *A Cancer Therapy: Results of Fifty Cases.* Bonita, CA: Gerson Institute. 1990.

49. Finley JW, Bogardus GM. Breast cancer and thyroid disease. *Quart Rev Surg Obstet Gynec* 1960;17:139–147.

50. Ghent W, Eskin B, Low D, et al. Iodine replacement in fibrocystic disease of the breast. *Can J Surg* 1993;36:453–460.

51. Flechas JD. Orthoiodosupplementation in a primary care practice. *The Original Internist* 2005;12:89–96.

52. Eskin BA, Grotkowski CE, Connolly CP, et al. Different tissue responses for iodine and iodide in rat thyroid and mammary glands. *Biol Trace Elem Res* 1995;49:9–19.

53. Brownstein D. *Iodine: Why You Need It and Can't Live Without It.* West Bloomfield, MI: Alternative Press, 2009.

54. Eskin BA, Bartuska DG, Dunn MR, et al. Mammary gland dysplasia in iodine deficiency. Studies in rats. *JAMA* 1967; 200:691–695.

55. Eskin BA. Iodine metabolism and breast cancer. *Trans N Y Acad Sci* 1970;32:911–947.

56. Eskin BA. Iodine and mammary cancer. *Adv Exp Med Biol* 1977;91:293–304.

57. Wiseman RA. Breast cancer hypothesis: a single cause for the majority of cases. *J Epidemiol Community Health* 2000; 54:851–858.

58. Finley JW, Bogardus GM. Breast cancer and thyroid disease. *Quart Rev Surg Obstet Gynec* 1960;17:139–147.

59. Kapdi CC, Wolfe JN. Breast cancer. Relationship to thyroid supplements for hypothyroidism. *JAMA* 1976;236:1124–1127.

60. Lakshmy R, Rao PS, Sesikeran B, et al. Iodine metabolism in response to goitrogen induced altered thyroid status under conditions of moderate and high intake of iodine. *Horm Metab Res* 1995;27:450–454.

61. Nuñez-Anita RE, Arroyo-Helguera O, Cajero-Juárez M, et al. A complex between 6-iodolactone and the peroxisome proliferator-activated receptor type gamma may mediate the antineoplastic effect of iodine in mammary cancer. *Prostaglandins Other Lipid Mediat* 2009;89(1–2):34–42.

62. Jakab F, Shoenfeld Y, Balogh A, et al. A medical nutriment has supportive value in the treatment of colorectal cancer. *Br J Cancer* 2003;89:465–459.

63. Demidov LV, Manziuk LV, Kharkevitch GY, et al. Adjuvant fermented wheat germ extract (Avemar) nutraceutical improves survival of high-risk skin melanoma patients: a randomized, pilot, phase II clinical study with a 7-year follow-up. *Cancer Biother Radiopharm* 2008;23:477–482.

64. Sukkar SG, Cella F, Rovera GM, et al. A multicentric prospective open trial on the quality of life and oxidative stress in patients affected by advanced head and neck cancer treated with a new benzoquinone-rich product derived from fermented wheat germ (Avemar). *Mediterr J Nutr Metab* 2008;1:37–42.

CARDIOVASCULAR DISEASE

O N NOVEMBER 19, 1992, the daily New York newspaper *Newsday* carried a report that vitamin E had decreased the risk of heart disease between one-third and one-half. The studies reported were conducted at the Harvard School of Public Health. In one study, Dr. Meir Stampfer found that, during an eight-year follow-up, women who had taken at least 100 international units (IU) of vitamin E daily for two years had a 46 percent lower risk of having a heart attack. This was based on a population study involving 87,245 women. The second study, on men, by Dr. Eric Rimm, based upon 51,529 subjects, showed a 37 percent lower risk. They found that there was not enough vitamin E in food; Dr. Stampfer was so convinced by the data he began taking the vitamin himself.

These findings, of course, are not surprising to anyone familiar with the history of vitamin E and heart disease. In the late 1940s, Drs. Wilfrid and Evan Shute began to treat large numbers of patients with megadoses of vitamin E, usually above 800 IU daily. Their clinic eventually had experience with perhaps 30,000 patients who came from all over North America to receive their treatment. Their work was a model of clinical research, but the idea was so novel that their work was discounted entirely and they were considered quacks for recommending these doses for a disease "known" not to be a vitamin deficiency disease. Fifty years ago, about the time they began their studies, hardly anyone knew what vitamin E was, and it was not considered important or relevant.

Today, 40 percent of all deaths are caused by heart disease. Each day 2,000 people, or about 750,000 persons per year, die from heart disease. Let us assume that the Stampfer/Rimm reduction in risk is exaggerated, and that in reality there was, say, only a 10 percent reduction. This means that each year about 75,000 fewer people would have died, saving some 200 patients daily. It is difficult to calculate overall how many would have been saved if the medical profession had done its duty and examined the vitamin E claims in 1950 instead of waiting until 1992.

The medical establishment consoles itself by claiming that the onus for proving new findings is on the original investigator. This is merely an excuse for doing nothing. The true cost in human lives is enormous, especially when the suggested treatments that you'll read about here—not only for vitamin E but also for vitamin C, niacin, magnesium, and other important nutrients—are safe, economical, and, in the opinion of doctors who follow these treatments, so effective.

— ABRAM HOFFER, *JOM* 1992 (updated by A.W.S.)

TERMS OF CARDIOVASCULAR DISEASE

APOPROTEIN A. Apo(a) is the main protein component of high-density lipoproteins (healthy cholesterol) particles.

ARRHYTHMIA. Irregular heartbeat.

ATHEROSCLEROSIS. Fatty deposits along blood vessel walls, resulting in a hardening and narrowing of artery walls.

CHOLESTEROL. A waxy, fat-like substance manufactured by the body and present in all cells of the body. It is also found in meat and other animal foods, but not plant foods. Cholesterol is transported in the bloodstream by lipoproteins.

CORONARY ARTERIES. The arteries that supply blood to the heart.

CORONARY HEART DISEASE. Atherosclerosis of the coronary arteries; coronary artery disease.

EMBOLUS. A piece of tissue or air that becomes trapped in a blood vessel, obstructing the flow of blood.

ENDOTHELIUM. Cells that line and protect the inside portion of the arteries and vessels that are exposed to the blood stream.

FOAM CELLS. Components of atherosclerotic plaque.

HYPERCHOLESTEROLEMIA. High cholesterol.

LIPOPROTEIN. Types of lipoprotein include high-density lipoproteins (HDL), which prevent atherosclerosis; low-density lipoproteins (LDL), which promote atherosclerosis; and very-low-density lipoproteins (VLDL), which are considered the most harmful.

LIPOPROTEIN(A). Lp(a) is a cholesterol-carrying protein closely related to low-density lipoprotein.

PLATELET AGGREGATION. The tendency of blood platelets to stick together, promoting clot formation.

THROMBOEMBOLISM. The formation of a clot in a blood vessel; also called thrombosis.

TRIGLYCERIDES. One of the blood fats involved in cardiovascular disease; triglycerides bind to proteins to form the high- and low-density lipoproteins.

AN ORTHOMOLECULAR THEORY OF HUMAN HEALTH AND DISEASE
by Linus Pauling, PhD, and Matthias Rath, MD

During the last half century many researchers have suggested that the usually recommended intake of ascorbate (vitamin C) is not enough to put people in the best of health. The arguments were strengthened in 1967 by the biochemist Irwin Stone, who stated that almost all human beings suffer from the genetic disease hypoascorbemia and that the optimum intake of vitamin C, providing the best of health and the greatest control of disease, is 50 or more times the Recommended Dietary Allowance (RDA) of 60 milligrams (mg) per day for an adult.[1] In 1972, in his book *The Healing Factor: Vitamin C Against Disease*,[2] Dr. Stone discussed over 500 published papers in which the authors reported the value of high doses of ascorbate in preventing and treating about 100 diseases. Stone's discussion was repeated and extended somewhat by Linus Pauling,[3,4] and much additional evidence about the value of a high intake of ascorbate in the prevention of disease, and as an adjunct to appropriate conventional therapy in the treatment of disease, has been published during the last 20 years. The discovery by Rath and others[5,6] that atherosclerotic plaques are formed by lipoprotein(a) [Lp(a)] rather than by low-density lipoprotein (LDL), and our recognition of the connection of Lp(a) and its apoprotein Apo(a) with ascorbate,[7] have led us to investigate the evidence about the relation between the concentration in the blood of Lp(a) and the intake of ascorbate in achieving the best of health, with the greatest amount of control of disease. We have reached the conclusion that an optimum intake of ascorbate and an optimum level of Lp(a) are both required for the best of health, and that the basic risk factors for nearly all diseases may well be these two substances.

The Ascorbate-Apo(a) Connection

Ascorbate is an important hydroxylating agent. It is required for the synthesis of procollagen to collagen and of proelastin to elastin and is used up in these reactions. Accordingly, ascorbate deficiency results in weakness of vascular walls, which are not sufficiently strengthened by the deposition of collagen and elastin. The fact that Lp(a) is found in good amounts mainly in the blood of animal species that do not synthesize ascorbic acid suggested to us[7] that Apo(a) is a surrogate for ascorbate, serving to rectify some of the problems caused by ascorbate insufficiency; in particular, deposition of Lp(a) on the vascular wall can strengthen the blood vessels and stabilize connective tissue throughout the body.

The loss of the ability of primates to synthesize vitamin C occurred in the common ancestor of humans and other primates at a time about 40 million years ago, and the genetic change resulting in the synthesis of good amounts of Apo(a) occurred somewhat later. Lp(a) is an unusual bodily constituent in that its concentration in the blood of a person varies 1,000-fold, from less than 1 mg per deciliter (dL) to more than 100 mg/dL. We suggest that this great variation is the result of the short time that has passed since the need for Lp(a) developed: there has not been time enough for the evolutionary processes to occur that would stabilize the rate of synthesis of Apo(a) to strengthen the blood vessels and normalize the connective tissue, whereas others overshoot the mark and deposit atherosclerotic plaques. Apo(a) is synthesized in the liver, where it attaches itself to Apo(b), the main protein component of low-density lipoprotein ("bad") cholesterol, and takes up lipids to form the Lp(a) particles to be transported to the sites of requirement.

Ascorbate and Lp(a) in Relation to Health and Disease

There is now no doubt that the optimum intake of ascorbate—much greater than the RDA—leads to improved health and greater control of diseases. The relation between ascorbate intake and cardiovascular disease mortality has been discussed in

From the *J Orthomolecular Med* 1991;6(3&4):135–138.

our earlier paper.[8] Published epidemiological papers showing a correlation of increased mortality with decreased ascorbate intake or decreased ascorbate plasma level include not only cardiovascular disease but also cancer, diabetes, and many other diseases. We shall not give references to the many papers in this field, which support the conclusions reached earlier by Stone, Pauling, and others. There are also many published reports of studies showing that high levels of Lp(a) are correlated with an increased risk for many diseases. An important early investigation is that by Rhoads and others.[9] They found the risk for heart attack to be much greater for those subjects whose Lp(a) level was in the top quartile (20–72 mg/dL) than for those in the third quartile (11–20 mg/dL). It is interesting that they reported also that the risk for the quartiles (0–11 mg/dL) was found to be larger than for the third quartile. Our interpretation of these observations is that the optimum Lp(a) level is 11–20 mg/dL. People with lower values are at increased risk because they do not have enough Lp(a) to rectify the damage done by the ascorbate insufficiency and those with the high values have too much Lp(a), causing atherosclerotic plaque formation and other deleterious consequences. In another study,[10] a significant association was found between high levels of Lp(a) (>17 mg/dL) and the incidence of both coronary heart disease and cerebral infarction (stroke). In a recent study of patients with angiographically documented coronary heart disease compared with control patients free of cardiovascular disease, it was found that the Lp(a) level for the patients was significantly higher than for the controls.[11]

With respect to cancer, we quote Wright and others,[12] who refer to several earlier studies about cancer in relation to Lp(a). Wright et al. report that 48 percent of their sample of cancer patients had Lp(a) levels greater than 35 mg/dL, considerably higher than the 20 percent for normal blood donors and the 29 percent of hospitalized control patients with cardiovascular disease.

Insulin-dependent diabetes patients are at high risk for cardiovascular disease. This fact may be explained by the observation[13] that improved glycemic control leads to a decrease in the Lp(a) level in patients with insulin-dependent diseases. Among other diseases associated with elevated Lp(a) levels include membranoproliferative glomerulonephritis (a kidney disorder).[14] Patients with chronic renal disease treated by hemodialysis tend to have much higher Lp(a) levels (>30 mg/dL) than controls (10 mg/dL).[15] These investigators mention that this fact may explain the development of atherosclerosis in these patients.

The observation that the Lp(a) level increases after an acute attack of a myocardial infarction and also after a surgical operation suggests that it is functioning as an acute-phase protein.[16,17] The discovery that Apo(a) (not LDL) is found in sperm and other tissues suggests that this glycoprotein has functions in addition to forming Lp(a) and that the presence of some Apo(a) in these tissues may contribute to good health and the control of disease by mechanisms that have not yet been discov-

IN BRIEF

Orthomolecular substances are substances normally present in the human body. Many of them (vitamins, essential minerals, essential amino acids, essential fats) are obtained only exogenously, as foods or dietary supplements, and thousands of others (coenzyme Q10, L-carnitine, apoprotein[a], and other proteins) are synthesized in the cells of the human body. Optimum health and optimum resistance to disease are achieved when all of these substances are present in the optimum amounts. The intake of most of the vitamins is less than optimum, and endogenous synthesis of many substances occurs at less than the optimum rate; the intake of supplementary amounts of these substances can lead to improvement in health. Some regulation of the rates of synthesis and the functioning of macromolecules such as proteins can also be achieved. The evidence indicates that ascorbate insufficiency is the most important cause of poor health, with the blood level of apoprotein(a) also contributing, as well as insufficiencies in some other vitamins and some endogenous substances. Measures to achieve the optimum levels of the most important orthomolecular substances can be taken to improve health and control disease.

ered. We have now obtained immunological evidence that Lp(a) is present in the plasma of guinea pigs, rabbits, sheep, goats, and a few other animal species. The concentrations are, however, much lower than the average for human plasma.

Endogenous Substances

In 1968, one of us published a detailed physiochemical analysis of the process of synthesis of endogenous substances.[18] It was shown in general that the concentration that is optimum for endogenous production is less than the optimum that would be reached if the substance were provided exogenously, without the organism having to do work and use materials for its production. Accordingly, an improvement in health may be achieved by supplementary intake of endogenous substances. Two examples are coenzyme Q10 (CoQ10) and L-carnitine, each of which, taken as an oral supplement, improves muscular strength, with special value in cardiac insufficiency. The concentration of a protein is not easily increased, usually injection is required. The effectiveness of many enzymes can, however, be augmented by increasing the intakes of the corresponding coenzymes.

Unified Concept of Occurrence and Control of Disease

A high intake of tocopherol (vitamin E) is reported to be of value in controlling cardiovascular disease and cancer, and, especially because of its function as a fat-soluble antioxidant, probably of other diseases as well. Also, niacin (vitamin B3) in increased intake decreases the mortality from cardiovascular disease and cancer. Other orthomolecular substances in increased intake may also contribute to the improvement of health, especially those that serve as coenzymes. It is our opinion, however, that the primary cause of early incidence of and death from most diseases is the poor health that results from insufficiency of ascorbate. An example is the fact that atherosclerotic plaques usually occur at lesions in the vascular wall, and that the occurrence of these lesions can be attributed to the weakness of the wall resulting from the decreased rate of synthesis of collagen and elastin caused by an insufficiency of ascorbate. Because a high level of Lp(a) is the largest risk factor for cardiovascular disease, the principal cause of death in many parts of the world, and is correlated also with mortality from other diseases, we associate Lp(a) with ascorbate in our unified concept of the occurrence and control of all diseases. The unified concept is that a low intake of vitamin C and a high level of plasma Lp(a) result in poor health of human beings and an increased incidence of nearly all diseases, and that measures to rectify these factors can contribute to the control of nearly all diseases.

Rectification of vitamin C deficiency is rather simple. It usually consists of taking ascorbate regularly by mouth in amounts of several thousand milligrams per day, or, in severe illnesses, intravenously administering sodium ascorbate in large amounts, as much as 200,000 mg in 24 hours. The plasma level of Lp(a) is not so easily controlled. It is determined largely by genetic factors that regulate the rate of Apo(a) synthesis in the liver. This rate is decreased, however, by an increased intake of ascorbate. Moreover, we have observed in a preliminary tissue-culture study with human liver cells that an increased concentration of niacin also decreases the rate of Apo(a) synthesis, and other ways of controlling this rate may be discovered. Moreover, to the extent that a disease is related to plaque formation, much control may be achieved by the administration of inhibitors that block the binding of Lp(a) to the arterial wall, such as L-lysine.

CONCLUSION

There is much evidence that the optimum intake of vitamin C—the intake that would lead to the best health and the greatest effectiveness in the prevention and treatment of disease—is far greater than the RDA. People receiving only the RDA of vitamin C have weaker blood vessels and other tissues and organs because of the inability to synthesize the proper amounts of the structural proteins collagen and elastin to carry out other hydroxylation reactions at the optimum rates, and to provide the maximum protection that this antioxidant, the most important one in the human body, might provide. As a result of the impairment in health caused by vitamin C insufficiency, nearly every person suffers unnecessarily from premature incidence of disease and from suffering and death caused by disease. Consideration of all of the present evidence has led us to the conclusion that insufficiency of ascorbate is the principal cause of early incidence of and mortality from disease.

An important contributing factor is the high concentration of Lp(a) in the blood of many people, which leads to the development of plaques and to cardiovascular disease. Lp(a) and its apoprotein Apo(a) are so important in relation to health and disease that we have associated them with ascorbate in our formulation of a unified concept of health and disease. Other orthomolecular substances, such as vitamins B3 and E, and the amino acid L-lysine, may also be incorporated into our unified theory. The efforts to control disease suggested by this theory are to some extent to be considered as adjuncts to appropriate conventional methods, and to some extent as alternatives. Since episodes of illness are known to increase the rate of aging and decrease survival time, the relation of this theory to aging and survival time is obvious.

REFERENCES

1. Stone I. The genetic disease hyposcorbemia. *Acta Geneticae Medicae et Gemellologicae* 1967;16:52–60.

2. Stone I. *The Healing Factor: Vitamin C Against Disease.* New York: Grosset & Dunlap, 1972.

3. Pauling L. *Vitamin C and the Common Cold.* San Francisco: W.H. Freeman & Co, 1970.

4. Pauling L. *How to Live Longer and Feel Better.* New York: W.H. Freeman & Co, 1986.

5. Rath M, Niendorf A, Reblin T, et al. Detection and quantification of lipoprotein(a) in the arterial wall of coronary bypass patients. *Arteriosclerosis* 1989;9:579–592.

6. Beisiegel U, Niendorf AS, Wolf K, et al. Lipoprotein(a) in the arterial wall. *European Heart J* 1990;11:174–183.

7. Rath M, Pauling L. Hypothesis: Lipoprotein(a) is a surrogate for ascorbate. *Proc Natl Acad Sci USA* 1990;87:6204–6207.

8. Rath M, Pauling L. Solution of the puzzle of human cardiovascular disease: its primary cause is ascorbate deficiency, leading to the deposition of lipoprotein(a) and fibrinogen/fibrin in the vascular wall. *J Orthomolecular Medicine* 1991;6(3&4):125–134.

9. Rhoads CG, Dahlen G, Berg K, et al. Lp(a) as a risk factor for myocardial infarction. *Amer Med Assn* 1986;256:2540–2544.

10. Murai AS, Miyahara T, Fukimoto N, et al. Lp(a) lipoprotein as a risk factor for coronary heart disease and cerebral infarction. *Atherosclerosis* 1986;59:199–204.

11. Genest J Jr, Jenner JL, McNamara JR, et al. Prevalence of lipoprotein(a) [lp(a)] excess in coronary artery disease. *Amer J Cardiology* 1991;67:1039–1045.

12. Wright LC, Sullivan DR, Muller M, et al. Elevated apolipoprotein(a) levels in cancer patients. *Int. J. Cancer* 1989;43:241–244.

13. Haffner SM, Tuttle K, Rainwater DL. Decrease of lipoprotein(a) with improved glycemic control in IDDM subjects. *Diabetes Care* 1991;14:302–307.

14. Karadi I, Romics L, Palos G, et al. Lp(a) lipoprotein concentration in serum of patients with heavy proteinuria. *Clin Chem* 1989;35:2121–2123.

15. Parra HJ, Mezdour H, Cachera C, et al. Lp(a) lipoprotein in patients with chronic renal failure treated by hemodialysis. *Clin Chem* 1987;33:721.

16. Maeda S, Abe A, Seishima M, et al. Transient changes of serum lipoprotein(a) as an acute phase protein. *Atherosclerosis* 1989;78:145–150.

17. Etingin OR, Hajjar DP, Hajjar KA, et al. *Biol Chem* 1991 266:2459–2465.

18. Pauling L. Orthomolecular psychiatry. *Science* 1968;160:265–271.

A Unified Theory of Human Cardiovascular Disease Leading the Way to the Abolition of This Disease as a Cause for Human Mortality

by Matthias Rath, MD, and Linus Pauling, PhD

Until now therapeutic concepts for cardiovascular disease were targeting individual mechanisms or specific risk factors. In a paper last year, we presented ascorbate (vitamin C) deficiency as the primary cause of cardiovascular disease. We proposed that the most frequent mechanism leading to the development of atherosclerotic plaques is the deposition of lipoprotein(a) (Lp[a]) in the ascorbate-deficient vascular wall.[1,2] In the course of this work, we discovered that virtually every mechanism for cardiovascular disease known today can be induced by ascorbate deficiency. Besides the deposition of Lp(a), this includes such seemingly unrelated processes as foam-cell formation and decreased reverse-cholesterol transfer, and also peripheral angiopathies in diabetic or homocystinuric patients. We did not accept this observation as a coincidence.

Consequently, we proposed that ascorbate deficiency is the precondition as well as a common denominator of human cardiovascular disease. This far-reaching conclusion deserves an explanation; it is presented in this paper. We suggest that the direct connection of ascorbate deficiency with the development of cardiovascular disease is the result of extraordinary pressure during the evolution of humans. After the loss of the endogenous ascorbate production in our ancestors, severe blood loss through the scorbutic vascular wall became a life-threatening condition. The resulting evolutionary pressure favored genetic and metabolic mechanisms predisposing man to cardiovascular disease.

The Loss of Endogenous Ascorbate Production in the Ancestor of Man

With few exceptions all animals synthesize their own vitamin C by conversion from glucose. In this way they manufacture a daily amount of ascorbate that varies between about 1,000 and 20,000 milligrams (mg), when compared to the human body weight. About 40 million years ago, the ancestor of man lost the ability for endogenous vitamin C production. This was the result of a mutation of the gene encoding for the enzyme gulonolactone oxidase (GLO), a key enzyme in the conversion of glucose to ascorbate. As a result of this mutation, all descendants became dependent on dietary ascorbate intake.

The precondition for the mutation of the GLO gene was a sufficient supply of dietary ascorbate. Our ancestors at that time lived in tropical regions. Their diet consisted primarily of fruits and other forms of plant nutrition that provided a daily dietary vitamin C supply in the range of several hundred milligrams to several grams per day. When our ancestors left this habitat to settle in other regions of the world, the availability of dietary ascorbate dropped considerably, and they became prone to scurvy.

Fatal Blood Loss Through the Scorbutic Vascular Wall

Scurvy is a fatal disease. It is characterized by structural and metabolic impairment of the human body, particularly by the destabilization of the connective tissue. Vitamin C is essential for an optimum production and hydroxylation of collagen and elastin, key constituents of the extracellular matrix. Ascorbate depletion thus leads to a destabilization of the connective tissue throughout the body. One of the first clinical signs of scurvy is perivascular bleeding. The explanation is obvious: nowhere in the body does there exist a higher pressure difference than in the circulatory system, particularly across the vascular wall. The vascular system is the first site where the underlying

From the *J Orthomolecular Med* 1992;7(1):5–11.

destabilization of the connective tissue induced by vitamin C deficiency is unmasked, leading to the penetration of blood through the permeable vascular wall. The most vulnerable sites are the proximal arteries (the initial portion of the arteries branching off from the coronary arteries), where the systolic blood pressure is particularly high. The increasing permeability of the vascular wall in scurvy leads to petechiae (minor hemorrhaging) and ultimately hemorrhagic blood loss.

Scurvy and scorbutic blood loss decimated the ship crews in earlier centuries within months. It is thus conceivable that during the evolution of man periods of prolonged vitamin C deficiency led to a great death toll. The mortality from scurvy must have been particularly high during the thousands of years the ice ages lasted and in other extreme conditions, when the dietary ascorbate supply approximated zero. We, therefore, propose that after the loss of endogenous ascorbate production in our ancestors, scurvy became one of the greatest threats to the evolutionary survival of man. By hemorrhagic blood loss through the scorbutic vascular wall our ancestors in many regions may have virtually been brought close to extinction.

The morphologic changes in the vascular wall induced by vitamin C deficiency are well characterized: the loosening of the connective tissue and the loss of the endothelial barrier function. The extraordinary pressure by fatal blood loss through the scorbutic vascular wall favored genetic and metabolic countermeasures attenuating increased vascular permeability.

Ascorbate Deficiency and Genetic Countermeasures

The genetic countermeasures are characterized by an evolutionary advantage of genetic features and include inherited disorders that are associated with atherosclerosis and cardiovascular disease. With sufficient ascorbate supply, these disorders stay latent. In ascorbate deficiency, however, they

IN BRIEF

Until now therapeutic concepts for cardiovascular disease were targeting individual mechanisms or specific risk factors. On the basis of genetic, metabolic, evolutionary, and clinical evidence, we present here a unified pathogenetic and therapeutic approach. Ascorbate deficiency is the precondition and common denominator of human cardiovascular disease. Ascorbate deficiency is the result of the inability of man to synthesize ascorbate endogenously in combination with insufficient dietary intake. The invariable consequences of chronic ascorbate deficiency in the vascular wall are the loosening of the connective tissue and the loss of the endothelial barrier function. Thus human cardiovascular disease is a form of prescurvy. The multitude of mechanisms that lead to the clinical manifestation of cardiovascular disease are primarily defense mechanisms aiming at the stabilization of the vascular wall. After the loss of endogenous ascorbate production during the evolution of humans, these defense mechanisms became life-saving. They counteracted the fatal consequences of scurvy and particularly of blood loss through the scorbutic vascular wall.

These countermeasures constitute a genetic and a metabolic level. The genetic level is characterized by the evolutionary advantage of inherited features that lead to a thickening of the vascular wall, including a multitude of inherited diseases. The metabolic level is characterized by the close connection of ascorbate with metabolic regulatory systems that determine the risk profile for cardiovascular disease in clinical cardiology today. The most frequent mechanism is the deposition of lipoproteins, particularly lipoprotein(a) [Lp(a)], in the vascular wall. With sustained ascorbate deficiency, the result of insufficient ascorbate uptake, these defense mechanisms overshoot and lead to the development of cardiovascular disease. Premature cardiovascular disease is essentially unknown in all animal species that produce high amounts of ascorbate endogenously. In humans, unable to produce endogenous ascorbate, cardiovascular disease became one of the most frequent diseases. The genetic mutation that rendered all human beings today dependent on dietary ascorbate is the universal underlying cause of this disease. Optimum dietary ascorbate intake will correct this common genetic defect and prevent its deleterious consequences. Clinical confirmation of this theory should largely abolish cardiovascular disease as a cause for mortality in this generation and future generations of mankind.

become unmasked leading to an increased deposition of plasma constituents in the vascular wall and other mechanisms that thicken the vascular wall. This thickening of the vascular wall is a defense measure compensating for the impaired vascular wall that had become destabilized by vitamin C deficiency. With prolonged insufficient ascorbate intake in the diet, these defense mechanisms overshoot and cardiovascular disease develops.

The most frequent mechanism to counteract the increased permeability of the ascorbate-deficient vascular wall became the deposition of lipoproteins and lipids (fats) in the vessel wall. Another group of proteins that generally accumulate at sites of tissue transformation and repair are adhesive proteins such as fibronectin, fibrinogen, and particularly apoprotein(a) [Apo(a)]. It is therefore no surprise that Lp(a), a combination of the adhesive protein Apo(a) with a low-density lipoprotein (LDL) particle, became the most frequent genetic feature counteracting ascorbate deficiency.[1] Besides lipoproteins, certain metabolic disorders, such as diabetes and homocystinuria, are also associated with the development of cardiovascular disease. Despite differences in the underlying mechanism, all these mechanisms share a common feature: they lead to a thickening of the vascular wall and thereby can counteract the increased permeability in vitamin C deficiency.

In addition to these genetic disorders, the evolutionary pressure from scurvy also favored certain metabolic countermeasures.

Ascorbate Deficiency and Metabolic Countermeasures

The metabolic countermeasures are characterized by the regulatory role of vitamin C for metabolic systems determining the clinical risk profile for cardiovascular disease. The common aim of these metabolic regulations is to decrease the vascular permeability in ascorbate deficiency. Low-vitamin C concentrations therefore induce vasoconstriction and hemostasis (blood clotting) and affect vascular wall metabolism that encourages the atherosclerosis process. Toward this end, ascorbate interacts with lipoproteins, coagulation factors, prostaglandins (substances that help open up blood vessels), nitric oxide (a compound that helps relax blood vessels), as well as other cellular and extracellular defense measures in the vascular wall.

In the following sections we shall discuss the role of ascorbate for frequent and well-established mechanisms of human cardiovascular disease. In general, the inherited disorders described below are polygenic, having arisen from the interaction of a number

---

VITAMIN C AS COLLAGEN PRODUCER AND REPAIR NUTRIENT

A very important function of vitamin C in the body is its role in the production of collagen. Collagen is the most abundant protein in the body and forms into fibers that are stronger than iron wire of comparable size. These fibers provide strength and stability to all body tissues, including the arteries. Vitamin C is absolutely essential for the production and repair of collagen, and is destroyed during the process, so a regular supply of vitamin C is necessary to maintain the strength of body tissues. Severe deficiency of vitamin C causes the total breakdown of body tissue witnessed in scurvy. Linus Pauling believed that, although humans normally obtain sufficient vitamin C to prevent full-blown scurvy, they do not consume enough to maintain the strength of the walls of the arteries. He suggested that, of all the structural tissues in the body, the walls of the arteries around the heart are subject to the greatest continual stress. Every time the heart beats, the arteries are flattened and stretched, and this has been likened to standing on a garden hose thousands of times a day. Many tiny cracks and lesions develop and the artery walls become inflamed. Pauling believed that in the presence of adequate supplies of vitamin C this damage can be readily repaired and heart disease is avoided. However, in the absence of adequate levels of vitamin C, the body attempts to repair the arteries using alternative materials: cholesterol and other fatty substances, which attach to the artery wall.

Excerpted from the *Orthomolecular Medicine News Service*, June 22, 2010.

of genes. Their separate descriptions, however, will allow the characterization of the role of vitamin C on the different genetic and metabolic levels.

Apo(a) and Lp(a), the Most Effective and Most Frequent Countermeasure

After the loss of endogenous vitamin C production, Apo(a) and Lp(a) were greatly favored by evolution. The frequency of occurrence of elevated Lp(a) plasma levels in species that had lost the ability to synthesize vitamin C is so great that we formulated the theory that Apo(a) functions as a surrogate for ascorbate.[6] There are several genetically determined isoforms of Apo(a). They differ in structure (the number of kringle repeats) and in their molecular size.[7] An inverse relation between the molecular size of Apo(a) and the synthesis rate of Lp(a) particles has been established. Individuals with the high-molecular weight Apo(a) isoform produce fewer Lp(a) particles than those with the low-Apo(a) isoform.

In most population studies, the genetic pattern of high-Apo(a) isoform/low-Lp(a) plasma level was found to be the most advantageous and therefore most frequent pattern. In ascorbate deficiency, Lp(a) is selectively retained in the vascular wall. Apo(a) counteracts increased permeability by compensating for collagen, by its binding to fibrin, as an antioxidant, and as an inhibitor of plasmin-induced proteolysis (protein breakdown).[1]

Moreover, as an adhesive protein, Apo(a) is effective in tissue-repair processes.[8] Chronic vitamin C deficiency leads to a sustained accumulation of Lp(a) in the vascular wall. This leads to the development of atherosclerotic plaques and premature cardiovascular disease, particularly in individuals with genetically determined high-plasma Lp(a) levels. Because of its association with Apo(a), Lp(a) is the most specific repair particle among all lipoproteins. Lp(a) is predominantly deposited at predisposition sites, and it is therefore found to be significantly correlated with coronary, cervical, and cerebral atherosclerosis but not with vascular disease that affects the extremities.

The mechanism by which vitamin C supplementation prevents cardiovascular disease in any condition is by maintaining the integrity and sta-

bility of the vascular wall. In addition, ascorbate exerts in the individual a multitude of metabolic effects that prevent the exacerbation of a possible genetic predisposition and the development of cardiovascular disease. If the predisposition is a genetic elevation of Lp(a) plasma levels, the specific regulatory role of ascorbate is the decrease of Apo(a) synthesis in the liver and thereby a decrease of Lp(a) plasma levels. Moreover, ascorbate decreases the retention of Lp(a) in the vascular wall by lowering fibrinogen synthesis and by increasing the hydroxylation of lysine residues in vascular wall constituents, thereby reducing the affinity for Lp(a) binding.[1]

In about half of cardiovascular disease patients, the mechanism of Lp(a) deposition contributes significantly to the development of atherosclerotic plaques. Other lipoprotein disorders are also frequently part of the polygenic pattern predisposing the individual patient to cardiovascular disease.

Other Lipoprotein Disorders Associated with Cardiovascular Disease

In a large population study, Goldstein and others discussed three relatively frequent hereditary lipid disorders: familial hypercholesterolemia (very high cholesterol levels), familial hypertriglyceridemia (very high triglyceride levels), and familial combined hyperlipidemia (very high levels of a combination of blood fats).[9] Ascorbate deficiency unmasks these underlying genetic defects and leads to an increased plasma concentration of lipids (e.g., cholesterol, triglycerides) and lipoproteins (e.g., LDL, VLDL) as well as to their deposition in the impaired vascular wall. As with Lp(a), this deposition is a defense measure counteracting the increased permeability. It should, however, be noted that the deposition of lipoproteins other than Lp(a) is a less specific defense mechanism and frequently follows Lp(a) deposition. Again, these mechanisms function as a defense only for a limited time. With sustained vitamin C deficiency the continued deposition of lipids and lipoproteins leads to atherosclerotic plaque development and cardiovascular disease. Some mechanisms will now be described in more detail.

Hypercholesterolemia, LDL-Receptor Defect

A multitude of genetic defects lead to an increased synthesis and/or a decreased breakdown of cholesterol or LDL. A well-characterized although rare defect is the LDL-receptor defect. Ascorbate deficiency unmasks these inherited metabolic defects and leads to an increased plasma concentration of cholesterol-rich lipoproteins (e.g., LDL), and their deposition in the vascular wall. Hypercholesterolemia increases the risk for premature cardiovascular disease primarily when combined with elevated plasma levels of Lp(a) or triglycerides.

The mechanisms by which vitamin C supplementation prevents the exacerbation of hypercholesterolemia and related cardiovascular disease include an increased breakdown of cholesterol. In particular, ascorbate is known to stimulate 7-a-hydroxylase, a key enzyme in the conversion of cholesterol to bile acids and to increase the expression of LDL receptors on the cell surface. Moreover, ascorbate is known to inhibit endogenous cholesterol synthesis as well as oxidative modification of LDL.

Hypertriglyceridemia, Type III Hyperlipidemia

A variety of genetic disorders lead to the accumulation of triglycerides in the form of chylomicron remnants (lipid carriers), very low-density lipoproteins (VLDL), and intermediate-density lipoproteins (IDL) in plasma. Vitamin C deficiency unmasks these underlying genetic defects, and the continued deposition of triglyceride-rich lipoproteins in the vascular wall leads to cardiovascular disease development. These triglyceride-rich lipoproteins are particularly subject to oxidation, cellular lipoprotein uptake, and foam-cell formation. In hypertriglyceridemia, nonspecific foam-cell formation has been observed in a variety of organs.[10] Ascorbate-deficient foam-cell formation, although a less specific repair mechanism than the extracellular deposition of Lp(a), may have also conferred stability.

Vitamin C supplementation prevents the exacerbation of cardiovascular disease associated with high triglyceride blood levels, type III hyperlipidemia, and related disorders by stimulating lipoprotein lipases and thereby enabling a normal breakdown of triglyceride-rich lipoproteins.[11] Ascorbate prevents the oxidative modification of these lipoproteins, their uptake by scavenger cells, and foam-cell formation. Moreover, we propose here that, analogous to the LDL receptor, vitamin C also increases the expression of the receptors involved in the metabolic clearance of triglyceride-rich lipoproteins, such as the chylomicron-remnant receptor.

The degree of build-up of atherosclerotic plaques in patients with lipoprotein disorders is determined by the rate of deposition of lipoproteins and by the rate of the removal of deposited lipids from the vascular wall. It is therefore not surprising that vitamin C is also closely connected with this reverse pathway.

Hypoalphalipoproteinemia

Hypoalphalipoproteinemia is a frequent lipoprotein disorder characterized by a decreased synthesis of high-density lipoprotein (HDL) particles. HDL is part of the reverse-cholesterol-transport pathway and is critical for the transport of cholesterol and also other lipids from the body periphery to the liver. In ascorbate deficiency, this genetic defect is unmasked resulting in decreased HDL levels and a decreased reverse transport of lipids from the vascular wall to the liver. This mechanism is highly effective and the genetic disorder hypoalphalipoproteinemia was greatly favored during evolution. With vitamin C supplementation, HDL production increases[12] leading to an increased uptake of lipids deposited in the vascular wall and to a decrease of the atherosclerotic lesion. A look back in evolution underlines the importance of this mechanism.

During the winter seasons when our ancestor's ascorbate intake was low, they became dependent on protecting their vascular wall by the deposition of lipoproteins and other constituents. During spring and summer seasons, the ascorbate content in their diet increased significantly and mechanisms were favored that decreased the vascular deposits under the protection of increased ascorbate concentration in the vascular tissue. It is not unreasonable for us to propose that vitamin C can reduce fatty deposits in the vascular wall within a relatively short time. In an earlier clinical study, it was shown that 500 mg of dietary ascorbate per day can lead to a reduction of atherosclerotic deposits within two to six months.[13] This concept, of course, also explains why heart attack and stroke occur today with a much higher frequency in winter than during spring and summer, the seasons with increased vitamin C intake.

Other Inherited Metabolic Disorders Associated with Cardiovascular Disease

Besides lipoprotein disorders, many other inherited metabolic diseases are associated with cardiovascular disease. Generally these disorders lead to an increased concentration of plasma constituents that directly or indirectly damage the integrity of the vascular wall. Consequently, these diseases lead to peripheral angiopathies as observed in diabetes, homocystinuria, sickle-cell anemia,[14] and many other genetic disorders. Similar to lipoproteins, the deposition of various plasma constituents as well as proliferative thickening provided a certain stability for the ascorbate-deficient vascular wall. We illustrate this principle for diabetic and homocystinuric angiopathy.

Diabetic Angiopathy

The mechanism in this case involves the structural similarity between glucose and ascorbate and the competition of these two molecules for specific cell-surface receptors.[15,16]

Elevated glucose levels prevent many cellular systems in the human body, including endothelial cells, from optimum ascorbate uptake. Ascorbate deficiency unmasks the underlying genetic disease, aggravates the imbalance between glucose and ascorbate, decreases vascular ascorbate concentration, and thereby triggers diabetic angiopathy. Vitamin C supplementation prevents diabetic angiopathy by optimizing the ascorbate concentration in the vascular wall and also by lowering the insulin requirement.[17]

Homocystinuric Angiopathy

Homocystinuria is characterized by the accumulation of homocysteine and a variety of its metabolic derivatives in the plasma, tissues, and urine as the result of decreased homocysteine breakdown.[18] Elevated plasma concentrations of homocysteine and its derivatives damage the endothelial cells throughout the arterial and venous system. Thus, homocystinuria is characterized by peripheral vascular disease and thromboembolism. These clinical manifestations have been estimated to occur in 30 percent of the patients before the age of 20 and in 60 percent of the patients before the age of 40.[19] Vitamin C supplementation prevents homocystinuric angiopathy and other clinical complications of this disease by increasing the rate of homocysteine breakdown.[20]

Thus, vitamin C deficiency unmasks a variety of individual genetic predispositions that lead to cardiovascular disease in different ways. These genetic disorders were conserved during evolution largely because of their association with mechanisms that lead to the thickening of the vascular wall. Moreover, since ascorbate deficiency is the underlying cause of these diseases, vitamin C supplementation is the universal therapy.

The Determining Principles of This Theory

The determining principles of this comprehensive theory are summarized in the steps below.

1. Cardiovascular disease is the direct consequence of our lost ability to make ascorbate in combination with our low-dietary intake of vitamin C.

2. Ascorbate deficiency leads to increased permeability of the vascular wall by the loss of the endothelial barrier function and the loosening of the vascular connective tissue.

3. After the loss of endogenous vitamin C production, scurvy and fatal blood loss through the scorbutic vascular wall rendered our ancestors in danger of extinction. Under this evolutionary pressure over millions of years, genetic and metabolic countermeasures were favored that counteract the increased permeability of the vascular wall.

4. The genetic level is characterized by the fact that inherited disorders associated with cardiovascular disease became the most frequent among all genetic predispositions. Among those predispositions lipid and lipoprotein disorders occur particularly often.

5. The metabolic level is characterized by the direct relation between vitamin C and virtually all risk factors of clinical cardiology today. Vitamin C deficiency leads to vasoconstriction and hemostasis and affects the vascular wall metabolism in favor of atherosclerotic deposits.

6. The genetic level can be further characterized. The more effective and specific a certain genetic feature counteracted the increasing vascular permeability in scurvy, the more advantageous it became during evolution and, generally, the more frequently this genetic feature occurs today.

7. The deposition of Lp(a) is the most effective, most specific, and therefore most frequent of these mechanisms. Lp(a) is preferentially deposited at predisposition sites. In chronic ascorbate deficiency the accumulation of Lp(a) leads to the localized development of atherosclerotic plaques and to myocardial infarction and stroke.

8. Another frequent inherited lipoprotein disorder is hypoalphalipoproteinemia. The frequency of this disorder again reflects its usefulness during evolution. The metabolic upregulation (promotion) of HDL synthesis by ascorbate became an important mechanism to reverse and decrease existing lipid deposits in the vascular wall.

9. The vascular defense mechanisms associated with most genetic disorders are nonspecific. These mechanisms can aggravate the development of atherosclerotic plaques at predisposition sites. Other nonspecific mechanisms lead to peripheral forms of atherosclerosis by causing a thickening of the vascular wall throughout the arterial system. This peripheral form of vascular disease is characteristic for angiopathies associated with type III hyperlipidemia, diabetes, and many other inherited metabolic diseases.

10. Of particular advantage during evolution and therefore particularly frequent today are those genetic features that protect the ascorbate-deficient vascular wall until the end of the reproduction age. By favoring these disorders nature decided for the lesser of two evils: the death from cardiovascular disease after the reproduction age rather than death from scurvy at a much earlier age. This also explains the rapid increase of the cardiovascular disease mortality today from the fourth decade onward.

11. After the loss of endogenous vitamin C production, the genetic mutation rate in our ancestors increased significantly.[21] This was an additional precondition favoring the advantage not only of Apo(a) and Lp(a) but also of many other genetic countermeasures associated with cardiovascular disease.

12. Genetic predispositions are characterized by the rate of vitamin C depletion in a multitude of metabolic reactions specific for the genetic disorder.[22] The overall rate of ascorbate depletion in an individual is largely determined by the polygenic pattern of disorders. The earlier the ascorbate reserves in the body are depleted without being supplemented, the earlier cardiovascular disease develops.

13. The genetic predispositions with the highest probability for early clinical manifestation require the highest amount of vitamin C supplementation in the diet to prevent cardiovascular disease development. The amount of vitamin C for patients at high risk should be comparable to the amount of ascorbate our ancestors synthesized in their body before they lost this ability: 10,000–20,000 milligrams per day.

14. Optimum vitamin C supplementation prevents the development of cardiovascular disease independently of the individual predisposition or mechanism. Ascorbate reduces existing atherosclerotic deposits and thereby decreases the risk for heart attack and stroke. Moreover, vitamin C can prevent blindness and organ failure in diabetic patients, thromboembolism in homocystinuric patients, and many other manifestations of cardiovascular disease.

■ CONCLUSION

In this paper, we present a unified theory of cardiovascular disease. This disease is the direct consequence of our inability to synthesize vitamin C in combination with insufficient intake of vitamin C in the modern diet. Since ascorbate deficiency is the common cause of cardiovascular disease, vitamin C supplementation is the universal treatment for this disease. The available epidemiological and clinical evidence is reasonably convincing. Further clinical confirmation of this theory should lead to the abolition of cardiovascular disease as a cause of human mortality for the present generation and future generations of mankind.

REFERENCES

1. Rath, M, Pauling L. Solution of the puzzle of human cardiovascular disease: its primary cause is ascorbate deficiency, leading to the deposition of lipoprotein(a) and fibrinogen/fibrin in the vascular wall. *J Orthomolecular Med* 1991;6:125–134.

2. Pauling L, Rath M. Plasmin-induced proteolysis and the role of apoprotein(a), lysine, and synthetic lysine analogs. *J Orthomolecular Med* 1992;7:17–23.

3. Ginter E. Marginal vitamin C deficiency, lipid metabolism, and atherosclerosis. *Lipid Research* 1973;16:162–220.

4. Third Conference on Vitamin C, Annals of the New York Academy of Sciences 498 (BurnsJJ, Rivers JM, Machlin LJ, eds) 1987.

5. Pauling L. *How to Live Longer and Feel Better.* New York: W.H. Freeman & Co., 1986.

6. Rath M, Pauling L. Hypothesis: lipoprotein(a) is a surrogate for ascorbate. *Proc Natl Acad Sci USA* 1990;87:6204–6207.

7. Koschinsky ML, Beisiegel U, Henne-Bruns D, et al. Apolipoprotein(a) size heterogeneity is related to variable number of repeat sequences in its mRNA. *Biochemistry* 1990;29:640–644.

8. Rath M, Pauling L. Apoprotein(a) is an adhesive protein. *J Orthomolecular Med* 1991;6:139–143.

9. Goldstein JL, Schrott HG, Hazzard WR, et al. Hyperlipidemia in coronary heart disease. *J Clin Invest* 1973;52:1544–1568.

10. Roberts WC, Levy RI, Fredrickson DS. Hyperlipoproteinemia: A review of the five types, with first report of necropsy findings in type 3. *Arch Path* 1970;59:46–56.

11. Sokoloff B, Hori M, Saelhof CC, et al. Aging, atherosclerosis and ascorbic acid metabolism. *J Am Ger Soc* 1966;14:1239–1260.

12. Jacques PF, Hartz SC, McGandy RB, et al. Vitamin C and blood lipoproteins in an elderly population. *Ann NY Acad Sci* 1987:100–109.

13. Willis GC, Light AW, Gow WS. Serial arteriography in atherosclerosis. *Can Med Assoc J* 1954;71:562–568.

14. Pauling L, Itano HA, Singer SJ, et al. Sickle cell anemia, a molecular disease. *Science* 1949;110:543.

15. Mann GV, Newton P. The membrane transport of ascorbic acid. Second Conference on Vitamin C. *Ann NY Acad Sci* 1975;243–252.

16. Kapeghian JC, Verlangieri J. The effects of glucose on ascorbic acid uptake in heart endothelial cells: possible pathogenesis of diabetic angiopathies. *Life Sciences* 1984;34:577–584.

17. Dice JF, Daniel CW. The hypoglycemic effect of ascorbic acid in a juvenile-onset diabetic. International Research Communications System 1973;1:41.

18. Mudd SH, Levey HL, Skovby F. Disorders of transsulfuration. In: *The Metabolic Basis of Inherited Disease* edited by CR Scriver, Al Beaudet, and WS Sly. New York: McGraw-Hill, 1989, 693–734.

19. Boers GH, Smals AH, Trijbels FM, et al. Heterozygosity for homocystinuria in premature peripheral and cerebral occlusive arterial disease. *N Engl J Med* 1985;313:709–715.

20. McCully KS. Homocysteine metabolism in scurvy, growth and arteriosclerosis. *Nature* 1971;231:391–392.

21. Fraga CG, Motchnik PA, Shigenaga MK, et al. Ascorbic acid protects against endogenous oxidative DNA damage in human sperm. *Proc Natl Acad Sci USA* 1991;88:11003–11006.

22. Pauling L. Orthomolecular psychiatry. *Science* 1968;160:265–271.

INTRODUCTION OF NIACIN AS THE FIRST SUCCESSFUL TREATMENT FOR CHOLESTEROL CONTROL: A REMINISCENCE

by William B. Parsons, Jr., MD

My years of training in internal medicine at the Mayo Clinic in Rochester, Minnesota, began in 1950 and were interrupted by two years of active duty in the U.S. Naval Reserve, spent in San Diego, from spring 1953 to spring 1955. Back in Rochester for a fourth year of training, I was serving as a first assistant in the peripheral vascular service unit at St. Mary's Hospital for the summer quarter of 1955, when a series of incredible coincidences culminated in an event that changed my life. No one had any way of knowing at the time, but it also changed millions of lives around the world.

The staff consultant with the vascular service in August was Edgar V. Allen, a distinguished authority in the peripheral vascular field. Dr. Allen and his associates, Nelson Barker and Edgar Hines, had some years earlier written the bible of their specialty, *Peripheral Vascular Diseases*. Dr. Allen loved to teach. More often than not, when he met me and the four second assistants on the unit, he would suggest that we sit and chat for a while before starting morning rounds. We never objected, for from these informal sessions came some of the most memorable teaching of our training years.

On this particular morning our chat was interrupted by a knock on the door of the conference room by Dr. Howard Rome, chief of the section on psychiatry at the clinic, who was a duck-hunting buddy of Dr. Allen. He brought a surprising question: Would you be interested in hearing about a drug that reduces cholesterol levels? Skeptically (because there had been no successful drugs until then), we said that we would, of course, if there were such a drug. My mind quickly sorted through the short list of drugs that had been tried for this purpose. Thyroid had been tried but hadn't worked. Another agent, which had also failed, was a vegetable oil product, sitosterol, which one pharmaceutical company had marketed. I could think of no others.

The name of the drug surprised us, as Dr. Rome provided the few details he had. The preced-

ing evening he had had dinner with Dr. Abram Hoffer, a psychiatrist from Regina, Saskatchewan, who had been in Rochester to give a series of lectures on schizophrenia. For years, he told Dr. Rome, he had administered large doses of niacin (then often called nicotinic acid) to his schizophrenic patients, feeling that it had helped them. Learning of this, his former anatomy professor at University of Saskatchewan, Dr. Rudolf Altschul, had suggested that he measure cholesterol levels in patients receiving niacin. Altschul, who had done studies of atherosclerosis in cholesterol-fed rabbits, predicted that niacin would reduce cholesterol levels. When his prediction proved correct, the two teamed with laboratory director Dr. James Stephen to try the drug in other volunteers. Their brief observations showed that niacin did, in fact, reduce cholesterol levels in a short period of time.

Early Niacin Use

Niacin was originally known as a member of the vitamin B complex, which prevents the vitamin deficiency disease pellagra in humans and black tongue in dogs. It was in all the pharmacology textbooks and was well known to doctors. Niacin was notable mainly because its administration, usually in 50–100-milligram (mg) doses, was rapidly followed by flushing of the skin (redness of the skin of the face and neck, sometimes the whole upper body), accompanied by a very warm feeling, often with itching. For this reason, in vitamin preparations the closely related compound niacinamide was used because it had the vitamin activity without the flush. At that time niacin had practically no use in medicine other than its vitamin activity. Ear, nose, and throat doctors (otolaryngologists) sometimes recommended it for vertigo. Physicians sometimes hoped it might help patients who had experienced a thrombotic stroke. Mayo neurologists

From the *J Orthomolecular Med* 2000;15(3):121–126.

had studied this use, along with other agents alleged to dilate cerebral blood vessels, but found that there was really no benefit. They acknowledged that the flush might make the family think that something was being done, although there was little that could be done for a stroke in those days. The fact that it was very safe seemed to justify its use, albeit as a placebo in those instances.

Niacin was made in 50-mg or 100-mg tablets. Our first thought was that the doses used by the Canadians, 1,000 mg three or four times a day, would cause greater, intolerable flushing. Dr. Rome hastened to assure us that, according to Dr. Hoffer, flushing usually subsided in about three to four days and was no worse than with small doses. The Canadians had also briefly tried giving niacinamide. Although it caused no flush, it had failed to reduce cholesterol levels. Dr. Rome really had no further details, just these few important facts Dr. Hoffer had shared with him. It was evident that the Canadian originators had not performed a systematic trial to begin developing a useful method of treatment. Their specialties in psychiatry, anatomy, laboratory science were not conducive to a clinical trial. On rounds that morning, I told Dr. Allen that, although it sounded like a strange idea, we could easily test the claim that large doses of niacin could reduce cholesterol. In those days we did not have today's vascular surgery, which can sometimes bypass occluded leg arteries.[4] Therefore, we kept numerous patients in the hospital for weeks while we did everything medically possible to increase circulation, trying to heal ulcers on feet or legs. If our efforts failed and the leg became gangrenous, amputation was usually necessary, frequently above the knee. With so much at stake we often lavished weeks of hospital care, attempting to save a limb. One must remember that hospital charges at that time were reasonable.

Niacin/Cholesterol Trials

We customarily measured cholesterol and other blood lipids as part of our admission workup, even though we had no good method for improving abnormal lipids beyond altering diet. Then, as now, diet was a weak and often ineffective way to reduce elevated cholesterol levels. I told Dr. Allen

that I could recheck lipids on five or six patients with hypercholesterolemia, tell them about the new treatment, and see whether we could verify the Canadian observations. Dr. Allen gave his blessing and promptly forgot about it. I have always been grateful for his approval.

I found five patients on the unit with high cholesterol levels and a vascular status that would keep them hospitalized for several weeks. That afternoon, at the bedside of each patient I recited the fragmentary word-of-mouth report we had received and invited them to take part in a brief trial of a well-known drug, widely regarded as safe, to see whether it really did reduce cholesterol. I described the flush and assured them it would subside in a few days if our informant had been correct.

The patients agreed and began taking tablets (ten 100-mg tablets with each meal), after another baseline blood test. The flush lessened and disappeared in the first week, as predicted. So far so good. After one week I repeated the lipid studies and could not believe the striking reductions in cholesterol, triglycerides, and total lipids. In disbelief, I waited for the second week's results (as good or better) before showing the results to the others on the service. The initial hospital trial continued for four weeks, by which time it was apparent that a longer, carefully planned study was the next step.

The Mayo Clinic has a section just for care of Rochester residents. One of the young consultants in that section was my close friend, Dr. Richard Achor. He and Dr. Kenneth Berge (whom I hadn't met until then because he joined the staff during my two-year absence) had a list of patients with hypercholesterolemia, which they gave me to recruit volunteers. By telephone I obtained 18 participants for at least 12 weeks of study, using niacin in 1,000-mg doses with meals and measuring cholesterol weekly.

Laboratory scientist Dr. Bernard McKenzie brought a unique contribution to the study. His laboratory had been separating cholesterol fractions by a technique known as electrophoresis, giving us a means of determining beta-lipoprotein cholesterol (now LDL cholesterol) and alpha-1-lipoprotein cholesterol (now HDL cholesterol). Preliminary studies had shown that a high ratio of LDL to HDL cholesterol often led to premature heart attacks. We incorporated his testing into our study.

The results were just as impressive as in the preliminary hospital observations. There were marked cholesterol reductions in the first week in many, if not most, participants. Not only that, but the cholesterol fraction was the site of major reduction, accompanied by an increase in the fraction.

My Mayo colleagues encouraged me to report this promising new treatment before leaving Rochester in April 1956 to practice with a Madison, Wisconsin, clinic. The paper I presented at a staff meeting was published in June in the *Proceedings of the Staff Meetings of the Mayo Clinic*,[1] the prestigious journal with worldwide circulation, which has since then has shortened its name to *Mayo Staff Proceedings*.

At the time I realized that I was reporting the first successful cholesterol-lowering drug in history. My enthusiasm was tempered by the knowledge that it would have to be studied in many people for years just to show that it remained effective, that it was safe in prolonged use, and that reducing cholesterol would, as we hoped, reduce atherosclerosis and prevent its disastrous complications.

A Fortuitous Chain of Events

Something I did not even consider at the time was the incredible series of coincidences that led to my first studying niacin's effect. Only later, in the 1970s, increasingly in the 1980s, and reaching a peak in the 1990s, did I fully realize that these circumstances came together like a string of beads to provide their eventual result bringing niacin to the attention of the medical world. If the scenario had developed in a slightly different way, the chain of events would have been broken, altering its conclusion.

A Lecture

To begin with, suppose Dr. Hoffer had not gone to Rochester just then to speak, after he and his colleagues had made some brief, unstructured observations, which showed niacin's promise in cholesterol control. Suppose on his last evening in Rochester he had not sat with Howard Rome. Before becoming a psychiatrist, Rome had been a board-certified internist. He was especially interested in medications because chlorpromazine

(Thorazine), then a new breakthrough drug, had begun to get people out of mental hospitals, introducing a new era of pharmacotherapy in psychiatry. What if Hoffer had dined with one of the analytical psychiatrists instead of Rome? Suppose Dr. Rome had not been on the St. Mary's Hospital service that month. And suppose that, even if he had, the peripheral vascular service section had been headed at that time by any other consultant instead of his duck-hunting buddy, Ed Allen. Would Rome have burst in and shared the news of niacin so readily? Suppose it had not been my quarter as a first assistant on the unit. No one else in the room on that August day, all bright and capable fellows of the Mayo Foundation, decided to confirm the Canadian observations.

But all these events did come together just as though planned, resulting in the Mayo study already described. What ensued in the following years made me more and more certain: it was meant to be!

The Mayo publication was important because it reported to its wide circulation the first systematic study, including the favorable results in the cholesterol fractions. Altschul, Hoffer, and Stephen had earlier published a letter to the editor of the *Archives of Biochemistry and Biophysics*,[2] which might have been overlooked by clinical investigators and never implemented.

I first presented the updated Mayo report at the November 1956 meeting of the American Society for the Study of Arteriosclerosis (ASSA), its first airing at a national meeting. (The ASSA later became the Council on Arteriosclerosis of the American Heart Association.) I first met Dr. Rudolf Altschul at their November 1957 meeting, saw him at any subsequent ASSA meetings he attended, and contributed a chapter to his book[3] on what was then known about niacin, which he was editing when he died in 1963. Of current interest, I recall his talk at the 1957 or 1958 meeting about his rabbit work, in which he showed that niacin strikingly reduced the foam-cell content of atherosclerotic plaques. This is now especially significant in view of the emphasis in recent years on rupture-prone plaques as a cause of sudden arterial occlusion (blockage), even when the narrowing is no more than 50 percent of the arterial diameter.

A Phone Call

I had never met Abram Hoffer when in 1990 we had a momentous telephone conversation that convinced me more than ever about my meant-to-be hypothesis. Something told me that summer to contact him. I learned that he had been in Victoria since 1976. Somehow he knew that I had been with Armour Pharmaceutical Company in Phoenix (1974–1978) after moving from Madison and before starting solo practice in Scottsdale. He had probably seen my address on one of the few papers I had published during those years.

The story of how niacin came to be tested in hypercholesterolemia was stranger than I had expected. In 1952, Hoffer had experienced some bleeding from the gums, for which he had taken vitamin C without benefit. He had already been using niacin for schizophrenic patients and decided to take 3,000 mg daily to see how the flush felt. His gums improved. He reasoned that niacin had promoted rapid healing in gums that had been affected by chronic malocclusion and, with age, had not been healing as well as in earlier years.

Dr. Hoffer's use of niacin in schizophrenia began in 1952, at which time he was using 3,000–6,000 mg per day, as well as niacinamide. He called his work the first double-blind psychiatric study ever performed. In the mid-1950s he lived and practiced in Regina. Dr. Altschul, who had been Hoffer's professor of anatomy in medical school at Saskatoon, had been doing oxidation experiments, exposing rabbits to ultraviolet light and to increased concentrations of oxygen in inspired air to see whether these measures would somehow alter cholesterol deposition in arteries.

On one occasion Professor Altschul sought to arrange a trial in humans for his idea that exposure to ultraviolet light might reduce cholesterol levels. He contacted his former student, Abram Hoffer, who was director of research for the province, and asked for his help in setting up such a study at Saskatchewan Hospital, a 1,600-bed mental hospital in Weyburn. They planned a joint visit to the hospital for this purpose. Dr. Altschul took a train to Regina, and together they drove to Weyburn, 71 miles away.

During the drive they talked about their individual interests. Altschul expressed his opinion that atherosclerotic plaques developed because of injury to the innermost lining of the blood vessels called the intima. He went on to speculate that the intima was not healing fast enough. Hoffer suggested a trial of niacin, based on his personal experience with bleeding gums.

In our telephone conversation, Hoffer told me that, when he made his suggestion, Dr. Altschul didn't know what niacin was! Having received large quantities of niacin and niacinamide for his work, Hoffer gave a pound of niacin powder (450,000 mg) to his former anatomy professor, who then fed it to rabbits whose blood cholesterol had been elevated to very high levels by dietary maneuvers well known to animal researchers. How he knew how much niacin to use is among the bits of information still lacking, but apparently niacin reduced the blood cholesterol levels within days. Hoffer reported that Altschul then phoned him, excitedly shouting, "It works! It works!"

Until that conversation in September 1990, I had never known who Jim Stephen was. Hoffer explained that he was the chief pathologist and laboratory director at the hospital in Regina where Hoffer practiced.

With his permission, in 1954, Hoffer did a two-day study, giving niacin to about 60 patients who demonstrated a reduction in their cholesterol levels. Altschul, Hoffer, and Stephen then wrote their letter (mentioned earlier) to the editor of *Archives of Biochemistry and Biophysics*.[2] Hoffer's story ended where mine had begun. In August 1955, he went to Rochester, invited by the Mayo Foundation to give a series of three lectures on schizophrenia. He confirmed that on his last night in town the section on psychiatry had taken him to dinner, where he happened to sit with Howard Rome. Tired of talking about schizophrenia, he mentioned his niacin experience. Hoffer's incredible series of coincidences merged with mine. Bringing niacin's striking cholesterol-reducing properties to the attention of the medical world was meant to be.

In our phone conversation, I picked up the story and told Hoffer of the chain of events that

374

had brought his information to me and resulted in my decision to do further studies.

A Meeting

In the fall of 1997, a medical association in Victoria to which Dr. Hoffer belongs invited me to speak to them and the public about my work with niacin and my forthcoming book, *Cholesterol Control Without Diet! The Niacin Solution* (1998).[4] This was the pilgrimage I had always envisioned to meet Dr. Hoffer. We used it for a dual purpose, which included beginning the promotion for the book. I finally met Abram Hoffer in person for the first time in the driveway of the Empress Hotel in Victoria, on November 11, 1998, more than 43 years after my first use of niacin for high cholesterol. It was his 80th birthday. Later that evening over dinner we reviewed the circumstances that had brought us together and all that niacin had come to mean to doctors and their patients around the world. We hoped that my book would teach patients the importance of niacin's distinctive advantages not shared by any other cholesterol-control drugs, and also would show doctors how to become proficient at using niacin.

I have always been happy to share with the Canadian originators whatever credit there may be for pioneering the use of niacin for cholesterol control and for its eventual reduction of heart attacks (24 percent), strokes (26 percent), cardiovascular surgery (46 percent), and deaths (11 percent, adding a mean of 1.63 years of life to men, ages 30 to 65, with one or more preceding heart attacks).[5] Without their vision and Hoffer's taking their observations to the Mayo Clinic, I would not have been able to perform the first systematic study and follow it with further research in Madison, leading to the Coronary Drug Project's demonstration of niacin's preventive effects in cardiovascular disease.[6] Dr. Hoffer has correctly said that while pioneers in many fields argue about precedence, we are friends who readily acknowledge each other's roles in starting niacin research. Clearly, it was meant to be.

REFERENCES

1. Parsons WB Jr., Achor RWP, Berge KG, et al. Changes in concentration of blood lipids following prolonged administration of large doses of nicotinic acid to persons with hypercholesterolemia: preliminary observations. *Proc Staff Meet Mayo Clinic* 1956;31:377–390.

2. Altschul R, Hoffer A, Stephen JD. Influence of nicotinic acid on serum cholesterol in man. *Arch Biochem & Biophys* 1955;54:558–559.

3. Altschul R. *Niacin in Vascular Disorders and Hyperlipidemia.* Springfield, IL: Charles C. Thomas, 1964.

4. Parsons WB Jr. *Cholesterol Control Without Diet! The Niacin Solution.* Scottsdale, AZ: Lilac Press,1998.

5. Coronary Drug Project Research Group. Clofibrate and niacin in coronary heart disease. *JAMA* 1975;231:360–381.

6. Canner PL, Berge KG, Wenger NK, et al. for the Coronary Drug Project Research Group. Fifteen-year mortality in Coronary Drug Project patients: long-term benefit with niacin. *J Am Coll Cardiol* 1986;8:1245–1255.

ORTHOMOLECULAR MEDICINE AND HEART HEALTH: UNMASKING THE MAGNESIUM LINK TO MULTIPLE RISK FACTORS FOR CARDIOVASCULAR DISEASE

by Aileen Burford-Mason, PhD

Cardiovascular disease is a major cause of disease and death in industrialized countries, and an increasing concern in developing countries. Independent risk factors frequently coexist in the same individuals, and include high blood pressure, arterial calcification, high cholesterol, and heart rhythm abnormalities. Drug treatments for primary and secondary prevention target each risk factor separately. A growing problem, therefore, is the use of polypharmacy in individuals with cardiovascular disease, and the major challenge this creates for adverse reactions due to drug-drug interactions.[1]

In orthomolecular medicine the focus is different and aims to identify and correct potential nutritional deficiencies that may underlie multiple system dysfunctions. The various roles of vitamin D, omega-3 fats, antioxidants, and the B vitamins in heart health are all currently under investigation. A relationship between magnesium and risk of cardiovascular disease has long been proposed.[2] Variations in cardiovascular disease risk between different countries, and also between different areas of the same country, have been shown roughly to correlate with regional variations in the magnesium content of soil and water.[3] Diets rich in vegetables and fruits, nuts, seeds, and whole grains, currently recommended to reduce the prevalence of cardiovascular disease, are also coincidentally high in magnesium.[4]

Magnesium is a required cofactor for over 300 regulatory enzymes. Virtually all hormonal reactions depend on magnesium. Besides being directly required for specific enzymes, magnesium is indirectly involved in all enzymatic processes, since the energy-transporting molecule adenosine triphosphate (ATP) must be joined with the positive magnesium ion to be metabolically available. Magnesium status affects cholesterol levels, blood pressure, and arterial calcification, and deficiency is a known risk factor for atrial fibrillation (a common arrhythmia). A unifying hypothesis, therefore, as to why high blood pressure, high cholesterol, and other cardiovascular disease risk factors so often occur in the same individual may be inadequate intakes of this critically important mineral.

Magnesium and Cardiovascular Disease

Magnesium acts as a calcium antagonist, competing for calcium absorption and reabsorption in the kidneys,[5] as well as for calcium influx into cells. Because of this function magnesium has been dubbed "nature's physiological calcium channel blocker."[6] At least in animal models, adequate magnesium will prevent and even reduce calcification of arterial tissue and decrease injury to blood vessel walls.[7] Through its association with sodium, potassium, and calcium, magnesium is closely involved in maintaining cellular electrolyte (fluid and mineral) balance and adequate amounts of magnesium are needed to maintain normal levels of potassium.[8] Potassium is important for a regular heart rhythm.

Magnesium plays a pivotal role in the regulation of skeletal, cardiac, and smooth muscle relaxation following contraction.[9] Calcium needs to rise in muscle cells for contraction to occur. However, before relaxation can follow, calcium must be shifted either outside the cell or back into storage sites (sarcoplasmic reticulum) within the cell. This process depends on the availability of magnesium.[10] Inadequate magnesium intake will therefore impede relaxation of smooth and cardiac muscle and increase the risk of atrial fibrillation and high blood pressure, as well as coronary and cerebral vasospasm.[11]

Magnesium deficiency induces endothelial dysfunction in animal models and in cultured endothelial cells. The functional and structural integrity of

From the *J Orthomolecular Med* 2013;28(1):9–16.

the endothelium (the inner linings of the arteries) is critical in preventing atherosclerosis. Correcting magnesium homeostasis, or balance, has therefore been suggested as a useful and inexpensive intervention to prevent and treat endothelial dysfunction, and in turn, atherosclerosis.[12]

Magnesium and Cholesterol Regulation

Magnesium is required for the appropriate regulation of 3-hydroxy-3-methyl-glutaryl-CoA reductase (HMG-CoA reductase), the enzyme that controls cholesterol production, switching HMG-CoA activity on and off as needed. In this respect, magnesium overlaps in function with the widely used statin drugs, which work through inhibiting HMG-CoA.[13] However, continuous inhibition of cholesterol production would limit its availability for cell membrane synthesis and repair, as a precursor for sex and stress hormones, and for vitamin D. Lower circulating testosterone, which protects against cardiovascular disease risk in both men and women[14,15] has been reported in statin users (cholesterol-lowering drugs).[16] On the other hand, supplementing with magnesium has been shown to increase both free and total testosterone.[17]

Magnesium has anti-inflammatory properties, and magnesium deficiency magnifies both immune system and oxidative stress, with a consequent increase in systemic inflammation.[18] Inflammation is an initiating factor that stimulates a cascade of events resulting in endothelial dysfunction, thrombosis, and pro-atherogenic changes in lipoprotein metabolism. One study examined the effect of restricting 14 postmenopausal women to a magnesium intake of 33 percent of the Recommended Dietary Allowance (RDA), a level of intake not uncommon in those consuming Western-style diets. Magnesium restriction over a period of 78 days induced heart arrhythmias, increased serum glucose, urinary excretion of potassium and sodium, altered cholesterol homeostasis, and decreased levels of the antioxidant superoxide dismutase.[19]

Magnesium Deficiency

Magnesium deficiency may be due to the genetic inability to absorb magnesium, inherited renal magnesium wasting, or excretion of excessive amounts of magnesium due to stress or low nutritional intake.[20] Magnesium is maintained within a narrow range by the small intestine and kidneys. In response to high dietary intake of the mineral, kidney excretion increases. When intake falls, the small intestine and kidney both increase their fractional magnesium absorption. If magnesium depletion continues, bone stores help to maintain magnesium by exchanging part of their content with extracellular fluid.[21] Ongoing magnesium status therefore depends on the health of both organs: magnesium deficiency is a known complication of inflammatory bowel disease,[22] while serious kidney disease may result in hypermagnesemia (high concentrations of magnesium in the blood).[23]

In many Western nations dietary intake of magnesium is suboptimal. In Canada, for example, the estimated daily intake of magnesium in those consuming an average diet is between 200 and 300 milligrams (mg) daily,[24] whereas the RDA, which varies depending on age and sex, is 320 mg for females over 30 years of age, 400 mg in pregnancy and 360 mg during lactation, and for men over 30 is 420 mg. However, it has been suggested that the RDA underestimates daily needs and that 500 to 750 mg per day is more realistic.[25] In the United States, the 1999–2000 National Health and Nutrition Examination Survey found 79 percent of adults had magnesium intakes below the RDA.[26]

IN BRIEF

Magnesium deficiency has a major impact on the development and progression of cardiovascular disease. Magnesium deficits are induced by Western-style diets and genetic differences in magnesium needs, as well as the continuous depletion of magnesium by chronic stress and many commonly used drugs. This article outlines our current understanding of magnesium physiology and its effect on heart health, including its requirement for blood pressure and cholesterol control, and prevention of arrhythmias and tissue calcification.

Apart from chocolate, foods richest in magnesium are not prominent in the highly processed foods that most Westerners live on. (Foods relatively rich in magnesium include halibut and shrimp; whole-grain breads and oats; beans and legumes; leafy vegetables; seeds, and nuts.) Interestingly, consumption of dark chocolate has several beneficial effects on heart health, including a reduction in blood pressure, improvement of vascular function and glucose metabolism, and reduction of platelet aggregation (the first step in forming a clot), and adhesion.[27] Researchers usually assume that the benefits of chocolate are due solely to its antioxidant properties, and its contribution to enhancing magnesium intake is rarely considered.

Apart from diet, several medical conditions may influence magnesium status. Chronic diarrhea and vomiting results in magnesium deficiency,[28] and excessive urination (polyuria) associated with poorly controlled diabetes depletes magnesium stores.[29] Because of increased demand for magnesium by skeletal muscle under sustained exertion, intense or prolonged exercise will negatively affect magnesium status.[30] Excess alcohol intake[31] and commonly prescribed drugs, including many targeted at heart disease, like loop diuretics, such as furosemide (Lasix), and thiazide diuretics (water pills), deplete magnesium.

A drug safety announcement from the Food and Drug Administration (FDA) warned of magnesium depletion by proton pump inhibitors such as omeprazole (Prilosec), lansoprazole (Prevacid), and esomeprazole (Nexium). These commonly prescribed drugs are used to treat gastroesophageal reflux disease (heartburn). The alert listed warning signs of magnesium depletion, including leg cramps, muscle twitching and weakness, tremors, tetany, seizures, atrial fibrillation, and supraventricular tachycardia.[32] The FDA further stressed that this magnesium depletion might be exacerbated in those taking other drugs known to deplete magnesium, such as digoxin (Lanoxin) and diuretics, both commonly used in cardiovascular disease patients.

Calcium/Magnesium Balance, Stress, and Calcium Supplements

The shortfall between actual and recommended magnesium intake is further complicated by the widespread depletion of magnesium by stress.[33] Effect or hormones of the hypothalamic-pituitary-adrenal axis trigger a fall in intracellular magnesium levels, which results in an influx of calcium into neurons causing hyperexcitability. This, in turn, produces hypertonicity (tightness) in all types of muscle. Cardiac muscle and vascular smooth muscle are particularly reactive, since they must respond rapidly to sudden acute stress.[34] This reaction is a necessary preparation for the "fight or flight" response and under normal physiological conditions cells will return to their relaxed state once the emergency is past. However, under conditions of chronic stress, deficiency of magnesium relative to calcium will result in sustained contraction of skeletal, cardiac, and vascular smooth muscle.[35]

A dramatic shift in calcium to magnesium balance can be seen in modern diets. Unlike our hunter-gatherer forebears, modern diets are low in magnesium and, because of the ready availability and consumption of dairy products, are much higher in calcium. The combination of modern dietary changes, common use of magnesium-depleting drugs, high levels of stress in urban lifestyles, and increased intakes of calcium supplements to prevent osteoporosis would favor an elevation of intracellular calcium and a deficit of magnesium, thus increasing the threshold for skeletal, cardiac, and vascular smooth muscle contractility. In large cohort studies, consuming calcium supplements without reference to magnesium intakes has been

GOOD FOOD SOURCES OF MAGNESIUM

Pumpkin seeds: ½ cup supplies 350 mg

Chocolate (baking): 3.5 ounces supplies 295 mg

Mixed nuts: ½ cup supplies 150 mg

Black beans: 1 cup supplies 120 mg

Halibut: 3 ounces supplies 70 mg

shown to be associated with increased risks of heart disease in both men and women.[36,37]

Both simple magnesium deficiency and changes in the calcium/magnesium balance may therefore increase vulnerability to cardiovascular disease.

Testing and Functional Biomarkers of Magnesium Deficiency

Laboratory assessment of magnesium status is notoriously difficult.[38] Magnesium is not a static ion but moves between compartments and across membranes. A drop in serum magnesium is quickly normalized from bone or intracellular stores. Nor is magnesium fixed in red blood cells, which means that measuring magnesium by conventional standards (e.g, in the serum, plasma, or red blood cells) cannot reliably indicate an individual's magnesium status.

An alternative approach that requires no laboratory tests uses functional evidence of calcium/magnesium imbalance as a biomarker of magnesium status. Theoretically, inadequate tissue stores of magnesium should manifest as malfunctions of skeletal muscle, such as leg cramps or spasms (charley horse), muscle twitching, restless leg syndrome, and tight muscles. Imbalances will also be obvious in smooth muscle, resulting in physical signs of dysregulated lung function such as shortness of breath, wheezing or asthma, and perhaps frequent sighing.

The tone of the bladder is dependent on the calcium to magnesium balance and hyperactive bladders, especially at night when magnesium needs are highest, frequently respond well to magnesium supplementation. Magnesium's role in relaxing gastrointestinal smooth muscle has long been exploited in the treatment of functional constipation, especially in children.[39] Although there are a myriad of functional symptoms of magnesium deficiency, this simple questionnaire can be used to quickly identify a magnesium shortfall.

1. Do you get leg or foot cramps?

2. Are your shoulders frequently tight or tense at the end of the day?

3. Does your back ever go into spasm?

4. Do you ever experience muscle twitching, especially around the eye?

5. Do you suffer from wheezing or asthma, especially after exercise?

6. Do you experience any shortness of breath, for example, climbing stairs?

7. Do you sigh frequently?

8. Do you ever get palpitations or suffer from an irregular heartbeat?

9. Do you need to urinate frequently, especially at night?

10. Are you ever constipated?

Note: It is unlikely to suffer from all of these symptoms. However, all the symptoms that are present should resolve after appropriate magnesium supplementation.

Magnesium Supplementation

Except in the case of overt kidney failure where magnesium supplements are contraindicated, the most effective way to improve magnesium status is with oral supplementation. A standard dose of 5 mg per kilogram of body weight per day has been proposed.[40] However, individual needs for magnesium are hard to predict and vary from time to time even in the same individual, depending on stress levels, diet, and concurrent medications. A standard dose may therefore not achieve optimal outcomes in all individuals.

A tried-and-tested method for optimizing magnesium intake is to increase your intake to bowel tolerance, thus creating a positive magnesium balance. As noted above, a shortfall in magnesium will inhibit normal gastrointestinal peristalsis and result in sluggish bowel function. When increasing magnesium, it is important that the potential cathartic action does not overwhelm gastrointestinal capacity to absorb magnesium. A very gradual increase in magnesium (every three to four days), in small incremental doses (of approximately 50 mg of elemental magnesium) to generate one to two soft bowel movements daily achieves the best outcomes, as evidenced by the gradual disappearance of symptoms listed in the questionnaire above. Coincidentally, the central nervous system symptoms associated with magnesium deficits such as anxiety, fatigue, headaches, insomnia, and hyper-emotionality should also be somewhat relieved. Benefits may include improved mood, sleep, and energy levels.

The form of magnesium you use is very important. A large number of magnesium preparations are available. One of the best is magnesium citrate. Magnesium oxide has the highest concentration of elemental magnesium by weight but compared with the citrate salts of magnesium is not well absorbed.[41] Because of the impact of day-to-day stress and the continuous drain on magnesium stores by certain medications, dividing the dose between morning and evening achieves the best outcomes.

■ CONCLUSION

Magnesium deficits are induced by modern diets and several chronic health conditions and are difficult to detect using standard laboratory testing. And because of the mineral's continuous depletion by chronic stress and many commonly used medications, magnesium deficits are not simple to rectify. Poor magnesium status has profound implications for health in general but it has particular relevance to cardiovascular disease since it influences the manifestation of all the major risk factors. As knowledge of widespread magnesium undernutrition emerges and the considerable variations in magnesium needs across populations becomes clear, the need for magnesium replacement therapy in the prevention and treatment of cardiovascular disease should be a priority.

At a population level encouraging consumption of a diet that is unprocessed and in which approximately two-thirds of the energy is obtained from plant foods and one-third from animal products has been suggested for improving heart health.[42] This is similar in composition to the Dietary Approaches to Stop Hypertension (DASH) diet, which is high in fruits, vegetables, whole grains, and low-fat dairy products, and has been proven to lower blood pressure and cholesterol, and risk of heart failure and stroke. Assuming an energy intake of 2,100 calories, such a diet would contain approximately 1,100 mg of calcium and 800 mg of magnesium.[42]

While dietary reforms could increase magnesium intake and shift the calcium to magnesium balance to being more favorable upon heart health, individual variations in magnesium needs due to stress, individual genetics, or the concurrent use of magnesium-depleting drugs require a more rigorous approach.

The method of magnesium repletion described in this paper is one approach to customizing magnesium supplementation and is in line with our understanding of biochemical individuality, a concept enshrined within the principles of orthomolecular medicine.

REFERENCES

1. Fleg JL, Aronow WS, Frishman WH. Cardiovascular drug therapy in the elderly: benefits and challenges. *Nat Rev Cardiol* 2011;8:13–28.

2. Burch GE, Giles TD. The importance of magnesium deficiency in cardiovascular disease. *Am Heart* J 1977;94:649–657.

3. Karppanen H. Ischaemic heart disease: an epidemiological perspective with special reference to electrolytes. *Drugs* 1984;28(Suppl 1):17–27.

4. Hu FB, Willett WC. Optimal diets for prevention of coronary heart disease. *JAMA* 2002; 288:2569–2578.

5. Wei M, Esbaei K, Bargman J, et al. Relationship between serum magnesium, parathyroid hormone, and vascular calcification in patients on dialysis: a literature review. *Perit Dial Int* 2006;26:366–373.

6. Iseri LT, French JH. Magnesium: Nature's physiological calcium channel blocker. *Am Heart J* 1984;108:188–193.

7. LaRusso J, Li Q, Jiang Q, et al. Elevated dietary magnesium prevents connective tissue mineralization in a mouse model of pseudoxanthoma elasticum (Abcc6(-/-). *J Invest Dermatol* 2009;129:1388–1394.

8. Gums JG. Magnesium in cardiovascular and other disorders. *Am J Health Syst Pharm* 2004;61:1569–1576.

9. Ueshima K. Magnesium and ischemic heart disease: a review of epidemiological, experimental, and clinical evidence. *Magnes Res* 2005;18:275–284.

10. D'Angelo EK, Singer HA, Rembold CML. Magnesium relaxes arterial smooth muscle by decreasing intracellular Ca2+ without changing intracellular Mg2+. *J Clin Invest* 1992;89:1988–1994.

11. Iannello S, Belfiore F. Hypomagnesemia: a review of pathophysiological, clinical, and therapeutical aspects. *Panminerva Med* 2001;43:177–209.

12. Maier JA. Endothelial cells and magnesium: implications in atherosclerosis. *Clin Sci* (Lond), 2012;122:397–407.

13. Rosanoff A, Seelig MS. Comparison of mechanism and functional effects of magnesium and statin pharmaceuticals. *J Am Coll Nutr* 2004;23:501S–505S.

14. Saad F. Androgen therapy in men with testosterone deficiency: can testosterone reduce the risk of cardiovascular disease? *Diabetes Metab Res Rev* 2012; 28(Suppl 2):52–59.

15. Barrett-Connor E. Menopause, atherosclerosis, and coronary artery disease. *Curr Opin Pharmacol* 2013;12(2):186–191.

16. La Vignera S, Condorelli RA, Vicari E, et al. Statins and erectile dysfunction: a critical summary of current evidence. *J Androl* 2012;33:552–558.

17. Cinar V, Polat Y, Baltaci AK, et al. Effects of magnesium supplementation on testosterone levels of athletes and sedentary subjects at rest and after exhaustion. *Biol Trace Elem Res* 2011; 140:18–23.

18. Mazur A, Maier JA, Rock E, et al. Magnesium and the inflammatory response: potential physiopathological implications. *Arch Biochem Biophys* 2007;458:48–56.

19. Nielsen FH, Milne DB, Klevay LM, et al. Dietary magnesium deficiency induces heart rhythm changes, impairs glucose tolerance, and decreases serum cholesterol in post-menopausal women. *J Am Coll Nutr* 2007;26:121–132.

20. Mauskop A, Varughese J. Why all migraine patients should be treated with magnesium. *J Neural Transm* 2012;119:575–579.

21. Rude RK. Magnesium deficiency: a cause of heterogeneous disease in humans. *J Bone Miner Res* 1998;13:749–758.

22. Galland L. Magnesium and inflammatory bowel disease. *Magnesium* 1988;7:78–83.

23. Cunningham J, Rodríguez M, Messa P. Magnesium in chronic kidney disease stages 3 and 4 and in dialysis patients. *Clin Kidney J* 2012;5(Suppl 1):i39–i51.

24. Health Canada. Environmental and Workplace Health. Guidelines for Canadian Drinking Water Quality: Supporting Documents on Magnesium. Retrieved from: www.hcsc.gc.ca/ewh-semt/pubs/water-eau/magnesium/index-eng.php.

25. Littlefield NA, Haas BS. Is the RDA for magnesium too low? *FDA Science Forum* 1996; Abstract # C-13.

26. Ervin RB, Wang CY, Wright JD, et al. Dietary intake of selected minerals for the United States population:1999–2000. *Adv Data* 2004;341:1–5.

27. Sudano I, Flammer AJ, Roas S, et al. Cocoa, blood pressure, and vascular function. *Curr Hypertens Rep* 2012;14:279–284.

28. Rude RK. Magnesium deficiency: A cause of heterogeneous disease in humans. *J Bone Miner Res* 1998;13:749–758.

29. Rosanoff A, Weaver CM, Rude RK. Suboptimal magnesium status in the United States: are the health consequences underestimated? *Nutr Rev* 2012;70:153–164.

30. Buchman AL, Keen C, Commisso J, et al. The effect of a marathon run on plasma and urine mineral and metal concentrations. *J Am Coll Nutr* 1998;17:124–127.

31. Abbott L, Nadler J, Rude RK. Magnesium deficiency in alcoholism: possible contribution to osteoporosis and cardiovascular disease in alcoholics. *Alcohol Clin Exp Res* 1994;18: 1076–1082.

32. U.S. Food and Drug Administration. FDA Drug Safety Communication: low magnesium levels can be associated with long-term use of proton pump inhibitor drugs (PPIs). Retrieved from: www.fda.gov/drugs/drugsafety/ucm245011.htm.

33. Classen HG. Stress and magnesium. *Artery* 1981;9:182–189.

34. Weber KT, Bhattacharya SK, Newman KP, et al. Stressor states and the cation crossroads. *J Am Coll Nutr* 2010;29: 563–574.

35. Seelig MS. Consequences of magnesium deficiency on the enhancement of stress reactions; preventative and therapeutic implications. *J Am Coll Nutr* 1994;13:1429–1446.

36. Xiao Q, Murphy RA, Houston DK, et al. Dietary and supplemental calcium intake and cardiovascular disease mortality: The National Institutes of Health–AARP Diet and Health Study. *JAMA* 2013;173:1–8.

37. Bolland MJ, Grey A, Avenell A, et al. Calcium supplements with or without vitamin D and risk of cardiovascular events: reanalysis of the Women's Health Initiative limited access dataset and metaanalysis. *BMJ* 2011; 342:d2040.

38. Dewitte K, Stockl D, Van de Velde M, et al. Evaluation of intrinsic and routine quality of serum total magnesium measurement. *Clin Chim Acta* 2000;292:55–68.

39. Tatsuki M, Miyazawa R, Tomomasa T, et al. Serum magnesium concentration in children with functional constipation treated with magnesium oxide. *World J Gastroenterol* 2011;17:779–783.

40. Durlach J, Durlach V, Bac P, et al. Magnesium and therapeutics. *Mag Res* 1994;7:313–328.

41. Lindberg JS, Zobitz MM, Poindexter JR, et al. Magnesium bioavailability from magnesium citrate and magnesium oxide. *J Am Coll Nutr* 1990;9:48–55.

42. Karppanen H, Karppanen P, Mervaala E. Why and how to implement sodium, potassium, calcium and magnesium changes in food items and diet. *J Hum Hypertens* 2005;19(Suppl 3):S10–19.

VITAMIN E AND CARDIOVASCULAR DISEASES

Evidence supporting vitamin E's efficacy in preventing and reversing heart disease is strong. Two landmark studies published in the *New England Journal of Medicine*[1,2] followed a total of 125,000 men and women health care professionals for a total of 839,000-person study years. It was found that those who supplement with at least 100 IU of vitamin E daily reduced their risk of heart disease by 59–66 percent. The studies were adjusted for lifestyle differences (smoking, physical activity, dietary fiber intake, aspirin use) in order to determine the heart effect of vitamin E supplementation alone. Because a diet high in foods containing vitamin E as compared to the average diet further showed only a slight heart-protective effect, the authors emphasized the necessity of vitamin E supplementation.

The Power of E

Researchers at Cambridge University[3] in England reported that patients who had been diagnosed with coronary arteriosclerosis could lower their risk of having a heart attack by 77 percent by supplementing with 400 IU to 800 IU per day of the natural (d-alpha tocopherol) form of vitamin E.

Pioneer vitamin E researchers and clinicians Drs. Wilfrid and Evan Shute treated some 30,000 patients over several decades and found that people in average health received maximum benefit from 800 IU of the d-alpha tocopherol form of vitamin E. Vitamin E has been proven effective in the prevention and treatment of many heart conditions. "The complete or nearly complete prevention of angina attacks is the usual and expected result of treatment with alpha tocopherol" according to Wilfrid Shute, MD, a cardiologist. Shute prescribed up to 1,600 IU of vitamin E daily and successfully treated patients for acute coronary thrombosis, acute rheumatic fever, chronic rheumatic heart disease, hypertensive heart disease, diabetes mellitus, acute and chronic nephritis, and even burns, plastic surgery, and mazoplasia (degeneration of breast tissue). The reason one nutrient can cure so many different illnesses is because a deficiency of one nutrient can cause many different illnesses.

What Else This Vitamin Can Do

Vitamin E is a powerful antioxidant in the body's lipid (fat) phase. It can prevent LDL lipid peroxidation caused by free radical reactions. Its ability to protect cell membranes from oxidation is of crucial importance in preventing and reversing many degenerative diseases.

In addition, vitamin E inhibits blood clotting (platelet aggregation and adhesion) and prevents plaque enlargement and rupture. Finally, it has anti-inflammatory properties, which may also prove to be very important in the prevention of heart disease.

Among other things, vitamin E supplementation:

* Reduces the oxygen requirement of tissues;[4]
* Gradually melts fresh clots and prevents embolism;[5]
* Improves collateral circulation;[6]
* Prevents scar contraction as wounds heal;[5,7]
* Decreases the insulin requirement in about one-fourth of diabetics;[8]
* Stimulates muscle power;[9]
* Preserves capillary walls;[10]
* Reduces C-reactive protein and other markers of inflammation.[11]

Epidemiological evidence also suggests that a daily supplement of vitamin E can reduce the risk of developing prostate cancer and Alzheimer's disease.[12,13] If all Americans daily supplemented with a good multivitamin/multimineral plus extra vitamins C and E, it could save thousands of lives a month.

REFERENCES

1. Stampfer MJ. *N Engl J Med* 1993;328:1444–1449.

2. Rimm EB. *N Engl J Med* 1993;328:1450–1456.

3. Stephens NG. *Lancet* 1996;347:781–786.

4. Hove. *Arch Biochem* 1945;8:395.

5. Shute E. *Surg Gyn and Obst* 1948;86:1.

6. Enria F. *Arch per la Scienze Med* 1951;91:23.

7. Shute, et al. *Surg Gyn and Obst* 1948;86:1.

8. Butturini. *Gior di Clin Med* 1950;31:1.

9. Percival. *Summary* 1951;3:55.

10. Ames, Baxter, Griffith. *International Review of Vitamin Research* 1951;22:401.

11. Ridker PM. *N Engl J Med* 2000;342:836–843.

12. Ni J. *Biochem Biophys Res Commun* 2003;300(2):357–363.

13. Morris MC. *JAMA* 287(24):3230–3237.

Excerpted from the *Orthomolecular Medicine News Service*, March 23, 2005.

TREATMENT OF HYPERTENSION FROM AN ORTHOMOLECULAR MEDICINE STANDPOINT

by George D. O'Clock, PhD

High blood pressure (hypertension) is the most prevalent cardiovascular disease. Approximately 30 million Americans have been diagnosed with hypertension[1] and over 58 million Americans appear to be affected.[2] Within certain segments of the medical profession, blood pressure thresholds and definitions for hypertension vary. Often, a blood pressure reading between 140 and 160 systolic (upper number) and/or between 90 and 95 diastolic (lower number) is used as a "borderline" to identify the transition from an acceptable blood pressure level into the realms of hypertension.[3] Absolute hypertension occurs, once the 160/95 millimeters of mercury (mmHg) limits have been exceeded.[2]

The majority of people with hypertension have essential hypertension. In their case, the high blood pressure condition does not have an obvious cause.[3,4] Cardiac rate and cardiac output increase in some individuals with hypertension, but not all. However, an increase in total vascular peripheral resistance (pressure against the walls of the blood vessels) is a common characteristic of hypertension.

Experimental Procedure

Systolic/diastolic blood pressure and pulse rate were obtained for a number of individuals over a three-year period. One of the individuals was a 58-year-old male diagnosed with essential hypertension. Initially, his average systolic/diastolic blood pressure was approximately 176/104 mmHg with episodes exceeding 210/118 mmHg during periods of stress. Peak-to-peak systolic/diastolic blood pressure variations throughout the day of 60/18 mmHg were fairly common. An echocardiogram revealed hypertrophy (thickening) of the left ventricle. Records indicate that this person had an untreated high blood pressure problem for almost 16 years.

After recording blood pressure data for nine months, this individual accepted medication for his condition. Initially, this involved his taking a 5-milligram (mg) dose per day of the angiotensin-converting-enzyme (ACE) inhibitor enalapril (Vasotec). After taking the Vasotec prescription for eight days, his average blood pressure dropped to approximately 152/90 mmHg with peak-to-peak variations decreasing to 30/10 mmHg. Although further intervention was discussed, the hypertense individual would not accept an increase in ACE-inhibitor dosage and would not accept any other form of medication (such as beta blockers, calcium channel blockers, or diuretics). He preferred to try other means of blood pressure reduction through diet, stress control, exercise, and nutritional supplementation. There is some controversy concerning blood pressure variability and the impact of various kinds of activities and stress on blood pressure data. Part of this three-year study involved recording blood pressure variations that can occur with stress (family and work-related), diet, exercise, leisure-time activities, relaxation, and sexual activity for an individual who has hypertension.

From an orthomolecular medicine standpoint, the effect of various nutritional supplements (vitamins, minerals, soy products, herbs, etc.) on blood pressure and blood pressure variations is of significant interest. One very interesting feature concerning the various methods that lower blood pressure involves their combined (cumulative) effect. Information on the ability of the various methods to lower blood pressure in a coherent additive manner, or a noncoherent additive manner, is very important from a treatment expectations standpoint.

Mechanisms of Hypertension

One issue that must be addressed involves the mechanisms that might be associated with essential hypertension. As stated earlier, this condition may have a variety of causes.[4] However, conventional physiological and biochemical models have not been able to provide enough information to

From the *J Orthomolecular Med* 1998;13(2):74–84.

clearly define a cause for this disease. Blood pressure problems are often attributed to some form of malfunction in the renal (kidney) system. In some cases, aberrations in kidney function can produce inappropriate levels of renin secretion, higher levels of angiotensin II production, and increased aldosterone secretion—three hormones that influence blood vessel contraction, water balance, and all aspects of blood pressure. Essential hypertension is often responsive to treatment with ACE inhibitors. If this is the case one might ask: "Are there other medical paradigms that might be considered so that an 'obvious cause,' associated with the renal system, can be provided for some cases of essential hypertension?"

A possible link to one of the mechanisms of essential hypertension could be associated with Dr. Björn Nordenström's theory of biologically closed electric circuits (BCECs) and his description of vascular-interstitial closed electric circuits (VICCs).[5,6] Charge transport can occur over VICC pathways because blood vessels can function as relatively insulated cables providing a pathway for tissue fluids and moving charges to reach the capillaries.[7] After years of careful experimentation and analysis, Dr. Nordenström developed a theory involving continuous energy circulation and a corresponding electric/magnetic/electromagnetic field circulation in living systems. Field circulation is accompanied by the co-transport of charged molecules (ions and electrons) forming continuous electric currents in the human body. These currents are maintained within various BCEC pathways in the body involving blood, interstitial (extracellular) fluid, blood vessels, tissue, organs, and neuromuscular units. Nordenström realized that by augmenting various healing processes normally associated with BCEC systems in the human body, electrotherapeutic techniques could be developed to treat a variety of diseases including cardiovascular disease, cancer, and neuromuscular disorders. Nordenström essentially "closed the loop" with respect to electrical activity in living systems. He described a closed system of adaptive electrical circulatory systems that maintain and regulate various functions and promote healing processes.[8]

In the booklet *Hypertension Report*,[9] Dr. Julian Whitaker makes a statement, regarding the treatment of high blood pressure with diuretics, that blends quite well with Nordenström's BCEC theory. He writes, "Water alone is the best diuretic, so for goodness sake, do your best to increase daily water consumption. This approach increases urine production and replaces the need for medication. Water allows the body to function at maximum efficiency and supports the hydroelectric mineral salts that convey electrical currents throughout the body."

From the standpoint of "convey[ing] electrical currents throughout the body," Nordenström has measured endogenous electrical potential differences and electric currents between tissues and vascular components of the stomach, vena cava (arteries leading to the heart), aorta (arteries leading from the heart) and left/right ureters (passageways connecting the kidney and the bladder) of an anesthetized pig.[7] Current flow between organs and veins was observed for potential differences.

Nordenström's results indicate that VICC systems can respond to very small changes in energy state and they can be activated at very low electric potentials. Therefore, in the absence of any physical damage or biochemical aberrations, a hydroelectric imbalance in the renal system could activate a number of mechanisms that promote high blood pressure. For instance, changes in electric potential can produce electric field variations that can have an effect on the porosity of capillaries, the pH (alkalinity/acidity) of various body fluids, the movement of electrolytes (minerals that conduct electricity), and immune response.[5] Capillary porosity and electrolyte movement can be affected by changes in localized electric fields. Therefore, the filtration process provided by the glomerular capillaries of the kidney, along with mechanisms associated with various renal clearance rates, could be affected by the variations in potentials that occur between organs and various components of the renal system. In this case, BCEC theory and the VICC model could be the basis of a new medical paradigm that will help to explain some of the causes and mechanisms associated with essential hypertension.

Results: Blood Pressure and Pulse-Rate Characteristics

The blood pressure and pulse rate data for this 58-year-old male with hypertension was compared with data obtained for a 48-year-old female who was in good health, and a 17-year-old high school student who was in very good shape (actively engaged in swimming and bicycling). The systolic and diastolic blood pressures vs. pulse rate data for these individuals was plotted graphically to detect any irregularities in their cardiovascular characteristics and to identify significant differences in the slopes of the individual blood pressure vs. pulse-rate characteristics.

The higher systolic blood pressure levels found for the hypertense individual are most likely due to variations in cardiac output. The lower pressure levels of the hypertense individual's blood pressure characteristics would tend to indicate that it is more difficult to promote increases in cardiac output as average blood pressure increases. In this case, the arterial capacitance (flexibility of the vein) decreases at the higher blood pressure levels because of limitations on volume increases and elasticity with increased blood pressure. The sharp increase could be indicative of an abnormality associated with increase in arterial impedance. The arterial impedance increase at the higher blood pressure levels could be due to the combination of a reduction in arterial capacitance and an increase in resistance due to stress and turbulent blood flow. Certain forms of turbulence can be produced by large surges of ejected blood from the hypertensive individual's enlarged left ventricle. In addition, this nonlinear characteristic indicates that for larger and larger increments of heart rate, the incremental change in systolic blood pressure tends to decrease. This could be indicative of the arterial capacitance variations that promote orthostatic intolerance conditions sometimes associated with reno-vascular hypertension and essential hypertension.[10]

Increases in cardiac output generally raise the systolic blood pressure more than the diastolic.[3] For situations where the hypertense individual's blood pressure is increasing, the higher systolic blood pressures could be indicative of a higher peripheral resistance along with a higher cardiac output (cardiac rate). This resistance increase could be due to a number of interactive mechanisms including the effects of turbulent blood flow.

Blood Pressure Reduction: Initial Therapeutic Approach

Blood pressure data for this person was recorded daily for three years. Very pronounced cyclical variations were measured on a daily, weekly, and monthly basis, and a six-month cycle was also noticeable. The average (baseline) blood pressure for the hypertensive individual was approximately 170/103 mmHg, with very large blood pressure peak variations. After a full meal, this individual could suffer incremental blood pressure increases up to 45/20 mmHg. In addition, incidences of family- and work-related stress caused incremental blood pressure increases up to 40/15 mmHg. At times, blood pressure readings of 210/118 mmHg were observed at home, work, and at the doctor's office. During periods of reduced work, summer vacations, and work breaks, a consistent decrease in incremental blood pressure was recorded. From this data, it appears that the work environment contributes approximately 15/9 mmHg to this individual's hypertension problem. However, from the baseline data, it would appear that the work environment is not the primary cause of this person's high blood pressure problems.

As a first therapeutic step, this hypertensive agreed to increase his blood pressure medication, gradually progressing from 5 mg of Vasotec per day to 25 mg per day of lisinopril (Zestril), another ACE inhibitor. His average blood pressure had decreased to 150/90 mmHg on the Vasotec, with significantly lower blood pressure variations. Initially, some adverse effects were noted (diarrhea and fatigue), and these symptoms subsided after a week on the medication. Increasing the prescription by 50 percent produced an additional reduction in systolic blood pressure of approximately 7 mmHg. However, the increased intake of the drug caused a significant increase in fatigue along with coordination problems, dizzy spells, and depression. At this point, it was clear that the primary approach toward blood pressure control could have its share of health hazards if it was based on drug therapy alone.

Blood Pressure Reduction: From an Orthomolecular Approach

The initial approach toward blood pressure control involved diet. A lower intake of fat and refined sugar produced an incremental decrease of 15/6 mmHg in blood pressure over a period of three weeks. However, blood pressure variations remained high.

One of the simplest and most effective therapeutic approaches involved the combination of a significantly higher water intake and supplementation with lecithin (3,600 mg/day) and L-carnitine (500 mg/day). Increasing water intake can help to promote a better hydroelectric and sodium-potassium balance in the renal system. Lecithin (phosphatidylcholine) will promote the synthesis of acetylcholine, a neurotransmitter that tends to reduce blood pressure. L-carnitine is

"Niacin is not liver toxic. Niacin therapy increases liver function tests. But this elevation means that the liver is active. It does not indicate an underlying liver pathology. Dr. Bill Parsons discussed this extremely well in his book on niacin, Cholesterol Control Without Diet. *I personally have been on 1,500–6,000 milligrams daily since 1955. The biggest danger of taking niacin is that you live longer. One of my patients is 112. She does cross-country skiing and has been on niacin for 42 years. The fear doctors have of niacin is not based on data or facts and, like any myth, is very hard to eradicate."*

—ABRAM HOFFER

important in the oxidation of fatty acids and is sometimes described as an oral chelating agent. The combination of these three substances promoted an incremental blood pressure reduction of 16/8 mmHg over a period of 12 days. One of the interesting characteristics associated with this approach involves a three-day lag before any noticeable response is observed. The hypertense individual also noticed that the nocturnal reduction in his systolic and diastolic blood pressure began to return. Prior to this, his blood pressure was often higher in the morning than it was the evening before. In addition, previous to this, his systolic blood pressure incremental increases were often quite high ($\geq$45 mmHg) after eating a full meal. After the water/lecithin/L-carnitine combination was implemented, incremental increases in systolic blood pressure were significantly lower ($\leq$25 mmHg) after eating a full meal.

In many cases, exercise and weight lifting (in moderation) are recommended for blood pressure control. This particular hypertense individual tried a number of exercise programs and found them to be beneficial in a number of areas (including an increase in energy and a greater ability to sleep), but very little reduction in blood pressure was observed with exercise. In fact, often, when he was exercising the most, these were the time periods when his average blood pressure readings were at their higher levels.

A variety of supplements were taken in order to promote cardiovascular conditioning and reduce blood pressure. These supplements included beta-carotene (20,000 IU/day), calcium/magnesium (600/300 mg/day), vitamin-B complex, niacin (300 mg/day), flaxseed oil (500 mg/day), coenzyme Q10 (60 mg/day), zinc picolinate (30 mg/day), gingko biloba (100 mg/day), bilberry extract (250 mg/day), horse chestnut extract (400 mg/day), and potassium (100 mg/day). The most pronounced effect observed with this combination was a 10 mmHg reduction in diastolic blood pressure (indicating a reduction in total peripheral resistance). There was no significant reduction in systolic blood pressure (indicating a minimal effect on cardiac rate or blood volume). Also, no additional decrease in diastolic blood pressure was observed for this individual when these supplements were increased.

Another factor in blood pressure control involves the reduction of cholesterol and triglycerides. A number of nutritional supplements were taken each day by the individual with hypertension in an attempt to reduce his total cholesterol level (223 mg per deciliter [dL]) and triglyceride level (208 mg/dL). The list of supplements included cayenne pepper (40,000 heat units/day), omega-3 fish oil (500 mg/day), vitamin C (1,000 mg/day), L-carnitine (500 mg/day), pycnogenol (100 mg/day), vitamin E (800 IU/day), L-lysine (500 mg/day), garlic (400 mg/day), selenium (200 micrograms [mcg]/day), inositol (150 mg/day), licorice root, and L-arginine (100 mg/day). Within a year, his cholesterol level decreased to 177 mg/dL and his triglyceride level decreased to 131 mg/dL. The cholesterol and triglyceride reduction did not seem to produce significant reductions in average blood pressure levels. However, some reduction in day-to-day incremental blood pressure variations was observed over that time.

In the analysis of the various items that increase and decrease blood pressure, the three-year study strongly indicates that one must be very careful not to use coherent addition in the analytical approach. For instance, assume a certain supplemental herb, by itself, reduces systolic blood pressure by 10 mmHg. Assume another nutritional supplement, by itself, also reduces systolic blood pressure by 10 mmHg. When the two supplements are combined, the total reduction in systolic blood pressure will not be 20 mmHg. In this case, the process of non-coherent addition is more applicable. When the two supplements are combined, the total reduction in systolic blood pressure will be closer to 14 mmHg. Combining substances that reduce blood pressure does produce a cumulative effect. However, under the constraints of non-coherent addition, the substances that have the smaller effects do not accumulate as efficiently as one would expect when they are combined with substances that produce more pronounced reductions in blood pressure.

CONCLUSION

Blood pressure reduction for individuals with hypertension is strategically important, not only for cardiovascular health, but also from the standpoint of minimizing kidney damage. However, blood pressure medications appear to have their own complications and dangers. Certain diuretics can deplete potassium and magnesium levels and increase cholesterol and triglyceride levels. They can cause digestive stress, muscle spasms, problems with kidney dysfunction, and anemia along with increasing the risk of heart attack and cardiac arrhythmias.[11,12] Beta blockers can promote impotence, fatigue, depression, and congestive heart failure in susceptible patients.[11,13] Calcium channel blockers can weaken the heart and damage the liver.[11,13] Adverse consequences associated with ACE inhibitors are generally not quite as severe as those associated with other medications. However, the attempt to go off the ACE inhibitor can produce a very significant rebound effect. In this case, the blood pressure goes to a higher level than it was previously. Clearly, alternative forms of blood pressure control are desirable, especially from a long-term standpoint.

Often, diet and control of the work environment will be recommended as primary therapeutic approaches toward the treatment of high blood pressure. The results of this three-year study on hypertension indicate that focusing on a recommendation like this may not be the best approach for some people afflicted with hypertension. In most cases, blood pressure problems have underlying physiological reasons, and the physiological deficiencies must be corrected. For older people, there are usually a large number of interactive deficiencies that must be addressed.

The hypertense individual in this three-year study has a number of interrelated health problems that are contributing to his high blood pressure condition. First of all, based on his responses, he is obviously dehydrated. This is a very common problem in many older people and is often the root cause for a variety of health problems ranging from cardiovascular disease to lower back pain.[9] Referring to Whitaker's statement and Nordenström's BCEC/VICC model of the renal/vascular system, deficiencies in the body's hydroelectric system can promote aberrations in the electric potentials between various VICC components (ureters, blood vessels, other organs). Small variations in these potentials can have a significant influence in filtration processes, electrolyte balance, and renal clearance rates. This model appears to be appropriate for the essential hypertension condition, and it would appear that, for many individuals, water intake is one of the first primary items to address for the treatment of essential hypertension. Electrical imbalances in the renal system could contribute to a hypertension problem that eventually damages the renal system, which will produce additional complications for the high blood pressure condition.

Along with increased water intake, it would also appear that essential hypertension problems could be addressed by recommending a certain amount of lecithin and L-carnitine supplementation. L-carnitine is biosynthesized in the liver. Any decreased liver function, often associated with aging processes, could require supplementation of this amino acid.

The second primary item to be addressed involves the high diastolic blood pressure levels. The cardiovascular system is under the influence of the diastolic pressure for most of the cardiac cycle. The total peripheral resistance is indicated by the diastolic pressure, and diastolic pressures of 104 to 118 mmHg are unacceptable. Nutritional supplementation included vitamin A, calcium/magnesium, vitamin-B complex, niacin, flaxseed oil, coenzyme Q10, zinc picolinate, gingko biloba, bilberry extract, horse chestnut, and potassium would appear to be the next step in the therapeutic process to reduce total peripheral resistance and help to promote renal system electrolyte balance.

The third item is partially addressed in the first two items. It involves long-term remediation of cholesterol and triglycerides contributing to overall cardiovascular health and the minimization of extremes in blood pressure incremental variations. Once cardiovascular and renal health problems have been addressed, appropriate, safe, and realistic exercise and work environment control programs can be incorporated.

REFERENCES

1. US Dept. of Commerce. *Statistical Abstracts of the United States*, 116th ed. Washington DC: Bureau of the Census, 1996.

2. US Dept. of Health and Human Services. *Detection, Evaluation and Treatment of High Blood Pressure.* Washington, DC: NIH Publication # 89–1088, 1989.

3. Fox SI. *Human Physiology.* 3rd ed. Dubuque, IA: Wm. C. Brown, 1990.

4. Rushmer R. *Cardiovascular Dynamics.* 2nd ed. Philadelphia, PA: W.B. Saunders, 1961.

5. Nordenström BEW. *Biologically Closed Electric Circuits.* Stockholm, Sweden: Nordic Medical Publications, 1983.

6. Nordenström BEW. Neurovascular activation requires conduction through vessels. *Physiol Chem Phys & Med NMR* 1989;21:249–256.

7. Nordenström BEW. An additional circulatory system: vascular-interstitial closed electric circuits (VICC). *J Biol Phys* 1987;15:43–55.

8. O'Clock GD. The effects of in vitro stimulation on eukaryotic cells: suppression of malignant cell proliferation. *J Orthomolecular Med* 1997;12:173–181.

9. Whitaker J. *Hypertension Report.* Potomac, MD: Phillips Publishing, 1997.

10. Jocob G, et al. Relation of blood volume and blood pressure in orthostatic intolerance. *Am J Med Sci* 1998;315:95–100.

11. Whitaker J. *Health and Healing* 1993;3:6–7.

12. *Physician's Desk Reference.* 50th ed. Montvale, NJ: Medical Economics, 1996.

13. Hardman JG, Limbird LE. *The Pharmacological Basis of Therapeutics.* 9th ed. New York: McGraw-Hill, 1996.

CHOLESTEROL-LOWERING DRUGS FOR EIGHT-YEAR-OLD KIDS?
AMERICAN ACADEMY OF PEDIATRICS URGING "McMEDICINE"

by Andrew W Saul, PhD

Two-thirds of North America is overweight or obese. Our kids are getting fatter too. And these children's cholesterol is going up so fast that the American Academy of Pediatrics (AAP) wants kids as young as eight years of age to take cholesterol-lowering drugs.[1] But before you let any pediatrician put your child on drugs, check what may be a reason behind the recommendation: money. American Academy of Pediatrics projects receive cash from drug companies, including Abbott, AstraZeneca, Dermik, McNeil, Merck, PediaMed, and Sanofi-Aventis. The AAP also receives money from PepsiCo and McDonalds.[2] No wonder they support putting your kids on drugs. Statins for second graders? Sure! Do you want fries with that?

The money flows freely too. The AAP, with 60,000 pediatrician members, is a business. To see just what kind of business they do, look at the program for their October 2008 conference in Boston: "The AAP 2008 Exhibition Hall is *Sold Out*." (Their emphasis.)[3] Sponsoring the Welcome Reception will cost you $150,000. Your drug company can sponsor the convention's shuttle buses for a mere $50,000. But the real deal is this: for $150,000, your drug company can sponsor the AAP magazine, *Healthy Children*, "distributed to physicians' rooms at AAP conference hotels" and "for placement in waiting rooms for availability to parents." You even get two full-page ads, including the back cover.[4]

Drugs Are Not the Answer

Drugs are not the answer . . . unless you are a drug company. The cholesterol-lowering drug Lipitor is the best-selling drug on the planet. Yet it is well established that cardiovascular disease is not caused by a failure to take enough pharmaceuticals as a child. It is a lifestyle disease. If a person will not change their lifestyle, their doctor should prescribe niacin (vitamin B3), the most effective way to lower cholesterol and triglycerides and raise beneficial HDL. It is also the cheapest way. But most important, it is by far the safest way. The president of the American College of Cardiology, Dr. Steven E. Nissen, said, "Niacin is really it. Nothing else available is that effective."[5] Additional protection against cardiovascular disease comes from supplementing the diet with vitamin E, vitamin C, and the amino acid L-lysine.

Cholesterol-lowering drugs can produce serious side effects in adults. This risk is even greater for the still-developing bodies of children. Side effects of cholesterol-lowering drugs include fever, liver damage, muscle pain, rhabdomyolysis (muscle breakdown), memory loss, personality changes, irritability, headaches, anxiety, depression, chest pain, acid regurgitation, dry mouth, vomiting, leg pain, insomnia, eye irritation, tremors, dizziness, and even more. If you check the *Physician's Desk Reference*, you'll see the whole disturbing list.

Reality Check

It is high time for a reality check. Obesity comes from lack of exercise. Obesity comes from high-fat, high-sugar diets. "Childhood obesity is almost completely preventable," says cardiologist Dr. Dean Ornish. "We don't have to wait for a new drug or technology; we just have to put into practice what we already know. What's changed is our diet and lifestyle. If we caused it, we can reverse it."[4] A typical teenage boy drinks 20 ounces of soda a day. "Even chocolate milk gets a thumbs-up from dentists, who would rather see a child drink flavored milk than none at all," commented the *New York Times*.[5] "Most experts agree that Americans' increasingly sedentary lifestyle and fondness for fast food contributed to the nation's growing girth," says PBS-*Frontline*. But then, "Nobody ever got rich marketing self-control."[6]

But many have gotten rich marketing drugs, and now the American Academy of Pediatrics is there to help them get even richer. For shame. Kids need to eat right and exercise. If they need help lowering cholesterol, give them a safe vitamin, not a dangerous prescription drug. And send them out to run around and play.

REFERENCES

1. Tanner L. *Associated Press*. www.aap.org/donate/FCF honorroll.HTM.

2. AAP. Available at www.aap.org/donate/FCFhonorroll.HTM.

3. AAP Exhibitor information. Available at http://s23.a2zinc.net/ clients/aap/nce2008/public/e_exhibitorhome.aspx?sortmenu=1 01000&TopNavType=2.

4. AAP. Available at www.aap.org/nce/08Downloads/Sponsor shipOpportunities08AAPNCE.pdf

5. Mason M. *NY Times*, Jan 23, 2007.

6. PBS *Frontline* presentation. Diet Wars. Available at www.pbs.org/wgbh/pages/frontline/shows/diet/view.

Excerpted from the *Orthomolecular Medicine News Service*, August 18, 2008.

NUTRITIONAL TREATMENTS FOR HYPERTENSION
by Eric R. Braverman, MD, and Ed Weissberg

Over the last 15 years, medicine has gone through a revolutionary change. The medical dictum was that nutrition and lifestyle made no contribution to chronic disease. Medicine has done a complete turnaround and has started a war against bad lifestyle habits like smoking, fat consumption, inactivity, and other harmful behaviors. Modern medicine has accepted its responsibility to direct the lifestyles of people toward health. Possibly no movement other than orthomolecular medicine was shouting like a voice in the wilderness before the rest of the profession identified the important role of nutrition. Indirectly, and often directly, orthomolecular physicians and scientists have heralded the way for the complete nutrition revolution in the United States. This nutritional revolution is most evident in the transformation of the American doctor's treatment of hypertension. More than any other illness, it is now accepted by mainstream medicine that nutritional and dietary factors and therapies should be utilized by physicians in treating hypertension.

Epidemiology

High blood pressure (hypertension) is clinically defined as systolic blood pressure greater than 140 mmHg and/or diastolic blood pressure greater than 90 mmHg. It is a leading problem in the United States, where nearly 20 percent of Americans are affected by this disease.[53,54] The condition afflicts over 60 million Americans and contributes to 1 million deaths per year, adding 18 billion dollars per year to U.S. health expenditures.[55] Genetic, psychological, and environmental factors play a role in hypertension. In 1975, over half (54 percent) of all United States deaths were from cardiovascular disease. Hypertension is the most significant and preventable contributing factor and is associated with an increased risk of heart failure, kidney failure, and stroke.[56]

Five percent of all hypertension has been classified as "secondary," that is, associated with some other disease. Ninety-five percent of hypertension is classified as "primary" or "essential" and is related to stress, nutrition, and other lifestyle factors.[67,96] Most hypertension cases are probably due to arteriosclerosis. Patients with sustained high blood pressure show increased resistance to blood flow (peripheral resistance). This is possibly due to a decrease in the number of blood vessels and increased blood viscosity. The physician should treat only after making an acceptable benefit/risk ratio, and then involve the patient in his/her treatment.[70]

Treatment

Our paper is devoted to the nutritional treatment of essential hypertension. This is a very successful program and should be the first approach to hypertension. A whole array of symptoms and effects manifest themselves with the usage of standard hypertensive pharmacological therapy.[72] Any regimen for hypertension may have detrimental effects on the cerebral functioning of the aged.[73] Approximately, 30–50 percent of elderly patients experience side effects from antihypertensive therapy.[74] Rapid treatment of hypertension in the elderly can cause quick drops in blood pressure and possibly lead to stroke.[75] Antihypertensive drugs have been postulated to be related to the genesis of acute, as well as chronic pancreatitis.[76] Drug therapy for mild hypertension (140–150/90–100) will only help a small percentage of patients, and the side effects may far outweigh the potential gain.[52] Antihypertensive therapy should be matched to the underlying biochemical problems; this would give more efficacious therapy than the standard stepped-care approach.[77]

The financial cost of an antihypertensive regimen should be considered for long-term patient compliance.[78] The great many side effects of antihypertensive medications for treating mild hyper-

From the J Orthomolecular Med 1992;7(4):221–244.

tension has caused many cases of noncompliance and ineffective long-term therapy.[80] It is becoming apparent that drug regimens for the treatment of hypertension have become increasingly unsatisfactory to modern physicians. Even mild hypertension poses risks in the long run and should be treated.[81] This is where our nutritional and lifestyle program has a tremendous input.

The Dangers of Drugs

There are approximately five categories of drug treatments used to control high blood pressure: diuretics, beta blockers, alpha blockers, angiotensin-2 receptor blockers, and calcium channel blockers.

Diuretics

The most commonly used treatment for high blood pressure is diuretics, which have a large variety of side effects.[82–86] Diuretics, also known as water pills, help the kidneys get rid of sodium, thus reducing the volume of blood coursing through the bloodstream. Patients who receive diuretics as their sole therapy have an increased risk of mortality due to heart attack or sudden death.[84] Diuretics deplete magnesium and potassium.[83] Thiazide diuretic therapy in the elderly leads to almost 50 percent of the patients displaying hypokalemia (low blood potassium) or hypomagnesemia (low blood magnesium).[90] Further support for magnesium loss during diuretic therapy comes from Dyckner and Wester.[91] They demonstrate that 42 percent of patients with arterial hypertension had subnormal levels of magnesium. Potassium deficiency can usually be corrected, but the loss of magnesium is rarely addressed. Sodium increased, sodium-potassium-ATPase activity decreased, and potassium decreased when patients were studied who were receiving the diuretic hydrochlorothiazide (Microzide). Even at low doses, diuretics, like hydrochlorothiazide, will have adverse effects on serum lipid (fat) levels.[92] Serum cholesterol as well as other serum lipids are increased during treatment with diuretics. This includes triglycerides and LDL levels.[82] One study showed that with up to one year of treatment with diuretics, plasma cholesterol increased accordingly.[116] Diuretic drugs prescribed for hypertension also cause glucose intolerance (a prediabetic state associated with increased risk of cardiovascular disease) and raise glycohemoglobin (glucose bound to hemoglobin) concentrations. The side effects of diuretics are still disputed by some physicians.[93] Hollifield pointed out the problems of thiazide diuretics relative to potassium and magnesium metabolism, and ventricular ectopy (a cardiac arrhythmia).[94]

Beta Blockers

The second most commonly used therapy are beta blockers. Beta blockers allow the heart to beat more slowly and with less force. They have similar side effects as diuretics. Weinberger has pointed out undesirable serum lipid fractions in patients treated with beta blockers. At least 23 percent of all patients using beta blockers will develop a need for antidepressants.[95] Moreover, they have negative effects on muscular contractions, which can cause an increased risk of heart failure.[96] Miettinen suggested that patients on beta blockers had an increased risk of coronary heart attacks, as did patients on anticholesterol drugs or diuretics. Beta blockers, like most antihypertensive drugs, can cause sexual dysfunction.[80] Twenty-eight percent of patients on the beta-blocker timolol maleate (Blocadren)) experienced adverse reactions, which most commonly consisted of fatigue, dizziness, and nausea. Lipid-soluble beta blockers that cross the blood-brain barrier have been known to produce neurotoxic side effects as well as cold in the bodily extremities.[97] Long-term use of beta blockers, more than two to three years, is probably contraindicated for most patients.

Alpha Blockers

Alpha blockers such as clonidine (Catapres) have a significant amount of side effects, notably hypotension (low blood pressure), constipation, sedation, dry mouth, and dizziness. I have not found them to be particularly helpful in long-term treatment of hypertension.

Methyldopa and Angiotension

Methyldopa, for instance, seems to lower work performance and general well-being, as compared to other antihypertensive agents.[80] In the same study, methyldopa was compared to propranolol (Inderal) and captopril (Capoten) and rated worse in causing the following conditions: fatigue, sexual disorder, headache, neck pressure, insomnia, and nightmares. Up to 50 percent of patients on one of these three drugs experienced fatigue or lethargy; up to 30 percent had some form of sexual disorder; and over 10 percent had sleep disorder, nightmares, headaches, anxiety, irritability, palpitation, dry mouth, dizziness, nausea, and muscle cramps.[80] Captopril, an ACE inhibitor, stops the formation of angiotensin II, which narrow the blood vessels. It is one of the safer drugs for hypertension, wherein it does not affect a patient's glucose tolerance. Nevertheless, ACE inhibitors seem to affect trace elements significantly. Selenium and zinc are decreased and copper increased, which may be a problem in the psychologically sensitive.[99]

Calcium Channel Blockers

Calcium channel blockers are seen to be more efficient and give fewer side effects as compared to the traditional hypertension therapy of diuretics and/or beta blockers.[100] These drugs relax the blood vessel muscle. As such they work like vasodilators to widen blood vessels and increase blood flow. Vasodilators are frequently accompanied by headaches. Drugs like apresoline (Hydralazine) also produce depression in 10–15 percent of the patients taking it. Dopamine-metabolite inhibitors (i.e., methyldopa or Aldomet) are frequently linked with depression and other negative side effects. Hence, we have found virtually all drug regimens have side effects significant enough to warrant searching for other modalities.

It appears that once drug regimens are opted for, drug therapies will spiral. However, the Framingham Heart Study, an ongoing cardiovascular study, indicates that a certain small percentage of formerly treated hypertensives maintain normal blood pressure when treatment is stopped. After abrupt withdrawal from antihypertensives, blood pressure usually rebounds.[108] The need for drugs continues to increase. This is why a suitable nutritional program is necessary. Ironically, it has come from publications such as the *Annals of Internal Medicine* and the *American Medical Association (AMA) News* to suggest that dietary changes and not drugs are the best option.[103,109] The focus of treatment in hypertension should move towards elimination of pharmacological side effects and reduction of risk factors for coronary heart disease.[110] An article in the *Journal of the American Medical Association*[111] states that "Nutritional therapy may substitute for drugs in a sizeable portion of hypertensives, and if drugs are still needed it can lessen some unwanted biochemical effects of drug treatment." A study in Finland where people restructured their diet found that the mortality from coronary heart disease decreased up to 49 percent in some segments of the population. In hypertensive therapy, more than any other aspect of medicine, the role of dietary factors has entered into orthodox medical thinking.

Lifestyle Considerations

Numerous lifestyle factors have been identified in hypertension by McCarron and colleagues.[112] A study in New York City, where schoolchildren maintained ideal weight, decreased total and saturated fat, cholesterol, and sodium (salt) while increasing consumption of complex carbohydrates and fibers, showed improved blood pressure, plasma cholesterol, body mass index, and overall cardiovascular fitness. Even men with a genetic history of familial hypercholesterolemia can greatly reduce cardiovascular risks by eating a low-fat diet, doing regular aerobic exercise, strictly avoiding cigarettes, and monitoring blood pressure and blood cholesterol.[116]

The sympathetic nervous system, which is activated by stress, isometrics (a type of strength-training exercise), and other stressors, plays an important role in creating hypertension.[113] It has become increasingly clear that lifestyle changes can reduce excess catecholamine (epinephrine, dopamine) levels, which are potentially harmful chemicals when inappropriately distributed in the body and increase under stress.[136,137] Nicotine from cigarette smoking causes small blood vessels to constrict, blocks the useful effects of antihypertensive medicines, and is associated with a type of very high blood pressure that comes suddenly called malignant hypertension. A reduction of blood pressure was found with exercise when hypertensive rats were given the opportunity to do so.[133] A cold environment might correlate with higher blood pressure levels. Differences between winter and summer blood pressure may be predictive of future hypertension. There is some evidence that the roots of hypertension are found in early childhood and preventive attention should begin as early as adult blood pressures are achieved.

Weight Considerations

Obesity is the number-one lifestyle factor related to hypertension and probably overall health and longevity. Therefore weight loss is an essential part of a high blood pressure regimen.[120] We do not, however, recommend appetite suppressants. One of these, phenylpropanolamine, can induce significant hypertension. Obesity is a major cardiovascular risk factor having a very complex socioeconomic, cross-cultural interrelationship with various other risk factors. One study established that long-term changes in blood pressure correlate with decreases in body weight.[121] Hypertension has been shown to be directly proportional to obesity and glucose intolerance.

Diet and exercise such as walking, swimming, and biking have beneficial effects on blood lipid levels. We always encourage our patients to exercise, if capable. Exercise has been shown not to depress appetite but rather help to control it and is almost essential in a weight-loss plan for hypertension. Simple exercise such as walking or swimming can add years to one's life. In a study where energy expenditure per week approached 3,500 calories, illness also decreased significantly.

Seventh-day Adventist lacto-vegetarians were compared with omnivorous Mormons theoretically matching groups for effects of religiosity and abstention from alcohol, tobacco, and caffeine. The lacto-vegetarians had lower blood pressure, even after adjusting for the effects of weight. "Long-term adherence to a vegetarian diet is associated with less of a rise of blood pressure with age and a decreased prevalence of hypertension. Specific mechanisms and nutrients involved have not been clarified."[30]

Psychosocial and Environmental Considerations

Psychological, emotional, and environmental factors play a large role in cardiovascular disease, and this knowledge can be used to complement treatment regimens. Psychosocial and behavioral modification techniques are safe and somewhat effective in hypertension therapy. Feedback monitoring of blood pressure at intervals of several weeks was shown to be as effective as relaxation and biofeedback. Cranial electrotherapy stimulation, a stress- and anxiety-reduction technique, also probably lowers blood pressure.

An Australian study showed that after adjustment for different variables, the level of education was inversely related to blood pressure levels. Learning and education correlates with better lifestyle and lower blood pressure.

Dietary Considerations

Serum cholesterol correlates very closely to blood pressure levels and helps to identify the segment of the population in need of treatment. Elevated serum cholesterol above 240 milligrams per deciliter (mg/dL) is the single, most important risk factor in coronary heart disease. In a study with more than 360,000 men, cardiovascular mortality rises steadily with increasing serum cholesterol levels (718 mg/dL). Aggressive dietary modifications are very useful to lower blood cholesterol levels, which are linked to atherosclerotic vascular disease and coronary artery disease. Elevated serum and arterial cholesterol is a major entity in hypertension and cholesterol and can be reduced by dietary fibers such as bran and pectin. The positive role of fiber in reducing cholesterol is further supported by Fletcher and Rogers.[122] Dietary fibers contained in foods such as carrots and other vegetables lower body cholesterol levels by binding bile salts that mix with fats to help digest them. Dietary fiber has an important moderating effect on serum cholesterol. Insoluble dietary fibers such as guar gum and pectin have been shown to be hypocholesterolemic (cholesterol-lowering) and hypertriglyceridemic (triglyceride-raising) substances.

High-quality fresh and whole-food sources of oils and animal products are important. Fatty acids (including polyunsaturated fats and cholesterol) are susceptible to degradation by oxidation and free radical reactions. Studies on animals show the resultant oxycholesterols have atherogenic properties. Powders of egg and moldy cheeses (found in many fast foods) are especially susceptible.

Serum cholesterol and changes in serum cholesterol were correlated to consumption of fats. However, serum cholesterol levels are not significantly related to dietary cholesterol in conjunction with a diet rich in polyunsaturated fats. Egg intake coupled with a diet low in other saturated fats (found primarily in animal products) and high in polyunsaturated fats does not significantly raise blood cholesterol. Polyunsaturated fats (abundant in corn, soybean, safflower, and sunflower oils) can be used to lower total serum cholesterol and to raise healthy high-density lipoproteins (HDLs), and thus can help to prevent atherosclerosis.

Animal studies suggest that sucrose (found in cane sugar and some fruits and vegetables) has the effect of raising blood pressure. At high levels of carbohydrate consumption (50–80 percent) increased blood pressure is also noted.[50] Kannel pointed out that the dietary factors in hypertension may relate to the excess calories of saturated fat intake as well as high cholesterol and salt intake.[120]

Fruits, vegetables, whole grains, and low-fat dairy items protect against hypertension. An epidemiological study showed that one Chinese group with a history of hypertension had a high intake of added salt to their milk and tea and consumed little starchy foods, fresh fruits, and vegetables. Consumption of proteins, animal fats and animal products, sucrose, fructose, refined foods, and high daily energy content of food were directly related to congestive heart disease morbidity, arteriosclerosis, myocardial infarction, and arteriosclerosis mortality, whereas consumption of vegetable oils, starch, soluble and insoluble fiber, vegetables, and fruit shared an inverse correlation.

Hypertensive patients may have impaired glucose tolerance, especially when treated with diuretics. Glucose tolerance tests in hypertensive patients are frequently abnormal. A high-carbohydrate (sucrose) diet has been shown to induce sodium retention. Sucrose or glucose can mediate a sodium retention effect, and, thus, through this retention of sodium, raise systolic blood pressure. A diet high in sucrose will raise blood pressure in animals significantly, possibly due to a relative decrease in potassium intake. Glucose intolerance, obesity, and blood pressure are tightly interrelated, so a derangement in one will cause problems in the others.

Significant decreases in the consumption of calcium, potassium, vitamin A, and vitamin C have been identified as nutritional factors that distinguish hypertensive from normotensive (normal blood pressure) subjects. Calcium intake was the most consistent factor in hypertensive individuals. Previous reports showed a significant negative correlation between water hardness and mortality rates. A study comparing the twin Kansas cities in the United States showed the opposite to hold true; hard-watered Kansas City, Kansas, had more cardiovascular problems including a 10-fold higher serum cadmium level. Coffee has been shown to increase coronary heart disease risk by almost 250 percent. Smoking and hypertension are the two main risk factors for coronary artery disease. Youngsters who smoke even less than one pack of cigarettes per day increase blood cholesterol and triglycerides.

Harlan and others have suggested that alcohol plays a role in hypertension.[160] Moderate use of alcohol may lower blood pressure, but excessive use may elevate it. At moderate levels of one drink per day, alcohol has been shown in some cases to be protective against coronary artery disease. Alcohol in large doses may lead to rhythmic disturbances in the electrophysiology of the heart. Alcohol use may lead to depression and increase carbohydrate consumption, which will lead to hypertension.

In light of these findings, we recommend the following dietary guideline to most of our hypertensive patients: a low-sodium, low-saturated fat, and low-refined carbohydrate intake, with high-vegetable intake from the starch group (like potatoes, peas, and corn), and a high-salad and protein intake (particularly from fish). Simple sugar, alcohol, caffeine, nicotine, and refined carbohydrates should be reduced drastically or eliminated.

Nutritional Substances as Pharmacological Low-Blood Pressure Agents

In treating high blood pressure, it is important to consider the use of dietary supplements. Each of the nutrients below has a role in the nutritional control of hypertension and can be of great benefit in a patient's hypertension therapy.

Fish Oil and Essential Fatty Acids

Numerous researchers have suggested that saturated fats can raise blood pressure, while Singer and colleagues[145-147] have suggested the potential blood pressure–lowering effect of fish oil. As pointed out earlier, polyunsaturated fats can be used to lower total serum cholesterol and to raise HDL level, and thus can help to prevent atherosclerosis. Dietary fat modifications, such as an increase in polyunsaturated to saturated fat ratio and an overall decrease in percentage of fat in the diet, lower blood pressure and have favorable effects on serum lipid levels. Greenland and Icelandic Eskimos whose diet is rich in saturated fats have a much lower incidence of coronary heart disease than controls because of high fish consumption. An inverse relationship was found with fish consumption and twenty-year mortality from coronary heart disease. Those who consumed 30,000 mg or more of fish per day had a 50 percent lower cardiac mortality rate than those who did not. Fish oils (an especially rich source of omega-3 fatty acids) reduce high levels of plasma lipids, lipoproteins, and apolipoproteins in patients with hypertriglyceridemia. They also have effects on serum lipid levels in healthy humans. Eicosapentaenoic acid, or EPA (the omega-3 component most commonly found in fish oil), lowers abnormal blood lipid levels and decreases blood viscosity. Fish oil like niacin raises HDL and reduces risk from heart disease. Atherosclerosis formation is a very complex problem and may be related to an intracellular deficiency in essential fatty acids. Halberg[155] suggests that dietary lipid controls may be even more important than salt restriction in the control of hypertension.

Mogenson and Box[143] and Puska and colleagues[156] have suggested that two polyunsaturated fatty acids, linoleic acid, an omega-6 fatty acid especially plentiful in safflower oil, and gamma-linolenic acid, an omega-3 fatty acid found in evening primrose oil, can be extremely useful in the treatment of hypertension. Dietary supplementation with linoleic acid, gamma-linolenic acid, or other polyunsaturated fatty acids is of use in controlling hypertension. These agents lower blood pressure and have both a diuretic effect (particularly linoleic acid and gamma-linolenic acid) and a prostaglandin E-2 (PGE2, a pro-inflammatory substance) inhibitory effect. A diet high in linoleic acid lessened a rise in blood pressure in nephrectornized rats. Linolenic acid is helpful in the treatment and prevention of hypertension probably due to its conversion to prostaglandins and/or other vascular regulators. Linoleic and linolenic acids are both prostaglandin precursors and are useful in hypertension therapy.[84]

Cis-linoleic acid is converted to gamma-linolenic acid and eventually to the anti-inflammatory prostaglandin E (PGE), which is a vasodilator and inhibitor of platelet aggregation.[122] Smith and Dunn[141] of Case Western Reserve University in Cleveland, Ohio, did at least eight different studies where safflower oil, linoleic acid, cod liver oil, and EPA all lowered blood pressure significantly. Fish oils, especially the omega-3 fatty acids, have been shown to decrease risk of coronary heart disease. A diet high in fish or fish oil supplementation is recommended in patients with increased risk of coronary heart disease. In doses of up to 16,500 mg, fish oil has been shown to significantly lower blood pressure and cardiovascular risk factors.[157]

Omega-3 fatty acids prevent elevated triglycerides induced by carbohydrates by blocking the triglyceride-carrying very-low-density lipoproteins (VLDLs) and triglyceride metabolism. Angina patients showed a lower ratio of EPA to arachidonic acid, a pro-inflammatory substance. The authors of the study consider this a new cardiovascular risk factor. Six thousand milligrams of fish oil per day lowered VLDL and raised HDL, while greatly decreasing plasma triglycerides and cholesterol. A diet high in fish as compared to one high in cold cuts or meat lowered serum cholesterol, blood pressure, and raised HDL. Fatty acids, especially linoleic, oleic, and arachidonic acids, have been shown to reduce angiotensin receptor affinity. An olive oil-rich diet has been shown to decrease non-HDL cholesterol, while leaving triglyceride levels constant. EPA in the form of cod liver oil or mackerel is an excellent polyunsaturate and lowers cardiovascular risk factors.[145]

Hence, all our patients were treated with EPA (fish oils), linoleic acid (safflower oil), or gamma-linolenic acid (evening primrose oil), or all three.[141] Dietary fatty acid intake is of particular importance in relation to blood pressure when weight reduction is occurring, as is the case with our patients.

Calcium

Numerous studies suggest that calcium may have an important role in hypertension.[54] An oral calcium load has been shown to decrease systolic and diastolic blood pressure, elevate PGE2, decrease parathyroid hormone, decrease norepinephrine, and decrease vitamin D. Hypertensive patients showed significant deficiencies in dietary calcium, potassium, vitamin A, and vitamin C with calcium being the most consistent dietary risk factor for hypertension.[54] Preliminary reports show that oral calcium supplements (1,000–2,000 mg/ day) lower blood pressure in some patients, particularly in young adults, possibly more so in women. However, manipulation of dietary calcium may not be very useful in older women. Oral calcium carbonate administration also seems to have an effect on mild hypertensives. Calcium citrate is probably the best therapy.

In one study, calcium supplementation reduced blood pressure in young adults. Calcium supplementation of up to 1,000 milligrams has been shown to lower blood pressure in mild to moderate hypertension.[54] Furthermore, surveys have shown a positive relationship between blood pressure and serum calcium levels. Acute elevation of circulating calcium levels during elevation of blood pressure, chronic hypercalcemia (too much calcium in the body), or hyperthyroidism (overactive thyroid), and vitamin D intoxication are all associated with increased chronic hypertension. Calcium supplementation may

lower elevated blood pressure by increasing natriuresis (sodium excretion). Three clinically paradoxical findings in the relationship of calcium and hypertension arc as follows: calcium mediates vascular smooth muscle (the layer in arterial wall that allows the vessel to relax and constrict); calcium channel blockers lower blood pressure; and increased calcium intake can also relieve hypertension.[54] A recent hypothesis says that there is a circulating plasma factor that increases intracellular platelet coagulation in hypertension.

In contrast, several studies have shown that calcium can be a factor in elevating hypertension. Therefore, we use calcium sparingly except in the case of a woman suspected of having osteoporosis or in cases of normal plasma, ionized calcium, or red blood cell calcium.[7,38,54]

Magnesium

Magnesium, in contrast to calcium, is well known to lower blood pressure and has been used in the treatment of hypertension in pregnancy for a number of decades.[91] Magnesium, calcium, phosphorus, potassium, fiber, vegetable proteins, starch, vitamin C, and vitamin D showed an inverse relationship with blood pressure, with magnesium's correlation being the strongest.[126]

Magnesium is a vasodilator and at high levels can cause low blood pressure. The use of various nutritional substances as pharmacological agents for hypertension has produced many success stories. Nevertheless, magnesium therapy has been instituted for hypertension to combat a deficiency state often inflicted by diuretic usage. In a study with Finnish ewes, hypomagnesium (low blood magnesium) was correlated with hypertension. Magnesium deficiency may relate to high blood pressure by increasing microcirculatory changes or microcirculatory arteriosclerosis. Direct lowering of blood pressure with magnesium in patients with high blood pressure has been demonstrated by Dyckner and Wester.[91] Magnesium works like a calcium channel blocking drug such as Verapamil or Diltiazem.

Research also has suggested that magnesium supplements have a valuable effect on diabetic and hypertensive rats. Magnesium's use has been documented in cardiac situations, such as arrhythmias due to magnesium depletion and heart attacks due to decreases in potassium. Magnesium may be an important prophylaxis in hypertensive patients prone to arrhythmia. Untreated hypertensives showed lower levels of magnesium, which strongly correlates to systolic and diastolic blood pressure. Studies have found that hypertensive patients using diuretics had a magnesium level of 1.79 mg to 100 milliliters (ml) compared to nonhypertensive patients with 1.92 mg to 100 ml, a significant difference. Magnesium is also low in mononuclear cells in intensive cardiac patients. Type A personalities have been shown to lose magnesium under stress and thus show a correlation to their behavioral tendency to eventually develop hypertension, coronary artery disease, and coronary vasospasms.[161] Further support for magnesium's use in hypertension treatment is documented by Wester and Dyckner,[91] who claim that magnesium acts by vasodilation or by sodium-potassium-ATPase metabolism, which supplies energy to every cell in the body. Magnesium metabolism was abnormal in spontaneously hypertensive rats.

Sulfur Amino Acids

A study by Ogawa and colleagues[164] suggested that decreases in plasma taurine and methionine were significant in patients with essential hypertension. Taurine may lower blood pressure. Furthermore, all sulfur amino acids (methionine, cysteine, and taurine) lower heavy metals that are often factors in hypertension. In our study we found a trend toward decreases in plasma cysteine probably due to B6 deficiency. Hence, most of our patients with hypertension receive supplemental sulfur-amino acid treatment. Three thousand milligrams of taurine daily could elevate blood taurine levels two to three times normal. We consider this an appropriate level to reach for hypertensives.

Sodium and Potassium

The role of dietary sodium (salt) in hypertension is long-standing and well known. It has been suggested that the average person consumes 10,000–12,000 mg of sodium per day, which should be reduced to 2,300 mg per day. This can be counter-balanced by increasing potassium intake, which may lower blood pressure. A higher ratio of potassium to sodium has been shown to lower moderately high blood pressure. Potassium therapy is useful in lowering blood pressure induced by diuretic-induced hypercalcemia (high blood calcium). An inverse relationship between serum potassium and blood pressure was shown by Luft and others.[49] High potassium intake greatly reduced brain hemorrhages, heart attacks, and death rate in spontaneous hypertensive rats. A high potassium intake may help to alleviate high blood pressure, the leading risk factor for smokers.

The hazards of high sodium intake are beyond hypertension and include gastric cancer. Dietary sodium affects urinary calcium and potassium excretion in men with regular blood pressure and differing calcium intakes. Anderson[159] suggested that stress and salt are cyclical, meaning that increased salt intake produces stress and craving salt is a sign of stress. Dietary sodium and copper have long-term effects on elevating blood pressure in the Long-Evans group of rats. Decreased sodium intake can decrease stress.[103]

Some essential hypertensives have a low sodium to potassium and/or a high lithium to sodium counterpart. One study shows that hypertension in spontaneous hypertensive rats is caused by a circulating hypertensive agent produced by the kidneys and adrenals whose secretion can be suppressed by salt depletion. Hence, all of our patients are asked to restrict sodium as completely as possible and to use a salt substitute. We suggest to all our patients that they use high-potassium salt substitutes.

Trace Elements

Numerous studies have suggested that elevations in serum copper can raise blood pressure. Excess dietary copper can increase systolic blood pressure in rats. Elevations in serum copper and cadmium have been found in smokers, which may be the reason why they have elevated blood pressure, according to Kromhout and others.[152] Serum copper was inversely related to HDL level.[152] Contraceptive pill users have elevations in serum copper and elevations in arterial pressure. Patients who suffered from heart attacks had decreased levels of zinc and iron but increased nickel levels. Hypertensive subjects that use diuretics have significantly higher serum copper levels. Increased serum copper has a role in primary or pulmonary hypertension (a condition caused by increased pressure in the lung's pulmonary artery). Zinc lowers serum copper and may actually lower blood pressure. Higher dietary zinc intake has been associated with lower blood pressure.[128] Zinc is depleted by diuretics.

Increased red blood cell content of zinc in essential hypertension has been found by Henrotte and others.[161] Zinc is a well-known antagonist of heavy metals such as cadmium and lead, which even in chronic dosages has been found to elevate blood pressure. Hence, all our hypertensive patients receive zinc to lower copper, lead, cadmium, and manganese. Studies suggesting that subacute elevations in cadmium and lead have a role in the elevation in blood pressure have been done by Staessen and others, and the *AMA News*.[109,163]

Blood lead levels, which are elevated in chronic alcoholism, have been correlated with increases in blood pressure. The correlation of blood lead to blood pressure is stronger for systolic than diastolic blood pressure.[152] An over-abundance of lead can lead to a form of hypertension with renal impairment. Further evidence for a relationship between blood lead levels and blood pressure has been presented. Serum zinc levels were significantly lower for older hypertensive women and older men with high systolic readings.[160] Elevations of lead and cadmium with decreases in zinc are a factor in many inner-city patients with hypertension. Plasma zinc levels were significantly lower in patients having coronary heart disease risk factors. Furthermore, it has been shown that vitamin C in combination with zinc may be an even more effective way of reducing subacute levels of lead and cadmium. We have had every patient follow a treatment plan that included zinc therapy.

PHYSICIAN'S REPORT:
IMPROVEMENT OF ARTERIAL STIFFNESS BY MULTINUTRIENT SUPPLEMENTATION
by P. A. Öckerman, MD, PhD

Nutrients like amino acids,[1] fatty acids,[2] vitamins,[3-6] trace elements,[7] minerals[8] and antioxidants,[9] as well as food extracts,[10] and nutritional[11-14] and lifestyle interventions[15] have in some studies been found to diminish risk factors for cardiovascular disease. Often a more critical conclusion has been drawn.[16] With the advent of new evaluation methods, such as aortic arterial stiffness and endothelial function, it has become easier to evaluate the potential impacts of specific interventions like broad-spectrum nutrients upon cardiovascular disease risk factors.

Patient Profiles
All patients were thoroughly examined and diagnosed in the ordinary medical system before seeking advice from an integrative medicine out-patient clinic, where they were routinely tested for aortic arterial stiffness (via measuring pulse-wave velocity) and endothelial function (via measuring augmentation index) by an arteriograph, a special type of magnetic resonance imaging (MRI) scan. Patients had many different diagnoses and were on many different types of medications. Smokers and cancer patients were excluded from participating in this study. Selected patients were offered treatment with multinutrient supplementation if their pulse-wave velocity and augmentation index values indicated a possible problem. In total, 85 patients participated, ranging in age from 44 to 91, with a mean age of 67.1 years. A total of 51 females and 34

males completed treatment for two months. Measurements were taken of pulse-wave velocity and augmentation index at pretreatment time and after two months of treatment.

Treatment

The patients were prescribed the following multinutrient interventions:

- Broad-spectrum multivitamin and mineral supplement with the antioxidants: 6 tablets per day

- Pollen extract: 1,000 milligrams (mg) per day

- Vitamin C: 2,000 mg per day in tablet form

- L-arginine: 2,250 mg per day

- N-acetylcysteine: 400 mg per day

- Fish oil: 2,000 mg per day

- Extra minerals: Potassium (367 mg/day), magnesium (167 mg/day), and calcium (317 mg/day)

- Probiotic preparation: 5 milliliters per day containing *Lactococcus lactis*, *Lactobacillus rhamnosus*, inulin, and dried powder of blueberries

Results

In 85 patients, multinutrient supplementation produced highly significant improvements in aortic pulse-wave velocity (i.e., aortic artery stiffness) and augmentation index (i.e., peripheral artery stiffness and function) in two months. Improvement was seen for pulse-wave velocity in 87.1 percent and for augmentation index in 88.2 percent of patients. Values for augmentation index decreased from +5.2 to -14.1 and for pulse-wave velocity from 12.0 to 10.0 meters per second. Pulse-wave velocity values can be expressed as a decrease of the biological age of the aorta. In this case, it is 92.9 years to 63.2 years, a very substantial decrease of 29.7 years.

Discussion

Most studies that have evaluated nutrients in the prevention and treatment of cardiovascular disease have used single nutrient interventions. The results of such studies have most often been negative. The background for the approach in the present study was that multi-nutrient supplementation might afford synergistic effects, and therefore prevent negative results due to incipient nutrient deficiencies. This philosophy was derived from the fact that a diet rich in antioxidants counteracts oxidative stress, but single antioxidants might not. Also, it is general knowledge that antioxidants in combination possess synergistic effects while single antioxidants might not. The mechanisms behind the therapeutic effects induced by multiple nutrients are most certainly complex. The addition of essential nutrients, that might be wanting, would help to restore adequate or "healthy" endothelial function. Vitamin C and other antioxidants counteract oxidation of cholesterol moieties (e.g., low-density lipoprotein cholesterol) but also diminish free radical activity, since oxidative stress is a well-known cardiovascular disease risk factor. Chronic low-grade inflammation, common to cardiovascular disease, rheumatoid arthritis, and other degenerative diseases, might also be counteracted by judicious nutritional supplementation. Since multiple nutrient preparations appear to diminish inflammation, they might be of value in other diseases in which an increased risk of cardiovascular disease has been demonstrated.[16]

REFERENCES

1. Heffernan KS. *J Cardiovasc Pharmacol Ther* 2010;15:17–23.
2. Lavie CJ. *J Am Coll Cardiol* 2009;54:585–594.
3. Rasool AH. *Arch Pharm Res* 2008;31:1212–1217.
4. Jablonski KL. *Hypertension* 2011;57:63–69.
5. Chacko SA. *Am J Clin Nutr* 2011;94:209–217.
6. Rumberger JA. *Nutr Res* 2011;31:608–615.
7. Lubos E. *Atherosclerosis* 2010;209:271–277.
8. Chacko SA. *Am J Clin Nutr* 2011;93:463–473.
9. Riccioni G. *J Biol Regul Homeost Agents* 2010;24:447–452.
10. Koyama N. *Br J Nutr* 2009;101:568–575.
11. Stamatelopoulos K. Curr *Opin Clin Nutr Metab Care* 2009;12: 467–473.
12. Riccioni G. *Expert Rev Cardiovasc Ther* 2008;6:723–729.
13. Gregory SM. *Nutr Rev* 2011;69:509–519.
14. Riccioni G. *Eur J Cardiovasc Prev Rehabil* 2009;16:351–357.
15. Ford ES. *Arch Intern Med* 2009;169:1355–1362.
16. Buhr Gand Bales CW. *J Nutr Elder* 2009;28:5–29.
17. Wållberg-Jonsson S. *Scand J Rheumatol* 2008;37:1–5.

From the *J Orthomolecular Med* 2011;26(4):159–612

Vitamin B6

It has been established by Dakshinamurti and others[162] that pyridoxine (vitamin B6) deficiency has a role in hypertension. Vitamin B6 inhibits platelet aggregations through its metabolite pyridoxal-5'-phosphate.[144] Pyridoxine deficiencies, which can cause serotonin and GABA deficiencies (neurotransmitters involved in blood pressure regulation) as well as general increases in sympathetic nervous system stimulation, can cause blood pressure to become elevated. Besides being a cofactor for transamination (moving amino acids), vitamin B6 seems to relieve edema and swelling and thus has mild diuretic properties; therefore, all of our patients receive pyridoxine.

Niacin

Niacin (vitamin B3), possibly because of its flushing or vasodilating properties, can lower blood pressure and significantly raise HDL, which is frequently reduced in hypertensive patients (Hoeg,1984). Niacin administration is a very effective agent against an increased level of LDL in patients with type II hyperlipoproteinemia (a disorder associated with earlier cardiovascular disease). Niacin has also been shown to reduce the average numbers of lesions per subject and block new plaque formation. Niacin, when used alone or in conjunction with the drug colestipol (Colestid), can effectively lower cholesterol and triglyceride levels to the normal physiological range (*J Lipid Res*, 1981). Niacin is used as an adjunct therapy in our treatment.

Selenium and Chromium

Serum selenium in patients who had had an acute heart attack was determined to be low before this condition occurred and not as a result. Further evidence for serum selenium levels and cardiovascular death correlation comes from the work of Virtamo and colleagues.[165] Chromium concentrations in aortas of patients dying from atherosclerotic disease were significantly lower as compared to a control group. Low plasma chromium was found in patients with coronary artery and heart diseases. Both selenium and chromium may have a role in the nutritional control of hypertension, at least in the protection from heart attack during a difficult dietary period.

Other Nutrients

Vitamin C stabilizes vascular walls and helps metabolism of cholesterol into bile acids. When elderly patients receive 3,000 mg of inositol (a member of the B family), their total blood lipid and cholesterol levels decreased.

Garlic has been shown to be of great benefit in hypertension therapy, raising HDL and lowering both total cholesterol and LDL. Garlic oil decreases platelet aggregation, serum cholesterol, and mean blood pressure, while it raises HDL. Thus, garlic has been shown to be an anti-atherosclerotic, antithrombotic, and an antihypertensive agent.

Vitamin E lowers cholesterol and effects prostaglandin synthesis, yet vitamin E, by clinical observation, raises blood pressure.

The hormone melatonin may have a role in regulating high blood pressure. One study has shown that nutritional and hormonal treatments can enhance the sodium-potassium-ATPase activity level and in turn helps to prevent or treat essential hypertension. Another study has shown estrogen given to postmenopausal women reduces heart attack risk.

Coenzyme Q10 has been found deficient in approximately 40 percent of hypertensives and has a possibly beneficial effect on blood pressure therapy.

Everyone with hypertension and/or a family history of it needs a dietary and nutritional regimen.

Biochemical Individuality/Genetic Differences

It is very important for both the physician and hypertension patient to realize that every human being is genetically and, thus, biochemically distinct. Dietary or drug regimens have different effects on different patients. The influence of diet on blood lipid levels is not predictable for each individual due to different genetic traits. Similarly, sodium restriction is generally recommended in an antihypertensive diet, and, in most cases, this reduces blood pressure through volume effects. Sodium restriction is beneficial for the majority of hypertensives. However, one epidemiologic study showed sodium restriction to be of no value in a small subgroup of the population at large (*Cardiology Observer*, 1987). Furthermore, in a small group of patients, sodium restriction actually increases the activity of the renin-angiotensin system (the enzyme system that regulates blood pressure and fluids) and thus raises blood pressure. According to Dr. Weinberger of Indiana University, Indianapolis, dietary sodium restrictions show a variety of responses due to genetic differences.

The dietary recommendations made in this paperwork work exceptionally well in a vast majority of the hypertensive population, but some trial and error might be needed to tailor the program to a patient's specific biochemical needs. Clinical judgment of which nutrient and diet to use can be refined by measuring, plasma fatty acids, plasma amino acid, red blood cell trace elements, and vitamin levels. Following test results for sedimentation rates (to detect inflammation), cholesterol, and fibrinogen (a blood-clotting protein) levels is also useful.

Treatment and Case Histories

At our clinic the typical person with hypertension is usually started on the following nutrient regimen: chromium (200 mcg/1x per day), CoQ10 (60–90 mg/1x per day), cysteine (500 mg/2x per day), fish oil (2,000 mg/2x per day), garlic (2x per day, preferably morning and evening), magnesium oxide (500 mg/2x per day), niacin (400 mg/2x per day), potassium (10–25 mg/1x per day), primrose oil (1,000 mg/2x per day), selenium (200 mg/1x per day), taurine (500 mg/2x per day), tryptophan (1,000 mg at bedtime), vitamin B6 (200 mg/1x per day), vitamin C (500 mg/2x per day), and zinc (15 mg/2x per day).

We usually suggest that all patients have an initial complete chemical screen before beginning this treatment. Based on the findings we adapt the nutrient regimen to the unique needs of each patient. Following are nearly a dozen case histories using this approach.

1. Removal of Multiple Drugs

G. F. is a 51-year-old male on multiple medications, weighing 265 pounds, with a 25-year history of smoking two packs of cigarettes per day. He stopped smoking three years ago. His blood pressure (BP) was between 150/100 and 140/100, with a pulse of 74. He was taking methyldopa (Aldomet), timolol (Blocadren), potassium chloride (Klotrix), hydrochlorothiazide for 10 years and using a nitroglycerin transdermal patch (Nitro-Patch) nightly. He was put on a weight-reducing, low-carbohydrate diet and started on a daily supplement regimen that included six multivitamins, vitamin B6 (500 mg), magnesium orotate (3,000 mg), garlic (1,440 mg), taurine (3,000 mg), evening primrose oil (3,000 mg), EPA (6,000 mg), magnesium oxide (1,500 mg), and four Klotrix (40 micrograms [mcg]. Blocadren was reduced to two tablets per day and Aldomet to one tablet. After one month, his BP was 144/104 (an increase in BP can occur in early reversal of drugs), weight 248. On 1/28 his BP was 120/88, weight 249; Aldomet was stopped and Blocadren was maintained. On 2/11 his BP was 140/90, pulse 78, and weight 235; Blocadren was reduced to one pill, but he still used Nitro-Patch. On 3/11 BP was 140/94, weight 226, and Blocadren was stopped; taurine was reduced to 2,000 mg and garlic to 960 mg. He was no longer on any medication except Nitro-Patch for BP. Klotrix was reduced to three tablets, and fish oil was switched to Mega-EPA, a more potent brand of EPA. On 4/10 his BP was 150/90, pulse 78, and weight 216. On 5/23 his BP was 130/70, pulse 80, and weight 214 pounds, and Nitro-Patch was stopped. Medication was reduced to four multivitamins, four garlic (60 mg), primrose oil (2,000 mg), fish oil (6,000 mg), and his antihypertensive formula was stopped. From 3/11 on, he was taking per day two zinc pills, magnesium oxide (1,000 mg, substituted for magnesium orotate), and niacin (1,000 mg). Safflower oil (2 tablespoons) per day was also prescribed from 3/11 on, and vitamin C (2,000 mg) per day from 4/10 on. Chromium (200 mcg) was taken from 5/22 on. Hence, this patient, through the use of meganutrient therapy, was completely removed from drugs. His BP remains stable at 130/70. He occasionally used vodka, coffee, and tea. His sex drive was increased gradually throughout the treatment, and exercise (walking) gradually increased.

2. Removal of Beta Blockers

A 42-year-old male, five foot ten, weighing 179.5 pounds, was on nadolol (Corgard) for two years, drinking two cups of coffee a day, with a high sex drive and craving for salt. His BP was 150/90 on 5/16, and he was started on multivitamins, vitamin B6 (500 mg) folic acid (200 mcg), vitamin B12 (250 mcg), magnesium orotate (3,000 mg), taurine (3,000 mg), garlic (1,500 mg), and primrose oil (3,000 mg). On 5/30 his BP was very good at 128/82. He was off Corgard, with a pulse of 86 and weight 173.

3. Removal of Beta Blockers

A 51-year-old female with a 10-year history of hypertension was presented to us for treatment. She weighed 150 pounds at five foot three, and was taking metoprolol (Lopressor, 50 mg/2x per day). She did not smoke or use alcohol or tea. On 5/23 her BP was 194/120, with a pulse of 116. She began taking multivitamins, two vitamin B6 (500 mg), folic acid (60 mg for atrophic vaginitis), magnesium orotate (3,000 mg), magnesium oxide (2,000 mg), taurine (3,000 mg), garlic (1,440 mg), and EPA (6,000 mg). She returned on 6/12 with BP 160/100, having gone three weeks without a migraine for the first time in years. Her regimen was adjusted to 50 mg of magnesium orotate, 3,000 mg of magnesium oxide, 2,000 mg of taurine, 600 mg of calcium carbonate, 3,000 mg of primrose oil, 100 mg of niacin, 200 mcg of chromium, and 200 mcg of selenium. She received instructions to go off 50 mg of Lopressor if there was improvement in two weeks. She returned drug free and her BP was 130/80. The rapid recovery of this patient was due to following the supplement protocol as well as a stricter diet, which consisted of fish (two times daily), meat (two to three times per week), safflower oil (3 tablespoons daily), and frequent use of ginger, garlic, and onions.

4. Removal of Diuretics

A 57-year-old male, five foot six, came to us for treatment in December with a BP of 160/100. He was taking Corgard, had a moderate sex drive, did not use caffeine, did not exercise, and had a 30-year history of hypertension. He was started on chromium (2 tablets/2x per day), vitamin C (1,000 mg/2x per day), zinc (10 mg), manganese (2 mg), selenium (200 mcg/morning), EPA (6,000 mg/day), taurine (500 mg/day), magnesium orotate (2,000 mg/day), and Corgard was reduced to 30 mg per day. On 1/8 niacin was added (timed-release evening), and his weight had fallen to 154 pounds, with BP 120/75. On 2/5 Corgard was reduced to half a pill every other day, and he was advised to stop it in two weeks. Safflower oil (1 tablespoon/2x per day) was added, zinc (50 mg/2x per day), dolomite (1 tablet/2x per day), and all medications remained stable. On 3/17 he was feeling light-headed and came in with a BP of 85/70 and a pulse of 90. His medication remained the same (he should have stopped Corgard 2/19), but the safflower oil was stopped. He returned on 4/1 with BP 132/62, pulse 62, and weight 149. Initially, his triglycerides were 256, cholesterol 190, and HDL fraction was 26 (high coronary risk). On 3/17 his triglycerides were normal at 153, with cholesterol of 176 and an HDL fraction of 41 with all drugs removed.

5. Removal of Diuretics

A 62-year-old female, five foot three, with a 15-year history of hypertension came to us for treatment. She had been treated daily for 20 years with chlorthalidone (Hygroton, 50 mg) and allopurinol (Zyloprim) because of gout induced by Hygroton. Her BP was 160/100 and her weight was 204. Hygroton was stopped, and she was put on a Dyazide (instead of a diuretic) every other day. She was then permitted no fried or salted foods and was asked to follow a low-carbohydrate diet. In July she was started on a multivitamin (1 tablet per day), chromium (200 mcg/2x per day), vitamin C (2,000 mg/2x per day), vitamin B6 (500 mg per day), taurine (1,000 mg per day), evening primrose oil (2,000 mg/2x per day), zinc (50 mg/2x per day), and safflower oil (1 teaspoon/2x per day). The diuretic was finally stopped on 12/9, and her medication was changed to multivitamin (1 tablet/2x per day), vitamin B-complex (50 mg at night), chromium (1 tablet/2x per day), niacin (500 mg/2x per day), vitamin C (1/2 teaspoon/2x per day), kelp (2 tablets as a salt substitute/2x per day), EPA (1,000 mg/2x per day), and taurine (500 mg). In the evening, she continued to take vitamin B complex (50 mg) and zinc (50 mg). On 4/30 her BP was 130/70, and she was without the use of diuretics and her vitamins were reduced gradually without elevation of blood pressure.

6. Fifteen-Year History of Hypertension

A 53-year-old male, five foot eleven, with a 15-year history of hypertension, was taking hydrochlorothiazide (Maxzide), Lopressor (300 mg), prazosin (Minipress, 20 mg), and Zyloprim (300 mg for the treatment of gout) each day. He had a moderate sex drive, drank two cups of coffee a day, and had as many as three to seven drinks per week. His BP was initially 130/85, pulse 66, and weight 209 pounds. He was started on a multivitamin (1 tablet), chromium (2 mcg/2x per day), niacin (400 mg/2x per day), vitamin B6 (500 mg), vitamin C/calcium/magnesium powder (1/2 teaspoon/2x per day), magnesium orotate (2 tablets of 500 mg/2x per day), taurine (2 tablets of 500 mg/2x per day), methionine (500 mg/2x per day), Mega-EPA (2,000 mg/2x per day), and zinc gluconate (1 tablet/2x per day). Maxzide was changed to every other day, and he was instructed to stop it if lightheadedness developed. He was put on a very low-carbohydrate diet that consisted primarily of protein and vegetables. On 5/6 he returned with BP of 118/78, pulse of 60, and weight of 196 pounds, During that period, Lopressor had been reduced to 100 mg twice a day, Minipress to 5 mg twice a day, and Maxzide was stopped based on BP readings that the patient had done at home on his machine. On 5/6 vitamin C was reduced due to diarrhea, but the other supplements were virtually the same but with general increases or additions of chromium (2 tablets of 200 mcg/2x per day), a multivitamin (2x per day), niacin (400 mg/3x per day), selenium (200 mcg), magnesium orotate (1 tablet, reduced due to diarrhea), Mega-EPA (3,000 mg/2x per day), primrose

oil (2x per day), and zinc (15 mg in morning, 30 mg in evening). On 5/27 the patient returned with BP of 120/80 and weight at 188. Most of the supplements remained the same with exception of the following. The patient had now gradually reduced Minipress to 5 mg per day, Lopressor to 100 mg every other day, methionine (100 mg/2x per day), niacin (2 tablets per day), chromium (2 tablets per day), and magnesium oxide was stopped due to diarrhea. To this regimen was added lithium (1 tablet in the evening), tryptophan (500 mg/2x per day), and an increase in the multivitamin to twice per day. On 6/25 the patient returned with weight of 184, BP of 110/80, and pulse 75. He was now put on a lower dosage of 50 mg of Lopressor per day. On 7/15 the patient was drug free and BP of 120/180 consistently over multiple readings.

7. Getting Off Diuretics

A 65-year-old female, five foot six, with a long history of hypertension, who had been treated with diuretics, with BP 170/110, pulse 102, weight 170, triglycerides 70, cholesterol 234, HDL 65, was presented to us and was placed on a low-carbohydrate diet and supplement regimen. This included chromium (1 tablet/2x per day), time-release niacin (1,000 mg/2 tablets at night), vitamin B6 (500 mg/1x morning), vitamin E (400 mg/2x per day), vitamin A (25,000 IU/1x morning), selenium (200 mcg/1x morning), EPA (3,000 mg/1x morning; 2,000 mg/ noon; 3,000 mg/evening) tyrosine (2,000 mg/morning), methionine (1,000 mg/morning), dolomite (2 tablets at bedtime), and zinc-manganese supplement (1 tablet/2x per day). The patient returned on 1/21 with BP 152/90, with a weight of 164, and was put on EPA and primrose oil (1,000 each/2x per day), vitamin C (2,500 mg/2x per day , safflower oil (1 teaspoon/2x per day). She then returned on 4/15 with BP 110/85 without medication, pulse 78, and weight of 162. Her BP is well controlled on this regimen and her caffeine consumption has been stopped.

8. Formerly Treated with Dyazide and Lopressor

A 45-year-old female, five foot five, treated with hydrochlorothiazide/triamterene (Dyazide) and metroprolol (Lopressor), had a BP of 130/80, weight 105, triglycerides 115, and cholesterol 178. She started with a multivitamin (1 tablet per day), chromium (200 mcg/1x morning), time-release niacin (400 mg/2x per day), vitamin B6 (500 mg/1x morning), methionine (500 mg/2x per day), tryptophan (1,000 mg before sleep), taurine (500 mg/1x morning), primrose oil (1,500 mg/2x per day), EPA (1,000 mg/2x per day), bone meal (1 tablet/2x per day), and zinc (15 mg/2x per day), Dyazide was reduced to two a day and one the next, and Lopressor was stopped. On 8/1 she was taking Lopressor every other day as well as Dyazide, with essentially the same regimen of vitamins. By 11/12 her BP was 110/80, pulse 80, and weight 109. She was off all BP medication. In sum, this patient highlights the growing effect of nutrients over time, with very little change in her diet except for the reduction of fried foods, caffeine, and white flour.

9. Taken Off Diuretics

A 59-year-old man, five foot eight, weighing 227, on hydrochlorothiazide (Maxzide) for 10 years, was presented to us with BP 120/90, pulse 60, triglycerides 298, and cholesterol 173. He was started on chromium (200 mcg/2x per day), vitamin C (500 mg/2x per day), vitamin B complex (500 mg/1x morning), beta-carotene (50 mg), selenium (200 mcg/1x morning), EPA (1,000 mg/2x per day), cysteine (100 mg/2x per day), dolomite (2 tablets/2x per day) pm, and a zinc-manganese supplement (1 tablet/2x per day). He was put on a high-vegetable, low-fruit, low-carbohydrate diet, and Maxzide was changed to 1 tablet every other day. He was put on safflower oil (2 teaspoons/2x per day) and taken off caffeine beverages. Due to lightheadedness, the patient had to stop Maxzide shortly thereafter. On 12/18 his BP was 120/90 without a diuretic, and his weight was up to 238. Vitamins were kept the same except for EPA, which was increased to 4,000 mg (2x per day), and taurine was started at 500 mg (2x per day). On 3/17 his triglycerides were normal at 153, with cholesterol of 176, and the HDL fraction was improved. By 5/14 his BP was 120/80, and his pulse was 60 without medication. His weight is

227, and he still continues to do well without medication, diuretic free, with reducing the vitamins by half the dose.

10. Ten-Year History of Hypertension

A 56-year-old female, five foot ten, and a 10-year history of hypertension. She drank one to two cups of coffee a day and was presented to us with a BP of 160/90, pulse 80, weight 185, triglycerides 154, and cholesterol 233, while taking one hydrochlorothiazide/triamterene (Dyazide) daily. She was started on a multivitamin (1 tablet per day), chromium (1 tablet/2x per day), time-release niacin (400 mg), vitamin B6 (500 mg/1x morning), taurine (500 mg 2x per day), Mega-EPA (1,000 mg/2x per day), magnesium oxide (1 tablet/2x per day), and primrose oil (1,000 mg/2x per day). She was presented on 5/20 with a BP of 140/84, after having stopped diuretics, with a weight of 181 pounds. She had not even begun magnesium or niacin. Later, she added this treatment and her BP was 120/80 and is well controlled.

11. On Diuretics for Twenty Years

An 80-year-old female, four foot eleven, on diuretics for 20 years, drinking four cups of coffee daily, had a BP of 200/98, pulse of 88, and weight of 114. She was started on a daily regimen of multivitamins, vitamin B6 (500 mg), calcium pantothenate (2,000 mg), zinc (1 tablet), manganese (1 tablet), magnesium orotate (3,000 mg), calcium orotate (1,500 mg), taurine (3,000 mg), and tyrosine and dhyphenylalanine (3 tablets each). On 1/23 her BP was 180/90, pulse 78, and she was removed from diuretics. Medication was changed to four multivitamins per day, calcium (1,000 mg), zinc (15 mg/2x per day), manganese was stopped, evening primrose oil (2,000 mg) was added, vitamin C (3,000 mg), and fish oil as EPA (2,000 mg). On 2/20 her BP was 174/80, pulse 76, and weight was stable at 113. Taurine was reduced to 1,000 mg, evening primrose oil increased to 3,500 mg, vitamin C increased to 5,000 mg, and fish oil to 3,000 mg. On 3/21 her BP was 150/90, pulse 76, and weight was 116. One tablespoon of safflower oil was added with magnesium (1,000 mg). On 4/18 her BP was 150/80, pulse 76, and weight 114.

■ CONCLUSION

In summary, it appears that meganutrient therapy can replace much drug treatment, although there may be some difficulty in the age group of 75 and older, due to a more advanced stage of the disease, and in individuals who are taking two or more drugs. Catching the disease early and treating with the orthomolecular approach is the best answer. Treating hypertension can be an art and can require thyroid function tests, 24-hour free cortisol/renal scan, intravenous pyelography (IVP), 24-hour urine steroids, and plasma renin for the patients who do not respond to either drug or nutrient regimens. At this point we have had an extremely high success rate using meganutrients, which have emphasized large dosages of magnesium (particularly in oxide form), large dosages of EPA (up to 7,000 mg), large dosages of evening primrose oil (2,000–3,000 mg), safflower oil, vitamin-B complex (500 mg), niacin (up to 2,000 mg), taurine (up to 3,000 mg), methionine (up to 1,000 mg), zinc (up to 60 mg), and garlic (up to 1,500 mg).

Although the number of nutrients replacing drugs can be an enormous amount, we have seen no significant side effects other than diarrhea from taking large doses of vitamin C and/or magnesium. Patients claim to feel better, do better, feel good about being drug free, and have far fewer side effects than any other regimen so far reported. Orthomolecular treatment of hypertension through diet and nutrients has arrived as a documented and successful approach.

REFERENCES

1. Patki SS, Singh Jagmeer, Gokhale SV, et al. Efficacy of potassium and magnesium in essential hypertension: ad double blind, placebo controlled, crossover study. *BMJ* 1990;301:521–523.

2. Goldenberg K, Tomlinson FK. Use of a predictor for total body potassium content: application to nutrition and hypertension. *Journal of Medicine* 1988;19:215–227.

3. Saito K, Hattori K, Omatsu T, et al. Effects of oral magnesium on blood pressure and red cell sodium transport in patients receiving long-term, thiazide diuretics for hypertension. *Am J Hypertens* 1988;1:71S–74S.

4. Boulos BM, Smolinski AV. Alert to users of calcium supplements as antihypertensive agents due to trace metal contaminants. *Am J Hypertens* 1988;137S–142S.

5. Weber MA, Cheung DG, Graettinger WF, et al. Characterization of antihypertensive therapy by whole-day blood pressure monitoring. *JAMA* 1988;259:3281–3282.

6. Eid H, Champlain JD. Effects of chronic dietary lithium on phosphatidylinositol pathway in heart and arteries of DOCA-salt hypertensive rats. *Am J Hypertens* 1988;1:64–66.

7. Kesteloot H, Joosens JV. Belgian Interuniversity research on nutrition and health relationship of dietary sodium, potassium, calcium, and magnesium with blood pressure. *Hypertension* 1988;12:594–599.

8. Koopman H, Spreeuwenberg C, Westerman RF, et al. Dietary treatment of patients with mild to moderate hypertension in a general practice: a pilot intervention study. (2) Beyond three months. *J Hum Hypertens* 1990;4:372–374.

9. Koopman H, Spreeuwenbeg C, Westerman RF, et al. Dietary treatment of patients with mild to moderate hypertension in a general practice: a pilot intervention study. *J Hum Hypertens* 1990;4:368–371.

10. Spence DJ, Manuck SB, Munoz C, et al. Hemodynamic and endocrine effects of mental stress in untreated borderline hypertension. *Am J Hypertens* 1990;3:859–860.

11. Troisi JR, Weiss ST, Segal RM, et al. The relationship of body fat distribution to blood pressure in normontensive men: the Normative Aging Study. *Int J Obesity* 1990;14:515–525.

12. Iacono JM, Dougherty RM, Puska P. Dietary fat and blood pressure in humans. *Klin Wochenschr* 1990;68:23–32.

13. Levinson PD, Iosiphidis AH, Saritelli AL, et al. Effects of n-3 fatty acids in essential hypertension. *Am J Hypertens* 1990;3:754–760.

14. Seelig CB, Neb O. Magnesium deficiency in two hypertensive patient groups. *Magnesium Deficiency* 1990;83:739–742.

15. Sauter A, Rudin M. Calcium antagonists for reduction of brain damage in stroke. *J Cardiovasc Pharm* 1990;15:S43–S47.

16. Jula A, Ronnemaa T, Rastas M, et al. Long-term nonpharmacological treatment for mild to moderate hypertension. *J Intern Med* 1990;227:413–421.

17. Digiesi V, Cantini F, Brodbeck B. Effect of coenzyme Q on essential arterial hypertension. *Curr Therap Res* 1990;47:841–845.

18. Mills DE, Prkachin KM, Harvey KA, et al. Dietary fatty acid supplementation alters stress reactivity and performance in man. *J Hum Hypertens* 1989;3:111–116.

19. Hui R, St. Louis J, Falardeau P. Antihypertensive properties of linoleic acid and fish oil omega-3 fatty acids independent of the prostaglandin system. *Am J Hypertens* 1989;2:610.

20. Picketing TG, et al. How common is white coat hypertension? *JAMA* 1988;259:225–228.

21. Drayer J. The future of ambulatory blood pressure monitoring primary care technology. *May–June*, 1985.

22. Dipette DJ, Greilich PE, Nickols GA, et al. Effect of dietary calcium supplementation on blood pressure and calciotropic hormones in mineralocorticoid-salt hypertension. *J Hypertens* 1990;8:515–516.

23. Salvaggio A, Periti M, Miano L, et al. Association between habitual coffee consumption and blood pressure levels. *J Hypertens* 1990;8:585–586.

24. Steiner A, Oertel R, Battig B, et al. Effect of fish oil on blood pressure and serum lipids in hypertension and hyperlipidaemia. *J Hypertens* 1989;7:S73–S76.

25. Ashry AE, Heagerty AM, Ollerenshaw JD, et al. The effect of dietary linoleic acid on blood pressure and erythcyte sodium transport. *J Hum Hypertens* 1989;3:9–15.

26. Baksi SN, Abhold RH, speth RC: Low-calcium diet increases blood pressure and alters peripheral but not central angiotensin II binding sites in rats. 1989;7:423–424.

27. Trachtman H, Del Pizzo R, Rao P, et al. Taurine lowers blood pressure in the spontaneously hypertensive rat by a catecholamine independent mechanism. Am *J Hypertens* 1989;2:909–912.

28. Oberman A, Wassertheil-Smoller S, Langford HG, et al.: Pharmacologic and nutritional treatment of mild hypertension: changes in cardiovascular risk status. *Ann Intern Med* 1990;112:89–95.

29. Treiber FA, Musante L, Riley W, et al. The relationship between hostility and blood pressure in children. *Behavioral Medicine* 1989;173–178.

30. Rouse IL, Beilin LJ, Armstrong BK, et al. Vegetarian diet, blood pressure and cardiovascular risk. *Aust NZ J Med* 1989; 14:439–443.

31. Kaplan NM. The potential benefits of nonpharmacological therapy. Am *J Hypertens* 1990;3:425–427.

32. El Zein M, Areas JL, Knapka J, et al. Excess sucrose and glucose ingestion acutely elevate blood pressure in spontaneously hypertensive rats. Am *J Hypertens* 1990;3:380–386.

33. Pollare T, Lithe H, Berne C. Insulin resistance is a characteristic feature of primary hypertension independent of obesity. *Metabolism* 1990;39(2):167–174.

34. Geiger H, Bahner U, Heidland A. Does cadmium contribute to the development of renal parenchymal hypertension? *Journal of Artificial Organs* 1989;12(11):733–737.

35. Grimm RH Jr, et al. The influence of oral potassium chloride on blood pressure in hypertensive men on a low sodium diet. *N Engl J Med* 1990;322(9).

36. Kaplan NM, Ram CVS. Potassium supplements for hypertension. *N Engl J Med* 1990;322(9).

37. Dawson JA, et al. HIV in intravenous drug users. *N Engl J Med* 1990;322(9).

38. Cappuccio FP, Siani A, Strazzullo P. Oral calcium supplementation and blood pressure: an overview of randomized controlled trials. *J Hypertens* 1989;7:941–946.

39. Rinner MD, Spliet-van Lar L, Kromhout D. Serum sodium, potassium, calcium and magnesium and blood pressure in a Dutch population. *J Hypertens* 1989;7:977–981.

40. Lawton WJ, Fitz, AE, Anderson EA, et al. Effect of dietary potassium on blood pressure, renal function, muscle sympathetic nerve activity, and forearm vascular resistance and flow in normotensive and borderline hypertensive humans. *Circulation* 1990;81:173–184.

41. Marraccini P, Palombo C, Giaconi S, et al. Reduced cardiovascular efficiency and increased reactivity during exercise in borderline and established hypertension. Am *J Hypertens* 1989;2:913–916.

42. Hoffman CJ. Does the sodium level in drinking water affect blood pressure levels? *Perspectives in Practice* 1988;88(11):1432–1435.

43. Morris CD, Bennett IS, McCarron DA, et al. Div. of Neph., Oregon Hlth. Sci. Univ., Portland OR. The relationship of blood lead to blood pressure is continuous and grade. *American Society of Hypertension* 1989;2:26A #1101.

44. Lind L, Wengle B, Ljunghall S. Blood pressure is lowered by vitamin D (alphacalcidol) during long-term treatment of patients with intermittent hyperalcaemia: a double-blind, placebo-controlled study. *Current Contents* 1988;16(2):37.

45. Murakami E, Hiwada K, Kokubu T. The role of brain glutathione in blood pressure regulation. *Japanese Circulation Journal* 1988;52:1299–1300.

46. Radack K, Deck C. The effects of omega-3 polyunsaturated fatty acids on blood pressure: a methodologic analysis of the evidence. *J Am Coll Nutr* 1989;8(5):376–385.

47. Bak AA, Grobbee DE. Abstinence from coffee leads to a fall in blood pressure. *J Hypertens* 1989;7(suppl. 6):S260–S261.

48. Stamler R, Stamler J, Gosch FC, et al. Primary prevention of hypertension by nutritional-hygienic means. *JAMA* 1989;262:1801–1807.

49. Luft FC, Miller JZ, Lyle RM, et al. The effect of dietary interventions to reduce blood pressure in normal humans. *J Am Coll Nutr* 1989;8(6):495–503.

50. Abu Hamdan D, Desai H, Sondheimer J, et al. Taste acuity and zinc metabolism in captopril (cp)-treated male hypertensive patients. *American Society of Hypertension*, May 16–21, 1987.

51. Anavekar SN, Drummer OH, Louis WJ, et al. Evaluation of Tertatolol, a New B-adrenoceptor antagonist as an antihypertensive agent. Am *J Hypertens* May 16–21, 1987.

52. Chobanian AV. Antihypertensive therapy in Evolution. *New Eng J Med* 1986;514(26):1701–1702.

53. Kaplan NM. *Hypertension: Understanding Your High Blood Pressure.* New York: JB Lippincott Co, 1984.

54. McCarron DA. Dietary Calcium as an antihypertensive agent. *Nutr Rev* 1984;42(6).

55. Laragh JH. *Disarming a Silent Killer.* Chicago: World Book, 1987, 124–137.

56. Frohlich ED. Hypertension—evaluation and treatment: why and how. *Hypertension* 1986;80(7):28–46.

57. Check WA. Interdisciplinary efforts seek hypertension causes, prevention, therapy in blacks. Medical News and Perspectives. *JAMA* 1986;256(1):11–17.

58. Harburg E, Gleibermann L, Harburg J. Blood pressure and skin color: Maupiti, French Polynesia. *Human Biol* 54(2):283–298.

59. Schachter J, Kuller LH, Perfetti C. Heart rate during the first five years of life: relation to ethnic group (black or white) and to parental hypertension. *Amer J Epidemiol* 1984; 119(4):554–563.

60. Tyroller HA, James SA. Blood pressure and skin color. *Amer J Pub Health* 1978;68(12):1170–1172.

61. Williams L. Stress of adapting to white society cited as major cause of hypertension in blacks. *Wall Street J* May, 28, 1986, 1.

62. Daughterty SA, Berman R, Entwisle G et al. Cerebrovascular events in the hypertension detection and follow-up program. *Prog Cardiovas Dis* 1986;Suppl. 1:63–72.

63. Doheny K. Hypertension: no longer just an adult disease. *Nutr Health Rev* Spring 1986:7.

64. Golan M, Barav Z, Levin N. Nutritional status of the elderly. Program and Abstracts. 2nd International Conference on Diet and Nutrition. Jerusalem, 14–16 September 1986.

65.Weigley ES: Nutrition and the older primigravida. *J Am Diet Assoc* 1982;82(5):529–530.

66. Burch PRJ. Blood pressure and mortality in the very old. *Lancet* 1983:852.

67. Davidman M and Opsahl J. Mechanisms of elevated blood pressure in human essential hypertension. *Med Clin N Amer* 1984;68(2):301–320.

68. Bravo EL. Secondary hypertension: a streamlined approach to diagnosis. *Postgrad Med* 1986;80(1):139–151.

69. Messereli FH: Essential hypertension: matching pathophysiology and pharmacology. *Postgrad Med* 1987;81(2):165–180.

70. Bass MJ. Effective management of Hypertension. *Med Aspects Human Sesual* 1987:171.

71. Dimitriou R, De Gaudemaris R, Debru JL, et al. Data on the echocardiogram, pressure profile during exertion, and ambulatory blood pressure measurements in borderline arterial hypertension. *Arch Mai Coeur* 1977;11:1162–1166.

72. Curb JD, Maxwell MH, Schneider KA, et al. Adverse effects of antihypertensive medications in the Hypertension Detection and Follow-up Program. *Prog Cardiovas Dis* 1986;29(3):73–88.

73. Middleton RSW. Anti-hypertensive therapy in the elderly and its effects on cerebral function. *Mech Age Devel* 1984;28:229–236.

74. Gifford RW. Statement on hypertension in the elderly. *JAMA* 1986;256(1):71–74.

75. Jansen PAF, Schulte BPM, Meyboom RHB, et al. Antihypertensive treatment as a possible cause of stroke in the elderly. *Age and Ageing* 1986;15(3):129–138.

76. Weaver GA. Do antihypertensive agents cause chronic pancreatitis? *Clin Gastroenterology* 1987;9(1):8.

77. Frohlich ED. Initial therapy for hypertension. *Hospital Practice* 1987:89–96.

78. Sahler CP. Antihypertensive therapy and quality of life. *New Eng J Med* 1987;52:1.

79. Labarthe DR. Mild hypertension: the questions of treatment. *Ann Rev Public Health* 1986;7:193–215.

80. Croog SH, et al. The effects of antihypertensive therapy on the quality of life. *New Eng J Med* 1986;314:1657–1664.

81. Schoenberg JA. Mild hypertension: the rationale for treatment. *Amer Heart J* 1986;112(4):872–876.

82. Ames RP. Coronary heart disease and the treatment of hypertension: impact of diuretics on serum lipids and glucose. *J Cardiovas Pharmacol* 1984;6:S466–S473.

83. Reyes AJ and Leary WP. Diuretics and magnesium. *Magnesium Bulletin* Apr 1984:87.

84. Morgan T, Adam W, Hodgson M. Adverse Reactions to Long-Term Diuretic Therapy for Hypertension. *J Cardiovas Pharmacol* 1984;6:S269–S273.

85. Weinberger MH. Antihypertensive therapy and lipids. *Arch Intern Med* 1985;145:1102.

86. Kaplan NM. Problems with the use of diuretics in the treatment of hypertension. *Amer J Nephrol* 1986;6(l):l–5.

87. Papademetriou V, Price M, Johnson E, et al. Early changes in plasma and urinary potassium in diuretic-treated patients with systemic hypertension. *Amer J Cardiol* 1986;48:12D–15D.

88. Phan HT. Hypertension, part II: treatment with diuretics. *Dialysis and Transplantation Today* Oct 1986:573–580.

89. Pickering TG. Pathophysiology of systemic hypertension. *Amer J Cardiol* 1986;58:12D–15D.

90. Petri M, Cumber P, Grimes L, et al. The method effects of thiazide therapy in the elderly: a population study. *Age and Ageing* 1986;15(3):150–156.

91. Dyckner T, Wester PO. Effect of magnesium on blood pressure. *Brit Med J* 1983;286:1857–1849.

92. McKenney JM, Goodman RP, Wright JT, et al. The effect of low-dose hydrochlorothiazide on blood pressure, serum potassium, and lipoproteins. *Pharmacology* 1986;6(4):179–184.

93. Freis ED: The cardiovascular risks of thiazide diuretics. *Clin Pharmacol Therapeut* 1986; 39(3):239–243.

94. Hollifield JW. Thiazide treatment of hypertension: effects of thiazide diuretics on serum potassium, magnesium, and ventricular ectopy. *Amer J Med* 1986;80(4A):8–12.

95. Avorn J, Everitt DE, Weiss S. Increased antidepressant use in patients prescribed b-blockers. *JAMA* 1986;255(3):357–360.

96. Chobania AV. Hypertension. *Clinical Symposia* 1982;34(5).

97. Thadani U. Beta blockers in hypertension. 242 nutritional treatments for hypertension. *Amer J Cardiol* 1983;52(9):10D–15D.

98. Veiga RV, Taylor RE. Beta blockers, hypertension, and blacks: is the answer really in? *J Nat Med Assoc* 1986;78(9):851–856.

99. Braverman ER, Pfeiffer CC. Essential trace elements and cancer. *J Orthomolecular Psych* 1982;11(1):28–41.

100. Tarazi RC, Fouad-Tarazzi M. Current therapy, present limitations and future goals for systemic hypertension. *Am J Cardio* 1986;58:3D–7D.

101. Simon G, Wittig VJ, Cohn JN. Transdermal nitroglycerin as a step 3 antihypertensive *Drug Clin Pharm Ther* 1986;40:42–45.

102. Lesser F. The costs of treating high blood pressure. *New Scientist* Jul 1985.

103. Kaplan NM. Non-drug treatment of hypertension. *Ann Intern Med* 1985;103(3):359–373.

104. Grimm RH: Should mild hypertension be treated? *Med Clin N Amer* 1984;68(2):477–490.

105. McAlister NH. Should we treat "mild" hypertension? *JAMA* 1983;249(3):379–382.

106. Amery A, Brixko R, Clement D, et al. Efficacy of antihypertensive drug treatment according to age, sex, blood pressure, and previous cardiovascular disease in patients over the age of 60. *Lancet* 1986:589–592.

107. Dannenberg AL, Kannel WB. Remission of hypertension. *JAMA* 1987;257:1477–1483.

108. Greenberg G. Course of blood pressure in mild hypertensives after withdrawal of long term antihypertensive treatment. *Brit Med J* 1986;293:988–992.

109. *American Medical News*. Dietary changes best for cutting heart disease. Apr 1986, 23.

110. Weinberger MH. Treatment of hypertension in the 1990s. *Amer J Med* 1987;82(Suppl. 1A):44–49.

111. Stamler R, Stamler J, Grimm R, et al. Nutritional therapy for high blood pressure. *JAMA* 1987;257(11):1484–1491.

112. McCarron DA, Morris CD, Henry HJ, et al.: Blood pressure and nutrient intake in the United States. *Science* 1984;224:1392–1398.

113. Tuck ML. The sympathetic nervous system in essential hypertension. *Am Heart J* 1986;112:887.

114. Herman JM. Psychoso matische therapies bei hypertonic. *Munch Med Wschr* 1986;128(49):869–872.

115. M'Buyamba-Kabangu JR, Fagard R, Lijnen P, et al. Blood pressure and urinary cations in urban Bantu of Zaire. *Amer J Epidemiol* 124(6):957–968, 1986.

116. Williams RR, et al. Evidence that men with familial hypercholesterolemia can avoid early coronary death. *J Amer Med Assoc* 1986;255(2):219–224.

117. Zhao GS, Yuan XY, Gong BQ, et al. Nutrition, metabolism, and hypertension: a comparative survey between dietary variables and blood pressure among three nationalities in China. *J Clin Hypertens* 1986;2(2):124–131.

118. Artemov AA. Correlation between chronic non-infectious diseases of the cardiovascular system and nutritional factors. *Ter Arkh* 1985;57(10):117–120.

119. Altmann J, Komhuber AW, Komhuber HH. Stroke: cardiovascular risk factors and the quantitative effects of dietary treatment on them. *Eur Neurol* 1987;26:90–99.

120. Garrison RJ, Kannel WB, Stokes J, et al. Incidence and precursors of hypertension in young adults: the Framingham Offspring Study. *Pre Med* 1987;16:235–251.

121. Dornfeld LP, et al. Obesity and hypertension: long-term effects of weight reductions on blood pressure. *Inter J Obesity* 1985;9:381–389.

122. Fletcher DJ, Rogers DA. Diet and coronary heart disease. *Postgraduate Medicine* 1985;77(5):319–325.

123. Kannel WB. Nutritional contributors to cardiovascular disease in the elderly. *JAGS* 1986;34:27–38.

124. Kritchevsky D. *Atherosclerosis and Nutrition: Advances in Nutritional Research.* London: Plenum Press, 1979.

125. Ullrich IH, Peters PJ, Albrink MJ. Effects of low-carbohydrate diets in either fat or protein on thyroid function, plasma insulin, glucose, and triglycerides in healthy young adults. *J Amer Coll Nutr* 1985;4:451–459.

126. Joffres MR, Reed DM, Yano K. Relationship of magnesium intake and other dietary factors to blood pressure: the Honolulu Heart Study. *Am J Cli. Nutr* 1987;45:469–475.

127. Green EM, Perez GO, Hsia SL, et al. Effect of egg supplements on serum lipids in uremic patients. *J Amer Dietetic Assoc* 1985;85(3):355–357.

128. Pfeiffer CC. *Mental and Elemental Nutrients.* New Canaan, CT: Keats Publishing, 1975.

129. Blankenhorn DH. Two new diet-heart studies. *New Eng J Med* Mar. 28, 1985.

130. Dyerberg J. Linolenate-derived polyunsaturated fatty acids and prevention of atherosclerosis. *Nutr Rev* 1986;44(4):125–133.

131. Garrone G. Emotions et troubles psychosomatiques cardiovasculaires. *Schweizerischie Medizinische Woshenschrift* 1984;114:1819–1821.

132. Affarah HB, Hall WD, Heymsfield SB, et al. High-carbohydrate Diet: antinatriuretic and blood pressure response in normal men. *Amer J Clin Nutr* 1986;44:341–348.

133. Fregly MJ. Effect of an exercise regimen on development of hypertension in rats. *J Appl Physiol* 1984;56(2):381–387.

134. Woo R, Pi-Sunyer F: Effect of increased physical activity on voluntary intake in lean women. *Metab V* 1985;34:836–841.

135. Paffenbarger RS, et al. Physical activity, all-cause mortality, and longevity of college alumni. *New Eng J Med* 1986;314(10):605–613.

136. Eliasson K, Sjoquist B. Urinary catecholamine metabolites in borderline and established hypertension. *Acta Med Scand* 1984;216:369–375.

137. Masuo K, Ogihara T, Kumahara Y, et al. Increased plasma norepinephrine in young patients with essential hypertension under three sodium intakes. *Hypertens* 1984;6:315–321.

138. Floras JS. Effects of various beta-blockers on hypertension. *Cardiology Board Rev* 1986;3(2):83–90.

139. Gruchow HW, Sobocinski KA, Barboriak JJ, et al. Alcohol, nutrient intake, and hypertension in U.S. adults. *JAMA* 1985;253(11):1567–1570.

140. Sacks FM, Marais GE, Handysides G, et al. Lack of an effect of dietary saturated fat and cholesterol on blood pressure in normotensives. *Hypertension* 1984;6:193–198.

141. Smith MC, Dunn MJ. The role of prostaglandins in human hypertension. *Hypertension and the Kidney: Proceedings of a Symposium*, 1985.

142. Iacono JM et a. Studies on the effects of dietary fat on blood pressure. *An Clin Res* 1984;16(4):116–125.

143. Mogenson GJ, Box BM. Physiological effects of varying dietary linoleic acid in spontaneously hypertensive rats. *Ann Nutr Metb* 1982;26:232–239.

144. Fletcher DJ, Rogers DA. Diet and coronary heart disease. *Postgraduate Medicine* 1985;77(5):319–325.

145. Singer P, et al. Clinical studies on lipid and blood pressure lowering effect of eicosapentaenoic acid-rich diet. *Biomed Biochim Acta* 1984;43:421–425.

146. Knapp HR, et al. In vivo indexes of platelet and vascular function during fish-oil administration in patients with atherosclerosis. *New Eng J Med* 1986;314:937–942.

147. Nestel PJ. Fish oil accentuates the cholesterol induced rise in lipoprotein cholesterol. *Amer J Clin Nutr* 1986;43:752–757.

148. Blankenhorn DH. Two new diet-heart studies. *New Eng J Med* Mar 28, 1985.

149. Dyerberg J. Linolenate-derived polyunsaturated fatty acids and prevention of atherosclerosis. *Nutr Rev* 1986;44(4):125–133.

150. Vartiainen E, et al. Effects of dietary fat modifications on serum lipids and blood pressure in children. *Acta Paediatr Scand* 1986;75:396–401.

151. Bang HO, Dyerberg J, Nielsen AB. Plasma lipid and lipoprotein pattern in greenlandic west coast Eskimos. *Lancet* 1971;7701(1):1143–1146.

152. Kromhout D, Bosschieter EB, Coulander CL. The inverse relation between fish consumption and 20-year mortality from coronary heart disease. *New Eng J Med* 1985;312(19).

153. Von Lossonczy TO, et al. The effect of a fish diet on serum lipids in healthy human subjects. *Amer J Clinic Nutr* 1978;31:1340–1346.

154. Verheugt FWA, Schouten JA, Eeltink JC, et al. Omega-3 polyunsaturated fatty acids in the treatment of angina pectoris: effect on objective signs of exercise-induced myocardial ischemia. *Current Ther Res* 1986;39(2):208–209.

155. Halberg M. Lipid, not salt control to trim blood pressure? *Hospital Tribune* Oct. 5, 1983.

156. Puska P, et al. Dietary fat and blood pressure: an intervention study on the effects of a low-fat diet with two levels of polyunsaturated fat. *Preventive Medicine* 1985;14:573–584.

157. Norris PG et al. Effect of dietary supplementation with fish oil: systolic blood pressure in milk essential hypertension. *Brit Med J* 1986;293:104–105.

158. O'Brien OMS et al. The effect of dietary supplementation with linoleic acid and linolenic acid on the pressor response to angiotensin ii: a possible role in pregnancy-induced hypertension? *Brit J Pharmacol* 1985;19(3):335–342.

159. Anderson DE. Interactions of stress, salt, and blood pressure. *Annu Rev Physiol.* 1984;46:143–153.

160. Harlan WR, et al. Blood pressure and nutrition in adults: the National Health and Nutrition Examination Survey. *Am L Epidemiol* 1984;120:17–28.

161. Henrotte JG, et al. Blood and urinary magnesium, zinc, calcium, free fatty acids and catecholamines in type A and type B subjects. *J Am Coll Nutr* 185;4(2):165–172.

162. Dakshinamurti K, Paulose CS, Packer S, et al. Hypertension in pyridoxine deficiency. *Hypertens* 1986;4(5): S174–S175.

163. Staessen J, Bulpitt CJ, Roels H, et al. Urinary cadmium and lead concentrations and their relation to blood pressure in a population with low exposure. *Br J Ind Med* 1984;41(2):241–248.

164. Ogawa M, et al. Decrease of plasma sulfur amino acids in essential hypertension. *Jpn Circ J* 1985;49(12):1217–24.

165. Virtamo J, et al. Serum selenium and the risk of coronary heart disease and stroke. *Am J Epidemiol* 1985;122(2):276–82.

NIACIN BEATS STATINS

by Andrew W. Saul, PhD

Cholesterol-lowering statin drugs can produce serious side effects. Statin side effects may include liver damage, elevated CPK (creatine kinase) and/or muscle pain, aches, and muscle tenderness or weakness (myalgia), drowsiness, myositis (inflammation of the muscles), rare but potentially fatal kidney failure from rhabdomyolysis (severe inflammation of muscle and muscle breakdown), memory loss, mental confusion, personality changes or irritability, headaches, insomnia, anxiety, depression, chest pain, high blood sugar and type 2 diabetes, acid regurgitation, dry mouth, digestive problems such as bloating, gas, diarrhea or constipation, nausea and/or vomiting, or abdominal cramping and pain, rash, eye irritation, tremors, dizziness, and more.

What a list. Well, this is America, and you have the right to remain sick. Evidently you also have the right to be continually bombarded with exhortations to take statins, and to give them to your children as well. However, you also have the right to refuse drugs, and you have available nutrition-based alternatives.

Say No to Statins

Here are researchers and physicians who say "no" to statins, and their reasons why:

- W. Todd Penberthy, PhD: "Niacin raises good high-density lipoprotein (HDL) cholesterol more than any known pharmaceutical, while simultaneously lowering total cholesterol, triglycerides, and the most pathogenic form of cholesterol-associated very low-density lipoprotein (VLDL). Niacin is frequently the gold standard control used for basic research experiments using animal models of atherosclerosis. In clinical trials, when niacin has been compared to other marketed drugs it has led to most undesirable effects for business, but most therapeutically beneficial effects for the fortunate patients" (from *Niacin: The Real Story*, Basic Health Publications, 2011).

- Robert G. Smith, PhD: "Although statins can lower cholesterol, they do not greatly reduce the risk of heart disease for most people. A much more effective treatment to prevent heart disease is vitamin C taken to bowel tolerance (3,000–10,000 mg/day in divided doses), vitamin E (400–1,600 IU/day), niacin (800–2,000 mg/day in divided doses), magnesium (300–600 mg/day, divided doses), along with an excellent diet that includes generous servings of leafy green vegetables and only moderate amounts of meat" (pers. comm., 2013).

- **Thomas E. Levy, MD, JD:** "The lower your cholesterol goes, the greater your risk of cancer, as cholesterol is a protective agent against toxins. Efforts to lessen the chances of morbidity and mortality of one major disease (coronary artery disease) should not substantially increase the chances of morbidity and mortality from another disease (cancer)" (pers. comm., 2013).

- **Abram Hoffer, MD, PhD:** "Niacin is effective in decreasing the death rate of patients with cancer by protecting cells and tissues from damage by toxic molecules or free radicals. In the body, niacin is converted to nicotinamide adenine dinucleotide (NAD), used by the body to catalyze the formation of ADP-ribose. When the long chains of DNA are damaged, poly (ADP-ribose) [polymerase] helps repair it by unwinding the damaged protein. Poly (ADP-ribose) [polymerase] also increases the activity of DNA ligase. This enzyme cuts off the damaged strands of DNA and increases the ability of the cell to repair itself after exposure to carcinogens" (from *Niacin: The Real Story*, Basic Health Publications, 2011).

- **Ralph Campbell, MD:** "You have likely heard about the conclusions from Cleveland Clinic gathering of heart specialists. Their objective was to zoom in on low-density lipoprotein (LDL) level as it relates directly to heart disease. No mention of LDL/HDL ratio or of triglyceride levels. Again, niacin got very little recognition. The panel was made up of many with financial ties to industry, but 'it is practically impossible to find a large group of outside experts who have no relationship to industry.' This was followed (yes, actually) by stating the new guidelines are based on solid evidence and that the public should *trust* them" (pers. comm., 2013).

- **Carolyn Dean, MD, ND:** "The mineral magnesium is the natural way that the body has evolved to control cholesterol when it reaches a certain level, whereas statin drugs are used to destroy the whole process. If sufficient magnesium is present in the body, cholesterol will be limited to its necessary functions— the production of hormones and the maintenance of membranes—and will not be produced in excess" (from *The Magnesium Miracle*, Ballantine Books, 2006).

- **Jorge Miranda, PharmD:** "Statin drugs are one of my favorite examples of a sickening drug. A fixation on cholesterol fails to address the importance of correcting the excessive oxidation of LDL and fails to recognize the importance of correcting many other contributing risk factors such as homocysteine, Lp(a), and C-reactive protein. It is important to recognize that the reason we form cholesterol is because it's needed to form cell membranes, the eye's lens, hormones, and many other molecules including coenzyme Q10 (CoQ10), an energy-producing molecule. Decreasing cholesterol decreases CoQ10, which means less energy for a multitude of functions. The result can be neurologic disease and even cancer" (pers. comm., 2013).

- **William B. Grant, PhD:** "Statin use reduces CoQ10 concentrations and leads to myopathy (muscle weakness), which can lead to heart failure. Those taking statins should be aware of this problem and consider taking CoQ10 supplements" (pers. comm., 2013).

- **Damien Downing, MBBS, MSB:** "Statins overall succeed in reducing the risk of coronary events by about 17 percent—but that is *relative* risk. Taking a statin each day actually lowers one's chance of an event by about 0.16 percent—that is the absolute risk. But these figures are not lives saved; recent meta-analysis found only a non-significant reduction in mortality of 7 per 10,000 patient-years, or 0.07 percent. The difference between statins' effects on relative risk and absolute risk is about two orders of magnitude. Just ask any person in the street whether a reduction of 0.16 percent in the risk of a coronary event is 'significant,' and whether it warrants taking statins. Unpleasant muscular side effects occur in up to 10 percent of statin-takers, which may rise to 25 percent if the person exercises; this is unhelpful to anybody seeking to improve their cardiovascular health. But because the primary threshold for acceptance under 'evidence-based medicine' is statistical significance, we are to accept that the benefit of statins has been proven. Data on worldwide sales of statins currently run at approximately $30 billion per year" (pers. comm., 2013).

Perhaps this helps explain the massive media blitz favoring statins. But drugs are not the answer, unless you are a drug company.

Excerpted from the *Orthomolecular Medicine News Service*, November 14, 2013.

THE ROLE OF HOMOCYSTEINE IN HUMAN HEALTH
by K. J. McLaughlin, DC

For the last two decades, the modus operandi of most health-care providers managing their patients with atherosclerosis was to prescribe cholesterol-lowering drugs. It would seem that this essential sterol has been inadvertently implicated for the epidemic of atherosclerotic and thromboembolic disease, which has permeated our society and overburdened our health-care system.

The most popular pharmaceutical management tool has been the statin class of cholesterol-lowering drugs. These drugs are HMG-CoA reductase inhibitors and function to interfere with cholesterol syntheses in the liver.[1] These drugs are widely prescribed to treat heart disease with the underlying presumption being that cholesterol is the definitive cause of coronary artery stenosis (narrowing of the coronary arteries). Despite their questionable safety and the fact they deplete the myocardium (heart muscle) of coenzyme Q10 (potentially increasing the risk of cardiac mortality), they continue to be one of the most frequently prescribed drugs. As the body of evidence regarding this controversial subject in cardiac management has continued to expand, clinicians are considering other factors that may be more important with regard to prevention and management of cardiovascular disease. Some of these concepts relate to the inappropriate intake or metabolism of fatty acids, endogenous or exogenous lipid peroxidation, lipid or triglyceride reactivity to dietary stimuli, unchallenged free-radical activity, and various nutrient deficiencies. The most frequently cited of which include vitamin C, vitamin E, coenzyme Q10, magnesium, carotenoids, selenium, L-carnitine, zinc, and B-complex nutrients. Subclinical deficiencies of these nutrients are more prevalent than previously realized, and they all subsequently play an important role in human health in many different ways.

Importance of Homocysteine

In recent years, another important element in the genesis of atherosclerotic vascular disease has become manifest, that being elevated serum levels of homocysteine. The role of homocysteine as a causative factor in the development of vascular pathology was proposed by Dr. Kilmer McCully in 1969.[2] Homocystinuria, the rare genetic disorder frequently associated with advanced occlusive arterial disease (widespread atherosclerosis), elevated plasma homocysteine levels, and premature death from advanced cardiovascular disease, was used to link elevated homocysteine levels to vascular pathology.[3] This disease was known to be caused by an inherent lack of enzymic activity in the liver (cystathione synthetase), which is required to metabolize homocysteine into less harmful metabolites.[4]

Homocysteine is a sulfur-containing amino acid and a direct metabolic byproduct of methionine metabolism. Homocysteine is typically measured as serum total homocysteine. However, this measurement also accounts for the oxidized components, homocysteine and cysteine-homocysteine. Total protein or methionine intakes may not correlate to blood levels of homocysteine. However, a single dose of methionine (100 milligrams per kilogram [mg/kg] of body weight) has been shown to elevate homocysteine levels and is frequently utilized to assess homocysteine metabolism.[5] Normal fasting plasma homocysteine levels are considered to be between 5 and 15 micromoles per liter (μM/L). Hyperhomocysteinemia is considered when the concentrations of homocysteine are above 15 μM/L.[6]

There are several key nutrients that function as cofactors in the metabolism of methionine and homocysteine. Folic acid and cyanocobalamin (vitamin B12) directly affect the activity of the enzymes methylenetetrahydrofolate reductase and methionine synthase. Pyridoxine (vitamin B6) is a cofactor for the enzyme cystathionine-B-synthase. These metabolic pathways control the accumulation of homocysteine, which has a deleterious effect upon vascular endothelial cells. Errors in this enzymic cascade may be due to a mutated gene,

From the *J Orthomolecular Med* 2001;16(1):33–39.

which has been identified by Dr. Rima Rosen of McGill University, but, more commonly, errors in homocysteine metabolism are closely linked to deficiencies in specific nutrients, particularly vitamins B6, B12, and folic acid.[2] Like cholesterol, homocysteine is necessary to the human organism; if the appropriate cofactors are present it will convert to cysteine, adenosine triphosphate (ATP), and S-adenosylmethionine (SAMe).

Homocysteine and Development of Cardiovascular Disease

Some speculation has arisen regarding limiting the intake of protein foods high in methionine. Not only is this idea inappropriate because of the importance of methionine in protein or amino acid metabolism (cartilage, carnitine, taurine), but this solution does not address the underlying problem of excessive homocysteine accumulation, which is attributable to deficiencies in key nutrients, necessary for its enzymatic conversion. The relationship between homocysteine and B vitamins is quite close. In fact, it has been suggested that homocysteine levels could reliably be used as a physiological marker to evaluate nutrient status.[2] This relationship and how it relates to cardiovascular disease is also very revealing. The use of synthetic hormones, smoking, and alcohol deplete tissue stores of vitamins B6, B12, and folic acid. It would subsequently not be surprising that these groups would have higher levels of homocysteine and a concurrent increased incidence of heart disease. Elevated levels of homocysteine have been identified in 21 percent of patients with coronary artery disease (atherosclerosis of the coronary arteries), 24 percent of patients with cerebrovascular disease (atherosclerosis of the cerebral arteries), and 32 percent of patients with peripheral vascular pathology (atherosclerosis in the arteries in the arms and legs). Some researchers have indicated that homocysteine levels are up to 40 times more predictive than total serum cholesterol in assessing cardiovascular disease risk.[2]

Homocysteine is thought to be one of the early factors predisposing one to the development of the atherosclerotic lesion by injuring vascular endothelium.[7] Typical studies have indicated that patients with arterial occlusive disease and hyperhomocysteinemia show elevated levels of endothelium-derived proteins such as thrombomodulin, von Willebrand factor, and tissue-type plasminogen activator.[7] These proteins are secreted by damaged endothelial cells resulting from constant free-radical exposure produced by homocysteine. Many of these studies have used various B vitamins to lower homocysteine and endothelium-derived proteins.[7] Other studies have directly linked low levels of B nutrients to homocysteinemia and low levels of tissue folate to increased coronary artery risk.[8] Other reports have linked elevated homocysteine levels with an increased, independent risk of atherogenesis and thromboembolism.[9,10] Studies have linked homocysteine with the promotion of lipid peroxidation, interference with platelet aggregation, and fibrin metabolism.[11]

Certainly, circulating plasma lipids play an important role in the development of atherosclerotic lesions. Oxidation of intra- or extracellular endothelial low-density lipoproteins (LDLs) is known to be one of the earliest lesions that develops in endothelial tissue.[17] It has also been postulated that homocysteine enhances lipoprotein(a) adherence to fibrin, an inherent mechanism by which damaged endothelium tries to repair itself.[12] Endothelial tissue continuously secretes nitric oxide, which relaxes the smooth muscle cells that line the vascular wall. Damaged endothelial cells can also secrete vasoconstrictor factors (endothelin-1) and factors that affect the growth of smooth muscle cells, vascular permeability, and vascular adhesive capability.[13] Other reports indicate that hyperhomocysteinemia is associated with impaired endothelium-dependent vasodilation in humans.[14] Some other studies have shown vascular wall damage caused from high homocysteine levels attributable to increased endothelial levels of thiolactone and low levels of oxidase.[15,16] These factors are associated with higher levels of oxidative stress within endothelial tissue. There are other theories pertaining to the mechanism by which homocysteine inflicts chemical harm upon vascular structures. Another plausible explanation may involve the enhanced secretion of cholesterol and apolipoprotein B (a lipid required to form LDL) following elevated levels of homocysteine.[23] Chronic, elevated levels of homocysteine also have an impact upon cellular methylation reactions involving DNA, RNA, various proteins, and phospholipids. Excessive levels of homocysteine negate the enzyme S-adenosylhomocysteine hydrolase, which causes excessive binding of S-adenosylhomocysteine to active cellular methyltransferase sites.[18]

Regulating Homocysteine

There exists a multitude of evidence to indicate that high levels of homocysteine are a major risk factor in the development of vascular pathology.[19–23] There is also a great deal of evidence to suggest that the addition of vitamins B6 (100 mg), B12 (1 mg), and folate (5–15 mg) to the diet in a supplement form can normalize high levels of circulating homocysteine. Studies indicate that test subjects are frequently deficient in the essential nutrients that regulate homocysteine metabolism.[24–29] Using supplements such as B vitamins (B6, B12, folate) and trimethylglycine, which remethylates homocysteine into methionine and S-adenosylmethionine, is clinically prudent. Choline and zinc are also required to remethylate homocysteine and should also be considered.[30–34]

Plasma concentrations of homocysteine increase with age, male gender, impaired renal function, nutrient deficiency, and genetic factors. The odds ratio for coronary artery disease has been estimated to be 1.4 for every (.5 µmol/L) increase in total plasma homocysteine.[35] That confers a 6–7 percent increase in risk for having a stroke or heart attack for every 1 µmol/L increase in total homocysteine.[36] With an increase in each tertile intake of vitamins B6, B12, and folate, a concomitant decrease in homocysteine of .4–.7 µmol/L is produced.[37] This chemical relationship has caused an interest in increasing vitamin fortification of our current food supply, more specifically with folic acid.[38]

There have been several large studies indicating that elevated homocysteine levels can lead to vascular disease. A large, European trial, published in the June 1997 *Journal of the American Medical Association* indicated that adults had 2.2 times higher risk of developing vascular disease if their plasma homocysteine levels were in the top one-fifth of the normal range compared with those in the bottom four-fifths. This risk was independent of other risk factors but was higher in smokers and those with hypertension. A Norwegian study, which appeared in the July 1997 *New England Journal of Medicine*, indicated that the risk of death in patients with coronary artery disease was proportional to plasma total homocysteine levels. The risk rose from 3.8 percent in those with the lowest levels (below 9 µmol/L) to 24.7 percent with the highest levels (above 15 µmol/L). These studies and many more like them indicate the need for regular testing for homocysteine levels so that appropriate risk factors can be properly assessed. Total plasma homocysteine status may also be used as a sensitive tool to assess red blood cell folate status.[35]

Professor Rene Malinow from the Oregon Regional Primate Research Center has stated in his study published in the *New England Journal of Medicine* that folic acid intake (between .2 and 5 mg per day) may be necessary to lower homocysteine levels and prevent an estimated 50,000 heart attacks per year in the United States. Dr. Malinow indicated that levels of vitamin fortification need to be at levels higher than the current government recommendation. Food and Drug Administration (FDA) guidelines for nutrient quantity were found to be insufficient at lowering homocysteine levels. A level of at least 0.4 mg (400 micrograms) of folic acid per day is considered the minimum dose required.

It has been estimated that a 25 percent reduction in homocysteine can be achieved with mean supplementation of .5–5.7 mg of folic acid, and an additional 7 percent reduction has been observed after the addition of vitamin B12 (.02–1 mg/day, mean .5 mg).[36] Other studies have shown that vitamin B6 can reduce homocysteine levels following a methionine load by 25 percent, and 22 percent utilizing dosages of 50–250 mg per day.[37–42] A combination of nutrients including folic acid, vitamin B6, and vitamin B12 was very effective at reducing homocysteine levels in patients with moderate or intermediate hyperhomocysteinemia.[43] However, increasing vitamin intake from food sources (1 mg of folic acid, 12.2 mg of B6, and 50 mcg of B12 per day) did not maintain normalized homocysteine levels previously attained by supplements.[44] The daily use of fortified cereals containing 499 and 650 mcg of folic acid per serving and the RDA of other vitamins reduced homocysteine by 11 percent and 14 percent, respectively.[45] Observational studies have indicated that the users of multivitamin supplements have lower homocysteine levels and also have higher concentrations of plasma folic acid, and vitamins B6 and B12 than non-users.[46]

The relationship between homocysteine and protein intake is rather obscure. A University of Iowa study indicated that high levels of protein in the diet can elevate homocysteine levels by increasing the methionine load. (Methionine, an essential amino acid, is not synthesized in the body and so must be obtained from food sources or supplements.) Dr. William Haynes indicated that increasing levels of methionine accompanied by a diet low in folic acid may cause blood vessel dysfunction. Haynes also stated the effect of vitamin C on large and small vessel function following methionine load. The addition of 2,000 mg of vitamin C rapidly improved large and small vessel function. Other reports have not supported this relationship between protein consumption and homocysteine levels.[47]

There are various methods by which homocysteine levels are controlled within the body. The most common pathway is the remethylation process by which methyl groups (CH3) are donated to homocysteine to ultimately produce methionine and S-adenosylmethionine. This can be accomplished by using trimethylglycine (betaine) (500–9,000 mg/day), vitamin B12 (1,000–3,000 mcg/day), folic acid (800–5,000 mcg/day), and zinc (30–90 mg/day). Choline is also considered a methyl donor, but it does not require the other nutrients to methylate homocysteine. Choline only functions as a methyl donor in the liver and kidneys, not in other organs such as the brain and heart.[48]

The other pathway involves trans-sulfuration of homocysteine into cysteine and glutathione. This pathway is dependent upon adequate levels of vitamin B6. The subsequent levels of vitamin necessary to control homocysteine are dependent upon other nutrient levels (folate and B12) and methionine intake. Supplementation with vitamin B6 (100–600 mg) per day is usually adequate. Those requiring greater amounts may have a genetic deficiency in the cystathionine-B synthase enzyme, which regulates the trans-sulfuration pathway.[48] At the University of Michigan, Dr. Rowena Matthews discovered how folates lower high homocysteine levels. Her findings indicated that folic acid assists the binding of flavin adeninedinucleotide (FAD) to the enzyme methylenetetrahydrofolate reductase. This enzyme is essential in catalyzing the conversion of homocysteine to methionine. Trimethylglycine is thought to stimulate activity of the enzyme betaine-homocysteine methyltransferase in the liver.[49]

The risk of stroke or heart attack is increased following mild elevations in homocysteine. It appears that there is no "safe" normal range of homocysteine concentration. Studies indicate that homocysteine levels above 6.3 µmol/L cause a steep, progressive increased risk of heart attack. A study published in the *American Journal of Epidemiology* indicated that each 3-unit increase in homocysteine equates to a 35 percent increase in risk of heart attack.[49] A recent study published in Acta Cardiologica indicated that the average American's homocysteine level is 10 mg µmol/L. It appears a safer range one would want to achieve would be below 6.3 µmol/L of blood.[49] Scientists like Dr. Richard Macko of the Baltimore Veterans Administration Medical Center has indicated the research illustrates that there is a clear risk associated to even small increases in homocysteine levels. Macko found that lowering homocysteine levels with B vitamins decreased levels of markers indicative of vessel wall damage and decreased the risk of stroke and heart attack. A study published in the August 1999 issue of *Stroke* indicated that younger women who had the highest levels of homocysteine had double the increase in risk of stroke compared to women with lower levels. Dr. Steven Kittner, who headed the study indicated that the potential to improve public health and reduce the risk of stroke and other forms of cardiovascular disease by using nutritional intervention is significant. It should also be mentioned that elevated homocysteine levels have been closely linked to altered DNA repair, Alzheimer's disease, chronic fatigue syndrome, and rheumatoid arthritis.[48–49]

In the January 1999 issue of *Circulation*, the American Heart Association Science Advisory urged physicians to begin screening of high-risk patients with a personal or family history of vascular disease. Unfortunately, other than suggesting that people increase their intake of foods high in B vitamins, they did not advise the use of supplements. However, certain physicians like Dr. A. DeMaria, who is the associate editor for *Health News*, recommends that everyone who has heart disease or is at increased risk take a multivitamin supplement containing all the B vitamins. This kind of advice is, unfortunately, rarely given despite the evidence that this inexpensive procedure could save thousands of lives and millions of dollars.

Checking Homocysteine Levels

The advice regarding screening is also contradictory. One report indicated that cases of multiple failed angioplasty are more likely related to high homocysteine levels than elevated LDL. In one such case, although LDL was within normal limits, homocysteine was 30 μmol/L. No wonder this expensive, invasive procedure sometimes proves ineffective. Elevated homocysteine should also be suspected if vascular pathology is apparent and standard blood tests prove unrevealing. Anyone who has cardiovascular disease or is at increased risk should have their homocysteine levels checked annually, especially if they are considering surgery. Patients with a family history of Alzheimer's disease, lupus, diabetes, or other chronic disease are also advised to have their homocysteine levels evaluated. Those who are taking supplements to control or lower homocysteine levels also need to have regular measurements taken to gauge therapeutic efficacy.[50] Appropriate nutritional management including adequate supplement dosages can then be evaluated, and the subsequent benefit maintained.

Although the test for homocysteine is not considered inexpensive, the subsequent reduction in homocysteine from treatment is effective and safe. Therefore, regular screening for elevated homocysteine levels and concurrent treatment with appropriate vitamin supplementation should be considered as one of the most important measures that a clinician could implement to significantly lower the risk of developing potentially life-threatening degenerative disease attributable to chronic homocysteinemia.

REFERENCES

1. Mindell E. *Prescription Alternatives.* New Canaan, CT: Keats Publishing, 1998, 168–172.

2. Gordon F. It is homocysteine that we do not want same to turn into? It may without B12 and folic acid. *Web MD Health*, Feb 3, 2000:1–5.

3. Pinkowish M. New CAD risk factors: interesting but how useful? *Web MD Health*, May 26, 2000:1–14.

4. Robinson K, Mayer E, Jacobson DW. Homocysteine and coronary artery disease. *Clev Clin J Med* 1994;61(6):438–450.

5. Shimakawa T, Nieto F J, Malinow MR, et al. Vitamin intake: A possible determinant of plasma homocysteine among middle-aged adults. *Ann Epidemiol* 1997;7:285–293.

6. Kang SS, Wong PWK, Malinow MR. Hyper-homocysteinemia as a risk factor for occlusive vascular disease. *Ann Rev Nutr* 1992;12:279–298.

7. Vanden Berg M, Boers GH, Franken DG, et al. Homocysteinemia and endothelial dysfunction in young patients with peripheral arterial occlusive disease. *Eur J Clin Invest* 1995;25(3):176–181.

8. Ubbink JB. Vitamin nutrition status and homocysteine: An atherogenic risk factor. *Nutr Rev* 1994;52(11):383–387.

9. Janssen MJ, Vanden Berg M, Stehouwer CD, et al. Homocysteinaemia: A role in accelerated atherogenesis of chronic renal failure? *Neth J Med* 1995;46(5):224–251.

10. Vanden Berg M, Boers GHJ. Homocystinuria: what about mild hyperhomocysteinaemia? *Postgrad Med J* 1996;72/851:513–518.

11. Piolot A, Nadler F, Parez N, et al. Homocysteine: Relation with ischemic vascular diseases. *Revue de Medecine Interne* 1996;1711:34–45.

12. DeMaria A. *Maturitas* 1996; 23/Suppl:S47–S49.

13. Haller H. Endothelial function: general considerations. *Drugs* 1997;53/Suppl:1–10.

14. Tawako A, Omland T, Gerhard M, et al. Hyper-homocysteinemia is associated with impaired endothelium-dependent vasodilation in humans. *Circulation* 1997;95(5):1119–1121.

15. Jakubowski H, Zhang L, Bardequez A, et al. Homocysteine, thiolactone and protein homocysteinylation in human endothelial cells: Implications for atherosclerosis. *Circ Res* 2000;87(1):45–51.

16. Chenn Lui Y, Greiner CD, et al. Physiologic concentrations of homocysteine inhibit the human plasma GSH peroxidase that reduces organic hydroperoxides. *J Lab Clin Med* 2000;136(1):58–65.

17. Choy PC, Mymin D, Zhu Q, et al. Atherosclerosis risk factors: the possible role of homocysteine. *Mol Cell Biochem* 2000;207(1-2):143–148.

18. Yi P, Melnyks, Pogribera M, et al. Increase in plasma homocysteine associated with parallel increases in plasma S-adenosylhomocysteine and lymphocyte DNA hypomethylation. *J Biol Chem* Jul 6, 2000.

19. Graham IM, Daly LE, Refsum HM, et al. Plasma homocysteine as a risk factor for vascular disease: the European Concerted Action Project. *JAMA* 1997;277(22):1775–1781.

20. D'Angelo A, Mazzola G, Crippal, et al. Hyper-homocysteinemia and venous thromboembolic disease. *Haematologica* 1997;82(2):211–219.

21. Duell PB, Malinow MR. Homocysteine: an important risk factor for atherosclerotic vascular disease. *Curr Opin Lipidol* 1997;8(1):28–34.

22. Grobbee DE, Ueland PM, Refsum H. Plasma total homocysteine, B vitamins, and risk of coronary atherosclerosis. *Arterioscler Thromb Vasc Biol* 1997;1715:989–995.

23. Robinson K. Hyperhomocysteinemia confers an independent increased risk of atherosclerosis in end-stage renal disease and is closely linked to plasma folate and pyridoxine concentrations. *Circulation* 1996;94/11:2743–2748.

24. Fenech MF, Dreosfi IE, Rinaldi Jr. Folate, vitamin B12, homocysteine status and chromosome damage rate in lymphocytes of older men. *Carcinogenesis* 1997;2:1329–1336.

25. Bostom AG. High dose B-vitamins treatment of hyperhomocysteinemia in dialysis patients. *Kidney Int* 1996;49(11):147–152.

26. Toborek M. Dietary methionine imbalance, endothdial cell dysfunction and atherosclerosis. *Nutr Res* 1996;16(7):1251–1266.

27. Sobra J. Hyperhomocysteinemia. *Cas Leck Cesk* 1996;135(9):266–267.

28. Charweau P, Chadefaux B, Coude M et al. Long-term folic acid (but not pyridoxine) supplementation lowers elevated plasma homocysteine level in chronic renal failure. *Min Electrolyt Metab* 1996;22(1–3):106–109.

29. Mayer EL, Jacobsen DW, Robinson K. Homocysteine and coronary atherosclerosis. *JAM Coll Cardiol* 1996;(3):517–527.

30. Bottiglieri T. Folate, vitamin B12, and neuropsychiatric disorders. *Nutr Rev* 1996;54(12):382–390.

31. Malinow MR, Duell PB, Hess DL, et al. Reduction of plasma homocysteine levels by breakfast cereal fortified with folic aid in patients with coronary heart disease. *N Eng J Med* 1998;338(15):1009–1015.

32. Ubbink JB, Vermaak WJ, Van der Merwe A, et al. vitamin B12, vitamin B6, and folate nutritional status in men with hyperhomocysteinemia. *Am J Clin Nutr* 1993;57(1):47–53.

33. Robinson K, Mayer EL, Miller DP et al. Hyperhomocysteinemia and low pyridoxal phosphate: common and independent reversible risk factors for coronary artery disease. *Circulation* 1995;1992:(10):2825–2830.

34. Vehoef P, Stampfer MJ, Baring JE, et al. Homocysteine metabolism and risk of myocardiol infarction: relation with vitamins B6, B12, and folate. *Am J Epidemiol* 1996;143(9):845–859.

35. Andreotti F, Burzotta F, Mazza A, et al. Homocysteine and arterial occlusive disease: a concise review. *Cardiologia* 1999;44(4):341–345.

36. Bots ML, Laimer LJ, Lindemans, et al. Homocysteine and short-term risk of myocardial infarction and stroke in the elderly: the Rotterdam Study. *Arch Intern Med* 1999;159(1):38–44.

37. Shimakawa T, Nieto FJ, Malinow MR, et al. Vitamin intake: a possible determinant of plasma homocysteine among middle-aged adults. *Ann Epidemiol* 1997;4:285–293.

38. Tucker KL, Mahnken B, Wilson PW, et al. Folic acid fortification of the food supply: potential benefits for the elderly population. *JAMA* 1996;276(23):1879–1885.

39. Bottiglieri T, Laundry M, Crellin R, et al. Homocysteine, folate, methionine and monoamine metabolism in depression. *J Neurol Neurosurg Pychiat* 2000;69(2):228–238.

40. Lowering blood homocysteine with folic acid based supplements: meta analysis of randomized trials. *Homocysteine Trialists Collaboration* 1998:316:894–898.

41. Franken DG, Boers GH, Bloom HJ, et al. Treatment of mild hyperhomocysteinemia in vascular disease patients. *Arterioscler Throm* 1994;14:465–470.

42. Boston AG, Gohh RY, Bearbeu AJ, et al. Treatment of homocysteinemia in renal transplant recipients: a randomized placebo-controlled trial. *Ann Intern Med* 1997;127:1089–1092.

43. Ubbink JB, Becker PJ, Vermaak WJ, et al. Results of B-vitamin supplementation study used in a prediction model to define a reference range for plasma homocysteine. *Clin Chem* 1995;41:1033–1037.

44. Ubbink JB, Van der Merwe A, Vermaak WJ, et al. Hyperhomocysteinemia and the response to vitamins supplementation. *Clin Invest* 1993;71:993–998.

45. Malinow MR, Duell PB, Hess DL, et al. Reduction of plasma homocysteine level by breakfast cereal fortified with folic acid in patients with coronary heart disease. *N Engl J Med* 1998;338:1009–1015.

46. Malinow MR, Nieto FJ, Kruger WD, et al. The effects of folic acid supplementation on plasma total homocysteine are modulated by multivitamin use and methylenetetrahydrofolate reductase genotypes. *Arterioscler Thromb Vasc Biol* 1997;17:1157–1162.

47. Stolzenberg-Solomon RZ, Miller ER, Maguire M, G, et al. Association of dietary protein intake and coffee consumption with serum homocysteine concentration in an older population. *Am J Clin Nutr* 1999;69(3):467–475.

48. *Disease Prevention and Treatment.* 3rd ed. Hollywood, FL: Life Extension Foundation, 2000;70–72:348–353.

49. Wizman V. Is TMG, SAM-e for the poor? *Web MD Health* 1999;12/15:1–2.

50. American Heart Association recommends homocysteine testing in high-risk patients. *Doctor's Guide,* June 5, 1999.

ASCORBATE SUPPLEMENTATION REDUCES HEART FAILURE
by Andrew W. Saul, PhD, and Robert G. Smith, PhD

New research has reported that risk of heart failure decreases with increasing blood levels of vitamin C.[1] Persons with the lowest plasma levels of ascorbate had the highest risk of heart failure, and persons with the highest levels of vitamin C had the lowest risk of heart failure.

According to the U.S. Centers for Disease Control (CDC) and Prevention, there are about 600,000 deaths from heart disease each year.[2] This is an enormous number. The definition of heart failure used by the study authors was on the basis of drugs prescribed, which would include all forms of heart disease that cause death. This agrees well with the CDC definition.

Specifically, the study found that each 20 micromole/liter (μmol/L) increase in plasma vitamin C was associated with a 9 percent reduction in death from heart failure. That works out to 54,000 fewer deaths from heart failure for each increase in 20 μmol/L plasma vitamin C. If everyone took high enough doses of vitamin C to reach the highest quartile (80 μmol/L), that would work out to approximately 216,000 fewer deaths per year. Just from taking vitamin C.

What Is Heart Failure?

The heart muscle fails for many reasons. As we get older, it weakens and may not get enough nutrients to keep it healthy. A severe heart attack, that does not kill the patient but has caused significant damage to the heart muscle, may leave the heart in a very weakened state. Long-standing or acute high blood pressure can put a massive strain on the heart and cause it to fail. An abnormal beating of the heart such as a very fast heart rate, an irregular beat, or a lot of missed beats will result in a less effective pumping and eventual failure. Anemia will make the heart pump harder and faster in an attempt to deliver enough oxygen to the organs. The valves in the heart that direct blood flow are made up of an important fibrous strengthening tissue called collagen. Weakness or tearing of these valves can cause the blood to flow backwards, making the heart pump very inefficiently and eventually causing it to fail. When the heart muscle begins to fail, there is a buildup of carbon dioxide and waste products, resulting in weakening of the kidneys and liver. Eventually, fluid builds up in all the organs and the person presents with severe fatigue, shortness of breath (from fluid in the lungs), and swelling of the ankles.

Viruses and other microorganisms can attack the heart and weaken the heart muscle cells permanently by causing viral myocarditis. As the heart muscle cells get older, they may require more energy to work and a greater level of protection from free radical damage. Nutrients such as magnesium, orotic acid, coenzyme Q10, acetyl L-carnitine, and others may be required. Toxins, chemotherapeutic drugs, alcohol, and deficiencies of some nutrients such as selenium may cause the heart to increase the size of its cells to compensate for the weakness. An enlargement of the heart muscle is called cardiomyopathy. These hearts are much more likely to fail.

Medical treatment of cardiac failure uses drugs that open the arteries, reduce blood pressure, and force the excessive fluid out of the body (diuretics). Drugs known as ACE inhibitors improve quality of life and survival. Diet, fluid and salt restriction, and tolerable exercise are essential. For the most severe cases, a heart transplant may be required.

How Much Vitamin C Is Needed?

Many of these treatments, however, have significant side effects. For example, treatment with diuretics to remove excess fluid will tend to lower the plasma vitamin C level and exacerbate the causes of cardiac failure.

Excerpted from the *Orthomolecular Medicine News Service*, November 22, 2011.

It takes less vitamin C than you may have thought. To achieve a plasma level of 80 μmol/L, and thereby reduce deaths by 216,000 per year, requires a daily dosage of about 500 milligrams (mg) of vitamin C. This is only one or two tablets per day, costing less than 10 cents.

Taking 3,000–8,000 mg per day, in continued divided doses, can achieve a plasma level twice as high (160 μmol/L). This much C could save an additional 216,000 lives as it is an additional 80 μmol/L, assuming the relationship holds.

We can go still higher, and without intravenous administration. Taking 1,000 mg of oral vitamin C per hour for 12 hours (12,000 mg/day) will result in a plasma level of about 240 μmol/L. A single 5,000-mg dose might take you to a peak of 240 μmol/L, but only for about 2 to 4 hours after the intake. That is why the dosage needs to be spread out: better absorption, gradual excretion, higher plasma levels . . . and better results.

CONCLUSION

Optimizing vitamin C intake optimizes the health of a person taking it. This includes people with potentially life-threatening disorders. It is a simple, cheap, effective, and safe therapy. Vitamin C is no longer a "controversial" therapy. It is an ignored therapy. It is time for the medical profession to fully awaken to what this recent study confirms: higher vitamin C intakes mean less heart failure. That means that higher vitamin C intakes mean fewer deaths. 200,000 per year fewer.

With just two vitamin C tablets per day.

REFERENCES

1. Pfister R, Sharp SJ, Luben R, Wareham NJ, Khaw KT. Plasma vitamin C predicts incident heart failure in men and women in European Prospective Investigation into Cancer and Nutrition-Norfolk prospective study. Am Heart J, 2011;162:246–253.

2. CDC. Leading causes of death. "FastStats." Available at www.cdc.gov/nchs/fastats/lcod.htm.

DEPRESSION AND ANXIETY

BASICALLY, MODERN PSYCHIATRISTS HAVE two main treatment functions: they prescribe drugs—tranquilizers or antidepressants; and they may also do psychotherapy or counseling. Over the past 100 years, psychiatric conditions that were almost exclusively treated in mental hospitals have disappeared from psychiatry because they were treated successfully by general practitioners. However, if modern physicians did their job effectively, there would be no need to consider replacing them with their more biochemically oriented colleagues.

The results of modern drug treatment are not very good compared to what was obtained before. We need better treatment. Orthomolecular treatment is not new, but it is an awful lot better than merely allowing patients to vegetate on antidepressants. Yet practitioners seem to be content with a very dismal long-term drug response rate while they wait for the miracle—the drugs that will actually cure their patients, without side effects. Each year we hear the announcement of new, ever more expensive drugs, with little evidence they have any major impact on the problem as a whole. But how long can patients wait? A year in the life of a depressed person can be like an eternity. Patients and their families do not have the luxury of waiting for the day when psychiatry will at last start treating their patients properly. Modern psychiatry has not been very good at treating depression.

I do not know of a single pharmaceutical chemical that has ever cured anything, even though some of them are useful in ameliorating the discomfort of the disease. The answer to depression will come from recognizing more clearly its causes and biochemistry and dealing with them, as is done in orthomolecular psychiatry.

Physicians have been struggling for decades with the drug dilemma, which they are aware of but have not clearly faced. Very simply it is this: when one uses a drug, one converts one mental illness into another. Antidepressants alleviate many symptoms and make life more comfortable for the patient and for their families, as well as for hospitals and their staff. As the patient begins to recover, she or he becomes more normal. However, antidepressants given to normal people make them psychotic. If a drug makes a well person sick, how can it make a sick person well?

Patients prefer to be normal. They do not prefer one set of problems over the other, but they have no choice and have to accept side effects in order to be freed of elements of their original problem. The modern solution is to keep them swinging between the extremes. In most cases, depression returns. But with orthomolecular treatment patients are offered a real choice, the choice of becoming and remaining well. The large doses of nutrients and the diet will maintain the patient in good health. One can combine the rapid effect of the drugs with the slow curative effect of the nutrients. As the patient begins to recover, one slowly reduces the dose of the drugs, and this time instead of becoming psychotic from the drug they remain well as the nutrients take over. By recovery I mean that they are free of signs and symptoms, they are getting along reasonably well with their family and with the community, and they pay income tax. They are working, or they are graduating and getting ready to work. Patients pay income tax because they are well enough to work.

— ABRAM HOFFER, *JOM* 1996

TERMS OF DEPRESSION AND ANXIETY

ADENOSINE TRIPHOSPHATE (ATP). The main energy molecule used to fuel most body processes and functions.

AFFECTIVE DISORDER. Mood disorders such as depression, bipolar, and anxiety.

BENZODIAZEPINES. Standard antianxiety drugs, which include alprazolam (Xanax), clonazepam (Klonopin), and lorazepam (Ativan), work by mimicking the actions of gamma-aminobutyric acid in the brain.

BIPOLAR DEPRESSION. Sometimes called manic-depressive illness, characterized by dramatic oscillations between feelings of depression and euphoria.

DYSTHYMIA. A mild form of depression with chronic symptoms that can persist for years.

GAMMA-AMINOBUTYRIC ACID (GABA). The main neurotransmitter in the brain that inhibits nerve transmission and calms nerve activity.

HOMOCYSTEINE. An amino acid that is produced in the body in the course of methionine metabolism.

METHYLATION. A process, central to mood control, among other functions, in which a molecule donates one of its methyl groups to another substance in the body.

NEUROTRANSMITTER. A chemical used to carry messages throughout the brain's network of cells. Neurotransmitters most commonly associated with moods are dopamine, serotonin, and noradrenaline (norepinephrine).

SELECTIVE SEROTONIN-REUPTAKE INHIBITORS (SSRIS). The primary pharmaceutical treatment for depression. SSRIs such as fluoxetine (Prozac), sertraline (Zoloft), and paroxetine (Paxil) raise the levels of the neurotransmitter serotonin outside and between nerve cells, thus improving mood; they are associated with numerous side effects, including sexual dysfunction, digestive complaints, and, in children and adolescents, increased suicide risk.

SEROTONIN. One of the brain's principal neurotransmitters, responsible for regulating mood; low levels can lead to depression.

TRYPTOPHAN. An amino acid obtained from the diet that is necessary for the production of vitamin B3 and is used by the brain to produce serotonin.

UNIPOLAR DEPRESSION. Episodic depression so debilitating that it becomes difficult for the sufferer to perform the basic tasks of daily life; also referred to as major depression.

VITAMIN B3 FOR DEPRESSION
by Jonathan E. Prousky, ND

The most commonly cited uses of vitamin B3 (also called niacin or niacinamide) are for the treatment of pellagra. Pellagra is a disease caused by a cellular deficiency of the nicotinamide coenzymes due to inadequate dietary supply of the protein amino acid tryptophan and vitamin B3. It is characterized by skin problems, diarrhea, dermatitis, and mental symptoms such as mania and dementia. The adult intake of vitamin B3 necessary to prevent pellagra is around 20 milligrams (mg) per day. The body can manufacture approximately 1 mg of niacin equivalents from 60 mg of tryptophan obtained mostly from dietary protein. This makes it rather difficult to develop frank pellagra in affluent, industrialized countries where food supply is seldom scarce unless there are mitigating factors like disease (anorexia nervosa, hypothyroidism, and alcoholism),[1-6] medication-induced nutrient depletion (the use of anticonvulsants),[7,8] or from a lack of food intake (homelessness and undernutrition).[9,10]

While it is not common practice to use vitamin B3 for medical reasons unless pellagra has been identified, orthomolecular practitioners have been using vitamin B3 therapeutically for more than 50 years to treat numerous neuropsychiatric conditions. One of the first publications documenting the need for vitamin B3 occurred in the early 1940s when the late Dr. William Kaufman of Connecticut detailed its use as a treatment for a syndrome that he termed, "aniacinamidosis."[11] Kaufman's description of aniacinamidosis is practically indistinguishable from the modern clinical presentations of anxiety and mood disorders. He describes it as being marked by feelings of anxiousness, impatience, irritability, and low self-esteem; indecisiveness; loss of interest in work family and friends; withdrawal and fear of unfamiliar people, ideas, or situations; difficulty sleeping; and prolonged sadness without apparent cause. The treatment of this syndrome could not be ameliorated by dietary modifications but required between 150–350 mg of niacinamide each day to reverse its clinical manifestations.[11]

One decade later, Dr. Abram Hoffer of Saskatchewan, Canada, along with his team of investigators, conducted a total of six double-blind, randomized, controlled clinical trials involving schizophrenic patients from 1953 to1960. These trials demonstrated that vitamin B3 doubled the recovery rate of acute schizophrenic patients, and also reduced patients' reliance upon the healthcare system.[12] These studies did not, however, show a favorable response among chronic schizophrenic patients who were ill longer than one year. When Hoffer reviewed this problem more substantially, he discovered that the treatment duration was not long enough to have produced adequate results. Chronic patients required vitamin treatment for five or more years in order to derive observable benefits.[13-15]

From the 1950s until Hoffer's death in 2009, he elucidated numerous additional therapeutic uses of vitamin B3 for the treatment of various neuropsychiatric conditions. Some of Hoffer's reports included those involving children with learning and behavioral issues,[16,17] dementia of both the Alzheimer's and non-Alzheimer's type,[18-20] Huntington's disease,[21-23] and the starvation-stress syndrome (similar to post-traumatic stress disorder).[24] While Hoffer was prolific in his writings about the therapeutic uses of vitamin B3 and other nutrients, he did not author (to my knowledge) a single report documenting the merits of vitamin B3 for the treatment of depression. He merely alluded to it when discussing the psychiatric and somatic complications of having a dependency on vitamin B3. He did, however, report on the relationship between chronic allergies and depression, and the need for allergy treatment as an effective antidepressant strategy.[25,26]

Like Hoffer, I have not considered vitamin B3 to be an effective antidepressant and have typically prescribed other treatments, such as omega-3 essential fatty acids, 5-hydroxytryptophan (5-

From the *J Orthomolecular Med* 2010; 25(3):137–146.

HTP), tyrosine, rhodiola, and St. John's wort extract to augment mood. While on parental leave during November 2009, my clinical shift was spearheaded by one of my colleagues who recommended fairly significant doses of no-flush niacin to treat a patient's depression. In January 2010, the patient returned for a visit on my clinical shift, and much to my surprise her long-standing depression had resolved.

Case Presentation

The patient was a 47-year-old female who came to the Robert Schad Naturopathic Clinic on October 21, 2009. She had a 27-year history of both anxiety and depression. When she was 20 years old she moved away from her home due to the stress imposed by her mother's bipolar disorder. As a result, the patient became depressed, which was further complicated by the challenges of taking care of her teenage sister. The patient referred to this as her "subclinical" depression that had lasted her entire adult life. Her father had mental health issues of his own, for he had depression and was a heavy social drinker. The patient reported suicidal thoughts on and off since being depressed. She also tried numerous antidepressant medications and found them to be ineffective, while also having the unfortunate side effect of increasing thoughts of suicide. She was currently taking 0.5 mg of lorazepam (Ativan) daily and 7.5 mg of zopiclone (Imovance) at bedtime to help with sleep. Her affect was depressed and flat. Her diagnosis was consistent with dysthymic disorder. On October 28, she returned for a second visit and was prescribed 3,000 mg of no-flush niacin (inositol hexaniacinate/hexanicotinate), 300 mg of the amino acid gamma-amino butyric acid (GABA), and a probiotic to improve overall health.

On November 24, the patient returned for a third visit. With the 3,000 mg of no-flush niacin, she felt better overall, more calm, more balanced, and reported no anxiety attacks as well. Her affect was normal and she even smiled during the intake. The no-flush niacin was increased to 6,000 mg in divided doses daily. On January 5, 2010, she returned for a fourth visit and was on my clinical rotation. She reported an absence of depression. There was even a marked improvement in her premenstrual depression that apparently plagued her as well. As of the latest entry in her chart, dated March 22, 2010, her dysthymia was noted to be in clinical remission presumed to be the result of the no-flush niacin. While it cannot be ascertained if the GABA (which acts as a neurotransmitter) and the probiotic helped in reducing this patient's depression, the patient did attribute her mood improvement to the no-flush niacin.

Review of the Literature

While this case is not very compelling, it did make me consider the possible antidepressant effects that vitamin B3 might possess. As a result, I conducted a search for articles describing the use of vitamin B3 for depression. To be included in my

IN BRIEF

While on parental leave during November 2009, my clinical shift was spearheaded by one of my colleagues who recommended fairly significant doses of inositol hexaniacinate (a form of niacin) to treat a patient's depression. In January 2010, the patient returned for a visit on my clinical shift, and much to my surprise her long-standing depression had resolved. As a result, I conducted a search for articles describing the use of vitamin B3 for depression. Six articles were found to meet the inclusion criteria and were included in this review. There is evidence that niacin and niacinamide (in combination with tryptophan) might be effective for the treatment of depression. Hypothetical reasons for niacin's effectiveness include its vasodilatory properties, while the mechanisms responsible for the effectiveness of niacinamide involve its ability to inhibit tryptophan pyrrolase and possibly protect neurons from damage. The side effect profiles of niacin and the niacinamide-tryptophan combination are also discussed. Even though the mechanisms of action for niacin and niacinamide have not been substantiated from well-conducted controlled clinical trials, these forms of vitamin B3 appear to have beneficial effects on depression.

final review the articles had to 1) report on the use of vitamin B3 for depression either alone or in combination with other medicines, and 2) describe the method of vitamin B3 administration. A total of eight potential eligible articles were screened. Of these, six articles were found to meet the inclusion criteria and were included in this review.[29-34] Following is a summary of the articles demonstrating the effectiveness of vitamin B3 for the treatment of depression.

Article 1: Case Series Study with 15 Patients with Various Types of Depression

All patients were given niacin as an adjunct to psychotherapy. Intravenous niacin (300–400 mg) was given to 10 patients, followed by oral niacin. Five other patients were given niacin orally and never did receive an initial intravenous dose. All patients received gradually increasing doses of niacin before meals until they reached 900 mg daily, but one patient reached 2,500 mg daily. All patients were maintained on their maximum dose for 7 to 10 days, and then the dose was gradually tapered. The average duration of niacin treatment varied from two to six weeks.[30]

The outcome: 14 of the 15 patients exhibited subjective and objective improvement following the use of niacin in conjunction with psychotherapy.

Article 2: Case Series Study with 16 Patients with Various Types of Depression

Eleven patients were given 400–600 mg of niacin daily for the first week, then 900 mg daily for the first week, then 900 mg daily for two weeks in divided doses. Treatment was then terminated abruptly. Five patients were given identical-looking placebo pills and no niacin in the same manner to the patients that were given niacin. Nightly sedatives were also prescribed to patients when necessary.[31] The outcome: no benefit was observed.

Article 3: Case Series Study with 100 Patients with a Mixture of Depressive and Anxiety Symptoms

Patients were given a combination of niacin and phenobarbital (Solfoton) in tablet form or elixir. Each tablet of the elixir contained 100 mg of niacin and 8 mg of phenobarbital. All patients received increasing daily dosages of the combination until 900 mg of niacin and 72 mg of phenobarbital was reached on day 15. From day 16 to day 21, daily doses of the combination were reduced to 450 mg of niacin and 36 mg of phenobarbital. Presumably, the combination was discontinued after day 21. The outcome: 4.5 percent of patients reported definite improvement, 34.0 percent reported some improvement, 13.2 percent reported no improvement, and 5.4 percent discontinued treatment.[32]

Article 4: Human Pilot Open-Label Trial with 27 with Unipolar Depression

Patients randomly assigned to two groups: Group 1 received two electroconvulsive therapy (ECT) treatments unilaterally weekly with a minimum of eight; Group 2 received 3,000 mg of niacinamide daily. Thirteen patients in Group 1 completed the trial, while 12 patients in Group 2 completed the trial. The Beck self-rating scale for depression was used the day before the trial began, and then on days 3, 7, 10, 14, 17, 21, 24, and 28. The average Beck score for Group 1 was 25.6, and the average Beck score for Group 2 was 24.4. The outcome: Group 2 improved more than Group 1 on day 10 (Beck scores: group 1, 16.8 and group 2, 15.2). By day 21, the results achieved statistical significance (Beck scores: group 1, 8.8 and group 2, 3.7). Scores for each group on day 28 were almost identical.[33]

Article 5: Human Pilot Open-Label Trial with 11 Newly Admitted Depressed Patients with Primary Affective Disorder

Patients received tryptophan-niacinamide combination for four weeks. Patients were given 2,000 mg of L-tryptophan and 500 mg of niacinamide during week 1, and then gradually increased to 6,000 mg of L-tryptophan and 1,500 mg of niacinamide at the start of week 3. All patients received diazepam (Valium) if needed for insomnia or agitation. The mental status of patients was scored before treatment, and on days 7, 14, 21, and 28, on a modified Hamilton Depression Rating Scale, and a Clinical Global Impression Scale of Severity (CGI). In addition, the Beck Depression Inventory was completed at the same intervals. The outcome: There were statistically significant improvements (i.e., reductions) in the mean scores of all patients among all the inventories used. The average Hamilton score went from a 33.7 on day 0 to a 20.5 on day 28. The Beck score went from a 33.1 on day 0 to 20.9 on day 28. The CGI went from a 7.2 on day 0 to 4.5 on day 28. On the basis of percentage improvement on the Hamilton scale, there were three marked-responders (50 percent or more), four moderate responders (25–49 percent), and four non-responders (less than 25 percent).[29]

Article 6: A Controlled Study of 25 Newly Admitted Severely Depressed Patients

All medications were administered under double-blind conditions for a period of four weeks. Eight patients received the tryptophan-niacinamide combination for four weeks. They were given 2,000 mg of L-tryptophan and 500 mg of niacinamide during week 1, and then gradually increased to 6,000 mg of L-tryptophan and 1,500 mg of niacinamide at the start of week 3. Eight patients were given a single dose at bedtime of 75 mg of imipramine (Tofranil) for week 1, which was increased to 225 mg at the start of week 3. Nine patients were given the tryptophan-niacinamide-imipramine combination using the same daily dosages described above. Throughout the study, the tryptophan-niacinamide group received imipramine placebo and the imipramine group received tryptophan placebo and niacinamide. All patients received diazepam (Valium) if needed for insomnia or agitation. The mental status of patients was scored before treatment, and on days 7, 14, 21, and 28, on a modified Hamilton Depression Rating Scale, and a CGI of Severity of Depression. In addition, the Beck Depression Inventory was completed on the specified days. The outcome: superior results occurred among patients in the imipramine group and in the tryptophan-niacinamide-imipramine group. However, if bipolar patients were excluded from the analysis (seven patients), then there were no differences in the therapeutic efficacy of the three treatment unipolar patients.[34]

Discussion

The results of this review indicate that vitamin B3 may have a therapeutic effect on depression. The quality of the evidence at this point, however, is only hypothesis-generating, and randomized trials are required to determine the clinical implications of this novel treatment.

Given these limitations, it is still important to comment on the biochemical and physiological mechanisms that might account for some of the positive results that were reported. For the studies in which niacin was used alone (article 1) and in combination with phenobarbital (article 3), the mechanism believed to produce its antidepressant benefits was cerebral vasodilation. Niacin causes peripheral vasodilation and skin flushing by inducing the production of prostaglandin D2 (PGD2) in the skin, leading to a marked increase of its metabolite, PGF2, in the plasma.[35] When niacin is administered orally in amounts of 500 mg or topically via a 6-inch patch of aqueous methylnicotinate on the forearm, PGD2 is markedly released in the skin and its metabolite appears in high amounts in the plasma.[35,36] It is not known if PGD2 causes vasodilation of the intracranial arteries, but niacin's ability to abort acute migraine headaches suggests that this might be what is occurring.[37] Old reports cited by Bicknell and Prescott[38] demonstrate that niacin does indeed cause vasodilation of the cerebral and spinal vessels, and that intravenous administration increases the rate of intracranial blood flow in human beings for 20 to 60 minutes without any significant change in blood pressure. Other published data pertaining to niacin's effects on cerebral vasodilation has been equivocal.[39–42] Based on the results of these reports, it appears that intravenously administered niacin might increase cerebral blood flow, but more studies are warranted. Unfortunately, to date, there have no reports examining the effects of orally administered niacin upon cerebral blood flow in human or animal subjects.

If intravenous and oral niacin do increase cerebral blood flow, this therapeutic benefit might be important since there are studies that have documented reduced cerebral blood flow in depressed patients and improved cerebral blood flow following treatment. Presumably, increasing brain perfusion would benefit depression. In a study of patients with late-life depression (55 years of age or older), reduced cerebral blood flow was increased in certain brain areas following a mean of 13.7 weeks of pharmacotherapy.[43] Specifically, reduced cerebral blood flow increased (improved) in the left dorsolateral prefrontal cortex to precentral areas and in the right parieto-occipital regions (parts of the brain that govern moods). In another study, patients with refractory depressive disorder (treatment-resistant depression) had alterations in regional perfusion in specific brain areas (decreased activity of the bilateral prefrontal areas) that differed from patients having non-refractory depressive disorder.[44]

A more compelling study evaluated cerebrovascular reactivity (CVR) following stimulation by medication with acetazolamide (Diamox) in a healthy control group and a depressed group of patients.[45] CVR reflects the capacity of blood vessels to dilate and is a vital mechanism that enables constant cerebral blood flow. The group of acutely depressed patients had a more significant reduction in their CVR values compared to healthy controls. On follow-up 21 months later when the depressed patients had received treatment and were in remission, their CVR had significantly improved, whereas the CVR values of the control group remained unchanged. Another study demonstrated that 81.5 percent of patients with depressive disorders had reduced cerebral blood perfusion as measured by single-photo emission computed tomography (SPECT) imaging.[46] SPECT is a type of nuclear imaging test that can show what areas within the brain are more or less active. In a study evaluating CVR in 16 patients with unipolar depression, their CVR was reduced during the depressive phase of their illness and increased in most of the depressed patients when in remission.[47] Based on the data cited here, it appears that depression is marked by reduced cerebral blood flow and that improvement is characterized by increased (or normalized) cerebral blood flow. These findings suggest that niacin might hypothetically have the capacity to increase

cerebral blood flow and therefore assist in ameliorating depression.

Another biochemical mechanism that might account for the antidepressant benefits of vitamin B3 involves the use of niacinamide in combination with tryptophan.[29,33,34] Niacinamide functions as an inhibitor of the liver enzyme, tryptophan pyrrolase, which prevents the metabolism of tryptophan.[29] When tryptophan is administered in combination with niacinamide, more tryptophan enters into the brain.[48] This would have the therapeutic benefit of increasing the production of 5-HTP (created in the body from tryptophan), and subsequently increasing the production of the mood-elevating serotonin neurotransmitter. This makes the niacinamide-tryptophan combination a therapeutically attractive intervention for the treatment of depression. Niacinamide also provides protection against neuronal and vascular injury.[49] While the mechanisms that account for these unique therapeutic properties are very complex and require further delineation, niacinamide might provide some antidepressant benefit by reducing neuronal damage because it protects against anoxia (low oxygen levels) and degeneration of nitric oxide, a molecule that modulates neurotransmitter signals involved with mood.[49] Niacinamide also alters tryptophan metabolism to increase serotonin synthesis while limiting the formation of kynurenines (metabolites of tryptophan).

With respect to dosing, it makes sense to use niacin alone or in combination with antidepressant medications. Since skin flushing is an important aspect to the putative therapeutic benefits of niacin, the daily dose should be low enough so that flushing is not significantly lessened. The daily dose should also be kept low since 900 mg was the dose most often used (except in one patient whose daily dose was 2,500 mg) in the cited studies. I speculate that there might be a relationship between the skin flushing (peripheral vasodilation) induced by niacin and cerebral vasodilation. When niacin is administered at 1,000 mg (or more) three times daily, the flushing is dramatically reduced after the first few days of use by depleting PGD2 and other metabolites in the skin. Therefore, lower daily doses of niacin would presumably be more therapeutic than daily doses that deplete PGD2 and other metabolites in the skin. I recommend that patient's take 100–300 mg of niacin about 15 to 20 minutes before meals three times daily. A patient's tolerance (or intolerance) to niacin's cutaneous effects might require dose adjustments. Preparations that produce no flushing, such as inositol hexaniacinate or niacinamide, or those that significantly lessen the flushing, such as timed-, sustained-, or slow-release preparations, would presumably be less effective than niacin at increasing cerebral blood flow. A 28- to 42-day trial seems appropriate since this approximates the duration of niacin treatment that was reported to be beneficial in the cited studies. If niacin does indeed benefit a patient, it might be necessary to prolong treatment for four to six months or several years depending on a patient's stability and functional capacities. Side effects such as headache, nausea, and/or vomiting are possible and patients should be informed that they are usually temporary.

When treating depression with niacinamide, it should be used in combination with tryptophan. In the studies that used this combination (articles 5 and 6), the niacinamide-tryptophan was administered twice daily and away from food. Taking this combination in the morning and prior to bed is an effective dosing strategy. The initial dose of this combination should be 500 mg of niacinamide and 1,000 mg of tryptophan twice daily, which should be doubled over several weeks of use. The daily dose of tryptophan does not need to exceed 4,000 mg and the daily dose of niacinamide does not need to exceed 1,500 mg to obtain an effective antidepressant effect. Doses of tryptophan above 4,000 mg are unlikely to provide additional benefit for unipolar depression, but for bipolar depression the daily dose of tryptophan should exceed 4,000 mg to be effective.[34] Older adult patients do not need as much niacinamide as do younger adult patients since they have less tryptophan pyrrolase activity.[29] For older patients the daily amount of niacinamide does not need to exceed 1,000 mg, but for younger adult patients the daily amount might need to exceed 1,500 mg to enable the accumulation of free plasma tryptophan in the blood, and consequently increase cerebral serotonin.[29] Trying

this combination for 28 days seems appropriate since this approximates the duration of treatment that was reported in the cited studies. Consideration to increase treatment duration should be discussed with patients who have a positive treatment response, for it can take four to six months of treatment or even years before there is clinically significant improvement in a patient's stability and functional capacities. Side effects from this combination are usually not severe, but patients can experience mild rigidity, mild tremor, dry mouth, constipation, nausea, vomiting, dizziness, fainting, anorexia, heartburn, and increased thirst. A rare side effect is serotonin syndrome (too much serotonin due to the tryptophan), which can be severe.

CONCLUSION

Even though vitamin B3's mechanisms of action have not been substantiated from rigorous controlled clinical trials, it does appear to have beneficial effects upon depression. Oral niacin is believed to increase cerebral blood flow and decrease depression. Intravenous niacin has some supportive data demonstrating that it might increase cerebral blood flow, but data on oral niacin and cerebral blood flow is lacking. Niacinamide in combination with tryptophan has more robust data demonstrating an effective antidepressant response among patients with unipolar depression. The niacinamide-tryptophan combination increases serotonin levels within the brain, but niacinamide by itself might possess antidepressant effects.

REFERENCES

1. Prousky JE. Pellagra may be a rare secondary complication of anorexia nervosa: a systematic review of the literature. *Altern Med Rev* 2003;8:180–185.

2. Hawn LJ, Guldan GJ, Chillag SC, et al. A case of pellagra and a South Carolina history of the disorder. *J S C Med Assoc* 2003;99:220–223.

3. Prasad PVS, Babu A, Paul EK, et al. Myxoedema pellagra—a report of two cases. *J Assoc Physicians India* 2003;51:421–422.

4. Wallengren J, Thelin I. Pellagra-like skin lesions associated with Wernicke's encephalopathy in a heavy wine drinker. *Acta Derm Venereol* 2002;82:152–154.

5. Pitsavas S, Andreou C, Bascialla F, et al. Pellagra encephalopathy following B-complex vitamin treatment without niacin. *Int J Psychiatry Med* 2004;34:91–95.

6. Sakai K, Nakajima T, Fukuhara N. A suspected case of alcoholic pellagra encephalopathy with marked response to niacin showing myoclonus and ataxia as chief complaints. *No To Shinke* 2006;58:141–144.

7. Lyon VB, Fairley JA. Anticonvulsant-induced pellagra. *J Am Acad Dermatol* 2002;46:597–599.

8. Kaur S, Goraya JS, Thami GP, et al. Pellagrous dermatitis induced by phenytoin. *Pediatr Dermatol* 2002;19:93.

9. Kertesz SG. Pellagra in 2 homeless men. *Mayo Clin Proc* 2001;76:315–318.

10. Prakash R, Gandotra S, Singh LK, et al. Rapid resolution of delusional parasitosis in pellagra with niacin augmentation therapy. *Gen Hosp Psychiatry* 2008;30:581–584.

11. Kaufman W. *The Common Form of Niacin Amide Deficiency Disease: Aniacinamidosis.* Bridgeport, CT: Yale University Press, 1943.

12. Hoffer A. *Adventures In Psychiatry. The Scientific Memoirs of Dr. Abram Hoffer.* Caledon, ON: KOS Publishing, 2005; 50–99.

13. Hoffer A. Vitamin B3 & Schizophrenia. *Discovery, Recovery, Controversy.* Kingston, ON: Quarry Press, 1998, 28–76.

14. Hoffer A. Chronic schizophrenic patients treated ten years of more. *J Orthomolecular Med* 1994;9:7–37.

15. Hoffer A, Prousky J. Successful treatment of schizophrenia requires optimal daily doses of vitamin B3. *Altern Med Rev* 2008;13:287–291.

16. Hoffer A. Vitamin B3 dependent child. *Schizophrenia* 1971;3:107–113.

17. Hoffer A. *Healing Children's Attention & Behavior Disorders.* Toronto, ON: CCNM Press, 2004.

18. Hoffer A. *Niacin Therapy in Psychiatry.* Springfield, IL: Charles C Thomas, 1962, 72–93.

19. Hoffer A. A case of Alzheimer's treated with nutrients and aspirin. *J Orthomolecular Med* 1993;8:43–44.

20. Hoffer A. Vitamin B3: niacin and its amide. *Townsend Lett* 1995;147:30–39.

21. Hoffer A. Megavitamin therapy for different cases. *J Orthomolecular Psych* 1976;5:169–182.

22. Hoffer A. Latent Huntington's disease–response to orthomolecular treatment. *J Orthomolecular Psych* 1983;12:44–47.

23. Hoffer A. Huntington's disease: a follow-up. *J Orthomolecular Psych* 1984;13:42–44.

24. Hoffer A. Vitamin B3 dependency: chronic pellagra. *Townsend Lett* 2000;207:66–73.

25. Hoffer A. Obsessions and depression. *J Orthomolecular Psych* 1979;8:78–81.

26. Hoffer A. Allergy, depression and tricyclic antidepressants. *J Orthomolecular Psych* 1980;9:164–170.

27. Sherrill D. Nicotinic acid in the treatment of certain depressed states. *J Bowman Gray School Med* 1950;8:137–144.

28. Chouinard G, Young SN, Annable L, et al. Tryptophan-nicotinamide combination in depression. *Lancet* 1977;1 (8005):249.

29. Chouinard G, Young SN, Annable L, et al. Tryptophan-nicotinamide combination in the treatment of newly depressed patients. *Commun Psychopharmacol* 1978;2:311–318.

30. Washburne AC. Nicotinic acid in the treatment of certain depressed states: a preliminary report. *Ann Intern Med* 1950;32:261–269.

31. Tonge WL. Nicotinic acid in the treatment of depression. *Ann Intern Med* 1953;38:551–553.

32. Thompson LJ, Proctor RC. Depressive and anxiety reactions treated with nicotinic acid and phenobarbital. *N C Med J* 1953;14:420–426.

33. MacSweeney DA. Letter: treatment of unipolar depression. *Lancet* 1975;2(7933):510–511.

34. Chouinard G, Young SN, Annable L, et al. Tryptophan-nicotinamide, imipramine and their combination in depression. A controlled study. *Acta Psychiatr Scand* 1979;59:395–414.

35. Morrow JD, Parsons WG 3rd, Roberts LJ 2nd. Release of markedly increased quantities of prostaglandin D2 in vivo in humans following the administration of nicotinic acid. *Prostaglandins* 1989;38:263–274.

36. Morrow JD, Awad JA, Oates JA, et al. Identification of skin as a major site of prostaglandin D2 release following oral administration of niacin in humans. *J Invest Dermatol* 1992; 98:812–815.

37. Prousky J, Seely D. The treatment of migraines and tension-type headaches with intravenous and oral niacin (nicotinic acid): systematic review of the literature. *Nutr J* 2005;4:3.

38. Bicknell F, Prescott F. *The Vitamins In Medicine.* 3rd ed. Milwaukee, WI: Life Foundation for Nutritional Research, 1953, 346.

39. Scheinberg P. The effect of nicotinic acid on the cerebral circulation, with observations on extra-cerebral contamination of cerebral venous blood in the nitrous oxide procedure for cerebral blood flow. *Circulation* 1950;1:1148–1154.

40. Nagornaia GV, Gaevyi. MD. Effect of complamine and nicospan on the cerebral blood flow and its regulation in changes in blood pressure [in Russian]. *Farmakol Toksikol* 1985; 48:55–59.

41. Jordaan B, Oliver DW, Dormehl IC, et al. Cerebral blood flow effects of piracetam, pentifylline, and nicotinic acid in the baboon model compared with the known effect of acetazolamide. *Arzneimittelforschung* 1996;46:844–847.

42. Oliver DW, Dormehl IC, Louw WK. Non-human primate SPECT model for determining cerebral perfusion effects of cerebrovasoactive drugs acting via multiple modes of pharmacological action. *J Neurol Sci* 2005;229–230:255–259.

43. Ishizaki J, Yamamoto H, Takahashi T, et al. Changes in regional cerebral blood flow following antidepressant treatment in late-life depression. *Int J Geriatr Psychiatry* 2008;23:805–811.

44. Lui S, Parkes LM, Huang X, et al. Depressive disorders: focally altered cerebral perfusion measured with arterial spin-labeling MR imaging. *Radiology* 2009;251:476–484.

45. Lemke H, de Castro AG, Schlattmann P, et al. Cerebrovascular reactivity over time-course – from major depressive episode to remission. *J Psychiatr Res* 2010;44:132–136.

46. Banas A, Lass P, Brockhuis B. Estimation of cerebral perfusion among patients with eating disorders, neurotic and depressive disorders [in Polish]. *Psychiatr Pol* 2009;43:329–340.

47. Vakilian A, Iranmanesh F. Assessment of cerebrovascular reactivity during major depression and after remission of disease. *Ann Indian Acad Neurol* 2010;13:52–56.

48. Badawy AA, Evans M. Letter: tryptophan plus a pyrrolase inhibitor for depression. *Lancet* 1975;2(7940):869.

49. Lin S-H, Chong ZZ, Maiese K. Nicotinamide: a nutritional supplement that provides protection against neuronal and vascular injury. *J Med Food* 2001;4:27–38.

50. Oxenkrug GF. Metabolic syndrome, age-associated neuroendocrine disorders, and dysregulation of tryptophan-kynurenine metabolism. *Ann NY Acad Sci* 2010;1199:1–14.

PHYSICAN'S REPORT:
INSANITY OR HYPOGLYCEMIA: A CASE HISTORY
by Harlan O. L. Wright, DO

Approximately two years ago a man called the office to talk to me about his wife, age 50. There was obvious anxiety and even a hint of desperation in his voice. He wanted an opinion as to whether or not I could help his wife. He started by saying that I was his last hope. If I could not help her she was going to have to be put in the state mental institution. With great emotion, he told the following story.

Patient Profile

Betty (not her real name) had always been a very vivacious, outgoing, and upbeat personality until approximately three years ago when she began to show signs of fatigue and irritability, and to have spells of mild depression. This went on for about two years, becoming a little worse all the time. She finally went to see her gynecologist who found that she was having "female problems" because of a fibroid uterus and advised that she have a hysterectomy and her ovaries removed. The surgery didn't improve her feelings of fatigue and depression as it was thought that it would. She was put on hormone supplementation, which helped for a while. However, Betty's condition gradually deteriorated. Her symptoms began to become more severe and more numerous, including complete fatigue, mental confusion, a feeling of tightness and tenseness in her chest, constantly cramping leg muscles, spells of panic and tachycardia, fainting spells, and deepening depression.

Her gynecologist referred her to an internist who did exhaustive studies on her blood, finding nothing that he considered significant. X-rays and complete cardiology studies revealed mitral valve prolapse. Her symptoms were assumed to be coming from the mitral valve prolapse and the resulting anxiety. She was put on alprazolam (Xanax), procainamide (Procan SR), nortriptyline (Pamelor), and levothyroxine (Synthroid). These medications made her even more lethargic and mentally inadequate and she became hallucinatory at times and out of touch with reality. She was then referred to the psychiatric ward of a hospital where several psychiatrists examined her and experimented with other antidepressants.

Betty's husband was finally told (within hearing of the patient) that she should be put in the state mental hospital and that she would finally end up committing suicide!

All of these happenings, in and out of doctor's offices and hospitals, occurred over a period of one-year post surgery. It was at this point that a family friend, whom I had helped with a similar problem, suggested that he call me.

Examination

Betty's husband was told to get copies of all the laboratory work that had been performed and we arranged to see her immediately. When she walked into the office I observed an extremely morose and expressionless woman with very attractive facial features, weighing 130 pounds. She sat in the chair next to my desk very depressed and withdrawn, displaying very hostile behavior and obviously not wanting to answer questions. She expressed the feeling that all of her troubles were her own fault and that God was punishing her for some reason.

Her past dietary history had been one of an average diet with frequent binges on sweets and eating lots of chocolates.

Notable findings on examination revealed a deeply grooved tongue in the center line, white spots on her fingernails, a very irregular heartbeat, several upper thoracic rib lesions, and very tender trigger points on both occipital ridges.

The laboratory findings were essentially normal with one notable exception. Her five-hour glucose tolerance test was highly abnormal and so typical of a very advanced case of reactive hypoglycemia that I could not understand how any thinking doctor could dismiss it as insignificant. Fasting blood sugar was a normal 105 milligrams (mg) percent; at 1/2 hour, 184 mg; at 1 hour, 168 mg; at 2 hours, 122 mg; at 3 hours, 106 mg; at 4 hours, 82 mg; and at 5 hours, 65 mg. The test should have been continued since the blood sugar was still dropping rapidly but any further figures would have been of only academic interest as the diagnosis of reactive hypoglycemia should have already been made! Such wide variations in blood sugar (or any other of the body's essential nutrients) cannot be tolerated by nature and severe symptoms result.

Treatment

I started treatment of this patient on June 2, 1989, by putting her on a good nutritious diet of unrefined foods with absolutely no refined foods of any kind. She was given the following supplements as needed to correct her obvious deficiencies: vitamin B complex (as evidenced by her badly fissured tongue), magnesium (as evidenced by her irregular heartbeat), magnesium and calcium (as evidenced by her leg cramps), large doses of niacinamide (as evidenced by her depression and mental confusion), vitamin C in megadoses (as evidenced by her bleeding gums and her adrenal cortex weakness), and zinc (as evidenced by the white areas on her nails and her poor glucose metabolism). She was given intensive intravenous infusions of these same substances. She was treated with osteopathic manipulative therapy to stimulate the pancreas and adrenal glands, and to correct the numerous thoracic and cervical bony lesions that were causing much of the discomfort in her chest and head.

On June 5, Betty was already beginning to show improvement. Her attitude was much improved and she even smiled a time or two. Her leg cramping was also improved. By June 11, she was having no more fainting spells and was beginning to think and communicate clearly. She was smiling a great deal on this visit. On June 22, Betty was taken off some of the Xanax. On each visit she was given the hands-on therapy and intravenous vitamin therapy, along with the assurance that she was going to get completely well. By this time I was seeing the patient only every week or so and she continued to make progress. By August 1, she was riding her bicycle and expressing some of her old enthusiasm for life. On September 7, she had just returned from a vacation in California and was doing extremely well and expressed gratitude for getting back her life again. By October 31, Betty was off all mind-altering drugs including Xanax! I have treated her very little since October 1989. She still comes in for general care but no longer needs treatment as far as her "insanity" is concerned. She is again a vibrant and wonderful woman who is thoroughly enjoying life. The only lingering effects of Betty's long suffering with her "mental illness" is the understandable resentment that her real problem wasn't discovered and treated by the numerous specialists she had consulted so that she wouldn't have had to go through a year of "hell" before she got help.

Comments

This is a perfect example of some of the serious problems in the allopathic professions today. We are being taught to depend on high-tech methods of diagnosis and then to prescribe drugs that are foreign to the human body, rather than to practice the original precepts of health. When are we going to start listening to the patient and using our reasoning power and common sense to help people overcome their self-induced and doctor-induced illnesses by helping the body help itself.

From the *J Orthomolecular Med* 1994:9(4):244–245.

THE EFFECT OF FOLIC ACID AND B12 ON DEPRESSION: 12 CASE STUDIES

by Joseph A. Mitchell, PhD

Recent research has indicated a connection between certain nutritional deficiencies and depression.[1] Deficiencies in folic acid and cyanocobalamin (vitamin B12) in the system can result in raised concentrations of plasma homocysteine due to the failure of methylation of the homocysteine from the lack of missing nutritional components.[2] Failure to methylate homocysteine can impair neurotransmitter metabolism.[1] Adequate levels of neurotransmitters in the brain like serotonin, dopamine, and noradrenaline (norepinephrine) are required for emotional well-being.[3] Given the widely held anecdotal belief that modern society is nutritionally deprived, there appears to be initial scientific evidence to suggest an empirical connection between the lack of proper nutrition and the growing prevalence of depression in the general population.[4]

In the mid- to late-1990s, the World Health Organization (WHO) ranked depression as the fourth most important disorder to address clinically, as the prevalent likely cause of disability and mortality.[5] By 1999, depression had become the number one cause of disability.[4] Treatment efficacy with antidepressant medications has stalled at 50 percent, while the use of placebos in experimental research has as nearly an effective treatment outcome at 32 percent.[6] Some researchers noted that this effect could be directly related to the rise in total homocysteine in our patients, indicating a failure of methylation of homocysteine to methionine due to a shortage of supply of methyl groups from methyl folate or, more rarely in depressed patients, lack of the vitamin B12 cofactor for the methylation reaction.[2]

Early research indicated that 56 percent or more of persons with affective disorders had a folate deficiency.[7] A more recent study indicated that people with B12 deficiency were 70 percent more likely to have symptoms of severe depression than those without the deficiency.[8] Speculation regarding the effect of nutritional deficiencies on mood appears stable across nationalities,[8] across ethnicity,[9,10] and even gender.[10,11]

Problem Statement

There appears to be a higher incidence of dysthymic presentations appearing in modern counseling agencies than in previous times.[4] The prevalence of depression in the overall population is approximately "5–8 percent . . . [but] later life depression is estimated to be 15 percent."[6] With only a few notable exceptions, a discussion of the effect of nutritional deficiencies on affect and behavior are nearly missing from modern research, despite the fact that the two constructs have been closely linked together in past research.[12,13,14] In addition, there is evidence to suggest that there is a mild to moderate correlation between nutritional problems in individuals and their subsequent presenting mood disruptions.[15,16]

It is important to recognize that if nutritional deficiencies are causal to symptoms of depression then the likelihood of an actual cure for the symptoms of depression with antidepressant medication, or with talk therapy for that matter, is very low. Since folic acid and vitamin B12 deficiencies have been identified as highly probable in affecting other neuropsychiatric disorders,[2] and vitamin B12 deficiency has been related to histadelic (or high histamine) related schizophrenia-like symptoms,[17] this research was designed to address the question of whether these specific deficiencies are related to symptoms of depression, and whether or not the symptoms can be corrected with a nutritional supplement. Since "folic acid deficiency is one of the most common nutritional deficiencies in the world,"[18] it is indeed time to re-explore to what exact extent the nutritional supplements folic acid and vitamin B12 can be employed to alleviate symptoms of depression.

From the *J Orthomolecular Med* 2007;22(4):183–192.

Significance of the Study

If indeed the symptoms of depression can be stabilized with a common vitamin or nutritional supplement, then the need for an unnecessary invasive allopathic medication could be reduced. While it is prudent to be cautious when exploring alternatives to conventional medicines for the treatment of depression,[19] the need to explore the effect of proper nutrition on negative affective states is overdue. If symptoms of depression can be corrected with non-invasive, orthomolecular treatment such as a nutritional supplement rather than a synthesized medication, the implications for modern medicine would be staggering. Further, if some forms of depression are resistant to antidepressant medication due to the lack of proper nutrition, then too, talk therapy will be futile in the face of the nutritional deficiency. This is a significant issue to address, research, and resolve in terms of professional counseling therapy, psychiatry, and even general practice medicine.

Given that a growing number of people are being prescribed antidepressant medications (that at best work for only 50 percent) and that a number of mood disorder symptoms are likely attributable to some form of nutritional deficiency, it then becomes imperative to determine if symptoms of depression can be reduced with a nutritional supplement rather than having to treat the depression with a medication. Currently, the American Psychiatric Association (APA) defines dysthymic disorder in the *Diagnostic and Statistical Manual of Mental Disorders* (DSM-IV)[20] as a cluster of symptoms that include changes in appetite, changes in sleep patterns, decreased energy, reduced self-esteem, cognitive disruptions, and feelings of hopelessness. There are also severity and longitudinal specifiers in the DSM-IV, as well as other specific criteria to clarify a differential diagnosis. Given the need to clinically assess the physical status of the client, as well as the mental and experiential conditions present with his or her depression, combined with the growing body of evidence that symptoms of depression can be linked with physical causes, it is difficult to understand why the notion of proper nutrition is overlooked in the DSM-IV as a potential causal property of dysthymic affect.

Research Question and Definition of Terms

The research question to be considered is: To what extent will individual symptomatic levels of depression be impacted by the inclusion of a nutritional supplement in the diet? The independent variable identified for this study was the incorporation of folic acid and vitamin B12 into the diets of the case study group. The dependent variable was the concept measured by testing instruments used (i.e., reported level of depression). The definitions for the following terms are taken from *Dorland's Illustrated Medical Dictionary*,[21] except for the chemical compound structures, which are taken from *Webster's New World Dictionary*.[22]

• Folic acid ($C19H19N7O6$) is a water-soluble vitamin that helps regulate the level of homocysteine in the blood and is required for methylation of homocysteine.[21,22]

• Vitamin B12 ($C63H88CoN14O14P$) is a water-soluble, endogenously obtained vitamin that participates in coenzyme-catalyzed reactions and methyl group transfers. It is required for the methylation of homocysteine as is folic acid, but to a lesser degree.

• Homocysteine, which is formed after the digestion of protein-rich foods, is a necessary but toxic amino acid. Abnormally high levels in the blood are believed to produce cardiovascular disease, stroke, atherosclerosis, complications in preg-

IN BRIEF

Nutrition plays a vital role in human behavior not just in terms of manifest physical processes but, in particular, nutrition has an impact on individual cognitive and emotional processing. Lack of nutrition or, more specifically, the lack of proper nutrition, is thought to have an adverse effect on mood. These 12 case studies will explore to what extent incorporating a nutritional supplement into a client's diet impacts the symptoms of persons afflicted with depression.

nancy, and disturbances in mood. Excesses are caused either by improper nutrition or by the genetically inherited disorder homocystinuria.

• Methionine (C5H11NO2S) is an exogenously obtained, sulfur-containing essential amino acid used in the production of protein. Methionine reacts with adenosine triphosphate (ATP), the main energy molecule used in most bodily processes, to produce S-adenosylmethionine (SAMe), a potent donor of methyl groups in the synthesis of norepinephrine. Methylation is the process by which enzymes are catalyzed to regulate protein functions, and results in the conversion of cytosine to 5-methlycytosine, a methyl group contributor.

• Serotonin (C10H12N2O), a neurotransmitter formed from the essential amino acid tryptophan, helps regulate cyclic physical processes and mood. Serotonin constricts the blood vessels, helps to contract smooth muscle tissue, and is important both as a hormone and as a neurotransmitter.

• Norepinephrine (C8H11NO3), also referred to as noradrenaline, is an adrenaline-related neurotransmitter and hormone that belongs to a class of endogenous chemicals known as catecholamines, which control heart rate and blood pressure, and stabilize mood. Norepinephrine is secreted by the adrenal glands, is used by the body to constrict blood vessels and stop bleeding, and is liberated at nerve endings to help transmit nerve impulses.

Assumptions and Limitations

Based on the growing number of peer-review journal articles, which support the notion that folic acid and cyanocobalamin have a direct influence on homocysteine levels, and thus on depression, it was assumed that each of the participants had an equal level of plasma homocysteine. Limitations of the study would thus include the problem of defining whether or not the participant's blood plasma homocysteine levels were abnormal. To test each participant would have been financially prohibitive, and thus each participant was treated as having equal levels. Since the purpose of this research was only to determine at what level the nutritional supplement impacted levels of depression (rather than homocysteine levels), the results would still be

generalizable and transferable to larger populations with depression. Additionally, since the study could not be held in a completely controlled environment there could be other nuisance or confounding variables that affected the outcome of the research, thus providing another limitation to the study. The participants of the research were in outpatient therapy at the time of the study, and thus the separation of treatments (i.e., nutritional supplement and talk therapy) could not be established.

Case Study Group

The sample consisted of twelve adults (four men and eight women) who were attending outpatient therapy at a local mental health agency. Their ages ranged from 29 to 59, and each of the participants had a diagnosis of dysthymic disorder. Each participant was provided with informed consent prior to the research, and each participant volunteered for the study.

Nutritional Supplements

The nutritional supplements used in this study were folic acid and vitamin B12 in the following dosages. Folic acid was taken in an 800-microgram (mcg) tablet once per day in the morning. Vitamin B12 was used in 500-mcg tablets twice per day, once in the morning with the folic acid, and again at noon. Any participant in the study who was prescribed an antidepressant medication prior to the research remained on the medication throughout the trial.

Instrumentation

The instruments used to measure the levels of depression in the sample were the Beck Depression Inventory-II (BDI-II)[23] or the Symptom Checklist-90-Revised.[24] The BDI-II is a 21-item, forced-choice, self-reporting instrument for the assessment of symptoms and attitudes of depression quite similar to the criteria set forth by the APA. The Symptom Checklist-90-Revised (SCL-90-R) is a 90-item, forced-choice, self-reporting instrument designed to assess a broad spectrum of symptoms, with one subscale that specifically evaluates depression. Validity of the SCL-90-R is high.

Case Studies

Richard, a 56-year-old Caucasian male, presented for treatment with depression and anger management issues. He reported not having any satisfaction with life and felt "moody" and angry all the time. His initial SCL-90-R depression subscale score was significantly elevated indicating clinical depression. A six-week retest after beginning the treatment with folic acid and vitamin B12 indicated the continued presence of clinical depression but the reduction of depressive symptoms and affective distress in Richard was evident.

Linda, a 45-year-old Caucasian female, presented for treatment with a high to moderate level of depression. She was referred by her primary health-care physician after the prescribed antidepressant medication paroxetine (Paxil) had failed to control her symptoms in a six-month follow-up. She presented as emotionally unstable, ruminating, and reported being barely able to control her emotions in public or at home. Linda continued to take her medication during the trial, and her six-week retest after beginning treatment with folic acid and vitamin B12 indicated a significantly reduced score on the BDI-II, placing her level of depression in the minimal range after treatment.

Arthur, a 52-year-old Caucasian male, presented with clinical depression and mild anxiety, and stated that he would not take antidepressant medication if prescribed. He reported being agitated and feeling "down" most of the time. His initial SCL-90-R score indicated the presence of mild depression. After beginning the folic acid and vitamin B12 treatment, he left outpatient treatment after only four weeks, stating that he no longer felt depressed or anxious, and felt as if he no longer needed therapy. Unfortunately, no test-retest information is available for this case, but Arthur's subjective report of reduced symptoms of depression can be accepted anecdotally.

Alicia, a 52-year-old African-American female, presented as clinically depressed with strong seasonal affective features. She was referred by her primary health-care physician after the prescribed antidepressant medication bupropion (Wellbutrin) had failed to control her symptoms in a nine-month follow-up with her doctor. She reported feeling sad most of the time, was crying at random intervals for nonspecific reasons, and had begun isolating herself from her family and friends. Her initial SCL-90-R results indicated a significant level of depression. Alicia continued to take her medication during the trial, and her retest after six weeks on folic acid and vitamin B12 indicated a significant reduction in symptoms. It should be noted that this trial took place during the season of her primary affective distress.

Karl, a 59-year-old Caucasian male, came to treatment suffering from chronic severe depression. Karl was referred to psychotherapy by his primary health-care physician after the prescribed antidepressant medication Wellbutrin had failed to control his symptoms after one year. Karl reported being sad and lethargic most of the time, and "angry at the world" the rest of the time. His initial SCL-90-R depression subscale score indicated a significant level of depression. Karl also continued to take his medication during the trial, and his retest after six weeks on folic acid and vitamin B12 indicated a reduced level of depression. His retest score on the SCL-90-R still indicated a clinical level of depression, but the reduction of symptoms from beyond the third standard deviation to just beyond the second is important.

Nancy, a 35-year-old Caucasian female, came to therapy suffering from short-term severe depression and a high level of situational stress. She reported having intense mood swings, uncontrollable emotional outbursts, feeling "burned out," and a very low tolerance to frustration. Her initial BDI-II score confirmed the presence of a severe level of depression. Nancy attended only a few therapy sessions during the trial, but her retest after six weeks on folic acid and vitamin B12 still indicated a significant reduction in her scores.

John, a 49-year-old Caucasian male, presented with short-term clinical depression that he attributed to ongoing circumstantial life events. His initial BDI-II score indicated a high-mild level of depression, bordering on moderate depression. John also only attended a few therapy sessions during this trial, and his retest after six weeks on folic acid and vitamin B12 did indicate a substantial reduction in his scores. These last two cases are especially important because they are less affected by other confounding variables than the rest, and yet both cases still resulted in a reduction of symptoms.

Alexia, a 52-year-old Caucasian female, presented with chronic clinical depression confounded by multiple psychosocial stressors. She was referred by her primary health-care physician for psychotherapy after the prescribed antidepressant medication escitalopram (Lexapro) had failed to control her symptoms in a one-year follow-up. She reported crying constantly, a general loss of interest in things she used to enjoy, and was extremely labile at intake. Her initial BDI-II score confirmed a severe level of depression. She continued to take her medication during the trial, and her retest after six weeks on folic acid and B12 indicated a significant reduction in reported symptoms measured by the BDI-II.

Barbara, a 47-year-old Caucasian female, presented with chronic clinical depression referred by her primary health-care physician for therapy after the prescribed antidepressant medication (Paxil) had failed to control her symptoms in a one-year follow-up. She reported being unable to control her mood, that she was crying constantly, and, observationally, she was emotionally unstable at intake. Her initial BDI-II score confirmed the presence of a severe level of depression and her initial SCL-90-R score was also elevated. She continued to take her medication during the trial, and her six-week retest after beginning the treatment with folic acid and vitamin B12 indicated reduced scores and reduced symptoms.

Helen, a 37-year-old Caucasian female, was referred by her primary health-care physician for psychotherapy after the prescribed antidepressant medication sertraline (Zoloft) had failed to control her symptoms in a six-month follow-up. Despite the use of her medication, she reported being sad, fatigued, and angry most of the time. Helen's initial BDI-II score placed her level of depression in the severe range. She continued to take her medication during the trial, and her six-week retest after beginning the treatment with folic acid and vitamin B12 indicated decreased symptoms.

Jessica, a 29-year-old Caucasian female, presented with long-term chronic depression. She also had been referred by her primary health-care physician for psychotherapy after the prescribed antidepressant medication fluoxetine (Prozac) had failed to control her symptoms in a nine-month follow-up. Despite the use of her medication, she reported feeling extremely sad and agitated most of the time, with accompanying fatigue. Her initial BDI-II score placed her level of depression in the severe range. She continued to take her medication, and her retest after six weeks on folic acid and vitamin B12 indicated a reduction in scores for the BDI-II and the SCL-90-R.

Lastly, Roxanne, a 45-year-old Caucasian female, presented with long-term chronic depression. She was self-motivated to enter outpatient treatment after her antidepressant medication Paxil reportedly began to "lose its effect" in controlling her symptoms. She reported feeling disconnected from herself, as if a "black cloud" or a "void" was around her at all times. Roxanne's initial SCL-90-R depression subscale score was elevated. She continued to take her medication during the trial, and her retest after six weeks on folic acid and vitamin B12 indicated a decrease in reported symptoms of depression.

Discussion

The scores of each of the participants indicated a reduction in reported levels of symptoms of depression. The findings of this research are limited based on the small size of the case study sample. However, the results are also important in terms of adding to the knowledge base regarding the potential benefits of folic acid and vitamin B12 supplements in the treatment of depression. In some cases, the effect of the supplements still failed to reduce symptoms below clinically diagnosable levels, but, in those cases, antidepressants had also previously failed to reduce those symptoms. Given that the greatest effect appeared in the participants who were already on antidepressant medication without relief from their symptoms, one can infer that it was the effect of the supplements rather than the effect of the medications that were responsible for the reduction in the participant's symptoms.

■ CONCLUSION

The results of this research indicated that folic acid and vitamin B12 nutritional supplements did indeed play a significant role in decreasing the symptoms of depression reported by the participants.

REFERENCES

1. Bottiglieri T, Laundy M, Crellin R, et al. Homocysteine, folate, methylation, and monoamine metabolism in depression. *J Neurol Neurosur Ps* 2006;69:228–232.

2. Bottiglieri T. Folate, B12, and neuropsychiatric disorders. *Nutr Rev* 1996; 54:382–390.

3. Deng G, Cassileth BR. Integrative oncology: complementary therapies for pain, anxiety, and mood disturbance. *CA Cancer J Clin* 2005;55:109–116.

4. Comer RJ. *Abnormal Psychology.* 5th ed. New York: Worth, 2004.

5. Murray CJ, Lopez, AD. Global mortality, disability, and the contribution of risk factors: global burden of disease study. *Lancet* 1997;349:1436–1442.

6. Coppen A, Bolander-Gouaille C. Treatment of depression: time to consider folic acid and vitamin B12. *J Psychopharmacol* 2005;19:59–65.

7. Shorvon S, Carney MWP, Chanarin I, et al. The neuropsychiatry of megaloblastic anaemia. *Brit Med J* 1980;281:1036–1038.

8. Tiemeier MJ, van Tuijl HR, Hofman A, et al. Vitamin B12, folate, and homocysteine in depression: The Rotterdam study. *Am J Psychiat* 2002;159:2099–2101.

9. Lindeman RD, Romero LJ, Koehler KM, et al. Serum vitamin B12, C, and folate concentrations in the New Mexico Elder Health Survey: correlations with cognitive and affective functions. *J Am Coll Nutr* 2000;19:68–76.

10. Ramos MI, Allen LH, Haan MN, et al. Plasma folate concentrations are associated with depressive symptoms in elderly Latina women despite folic acid fortification. *Am J Clin Nutr* 2004;80:1024–1028.

11. Tolmunen T, Hintikka J, Voutilainen S, et al. Association between depressive symptoms and serum concentrations of homocysteine in men: a population study. *Am J Clin Nutr* 2004;80:1574–1578.

12. Christensen L. Implementation of dietary intervention. *Prof Psychol-Res Pr* 1991; 22:503–509.

13. Christensen L. Issues in the design of studies investigating the behavioral concomitants of foods. *J Consult Clin Psych* 1991;59:874–882.

14. Lozoff B. Nutrition and behavior. *Am Psychol* 1989;44:231–236.

15. Christensen L, Redig C. Effect of meal composition on mood. *Behav Neurosci* 1993;107:346–353.

16. Williams PG, Surwit RS, Babyak MA, et al. Personality predictors of mood related to dieting. *J Consult Clin Psych* 1998;66:994–1004.

17. Hoffer A. *Orthomolecular Treatment for Schizophrenia.* Los Angeles: Keats Publishing, 1999.

18. Fugh-Berman A, Cott JM. Dietary supplements and natural products as psyhotherapeutic agents. *Psychosom Med* 1999;61:712–728.

19. Bassman L, Uellendahl G. Complimentary/alternative medicine: ethical, professional, and practical challenges for psychologists. *Prof Psychol-Res Pr* 2003;34:264–270.

20. American Psychiatric Association. *Diagnostic and Statistical Manual of Mental Disorders.* 4th ed. Washington, DC: self-published, 2000.

21. *Dorland's Illustrated Medical Dictionary.* 30th ed. Philadelphia: WB Saunders, 2003.

22. *Webster's New World Dictionary on Power CD* (version 2.11). Dallas, TX: Zane Publishing, 1994.

23. Beck AT, Steer RA, Brown GK. *Beck Depression Inventory Manual.* 2nd ed. San Antonio, TX: Psychological Corporation, 1996.

24. Derogatis LR. *Symptom Checklist-90-R: Administration, Scoring, and Procedures Manual.* Minneapolis, MN: National Computer Systems, 1994.

25. Beck AT. *Beck Interpretrak* [computer software]. San Antonio, TX: Psychological Corporation, 2000.

SUPPLEMENTAL NIACINAMIDE MITIGATES ANXIETY SYMPTOMS: THREE CASE REPORTS

by Jonathan E. Prousky, ND

Anxiety disorders are very prevalent conditions treated by primary care providers. In a recent survey of 2,316 randomly selected patients (ages eighteen and older) seen by general practitioners, 42.5 percent of all patients had evidence of a psychiatric disorder.[1] In the same survey, anxiety disorders were found in 19 percent of all patients. In a survey of 88 outpatients in an internal medicine clinic, 30 percent of patients had mixed anxiety features, 33 percent had generalized anxiety symptoms, almost half reported obsessive-compulsive personality symptoms, and about one-quarter had marked levels of worry.[2] The investigators concluded that anxiety disorders are more common in primary care settings than what had been previously reported.

Anxiety Disorders

Anxiety disorders are classified into various categories such as obsessive-compulsive disorder (OCD), panic disorder (PD), social phobia/social anxiety disorder (SAD), and generalized anxiety disorder (GAD). This report will not differentiate the various categories of anxiety disorders as described in the *Diagnostic and Statistical Manual of Mental Disorders*.[3] Considering their high prevalence, it is paramount that effective treatments are offered to patients due to the obvious suffering that accompanies anxiety disorders. Heart racing, muscular tension, sweating, flushing, nervousness, constant worry, and panic characterize some of the debilitating symptoms of anxiety disorders. It is unfortunate that many patients seeking standard (mainstream) treatment for anxiety disorders remain untreated and underdiagnosed many years after their initial diagnoses, leading to unremitting impairment in functional status and quality of life.[4]

I evaluate and treat patients every day suffering from unremitting anxiety symptoms. In my efforts to mitigate their anxiety, I have been prescribing the amide of niacin (known as niacinamide). Both niacin and niacinamide are commonly referred to as vitamin B3. The biochemistry of vitamin B3 is well known in that it is involved in some 200 enzymatic reactions within the human body. Its active forms or its coenzymes (enzyme cofactors) are both nicotinamide adenine dinucleotide (NAD) and nicotinamide adenine dinucleotide phosphate (NADP). Vitamin B3 can be absorbed directly from the stomach, but most of its absorption occurs within the small intestine. The liver contains the most concentrated amounts of the nicotinamide coenzymes, but all metabolically active tissues require these vital metabolic products.

The most common uses of niacinamide and niacin are for the treatment of pellagra. Pellagra is a disease caused by a cellular deficiency of the nicotinamide coenzymes due to inadequate dietary supply of tryptophan and vitamin B3 (as either niacin or niacinamide). Diarrhea, dermatitis, and dementia characterize this deficiency disease. Although it is not usually fatal, when the three Ds are present, death can occur. The adult intake of vitamin B3 necessary to prevent pellagra is 20 milligrams (mg) per day. The body can manufacture approximately 1 mg of niacin equivalents from 60 mg of tryptophan obtained mostly from dietary protein sources. This conversion makes it rather difficult to develop frank pellagra in affluent, industrialized countries. Rare forms of pellagra, however, do occur. Pellagra has been found among people with anorexia nervosa,[5] hypothyroidism,[6,7] alcoholism,[8,9] homelessness,[10] and in those taking anticonvulsant medications.[11,12]

Here, I report on three cases where the use of large pharmacological doses of niacinamide considerably improved the symptoms of anxiety.[13] In each of the cases, frank symptoms of pellagra were absent, even though neuropsychiatric and gastrointestinal manifestations were present. Niacinamide's therapeutic mechanism of action was

From the *J Orthomolecular Med* 2005;20(3):167–178.

likely related to the correction of subclinical pellagra, the correction of an underlying vitamin B3 dependency disorder, niacinamide's benzodiazepine-like effects, its ability to increase the production of serotonin, or its ability to modify the metabolism of blood lactate (lactic acid).

Case #1

An 11-year-old female first presented to my office on November 10, 2003. Her chief complaints were nervousness, anxiety, and excessive worrying. The onset of her symptoms occurred when her father tragically died in September 2003. The patient reported anxiety when she had to sit for examinations and when she was around her classmates. The most concerning symptom was her fear of being kidnapped, which was instigated by a well-publicized kidnapping of a young Asian girl in the city where she lives. She also reported having approximately two panic attacks each month since September for which she had learned to deal with them by "leaving the situation to get air." Other symptoms that were reported included some facial acne, frequent blushing, stomachaches, and sweatiness. Her past medical history was unremarkable, except for asthma that was diagnosed approximately one year earlier. A complete physical examination was performed and all findings were within normal limits. The only notable sign was some acne along her cheeks and chin. She was diagnosed with panic disorder, with some elements of social phobia. She was prescribed a daily multiple vitamin/mineral preparation, zinc (25 mg), pyridoxine (100 mg), magnesium (400 mg), and niacinamide (500 mg) twice daily.

A follow-up appointment occurred on December 13, 2003. The patient reported a slight improvement with her anxiety. She did not like taking all the supplements and agreed to continue with just the multiple vitamin/mineral preparation, zinc, and niacinamide. She also agreed to increase the dose of niacinamide to 1,000 mg twice daily. No side effects were reported.

A second follow-up occurred on February 7, 2004. The patient, now 12 years old, reported a striking improvement with her anxiety. She did not always take her pills daily but was happy with the results. Her panic attacks completely stopped and her acne was much improved as well. In a recent email from the patient, she reported to be taking only the 1,000 mg of niacinamide twice daily. Her anxiety remained much improved and was no longer interfering with her ability to engage in a regular life.

Case #2

A 28-year-old female came to my private practice with a chief complaint of generalized anxiety disorder on May 10, 2004. She had been struggling with this anxiety disorder for the past twelve years. She is a high school teacher and noted that her anxiety was more pronounced during the academic year. Her anxiety was worse in the morning with symptoms of frequent muscular tension, the passing of flatus, and chest pain. She reported a fear of smelling when she needed to expel gas. The anxiety also made it difficult for her to concentrate and focus on things. When she experienced anxiety symptoms, she would feel the need to isolate herself from others. The same isolating need

IN BRIEF

The purpose of this report is to highlight the potential of niacinamide for the treatment of anxiety disorders. Three patients were prescribed large pharmacological doses of niacinamide (2,000–2,500 mg per day). Each of the patients had considerable relief from their anxiety when regularly using niacinamide. The possible biochemical reasons for niacinamide's effectiveness might be related to the correction of subclinical pellagra, the correction of an underlying vitamin B3 dependency disorder, its benzodiazepine-like effects, its ability to raise serotonin levels, or its ability to modify the metabolism of blood lactate (lactic acid). Adverse effects did not occur with these doses, but nausea and vomiting can occur when doses as high as 6,000 mg per day are used. These positive case reports suggest that niacinamide might be helpful for the treatment of anxiety disorders.

would also occur when she simply thought about possibly feeling nervous and expelling gas. She also reported fears of embarrassment and worried about being criticized from others. She had been on paroxetine (Paxil) for one year but had not noticed any improvement. She reported feeling depressed due to the anxiety and would get apathetic when her anxiety was at its worst. Baths, lying in bed, walking, and exercising helped to slightly reduce her anxiety. She was unable to correlate any of her symptoms with foods. This patient also had a history of thrombocytopenia (low platelet count) for the past five years for which she was being regularly monitored by her family physician. She did report easy bruising but did not have any history of widespread bruising and bleeding. The rest of her past medical history was unremarkable.

Physical examination revealed a well-nourished woman with normal vital signs. All her systems were within normal limits. She was subsequently diagnosed with generalized anxiety disorder with some social phobia, and thrombocytopenia. Lab tests were requisitioned and she was prescribed niacinamide at an initial dose of 500 mg three times daily for three days, and then was instructed to increase it to 1,000 mg every morning, 500 mg at lunch, and 1,000 mg at dinner. She was also prescribed 5-hydroxytryptophan (5-HTP) at a dose of 100 mg twice daily for her mild depression, and 2,000 mg of vitamin C to be taken daily for the thrombocytopenia.

The patient had a follow-up appointment on May 31, 2004. She had difficulty swallowing the niacinamide pills due to their bitter taste. Despite this, she was taking the recommended dose of 2,500 mg per day. Her anxiety was much improved and she experienced only three minor panic attacks since the initial visit. Prior to the treatment her anxiety was chronic, occurring daily, with the sensation or need to pass gas. The patient continued to complain of depression, which she felt was more pronounced prior to menses. Her complete blood count was normal, except that her platelets were low at a value of 79. The patient was unsure if the treatments were working due to her time away from teaching. We agreed that she

would discontinue all prescribed treatments except for the vitamin C until June 14, 2004. After this date, the patient would resume the 5-HTP and niacinamide, and would begin taking vitamin B6 (250 mg) and magnesium (400 mg). The vitamin B6 (pyridoxine) and magnesium were prescribed for the premenstrual symptoms of depression.

On June 4, 2004, I received an urgent telephone call from the patient. Since discontinuing the prescribed treatments on June 1, her anxiety symptoms returned promptly and she had difficulty functioning. She agreed to resume only the niacinamide tablets.

On July 2, 2004, the patient emailed me with an update. She discontinued all the prescribed treatments except for the niacinamide. She found her anxiety and depression to be much relieved due to being at home and not teaching during the summer months. When she felt anxiety she would take niacinamide and it would help. In her words, "I take the niacinamide and I'm fine afterwards."

Case #3

A 42-year-old female first presented to my private practice on May 16, 2004, for chief complaints of constipation and anxiety. About three weeks ago her father had been diagnosed with advanced carcinoma of the stomach. For three days following his diagnosis, the patient experienced very soft stools once or twice daily. For her entire life she had been constipated, requiring regular laxatives in order to have a daily bowel movement. The patient reported additional gastrointestinal symptoms of bloating, gas, and right-sided abdominal pain. She had taken fiber therapy in the past but had never stayed on it long enough to see the benefits. She was not concerned about the constipation since she had been having at least one to two soft stools per day.

Since her father's diagnosis she had been feeling very anxious with symptoms of shakiness, light-headedness, numbness of the extremities, and balance problems. Her medical doctor had her do a 24-hour Holter monitor and the results were normal. She was unable to correlate her anxiety with feelings of hunger. In the past, she would have the same kind of anxiety symptoms when stressful events occurred. Her medical doctor felt that the patient's anxiety was related to hyperventilation. On physical examination, the patient was well nourished, slightly overweight, with normal blood pressure and normal heart sounds. All other systems were within normal limits. Even though her mother currently has heart disease, the rest of her family history was unremarkable. She was diagnosed with panic attacks, dyspepsia (possible irritable bowel syndrome), and mild obesity. She was advised to continue with her liquid multiple vitamin/mineral preparation, take 500 mg of niacinamide three times each day for two days, and was told to increase the dose to 1,000 mg twice daily. Two capsules of lactobacillus acidophilus were prescribed every morning upon rising.

A follow-up visit occurred on May 26, 2004. The patient felt a little better during the first week on niacinamide. However, she felt jittery and related this to her father's grim prognosis. Her sleep was unaffected, even though she did wake up once each night to go to the bathroom. Overall, she felt much more under control. She was advised to increase the niacinamide to 1,000 mg three times each day.

On July 12, 2004, she came in for another visit. She cut back on the niacinamide since she felt that it caused her to have feelings of not being present. Instead of 3,000 mg daily she lowered the dose to 2,000 mg per day. Her constipation was not a problem and she was having one bowel movement daily. Her anxiety was much improved on this dose and the previous shakiness had completely resolved. In fact, she had not experienced any episodes of shakiness since the last visit. She was told to continue the prescribed treatments and to take a B-complex vitamin preparation and 1 mg of folic acid each day.

Subclinical Pellagra

These three case reports and an additional case report by this author[14] demonstrate that niacinamide is capable of reducing symptoms of anxiety. All the patients responded favorably to large pharmacological doses of niacinamide (2,000–2,500 mg per day or as needed). These amounts were much greater than the amounts of vitamin B3 or

protein (containing tryptophan) that would be necessary to prevent full-blown pellagra. The initial symptoms of pellagra tend to involve the gastrointestinal system, which are known to precede the dermatological ones.[15] In these three patients, the gastrointestinal symptoms formed part of their clinical presentation. It was impossible to determine if these symptoms preceded their anxieties or neuropsychiatric symptoms. In case #3, the patient reported a long-standing history of constipation many years before the onset of acute anxiety. In the other two cases, the patients had anxiety symptoms with mild gastrointestinal manifestations. The patient in Case #1 had stomachaches when she felt anxious, and in Case #2 the patient passed gas when she experienced anxiety.

It appears that these patients did have pellagra-like symptoms primarily involving the neuropsychiatric system. One of the earliest reports describing the psychological patterning of central nervous system impairments due to an inadequate supply of niacinamide came from the work of Dr. William Kaufman.[16] He used the term "aniacinamidosis" to denote a deficiency state that could not be ameliorated by dietary modifications but required daily pharmacological doses (150–350 mg) of niacinamide to reverse its clinical manifestations. Some of the psychological symptoms associated with aniacinamidosis are similar to the symptoms exhibited by the patients in these case reports.

Dr. Glen Green, in his paper on subclinical pellagra, noted that mental symptoms occurred in patients without frank deficiency of vitamin B3.[17] Similarly, Dr. Abram Hoffer reported that the earliest symptoms of pellagra in its subclinical form manifest as modern mood disorders (e.g., anxiety, depression, fatigue, and vague somatic complaints), followed by the development of other symptoms.[18] It is evident that subclinical pellagra can present with symptoms primarily affecting the neuropsychiatric system, yet the reasons for its genesis remain unknown. One possible explanation might involve a phenomenon known as a localized cerebral deficiency disease. Dr. Linus Pauling discussed the possibility of having grossly diminished cerebrospinal fluid (CSF) concentrations of a vital substance, while its concentration in the blood and lymph remained essentially normal.[19] This localized cerebral deficiency, according to Pauling, might occur from decreased rates of transfer (i.e., decreased permeability) of the vital substance across the blood-brain barrier, an increased rate of destruction of the vital substance within the CSF, or from some other unknown factor.[19] If the serum and CSF were to be examined for micronutrient status, extreme perturbations between these compartments might demonstrate the presence of a localized cerebral deficiency. For example, in a study involving 49 patients with organic mental disorders, deficient CSF levels of vitamin B12 were found in 30 of the patients.[20] When the serum levels of vitamin B12 were tested, normal values were found in 45 of them, indicating a marked difference between both compartments. Given that serum levels of vitamin B12 can be normal yet deficient in the CSF, other micronutrients (such as vitamin B3) might follow a similar pattern of deficiency if the CSF and serum were to be respectively analyzed. The correction of subclinical pellagra might be one of the reasons for niacinamide's effectiveness.

Vitamin B3 Dependency as a Result of Enzymatic Defects

The patients' positive responses to niacinamide suggest that this vitamin might have corrected an underlying vitamin B3 dependency disorder. A vitamin B3 dependency denotes an increased metabolic need for the vitamin. Its cause is unknown, but it has been purported to result from a combination of malnutrition and long-term environmental-genetic stresses that disrupts the conversion of dietary tryptophan into a sufficient amount of vitamin B3.[18] Over time, this disruption would impair all the biochemical processes dependent on a constant supply of the nicotinamide coenzymes. In order to sustain adequate health it would be necessary to obtain a daily intake of vitamin B3 in amounts far greater than what could be accomplished from dietary sources alone.[21] This is not so unreasonable since many enzyme systems within the body require large pharmacological doses of vitamins to remedy defects in the synthesis of vital

metabolic products to sustain adequate health. Pauling reported that "mental disease is for the most part caused by abnormal reaction rates, as determined by genetic constitution and diet, and by abnormal molecular concentrations of essential substances."[19] He described how megavitamin therapy would be necessary for the optimal treatment of mental disease since the saturating capacity would be much greater for defective enzymes that have diminished combining capacity for their respective substrates. In other words, an enzyme-catalyzed reaction could be corrected when high doses of a particular micronutrient are provided.

Pauling's ideas were later confirmed by Laraine Abbey who found various B-vitamin dependent enzymopathies in 12 patients with agoraphobia.[22] All of Abbey's patients required 200–500 mg of the various B-complex factors in order to resolve both the associated enzymatic defects and symptoms of their anxiety and panic. [For more on Abbey's findings, see the article "Agoraphobia: A Nutritionally Responsive Disorder" later in this chapter.] In a more recent report, the need for large pharmacological doses of micronutrients were deemed necessary as a means to increase coenzyme concentrations and to correct defective enzymatic activity in some 50 human genetic diseases.[23] Surely, there must be a certain percentage of patients who would be responsive to large pharmacological doses of vitamin B3 to correct both the disordered biochemistry and the resulting neuropsychiatric manifestations; presumably, the result of defective enzymatic activity.

Benzodiazepine-Like Properties

Additional reasons for niacinamide's effectiveness likely have to do with its benzodiazepine-like effects. In a previous review of the literature by Hoffer, both niacin and niacinamide were shown to have some sedative activity and were able to potentiate the action of sedatives, anticonvulsant medications, and certain tranquilizers.[24] In a recent case report by this author, a review of the literature was undertaken to determine the biological mechanism for niacinamide's sedative-like effects.[14] It appears that both the benzodiazepines and niacinamide exert similar tranquilizing effects through the modulation of neurotransmitters commonly unbalanced in anxiety.[25–30]

Niacinamide might also be helpful when weaning patients off their benzodiazepine medications. Benzodiazepine withdrawal symptoms include tinnitus, involuntary movements, tingling in the extremities, perceptual changes, and confusion. Twenty-eight patients who had been abusing flunitrazepam (Rohypnol) for at least six months were abruptly taken off the drug.[31] The patients were randomly assigned to receive intravenous nicotinic acid (3,000 mg per day over the first 48 hours, followed by 1,500 mg over the following 48 hours), or a placebo (glucose solution alone). Although blinding was not specified, patients who received the nicotinic acid had significantly fewer withdrawal symptoms than those who received the placebo. These results suggest that intravenous administration of nicotinic acid can reduce withdrawal symptoms in patients withdrawing from flunitrazepam. Even though intravenous nicotinic acid would achieve higher blood concentrations than oral niacinamide, both nutrients are forms of vitamin B3, and, therefore, the infused and oral methods might similarly help to withdraw patients from their benzodiazepine medications.

Serotonin Synthesis

Another biochemical reason for niacinamide's tranquilizing effects might have to do with the vital role that it has upon the synthesis of serotonin. For example, in a patient with anorexia nervosa, an insufficient supply of vitamin B3 or protein resulted in reduced urinary levels of the serotonin breakdown product, 5-hydroxy-indolacetic acid (5-HIAA).[32] The authors of this report postulated that a deficiency of vitamin B3 disrupted the kynurenine pathway, resulting in tryptophan being diverted to the kynurenine pathway, making less tryptophan available for the synthesis of serotonin. By contrast, the use of pharmacological doses of vitamin B3 can increase the production of serotonin.[33] In a rat study, the administration of 20 mg of niacin resulted in increased levels of 5-HIAA.[34] Taking pharmacolog-ical doses of niacinamide (or any other form of vitamin B3) would increase the production of serotonin, by diverting more tryptophan available for serotonin synthesis. Niacinamide's therapeutic ability to increase serotonin production might explain why it was successful in reducing the anxiety symptoms of the three patients.

Modulation of Blood Lactate

The final biochemical reason for niacinamide's favorable effect might have to do with its ability to modulate the metabolism of blood lactate (lactic acid). All of the patients in the case reports experienced frequent panic attacks in addition to their other anxiety symptoms. Lactate sensitivity or an increased responsiveness to lactate might have caused some of their anxiety symptoms. Only one of the patients (Case #3) appeared to have hyperventilation as part of her clinical presentation. All of them had a therapeutic response to niacinamide, demonstrating its ability to reduce panic attacks. Abbey suggested that an insufficient supply of the coenzyme NAD would inhibit the conversion of lactate back to pyruvate (a molecule used in the production of cellular energy), which would contribute to a high lactate-to-pyruvate ratio and therefore to anxiety.[22] In 3 out of 12 patients, Abbey found deficient levels of urinary N1 methylnicotinamide (indicating deficient intake of niacinamide) normalized when large pharmacological doses of B-complex vitamins were provided, to which she conjectured that an excess of NAD was required to drive the conversion of lactate to pyruvate. Buist also hypothesized that anxiety neurosis is associated with elevated blood lactate and an increased lactate-to-pyruvate ratio to which effective treatment requires increasing niacin status (i.e., increasing NAD levels) through supplementation.[35]

The formation of lactate by the enzyme, lactate dehydrogenase, is the final product of anaerobic glycolysis. Niacinamide supplementation might result in an increased conversion of lactate to pyruvate, thus reversing the equilibrium of the pyruvate to lactate reaction. For example, when a patient with mitochondrial encephalopathy, myopathy, lactic acidosis, and stroke-like episodes (MELAS) was treated with 1,000 mg of niacinamide four times daily, large reductions (50 percent or more) in blood lactate and pyruvate concentrations occurred by the third day of treatment.[36] Large pharmacological doses of niacinamide appear to be capable of reducing blood lactate and pyruvate concentrations.

Patients with panic attacks likely have a greater demand placed upon anaerobic glycolysis due to the rapidity or shallowness of breathing that so often accompanies their anxiety attacks.

Therefore, a greater amount of NAD obtained by means of niacinamide supplementation might help the tissues of the body, including the central nervous system, to readily oxidize lactate (obtained from the blood) to pyruvate, and consequently mitigate panic attacks and hyperventilation (if present).

Prescribing Instructions

In terms of proper dosing, most patients require a minimum of 2,000–4,500 mg per day to achieve therapeutic results. These dosages were derived from the work of Hoffer, who recommended 1,500–6,000 mg of niacinamide per day for all patients with psychiatric syndromes.[21] Patients usually experience relief of their symptoms within one month of taking the medication (personal observation). The three patients tolerated the large pharmacological doses of niacinamide very well. Only one patient needed to reduce her dose from 3,000 mg per day to 2,000 mg per day due to feelings of not being present (perhaps de-realization). The 28-year-old patient had problems swallowing the niacinamide tablets. For this reason, it might be necessary to switch some patients to capsules or powder forms of niacinamide.

Large pharmacological doses of niacinamide (1,500–6,000 mg per day) have been safely used in children and adolescents for extended periods of time without any adverse side effects or complications.[37,38] The most common side effect with niacinamide is sedation,[39] but dry mouth and nausea have been the most common side effects that I have observed among some of my patients. I never

exceed 6,000 mg per day of niacinamide since most patients will develop nausea and sometimes vomiting on this dose.[21] There is hardly any need to go above 4,500 mg per day when treating anxiety. If nausea does occur, decreasing the dose by 1,000 mg usually corrects the problem.

CONCLUSION

Large pharmacological doses of niacinamide were effective in relieving the symptoms of anxiety in these three patients. Even though niacinamide's mechanisms of action have not been substantiated from controlled clinical trials, this agent does appear to have a wide spectrum of beneficial effects upon anxiety disorders. Niacin's ability to mitigate symptoms of anxiety, exert benzodiazepine-like properties, increase production of serotonin, as well as possibly correct longstanding deficiencies in vitamin B3—and all without the negative side effects of mainstream anti-anxiety medications, drugs—may perhaps make it a more effective agent than current contemporary medications for the treatment of anxiety disorders.

REFERENCES

1. Ansseau M, Dierick M, Buntinkx F, et al. High prevalence of mental disorders in primary care. *J Affect Disord* 2004;78: 49–55.

2. Sansone RA, Hendricks CM, Gaither GA, et al. Prevalence of anxiety symptoms among a sample of outpatients in an internal medicine clinic: a pilot study. *Depress Anxiety* 2004;19: 133–136.

3. *Diagnostic and Statistical Manual of Mental Disorders.* 4th ed. Washington, DC: American Psychiatric Association, 2000.

4. Colman SS, Brod M, Potter LP, et al. Cross-sectional 7-year follow-up of anxiety in primary care patients. *Depress Anxiety* 2004;19:105–111.

5. Prousky JE. Pellagra may be a rare secondary complication of anorexia nervosa: a systematic review of the literature. *Altern Med Rev* 2003;8:180–185.

6. Hawn LJ, Guldan GJ, Chillag SC, et al. A case of pellagra and a South Carolina history of the disorder. *J SC Med Assoc* 2003;99:220–223.

7. Prasad PVS, Babu A, Paul EK, et al. Myxoedema pellagra: a report of two cases. *J Assoc Physicians India* 2003;51:421–422.

8. Wallengren J, Thelin I. Pellagra-like skin lesions associated with Wernicke's encephalopathy in a heavy wine drinker. *Acta Derm Venereol* 2002;82:152–154.

9. Pitsavas S, Andreou C, Bascialla F, et al. Pellagra encephalopathy following B-complex vitamin treatment without niacin. *Int J Psychiatry Med* 2004;34:91–95.

10. Kertesz SG. Pellagra in 2 homeless men. *Mayo Clin Proc* 2001;76:315–318.

11. Lyon VB, Fairley JA. Anticonvulsant-induced pellagra. *J Am Acad Dermatol* 2002;46:597–599.

12. Kaur S, Goraya JS, Thami GP, et al. Pellagrous dermatitis induced by phenytoin. Pediatr *Dermatol* 2002;19:93.

13. Prousky JE. Orthomolecular treatment of anxiety disorders. *Townsend Lett* 2005;259:82–87.

14. Prousky JE. Niacinamide's potent role in alleviating anxiety with its benzodiazepine-like properties: a case report. *J Orthomolecular Med* 2004;19:104–110.

15. Hegyi J, Schwartz RA, Hegyi V. Pellagra: dermatitis, dementia, and diarrhea. *Int J Dermatol* 2004;43:1–5.

16. Kaufman W. *The Common Form of Niacinamide Deficiency Disease: Aniacinamidosis.* Bridgeport, CT: Yale University Press, 1943.

17. Green RG. Subclinical pellagra among penitentiary inmates. *J Orthomolecular Psychiat* 1976;5:68–83.

18. Hoffer A. Vitamin B3 dependency: chronic pellagra. *Townsend Lett* 2000;207:66–73.

19. Pauling L. Orthomolecular psychiatry: varying the concentrations of substances normally present in the human body may control mental disease. *Science* 1968;160:265–271.

20. van Tiggelen CJM, Peperkamp JPC, Tertoolen JFW. Vitamin B12 levels of cerebrospinal fluid in patients with organic mental disorders. *J Orthomolecular Psychiat* 1983;12:305–311.

21. Hoffer A. Vitamin B3: niacin and its amide. *Townsend Lett* 1995;147:30–39.

22. Abbey LC. Agoraphobia. *J Orthomolecular Psychiat* 1982;11:243–259.

23. Ames BN, Elson-Schwab I, Silver EA. High-dose vitamin therapy stimulates variant enzymes with decreased coenzyme binding (increased Km): relevance to genetic diseases and polymorphisms. *Am J Clin Nutr* 2002;75:616–658.

24. Hoffer A. Nicotinic acid and niacinamide as sedatives: niacin therapy. In: *Psychiatry.* Springfield: Charles C Thomas, 1962, 24–31.

25. Möhler H, Polc C, Cumin R, et al. Nicotinamide is a brain constituent with benzodiazepine-like actions. *Nature* 1979;278:563–565.

26. Slater P, Longman DA. Effects of diazepam and muscimol on GABA-mediated neurotransmission: interactions with inosine and nicotinamide. *Life Sci* 1979;25:1963–1967.

27. Kennedy B, Leonard BE. Similarity between the action of nicotinamide and diazepam on neurotransmitter metabolism in the rat. *Biochem Soc Trans* 1980;8:59–60.

28. Lapin IP. Nicotinamide, inosine and hypoxanthine, putative endogenous ligands of the benzodiazepine receptor, opposite to diazepamare much more effective against kynurenine-induced seizures than against pentylenetetrazol-induced seizures. *Pharmacol Biochem Behav* 1981;14:589–593.

29. Markin RS, Murray WJ. Searching for the endogenous benzodiazepine using the graph theoretical approach. *Pharm Res* 1988;5:408–412.

30. Akhundov RA, Dzhafarova SA, Aliev AN. The search for new anticonvulsant agents based on nicotinamide. *Eksp Klin Farmakol* 1992;55:27–29.

31. Vescovi PP, Gerra G, Ippolito L, et al. Nicotinic acid effectiveness in the treatment of benzodiazepine withdrawal. *Curr Ther Res* 1987;41:1017–1021.

32. Judd LE, Poskitt BL. Pellagra in a patient with an eating disorder. *Br J Dermatol* 1991;125:71–72.

33. Gedye A. Hypothesized treatment for migraine using low doses of tryptophan, niacin, calcium, caffeine, and acetylsalicylic acid. *Med Hypotheses* 2001;56:91–94.

34. Shibata Y, Nishimoto Y, Takeuchi F, et al. Tryptophan metabolism in various nutritive conditions. *Acta Vitamin Enzymol* 1973;29:190–193.

35. Buist RA. Anxiety neurosis: the lactate connection. *Int Clin Nutr Rev* 1985;5:1–4.

36. Majamaa K, Rusanen H, Remes AM, et al. Increase of blood NAD+ and attenuation of lactacidemia during nicotinamide treatment of a patient with MELAS syndrome. *Life Sci* 1996;58:691–699.

37. Hoffer A. Vitamin B3 dependent child. *Schizophrenia* 1971;3:107–113.

38. Hoffer A. *Dr. Hoffer's ABC of Natural Nutrition for Children.* Kingston, ON: Quarry Press, 1999.

39. Werbach MR. Adverse effects of nutritional supplements. In: *Foundations of Nutritional Medicine.* Tarzana, CA: Third Line Press, 1997:133–160.

NIACINAMIDE'S POTENT ROLE IN ALLEVIATING ANXIETY WITH ITS BENZODIAZEPINE-LIKE PROPERTIES: A CASE REPORT

by Jonathan E. Prousky, ND

Anxiety disorders are the most common psychiatric disorders in the United States.[1] Anxiety disorders are extremely debilitating for the suffering individual, disrupting one's ability to engage in a full, functional life. The consequences of anxiety are profound emotional, occupational, and social impairments. Some of the common physical (somatic) symptoms of anxiety are difficulty breathing, facial flushing, excessive sweating, muscle tension, and tachycardia. The typical emotional symptoms of anxiety are not independent of the somatic manifestations, but present as agitation, irritability, fearfulness, feelings of "impending doom," nervousness, and shyness. Most patients with anxiety disorders seek help from a primary care physician rather than a psychiatrist[2] and commonly report their health as poor,[3] smoke cigarettes, and abuse other substances.[4] These patients have an increased chance of developing chronic medical illnesses such as obstructive pulmonary disease, diabetes, and hypertension compared to the general population.[5] When they do acquire a medical illness it is often prolonged as a result of the anxiety.[4]

The conventional approach involves cognitive therapy and relaxation for mild anxiety.[6] More serious cases of anxiety often require pharmacologic treatment with benzodiazepines, selective serotonin reuptake inhibitors (SSRIs), or other mood elevators such as buspirone (BuSpar), imipramine (Tofranil), or trazodone (Desyrel).[6] Here, I report on a case where psychological therapy, SSRIs, buspirone, and numerous natural agents were ineffective in the treatment of severe anxiety. The only medications that completely resolved this patient's anxiety were benzodiazepines. In an effort to wean off the benzodiazepine, the patient took increasing doses of niacinamide. As demonstrated in the following case report, niacinamide was effective for addressing the benzodiazepine withdrawal symptoms and managing anxiety.

Case Report

A 33-year-old Caucasian male presented with a history of anxiety for the past 20 years. When the patient was 13, his homeroom teacher would embarrass him every week by having him stand up in front of the class and remain as such until he was noticeably red in the face, at which point the teacher would comment about how red he was. The entire class would laugh at this. Over time, this patient became increasingly nervous and fearful about social situations and involvement in activities that could draw attention to him. Throughout junior high and high school, the patient would have pronounced anxiety and panic when making presentations and conversing with his peers, friends, or girls. Typically his symptoms were facial flushing, profuse sweating, increased heart rate, muscle tension, burning in the stomach, and the need to get away.

These symptoms persisted throughout university and, when the patient was 22, he finally sought professional help for his anxiety. The clinical psychologist diagnosed the patient with social phobia, panic disorder, and mild agoraphobia. The patient underwent once- or twice-weekly sessions of psychodynamic and cognitive-behavioral therapy for the next six months. During this time the patient's symptoms improved only slightly, but the patient somehow convinced the psychologist that he was completely cured and that therapy was no longer necessary.

By the time he was 24 years old, he entered medical school and his anxiety worsened. He was so upset by his inability to just "go with the flow," or "feel comfortable in [his] own skin" that he again sought the help of a psychiatrist. This time the psychiatrist assessed and diagnosed him with social phobia, panic disorder, dysthymia, and mild agoraphobia. He was started on 50 milligrams

From the *J Orthomolecular Med* 2004;19(2):104–110.

(mg) of sertraline (Zoloft) daily. After the first two weeks the patient's anxiety slightly improved, but he had noticeable side effects from the medication such as lethargy, apathy, and anorgasmia. By four weeks of use, the Zoloft seemed to work fairly well, as the patient had some days without any anxiety. His dose of Zoloft was increased to 100 mg daily. The patient was also put on 5 mg of BuSpar three times each day. After three months of use, the patient had no significant improvement and his anxiety symptoms continued to be debilitating. He found his tendency to avoid social situations increased due to severe fears of blushing. He also avoided interactions with his professors and peers as much as possible. He preferred to stay at home and only go out when necessary. At this point he discontinued both the Zoloft and BuSpar due to their ineffectiveness.

From age 25 to 28, the patient investigated a variety of natural approaches for the treatment of his anxiety. From his readings, he decided to take the following nutrients daily: vitamin C (6,000–12,000 mg), vitamin E (800 IU), zinc (50 mg), vitamin B-complex (containing 100 mg of each major B vitamin), calcium (1,000 mg), and magnesium (400 mg). Although he followed this plan diligently, his anxiety did not lessen. By the time the patient was 28, he had also tried St. John's wort, adrenal extract, constitutional homeopathic medicine, and amino acids such a gamma-aminobutyric acid (GABA), inositol, and L-taurine. None of these natural approaches helped.

From the ages of 29 to 33, he then experienced success with prescribed benzodiazepine medication.

When he turned 33, he did somewhat of a literature search on anxiety and found intriguing information on niacinamide. He informed his psychiatrist of his plan to wean himself off medication and take niacinamide. The psychiatrist encouraged the patient to do so but wanted the patient to contact him if he were to experience withdrawal symptoms such as recurrent anxiety, insomnia, and irritability. For the first week, the patient took 0.5 mg of clonazepam (Klonopin) every morning along with 500 mg of niacinamide, 500 mg of niacinamide at lunch, and 1,000 mg at bedtime. He experienced no recurrences of his anxiety or insomnia during the first week of weaning. In the second week, the patient discontinued the medication and took 1,000 mg of niacinamide in the morning, 500 mg at lunch, and 1,000 mg at bedtime. The patient felt great and could not distinguish between taking Klonopin and niacinamide. The patient was completely free of benzodiazepine medication as of August 1, 2002. The psychiatrist was so impressed with the outcome and commented that it gave him hope that a patient could actually go off benzodiazepine medication and not chronically depend on them.

As of November 7, 2003, this 34-year-old patient has been able to practice as a doctor without any impairments or restrictions and continues to do very well approximately 15 months after stopping the Klonopin. He no longer feels that anxiety is a problem and believes that the niacinamide is equally as effective as benzodiazepine medication but is potentially safer to take for long-term use.

IN BRIEF

Anxiety disorders are extremely debilitating and are the most common psychiatric disorders in the United States. The conventional approach to severe anxiety involves pharmacotherapy with benzodiazepines, selective serotonin reuptake inhibitors (SSRIs), or other medications. A case report demonstrated that the use of 2,500 mg of niacinamide (nicotinamide) per day ameliorated severe anxiety in a 34-year-old male patient. It appears that niacinamide has therapeutic properties similar to the benzodiazepines. Niacinamide might exert its effects through its modulation of neurotransmitters that are commonly unbalanced in those areas of the brain associated with anxiety. Niacinamide might also reduce anxiety by shunting more tryptophan toward the production of serotonin and/or by simply correcting a vitamin B3 dependency. The use of niacinamide for extended periods of time appears to be safe, but very high doses cause nausea and vomiting.

Discussion

It is of no surprise that this patient benefited tremendously from the benzodiazepines. It appears that niacinamide has similar sedative-like properties to that of the benzodiazepines. This is supported by the fact that the patient did not feel any difference, in terms of response and effectiveness, between the benzodiazepines and niacinamide. He was able to switch with little difficulty from the daily use of a benzodiazepine to niacinamide. Furthermore, during the transition he did not experience common withdrawal symptoms such as insomnia, recurrent anxiety, or panic attacks. However, unlike the benzodiazepines, the pharmacologic data pertaining to the anti-anxiety properties of niacinamide are not well known since its precise mechanisms of action upon the central nervous system have yet to be conclusively determined.

It appears that niacinamide does possess pharmacologic properties that are similar to benzodiazepines. A 1992 study found that niacinamide and its analogs possessed properties similar to benzodiazepines at various zones of the cerebral cortex (the area largely responsible for higher brain functions) by influencing the GABAergic system.[7] While it is impossible to conclude that the effects of niacinamide are due to its interaction upon the benzodiazepine receptor, it does appear to influence neurotransmitter metabolism in a manner that is comparable to benzodiazepines by a route as yet undetermined.[8,9]

More case reports, research, and rigorous controlled trials are needed to properly evaluate niacinamide's therapeutic effectiveness, safety, and mechanisms of action for the treatment of anxiety. In light of the positive results accomplished from using megadoses of niacinamide in this case report, perhaps this nutritional agent is indicated for the management of anxiety.

An anxiety sufferer writes . . .

"I have coped for years with regular panic attacks and severe depersonalization episodes and have 'done' the therapist routine (more than 15 different therapists in the course of 20 years). This summer and fall I went through a period where the attacks were coming every few days and might last for days. Finally, in desperation, I started taking B-complex vitamins two to three times daily, vitamin C to help with the metabolism of tryptophan-rich foods (which I have tended to crave without knowing why), and daily doses of lecithin (2–4 tablespoons/day). The change feels almost miraculous. I still have episodes, but they are much more manageable. I can maintain some sane perspective and can see them as episodes rather than as some unbearable state that feels like it will go on forever. I am convinced that the nutritional substances are making the difference."

Source: Personal communication (AWS), 2005

REFERENCES

1. Kessler RC, McGonagle KA, Zhao S, et al. Lifetime and twelve-month prevalence of DSM-III-R psychiatric disorders in the United States: results from the National Comorbidity Survey. *Arch Gen Psychiat* 1994;51:8–19.

2. Shear MK, Schulberg HC. Anxiety disorders in primary care. *Bull Menninger Clin* 1995;59:A73–85.

3. Katon WJ, Von Korff M, Lin E. Panic disorder: relationship to high medical utilization. *Am J Med* 1992;92: 7S-11S.

4. Shader RI, Greenblatt DJ. Use of benzodiazepinein anxiety disorders. *New Engl J Med* 1993;328:1398–1405.

5. Wells KB, Golding JM, Burnam MA. Psychiatric disorder in a sample of the general population with and without chronic medical conditions. *Am J Psychiat* 1988;145:976–981.

6. Gliatto MF. Generalized anxiety disorder. *Am Fam Physican* 2000;62:1591–1600, 1602.

7. Akhundov RA, Dzhafarova SA, Aliev AN. The search for new anticonvulsant agents based onnicotinamide. *Eksp Klin Farmakol* 1992;55:27–29 [in Russian; abstract only].

8. Hoffer A. Vitamin B3 and schizophrenia. *Townsend Lett* 2001; 213:20–23.

9. Paterson ET. Vitamin B3 and liver toxicity. *Townsend Lett* 2001; 207:23.

A BIOCHEMIST'S EXPERIENCE WITH GABA

by Phyllis J. Bronson, PhD

Gamma-aminobutyric acid (GABA) is a biochemical molecule that has a profound effect on the central nervous system (CNS). While other amino acids act on the CNS (e.g., L-taurine has a calming effect on the amygdala, part of the limbic system, involved with behavior and emotion), GABA is unique, in that it is both an amino acid and neurotransmitter. Biochemically, the root of anxiety is an overfiring of nerves, leading to a feeling of being overwhelmed. Often, when the receptors for the CNS are filled with GABA, this overfiring stops and anxiety can be assuaged.

GABA's Mechanism of Action

While the mechanism of action of GABA is not completely understood, it appears to act on the CNS directly without crossing the blood-brain barrier. In the CNS, the GABAA receptor (often referred to as GABAAR) is inhibitory, meaning that when GABA binds to it, the result is a calming effect on the body. The GABAAR is a pentameric (i.e., five-sided) structure comprised of combinations of alpha and beta subunits. Each subunit in turn is comprised of four trans-membrane spanning alpha helices, which pass through and form a central chloride ion channel. The active site (binding site for GABA) is the alpha-4 subunit, which is located between the alpha and beta subunits. When two GABA molecules bind together in this site, the molecule opens the channel and allows chloride ions to flow. This hyperpolarization results in neuroinhibition, or a sensation of calm. All of this is done without the GABA molecule actually crossing the blood-brain barrier.

The GABAAR also contains several allosteric-binding sites, which are the target of many current anti-anxiety medications, such as benzodiazepines, barbiturates, ethanol, and some neuroactive steroids. When these molecules bind to the allosteric sites of the GABAAR, the receptor again changes shape and opens the chloride channels.[1] These drugs work by further enhancing chloride influx.[2] By changing the shape of the GABAAR, these drugs might also inhibit the ability of endogenous GABA in the body to bind to the active site of the molecule, thus interfering with the body's natural ability to balance neurotransmitters. This may be the basis for some of the addictive properties of these drugs.

GABA Modulation

While GABA affects both men and women, the reproductive hormones progesterone and estradiol are both major modulators of this process, leading to the hypothesis that GABA may function somewhat differently in women than in men. Progesterone produces a breakdown product, allopregnanolone, which enhances the calming effect of GABA. Current research suggests that in the presence of allopregnanolone, GABA binds more easily to the alpha-4 subunit of the GABAAR. Without enough allopregnanolone, GABA does not bind as easily, and this leads to many of the symptoms of progesterone deficiency including severe anxiety, premenstrual syndrome, and postpartum depression.[3]

It is also postulated that hypothalamic cells treated with estradiol (the most potent form of estrogen) will respond to GABA as excitatory rather than inhibitory.[4,5] In my work, I believe that the balance between estrogen and progesterone is critical, and this is one example where upsetting that balance can lead to many problems for women. I have worked with a number of women who are dealing with anxiety and other issues of perimenopause and have found GABA to be of key importance. Here, I present two patient cases that depict how GABA was used clinically to reduce their anxiety.

Case #1

Elaine was an architecture professor at a prestigious design school. For years she had assumed

From the *J Orthomolecular Med* 2011;26(1):11–14.

she was simply a type-A personality. Then in her early 40s, she started experiencing panic attacks, periods when she felt that she could not get enough air. Her long-time internist prescribed venlafaxine (Effexor) and alprazolam (Xanax), which helped with the depression, but she felt like she was on a roller coaster of anxiety masked by an almost catatonic state as she steadily became dependent on these drugs. As she was in her 40s, the time of drug dependency correlated with stage two of perimenopause, which is marked by declining progesterone. She tried to reduce her alprazolam dependency but could not. She had repeated visits to the local emergency room, claiming to her family that she was having severe menstrual cramps, when in fact she was having acute anxiety.

She came to me on the recommendation of one of her emergency room doctors. I started her on a withdrawal protocol from the alprazolam, which had to be done slowly and carefully, and at the same time I gave her a powder-filled capsule of 750 milligrams (mg) of pharmaceutical grade GABA. She was instructed to mix the GABA in water and sip it over 10–20 minutes, which reduces possible side effects of skin flushing and neurologic tingling. Within half an hour, her level of calmness noticeably increased and she was astounded that she could feel that level of calmness without the feeling of being drugged. She was maintained on the 750 mg a day of GABA mixed in water. She was also prescribed bio-identical progesterone (not synthetic progestins found in birth control pills) to potentiate the therapeutic effects of GABA and reduce her perimenopausal symptoms. Doses of 750–1,000 mg of GABA, up to three times daily, are ideal for stopping panic attacks. Some clinicians use more but I have found higher doses to be unnecessary for most women, especially if

progesterone is used. (Men may need more than 750 mg a day, though not often). Higher daily doses of GABA appear to affect hyperpolarization more significantly.

I followed Elaine for over five years. She improved using a combination of hormones, GABA, and therapy. As Elaine got her anxiety under control, she was able for the first time, to get in touch with the much deeper depression and feelings of alienation that had been haunting her since early adolescence.

Case #2

In high school, Lilly struggled with extreme premenstrual syndrome, which caused severe, painful cramps, combined with powerful feelings of anxiety, and obsessive/compulsive thinking. This left her feeling as if her head were disconnected from her body. At times, she felt as if she was drowning in her emotional world. During her 20s, therapy helped but it was the later combination of biochemical support and talking about her feelings that allowed her to see life more clearly.

Lilly also had a curvy body, typical of women who tend toward estrogen dominance in their younger years (i.e., she had far more estrogen relative to progesterone). Many women at midlife and younger have serious deficits of progesterone that impact everything from irregular cycles to mood issues, leading to symptoms like irritability, anxiety, and an overt sharpness of the tongue.

Initially, Lilly responded well to bioidentical progesterone and 400 mg a day of GABA in a blend with other nutrients and herbs to potentiate its therapeutic effects such as magnesium (100 mg), glycine (100 mg), vitamin B6 (10 mg), glutamine (140 mg), passion flower herb powder (150 mg),

IN BRIEF

This paper examines the clinical applications of gamma-aminobutyric acid (GABA) for the treatment of anxiety, as well as the relationship between GABA and allopregnanolone (a metabolite of progesterone). For many years I have been involved in biochemical research of GABA, looking at its elemental structure as well as its permeability across the blood-brain barrier. While it is clear that GABA is helpful for the treatment of anxiety, the current laboratory evidence is insufficient to confirm the uptake and absorption of GABA into the brain, as it appears to act on the central nervous system directly without crossing the blood-brain barrier.

and *Primula veris officinalis* herb powder (150 mg). The combination of GABA and bioidentical progesterone helped Lilly immensely.

I have been following Lilly for many years now. I have observed similar curvy, big-breasted women as they move into perimenopause and menopause. While these women tend toward estrogen dominance and respond beautifully to progesterone when they are younger, as they age and get closer to late perimenopause, their cells demand more estrogen because that is what they were used to. As primary estradiol plummets, they experience a shift from anxiety to more of a flat affect. The estrone (a less powerful estrogen) goes up, the estradiol goes down, and brain fog and depression set in. This is why there is such a crucial need to manage anxiety in its early stage, since later the chemical changes precipitate a need for more estrogen. In Lilly's case, she responded well to progesterone when she was younger and then needed increased estrogen as she moved through menopause. GABA was an integral part of managing these physiologic transitions.

CONCLUSION

GABA is nature's way of calming the nervous system. I have found GABA to be extremely useful in the treatment of anxiety. It is a safe and non-addictive treatment with far fewer side effects commonly seen with traditional pharmacological agents. For women in perimenopause, its effectiveness is enhanced by the addition of bio-identical progesterone.

REFERENCES

1. McCarthy MM, Auger AP, Perrot-Sinal TS. Getting excited about GABA and sex differences in the brain. *Trends Neuroscience* 2002;25:307–312.

2. Von Bohlen, Halbach O, Dermietzel R. *Neurotransmitters and Neuromodulators: Handbook of Receptors and Biological Effects.* Weinheim, Germany. Wiley-VCH Verlag GmbH, 2002, 64–73.

3. Eisenman LN, He Y, Covey DF, et al. Potentiation and inhibition of GABAA receptor function by neuroactive steroids. In ed. Smith SS. *Neurosteroid Effects in the Central Nervous System: The Role of the GABA-A Receptor.* Boca Raton, FL: CRC Press, 2004, 95–118.

4. Perrot-Sinal TS, Davis AM, Gregerson KA, et al. Estradiol enhances excitatory gamma-amino butyric acid-mediated calcium signaling in neonatal hypothalamic neurons. *Endocrinology* 2001;142:2238–2243.

5. Clayton GH, Owens GC, Wolff JS, et al. Ontogeny of cation-Cl-cotransporter expression in rat neocortex. *Brain Res Dev Brain Res* 1998;109:281–292.

AGORAPHOBIA: A NUTRITIONALLY RESPONSIVE DISORDER
by Laraine C. Abbey, RN

Agoraphobia, the most debilitating of all phobias, is a complex psychophysiological disorder that manifests as severe anxiety and/or panic reactions, accompanied by a dread of being away from a "safe" place. The term agoraphobia is derived from the two Greek words *phobos*, meaning fear, and *agora*, meaning marketplace or place of assembly.[1] The incidence of this disorder is significant and appears to be rapidly increasing. When studied in 1969, approximately 1 out of 100 people had phobias disabling enough to seek professional help. The greatest percentage of phobias seen in clinical practice is agoraphobic.[2] The realization that agoraphobia could be highly responsive to dietary manipulation occurred when a few clients of mine recovered after instituting an individually determined nutritional regimen. I have seen more than 50 agoraphobics (AGPs) and hundreds of people suffering with anxiety. Such symptoms typically disappear or are markedly ameliorated via an orthomolecular approach.

Nutritional Assessment and Study Method

As part of my nutritional assessment I use a form called the Systems Review. It is a compilation of signs and symptoms that may be observed when various nutrients are undersupplied. The form contains a total of 286 items, which are reviewed and circled by the client if relevant. Among the items are such symptoms as headaches, anxiety, nausea, palpitation, dizziness, loss of balance, muscle tension, breathlessness, sense of impending doom, and so on. Symptoms pertaining to all organ systems are assessed. As a group, the AGPs have markedly more symptoms than my non-AGP clients. It was my contention that such symptoms are born of biochemical dysfunction and that biochemical function could be manipulated nutritionally.

In general, vitamin testing is deferred pending a trial of dietary manipulation (an optimal nutrition diet) with nonspecific broad-spectrum nutri-

tional support in the form of various dietary supplements. Progress is determined through client evaluation, a repeat of the Systems Review, and follow-up of abnormal tests. Note that many clients in this sample had not completed individualized vitamin testing.

The category of Total Recovery was reserved for those AGPs in whom all panic and/or anxiety attacks were absent and who had returned to normal mobility.

The Marked Improvement category was applied when anxiety attacks, panic episodes, and lack of mobility were significantly diminished from that experienced at the time of the initial intake interview. (No matter how improved, a client was not categorized as totally recovered unless totally free of panic attacks and fully mobile.)

The Slight Improvement category was applied to those AGPs who had a diminished number of symptoms and signs as per the Systems Review, which may or may not include diminution of the panic and/or phobic symptoms.

The No Improvement category is reserved for those AGPs who experienced little or no decrease in symptoms or signs on the Systems Review.

Follow-up visits generally occurred at six-week intervals. Many AGPs experienced marked improvement by the first six-week follow-up.

As a consequence of my belief that the source of various common and chronic symptoms suffered by people might rest with defective enzyme activity (known as an enzymopathy) from a long-term deficiency in the dietary intake micronutrient/macronutrient ratio, I decided to measure vitamin-dependent enzyme reactions before and after stimulation with their respective coenzymes. The following blood and urine tests were done as a group on all subjects tested to determine a deficiency:

From the *Orthomolecular Psych* 1982;11(4):243–259

- Thiamine (vitamin B1): Measured by transketolase activity in blood.

- Riboflavin (vitamin B2): Measured by glutathione reductase activity in blood.

- Niacin (vitamin B3): Measured by N1-methylnicotinamide in urine.

- Pyridoxine (vitamin B6): Measured by glutamic pyruvate transaminase (EGPT) index in blood.

- Folic acid: Measured by serum folate, and additionally in some cases by urinary forminoglutamic acid (FIGLU) excretion and hypersegmentation.

- Vitamin B12 (cyanocobalamin): Measured by serum vitamin B12 and methylmalonic acid (MMA) in urine.

In addition to testing for these vitamin deficiencies and their coenzymes, I tested for a client's serum albumin (albumin is a protein that helps carry nutrients through the blood) and metal toxicity (using hair analysis). Additional tests were performed on various clients as individually indicated, often including: iron and iron binding capacity; liver and kidney function tests; complete blood count (CBC); 24-hour urines for calcium, magnesium, phosphorus; free tryptophan (serum), and 24-hour urinary test of 5-hydroxyindoleacetic acid (a metabolite of serotonin) and pyridoxal-5-phosphate (active coenzyme form of B6).

Results

Among my 23-client AGP sample, 12 have been tested for B-vitamin disturbances. B vitamins are used as coenzymes (important components of enzymes) in almost every area of the body. All were found to have abnormalities. Disturbed thiamine metabolism was the most frequent abnormality (in 7 of 12 patients) with pyridoxine running a close second (in 6 of 12 patients).

Dramatic improvements were observed in 83 percent (or 19 of 23 patients) of the sample. Progress, as measured by the client evaluation and the Systems Review, is remarkable. In one client, 47 of her original 80 presenting symptoms were gone in six weeks. In another client, 28 symptoms out of an original 38 had disappeared, while 33 symptoms out of 44 were gone in another. One severely obsessive-compulsive agoraphobic, who at certain times wouldn't mobilize from a chair, was completely recovered when in three months 44 of her 48 symptoms vanished! Her depression score on the Hoffer-Osmond psychological test (a test used to help make a psychiatric diagnosis) was initially 13 on an 18-point scale. At a three-month follow-up her score was 1.

Discussion

It must be realized that these vitamin-dependent enzymopathies (enzyme problems) can reflect, or create, genetic alterations. Such enzyme defects are more than simple dietary deficiencies, as correction of enzyme activity required pharmacological, not dietary, levels of nutrients, typically in the range of 200–500 milligrams (mg) of the various B-complex factors. Vitamin-dependent genetic disease is gaining attention from geneticists since the incidence of such disorders is proliferating rapidly.[3,4] A. D. Hunt and associates are credited with the discovery of the vitamin-dependent disorders. They administered pharmacologic doses of pyridoxine to successfully eliminate seizures in two infant siblings. Forty other documented cases have been demonstrated and in all the inherited, and therefore genetic, character was established.[3,4]

IN BRIEF

Data presented in this paper indicate that agoraphobia might be called a somatopsychic disorder, (i.e., a nutritional-biochemical imbalance that creates an emotional effect). Agoraphobia was attended by multiple vitamin-dependent enzymopathies (enzyme problems) in all of 12 clients tested. A genetic relationship is suggested in that pharmacological nutrient levels were necessary to eliminate the enzymopathies and reverse the symptoms. The relationship of agoraphobia to disturbed metabolism is explored, particularly emphasizing carbohydrate metabolism. The response of agoraphobics to a nutritional-biochemical approach has been dramatically successful, often resulting in complete recovery. Recovery in this context is defined as elimination of panic reactions and normal mobility.

I'd like to emphasize that with considerable frequency I have observed evidence of defective enzyme activity where the coenzyme precursor (vitamin) was perfectly normal in serum and in fact, on some occasions, elevated. Elevations in serum vitamins may reflect a failure of the vitamin to be properly metabolized due to various enzymopathies beyond the absorption level. Thus, they accumulate in the blood. This has been observed in the relationship between vitamin B12 and folate. When a thiamine deficiency exists, vitamin B12 and folate levels often rise in serum. Administration of thiamine generally results in a drop in such abnormal serum vitamin levels (personal observation and verbal communication with Derrick Lonsdale).

As one example, I frequently observe methylmalonic aciduria (MMA; the inability to break down certain fats and proteins, resulting in a buildup of methylmalonyl CoA) in people with normal or high serum vitamin B12 levels, who respond to pharmacological doses of B12 orally with a decrease in symptoms and cessation of methylmalonic acid production. This may explain the so-called placebo effect of vitamin B12 in those people without pernicious anemia who insist they feel better on high doses of the vitamin. Vitamin B12 is the vitamin cofactor for methylmalonyl CoA mutase, the enzyme that drives the conversion of methylmalonyl CoA to succinyl CoA. In *Cobalamin: Biochemistry and Pathophysiology* (1976),[5] Bernard Babior states that MMA is noted as a reliable and sensitive indicator of vitamin B12 deficiency, "except in the rare cases in which it is due to an inborn error of metabolism." My data suggest that the inborn error of metabolism, to which he refers, is anything but rare. I frequently see MMA without serum B12 depletion, which is indicative of enzymopathy, not simple deficiency.

All AGPs tested suffered multiple vitamin-responsive enzymopathies. Three patients had more than one enzymopathy, 10 had more than two enzymopathies, and 21 had more than three. Further establishing the genetic connection is a familial trend reported by some AGPs. In one family, grandma, daughter, and granddaughter all had it. In another, mother and daughter suffered.

Disturbances in Thiamine Metabolism

The idea that agoraphobia might be a sequel to disturbed carbohydrate metabolism presented itself when I noted that many of the symptoms suffered by AGPs were identical to those commonly presented in hypoglycemia. The characteristically excessive and diverse symptoms that hallmark the AGP syndrome (breathlessness, nervousness, dizziness, chest pain, rapid heart rate, excessive sweating, etc.) are reminiscent in nature and scope to those commonly experienced by hypoglycemics. The theory that agoraphobia might represent a sequel to disturbed carbohydrate metabolism began to take shape.

The dietary and laboratory data were consistent with the possibility of disturbed carbohydrate metabolism. As a group, the diets of AGPs are among the worst I've ever seen. There are exceptions, but by and large the majority virtually subsist on "foods" consisting primarily of refined carbohydrates with large amounts of caffeine. The average American derives roughly one-third of his or her calories from refined grains or white flour products. Such products, devoid of the bran and germ of the grain, are on average 80 to 85 percent deficient in minerals and trace elements, and significantly lacking in some vitamins as well.[6] Based on national consumption studies, refined sugars supply one-sixth of our daily calories—most of which are found in processed foods as an additive. Sugar is devoid of all micronutrients.[6,7] Thus, an average American gets a full 50 percent of his or her calories from refined sugar and refined flour, which contains only 15 to 20 percent of its original mineral content. Many of the AGPs I see get up to three-fourths of their calories from processed foods—usually junk carbohydrates.

Consumption of such refined carbohydrates creates enzymopathies by virtue of the lack of micronutrients in such foods. Enzymes are essential for digesting food and such enzymopathies result in disturbances of carbohydrate, protein, and fat metabolism. Enzyme systems incorporate coenzymes and metal ions, which are derived respectively from dietary vitamins, minerals, and trace elements. These latter items, collectively known as the micronutrients, are depleted in processed foods in general, and in sugar and white flour in particular. It is important to understand that for optimal biochemical function beyond a certain minimal level, the requirement for various micronutrients is not a fixed numerical value, but rather a range, in that the levels of various micronutrients are needed in proportion to the amount of a given macronutrient (carbohydrate, protein, fat) upon which the micronutrient-dependent enzymes must act.

One dramatic example of a disturbance in macro- vs. micronutrient ratio was reported by pediatric geneticist and noted thiamine researcher Dr. Derrick Lonsdale at the Cleveland Clinic in Ohio.[8] Thiamine-deficient chow was fed to two groups of animals. One group was permitted to feed naturally, while the other group was force-fed the thiamine-deficient ration. The force-fed group actually died faster than the others (unpublished address to the Society for Orthomolecular Medicine, East, 1978). Symptomology and ultimately clinical disability may result from a decrease in enzyme-product formation or from the toxic effects of accumulated substrate (compound) as a sequel to enzymopathy.

The relationship of vitamin B1 to carbohydrate metabolism was first established by Peters in 1930.[9] Wendel and Beebe studying glycolytic activity (the metabolism of glucose for energy) in schizophrenia reported on the association of anxiety with lactic acid production in neurosis.[10] During a glucose tolerance test (GTT), it had been observed that symptoms of anxiety became prominent when the blood glucose dropped below the fasting level. The researchers decided to measure blood lactate, pyruvate, and adenosine triphosphate (ATP) concentrations during the GTT. Their observations were most interesting. Lactate concentrations were markedly increased during the third, fourth, and fifth hours following the post-glucose challenge in anxiety-prone patients, but not in the non-anxiety psychiatric patients.[10] Further, with respect to pyruvate concentrations, only the anxiety patients showed a high production of lactate in relation to pyruvate or a high lactate ratio.[10] ATP concentrations were significantly lower in the blood of anxiety patients in the first, second, and third hours following a glucose challenge, whereas non-anxiety patients had no change.

Alterations in blood lactate, pyruvate, ATP, and the lactate/pyruvate ratio indicate a profound disturbance in transformation of chemical to kinetic energy in the anxiety-prone patients.[10] In such patients symptoms of anxiety may occur when there is a requirement to mobilize energy rapidly. Since these patients exhibit a marked shift from aerobic to anaerobic metabolism, their production of energy is markedly reduced. The relationship between lactic acid and anxiety has been explored by a number of researchers other than Beebe and Wendell. Pitts and McClure reported on the experimental production of anxiety attacks in patients suffering anxiety neurosis by blood infusions of the lactate ion.[11] Patients reported they experienced symptoms from the lactate infusion that were identical to those they experienced in spontaneous anxiety attacks. In 1950, Cohen and White summarized the then-current knowledge of neurocirculatory asthenia also referred to as anxiety neurosis, neurasthenia, and effort syndrome.[12] The chief symptoms of anxiety neurosis are breathlessness, palpitations, nervousness, fatigability, headaches, irritability, dizziness, chest pain, paresthesias (tingling in the extremities), and episodes of extreme tearfulness referred to as anxiety attacks. The disorder is characterized by the appearance of many symptoms but few signs.[11] Blood lactate was found to be twice as high in neurocirculatory asthenia as in controls.[12] The researchers found many measurable abnormalities in the response of the anxiety patients to muscular work. These abnormalities, which included low oxygen consumption, are consistent with a defect in aerobic metabolism and a high anaerobic metabolism.[12] A characteristic of both disorders is breathlessness or air hunger, which is particularly evident in crowded or stuffy atmospheres. Cohen and White also noted that sufferers report avoidance of churches or movie theatres due to such smothering feelings. The overdevelopment of this avoidance pattern (phobia) in response to the various symptoms, classified as an anxiety reaction, is the essence of what differentiates agoraphobia from simple anxiety and panic reactions.

The researchers also noted differences in the tolerance for inspired carbon dioxide between normal subjects, and those with anxiety neurosis were observed.[12] The oft-described feeling of choking or smothering in crowded places led to a study in which increased percentages of carbon dioxide were inhaled by study subjects. Approximately 80 percent of the anxiety group experienced symptoms similar or identical to those experienced during anxiety attacks, including a feeling of fear. They concluded that under laboratory-induced, stress-striking biochemical abnormalities were noted in anxiety patients,[12] including elevated blood lactate levels, decreased tolerance for carbon dioxide, and decreased ventilatory capacity and oxygen consumption.

Not just subjective, but objective and quantitative abnormalities were demonstrated in response to various stimuli and stressors. In addition to those mentioned, additional abnormal responses were noted to pain, cold, noise, and anticipation in those patients classified as having anxiety neurosis.[12] These determinations appear to have been undiscovered or disregarded by the many clinicians who accept the premise that anxiety reactions are purely psychogenic (born of personality factors rather than somatogenic, deriving from biochemical factors).

Disturbances in Pyridoxine Metabolism

The formation of nicotinamide adenine dinucleotide (NAD), a compound that helps ignite energy production in the body, requires ATP, and ATP formation requires NAD, which is to say that the reactions are coupled.[10] Therefore, disturbances originating with either ATP or NAD synthesis will affect energy metabolism. Niacin, as a precursor of the NAD compound, is derived through diet directly and by conversion of pyridoxine-dependent enzymes from tryptophan, an amino acid.

Disturbances in tryptophan metabolism have been related to anxiety reactions. Formation of the neurotransmitter serotonin, also derived from tryptophan, depends on pyridoxine-dependent enzyme reactions. Animals depleted in serotonin have been used as experimental models of anxiety.[12] Disturbances in pyridoxine metabolism could therefore affect the formation of serotonin and/or niacin via the tryptophan pathway, both of which could ultimately manifest in anxiety. Obsessive-compulsive anxiety disorders have been successfully treated with tryptophan.[13] Since disturbances in pyridoxine metabolism could affect the formation of serotonin and/or niacin via the tryptophan pathway it too can contribute to anxiety.

Six of the twelve AGPs on which functional vitamin tests were carried out had disturbances in pyridoxine metabolism. A higher percentage may actually have vitamin B6 disturbance, as in later data, when measurements of pyridoxal-5-phosphate (the coenzyme form of B6) were done (in addition to the EGPT) more vitamin B6 dependencies were detected. Hoes and others reported on treatment of hyperventilation syndrome (HVS) with tryptophan and pyridoxine.[14] Among those patients with HVS demonstrating abnormal xanthurenic acid excretion, all responded clinically as well as by normalizing of the xanthurenic acid excretion to the administration of pyridoxine and tryptophan.

One of my clients, in whom abnormal pyridoxine metabolism was isolated, failed to respond to the orthomolecular program as anticipated. Upon rechecking her previously abnormal tests all were found to be normal, including the EGPT enzyme (this B6-activated enzyme was previously abnormal) for which she had been placed on 500 mg of vitamin B6 daily. After reviewing Dr. William Philpott's work on defective conversion of pyridoxal-5-phosphate, I decided to measure serum pyridoxal-5-phosphate additionally along with free tryptophan in the blood and the major serotonin breakdown product 5-hydroxyindoleacetic acid (5-HIAA) in a 24-hour urine before a tryptophan load. This was followed by another 24-hour urine for 5-HIAA after a 5,000-mg tryptophan load the next day.[15]

Results were most interesting. Serum free tryptophan was significantly elevated before the tryptophan load and serum pyridoxal-5-phosphate was almost nonexistent! Note this woman was taking 500 mg of vitamin B6 daily. After the tryptophan load there was a very small increase in 5-HIAA, which suggested that tryptophan was not being converted efficiently to serotonin. After beginning a supplement of the phosphorylated form of vitamin B6 (pyridoxal-5-phosphate), in addition to 1,000 mg of regular vitamin B6 and L-cysteine, there was a rapid reduction in her constant anxiety. She is now completely free of panic attacks and highly mobile. Pyridoxine is necessary to synthesis of the inhibitory neurotransmitter gamma-aminobutyric acid (GABA),[4,16] which appears to be intimately involved with the regulation of anxiety.

Thus, it can be seen how disturbances in thiamine, pyridoxine, and niacin biochemistry could participate in the genesis of anxiety through increased production of lactic acid relative to pyruvic acid, through failure to synthesize adequate brain serotonin, and possibly through underproduction of GABA.

Enzymopathy and Genetic Damage

Since enzyme synthesis is controlled genetically,[16] enzyme problems may reflect genetic change as a result of mutant genes. Genetic change need not manifest in gross metabolic defects or deformity.[17] Wagner and Mitchell state that "although mutation is a sudden event, it can produce almost any degree of effect from those barely detectable by known means to those too extreme for the cell to survive." Altered enzyme activity as may arise from dietary nutritional insufficiency will ultimately affect cell function. Thus the genetic code contained within the cell nucleus can be altered to produce partial genetic blocks often referred to as "leaky" genes.[18–20]

In my experience with a total of 136 highly symptomatic patients (comprised of agoraphobic and non-agoraphobic clients) on whom functional vitamin testing was performed, only five people failed to show abnormalities in any of those nutrients assayed. Five out of one hundred thirty-six! In all such clients, low megadose levels of B vitamins failed to correct the symptomatology and the enzymopathy. Pharmacological doses of vitamins, given for the individually determined abnormalities, eliminated or markedly reduced symptomology, and in all patients retested the enzymopathy

was corrected when the symptoms were eliminated. This suggests that partial blocks in some enzymes' activities are being compensated for with the addition of more coenzyme. This compensatory ability is often possible because many enzymes are not saturated with coenzyme under physiological conditions.[16,20]

Under certain circumstances, massive levels of vitamins (coenzyme precursors) can increase coenzyme synthesis, which in turn increases both the reaction rate (maximum velocity or Vmax) and the substrate concentration (Michaelis constant or Km) of an enzyme. Increasing the percentage of functioning apoenzymes will override a partial enzyme block and, by increasing the Vmax and Km, increase product formation. The fact that signs aren't always apparent or are of lesser number should make us no less concerned about reporting on the presence of symptoms since many researchers have commented that clinical or biochemical lesions may precede histologic changes (National Academy of Sciences, 1977).

The value and importance of orthomolecular therapy lies in minimizing the effects of genetic or biochemical damage and in preventing hereditary damage to offspring. Cotzias and others demonstrated in a strain of mutant mice with a congenital defect of manganese transport into the brain that the ataxia, which resulted from this defect, could be prevented in the mice by supplementing with much larger than normal dietary levels of manganese. Further, the pregnant mice in this mutant strain so supplemented gave birth to completely normal offspring, free of the genetic defect.[21]

The real concern that must be extracted from all this is that a population with increasing persistent symptoms and signs is suffering genetic damage and that such damage can result largely from dietary abuse, particularly in depletion of many vitamins, minerals, and trace elements as a consequence of consuming refined and processed foods, thereby disturbing the macronutrient-micronutrient ratio. This ultimately results in enzymopathies and finally genetic damage.

Thiamine, Neurotransmitters, and Agoraphobia

Thiamine biochemistry was abnormal in 7 out of 12 agoraphobics tested. Exploring the biochemistry of beriberi (a thiamine deficiency disease) may identify the metabolic factors related to agoraphobia, since there is a similarity of symptoms between the two disorders, many of which reflect neuronal dysfunction.

The most common enzymopathy observed among the agoraphobia test sample was the abnormal erythrocyte transketolase, the vitamin B1-dependent enzyme. As mentioned earlier, thiamine is required in proportion to the amount of carbohydrate consumed.[22] Large-scale consumption of refined carbohydrates, particularly sugar (which contains no thiamine) will create metabolic abnormalities associated with autonomic nervous system dysfunction. When reviewing the literature on beriberi,[9,23,24] I was amazed to discover that much of the symptomology was virtually the same in agoraphobia, although the signs were not identical. The nature and abundance of symptoms presenting in agoraphobia and hypoglycemia (also discussed earlier) are suggestive of autonomic nervous dysfunction. Beriberi has been described as the prototype of autonomic dysfunction.[22] Autonomic nervous system effects are best seen as vasomotor changes. It has been observed that injections of adrenaline caused an exaggerated response of the nervous system resulting in tachycardia (fast or irregular heart rate), elevated blood pressure, substernal oppression, nausea, and vomiting in beriberi patients.[23]

Cardiovascular symptoms are among the most important clinical signs in beriberi. Palpitations, dyspnea (shortness of breath) with exertion, and mental excitement are symptoms commonly described as part of the agoraphobia syndrome. Also noted in beriberi is vertigo and instability or ataxia,[23] sensory and motor nerve afflictions, respiratory symptoms in the form of dyspnea and digestive symptoms, including full sensation in epigastrum, heartburn, and constipation. Note again that such symptoms are classically described by the agoraphobic. In 1928, Kawatara found that blood lactic acid was increased in beriberi and in experimentally induced vitamin-B deficiency.[23] This was confirmed in the same year by Inawashiro, who emphasized that the increase in blood lactic acid was more striking upon physical exertion. Note that an increase in lactic acid upon exertion was reported by Cohen and White in their study of patients with anxiety neurosis. While agoraphobia, defective glucose metabolism, and beriberi are different disorders, they all demonstrate symptomology of disturbances in the glucose-oxidative pathway.

A relationship between thiamine depletion and serotonin metabolism has been examined and reported by Plaitakis and others in a short communication in the *Journal of Neurochemistry*.[25] Increased brain concentrations of 5-HIAA, a breakdown product of serotonin, were found in pyrithiamine-treated rats with no alteration of serotonin or tryptophan levels noted. Pyrithiamine is a vitamin B1 analog (a synthetic imposter). This suggested an increased turnover of serotonin in the brain of pyrithiamine-treated animals.

Due to this increased turnover of serotonin, any disturbances in serotonin metabolism would be aggravated by a thiamine deficiency. Niacin

A patient writes . . .

"I went to the doctor at age 18 and I was diagnosed with bipolar, depression, and anxiety. I was on Lamictal and Wellbutrin for two years, and I just wasn't seeing any improvement. Two weeks ago I changed my life. I changed my diet to unprocessed, whole foods and started taking a multivitamin, vitamin B12, and 300 milligrams of niacin a day. I feel like the person I've always wanted to be. I went out last week for the first time in a year. I've literally been too scared to leave the house, being bombarded with terrible social anxiety. It's all gone away. I feel more productive and energized then I ever have in my life."

Source: Personal communication (AWS), 2011

deficiency may lead to depression of serotonin synthesis since tryptophan will be diverted away from serotonin production to synthesize niacin. Both niacin and serotonin synthesis from tryptophan require B6-dependent enzyme reactions for their synthesis. Thus, disturbed pyridoxine metabolism can inhibit synthesis of serotonin and formation of niacin via the tryptophan pathway. In experiments by Plaitakis and coworkers in 1978, a selective inhibition of serotonin uptake was demonstrated only by cerebellar neuron receptors. Kinetic studies on pyrithiamine-treated rats in this study indicated a 50 percent decrease in the Vmax and a 40 percent decrease in the Km for serotonin. The uptake of GABA, glutamic acid, norepinephrine, and choline were not affected. This work suggests a selective involvement of serotonergic activity in the development of neurological manifestations following thiamine deficiency.

Glucose metabolism has a key position in the synthesis of the amino acid neurotransmitters glutamic acid, aspartic acid, and GABA.[26] Diminished pyruvate dehydrogenase activity may be critical for regions of the brain in which an excess of enzyme activity is minimal, since Reynolds and Blass had shown that pyruvate dehydrogenase activity is not evenly distributed in the brain.[26] Thus, alterations in amino acids and neurotransmitters may be the result of reduced pyruvate dehydrogenase activity in response to thiamine deficiency or dependency. Such alterations could lead to the neuronal dysfunction associated with disturbed thiamine biochemistry.

I'd like to emphasize the relationship of caffeine and disturbed carbohydrate metabolism to neurotransmission and ultimately agoraphobia. Most of the agoraphobics I've encountered have been heavy caffeine consumers in the form of coffee, tea, chocolate, and cola beverages. Caffeine stimulates the adrenal glands, thus raising the level of circulating hormones.[27] Lonsdale reported that blood pyruvate is increased as a response to adrenaline, thus stressing the oxidative pathways.[24] Note that as previously mentioned, in beriberi there is a hyper-response of the nervous system to injected adrenaline. Thus, caffeine may result in increased adrenaline, which in a thiamine-deficient dependent state, could result in further disturbance in oxidative metabolism with accumulations of lactate and pyruvate. In the biochemically impaired agoraphobic, any adrenal stimulant or stressor, including emotions and caffeine, may initiate a hyper-response of the autonomic nervous system—manifesting in symptomology that triggers or is characteristic of panic attacks.

"As the knowledge concerning the biochemical pathology of genetically determined metabolic disorders accumulates," write thiamine experts Gubler, Fujiwara, and Dreyfus, "important interrelationships between various vitamins, cofactors, and essential substances seem to emerge, further complicating an already obfuscated field."[28] Nonetheless, much can be done to correct faulty biochemistry and to ameliorate symptoms and signs. Even genetic changes can be reversed in some situations as reported by Cotzias.[29]

Agoraphobia, characterized by a tremendous number of symptoms and few signs, would appear to be a sequel to dysfunction of metabolism and most particularly carbohydrate metabolism. The multitudinous and diverse symptoms of agoraphobia, so much like those of early beriberi, accompanied by multiple vitamin-dependent enzyme defects suggest the need for a massive dietary overhaul.

Agoraphobia and Allergy

For many, the association of allergy and agoraphobia may appear an odd one at best. The avoidance and/or neutralization treatment of substances to which the agoraphobic is found to be allergic or hypersensitive often results in a rapid and dramatic reduction in the various agoraphobic symptoms. In some agoraphobics, avoidance of reactive substances is of primary importance in symptom relief, whereas, in other agoraphobics, defective nutrient metabolism is more central to their symptoms. Invariably, both areas are involved and in general both areas should be assessed unless attention to either aspect singularly resolves all symptoms.

Following are some of the outstanding examples of agoraphobics in whom substance reactivity was a major contributor (but not the only contributor) to their symptomology:

• N. W., Maryland: Intense anxiety experienced after ingesting milk . . . fully mobile and panic free.

• J. A., New Jersey: Exposure to dogs produced nausea and ataxia (lack of coordination), sugar and wheat resulted in pronounced anxiety, depression, and headaches . . . fully mobile and panic free.

• M. A., Ohio: Housebound from panic attacks and paranoid; total elimination of symptoms by elimination of daily 10-cup coffee habit . . . fully mobile and panic free.

• S. L., New Jersey: Severe obsessive-compulsive behavior, accompanying panic attacks at various times, wouldn't move from a chair . . . sugar, mushrooms, and squash primary allergens . . . significant symptom reduction following elimination of these foods . . . fully mobile and panic free.

• M. S., New Jersey: Severe panic attacks and eczema virtually produced at will by consumption of potatoes to which it was discovered he was allergic . . . fully mobile and panic free.

• E. G., Florida: Panic, sweats, irregular heartbeats produced by milk . . . much improved, still in process.

• S. A., New Jersey: Panic attacks, breathing difficulty, choking sensations determined to be provoked by exposure to yeast . . . fully mobile and panic free.

Substance reactivity may manifest in very diverse symptoms. An individual's target organ is a function of his biochemical individuality. Thus, various substances may produce gastrointestinal symptoms in one individual, cardiac irregularities in another, behavioral or mood problems in yet another, and so forth. The term "cerebral allergy" or "neuroallergy" is often applied to apparently emotional or mental symptoms induced by a reactive substance. The reader is referred to the work of Drs. Theron Randolph, Marshall Mandell, Doris Rapp, Joseph Miller, William Philpott, and others in the field of clinical ecology for further exploration and understanding of this phenomenon.

Some techniques for assessing allergy-hypersensitivity reactions include food avoidance and challenge testing, cytotoxic testing, provocative intradermal serial dilution titration (SDT) (Miller technique), and radio-allergo-sorbent (RAST) and paper radio-immuno-sorbent (PRIST) testing.

Case #1

On December 17, 1979, S. M., a 30-year-old agoraphobic woman, somewhat overweight at 130 pounds, five feet two, when first seen in my office, presented with daily headaches, dizziness, fatigue, chest pains, and numbness in her left arm. She suffered episodes of what she called "visual field shrinking," as well as "shakes" (which she referred to as "seizures"), and stated rapid movements would provoke these.

Medical evaluations had been done, which included neurological, cardiac, and psychiatric workups. The working diagnosis was severe anxiety, more specifically agoraphobia. She was in weekly treatment with a psychiatrist for her panic attacks and phobic condition. Due to the multiplicity and severity of her symptoms, her brother reported he often literally carried her into and out of her psychiatrist's office.

In addition to the previously mentioned symptoms, she had a large number of rather typical nutritional signs such as periodontal problems (bleeding and receding gums), muscle spasms, skin problems, poor hair quality, and so on.

Her self-image was very poor. Her response to the systems review question, "Do you like yourself?" was, "No, I always feel ugly and sick."

A required detailed three-day chronological food/symptom diary demonstrated very poor nutritional practices, such as large-scale consumption of foods high in sugar, fat, salt, and caffeine, including coffee and carbonated beverages. She was also a smoker.

Functional nutritional testing was done that demonstrated abnormal activity of the erythrocyte transketolase and erythrocyte glutamic pyruvate transaminase (EGPT) enzymes. This established a functional deficiency or dependency for thiamine and pyridoxine, respectively.

Hair analysis demonstrated low zinc, chromium, and iron.

She was also sent for a food allergy screening using the Bryan method of cytotoxic testing and was found to be multiply allergic. Of particular significance were mushrooms, rice, rye, tobacco, fructose, and Brussels sprouts. She had slight reactions to most foods tested.

She was placed on a nutritional regimen that included a rotational diet (no food repeated more than once in five days). All refined carbohydrates, caffeine, and tobacco were to be strictly eliminated. For general health purposes and due to her significant hypersensitivity reactions, she was also to avoid additives, preservatives, and chemicals as much as possible.

Her nutrient program consisted of special low-allergy vitamin brands free of soy, yeast, wheat, lactose, and corn, and other potential allergens. She was placed on a daily regimen that included a multivitamin, vitamin C (6,000 mg), thiamine (500 mg), pyridoxine (200 mg), folic acid (800 micrograms [mcg]/2x per day), vitamin E (400 IU), calcium (500 mg), magnesium (250 mg), chelated zinc (50 mg), chelated manganese (17 mg), chelated iron (30 mg), choline (1,000 mg), inositol (1,000 mg), and methionine (300 mg).

At the three-month follow-up she was dramatically improved. Visual blurring and focusing difficulties were gone as were her frequent ear infections. Her periodontal signs and symptoms were much improved. Her muscle spasms were gone. Persistent nasal stuffiness was gone. Chest pain, headaches, dizziness, lightheadedness, trembling hands, and numbness and tingling in her extremities were gone. The "visual field shrinking" and "shakes" were gone. Sluggishness and fatigue had disappeared. Her phobias were almost gone as was her anxiety. Occasional mild episodes would still occur at times in shopping malls or in cars. She evaluated herself as 95 percent improved. Happily her self-concept improved right along with the decline in her symptoms.

The abnormal enzymes were retested and found normal, establishing functional adequacy of thiamine and pyridoxine.

Provocative intradermal testing, particularly for petrochemical reactivity, was suggested due to a mild persistence of reactions in shopping malls and automobiles. However, she declined to pursue this as she was more than happy with her progress.

In September 1980, I watched her slim, beautifully tanned body rise to leave my office. Her eyes sparkled and her hair shone as she flashed a smile that said it all . . . the beauty of health.

Case #2

J. A., a very determined woman of 51, told me that I was her last hope. She handed me a two-page summary of her medical history pertinent to the agoraphobia and rather significant depressions. Repeat hospitalizations for depression had occurred. She'd had trials on many psychotropic drugs, none of which had helped her and some of which had provoked significant adverse reactions. She told of the hell her life had become and of the virtual prison that was once her home. She was mobilizing from her home in a limited way only when accompanied by her husband. The caring between her husband and herself, though obvious, was severely stressed. His dreams for travel during retirement appeared shattered. Pride in her once independent and optimistic nature now taken from her left her with one way out—suicide. She would give this approach every chance, but, if she continued in this spiral of depression, fear, and incapacitation, she stated she would terminate her life.

Thankfully, she had an immediate response to the elimination of all refined sugars, white flour, and caffeine. Her depression, although still present, had lifted significantly. She began to feel hopeful.

The Bryan method of cytotoxic testing was done. She was placed on a five-day rotary diet combined with initial avoidance of major offending foods.

She was placed on a broad-spectrum orthomolecular nutrition program. Digestive enzymes and bulking agents were included to successfully eliminate her chronic constipation. (She had been moving her bowels approximately once in four days.)

Initially, she was receiving a multivitamin (1x per day), calcium ascorbate powder (1,000 mg/3x per day), a vitamin B-100 complex with 400 mcg of folic acid (1x per day), vitamin E (400 IU/1x per day), choline (330 mg/2x per day), inositol (330 mg/2x per day), methionine (100 mg/2x per day), chromium (200 mcg/3x per day), chelated copper (2 mg/1x per day), chelated zinc (50 mg/1x per day), calcium (330 mg/1x per day), and magnesium (150 mg/1x per day).

Her progress was remarkable. Her depressions were dramatically reduced in both frequency and intensity. Anxiety was markedly diminished and she was mobilizing both with and without her husband with greater frequency.

She was very subject to food-related depressions. Even small diversions from her rotary diversified diet would manifest in major shifts and anxiety.

Due to food reactions and to a persistence of some disturbing symptoms, including a history of chronic vaginal infections as assessed by the systems review, it was decided that she would begin allergy testing and treatment by the provocative intradermal serial dilution titration technique (Miller technique). My procedure has been to have all of the individual's commonly eaten foods tested (foods normally consumed more frequently than once in five days), stressing foods that are difficult to rotate. At a minimum, the following foods are generally included in the testing: milk, corn, wheat, yeast, tomato, sugar beet and sugar cane, onion, soy, beef, and eggs. Many other foods are commonly tested such as potato, chicken, garlic, rice, peanut, orange, and so on.

Common inhalants and substances such as house dust, mites, molds, yeast, fungi like trichophyton, epidermophyton, and *Candida albicans* are tested routinely. Grasses, trees, and pollens are often tested based in part on history and seasonality of symptoms. Pets or animals are included when indicated by exposure.

Neutralization doses (end points) for each allergen, when determined, are generally combined in one vial and injected subcutaneously twice weekly. Patients with high end points for *Candida albicans* and/or significant histories of vaginal infections or cutaneous itching are generally treated with the fungus-suppressing agent Nystatin in addition to neutralization. Acidophilus (probiotic) capsules taken orally as well as added to a douche solution are also helpful.

J. A. had strong reactions to the *Candida albicans* skin test as suspected by her history of vaginal infections and hormonally related anxiety and depression. She was reactive to many other substances tested. She was placed on Nystatin (4x per day) and neutralization therapy.

J. A. responded beautifully to neutralization and Nystatin; so well, in fact, that even before all allergy testing had been completed, she was able to take an airplane trip from New Jersey to Florida for a 10-day vacation with her husband! To her delight, her last remaining symptom, a periodic feeling of light-headedness, accompanied by some mild ataxia, disappeared altogether during the trip, only to return again on arrival at her home.

Was it the air, the water, the plant life? Her last round of allergy tests told the story: it was her dog. Intradermal injection of dog extract produced immediate light-headedness and ataxia. Her end point for dog extract was higher than for any other allergen tested. The neutralization dose relieved the induced symptoms immediately. This reaction treatment response was reproduced three times to the amazement of all. Simultaneously with allergy testing and treatment, functional vitamin studies were done.

Tests identified multiple disturbances. The erythrocyte glutamic pyruvate transaminase (EGPT) index was high indicating a functional deficiency of vitamin B6. She was excreting methylmalonic acid (MMA) in her urine, indicating a functional deficiency of vitamin B12. Urinary levels of formiminoglutamic acid (FIGLU) were elevated and can occur with a functional deficiency of either vitamin B12 or folic acid. Therefore, assessment for FIGLU was performed after correcting the functional B12 deficiency as indicated by MMA elimination. Her vitamin program was adjusted to include more folic acid, vitamin B12, and vitamin B6. Due to yeast allergy she was switched to hypoallergenic yeast-free brands of vitamins. The previous vitamin abnormalities were all corrected, except urinary FIGLU, which was significantly reduced. Her dosage of folic acid was increased a second time and when recently encountered in a shopping mall she reported virtually the complete elimination of her nervousness and ataxia. She commented, "the extra folic acid made a notable difference within 48 hours."

On vitamin-mineral orthomolecular therapy,

dietary modification, and allergen neutralization injections, J. A. is now totally recovered. She is fully mobile and free of any panic attacks, independent, and happy again.

REFERENCES

1. Frampton M. *Overcoming Agoraphobia*. New York: St. Martin's Press, 1974, 15.

2. Burns, LE, Thopre, GL. The epidemiology of fears and phobias. *J Int Med Res* 1977;5(suppl 5):2–3.

3. Rosenberg LE. Vitamin-dependent genetic disease. In: *Medical Genetics* edited by J Kusick and R Claiborne. New York: H.P. Publishers, 1970, 73–78.

4. Rosenberg LE. Vitamin-responsive inherited diseases affecting the nervous system. In: *Brain Dysfunction in Metabolic Disorders* edited by F Plum. New York: Raven Press, 1974, 263–264.

5. Babior BM, ed. *Cobalamine Biochemistry and Pathophysiology*. New York: John Wiley & Sons, New York, 1976, 386–387, 410.

6. Schroeder HA. *The Trace Elements and Man*. Greenwich, CT: Devin-Adair, 1975.

7. Yudkin J. *Sweet and Dangerous*. New York: Bantam Books, 1972, 17.

8. Lonsdale D, Faulkner W, et al. Intermittent cerebellar ataxia associated with hyperpyruvic acidemia, hyperalaninemia, and hyperalanura. *Pediatrics* 1069;43(6):1025–1034.

9. Wolstenholme GEW, O'Connor M, eds. *Thiamine Deficiency: Biochemical Lesions and Their Clinical Significance*. Ciba Fdn Study Group, No 28. Boston: Little, Brown & Co., 1967

10. Pauling L, Hawkins D, eds. *Orthomolecular Psychiatry: Treatment of Schizophrenia*. San Francisco: W.H. Freeman & Co., 1973, 289, 293, 295.

11. Pitts FN, McClure JN. Lactate metabolism in anxiety neurosis. *N Engl J Med* 1967;277(25): 1329–1336.

12. Cohen, ME, White PD. Life situations, emotions and neurocirculatory asthenia. *Nerv and Ment Dis Proc* 1950;29:832–869.

13. Hoes M, Colla P, Folgering, H. Hyperventilation syndrome: treatment with l-tryptophan and pyridoxine; predictive values of xanthurenic acid excretion. *J Orthomolecular Psych* 1981;10(1):7–15.

14. Yaryura-Tobias J, Bhaganan H. L-tryptophan in the treatment of obsessive-compulsive disorders. *Am J Psychiatry* 1977; 134:11.

15. Philpott W. New Evidence Showing Lack of Conversion of Vitamin B-6 into the Active Coenzyme Form in Patients with Chronic Degenerative Disease. Presented at 14th Annual Mtg. Society for Clinical Ecology, San Diego, Oct 28, 1979.

16. Wurtman R, Wurtman, J, eds. *Nutrition and the Brain*. New York: Raven Press, 1980, 142.

17. Reed S. *Parenthood and Heredity*. New York: John Wiley & Sons, 1964.

18. Williams, RJ. *Biochemical Individuality*. Austin, TX: Texas Univ. Press, 1956.

19. Roe DA. *Drug-Induced Nutritional Deficiencies*. Westport, CT: AVI Publishing, 1978.

20. Goodhart RS, Shils ME, eds. *Modern Nutrition in Health and Disease*. Philadelphia: Lea & Febiger, 1980, 1193–1219.

21. Cotzias GC. *Geochemistry and the Environment: The Relation of Other Selected Trace Elements to Health and Disease*. Vol. 2. Washington: Nat Acad Sci, 1977, 32–34.

22. Lonsdale D, Shamberger R. Red cell transkeltolase as an indicator of nutritional deficiency. *Am J Clin Nutr*, 1980;33: 205–211.

23. Shimazono N, Katsura, E. Review of Japanese literature on beriberi and thiamine. *Vitamin B Research Com of Japan* 1965;51–52.

24. Lonsdale, D. Thiamine metabolism in disease. *CRC Crit Rev Clin Lab Sci*, Jan 1975.

25. Plaitakis A, Van Woert MH, Hwang E, et al. The effect of acute thiamine deficiency on brain tryptophan, serotonin and 5-hydrooxyindoleacetic acid. *J Neurochem* 1978;31:1087–1089.

26. Hamel E, Butterworth R, Barbeau A. Effect of thiamine deficiency on levels of putative amino acid transmitters in affected regions of rat brain. *J Neurochem* 1979;33:575–577.

27. Bolton S, Null G, Pressman AH. Caffeine: its effects, uses and abuses. *J Appl Nutr* 1981;33(1):35–53.

28. Gubler, C. Effect of thiamine deprivation and thiamine antagonists on the level of aminobutyric acid and 2-oxogiutarate metabolism in rat brain. *J Neurochem* 1974;22:831–836.

29. Cotzias, GC. *Geochemistry and the Environment: The Relation of Other Selected Trace Elements to Health and Disease*. Vol. 2. Washington: Nat Acad Sci, 1977, 32–43.

DRUG ADDICTIONS

YOU HAVE TO BE SICK FIRST before you can become an addict to heroin, cocaine, or any other drug. The underlying problem is poor nutrition. In nearly every case, the person's diet is so deficient in the B vitamins that eventually the addict develops a chronic state of pan-nutrient deficiency and nutrient dependency that only large doses of the correct nutrients can help. It follows that, if addicts are sick to begin with, the best treatment is to discover what that sickness is and deal with that first.

The conventional approaches to drug addiction using synthetic or semi-synthetic opioids, with or without concomitant behavioral and psychological therapy, have lacked long-term success. Symptoms may be ameliorated by pharmaceuticals, which provide some relief but at an enormous cost. Until the crucial nutritional needs of addicts are met, these approaches will continue to have little beneficial effect. This is why orthomolecular treatment works.

The evidence is in, as this chapter will show. Even so, today medical evidence is considered adequate only if it is double-blind tested, if it comes out of orthodox medical centers, and if the person making the claim is well-known. It does not mean that this standard is better—physician reports provide excellent evidence. In fact, half of the evidence published in medical journals is wrong, and doctors do not know which half that is. Orthomolecular physicians recognize that a large fraction of those suffering from substance abuse issues are ill due to physical factors. Drug addiction, so often portrayed as without cure, can indeed be treated with high-dose nutrient therapy. This may surprise many, anger a few, and, we hope, arouse your interest.

—ABRAM HOFFER AND ANDREW SAUL
The Vitamin Cure for Alcoholism, 2009 (updated by A.W.S.)

TERMS OF ADDICTION

BARBITUTATES. A class of drugs that act as depressants and cause relaxation and sleepiness.

DRUG DEPENDENCY. Physical need for a drug; abruptly reducing or stopping the medication causes withdrawal symptoms.

HALLUCINOGENS. A class of drugs that alter cognition and perception that includes such drugs as PCP (phencyclidine), also known as angel dust, and LSD (lysergic acid diethylamide).

HYPOASCORBEMIA. Human inability to synthesize vitamin C, leading to population-wide chronically low blood vitamin C levels; also called subclinical scurvy.

METHADONE. A legalized opiate medication that is used by many drug treatment programs to prevent withdrawal symptoms and reduce craving in opioid-addicted individuals.

OPIATES. A class of potent but highly addictive painkillers that includes prescription drugs such as codeine and morphine, as well as illegal narcotics like heroin.

REDOX. A term that refers to an oxidation-reduction reaction; the loss (oxidation) or gain (reduction) of electrons.

XENOBIOTIC. A substance foreign to the body.

ATTENUATION OF HEROIN WITHDRAWAL SYNDROME BY THE ADMINISTRATION OF HIGH-DOSE VITAMIN C

by Alexander G. Schauss, PhD

A search of the literature in the medical school library of the University of New Mexico over 40 years ago suggested that vitamin C (ascorbic acid) might block the neuromodulatory response of opioid receptors to opioids such as heroin, a highly addictive narcotic drug. This suggested the possibility that vitamin C therapy might be a novel approach able to help heroin addicts withdraw from narcotic dependence.

I grew up in a crime-ridden neighborhood on the upper west side of Manhattan, a borough of New York City, which at the time had the highest per capita use of heroin in the United States. The junior high school I attended was only three blocks from notorious "Needle Park," where one could observe an endless progression of drug transactions night and day. And it spilled over into our neighborhood. It was not uncommon to watch classmates inject themselves with heroin in bathrooms, stairwells, or the playground. After giving themselves a "fix" they entered a state of euphoria that made them oblivious to the opportunity education afforded them to get out of the "airtight cage" and find relief from whatever familial, societal, or genetic factors inspired them to use heroin two or three times a day, day after day.

The "airtight cage" that Joseph P. Lyford described in his study of New York's West Side, funded by the Center for the Study of Democratic Institutions, eloquently described the despair and suffering experienced by those living within the boundaries of its gang-riddled, corrupt, and crime-infested streets.[1] Lyford had grown up in the lower East Side section of Manhattan, a neighborhood given the notorious name, "Hell's Kitchen," that harbored generations of immigrants to "the promised land." Yet, when he moved into the cage to watch over a tenement building he had purchased, he found it difficult to block out the sirens and sounds that instilled fear and resentment. It did not take him long to realize that this was a different community, a far more insidiously dangerous neighborhood riddled by tragic episodes of crime and violence nestled among decomposing tenement buildings occupied by broken spirits seeking escape from hopelessness and despair.

Having witnessed firsthand the destruction that heroin wages on the minds and bodies of peers, it seemed that destiny might give me an opportunity to find a way to break the powerful life-destroying shackle of heroin addiction. A former heroin addict described how it is able to take over one's life with these words: "The first time you inject it, it is as if you are kissing the creator... It is safe to say that you will *never* feel that way again, although you will certainly try—to the point of losing everything—maybe even your life." What makes heroin so addictive is eloquently explained as follows:

"It's like warm golden sunshine flowing through your veins. It makes everything okay, and it makes everything beautiful, and it makes anything seem within your reach. Then you come down. And need more. And will do anything to get it. It's your best friend at first, and, when you still can quit, you'd never dream of it. Then at some point that is indefinable and inevitable, it turns on you. It grows fangs and claws, and it wants your soul. It lies to you and tells you that you aren't doing anything wrong. It makes you feel like you would rather die than spend another second without it. Then before you know it, your days are consumed with waking up dry heaving and so sick you want to die (provided you could sleep at all, which is dependent upon whether or not you had a shot before bed). Once you finally get a first hit of the day, then it's time to start really looking for something to get you by. You lie, scam, break the law, and sell your soul to get just barely enough to keep you out of bed. You take that last shot of the day and become filled with dread and exhaustion thinking

From the *J Orthomolecular Med* 2012; 27(4):189–197.

how you'll manage it tomorrow. Then you go to bed, only to wake up a few hours later because your muscles are twitching and cramping. You fight with yourself for ten minutes about whether or not to take that small hit you saved for morning, inevitably take it, and then wake up a few hours later, only to start all over again. And you'd rather die than live any other way."

Heroin

For at least 6,000 years, opium poppies have been cultivated to produce a crude opium base used to relieve pain, treat chronic coughs, as an anti-diarrheal, or to induce a mind state of temporary euphoria.

Heroin (diacetylmorphine) is derived from the seedpod of the poppy plant (*Papaver somniferum*). The Latin name for the species means "that which induces sleep," while *papaver* has its origin in the Greek word for sap. *P. somniferum* is as a controlled substance since it contains addictive benzyliso-quinoline alkaloids. In the United States, heroin is listed as Schedule I under the Controlled Substances Act; no prescriptions may be written for heroin as it has a high potential for abuse and there is no accepted medical use for it. Since it is twice as potent by weight as morphine, some European countries allow its use to relieve pain in terminal cancer patients. In Switzerland, heroin is prescribed in cases where heroin addicts have not responded to other forms of substance abuse treatment.

Heroin, morphine, codeine, and thebaine (paramorphine) are all derived from the sap of *P.*

somniferum. This sap is extracted from the egg-shaped seedpod of the plant by slitting the pod vertically in parallel strokes. As the sap oozes out of the pod it forms a golden to dark brown gum that is collected and bundled into cakes or balls. These bundles are then transported for refinement into drugs such as morphine.

In 1847, C. R. Wright, a British scientist, synthesized heroin by boiling acetic anhydride with morphine for several hours. More recent methods of production and purification use a relatively easy process used around the world capable of producing tons of heroin annually. For instance, 10 tons of cheap opium can be processed into one ton of heroin. In the late 1990s, a kilo of heroin cost between $100,000 and $120,000. Of the 430 tons of heroin produced globally in 1996, half found its way into the United States to be sold illegally to heroin addicts.[2] Heroin is typically diluted to reduce its potency and to increase profits by adding such substances as powdered milk, quinine, or sugar.

Most heroin sold in the streets of New York during the 1950s to 1970s had been repeatedly adulterated, or "cut" to the point that the purity sold was in the range of 2 to 10 percent, yet potent enough to produce a rush followed by a temporary state of euphoria. As the amount of heroin entering the United States increased in the 1980s, heroin's purity rose to 20 to 30 percent. Some addicts became so addicted to the drug that they spent $1,000 or $2,000 a day getting high. As the flood of

IN BRIEF

Heroin addiction is a serious health and social problem that afflicts societies around the world. Its addicting characteristics have been known for thousands of years. Derived from opium, obtained from the opium poppy (*Papaver somniferum*), heroin is highly addictive. Conventional approaches to heroin withdrawal involve the use of synthetic or semi-synthetic opioids, with or without concomitant behavioral therapy. A study conducted in New York City in the 1960s demonstrated that, by giving increasing doses of vitamin C (ascorbic acid) salts administered orally in water or juice during withdrawal, vitamin C blocked opioid receptors in the brain and attenuated withdrawal symptoms, encouraging heroin addicts to end their dependence on heroin. A 1978 field visit to Seattle, Washington, by officials of the National Institute for Drug Abuse and Alcoholism (NIDAA) at the U.S. National Institutes for Health (NIH), confirmed its effectiveness, yet the agency to date has failed to provide funding to support further research on this promising treatment modality. Despite serious reported side effects, pharmacotherapeutic approaches in the treatment of heroin-dependence prevail with support by NIDAA, while nutrient-based therapies that could help break the cycle of addiction are disregarded.

heroin produced in Central America, South America, and the Middle East, particularly Afghanistan, and smuggled into the United States increased, the street price for a fix dropped to $5 (a "nickel bag") while purity increased up to 80 or 90 percent.

The most common way heroin is used is by cooking it in a spoon until it turns into a liquid. This fluid is then drawn into a syringe. After locating a vein, usually somewhere on the arm, it is injected into the vein and enters the bloodstream. The "rush" addicts experience by this route of administration is almost instantaneous. If administered intramuscularly, the rush may take 6 to 8 minutes. Some addicts prefer to snort the drug or smoke it, which delays the rush by as much as 15 minutes. Regardless of the route of administration, heroin use can be highly addictive.

When addicts share hypodermic needles, they risk contracting hepatitis B or C and HIV. According to the Centers for Disease Control and Prevention, 32 percent of females and 24 percent of males with AIDS acquired the disease by injection drug use.[3] The risk of overdose, heart disease, particularly heart failure and pulmonary complications, along with kidney disease, are just some of the consequences associated with heroin addiction. Since heroin affects the immune system, and the body's ability to fight infections, diseases such as tuberculosis, and pneumonia, are not uncommon. Immune reactions to adulterants added to heroin to reduce potency have been correlated with the onset of osteoarthritis and rheumatoid arthritis.

Whether injected or inhaled, heroin crosses the blood-brain barrier, where it is converted to morphine and binds to opioid receptors. How strong the "rush" is experienced depends on the amount of heroin administered and the speed with which it alters neural pathways and affects opioid receptors.

Any disruption in use of the drug once addicted can lead to symptoms of withdrawal within hours after taking the last dose. This creates a craving for the drug to avoid withdrawal symptoms. If the drug is stopped for too long a period, severe muscle and bone pains, diarrhea, vomiting, constant restlessness, insomnia, and involuntary arm and leg movements will occur. In addition, sudden feelings of hypothermia associated with

goose bumps are experienced. When this happens the skin looks very much like that seen on the skin of a frozen turkey. This is where the term "cold turkey" comes from, as every addict goes through periods of needing blankets to avoid the acute onset of chills they experience from time to time as they go through withdrawal.

By the 1950s and '60s, going cold turkey was the only choice heroin addicts had if they chose not to use certain drugs to try and block withdrawal symptoms. Some of these drugs simply replaced one addiction for another. This led to methadone becoming a drug of abuse that was also sold on the streets, given its addictive properties.

Many risk factors increase the likelihood that the addict will return to their addiction. So it is not unusual to have an addict go through withdrawal numerous times.

Heroin Addiction

Recent studies suggest that complex factors involving genetic and psychosocial factors contribute to substance abuse. Genetic studies have reported that genetic variants may account for up to 60 percent of the risk associated with developing opioid dependence.[4–6]

Of particular interest is the effect of heroin abuse upon the body's redox state. A study of 137 heroin addicts found that they experienced damaging oxidative injury. It was found that in addicts the balance between the production of oxidation products and antioxidant activity was gravely imbalanced, with the lack of sufficient exogenous (external) vitamin C, vitamin E, as well as endogenous (internal) nitric oxide production, closely correlated with and contributing to the damage to DNA and cells during chronic states of oxidative stress. In another study of 114 heroin abusers and 100 healthy volunteers, it was found that the longer the duration of heroin abuse the more injury occurred from oxidative stress. This correlated with decreased levels of antioxidant vitamins C and E, and beta-carotene, along with diminished values for several endogenous antioxidants, including superoxide dismutase, catalase, and glutathione peroxidase.[8] The authors concluded that it was necessary "in abstaining from heroin dependence" that the heroin abuser "acquire sufficient quantities of antioxidants such as vitamin C, vitamin E, and beta-carotene."

None of this was known in 1969, when the author organized a clinical trial to see if high-dose vitamin C would be of any benefit to heroin addicts wishing to break their dependency during cold turkey withdrawal.

While attending the City University of New York in 1969, a clinical trial was conducted to test the theory that vitamin C (as sodium ascorbate) might block opiate receptors in the brain of heroin addicts and block or diminish the "rush" and subsequent euphoria experienced following intravenous injection of the drug.

The hypothesis was based on a series of experiments performed by this author at the University of New Mexico, based on the premise that opioids bind to specific opioid receptors, as originally proposed in 1954 by Beckett and Casy,[9,10] and that vitamin C can occupy those receptors, thereby blocking the neuromodulatory effect of the opioid.

Pilot Animal Studies

Guinea pigs share with humans an inability to synthesize vitamin C, based on mutations in the gulonolactone oxidase (GLO) gene, which codes for the enzyme responsible for catalyzing the last step in the biosynthesis of vitamin C.[11] This is why humans can get scurvy from a deficiency of vitamin C in the diet.

An exploratory study injected guinea pigs with 5 percent pharmaceutical pure heroin in sterile water daily until dependency was established. Thereafter, the solution was administered twice daily for one week. When administration was withdrawn, the response resulted in significant behavioral and locomotor changes, somewhat similar to the withdrawal syndrome seen in humans.

In the second experiment, guinea pigs were injected with the same dose after being pretreated for four days with vitamin C. It was observed that vitamin C attenuated some of the withdrawal symptoms seen in the first study, compared to controls.

Additional experiments were performed, each of which demonstrated the ability of vitamin C to diminish withdrawal symptoms.

These encouraging results suggested that an open label pilot study of the effect of high dose oral vitamin C in humans was warranted. With the assistance of the City University of New York, the study was approved in 1969, and a site selected.

Titration Protocol

Volunteers who had been addicts for at least five years, who had experienced cold turkey withdrawals at least three times, agreed to participate in the trial, following written consent. The study was conducted at an addiction treatment center in Harlem, a community within the borough of Manhattan, known for a high per capita rate of heroin addicts. Five or more times a day each volunteer drank a 6-ounce glass of diluted orange juice or apple juice containing various amounts of vitamin C (as sodium ascorbate).

Initially, compliance was poor, as the juice had an unpleasant salty taste. It was explained to the volunteers that the reason for the salty taste was that the vitamin C was bound to a salt, which tasted salty but also was non-acidic (as sodium ascorbate has a neutral pH). The ratio of fruit juice to water was 50:50. Addicts were told that they might experience diarrhea. Volunteers were instructed to report any symptoms to the nursing staff by phone or in person and could terminate participation in the study at any time. Participants were paid $5 a week to participate in the two-week study. They were also informed that the principal investigator (the author) wanted to determine if vitamin C could reduce any side effects experienced during withdrawal.

Participants reported that the primary reason for participating in the study was to get their addiction under control by eliminating dependence on the drug. Fearful of going through withdrawal by cold turkey, they were willing to see if the vitamin could reduce the symptoms during withdrawal. Records were kept on 20 addicts who volunteered and who met exclusion and inclusion criteria to participate in the study.

The question of how much vitamin C an addict could tolerate before reaching "bowel tolerance" turned out to vary. (When diarrhea occurred, the amount of vitamin C was decreased to a lower dose.) Over time it was observed that addicts heavily addicted to heroin could tolerate considerable amounts of vitamin C before reaching bowel tolerance.

The first step in the protocol is to go through vitamin C loading for at least three days before going through withdrawal. This titration phase is critical. This would allow the dose of vitamin C to gradually increase to an amount of the vitamin that could be frequently administered every few hours once withdrawal symptoms were anticipated. Nurses adjusted the dose of sodium ascorbate in juice depending on the participant's body weight, medical history, and frequency of daily heroin use. The protocol for an addict who met inclusion criteria might be as follows:

• Day 1 (three days prior to day of withdrawal): Drink 6 ounces diluted fruit juice (DFJ) containing 500–1,000 milligrams (mg) of sodium ascorbate (SA) every two hours until bedtime.

• Day 2: Drink DFJ with 1,000–2,500 mg of SA every two hours until bedtime.

• Day 3: Drink DFJ with 5,000–7,500 mg of SA every three hours until bedtime. Begin withdrawal at bedtime. If withdrawal symptoms occur during the night, DFJ with 5,000–7,500 mg of SA, administered when awake, and taken every two hours until symptoms abate.

• Day 4: DFJ with 2,500–5,000 mg of SA every two hours until bedtime. If symptoms occur during the night, DFJ with 2,500–5,000 mg of SA, administered when awake, and taken every two hours until symptoms abate.

• Day 5: DFJ with 1,000–2,500 mg of SA every two hours until bedtime. If symptoms occur during the night, DFJ with 1,000–2,500 mg SA, administered when awake, and taken every two hours until symptoms abate.

• Day 6: DFJ with 1,000 mg of SA every two hours until bedtime. If symptoms occur during the night, DFJ with 1,000 mg of SA, administered when awake, and taken every two hours until symptoms abate.

Upon learning of the study's success, Linus Pauling, PhD, informed Vic Pawlek, the director of a drug treatment center in Phoenix, Arizona, about the study. In 1972, Pawlek reported favorable results.[12] The center created a cocktail that included vitamin C (as an ascorbate) and niacin, the addition of which was suggested by Abram Hoffer, MD, PhD, who felt the addition of niacin would be beneficial.[13]

Jordan Scher, MD, an addiction specialist and psychiatrist who worked at the National Council on Drug Abuse and Methadone Maintenance Institute in Chicago, reported that large doses of vitamin C significantly reduced withdrawal symptoms when co-administered with methadone.[14]

Despite these promising observations in several states, advocacy for the use of vitamin C during withdrawal failed to gain ground within the substance abuse field, partially due to criticism and concerns about the use of "megavitamins." The use of drugs was heavily favored over dietary supplementation at the time, combined with the belief that taking more vitamins or minerals only produced "expensive urine," a belief some critics continue to espouse to this day.

In 1979, I gave a presentation on a quasi-experimental study we had conducted in King and Pierce Counties, Washington, at a medical conference held near Seattle. During the presentation the subject of vitamin C came up during which I mentioned the observations made on using vitamin C in New York a decade earlier. I pointed out that among the 20 addicts who complied with the protocol, each one reported very few symptoms commonly experienced during heroin withdrawal. Attending the conference and in the audience was Janice Keller-Phelps, MD, the medical director of the King County Center for Addiction Services (which includes the city of Seattle). Dr. Keller-Phelps is a substance abuse specialist, with considerable experience treating addicts. She had been a medical director in Maryland's correction system and participated in studies funded by the National Institute for Drug Abuse and Alcoholism (NIDAA) at the National Institutes of Health (NIH).

After completing the presentation, the moderator asked the audience if anyone had any questions or comments. She grabbed the microphone and insisted that the suggestion vitamin C could help heroin addicts during withdrawal was "total nonsense." In response I challenged her to try treatment for one month with any of the hard-core addicts in her program. I also pointed out that she had no proof it did not work. During a sidebar conversation at the end of the session, I provided her information on programs using vitamin C on the west coast of the United States that she could visit to see how the vitamin is used. She accepted the challenge.

Her first trip took her to Oakland, California, where she visited an addiction treatment clinic that has been using vitamin C. She also met with Michael Lesser, MD, in Berkeley, California, a psychiatrist. Dr. Lesser described the work of Dr. Irwin Stone and his theory as to why primates could not synthesize vitamin C, and explained his "hypoascorbemia hypothesis."[15–16] She then traveled to the other side of the Bay, not far from Stanford University, and met Dr. Stone. He shared with her his collaboration with Alfred Libby, PhD, using vitamin C. Dr. Stone also mentioned the pioneering work of Frederick R. Klenner, MD, who in the 1940s began experimenting with megadoses of sodium ascorbate up to 350–700 mg per kilogram (kg) of body weight each day in the treatment of a wide range of diseases. Drs. Libby and Stone published a paper in 1978 that described a pilot study

VITAMIN C AND DRUG WITHDRAWAL

"Cameron and Baird reported (in 1973) that the first five ascorbate-treated patients who had been receiving large doses of morphine or heroin to control pain were taken off these drugs a few days after the treatment with vitamin C was begun, because the vitamin C seemed to diminish the pain to such an extent that the drug was not needed. Moreover, none of these patients asked that the morphine or heroin be given to them—they seemed not to experience any serious withdrawal signs or symptoms."

From *Cancer and Vitamin C* by Ewan Cameron and Linus Pauling, 1981, p. xii.

they conducted using sodium ascorbate in the treatment of drug addiction.[17] She also spoke with Bernard Rimland, PhD, a Navy psychologist in San Diego, who had taken an interest in the use of megadoses of nutrients in the treatment of neurological disorders, including autism.

Nevertheless cautious, Dr. Keller-Phelps continued to contact other practitioners who had used vitamin C in their practice, while also reading such works as Dr. Stone's classic work on the vitamin, *The Healing Factor: Vitamin C Against Disease.*[18]

Soon after her return to Seattle, Dr. Keller-Phelps began using sodium ascorbate at the addiction treatment facility in King County. By August 1979, she reported "dramatic" success in attenuating the symptoms of heroin addicts, some of whom had been addicted to the drug and gone through multiple withdrawals for more than 25 years. Her opinion was that it was like "a cure to cancer" for addicts. I urged her to temper her enthusiasm by reminding her that addiction was complex and due to multiple factors, as she herself had pointed out at the conference.

After treating 30 hard-core addicts with sodium ascorbate, and convinced of its benefit, she contacted officials of NIDAA in Washington, DC. At the time, I was research director of the Institute for Biosocial Research at City University of Seattle. Dr. Keller-Phelps persuaded NIDAA to send a fact-finding team to Seattle to verify and confirm her observations. Her request was approved. Upon arrival in Seattle, the team of three officials spent four days conducting interviews with addicts who had gone through the vitamin C withdrawal program. By the third day, they had interviewed over two-dozen addicts who had successfully gone through withdrawal using the vitamin C protocol Dr. Keller-Phelps had adopted. On the last day of their visit, one of the officials told executives of the university, including Clifford Simonsen, PhD, dean of the graduate school, and a noted professor of criminology, that what they learned and observed seemed "irrefutable," and worthy of NIDAA's support.

Several months passed as we waited for NIDAA's report. Finally, Dr. Simonsen called NIDAA to speak with the officials who came to Seattle. They informed everyone listening to the call on the speakerphone that regrettably the agency could not endorse the treatment. It would be an understatement to say that we were dismayed and in a state of disbelief. How could this be? Why would the agency not fund independent controlled studies of this seemingly effective and safe treatment modality?

Confirmatory Studies

In 1992, a paper was published in *Neuroscience Letters* that reported chronic treatment with vitamin C (1,000 mg per liter (L), in drinking water for three days, or 200 mg/kg subcutaneously three times daily for three days) inhibits morphine withdrawal symptoms in guinea pigs.[19] The authors determined that chronic, but not acute, administration of vitamin C blocked opiate withdrawal symptoms.

In 2000, a paper was published by the University of Ioannina in Greece, reporting on the results of a study they conducted on the effect of oral administration of high-dose vitamin C during heroin withdrawal.[20] In the study, heroin abusers were given 5 mg/kg of body weight each day of vitamins C and E for at least four weeks. A control group of addicts was administered conventional medication consisting of diazepam (Valium) and an analgesic each day during the same time period.

Whereas 57 percent of the vitamin C- and E-treated subjects experienced a significant reduction in symptoms during withdrawal, only 7 percent of the control group experienced a reduction in symptoms. The authors of the study concluded, "The results indicate that high doses of ascorbic acid administered orally may ameliorate the withdrawal syndrome of heroin addicts. Further studies are needed in order to estimate the dose- and time-dependent effects of ascorbic acid treatment, and to clarify its mechanisms of action in the withdrawal syndrome."

As a footnote, eleven years after meeting Dr. Keller-Phelps, she authored a book that discussed her experience using vitamin C and other nutrients in the treatment and amelioration of substance abuse.[21]

NIDAA Priority: Pharmacotherapeutics

At the same time NIDAA's fact-finding team was visiting Seattle in 1969, the agency was studying a semi-synthetic opioid, buprenorphine (Buprenex), which binds to morphine receptors, in the treatment of heroin withdrawal. NIDAA also promoted the use of methadone (manufactured by Eli Lilly), a synthetic acyclic analog of morphine and heroin, for use by patients with opioid dependency, at risk of opioid withdrawal syndrome.

Interestingly, in 1990, NIDAA created the Medications Development Division, to focus on developing drug treatments for addiction. Four years later, in 1994, NIDAA formed an agreement with the original developer of buprenorphine to bring the drug to market.[22] Buprenorphine was subsequently approved by the FDA for use in the treatment of addiction, in 2002, and continues to be used for this purpose to this day.

NIDAA also advocates the use of other drugs to reduce the severity of withdrawal symptoms. Among the drugs given research support are: clonidine (Catapres) and lofexidine (Britlofex), both centrally acting alpha-2 adrenergic agonist, the first of which was launched in 1992 for symptomatic relief in patients undergoing opiate withdrawal, and later naltrexone (Vivitrol), an opioid receptor antagonist, primarily used in the management of alcohol and opioid dependence. These pharmacotherapies, along with buprenorphine, naloxone (Narcane), methadone and its analogues, dipipanone (Diconal) and dextromoramide (Palfium), continue to be commonly prescribed drugs used in the treatment of narcotic addiction withdrawal.

These drugs are also known to cause serious adverse events. A 1997 study of naltrexone-treated opioid addicts by the University of California, Los Angeles (UCLA), and the Matrix Center and Los Angeles Addiction Treatment Center, found that 13 of 81 subjects overdosed within a 12-month period, of which four died. Among the nine nonfatal overdoses, four involved suicide attempts. These serious adverse events were described by the authors of the study as "characteristic of subjects" taking naltrexone.[23] By contrast, a 1997 paper in the *Journal of the American Medical Association* evaluating the safety of naltrexone in a heterogeneous population of persons treated for alcoholism, noted "no new safety concerns," or deaths identified among the 865 patients enrolled in the program they studied.[24]

The side effects reported by UCLA associated with naltrexone aren't limited to its use during treatment but can also result in serious adverse events following withdrawal. The Australian National Evaluation of Pharmacotherapies for Opioid Dependence (NEPOD) study analyzed the results of 12 trials of pharmacotherapies for opioid dependence and found serious adverse events and deaths associated with the use of these drugs. They found that "individuals who leave pharmacotherapies for opioid dependence experience higher overdose and death rates."[25]

CONCLUSION

Opioid dependence is a serious social and health problem. According to the Centers for Disease Control and Prevention, National Center for Health Statistics, from 2004 to 2008, the estimated rate of emergency visits involving nonmedical use of opioid analgesics doubled from 49 per 100,000 to 101 per 100,000.[26]

Treating opioid dependence requires a multidimensional approach that involves extinguishing dependency, withdrawal (detox), and relapse prevention. Vitamin C therapy may be an effective modality to help patients withdraw from heroin addiction, and improve retention in treatment programs designed to break the cycle of addiction. Combining high-dose vitamin C therapy with other nutrient-based therapies should be considered.

NIDAA and similar agencies concerned with substance abuse need to provide funding and support studies of nutrient-based therapies to determine what their place should be in the armamentarium of treatment modalities used in helping patients recover from the addiction. Research should also focus on whether subclinical deficiencies of nutrients, such as vitamin C combined with genetic factors, increase the risk that someone exposed to addictive drugs such as heroin may develop an addiction.[27] Until such funding and support becomes available, it is encouraging to learn that others are studying whether vitamin C holds promise in treating other substances of abuse such as crack cocaine.[28]

Recent studies have examined the role of non-coding microRNA (genetic material) in understanding the molecular mechanism behind the debilitating effects of addiction. Morphine has been a target for such investigations. Studies reported on the regulation of miR-133b by morphine and its involvement in morphine addiction, along with the role of microRNA let-7[29] in the regulation of morphine receptors involved in the development of opioid tolerance,[30] are two examples of such investigations.

The role microRNAs, such as miR-133b and other non-coding RNAs, play in leading to addiction either by direct opioid regulation or by controlling neuropathways, as affected by vitamin C, would be an example of the kind of research NIDAA could fund in helping us to understand its mechanisms of action in attenuating heroin withdrawal syndrome without pharmacological intervention.

REFERENCES

1. Lyford JP. *The Airtight Cage: a Study of New York's West Side.* New York: Harper & Row, 1968.

2. The opium kings. Transforming opium poppies into heroin. *Frontline.* Retrieved from www.pbs.org/wgbh/pages/frontline/shows/heroin/transform.

3. National Institute on Drug Abuse. Treatment can work. Retrieved from archives.drugabuse.gov/about/welcome/about drugabuse/treatment.

4. Kreek MJ, Neilsen DA, Nutelmann ER, et al. Genetic influences on impulsivity, risk taking, stress responsivity and vulnerability to drug abuse and addiction. *Nat Neurosci* 2005;8:1450–1457.

5. Silberg J, Rutter M, D'Onofrui B, et al. Genetic and environmental risk factors in adolescent substance use. *J Child Psychol Psychiat* 2003;44:664–676.

6. Clarke TK, Ambrose-Lanci L, Ferraro TN, et al. Genetic association analyses of PDYN polymorphisms with heroin and cocaine addiction. *Genes Brain Behav* 2012;11:415–423.

7. Zhou J, SI P, Ruan Z, et al. Primary studies on heroin abuse and injury by oxidation and lipoperoxidation. *Chin Med J* (Engl) 2001; 114:297–302.

8. Zhou JF, Yan XF, Ruan ZR, et al. Heroin abuse and nitric oxide, oxidation, peroxidation, lipoperoxidation. *Biomed Environ Sci* 2000; 13:131–139.

9. Wood PL. Multiple opioid receptors in the central nervous system. *Neuromethods* 1986;4:329–363.

10. Beckett AH, Casey AF. Synthetic analgesics: stereochemical considerations. *J Pharm Pharmacol* 1954;6:986–1001.

11. Drouin G, Godin J-R, Page B. The genetics of vitamin C loss in vertebrates. *Curr Genomics* 2011;12:371–378.

12. Pawlak V. *Megavitamin Therapy and the Drug Wipeout Syndrome: An Introduction to the Orthomolecular Approach as a Treatment for After-Effects of Drug Use/Abuse.* San Francisco: Bolerium Books, 1975.

13. Hoffer A. Vitamin B3: niacin and its amide. Available at www.doctoryourself.com/hoffer_ niacin.html.

14. Scher J, Rice H, Kim S, et al. Massive vitamin C as an adjunct in methadone maintenance and detoxification. *J Orthomolecular Psych* 1976;5:191–198.

15. Stone I. Hypoascorbemia, the genetic disease causing the human requirement for exogenous ascorbic acid. *Perspect Biol Med* 1966;10:133–134.

16. Stone I. The genetic disease, hypoascorbemia: a fresh approach to an ancient disease and some of its medical implications. *Acta Genet Med Gemellol* (Roma), 1967;16:52–62.

17. Libby A, Stone I. The hypoascorbemia-kwashiorkor approach to drug addiction therapy: a pilot study. *Australas Nurses J,* 1978;7:4–8,13.

18. Stone I. *The Healing Factor: Vitamin C Against Disease.* New York: Grosset & Dunlap, 1972.

19. Johnston PA, Chahl LA. Chronic treatment with ascorbic acid inhibits the morphine withdrawal response in guinea-pigs. *Neurosci Lett* 1992;135:23–27.

20. Evangelou A, Kalfakakov V, Georgakas P, et al. Ascorbic acid (vitamin C) effects on withdrawal syndrome of heroin abusers. *In Vivo* 2000;14:363–366.

21. Keller-Phelps J, Nourse AE. *The Hidden Addiction and How to Get Free.* New York: Little, Brown, 2000.

22. National Institute on Drug Abuse. Heroin: abuse and addition. Available at www.drugabuse.gov/publications/research-reports/ heroin-abuse-addiction/what-are-treatments-heroin -addiction.

23. Miotto K, McCann MJ, Rawon RA, et al. Overdose, suicide attempts and death among a cohort of naltrexone-treated opioid addicts. *Drug Alcohol Depend* 1997;45:131–134.

24. Croop RS, Faulkner EB, Labriola DF. The safety profile of naltrexone in the treatment of alcoholism. Results from a multicenter usage study. *Arch Gen Psychiat* 1997;54:1130–1135.

25. Digiusto E, Shakeshaft A, Ritter A, et al. Serious adverse events in the Australian National Evaluation of Pharmacotherapies for Opioid Dependence (NEPOD). *Addiction* 2004;99:450–460.

26. Warner M, Chen LH, Makuc DM, et al. Drug poisoning deaths in the United States, 1980–2008. NCHS Data Brief 2011; 81:1–8.

27. Kreek MJ, Levran O, Reed B, et al. Opiate addiction and cocaine addiction: underlying molecular neurobiology and genetics. *J Clin Invest* 2012;122:3387–3393.

28. WeeksMD. Vitamin or heroin–your choice! Available at weeksmd.com/2008/11/vitamin-c-or-heroin-your-choice.

29. Rodriquez RE. Morphine and microRNA activity: is there a relation with addition? *Front Genet* 2012;3:223.

30. He Y, Wang ZJ. Leet-7 microRNAs and opioid tolerance. *Front Genet* 2012;3:110.

METHODOLOGY: USE OF ORTHOMOLECULAR TECHNIQUES FOR ALCOHOL AND DRUG ABUSE IN A POST-DETOX SETTING

by Alfred F. Libby, PhD, Oscar Rasmussen, PhD, Wesley Smart, Charles Starling, MD, Patricia Haas, Cortland McLeod, John J. Wauchope, and Hortensia Gutierrez

Information is extremely sparse regarding ortho-molecular techniques for treating drug addiction and alcoholism. The reason appears to be a general lack of interest rather than lack of ability. This indifferent attitude is not surprising since this lack of interest has pervaded all branches of medicine and science. Following the Civil War, when it was recognized there was a significant alcohol and drug problem, there have been only two major government supported programs for the treatment of drug addiction. It took 47 years to decide on a strategy to deal with the increasing drug problems in the United States. A decision was made to establish legal narcotic dispensing clinics as a deterrent to the ever-increasing problem and so during 1912 clinics were opened in Florida and Tennessee. There were some 44 of these clinics opened across the United States supplying legal heroin to addicts by 1920. The theory behind this thinking was that if the addict received his/her unadulterated medicinal opiate legally, at low cost or without charge, the black market opiate pushers could hardly support themselves by selling opiates solely to non-addicts and the market would dry up. That logic is as wrong today as it was wrong in 1912. A kid trying out his first experience with drugs does not buy it from a stranger—he obtains the drug from a so-called friend.

In 1920, the Narcotic Unit of the Treasury Department, predecessor of the Federal Bureau of Narcotics, launched a successful campaign to close these dispensing clinics as non-beneficial and unsuccessful.

The Harrison Narcotic Act

Now comes a second blunder in the thinking of those empowered to deal with this problem, and the one that set the stage, the thinking, and the misdirection the United States government has taken concerning drug addiction since 1914, an incredible 68 years! The Harrison Narcotic Act was an outgrowth of the Hague Convention of 1912, aimed primarily at solving the opium problems of the Far East, especially China. The Act did not appear to be a prohibition law; on its face it appeared to be merely a law for the orderly marketing of opium, morphine, heroin, and other drugs, in small quantities over the counter, and in larger quantities on a physician's prescription. There was a section in this Act that protected the rights of a physician to prescribe for his patients any of the aforesaid drugs. The provision protecting physicians contained a "gotcha" clause, however, that was unrecognized at the time of the legislation. In this section of the Act it stated that a physician could prescribe drugs for his patients "in the course of his professional practice only." This single phrase was then interpreted by law enforcement officers to mean that a physician could not prescribe opiates to an addict to maintain his addiction. Since addiction was not a disease, the argument went, an addict was not a patient and opiates dispensed to or prescribed for him/her by a physician were therefore not being supplied "in the course of his professional practice only." Thus, a law that was apparently intended to insure the orderly marketing of narcotics was converted into a law prohibiting the supplying of narcotics to addicts. It developed that many physicians were arrested under this interpretation by law enforcement officers, and some physicians were convicted and imprisoned. Even those physicians who escaped conviction had their careers ruined by the publicity. It appears that, because of this harsh treatment of the medical profession by law enforcement, the drug addiction population would be the ultimate losers because since 1914 the medical profession has maintained a strict "hands-off" policy.

From the *J Orthomolecular Psychiatry* 1982;11(4):277–288.

The physician of 1914 recognized the problem created by the interpretation of the Harrison Narcotic Act and foretold the future role of the physician as well as the drug addict when an editorial appeared in *American Medicine* just six months after the enactment with the following statement: "Narcotic drug addiction is one of the gravest and most important questions confronting the medical profession today. Honest medical men have found such handicaps and dangers to themselves and their reputations in these laws that they have as little to do as possible with drug addicts or their needs. The addict is denied the medical care he urgently needs; open, aboveboard sources from which he formerly obtained his drug supply are closed to him, and he is driven to the underworld where he can get his drug. Abuses in the sale of narcotics are increasing. A particularly sinister sequence is the character of the places to which addicts are forced to go to get their drugs and the type of people with whom they are obliged to mix. The most depraved criminals are often the dispensers of these habit-forming drugs. The moral dangers, as well as the effect on the self-respect of the addict, call for no comment. One has only to think of the stress under which the addict lives, and to recall his lack of funds, to realize the extent to which these afflicted individuals are under the control of the worst elements of society. One can clearly see the withdrawal of the medical profession from investigating more effective methods of treating a drug addict for fear of prosecution and imprisonment. Who could rightfully fault the medical profession for its attitude under the circumstances?

Now left free to operate, the "dope peddlers" established a national organization and the underground traffic in narcotic drugs began to flourish. The problems of drug addiction so increased that the then Secretary of the Treasury in 1918 appointed a committee to investigate the problem. The 1918 committee, like countless committees since, called for sterner law enforcement as a solution to the problem. The medical situation and predicament of the drug addict was still not understood, but the "dope peddlers" understood, and now heroin prices could be doubled and tripled to increase their profits because nothing was being done for the addict, except prosecution.

Stiffer Jail Sentences as a Deterrent

Many of the United States federal and state laws were passed to stiffen the penalties for narcotic offenses. The maximum penalty specified in the three 1909 federal laws was two years imprisonment. The 1914 Harrison Act increased this maximum to five years. In 1922, a maximum federal penalty of ten years imprisonment was enacted. In this same year, Canada added whippings and deportation to its penalties! Subsequently, state laws were stiffened to provide 20-year, 40-year, and even 99-year maximum sentences.

Life imprisonment and the death sentence were added to both federal and some state laws during the 1950s. By 1970, Congress had passed some 55 federal laws to supplement the 1914 Harrison Act. This number, however, is incomplete in one very significant respect. It excludes the Volstead Act (Alcohol Prohibition) of 1919, and the many subsequent laws designed to stamp out the drinking of alcohol between 1920 and 1933, when alcohol was also considered an illicit drug.

Armed with these stiffer penalties as deterrents enacted by Congress, it is easy to see how the judiciary and the entire police system began to, and still do today, look upon the drug addict as an arch criminal and enemy of society. Indeed, there has been one blunder after another committed in dealing with this patient population, and it continues to this very day. Some of the more enlightened individuals who were in a position to judge these oppressive techniques began to speak out. One such individual was August Vollmer, an outstanding police chief and authority on police administration. After watching the results and effects of the Harrison Act, Chief Vollmer wrote in 1936, 22 years after passage of this law, the following statement: "Stringent laws, spectacular police drives, vigorous prosecution, and imprisonment of addicts and peddlers have proved not only useless and enormously expensive as means of correcting this evil, but they are also unjustifiably and unbelievably cruel in their application to the unfortunate drug victims." Vollmer went on to state that "drug addiction, like prostitution, and like liquor, is not a police problem; it never has been and never can be solved by policemen. It is first and last a medical problem, and if there is a solution, it will be discovered not by policemen, but by scientific and competently trained medical experts, whose sole objective will be the reduction and possible eradication of this devastating appetite."

Robert S. de Ropp, PhD, biochemist, made this comment in 1957, "Just why the alcoholic is tolerated as a sick man, while the opiate addict is persecuted as a criminal, is hard to understand. There is, in the present attitude of society in the United States toward opiate addicts, much the same hysteria, superstition, and plain cruelty as has characterized the attitude of our forefathers toward witches. Prison sentences up to 40 years are now being imposed and the death sentence has been introduced. Perhaps one should feel thankful that the legislators have not yet reached the point of burning addicts alive. If one insists on relying on terrorism to cope with a problem which is essentially medical, one may as well be logical and 'go the whole hog.'"

Enter the "Enlightened" Age (1950s)

For the first time since the closure of the legal opiate clinics, a treatment program was outlined for the opiate addict. This technique was developed at the Federal Hospital in Lexington, Kentucky, using a synthetic narcotic developed by the Germans near the end of World War II named methadone hydrochloride. The first step in this technique is to transfer the patient from morphine or heroin, in relatively equal dosage amounts, to methadone hydrochloride. In order to detoxify the patient, the daily methadone dose is progressively reduced over a period of 10 days or so, until a zero dose is reached, then the patient is considered "detoxed."

It was during this period of time that Marie Nyswander, MD, was assigned to the Lexington Hospital as a psychiatrist for the U.S. Health Service. Coincidentally, at this same period of time, Vincent P. Dole, MD, a specialist in metabolic disease at the Rockefeller University, became interested in heroin addiction through his studies of obesity, which in some respects might be considered addiction to food. Dr. Dole wanted to investigate drug addiction as having a metabolic, biochemical origin. As an initial step, he reviewed the existing scientific studies. Dr. Dole located a good deal of literature, but there was one serious flaw; almost all of the American literature concerned itself with opiates in the test tube, laboratory animals, non-addicted volunteers, or imprisoned addicts. He learned that American physicians in general had divorced themselves from the problems of the addict in the street ever since the early waves of physician arrests under the Harrison Narcotic Act.

Through a series of events, Drs. Dole and Nyswander united early in 1964 to jointly begin a research project investigating drug addiction using Methadone as the vehicle. The two physicians developed their own techniques regarding detoxification and ultimately developed what is known today as daily methadone maintenance. On the basis of their detoxification experience and treatment of just six patients, Dr. Dole visited the New York Commissioner of Hospitals armed with these six case histories, depicting their detox results with methadone and asking for six hospital beds to continue with their research. The drug problem being so great in New York, the hospital commissioner ordered instead 20,000 beds and heavy financial support. One has to admire the care and concern they both had for the street addict. It was the first time in 50 years that physicians once again undertook the care of street addicts, and they must have felt they had made a wonderful contribution to a pitifully neglected segment of our society! One still has to wonder, though, in light of the Harrison Narcotic Act language, why Drs. Dole and Nyswander, the Commissioner of New York Hospitals, and the Eli Lilly Company, not to mention the many physicians still dispensing methadone hydrochloride, to this very day, were not and are not arrested and prosecuted. Law enforcement and the federal government apparently have turned their heads the other way when methadone entered the scene. While the federal government was so zealous in 1914 and 1915 prosecuting physicians, everyone was obviously so frustrated in dealing with the drug-addict population in 1964, the federal government and law enforcement officers, as well as the judiciary, overlooked what did and does appear to be a clear violation of the language of the Harrison Narcotic Act. In every sense of the word, methadone maintenance certainly and absolutely is prescribing opiates to an addict to maintain his addiction.

Dr. Dole is certainly correct in our view in his assessment that drug addiction is of metabolic and biochemical origins. We take a strongly similar view in light of our research that the metabolic and biochemical disruptions are most certainly one of the results of drug and alcohol addiction. When speaking of origins, one must strongly consider the possibility that poor nutritional habits developed through childhood, assisted tremendously to create these abnormal urges or desires in the first instance.

Exploding the Myth

Above all else in this study we wanted to demonstrate conclusively that there is an ongoing misconception concerning the alcoholic and most particularly the drug addict. The traditional concept of "test clean" means the patient is "clean" or free of the addictive substance in his/her body. In other words, if the patient gives a blood or urine sample to the authorities and the test results prove negative for drugs, then the patient is assumed to be free of the drug from his/her body and now the patient is totally detoxed and a candidate for rehabilitation. If the patient can "test clean" for drugs, therefore, the "gut craving" for drugs that remains *must* be one of psychological origins, or at least so the traditional therapists in the field of alcohol and drug addiction would have us believe.

Psychiatrists and psychologists, after testing these "drug-free" individuals, found they tested abnormally in the paranoid, schizophrenic perceptual, depression, suicide, and IQ areas; therefore, the erroneous conclusion was reached that this population was, and is, an emotionally and mentally deficient group. Because of this erroneous belief, the rehabilitation therapy treats this class of patients psychologically with combative, confrontive, semi-confrontive, aversion therapies, religious teaching, or with drugs that are more detrimental to the organ

systems than the drug the patient was recently taking. Nowhere in medicine are patients treated with such abusive and barbaric techniques.

Where have you heard of a carcinoma patient being treated with carcinoma cells, a pneumonia patient with pneumocci, a diabetic with sugar, a gonorrhea patient with gonococci, a comatose patient with secobarbital (Seconal)? This sort of "therapy" would not be tolerated; in fact, it would not go unpunished. Why then do we tolerate such abominable drugs as methadone, L-alpha-acetyl-methadol (LAAM), ethanol, Antabuse, Darvon, Darvon-H, electrical devices, and other barbaric devices to treat the infirm? Foul and abusive language is, for the most part, the order of the day. Shaving the hair off the head, being made to wear abusive and degrading signs, not being allowed to speak, sitting in a corner for hours on end, and there are many other unspeakable tactics used on a daily basis. Can this be rightfully called rehabilitation? These tactics are abusive, offensive, inhumane, and must be put to an end. Religiously oriented programs should share a burden of this guilt as well. They allow an individual to go through the rigors of "cold turkey" while feeding their souls only, instead of the entire biochemical system. As if these people didn't have enough problems already; now if they fail in this type of program, they've failed God also. It seems too heavy a burden to carry.

There are hundreds of programs for alcohol and drug addiction in the United States and elsewhere that subscribe to the idea that the patients either have to live together, work together, eat together, and sleep together or else they won't "make it" in society by themselves. This philosophy smacks of a throwback to prehistoric tribal life as opposed to an advancement in the treatment of these two malignancies that plague all corners of society. There are other programs that state categorically that if the patient is to "make it" he/she must listen to reassuring brethren sermons each evening of the week and, since this patient is not to be trusted, his/her family is brought into the fold for lectures also. This is not treatment—it is in the end analysis a complex transfer of the addictive process from one addiction to another, neither of which is ultimately beneficial to the majority of patients. While it is to be recognized that these types of "programs" were absolutely essential for all in the past, perhaps even for a minority in the present, clearly there is no plausible excuse for their continued existence in the future.

The word "patient" is used advisedly because all people afflicted with a drug or alcohol affliction will forever remain a "patient" untreated until he/she is decontaminated first.

The Decontamination Process and the Procedures Used for Physical Mental and Emotional Regeneration

It must be understood at the onset the techniques that were used in this study were for a post-detox setting and one that is *not* to be used for acute detoxification. The techniques we employ for acute detox from drugs and alcohol are considerably different and involve both oral and intravenous applications. Throughout the study a probation officer visited his charges weekly and collected urine specimens at unannounced times, to be examined for illicit drugs.

Prior to the commencement of treatment, the patients were spoken to on three separate occasions about the intended orthomolecular treatment to encourage their voluntary participation. At all times there was a great deal of skepticism on the part of the patients about the effectiveness of what could be done for them. These individuals were at this facility under court order as an alternative to jail or prison. They did not want to be there, nor were they inclined to be cooperative with any type or form of authority, no matter what its purpose. After three weeks of patient discussion, cajoling, and frank answers to their numerous questions, the skeptics were quieted. With this most difficult period over, everyone was now ready to proceed in unison with the study.

• **On May 24, 1980,** two days prior to initiation of treatment, the following tests were done in preparation: hair analysis, dietary evaluation form, health hazard appraisal, diagnostic health profile questionnaire, 35mm color slide of each patient, voice cassette recordings of each patient for drug history and voice levels, and preparation of patients' charts.

• **On May 25, 1980,** a 24-hour urine collection began for the vitamin C levels, quantitative amino acid fractionation, and the 24-hour urine cortisol levels.

• **On May 26, 1980,** the 24-hour urines were collected by the medical laboratory. Prior to breakfast, the laboratory crew drew blood samples for a chemistry screen (SMA 18), vitamin B12 levels, complete blood count (CBC), and venereal disease (VDRL) test. At exactly noon the nutritional program began. Each patient was given 5,000 milligrams (mg) of sodium ascorbate (vitamin C) in a cup of orange juice. They were also given three tablets of calcium complex with magnesium. This was continued in the same manner every two hours until 8:00 P.M.

• **On May 27, 1980,** at 9:00 A.M., continuation was made with 4,000 mg of vitamin C and one calcium complex (375 mg) with magnesium tablet (150 mg). At 11:00 A.M., each patient was given three tablets each of a multivitamin formula, a vitamin B complex (50 mg of each major B vitamin), plus three tablets of extra pantothenic acid (vitamin B5, 100 mg), and one tablet of extra thiamine (vitamin B1, 100 mg), with zinc (60 mg), as well as 4,000 mg of sodium ascorbate with one calcium tablet (375 mg) with magnesium (150 mg). At noon it was determined that all but three of the patients had experienced diarrhea, a state we believe to be *absolutely necessary* in order to decontaminate the body, as well as reinitiate normal peristalsis of the bowel. Of the three patients, one had a long history of chronic constipation; no explanation for number two; number three deserves special attention. This gentleman, a young man from Nicaragua had a right mastoidectomy to remove an infection from behind the eardrum in 1965. Approximately seven months ago he developed pain in his right ear.

• **In March 1980,** he had consulted an ear specialist who advised the young man, after examination and cultures, that he had a staphylococcus infection. The specialist placed him on 500 mg of ampicillin (an antibiotic), four times daily. He was also given a solution of acetic acid and advised to place two drops four times per day in his ear. This regimen had been followed for two months, with no real relief. At 1:00 P.M., 4,000 mg of sodium ascorbate were given and one calcium complex (375 mg) with magnesium (150 mg). The vitamins and minerals given at 11:00 A.M. were repeated at 3:00 P.M. and at 7:00 P.M. The sodium ascorbate was repeated at 5:00 P.M. At 8:00 P.M., blood pressures were taken with no adverse pressures noted.

• **On May 28, 1980,** eight patients complained of headaches on the previous day; therefore, the vitamins and minerals were reduced by two-thirds on this date. At 9:00 A.M., 4,000 mg of sodium ascorbate and one calcium complex (375 mg) with magnesium (150 mg) were given. At 11:00 A.M. and 5:30 P.M., one multivitamin formula, one multimineral formula, one vitamin B complex (50 mg of each major B vitamin), plus one tablet extra of pantothenic acid (100 mg) and thiamine (100 mg), with one zinc tablet (429 mg) were given. Headaches were not complained of; at 1:00 P.M. on this date, a second cassette recording was taken to record progress.

• **On May 29, 1980,** at 11:00 A.M., 1:00 P.M., and 7:00 P.M., 4,000 mg of sodium ascorbate and one calcium complex (375 mg) with magnesium (100 mg) were given with each dose. At 11:00 A.M. and 5:00 P.M., one multivitamin formula, one multimineral formula, one vitamin B complex (50 mg of each major B vitamin), plus one tablet extra of pantothenic acid (100 mg) and thiamine (100 mg), with one zinc tablet (429 mg) were given.

The young man with the chronic right ear infection finally had diarrhea on this date at 4:00 A.M. He stated he felt much better physically and mentally and could now sleep well for the first time since the infection developed. On this date it was decided to arrange an organized exercise program, as there was none, and none had ever been a part of the existing program prior to our arrival to conduct the study.

• **On May 30, 1980,** at 9:00 A.M. and 3:00 P.M., 4,000 mg of sodium ascorbate and one calcium complex (375 mg) with magnesium (150 mg) were given with each dose. At 8:00 A.M., 12:00 noon, and 5:00 P.M., one multivitamin formula, one multimineral formula, one vitamin B complex (50 mg of each major B vitamin), plus one tablet extra of

pantothenic acid (100 mg) and thiamine (100 mg), with one zinc tablet (429 mg) were given. The vitamin C was reduced to 8,000 mg on this day (down from a total of 12,000 mg per day), and the entire patient population reported that they felt fine. All vitamins were given with meals and there were no stomach complaints.

• **On May 31, 1980,** the same nutrient regimen as on May 30, 1980, was followed. At 3:00 P.M., a group discussion was held with the patient population, discussing the results obtained thus far into the program. Their responses and participation were enthusiastically overwhelming. Following the discussion, one patient said he no longer suffered from the deep depression that had always been so much a part of him. This 29-year-old male went on to state that he no longer had paranoia when anyone was walking directly toward him; he suffered the gripping fear that they were "coming to get him" and he would make a fist, preparing for a combative situation.

• **On June 1, 1980,** a Sunday, only two meals were served. At 11:00 A.M. and 6:00 P.M., one multivitamin formula, one multimineral formula, one pantothenic acid (100 mg), one thiamine (100 mg), and one zinc tablet (429 mg) were given. At 3:00 P.M., 6,000 mg of sodium ascorbate and one calcium complex (375 mg) with magnesium (150 mg) were given.

• **On June 2, 1980,** at 8:00 A.M., 12:00 noon, and 5:00 P.M., the patients were given one multivitamin formula, one multimineral formula, one vitamin B complex (50 mg of each major B vitamin), plus one tablet extra of pantothenic acid (100 mg) and thiamine (100 mg), and one zinc tablet (429 mg). At 11:30 A.M., they were given 6,000 mg of sodium ascorbate and one calcium complex (375 mg) with magnesium (150 mg). Two counselors indicated they noted improvement in their "caseload" of patient handwriting. Patients indicated their delight with the improved quality and varied diet.

• **On June 3, 1980,** at 9:00 A.M., 6,000 mg of sodium ascorbate and one calcium complex (375 mg) with magnesium (150 mg) were given. At 12:00 noon and 5:00 P.M., one multivitamin formula, one multimineral formula, one vitamin-B complex (50 mg of each major B vitamin) plus one tablet extra of pantothenic acid (100 mg) and thiamine (100 mg), and one zinc tablet were given. On this date, the first psychological retesting was done, indicating remarkable changes in the psychological profiles, as well as physical and emotional well-being.

• **On June 4, 1980,** a second phase of the program was initiated by the addition of 22,500 mg of 22 uniquely combined "free" amino acids. At 10:30 A.M., 2:00 P.M., and 7:00 P.M., 10 amino acid capsules containing 750 mg of amino acids in each capsule were given. With each application of amino acid capsules, one 500 mg of pyridoxine (vitamin B6) and one 10,000 IU of vitamin A (as fish oil) were given.

The rationale for the amino acid intake is due primarily to the severe deficiencies consistently observed over several years in the 24-hour urine amino acid assays. Drugs and alcohol create crippling nutritional deficiencies. The vitamin B6 is used to offset any deficiency of this critical vitamin as nonessential protein metabolism will not occur if a pyridoxine deficiency exists. Vitamin A is necessary whenever protein is given, as evidenced by the critical mistake made by UNICEF when feeding hungry children with powdered milk in South America during 1964. There is always an increased need for vitamin A whenever protein is used. In the case of the South American children, permanent eye damage and blindness occurred. When UNICEF returned four years later, the protein powder was fortified with vitamin A and no problem occurred.

At noon the patients were given one multivitamin, one multimineral, and one vitamin B complex (50 mg of each major B vitamin). At 5:00 P.M., they were given 6,000 mg of sodium ascorbate and one calcium complex (375 mg) with magnesium (150 mg).

On this date the patient with the chronic ear infection revisited the ear, nose, and throat specialist. The physician was amazed at how well the ear had suddenly healed, since the infection had been so resistant to treatment. The specialist discontinued the antibiotic as there was no further need and the only change in this man's lifestyle was vitamin C and the other previously mentioned nutrients.

This nutritional regimen was continued as described from June 5, 1980, until June 15, 1980. On June 16, 1980, a new routine was initiated. Sublingual vitamin B12 lozenges were added. The lozenges contained 1,000 mcg of cyanocobalamin, with no sugar additives, and were quickly soluble under the tongue. One tablet was given under the tongue three times a day for a period of the next 17 days. The daily routine from June 16, 1980, until July 2, 1980, was the following: one multivitamin, one multimineral, one vitamin B complex (50 mg of each major B vitamin), plus one tablet extra of pantothenic acid (100 mg), and one zinc tablet (429 mg) per day. In addition, 6,000 mg of sodium ascorbate and one calcium complex (375 mg) with magnesium (150 mg) were given per day.

• **On July 3, 1980,** blood chemistries were drawn for the second time and the third psychological testing was done. Once the testing was completed, this effectively ended the study, a total of 40 days.

With the accumulated data collected on each individual in the study, an analysis was made of the biochemical makeup and the chronic nutritional deficiencies each individual had due to the abuse of alcohol and/or drugs. An individual maintenance program was given to each patient along with recommendations, according to their prior eating habits, of foods to include or exclude in the future in order to maintain a happy, wholesome life without the abnormal cravings that nutritional deficiencies create.

■ CONCLUSION

Drug addiction has mushroomed and has overgrown its host, just as a bacterium will flourish when it becomes resistant to antibiotics. It is time to recognize and accept the fact that the present programs do not, will not, and cannot work in the treatment of any form of substance abuse.

Law enforcement agencies, following the enactment of the Harrison Narcotic Act, decided to become involved in drug addiction through their interpretation of the Act. All of their most intense efforts have failed to have any lasting effect on the problem of substance abuse and their failure ratio is worsening each day. Addicts are not basically criminals. They become criminals because of their dependence on the addictive substance. A diseased body does not respond to legislation.

Medicine's level of contribution has resulted in the branding of addicts as chronic and incurable. In other words, the addictive person must wear the brand of an alcoholic or drug addict forever. The addicts' treatment has, for the most part, been placed in the hands of psychiatrists and psychologists. Their treatment has proven almost totally ineffective. There have been a few voices in the past that suggested that the addict might really be sick. Despite this, the treatment has been symptomatically oriented and the basic disease proves it has been ignored.

Our study has shown that all addictions are biochemical and psychological diseases, but this study has clarified many questions about the basic pathological processes that are involved in this multiple disease process. This treatment is based on the fact that toxic contaminants must be removed before any treatment can be effective. Therefore, the initial phase is termed decontamination rather than detoxification, although either term is acceptable as long as one understands that contamination is the basic problem to deal with first. No drugs are involved and none need be involved as each drug, regardless of its effect, is a foreign substance that becomes a contaminate and may produce an even more serious condition. Therefore, decontamination, replacement, and maintenance are the three essential phases of our treatment.

Education of medical and social agencies as to the exact basic nature of the biochemistry involved in addiction must be our first goal. Once this is done, we can proceed to the second goal of a realistic research and a developmental phase. Our third and ultimate goal is to eradicate this problem. In order to reach this goal, it will require treatment, education, and research, which will develop to the final stage of prevention. Prevention of addiction by proper feeding and supplementation of all young individuals will make the manufacturer of addictive substances unprofitable; remove the market and the problem will eventually resolve itself.

Through this study it has been effectively demonstrated that toxic residues from alcohol and drugs do remain in the organ systems for an indeterminate period of time, and, until they are removed, effectively, there is no prolonged hope for the patient to stay "clean."

Postscript

This study was accomplished under most adverse conditions. We received little or no cooperation from the entire staff. The house physician expressed little or no interest in what was being attempted. As of this writing, two years after the fact, the physician has never asked to review even one test result. With the exception of one, all probation officers were contemptuous, suspicious, and outright hostile over our new approach for their charges. The probation officers at no time offered any form of encouragement to their post-detox, court-appointed charges for rehabilitation.

Volunteer patients had varying jail sentences ranging from six months to two years. All patients remained under the same rigidly controlled circumstances throughout the study. Each probation officer visited his charges weekly and collected urine specimens at unannounced times, to be examined for illicit drugs. No positive urines were reported during the study.

Due to the restrictions placed by the court on all patients, no follow-ups were contemplated nor pursued. We were able to quickly decontaminate and detoxify each patient, thus removing the "gut craving" for the addictive substances, leaving them mentally, emotionally, and physically in their best condition ever. We conducted the diagnostic workup, pretest, and post-test so that we have quantitatively comparable data on the psychological and chemical profiles. When all wellness criteria are met, the patients are discharged with more than sufficient data to take home with them in order to maintain their wellness.

MASSIVE VITAMIN C AS AN ADJUNCT IN METHADONE MAINTENANCE AND DETOXIFICATION

by Jordan Scher, MD, Harry Rice, MD, Suck-oo Kim, MD,

Ralph DiCamelli, PhD, and Helen O'Connor, RN

Scurvy, an ancient plague, was mentioned by Hippocrates as the cause of debility, bleeding gums, and hemorrhages. Cities under siege, as well as ships at sea, were often devastated by this progressive and indefinable entity. During the Crusades, St. Louis and all of his knights were said to have been defeated and captured because of scurvy. During the 1497–1498 voyage of Vasco de Gama, 100 of his crew of 160 died of scurvy, and, in 1577, a Spanish galleon was found adrift with all dead of the disease. A story goes that on one of Columbus' trips, a number of Portuguese sailors were put ashore to die of scurvy. However, on a return trip, these men were found to be alive and healthy since they had out of desperation and hunger eaten the local wild plants and fruits they found on the island, which subsequently came to be called Curacao, meaning "cure" in Portuguese.

Physiologically, the functions of vitamin C are still very much up in the air. Vitamin C has been implicated in cellular respiration, enzyme activation, carbohydrate metabolism, folic acid conversion to folinic acid, endocrine interactions, and collagen synthesis. Yet, our understanding of the effects of vitamin C upon such conditions as scurvy has not advanced much since that of the early sailors who accidentally discovered the empirical relationship between limes and the cure and prevention of the condition. Much of what happens in medicine, as most of us know, is often a matter of art, accident, lucky guess, intuition, or chance observation. And it may well be that the tale we will tell here falls in one or several of these categories.

In a series of papers, Irwin Stone[1,2] proposed a concept of hypoascorbemia (chronically low blood vitamin C levels) as a kind of human genetic insufficiency. It has, further, been known for some time that man, other primates, and the guinea pig are the only mammals known to be unable to synthesize ascorbic acid. Burns[3] has suggested that these species genetically lack the hepatic enzyme necessary to carry out the conversion of gulonolactone to ascorbic acid (vitamin C) because of a gene-controlled enzyme "deficiency." Linus Pauling in his book *Vitamin C and the Common Cold* (1970)[4] picked up the suggestion given by Stone, and following earlier studies by Cowan and others[5] suggested that vitamin C was essentially a specific preventative in the development of the common cold. Stone went further, in his book *The Healing Factor: Vitamin C Against Disease* (1972),[6] and indicated that this agent was mandatory in the prevention, mitigation, or cure of a great number of other conditions not readily accessible to more specific treatment.

It has been known for some time that there are individual variations in biochemical needs. A number of years ago, Professor Roger Williams wrote an important book, *Biochemical Individuality* (1956)[7], stipulating this fact. In it, he states: "Some inbred rats on identical diets excreted 11 times as much urinary phosphate as others . . . some voluntarily consumed consistently 16 times as much sugar as others . . . some appeared to need about 40 times as much vitamin A as others . . . some young guinea pigs required for good growth at least twenty times as much vitamin C as others."

In their book *The Doctor's Book of Vitamin Therapy*, Drs. Rosenberg and Feldzamen (1974)[8] report that in a group of geriatric patients with mild scurvy, 700 milligrams (mg) of vitamin C daily initiated improvement. However, despite regular checks for urinary vitamin C, it took three weeks for the ascorbic acid to appear in the urine. This is echoed by a report by E. S. Wagner[9] who found that, despite the usual claim that excess vitamin C is readily excreted, only about half appears in the urine. There seems, therefore, to be an unknown reservoir for storing the vitamin with which we have not been familiar before.

From the *J Orthomolecular Psych* 1976;5(3):191–198.

Food, Drug, and Environmental Allergies

Food allergies, ecological mental illness, and ecological allergies are various names for an unusual and rather poorly defined class of conditions that are of untold importance, yet which have a devastating effect on our society. All the contaminants, pollutants, preservatives, drugs, and other agents with which we are continually bombarded have been having a disastrous effect upon man, only barely currently recognized. As noted above, a number of studies and much clinical observation bear out the reality of the food and environmental allergic conditions that relate to none of the ordinary allergic conditions with which we are medically familiar. They do not generally produce hives and rashes, but their effects are very real nonetheless.

These hypersensitivity reactions have a rather characteristic history and effect. Generally speaking, the individual tends to progressively prefer exposure to the implicated agents. For example, he may be a chocolate addict, a potato-chip fiend, or some other chronic persistent user of the very agent that tends to, in the long run, produce the damage. Initially, these agents, whatever they may be, will be merely foods, or relatively innocuous substances. However, they will progressively take on the quality of becoming demand substances. That is, the individual will feel that he *must* have a smoke, or a cup of coffee, or whatever it may be to "get him started in the morning." This idea that the particular agent is stimulating is an accurate one, at least initially. However, as the hypersensitivity process progresses, a number of rather surprising effects will develop. The allergic and addicted individual, as well as developing the compulsive need for the offending agent, will begin to suffer a number of withdrawal effects in the absence of the agent. He will feel irritable, tense, and perhaps will begin to sweat and develop muscular tensions, joint pains, cold hands and feet, as well as tense and restless hands and feet. He will find that most of these symptoms will be alleviated initially by the use of whatever the sensitizing substance may be.

Should the individual persist in the chronic misuse of the particular agent, or agents, he may discover a number of additional symptoms beginning to develop as well. There will be a tendency toward acute and chronic exhaustion and tiredness, despite the use of what had previously been a stimulating and relieving agent. There will be a kind of brain fog, in which will occur problems of retention of recent events and experiences, as well as difficulty in holding, conceiving, and developing ideas, and in finding and using the right words. In most cases, there will be a progressively reduced level of effective functioning intellectually. There may also develop a number of physical symptoms, including reduced libido, impotence, constipation, cold clammy skin, inefficiency in finer movements of limbs, a general awkwardness, and any number of frequently called hypochondriacal complaints. For example, there may be headaches resembling migraines and pains in the chest, stomach, back, and other body parts. These will often call down the unfortunate medical epithet of "crock," and cause such patients to wander peripatetically from doctor to doctor and from nostrum to nostrum.

Unfortunately, many of these nostrums will include tranquilizers, amphetamines, barbiturates, sedatives, and even at times narcotics, as well as unnecessary operations for nonexistent conditions. There is a kind of conspiracy that condemns such patients in their desperate and fruitless perambulations from physician to physician and clinic to clinic, until they are finally called chronic neurotics or chronic psychotics. It has been due to the efforts of several heroic and generally insufficiently recognized specialists in this area that at least a number of these patients have been spared the necessity of perpetual and unhappy pursuit of their illness. This is particularly disturbing since such conditions are strikingly easy to diagnose and incredibly easy to treat.

Diagnosis is based largely on history. For example, a patient who is chronically exposed to a particular agent will usually be able to tell you so. He will say that he is addicted to, or constantly finds himself compelled to use, this or that food or substance. Or in taking a work or environmental history of him, you will find that he is persistently exposed to a petroleum product, a gas, or some other chemical substance. An example of this phenomenon received worldwide attention when allergist Ben Feingold reported on 25 hyperactive schoolchildren. These children, who were uncontrolled and uncontrollable at school and at home, he said, could be "turned on and off at will, just by regulating their diets." By restricting the amount of processed food containing artificial flavors and colors, such as hot dogs, soft drinks, and ice cream, he could completely control the hyperkinetic syndrome.[10]

Randolph and other specialists in this field diagnose such patients by putting them in the hospital on a distilled water diet initially in order to clear out the residues of the offending agents, which takes several days.[11] Once this is done, differing classes and types of foods and agents are progressively reintroduced into the patient's diet so that the offending agent will, when introduced, produce a replication of the symptoms at that time. The treatment is the soul of simplicity itself. Elimination of the disturbing agent will completely resolve the condition and eliminate all the symptoms.

What is curious about the phenomenon is that, initially, as stated above, the offending agent acts as a stimulant and the hypersensitive individual seems brighter, and more physically and emotionally content with himself. Therefore, he will be drawn back to the use and misuse of the agent until it begins to have its whole pathological effect. At that time, the initial stimulatory phase passes over so quickly, and the symptomatic and exhaustion phase takes over very fully. The patient is aware only of the pain, anguish, and disturbance of his mind and body that he cannot seem to shake off and that no one can seem to either diagnose or help him with.

Although it is impossible to estimate accurately the number of persons afflicted with this condition, surely it numbers in the many millions. The description we have given above, for example, certainly applies to the alcoholic, who number at least 10 million. It applies to the "foodaholic," whose numbers are vastly greater. It probably applies as well to the narcotic addict, who may number as many as a million. And with the tremendous increase in offending environmental and polluting agents, one must multiply the victims of these conditions many times over.

A Personal Experience

It is not infrequent for many physicians given to sophistication, skepticism, and a predilection for scientific methodology to doubt the reality of the symptom complex and the clinical phenomenology we have described. But it is at least the very personal experience of the lead author Jordan Scher, MD, to know quite intimately the effect of the food-allergic mechanism and its deleterious and devastating personal assault. Having discovered long ago the reality of these symptoms in the course of chronic and progressive excessive use of coffee and tobacco, he knows and can attest firsthand that these symptoms are all too real.

As a result of these discoveries and after a number of years of suffering the condition, Dr. Scher, who, unaided by medical assistance, which seemed as puzzled by his condition as was he, spontaneously discovered that the elimination of the offending agent completely cleared up the disturbing conditions. Thus, he was enabled to have a period of four or five years without the burden of these painful symptoms interrupting the course of his life. But as in all food-allergic and food-addicted patients, he was inevitably drawn back to the misuse of the offending agents, since he longed for and knew of the initial and satisfying stimulatory effects of them. Beginning again to enjoy the ecstasies, he very quickly moved into the phase of exhaustion and symptom production, a totally expected and predictable result.

Yet, as in many scientific discoveries, serendipity and accident were to have a role. A friend, who was caught up in the vitamin fad of the time, suggested Scher try some vitamin C. To his great amazement, after scarfing down a handful of vitamin C tablets, he very shortly noticed a distinct tendency toward alleviation and relief of the exhaustion, brain fog, and tension phenomena. It became possible to overcome for a considerable period of time, most, if not all, of the phenomena associated with his particular food-allergic coffee-addiction problem. In fact, he was able to go back to a progressively greater and greater amount of coffee misuse as he had done prior to the realization of the devastating symptomatic effects he had experienced previously. This relief was only made possible through the use of truly massive amounts of chewable vitamin C ingested by the handful almost continuously over the 24-hour period. Taking 20,000–50,000 mg per day was not unusual. Ultimately, the protective effects of the vitamin C seemed to diminish and be overcome by the more prominent and pervasive food-allergic symptoms, so that Scher was compelled again to completely abstain from the offending agent perhaps for the final time.

Vitamin C and Methadone

This purely serendipitous effect caused Dr. Scher to experiment with the use of massive vitamin C in other conditions that might be suggestive of food-, drug-, or environmental-allergic disturbances. He experimented with the use of large doses of vitamin C to resist the effects of alcohol in patients, as well as to reduce the degree of symptomatic tension and disturbance experienced in both the hangover phenomena and the recovery stage of acute and chronic alcoholic intoxication and alcoholism. An abstract of some of these findings was reported in an international alcoholism meeting in Liverpool, England, in August 1973. Not long after, we received a letter from Linus Pauling about these suggestions and reporting on an abstract of Ewan Cameron and G. M. Baird.[12]

Based on strictly empirical evidence, we have observed that patients in a state of narcotic withdrawal often show symptoms of irritability, muscular tensions, a tendency toward exhaustion, and other phenomena suggestive of both the food-allergic syndrome as well as the magnesium-depletion syndrome. We have also observed clinically that certain patients on methadone seem to react to it with a highly stimulating amphetamine-like effect, while others tend to be more sedated and suppressed. These are, of course, not the majority of methadone-maintained patients who, if they are not misusing other drugs, will generally be relatively "normalized" through the use of methadone. This also takes into consideration the inevitable slight high produced in the course of a total single daily dose administration and slight withdrawal some 18 to 24 hours later.

Methadone-maintained patients have a tendency toward constipation, reduced libido, and restless sleep. Based on the analogy of similar symptoms in the food-allergic patient, it was decided to administer megadoses of vitamin C with a suggested average of 5,000 mg per day to all methadone-maintained patients. Most patients who complained of these minimal side effects of methadone treatment were relieved of these and other annoying symptoms. For example, many methadone patients show low-grade irritability, and minor and discomforting emotionality, debility, and mood shifts. After taking vitamin C, these patients seemed to feel an enhanced sense of comfort and well-being.

Again, based on the analogy of using vitamin C to relieve the acute and chronic symptoms of food allergy, it was decided that ascorbic acid might well play an alleviating role in the process of detoxification and methadone withdrawal. As is well known, ascorbic acid has a role in oxidative processes; collagen synthesis; and muscular, vascular, and adrenal metabolism. It was therefore hypothesized that, since all of these areas seem to be implicated symptomatically in the process of detoxification, ascorbic acid may very well play a role here too.

Vitamin C as a Tranquilizer

Consequently, the same regimen is now a standard feature of our outpatient and inpatient detoxification process. Furthermore, it would appear that ascorbic acid has a moderating and tranquillizing influence on behavior and emotional states, so that it is of great assistance in managing patients who are in the process of detoxification. Early on, when we first began to use ascorbic acid, a double-blind program with the use of placebos was employed in patients in the withdrawal state, with minor methadone side effects, and in the process of detoxification. In each of these instances, it was clear that vitamin C had a marked effect in relieving the fatigue, tension, muscular pains and cramps, vasoconstriction and cold limbs, constipation, and impotence that occur. In all of these areas and conditions, there was relief in 60–70 percent of the cases, or more. Where the relief was least successful was in that of reduced libido and impotency, where the relief was found in about 50 percent of the cases. But restless sleep and the other symptoms mentioned above were distinctly alleviated in a considerable proportion of the cases so compared. It was therefore felt that vitamin C represented a clear addition to the armamentarium of narcotic addiction treatment on a clinical and statistical basis, despite the fact that we could not demonstrate biochemically or pharmacologically what the relief was based on.

The tranquillizing effect of vitamin C was a distinctive plus that had not been anticipated and is one to which we feel more attention should be paid. If vitamin C is a mild benign physiological tranquilizer, it might well stand in the stead of more powerful and possibly more disrupting or problematic pharmacologically tranquillizing agents as a first choice in mild anxiety states. In fact, it may be that many so-called mild anxiety states, as well as mild depressive states, may represent subacute hypovitaminosis (vitamin deficiency), or perhaps more specifically the hypoascorbemia to which Stone refers.[1,2] The other alternative is that many individuals suffering mild symptoms of the kind described above may be really reacting to some kind of environmental or food-allergic assault at a relatively low level, and about which they have no real concept. If this is the case, and if ascorbic acid can and may be used in a fashion in which we are describing here, many of these conditions could be somewhat alleviated in their early phases or controlled for a considerable period of time.

Unfortunately, as in Scher's anecdotal incident described earlier, it may well be that the ecological hypersensitivity may outrun and overcome the prophylactic effect of the ascorbic acid eventually with the result that the patient may have to omit the use of the offending agent altogether. Since ecological and environmental and food allergies are at this point so poorly understood, unfortunately many individuals suffering from them will not be so lucky as to be able to identify and eliminate the source of their problem. Only a much broader educational and awareness program will permit this vital necessity to occur in the future.

Vitamins and the FDA

There is today considerable discussion about the restriction by the Food and Drug Administration (FDA) of the general unprescribed use and overuse of poly- and megavitamins. There are very real economic interests involved in the forefront and behind the scene of this presumably scientific discussion. Should vitamins be limited in ready availability and restricted to what many would consider minuscule doses, this would certainly throw into turmoil many people deeply committed to personal megavitamin programs. Such restrictions, including the limitations of vitamins to a prescription-only basis, would also doubtless please the drug companies for whom it would mean untold millions in financial reward.

It is not our intention to get into this discussion and this argument here, but we do feel that there is a legitimate place and a legitimate use for megavitamin treatment in a rational way on a purely empirical basis. We feel that we have demonstrated the usefulness of this program to ourselves and our patients. We also feel that our practice of megavitamin therapy may be adopted usefully by those who are involved in methadone maintenance and detoxification programs elsewhere. We have not found any of the side effects others have claimed, such as stone formation, or any involvement at all with oxalic acid in the course of this use of ascorbic acid or the other vitamins cited.

Attention should be paid to the use of trace elements, but we have not seriously studied the effects or relationship of these to the problems of addiction. We do, however, recommend to our patients the use of kelp tablets, on general principles, since kelp is well known to have a rather adequate supply of all of the known trace elements.

Comment

In closing, we would like to make a plea for an acknowledgment of the serendipitous in medicine and science. Had it not been for Scher's personal experiences, these thoroughly salubrious uses of a common vitamin would not have been developed. And if we were to wait for absolute methodological confirmation and knowledge of why ascorbic acid operates as it does, we might have to wait a long time indeed. In fact, as is well known, we know little about how or why aspirin does what it does, or indeed exactly why narcotics such as morphine or methadone do what they do. So, let us hope that in the spirit of enlightened acceptance of what works—the true guiding light of medicine—we are able to accept this very practical and useful remedial measure for what it is worth in the treatment of the addictive process, methadone maintenance, withdrawal, and detoxification.

REFERENCES

1. Stone I. Genetic etiology of scurvy. *Acta Geneticae Medicae et Gemellologiae* 1966;15:345.

2. Stone I. Hypoascorbemia: the genetic disease causing the human requirement for exogenous ascorbic acid. *Perspectives in Biology and Medicine* 1966;10:133.

3. Burns JJ, Mosbach EH, Schulenberg, S. Ascorbic acid synthesis in normal and drug treated rats. *Jour Biol Chem* 1954;207:679.

4. Pauling, L. *Vitamin C and the Common Cold.* New York: W.H. Freeman & Co, 1970.

5. Cowan DW, Diehl HS, Baker AB. Vitamins for the revention of colds. *JAMA* 1942;120:1267.

6. Stone I. *The Healing Factor: Vitamin C Against Disease.* New York: Grosset & Dunlap, 1972.

7. Williams R. *The Biochemical Individuality.* New York: Wiley & Sons, 1956.

8. Rosenberg H, Feldzamen AN. *The Doctor's Book of Vitamin Therapy.* New York: G.W. Putman's Sons, 1974.

9. Wagner ES. A new tip on an old acid trip. *Med World News* 1973;52:14, 34.

10. Feingold BF. *Why Your Child Is Hyperactive.* New York: Random House, 1975.

11. Randolph T. *Human Ecology and Susceptibility to the Chemical Environment.* Springfield, IL: Chas C. Thomas, 1962.

12. Shute EV. *Alpha Tocopherol (Vitamin E) in Cardiovascular Disease.* Toronto, ON: Ryerson Press, 1956.

SUPPLEMENTS ACCELERATE BENZODIAZEPINE WITHDRAWAL: A CASE REPORT

by W. Todd Penberthy, PhD, and Andrew W. Saul, PhD

A middle-aged male had success rapidly reducing fast-acting alprazolam (Xanax) dosage by taking very high doses of niacin, along with gamma-aminobutyric acid (GABA), and vitamin C. The individual had been on 1 milligram (mg) per day of Xanax for two years, a moderate dose but of fairly long duration. As a result, he had been presenting with increased anxiety, personality changes, and ringing in the ears (tinnitus)—all side effects likely due to long-term Xanax use. Xanax and other benzodiazepines like lorazepam (Ativan), clonazepam (Klonopin), and diazepam (Valium) are some of the most commonly used drugs. In addition to their effects as anti-anxiety medications, they are also used as sedatives, anticonvulsants, and muscle relaxants. They are also highly addictive.

Typical withdrawal from these drugs would involve substitution medication and a 10 percent or so dose reduction per week over a matter of months. A fast withdrawal is a 12.5 to 25 percent reduction per week. On very high doses of niacin, vitamin C, and also GABA, this individual reported being able to cut the dose 60 percent down to 0.4 mg in one week. The dose was reduced by 90 percent (to 0.1 mg/day) in less than a month. He reported residual anxiety, but that it was substantially less than when fully medicated. After a total of five weeks on the following supplements, the individual's medication intake was zero.

Niacin doses were between 6,000 and 12,000 mg daily. The individual reported reduced anxiety when taking the highest levels of niacin. Bowel tolerance levels of vitamin C were taken daily along with 750 mg of GABA two to three times daily. The individual also drank a quart of beet/cabbage soup broth daily for the first week, and took 400 mg of magnesium citrate a day and 5,000 micrograms (mcg) of sublingual methylcobalamin (high-absorption B12) twice a week.

During the initial total withdrawal from Xanax, the patient experienced daily but manageable anxiety. He also reported occasional nausea, possibly attributable to the GABA, and almost certainly attributable to the extremely high niacin intake. He experienced increased frequency of urination, especially at night. Evening niacin doses as inositol hexaniacinate (a semi-sustained release, no-flush niacin) reduced nighttime urination. The individual used regular-flush niacin about three-quarters of the time; inositol hexaniacinate constituted the balance. Dosage was divided into eight to ten 1,000 mg such doses in 24 hours.

Niacin

Niacin is thought to modulate neurotransmitters that are commonly unbalanced in the brains of those with anxiety, and it may also alter the metabolism of Xanax.[1] A derivative of niacin known as nicotinamide adenine dinucleotide (NAD) can speed up the metabolism of toxic waste products arising from the metabolism of the foreign alprazolam molecule.[1-2] NAD is used in over 450 reactions by the body, which is more than any other vitamin-derived molecule. It is quite complicated, but the small list of the pathways that are dependent on it include drug/xenobiotic metabolism, steroid metabolism, glucose metabolism, energy production, and much more. Administering high doses of niacin increases the concentration of NAD, which then accelerates the rate of the drug-metabolizing reaction, ultimately clearing the drug from the body faster.

GABA

GABA seems likely to be a safer replacement to withdraw from as compared to simple weaning off benzodiazepines. GABA is one of the main inhibitory neurotransmitters in the brain. Oral GABA does not cross the blood-brain barrier, but yet oral ingestion of GABA still exerts the calming effect that is attributed to GABA activity.[3] While GABA receptors are primarily known for their central nervous system (CNS) locations and functions, there are also GABA receptors in the liver, immune cells, and lung cells, which can activate neurons that ultimately affect the CNS.[4] It is also likely that at high doses some GABA does get into the CNS.

Vitamin C

Because ascorbate in high doses is a strong antitoxin, it is considered to be an important inclusion.[5] Flu-like symptoms common in benzodiazepine withdrawal may be ameliorated with vitamin C. Ascorbate also protects and provides support for the liver.

Magnesium

Magnesium depletion is common in nearly all examples of people ingesting drugs.[6] Thus, it makes sense for one to additionally consider taking nightly Epsom salt baths and 400 mg of magnesium citrate daily (200 mg in the morning and 200 mg in the afternoon) to facilitate a smooth transition away from benzodiazepines.

Summary

Collectively this experience indicates that very high doses of niacin, GABA, and vitamin C, with moderate doses of magnesium, together may greatly speed detox and reduce withdrawal symptoms from Xanax and other benzodiazepines. Every person is different and this one experience may not be applicable to all. Xanax is a seriously addictive drug and withdrawal symptoms may be severe. Each person should work closely with their health-care provider.

REFERENCES

1. Prousky JE. *J Orthomol Med* 2004;19(2):104–110.

2. Prousky J. *Nutr J* 2005;4.

3. Bronson PJ. *J Orthomolecular Med* 2011;26:11–14.

4. Belelli D. *Nat Rev Neurosci* 2005;6(7): 565–575.

5. Levy T. *Vitamin C, Infectious Diseases, and Toxins: Curing the Incurable*. West Greenwich, RI: Livon Books, 2002.

6. Seelig MS. *The Magnesium Factor*. New York: Avery, 2003.

Excerpted from the *Orthomolecular Medicine News Service*, March 18, 2014.

THE HYPOASCORBEMIA-KWASHIORKOR APPROACH TO DRUG ADDICTION THERAPY: A PILOT STUDY

by Alfred F. Libby, PhD, and Irwin Stone, PhD

Drug addictions, like cancer, are terrifying conditions to the victims because of the feelings of hopelessness and abandonment generated by the rigors and general failure of orthodox "treatments."

Although crude opium addiction has a very long history, the large-scale addictive use of morphine salts, in this country, is generally dated from their use on wounded Civil War soldiers.

Following 1864, morphine addiction was realized to be an emerging socially significant problem; therefore searches were instituted to find less addicting drugs. The year 1890 saw the introduction of heroin. For about five more decades, to the year 1912, nothing was done to stop the rising tide of morphine and heroin users. The realization of that fact prompted in that year the organizing of legal opiate clinics, not to treat the addict, but to support the user's habit in an attempt to stem the rising crime rate and sales of black market drugs. These legal opiate clinics remained open until 1924 when they were closed down as dismal failures. It took until the mid-1950s, another fallow period of about 30 years, before another major attempt started, the methadone program, which has continued up to the present. This program embraces the concept of orally giving a legally addicting drug (methadone) in place of an illegal addicting drug (heroin).

The lack of success in handling drug addiction, until now, is due to placing the emphasis on the legal aspects of the problem, mainly that of the crime and punishment concept, and ignoring the mental and physical condition of the addicts and neglecting to treat the health and metabolic problems of the victims. Drug addicts suffer from severe metabolic dysfunctions and are very sick people. Any attempted solution to the drug addiction problem that fails to bring total health back to the addict is doomed to failure.

Drug Addiction and Genetic Disease

Drug addicts, like other humans, are born carrying a defective gene for the synthesis of the liver-enzyme protein, gulonolactone oxidase (GLO). According to Irwin Stone, this birth defect[1] causes a potentially fatal, but now easily correctable[2] genetic liver-enzyme disease called hypoascorbemia.[3] This "inborn error of carbohydrate metabolism" has destroyed the capability of the human liver to synthesize ascorbate [vitamin C] from blood glucose, and thus deprives mankind of this important mammalian mechanism for combatting stresses. The normal mammalian response to stress is to increase liver-synthesis of ascorbate as an antistressor and detoxicant to maintain biochemical homeostasis within the body.[4]

Most mammals carry the intact gene for GLO and normally produce, under conditions of little stress, about 10,000–20,000 milligrams (mg) of ascorbate per day per 70 kilogram (154 pounds) of body weight to take care of their daily physiological needs. A biochemical feedback mechanism evolved in the early mammals[5] that increased daily ascorbate production possibly three to fivefold under a variety of chemical and physical stresses. Humans, among the very few mammals deprived of this homeostatic protective mechanism, suffer more physiological damage from equivalent stresses unless exogenous (external sources) ascorbate is supplied. Thus a daily intake of 10,000–20,000 mg of ascorbate by a relatively unstressed adult human is not "excessively high," but well within the normal mammalian range. Under stress humans require about 30,000–100,000 mg or more a day to maintain health. The therapeutic use of mega levels of ascorbate has met with great success in the treatment of the viral diseases,[6,7] cancer,[8] and many other pathologies. The sub-subsistence, "homeopathic" daily intakes of ascorbate, recommended for the past 40 years by the nutritionists as "vitamin C" for humans, would barely suffice to keep the other mammals alive and

From the J Orthomolecular Psych 1977;6(4):300–308.

certainly not in good health. The wide acceptance of this erroneous nutritional hypothesis by modern medicine has only led to the continued persistence of chronic subclinical scurvy (CSS syndrome)[9,10] as our most widespread and insidious human disease at present.

Physiological Effects of Drug Addiction

The usual history of addiction follows this sort of pattern: future addicts are born with the genetic defect for GLO, and already at birth are suffering from CSS syndrome. The CSS syndrome usually continues throughout childhood, adolescence, and adulthood without much of an attempt at any significant correction. It has been our experience that all the addicts we have dealt with began their introduction into the drug culture at an early age; first beginning with marijuana, alcohol, barbiturates, PCP, LSD, and then on to heroin. They usually begin as a weekend "high," escalating into a daily habit from which they can't escape. Each of these stresses further depletes the already dangerously low body stores of ascorbate leading to the severe exacerbation of CSS syndrome already present. Adequate repletion of the body stores of ascorbate is nonexistent.

On drugs, the addicts lose their appetite for food. Food deprivation or restriction leads to severe protein and vitamin malnutrition. All the chronic addicts tested suffer from hypoaminoaciduria (a deficiency of amino acids). This has led us to regard a confirmed addict as suffering from a hypoascorbemia-kwashiorkor type of syndrome (a form of malnutrition caused by not getting enough vitamin C and protein), and our treatment procedure was designed as an intensive holistic approach for the full correction of these genetic and multi-malnutritional dysfunctions. The procedure is completely orthomolecular, and no foreign substance or toxic narcotic or drug is used.

Briefly, by fully correcting this hypoascorbemia-kwashiorkor syndrome, we are able to take the addicts off heroin or methadone, without the appearance of withdrawal symptoms. If during the period of full correction, they take a "fix," it is immediately detoxified or otherwise handled by the body so that no "high" occurs. It is like inject-

ing pure water provided the dosage of ascorbate is high enough. After a few days on the regimen, appetite returns and they start eating voraciously. They also have restful sleep. Restless sleep or no sleep at all are characteristic of heroin and methadone addiction.

"Full correction" in the addicts treated comprised giving them 25,000–85,000 mg of sodium ascorbate a day in spaced doses along with high intakes of the other vitamins, essential minerals, and high levels of predigested proteins. Sodium ascorbate is a non-bitter, buffered vitamin C in a highly soluble form. This is continued for four to six days, and then the dosages are gradually reduced to lower holding-dose levels that varied from about 10,000–30,000 mg per day. Both the therapeutic and the holding-dose levels may vary widely according to the clinical response of the particular addict being treated. The therapeutic dosage is usually slightly beyond the bowel tolerance level, held for 12 to 24 hours. Selection of proper dosage is based on clinical experience and observation, and responses of the patient. Bowel tolerance is a concept introduced by Robert Cathcart[7] for judging the toxicity of the pathology and the required dosage of ascorbate needed for treatment. Cathcart found the bowel tolerance increases with increased stresses on the organism. The general improvement in the well-being of the addicts within 12 to 24 hours after beginning sodium ascorbate detoxification is striking. It is demonstrated by improved mental alertness and visual acuity, better appetite, and often surprise by the addict that treatment is working without the use of another narcotic.

Some Recent Work on Ascorbate

We do not claim to be the first to suggest or to use ascorbate in the addiction problem, but we do claim to be the first to use sodium ascorbate properly to get these desired results. Ascorbate injected into rats at the rate of 100 mg per kg of body weight attenuated and abolished the narcotic effects of morphine.[11] Ascorbate's detoxification of a wide variety of inorganic and organic poisons was reviewed[4] and included Klenner's work on the successful mega-ascorbic treatment of barbiturate poisoning, snakebite, and black widow spider bites. It was also suggested in this review that megadoses of ascorbate be used in drug addiction.[4] Two interesting papers appeared in 1976, one from Thailand which showed that the sleeping time induced in rabbits by 15 mg of pentobarbital (a drug commonly used to euthanize animals) could be progressively reduced by increasing amounts of ascorbate injected five minutes prior to the pentobarbital. The sleeping times in minutes for ascorbate dosages of 0, 250 mg, 500 mg, and 750 mg were 50, 29, 27, and 23, respectively, and at 1,000 mg ascorbate the rabbits did not fall asleep at all.[12] The other paper[13] was originally presented in 1974 to the North American Congress on Alcohol and Drug Problems, by these authors from the National Council on Drug Abuse and the Methadone Maintenance Institute, and was entitled, "Massive Vitamin C as an Adjunct in Methadone Maintenance and Detoxification." These authors realized that scurvy played a large part in the drug abuse problem, but they only saw ascorbate as a means to reduce some of the side effects of methadone administration like constipation, loss of libido, and restless sleep. For this they used about 5,000 mg of ascorbic acid a day. It apparently never occurred to them that by switching to sodium ascorbate and increasing their dosage by a factor of 10, they could completely eliminate the ill-conceived methadone program with all its problems and at the same time have a simple, nontoxic, and elegant solution to the drug abuse problem.

Orthomolecular Procedure for the Hypoascorbemia-Kwashiorkor Syndrome

Originally in our early testing, when the addict came in we took a urine sample for the urinary spillover of ascorbate and a 24-hour specimen for a complete quantitative assay of individual amino acids and related constituents. The results were so consistently low on the amino acids, and with no spillover of ascorbate, that we no longer go to the expense or bother of these tests.

Once the narcotic intake is stopped, the addict is given the first dose of sodium ascorbate, high levels of multivitamins and minerals, and 9 tablespoons per day of a predigested protein preparation in divided doses. Since the addicts have a rather abnormal digestive system, it is an aid to direct absorption of the amino acids into the vascular system if the liquid amino acid dosage is held in the mouth as long as comfortable before swallowing. The total amount of ascorbate given a day will vary with the extent of the drug addiction. It is never less than 25,000 mg a day in spaced doses and can go to 85,000 mg or more per day. As a rough rule-of-thumb means of judging dosage: a $50/day habit needs 25,000–40,000 mg sodium ascorbate, $150–$200/day about 60,000–75,000 mg). Judging dosage comes with experience, and any errors should be on the high-dosage side because of ascorbate's extremely low toxicity and lack of side effects. The megadoses are continued for four to six days. During this time no withdrawal symptoms should be encountered (if any appear, increase the sodium ascorbate intake). Generally, in two or three days, appetite returns and most patients begin to eat well and have restful sleep for the first time since the chronic addiction began. One of the first observations to be made of the patient on this orthomolecular therapy is the rapid change in well-being; they feel good. The megadoses are then gradually reduced to holding dose levels of about 10,000 mg per day of sodium ascorbate and lower levels of the vitamins and minerals. The predigested protein is discontinued if the patients are eating well.

Typical Case Histories

Case #1

T. M., male, age 23. He had been using drugs for 10 years. At 15, T. M. used heroin for a weekend high. At the time our treatment was started, he was supporting a $100-a-day habit. He had tried, on several occasions, the hospital detoxification programs of methadone and liquid propoxyphene (Darvon). Each time this program of substituting another narcotic for the heroin failed to give him satisfactory relief. The first thing he did when he came out of the hospital was to inject heroin because of the insatiable craving and being sick from the methadone or liquid Darvon. On coming in, his urine was tested for urinary spillover of ascorbate and amino acids.

There was no urinary spillover, confirming the presence of hypoascorbemia and hypoaminoaciduria. He was given 25,000 mg of sodium ascorbate in 4,000-mg doses along with the vitamins, minerals, and the protein supplements. After three days on the regimen, he began eating and feeling so much better and thinking more clearly, stating that "I don't want to go stealing no more," and he began to have restful sleep. The ascorbate was reduced to 10,000 mg per day on the sixth day. T. M. has now been on this holding dose for about three months, and is completely drug free and has lost his "desire" for the drug. He has graduated from the Manpower program and is now gainfully employed for the first time in his adult life.

Case #2

A. C., male, age 24, began using heroin at age 15 and now had a habit costing between $150 and $200 a day. He had tried at least seven different hospitals for detoxification and was on methadone maintenance for three years. He still "fixed" with heroin, in order to take the methadone, as it upset his stomach and made him ill. "Methadone kills your insides," to quote the patient. He was such a skeptic of the value of our orthomolecular program that on a Sunday he first took 45,000 mg of sodium ascorbate and then in the space of five hours he "shot-up" $300 to $400 worth of heroin, and he felt no effect from this large amount of heroin. He continued on the ascorbate, 45,000 mg per day for 10 days, along with the vitamins, minerals, and protein supplement. Then the dosage was reduced to 10,000 mg of sodium ascorbate and continued for another 30 days. A. C. has moved out of the area, but, when last seen, he was drug free and had an extreme sense of well-being and a good attitude.

Case #3

F. F., male, age 35, had been on drugs for 23 years, the last seven on the methadone maintenance program. He suffered the typical symptoms of methadone: severe constipation, loss of sleep, loss of libido. He would take laxatives and enemas and still was unable to move his bowels. When he did have a bowel movement, the stool was so hard and impacted that he would "faint or blackout from the pain." He was given the sodium ascorbate at the rate of 25,000 mg per day for four days, then increased to 45,000 mg, and then after one day reduced to 10,000 mg. He is still on this dosage level one month later and was seen at this time. He was doing so well that his mental attitude was excellent, his appetite had returned, his bowel movements were normal without laxatives, and his sex drive is slowly returning. He was advised to remain on the holding doses and return in one month for another checkup. Methadone maintenance is much more difficult to deal with than heroin addiction due to the adverse metabolic effect methadone has on the body.

At the time this paper was written 30 out of 30 patients were successfully treated in this pilot study. This reported 100 percent rate of success is the same as that noted by Dr. Cathcart in his megascorbic therapy of the viral diseases: "it works every time," provided enough ascorbate is used.

Orthomolecular Treatment of Drug Overdose

Drug overdose is a common occurrence because of the wide variability in the potency of the illicit "street" drugs and the tendency among addicts to mix different drugs. This causes many deaths among addicts. The following orthomolecular treatment of overdose acts as an antidote and rapidly relieves the stricken addict: if the victim is unconscious, immediately but slowly inject 30,000 mg or more of sodium ascorbate intravenously; if he or she is conscious and can swallow and retain liquids, give about 50,000 mg of sodium ascorbate, dissolved in a glass of milk.

In one case, a mother brought in her 16-year-old son, who was totally "spaced out" on angel dust (street name for PCP). This boy was incoherent and totally out of tune with reality. He was given 30,000 mg of sodium ascorbate mixed in a glass of milk, and within 45 minutes he could hold a normal conversation. If he had been given 50,000 mg, it is likely he would have become rational sooner. With intravenous ascorbate, this recovery time could be cut down to minutes.

Discussion

This joint pilot study was started in January 1977 after a series of coincidences between the authors.

Both researchers had been working independently on the drug abuse problem for many years, Libby conducting occasional clinical tests on addicts since 1974 and getting exceedingly promising results, and Stone working on the theoretical, genetic, and biochemical background. We heard of each other's work in December 1976 and pooled our knowledge and experience. Stone had been trying unsuccessfully to get some clinical research started for over a decade. His latest and most discouraging attempt came in November 1976 when a megascorbic clinical research protocol was turned down by one of the top people in the field. In the refusal, the reviewer noted, "There is no evidence for usefulness of massive doses of vitamin C in *any* disorder (except scurvy) least of all in conditions associated with heroin addiction . . . massive doses of vitamin C are potentially toxic . . . there is no known scientific basis for thinking that vitamin C would be beneficial in methadone maintenance or detoxification."

If we had not regarded this authoritarian certitude as utter nonsense, this promising new therapy of drug addiction could have been again delayed for years. This prevailing attitude toward megascorbics, however, convinced us that the orthodox drug abuse agencies were not the proper means for starting or conducting exploratory clinical tests on megascorbics in drug abuse. We also realized that getting any support for clinical work involving megascorbics, the black sheep of orthodox funding agencies, would be next to impossible to obtain, and certainly impossible to obtain quickly. Libby's preliminary tests were so impressive and this work had been delayed for so long, that, in view of the poor record of achievement by orthodox medicine, we felt immediate action was demanded. We eliminated all the time-consuming funding red tape by simply operating on our own personal funds and time.

Even though this therapy utilizes sodium ascorbate, vitamins, minerals, and predigested protein, we believe that the main antinarcotic effect is due to the sodium ascorbate, and the other materials are necessary adjuncts. High levels of sodium ascorbate have analgesic properties as shown by the observations of Cameron and Baird[14] and Sac-

coman[15] in terminal cancer, and by Klenner[6] in the relief of pain of severe burns and snakebite.

In terminal cancer, the ascorbate analgesia was so good that the patients' heavy toxic morphine schedules were discontinued. Thus, high levels of sodium ascorbate mimic morphine and probably fit into the opiate receptor sites. The fact that these terminal cancer patients abruptly removed from their morphine showed no withdrawal symptoms was one piece of evidence that indicated our megascorbic treatment of drug addiction would be successful.

As previously noted, ascorbate is a general detoxicant for many different poisons, but its mode of action is mostly unknown. Klenner[6] points out, "Ascorbic acid can be lifesaving in shock. Twelve grams of the sodium salt given with a 50 cc syringe will reverse shock in minutes. In barbiturate poisoning and monoxide poisoning, the results are so dramatic that it borders on malpractice to deny this therapy." The detoxicating effect of sodium ascorbate on narcotics appears to be so rapid that this very rapidity seems to preclude a mechanism involving direct chemical attack on the narcotic molecule to convert it into some inactive derivative. Also it works on so many different types of narcotic molecules. A more compatible hypothesis would be to view the action as a competition for opiate receptor sites of the brain, wherein high levels of sodium ascorbate in the brain prevent the attachment and displace narcotic molecules already attached to these sites.

Brain Receptor Sites

The research of S. H. Snyder and coworkers on the binding of morphine-like substances to brain opiate receptor sites was recently reviewed. They have shown that the largest amount of binding occurs in cells from the very primitive limbic system deep within the brain.

They also showed that the very primitive hagfishes and sharks have as much opiate receptor-binding sites as the most advanced of the mammals, monkeys, and man. They found that the properties of these receptor sites in these early and most recent vertebrates were similar, indicating that few changes have been made during the course of about 400 million years of evolution. It is stated that, "This suggested that the opiate receptor is normally concerned with receiving some molecule that has remained the same throughout evolution . . . possibly a neurotransmitter which acts at these sites."[16] Also, the presence of high levels of sodium helps dislodge the narcotic from the receptor sites.

We speculate that these binding sites were evolved in the early vertebrates to concentrate and localize, from the very low concentrations existing in these animals, the electronically labile ascorbate molecules, which aid in neurotransmission. The fact that these sites bind narcotics is purely happenstance because of a possible similarity in molecular shape. There does not seem to be any obvious physiological evolutionary reason for concentrating narcotics in the nerve endings of this newly developing control system, whereas there may have been a great need to concentrate and obtain high levels of ascorbate at synapses to aid in efficient nerve impulse transmission. Ascorbate is a molecule that appears to have changed little in the last 400 million years and was present on the evolutionary scene long before the fishes appeared.[5] If this hypothesis is valid, then the receptor sites should be renamed "ascorbate receptors" instead of "opiate receptors." It should not be difficult to experimentally test the validity of these theoretical considerations.

■ CONCLUSION

Chronic drug addiction produces in the victims severe subclinical scurvy along with multivitamin and mineral dysfunction and protein deficiencies. The widely used methadone program for "treating" these sick people merely substitutes a legal narcotic for an illicit one, which only continues the severe biochemical stresses contributing to their illness. This pilot study regarded the addicts as suffering from a serious hypoascorbemia-kwashiorkor type of syndrome. Our procedure was designed to fully correct both the genetic defect causing the vitamin C deficiency and also the multi-malnutritional disturbances and protein deficiencies involved in the kwashiorkor. The treatment is entirely orthomolecu-

lar and inexpensive, is nontoxic, and uses no drugs or narcotics. It is rapidly effective in bringing good health to the addicts. In the 30 addicts tested in this pilot study, the results were excellent in all cases, and it would appear that this simple nontoxic procedure should serve as the basis for large-scale testing to develop a new program for freeing drug addicts of their addiction.

REFERENCES

1. Stone I. On the genetic etiology of scurvy. *Acta Genet Med Gemellol* 1966;15:345–350.

2. Stone I. Hypoascorbemia: a fresh approach to an ancient disease and some of its medical implications. *Acta Genet Med Gemellol* 1967;16:52–62.

3. Stone I. Hypoascorbemia: the genetic disease causing the human requirement for exogenous ascorbic acid. *Perspect Biol Med* 1966a;10:133–134.

4. Stone I. *The Healing Factor: Vitamin C Against Disease.* New York: Grosset & Dunlap, 1972, 157–158.

5. Stone I. The natural history of ascorbic acid in the evolution of the mammals and primates and its significance for present-day man. *J Orthomolecular Psychiatry* 1972;1(2–3):82–89.

6. Klenner FR. Significance of high daily intake of ascorbic acid in preventive medicine. *J Internat Acad Prev Med* 1974;1:45–69.

7. Cathcart RF. Vitamin C and viral disease. Talk presented at the Annual Meeting of the California Orthomolecular Medical Society, February 19, 1976, San Francisco.

8. Stone I. The genetics of scurvy and the cancer problem. *J Orthomolecular Psychiatry* 1976;5 (31):183–190.

9. Stone I. Hypoascorbemia: our most widespread disease. Bull Nat Health Fed 1972;18:(101):6–9.

10. Stone I. The CSS syndrome: a medical paradox. *Northwest Acad Prev Med* 1977;1(11):24–28.

11. Ghione R. Morphine spasm and C-hypervitaminosis. *Vitaminologia* (Turin) 1958;16:131–136.

12. Bejrablaya D, Laumjansook K. Effect of various doses of ascorbic acid upon pentobarbital. *J Med Assoc Thailand* 1976;59(4):188–189.

13. Scher J, Rice H, Suck-oo K, et al. Massive vitamin C as an adjunct in methadone maintenance and detoxification. *J Orthomolecular Psychiatry* 1976;5(3):191–198.

14. Cameron E, Baird GM. Ascorbic acid and dependence on opiates in patients with advanced disseminated cancer. *J Internat Res Communic* 1973;1(6):33.

15. Saccoman, WJ. Personal Communication, 1976.

16. Snyder SH. Opiate receptors and internal opiates. *Sci Amer* 1977;236(31):44–56.

THE USE OF ASCORBIC ACID AND MINERAL SUPPLEMENTS IN THE DETOXIFICATION OF NARCOTIC ADDICTS

by Valentine Free, MA, and Pat Sanders, RN

The process of drug withdrawal is a constant concern and fear of the addict or drug abuser. Withdrawal symptoms differ according to the individual and the drug(s) of abuse but are typically painful and anxiety producing. Methods commonly used in the past by clinicians and physicians to help alleviate drug withdrawal symptoms include a combination of symptomatic medications such as propoxyphene (Darvon), chlordiazepoxide (Librium), belladonna (Bellaphen), and chloral hydrate, methadone, codeine, and diazepam (Valium), and intensive psychotherapy. While these and other chemical combinations have long been employed as drug detoxification alternatives, many of them present harmful or uncomfortable side effects of their own. Methadone, the drug most often used in treatment programs, is a powerful addictive substance. Thus individuals working with drug addicts continue to search for more effective, safe methods to help make the withdrawal process an easier one, and to encourage a healthier lifestyle.

The San Francisco Drug Treatment Program's pilot study investigating the use of megavitamin therapy for the treatment of narcotic withdrawal began in December 1977, in response to our clients' need to find a more healthful alternative to standard chemical detoxification procedures. Megavitamin therapy using sodium ascorbate, ascorbic acid, calcium, and other mineral supplements was seen as a cost-effective, convenient, safe way to detoxify narcotic addicts and is also a way to address the poor nutritional habits of our client population.

Background and Rationale for Use of Megadoses of Ascorbic Acid

Since the discovery and synthesis of ascorbic acid in the early 1930s, a vast amount of medical research has been carried out on the physiologic effects of this substance and its possible uses as a therapeutic agent in various disease states.[1-10] In addition to being identified as vitamin C, the substance is known as ascorbic acid (and its salt sodium ascorbate). Ascorbic acid in small amounts of 10–60 milligrams (mg) is required in the human diet to prevent the end-stage deficiency state known as scurvy, but both ascorbic acid and sodium ascorbate have been shown to be of benefit in large doses (megadoses) in a great variety of pathologic conditions.[11,12] Medical research and clinical experience have yielded results that tend to support the following possible therapeutic effects of ascorbic acid: preventing heart disease by lowering blood cholesterol and preventing deterioration of arterial walls;[1] counteracting the side effects of hay fever and various allergic conditions;[13] helping relieve pain and decrease healing time in burn patients;[12,14] helping control leprosy;[15,16] combating urinary tract infections and inflammations;[1] preventing and/or ameliorating symptoms of the common cold;[2] promoting increased survival in terminal cancer patients with improvement in symptoms;[1] treating many viral diseases (especially hepatitis, mononucleosis, and viral pneumonia);[17] and enhancing the effectiveness of antibiotics in bacterial diseases.[18,19] These reports, published in respected professional journals, yield intriguing findings in view of the fact that megascorbate therapy has not been accepted by the traditional medical establishment.

These therapeutic effects have been more effectively demonstrated using doses of ascorbic acid many times in excess of the daily doses required in human nutrition to prevent scurvy. For example, in the treatment of viral hepatitis and pneumonia as much as 150,000-mg doses have been used orally and intravenously without evidence of adverse effects.[17]

From the *J Orthomolecular Psych* 1978;7(4):264–270.

The Application of Ascorbic Acid to the Detoxification of Narcotic Addicts

More pertinent to the San Francisco Drug Treatment Program pilot study is the recent study by Drs. Alfred Libby and Irwin Stone on the use of megadoses of ascorbic acid to detoxify heroin addicts.[20] They compiled dozens of case reports of heroin addicts whom they detoxified using ascorbic acid and/or sodium ascorbate in doses of 25,000–85,000 mg per day for the first few days, gradually tapering to a holding dose of approximately 10,000 mg per day. In addition, based on the theory that addicts are malnourished in general and protein deficient in particular, most of these patients were given high levels of multivitamins and minerals and a predigested protein preparation. The patients in this study almost uniformly reported a loss of craving for drugs while taking megascorbate. These patients were treated for one to two weeks in a residential setting, and then patients were discharged on holding doses of ascorbic acid for outpatient follow-up.

Possible side effects of megadoses of ascorbic acid are few. The most common and well documented is gastrointestinal distress with symptoms of heartburn, stomachache, diarrhea, and excess gas. These are generally dose dependent and are influenced by the concept of bowel tolerance, meaning that the dose that will cause gastrointestinal symptoms increases in proportion to how sick the patient is. For example, a person who might normally get diarrhea on 2,000 mg per day will be able to tolerate 50,000 mg per day or more if she or he has the flu. No long-term complications have been confirmed by researchers and clinicians who have been using megadoses of ascorbic acid in humans for up to 30 years.

Our pilot study, suggested by the research of Libby and Stone,[20] was initiated in December 1977 to examine the effects of megadoses of ascorbic acid in the outpatient detoxification of heroin addicts. Volunteers from the San Francisco Drug Treatment Program served as subjects for this study. The goals of the pilot study were to compare the effectiveness of the ascorbic acid detoxification procedure with symptomatic medications in alleviating withdrawal symptoms, and to determine the appropriateness of this detoxification approach in an outpatient setting.

Methodology

In order to more easily compare the effectiveness of the two detoxification procedures (ascorbic acid and symptomatic medications), three detoxification groups were established: 1) subjects using only the ascorbic acid procedure, 2) subjects using symptomatic relief medications, and 3) subjects using symptomatic relief medications for three days followed by the ascorbic acid procedure for the remainder of the detoxification period. At the point of intake, subjects were given the option of participating in one of the three detoxification groups and were assigned a counselor who dealt with clinical issues of concern during the patient's treatment period.

IN BRIEF

Since its inception in 1968, the San Francisco Drug Treatment Program has responded to the mental and physical health needs of narcotic addicts. The search for safer, cost-effective detoxification alternatives grew from the controversial use of methadone and propoxyphene napsylate (Darvon) and has led to an exploration of nontraditional methods of detoxification that would address the poor nutritional habits of narcotic addicts. The present pilot study investigated the use of megadoses of ascorbic acid as sodium ascorbate, multivitamins, and mineral supplements in the treatment of drug withdrawal symptoms. A total of 227 subjects were compared: 30 subjects utilizing the ascorbic detoxification procedure, 186 subjects utilizing symptomatic relief medications, and 11 clients utilizing a combination approach of ascorbic acid and symptomatic medications. The results indicate that the ascorbic acid procedure is slightly more effective than symptomatic medications in alleviating narcotic withdrawal symptoms, and that the combination approach shows the greatest reduction in symptoms. Findings indicate the suitability of this approach to an outpatient setting, pointing to its acceptance potential, success rate, and cost effectiveness.

All subjects received a routine physical examination from the medical director upon admission to the program. Following the examination, a symptom checklist was completed for each subject. The methods utilized in the daily recording of subject symptoms were subject report (subjective) and interviewer observation of symptoms (objective). All symptoms were tabulated daily for each client. Common symptoms of narcotic withdrawal, which were recorded, include runny eyes and nose, sweating, chills, muscle aches and pains, diarrhea, abdominal cramps, craving for drugs, loss of appetite, and difficulty sleeping. A client met regularly with an assigned counselor who dealt with clinical issues, such as the relationship of physical well-being to psychological health.

Subjects in all groups followed a 21-day detoxification protocol.

Group 1: Ascorbic Acid Procedure

The procedure for the group consisted of the following: sodium ascorbate or ascorbic acid, in crystalline form, dispensed in packets containing 24,000–48,000 mg every 24 hours for 5 to 7 days, tapering to 8,000–12,000 mg per day for 14 days. In addition, clients were given multivitamin and multimineral tabs (1x–3x per day) for 21 days, a calcium complex and magnesium tab (3x per day), and liquid protein (20 oz/3x per day) for 3 to 5 days. Individual dosages were dependent upon the symptom checklist report. Dosage sheets were maintained on each client.

Group 2: Symptomatic Medication Procedure

Symptomatic relief medications administered to subjects in this group consisted of the following: propoxyphene (65 mg/6x per day) for 21 days, Librium (10 mg/3x per day) for 21 days, chloral hydrate (1,000 mg per day at bedtime) for 7 days. Symptomatic medications were routinely administered in individual medication packets, and dosage levels were lowered gradually as withdrawal symptoms decreased during the 21-day detoxification period. Medication sheets were maintained on each subject depicting daily dosage levels.

Group 3: Combination Procedure

Subjects participating in this group were administered routine doses of symptomatic medications for three days. On the fourth day, subjects were given sodium ascorbate in doses determined by their number of subjective and objective withdrawal symptoms. Dosage levels were ascertained by the medical director and/or program nurse and were tapered during the remaining 18 days of the 21-day detoxification period according to subject need. These clients also received 1 multivitamin and multimineral tab (3x per day) for 21 days, and 1 calcium complex and magnesium tab (3x per day). Medication and dosage sheets were maintained for each client.

Discussion

The six-month pilot study has yielded data on 227 subjects, the total number of persons requesting detoxification services from this agency since December 1977. Of these 227 subjects, 30 clients utilized the ascorbic detoxification procedure, 186 subjects utilized symptomatic relief medications, and 11 clients utilized a combination approach of ascorbic acid and symptomatic medications. The most notable differences between groups occurred in the average age of subjects in Groups 1 and 3, which was slightly higher than that of the total program and of subjects in Group 2. On the average, those clients utilizing symptomatic medications were younger, reported larger daily habits, and had a shorter period of addiction than did subjects in either of the other groups. They remained in the detoxification phase of the program longer than the other subjects.

The majority of subjects in each group (about two-thirds) reported no prior treatment experiences (Group 1, 63 percent; Group 2, 66 percent; Group 3, 72 percent). The findings indicate a greater reduction in symptoms among ascorbic acid subjects in Groups 1 and 3, with the most dramatic reduction in subjects utilizing the combination approach (from 9 symptoms down to zero symptoms). It is interesting to note that while subjects in Group 2 reported minimal reduction in withdrawal symptoms (from 8 symptoms reduced to 6 or 7) from taking symptomatic medications, these subjects remained in detoxification treatment on the average of 17 days, compared to an average of 8 days and 10 days for Groups 1 and 3, respectively, who took the vitamins. In addition, clients in the ascorbic acid–taking Groups 1 and 3 reported the following subjective findings:

• **Increased energy:** The majority of subjects utilizing ascorbic acid reported a feeling of having increased energy while large amounts of ascorbic acid were used. Subjects reported this effect as neither positive nor negative.

• **Drug blockage:** Approximately 45 percent of those subjects utilizing ascorbic acid reported having used heroin, methadone, or some other drug while continuing with ascorbic acid doses. A majority (60 percent) reported a definite blockage effect thought to be caused by the ascorbic acid.

• **Loss of craving for drugs:** Four of the ascorbic acid subjects (10 percent) reported a loss of "craving" for drugs as a result of continued ascorbic acid ingestion. All four subjects have remained drug free since utilizing the ascorbic acid detoxification method (from two to six months). This loss of craving was not reported by Group 2, which was following the symptomatic medication procedure.

• **Side effects:** One subject reported slight nausea, which necessitated termination of this approach. One subject reported an observable rash after taking initial doses of ascorbic acid, also indicating a termination of this detoxification procedure.

Results

Although the pilot study presents only preliminary data with the usual control limitations of an outpatient detoxification setting, the results do offer some noteworthy observations concerning ascorbic acid as a narcotic detoxification alternative. The results obtained suggest that the ascorbic acid procedure is slightly more effective than symptomatic medications in alleviating narcotic withdrawal symptoms. Combined with symptomatic medications, this approach appears to offer more effective withdrawal relief and also a longer detoxification period than ascorbic acid alone. The

data presented supports the use of the ascorbic acid procedure in an outpatient setting. Subjects utilizing this approach report a greater reduction in symptoms over a shorter period of time, allowing more treatment time to be spent on clinical issues than with the detoxification phase.

CONCLUSION

The ascorbic acid procedure offers some distinct advantages to the more commonly used drug detoxification methods of symptomatic medications and methadone. Ascorbic acid and mineral supplements applied to narcotic withdrawal symptoms offers a cost-effective, nontoxic method that can easily lead into nutritional counseling and other health perspectives once the detoxification phase has been successfully completed.

Perhaps the most noteworthy observation to consider is the acceptance potential of the ascorbic acid detoxification alternative. Of the total number of subjects in the current pilot study, nearly one-fifth chose to utilize a procedure that was entirely new to them. Realizing the seriousness of a long-time drug abuser's fear of experiencing the "sick" of narcotic withdrawal, the number of subjects willing to risk trying a new detoxification alternative seems high indeed. It was apparent that as the current study continued the demand for this procedure grew, indicating an even greater number of subjects as the word spreads of this alternative and its effectiveness. Another factor that could influence patient acceptance to new alternatives is the ineffectiveness of more commonly used detoxification methods.

Patient reports of increased energy and a sense of well-being add to a greater self-esteem in newly detoxified individuals—factors that outpatient treatment can build on by encouraging the patient to deal more effectively with the home and community environments.

Further research is needed to fully explore this procedure as an effective narcotic detoxification alternative. Awareness of the necessity for monitored dosages of ascorbic acid and mineral supplements is advised, as well as a clear procedure for all experiments in an outpatient setting.

It is evident that with further more controlled research, the ascorbic acid procedure can be a healthy, cost-effective alternative for the detoxification of narcotic addicts.

REFERENCES

1. Stone I. *The Healing Factor.* New York: Grosset & Dunlap Publishers, 1972.

2. Pauling L. *Vitamin C and the Common Cold.* San Francisco, CA: W.H. Freeman & Co, 1970.

3. Ritzel G. Critical evaluation of vitamin C as a prophylactic and therapeutic agent in colds. *Heluetia Medica Acta* 1961;2:63–68.

4. Magne RV. Vitamin C in treatment of influenza. *El Dia Medico* 1963;35:1714–1715.

5. Shaffer CF. Ascorbic acid and atherosclerosis. *AJCN* 1970;23:27–30.

6. Holmes HN, Alexander W. Hayfever and vitamin C. *Science* 1942;96:497–499.

7. Holmes HN. Food allergies and vitamin C. *Annals of Allergy* 1943;1:235.

8. Schlegel et al. The role of ascorbic acid in the prevention of bladder tumor formation. *Transactions of the American Association of Genito-Urinary Surgeons* 1969;61:85–89.

9. Bartelheimer H. Vitamin C in the treatment of diabetes. *Die Medizinische Welt* 1939;13:117–120.

10. Hoffer A, Osmond H. Scurvy and schizophrenia. *Diseases of the Nervous System* 1963;24:273–285.

11. Stone I. On the genetic etiology of scurvy. *Acta Cenetiacae Medicae et Gemollogogiae* 1966;15:345–349.

12. Klasson DH. Ascorbic acid in the treatment of burns. *New York State Journal of Medicine* 1951:2388–2392.

13. Stacpoole, PW. Role of vitamin C in infectious disease and allergic reactions. *Medical Hypotheses* 1975;1(2):4345.

14. Klenner FR. Observations on the dose and administration of ascorbic acid when employed beyond the range of a vitamin in human pathology. *Journal of Applied Nutrition* 1971; 23:3–4.

15. Ferreira DL. Vitamin C in leprosy. *Publicacoes Medicas* 1950;20:25–28.

16. Floch H, Sureau P. Vitamin C therapy in leprosy. *Bulletin de la Societe de Pathologie Exotique et de Ses Filiales* 1952; 45:443–446.

17. Cathcart R. Using vitamin C to treat viral diseases. *Today's Living* 1977.

18. Gupta GC, Guha B. The effect of vitamin C and certain other substances on the growth of microorganisms. *Annals of Biochemistry and Experimental Medicine* 1941;1:14–26.

19. Sirsi M. Antimicrobial action of vitamin C on M. tuberculosis and some other pathogenic organisms. *Indian Journal of Medical Sciences* (Bombay) 1952;6:252–255.

20. Libby A, Stone I. The hypoascorbemia-kwashiorkor approach to drug addiction therapy: a pilot study. *J Orthomolecular Psych* 1977;6(4):300–308.

NIACIN FOR DETOXIFICATION: A LITTLE-KNOWN THERAPEUTIC USE
by Jonathan E. Prousky, ND

Niacin (vitamin B3) has a number of well-established clinical uses and the potential for additional clinical applications. While numerous medical conditions (arthritis, cancer, depression, cholesterol and other blood lipid problems, migraine and tension-type headaches, pellagra, and schizophrenia) potentially benefit from niacin supplementation, its therapeutic application for enhancing detoxification has not been systematically reviewed.

The use of niacin for the purpose of enhancing detoxification was popularized by L. Ron Hubbard (founder of the Church of Scientology) in 1977. He developed a comprehensive detoxification method using niacin and other treatments, which he referred to as "The Sweat Program."[1] Because this took many months to complete, Hubbard's detoxification method was refined to produce quicker results in treatment duration of about two to four weeks. The Hubbard regimen has evolved into a comprehensive treatment that removes lipid-stored xenobiotics containing illegal drugs (e.g., cocaine, heroine, and marijuana), legal drugs (e.g., aspirin and codeine), and chemicals used in the commercial, agricultural, and industrial industries. The current Hubbard regimen consists of aerobic exercise, prescribed sauna therapy, dietary modifications, vitamin and mineral supplementation, polyunsaturated oils supplementation, and niacin. The overarching mechanism of action of the Hubbard regimen is to enhance excretion by sweat or sebum (oil secretions by the skin), and to reduce problematic clinical manifestations.

Niacin is also used among individuals attempting to mask urine drug screens; presumably, a result of its favorable therapeutic effect upon liver detoxification. A simple search on Google using the terms, "niacin" and "masking urine drug testing," resulted in over 900,000 links (May 2011).

This article will focus on published studies and reports describing the use of niacin for stimulating detoxification, and on attempts to misuse niacin to mask urine drug testing.

Literature Search

A search for articles describing the uses of niacin for detoxification and masking urine drug screens was undertaken. To be included in the final review the articles had to 1) report on the use of niacin for detoxification, or for masking urine drug screens, either alone or in combination with other medicines; and 2) describe the method of administration. Twelve articles were found to meet the inclusion criteria and were included in this review.[2–13] Nine articles reported on the benefits of niacin as part of a detoxification program to eliminate fat-stored xenobiotics.[2–10] Three articles reported on the misuses of niacin to mask the results of urine drug testing.[11–13]

Use in Detoxification

The results of this review demonstrate that niacin, as a component of the Hubbard regimen, does augment detoxification by lowering the body burden of lipid-stored xenobiotics. The daily doses of niacin used during treatment were not typically reported in the summarized studies. In one study, the range used on adults was 800–6,800 milligrams (mg) per day (average being 3,285 mg per day) during treatment.[2] For a child in one of the reported studies, the dose of niacin used during treatment was 25–212 mg per day.[8] While the precise mechanism of action that niacin has upon liver detoxification has yet to be elucidated, several possibilities do exist. The initial reductions in liver-mobilized free fatty acids from taking niacin are followed by short-lived increases in the release of free fatty acids from the liver.[14,15] When niacin is combined with other therapies that facilitate extra-renal excretion (as in the Hubbard regimen), the niacin-induced release of free fatty acids might therefore liberate lipid-stored xenobiotics from the liver and allow their removal through the skin.

From the *J Orthomolecular Med* 2011;26(2):85–92.

Niacin supplementation also increases the production of nicotinamide adenine dinucleotide phosphate (NADPH), which supports both Phase 1 and Phase 2 detoxification pathways within the liver.[16] The Phase 1 pathway is composed mainly of the cytochrome P450 (CYP450) supergene family of enzymes and is by and large the first enzymatic defense against foreign compounds.[17] In Phase 1, toxins enter the enzymatic pathway to be deconstructed into smaller, more easily managed parts. NADPH serves as the main donor of reducing equivalents in xenobiotic oxidations by the CYP450 system and therefore serves a vital role in the Phase 1 pathway.[16,17] The Phase 2 pathway essentially transforms a xenobiotic into a water-soluble compound that can be excreted through the urine or bile.[17] Impaired detoxification is associated with diseases, such as Parkinson's disease, fibromyalgia, and chronic fatigue/immune dysfunction.[17] One of the advantages of the Hubbard regimen (as reported in many of the cited publications) was an improvement, and sometimes complete clearing, of chronic symptoms reflective of xenobiotic burden. The evidence therefore seems to support niacin's therapeutic role, and the other treatments of the Hubbard regimen, in normalizing or perhaps optimizing the detoxification pathways in the liver.

Outside of liver detoxification, the cutaneous skin reactions produced by niacin likely contribute to the removal of lipid-stored xenobiotics. Niacin causes vasodilation of the capillaries and cutaneous flushing by inducing the production of prostaglandin D2 (PGD2) in the skin, leading to a marked increase of its metabolite, 9[alpha], 11β-PGF2, in the plasma.[18] When niacin is administered orally in amounts of 500 mg or topically via a 6-inch patch of aqueous methylnicotinate on the forearm, PGD2 is markedly released in the skin and its metabolite appears in high amounts in the plasma.[18,19] With increased peripheral vasodilation, there would presumably be increased blood flow to the skin. When niacin is therefore combined with the other treatments in the Hubbard regimen, there would be enhanced sweating and removal of lipid-stored xenobiotics through the skin or sebum.

Misuse in Urine Drug Testing

With respect to niacin's role in masking the results of urine drug testing, the data from several published reports have not shown niacin to be capable of this. Not one individual has been able to "fool" urine drug testing by taking niacin. The only unfortunate outcome has been adverse drug reaction reports since the skin flushing and vasodilation that result from niacin require proper education and guidance prior to use. When individuals take niacin without proper instruction, they and their unknowing clinicians believe these overt reactions to be evidence of serious adverse drug reactions.

First-time users of niacin typically experience marked skin warming (a medically harmless niacin flush), which can last for 30 to 60 minutes and seem unpleasant, surprising, and even unsettling to the point that people may think they are

IN BRIEF

Niacin has a number of well-established clinical uses and the potential for additional clinical applications. To date, its therapeutic application for enhancing detoxification has not been systematically reviewed. The use of niacin for the purpose of enhancing detoxification was popularized by L. Ron Hubbard (founder of the Church of Scientology) in 1977. He developed a comprehensive detoxification method using niacin and other treatments to remove lipid-stored xenobiotics. Niacin is also used among individuals attempting to mask urine drug screens; presumably, a result of its favorable therapeutic effect upon liver detoxification. All published reports using niacin as part of a detoxification regimen are summarized in this manuscript, along with several reports of attempts to misuse niacin to mask urine drug testing. The results demonstrate that niacin, as a component of the Hubbard regimen, does augment detoxification by lowering the body burden of lipid-stored xenobiotics. With respect to niacin's role in masking the results of urine drug testing, the data from several published reports have not shown niacin to be capable of this.

having a severe allergic reaction. The take-home message here is simple: niacin cannot mask the results of urine drug testing, but it can easily lead individuals to seek emergency care for cutaneous reactions that are normally self-limiting and without serious clinical consequences.

CONCLUSION

Published reports about using niacin as part of the Hubbard regimen suggest that therapeutic doses of niacin can facilitate detoxification by reducing the burden of lipid-stored xenobiotics. Three reports have not shown niacin to be capable of masking the results of urine drug testing. Niacin might help to remove lipid-stored xenobiotics by inducing the release of free fatty acids from the liver, by supporting Phase 1 and Phase 2 detoxification pathways, and/or by cutaneous reactions and vasodilation that increase sweating. Future analysis and research into the capabilities of niacin to enhance the body's detoxification capabilities may clarify niacin's mechanism of action and encourage the further refinement of detoxification protocols.

REFERENCES

1. Hubbard LR. *Clear Body Clear Mind.* Los Angeles: Bridge Publications, 2002, 13–75.

2. Schnare DW, Denk G, Shields M, et al. Evaluation of a detoxification regimen for fat stored xenobiotics. *Med Hypotheses* 1982;9:265–282.

3. Schnare DW, Ben M, Shields M. Body burden reductions of PCBs, PBBs and chlorinated pesticides in human subjects. *AMBIO* 1984;13:378–380.

4. Schnare DW, Robinson PC. Reduction of the human body burdens of hexachlorobenzene and polychlorinated biphenyls [abstract]. *IARC Sci Publ* 1986;77:597–603.

5. Kilburn KH, Warsaw RH, Shields M. Neurobehavioral dysfunction in firemen exposed to polychlorinatedbiphenyls (PCBs): possible improvement after detoxification. *Arch Environ Health* 1989;44:345–350.

6. Tretjak Z, Shields M, Beckmann SL. PCB reduction and clinical improvement by detoxification: an unexploited approach? *Human Exper Toxicol* 1990;9:235–244.

7. Wisner RM, Shields M, Curtis DL, et al. Human contamination and detoxification: medical response to an expanding global problem. *Environ Physician* 1992;Spring:6,8,10.

8. Wisner RM, Shields M, Beckmann SL. Treatment of children with the detoxification method developed by Hubbard. Proceedings of the American Public Health Association: National Conference. San Diego, CA. 1995.

9. Tsyb AF, Parshkov EM, Barnes J, et al. Rehabilitation of a Chernobyl affected population using a detoxification method. Proceedings of the 1998 International Radiological Post-Emergency Response Issues Conference. Washington, DC, 1998.

10. Cecchini MA, Root DE, Rachunow JR, et al. Chemical exposures at the world trade center: use of the Hubbard sauna detoxification regimen to improve the health status of New York City rescue workers exposed to toxicants. *Townsend Lett Doctors Doctors Patients* 2006;273:58–65.

11. Paopairochanakorn C, White S, Baltarowich L. Hepatotoxicity in acute sustained-release niacin overdose [abstract]. *J Toxicol Clin Toxicol* 2001;39:516.

12. No author. Use of niacin in attempts to defeat urine drug testing–five states, Jan–Sept 2006. *Morb Mortal Wkly Rep* 2007;56:365–366.

13. Mittal MK, Florin T, Perrone J, et al. Toxicity from the use of niacin to beat urine drug screening. *Ann Emerg Med* 2007;50:587–590.

14. Carlson LA, Orö L, Ostman J. Effect of a single dose of nicotinic acid on plasma lipids in patients with hyperlipoproteinemia. *Acta Med Scand* 1968;183:457–465.

15. Nye ER, Buchanon B. Short-term effect of nicotinic acid on plasma level and turnover of free fatty acids in sheep and man. *J Lipid Research* 1969;10:193–196.

16. Sies H, Brigelius R, Wefers H, et al. Cellular redox changes and response to drugs and toxic agents. *Fundam Appl Toxicol* 1983;3:200–208.

17. Liska DJ. The detoxification enzyme systems. *Altern Med Rev* 1998;3:187–198.

18. Morrow JD, Parsons WG, Roberts LJ. Release of markedly increased quantities of prostaglandin D2 in vivo in humans following the administration of nicotinic acid. *Prostaglandins* 1989;38:263–274.

19. Morrow JD, Awad JA, Oates JA, et al. Identification of skin as a major site of prostaglandin D2 release following oral administration of niacin in humans. *J Invest Dermatol* 1992;98:812–815.

EYE DISEASES

THE EYE IS A DELICATE sensory organ exposed daily to bright light and environmental toxins. Light and toxins such as chemicals and smoke generate free radicals that cause damage in eye tissues. Therefore the eye is susceptible to degenerative diseases related to oxidative stress and aging.

In macular degeneration, oxidized products of metabolism gradually build up in a layer underneath the retina, eventually causing retinal detachment and blindness. In glaucoma, the intraocular pressure builds up due to oxidative stress, causing retinal axons entering the optic nerve to progressively die. In retinitis pigmentosa, rods die from a genetic abnormality and cones progressively die due to oxidative stress. In diabetic retinopathy, high blood sugar causes progressive damage to the retina.

High levels of antioxidants such as vitamins C and E in the body are associated with a lower incidence of these diseases, and oral administration of these and other antioxidants reduces oxidative stress and the disease risk. Success is dependent on a sufficient level of supplements taken over a sufficient duration of time. There is abundant evidence that many eye diseases can be effectively slowed or prevented using supplements of antioxidants and other essential nutrients at high enough doses.

— ROBERT G. SMITH, *JOM* 2010

TERMS OF EYE DISEASE

AQUEOUS HUMOR. The clear fluid inside the eye in front of the lens; poor outflow of aqueous humor may elevate pressure and damage the optic nerve at the back of the eye.

CATARACTS. A clouding of the lens inside the eye that gradually restricts vision.

GANGLION CELLS. Cells located in the retina that transmit signals representing different aspects of vision (contrast, color, motion) through the optic nerve to the brain.

GLAUCOMA. A progressive eye disease in which increased pressure in the eye causes nerve cells in the retina to die.

INTRAOCULAR. Inside the eye.

MACULA. Visual center of the retina that is required for reading and is primarily composed of cells that sense color (cone photoreceptors).

MACULAR DEGENERATION. A progressive eye disease in which photoreceptors near the center of the retina slowly die.

MITOCHONDRIA. Parts of cells where the energy molecule (ATP; adenosine triphosphate) is produced.

PHOTORECEPTORS. Light-sensing cells in the retina that convert photons of light into chemical and electrical signals.

RETINAL PIGMENT EPITHELIUM (RPE). A layer of cells attached to the retina, which is continually active in the nourishment and maintenance of the photoreceptors.

RETINITIS PIGMENTOSA. A group of night-blindness diseases related to age-related macular degeneration in which rod photoreceptors die, usually due in part to a genetic abnormality but with a nutritional component; this is often followed by the gradual death of cone photoreceptors and subsequently blindness.

VITREOUS HUMOR. Also known as vitreous jelly or vitreous body; the gel-like transparent liquid behind the lens that fills most of the eye.

NUTRITION AND EYE DISEASES
by Robert G. Smith, PhD

The eye is one of the most wondrous organs in the body because of its function, sight, but also because of its structure.[1] It is a sphere that maintains its shape with a higher pressure inside than outside. At the front of the eye, a clear protective coating called the cornea, nourished and lubricated by tears and a fluid inside the eye called the aqueous humor, allows our eyelids to quickly slide up and down. Behind the cornea and aqueous humor sits the iris, which can open and close its pupil like a camera lens diaphragm. Just behind the iris sits the lens, which is a transparent tissue analogous to a camera lens comprising cells containing a clear crystalline protein. Behind the lens, filling most of the eye, is a gel-like transparent liquid called the vitreous humor. Near the back of the eye, attached to the inner lining of the eyeball, sits the retina. The neurons in the retina convert the light into electrical impulses, which are carried by the axons of ganglion cells across the surface of the retina to the optic disc, where they exit the eyeball and become the optic nerve that carries visual impulses to the brain. The retina is attached to the pigment epithelium (RPE), a layer of cells that are continually active in the nourishment of the photoreceptors. At the back of the eye, behind the pigment epithelium sits the choroid, a plexus of blood vessels nourishing the pigment epithelium and retina.

Antioxidants

A variety of mechanisms cause damage to the biological machinery of life, and the eye is particularly susceptible because it is right at the surface of the body and is delicate. Although oxygen is necessary to efficiently metabolize food and provide energy, it also can cause damage when an oxygen molecule binds to biochemicals in a way that damages them, called oxidative stress. This can result in molecules with a free unbound and energized electron, known as free radicals, which are highly reactive.[2] Free radicals can bind to any of a cell's biochemicals, damaging them. Such oxidative stress can also be caused by bacterial or viral infec-

tions, toxins, physical damage (bruises), or free radicals generated by light. The body's main defense against such oxidative stress is antioxidants such as vitamin C, vitamin E, and glutathione.[3] Vitamin C is transported into cells where it helps to maintain a reducing environment in the cytoplasm (a gel-like substance surrounding a cell's nucleus). Vitamin C in the cytoplasm and nucleus can prevent free radicals floating among the biochemicals there from damaging the intricate metabolic pathways and its deoxyribonucleic acid (DNA). It can also regenerate other antioxidants such as vitamin E and glutathione. Vitamin E sitting in the lipid bilayer of the cell's membrane can prevent oxidation of its fatty acids and proteins. Thus, antioxidants are essential to prevent mutations in a cell's DNA and to keep our cells functioning normally, so they are crucial for life and health.[2] Vitamin C is also important beyond its role as an antioxidant, for it is necessary in the synthesis of collagen, a crucial component of the body's organs and vasculature. Further, some evidence suggests that vitamin E acts as a cell-signaling modulator to reduce damage in addition to its known antioxidant properties.[4,5]

Effects of Light on the Eye

The eye is the only part of the body besides the skin that is exposed to ultraviolet (UV) and blue light for long periods. Light rays that pass into the eye are damaging because the photons when absorbed can create free radicals that damage the essential proteins and DNA throughout the eye.[6] Although the cornea, lens, and retina are transparent, they all absorb a small amount of the light and thus are susceptible to damage over many years of exposure. This, of course, is one good reason to wear dark glasses and broad-brimmed hats outside. By reducing the high-energy light, especially UV and blue, you can greatly reduce your eyes'

From the *J Orthomolecular Med* 2010;25(2):67–76.

exposure to oxidative damage from light. Most of the UV light is absorbed in the cornea and lens,[6] but much of the blue light passes on to the retina, which has one of the highest metabolic rates of any tissue in the body. Because the retina contains a lot of polyunsaturated lipids and has a higher concentration of oxygen than most other tissues, it has one of the highest risks of oxidative damage.[7,8]

Mitochondria in the axons of retinal ganglion cells, necessary for the high metabolic rate, contain cytochromes (biochemicals) that can absorb light and generate free radicals, damaging the cell's metabolism and ability to recover from further oxidative stress.[2,7,9] The iris helps to prevent the light damage. Its pupil, the central open area that passes light, is controlled by the brain according to the light intensity outside (and our mood), and its pigment absorbs light. The pigment, a melanin molecule similar to the pigment in skin, is a dark brown color; people with blue eyes are at greater risk of damage because the blue color represents a lack of the light-absorbing pigment.

The eye can recover and regenerate to some extent from the chemical reactions caused by light. Photoreceptor pigment (opsin) is located in flat discs located in the outer segments of the photoreceptors at the back of the retina. Each opsin molecule contains retinal, a submolecule that is chemically modified (bleached) when it absorbs a photon, and must be regenerated. The bleached retinal is released by the opsin, and transported into the RPE cells, which regenerate it and transport it back to the photoreceptors. In addition, the photoreceptors slough off their oldest discs to allow them to be renewed. In a process called phagocytosis, the old discs at the photoreceptor tip are digested by the RPE.[10] New discs containing a fresh array of pigment molecules and enzymes are generated at the base of the photoreceptor's outer segment and move progressively outward. Interestingly, whenever we go out into sunlight, virtually all the pigment in our rod photoreceptors is bleached in a few seconds and must be regenerated before we can see again in the dark.[1] The pigment is regenerated using vitamin A (retinyl or carotene), which we must obtain from our food. This is the normal process of vision, and the eye is normally able to keep this up over our whole lifetime, as long as we keep eating enough carrots and dark green leafy vegetables.

But over years of exposure to sunlight, cells in the cornea, lens, and retina are damaged by photon absorption in other molecules besides the photoreceptor pigment. The energy in a blue or UV photon is great enough to break chemical bonds between atoms, and, thus, when a photon is absorbed, it can generate a free radical ready to attack any molecule nearby. After many decades spent outside in bright sunlight, the oxidative damage can build up and cause the cells to be dysfunctional or die.

Antioxidants and the Eye

Oxidative stress can overwhelm the eye's antioxidant defenses, and many lines of evidence suggest that oxidative stress such as light exposure is a major factor in age-related eye diseases.[6,7] Early studies showed that aging eyes derived a prompt (within two weeks) benefit in vision from 600 milligrams (mg) of supplemental vitamin C. The benefit was thought to be in the retina, optic nerve, and their vasculature[11] and was shown even for patients who did not have an acute vitamin C deficiency. The eye concentrates vitamin C by a factor of 25 over its level in the blood, which is thought to help the eye prevent damage caused by light.[12] The eye is also susceptible to other types of oxidative damage such as free radicals in the bloodstream caused by environmental toxins like smoke and pesticides. Smokers have lower vitamin C levels in the bloodstream and also in the eye, so they are at risk for eye diseases. Obesity is also a risk factor for eye disease, possibly due to increased oxidation of lipids (fats) and lower production of antioxidant compounds such as glutathione.[13] The carotenoids lutein and zeaxanthin, the principal phytochemicals in green leafy vegetables, are the primary constituents of the macular filter that removes blue light from traversing the retina. These are antioxidants and are thought to lessen oxidative stress in the macula, the central part of the retina. A diet supplemented with lutein and zeaxanthin is associated with lower risk for eye disease.[13] Vitamin E is known to be helpful in preventing oxidative stress to photoreceptors in vitro[14] and can lower intraocular pressure. Further, vitamin E and other antioxidants such as glutathione have synergistic effects.[15] These lines of evidence may all be related because vitamin C can regenerate vitamin E and other antioxidants to their reducing form. Recent evidence suggests that natural antioxidants concentrated in mitochondria are essential for preventing oxidative damage.[16] New antioxidants designed with properties that target mitochondria have been found to prevent damage in RPE cells, extend the life of mice, and prevent oxidative eye damage in dogs, cats, and horses.[8,17] Thus, abundant evidence suggests that antioxidants are important in preventing damage from free radicals in the eye.

Retinal Detachment

In a normal eye, the retina is only weakly attached to the pigment epithelium and can be easily separated by physical damage such as a blow to the eye or inflammation. In diseased retinas such as wet age-related macular degeneration or diabetic retinopathy (described below), the attachment is weakened so retinal detachment is more common. When this occurs, fluid may accumulate beneath the retina, progressively detaching a larger area from the pigment epithelium. Wherever the retina is detached for more than a few hours from the pigment epithelium, the photoreceptors start to degenerate, and, after a few days of detachment, the photoreceptors will start to die.[18] Once such damage has occurred, the remainder of the retinal neurons do not receive normal responses and will eventually degenerate and die as well. Thus, acute retinal detachment is a medical emergency, where quick treatment is very important to preserve sight. An ophthalmologist can save the retina by pulsing a laser to cause small spots of scar tissue in the retina and pigment epithelium that holds the retina in place at the back of the eye. Although good nutrition is important in recovering from a detached retina, taking adequate amounts of antioxidants throughout our lives is crucial to prevent the build-up of oxidative stress-induced damage that can cause retinal detachment.

Macular Degeneration

Macular degeneration is a progressive disease of the retina where photoreceptors slowly die near the center of the eye.[19] Age-related macular degeneration (AMD) is the leading cause of blindness in people ages 50 years or more worldwide.[20] In the "dry" form of AMD, cellular waste deposits called drusen and lipofuscin build up between retinal photoreceptors and the choroid. How or why these deposits build up is unknown. They are thought to be waste deposits caused by oxidative damage to the retina and pigment epithelium. In the "wet" form of AMD, new blood vessels grow from the choroid at the back of the eye, pushing the retina away from the choroid, tending to cause retinal detachment. Although a large risk factor for AMD is genetic, both forms are thought to be initiated by oxidative damage, consistent with a typical onset after age 50.

The single most important environmental risk factor for developing AMD is smoking, which causes oxidative damage in many tissues of the eye.[19,20] Several toxic chemicals present in smoke are known to induce cell death in the retinal pigment epithelium.[21] Other important risk factors are exposure to bright sunlight and inflammation.[19] Cumulative exposure to light is associated with AMD in people with low antioxidant levels.[22] Conversely, a diet with a low glycemic index, high in omega-3 fatty acids and antioxidants (vitamins C, E, zinc, and lutein/zeaxanthin), is associated with the lowest risk of drusen and advanced AMD.[23–27] The protective effect is thought to be greater when the antioxidants and other beneficial nutrients are taken at a sufficient level for a decade or more. Antioxidants can prevent oxidative stress-induced damage to arteries in the retina and choroid, which helps to prevent wet AMD. This benefit is thought to come from reducing free radicals.[28] A relatively low level of vitamin E, an average of 300 international units (IU) per day, produced a small reduction in the risk for AMD, but a greater effect was shown for those who also took multivitamins.[29] The levels of supplements necessary to achieve an optimal reduction in AMD are easy to get but are not contained in most multivitamin tablets.[30] The level of vitamins C and E in most eye studies has not been high by orthomolecular standards. For example, a vitamin C level of 500 mg per day or lower and a vitamin E level of 200–400 IU per day (the amounts typically used in studies) are considered low to minimal, and higher levels of these nontoxic antioxidants are very likely beneficial in the long term.

Night Blindness

A variety of problems with the eye can cause difficulty seeing at night. A reduction of contrast sensitivity from cataracts can cause low vision at night because glare from bright lights can obscure low-contrast details. Night-blindness from a lack of vitamin A to regenerate the rhodopsin pigment in the rod photoreceptors can be prevented with an adequate intake of vitamin A or carotene. Deterioration at the back of the eye generates waste products from oxidation of fatty acids (lipofuscin and drusen) that can cause night blindness symptoms and AMD. In some cases this has been cleared by application of polyphenols (plant-based antioxidants) that remove metal ions.[31] Many genetic diseases can cause rod photoreceptors or other retinal neurons to die or malfunction, causing night blindness. A common type of night blindness is caused by retinitis pigmentosa.

Retinitis Pigmentosa

Retinitis pigmentosa (RP) is a group of night blindness diseases related to AMD in which rod photoreceptors die, usually due to a genetic abnormality.[32] In a common form of RP, the cone photoreceptors survive but then progressively die, resulting in gradual blindness. This gradual cone death is thought to originate in part from oxidative stress due to free radicals generated by light, possibly through an effect on vasculature. The stress is thought to spread through oxidative damage to lipids.[33] Compared to rods the cones are scarcer and therefore use less oxygen. After the rods die in RP, the cones still receive the same amount of oxygenation from the choroidal blood vessels, so they are subject to increased oxidative stress. Antioxidants and omega-3 fatty acids can slow or prevent

this damage. Vitamin C reduces oxidative stress in photoreceptors due to bright light, but only when taken before the light exposure, implying that it directly prevents free radical formation by light.[34] In a mouse model of RP, a supplement of vitamins C, E, and other antioxidants reduced cone cell death.[35] Genetic manipulation of a RP model that increased expression of natural antioxidants in cones also prevents cone cell death.[36] Further, people with a genetic abnormality that prevents vitamin E uptake are prone to RP,[5,37] supporting the oxidative stress hypothesis. Painkiller drugs that affect mitochondrial function are thought to cause oxidative stress and this may contribute to RP and other ocular diseases.[38] Depending on which genes are affected, vitamin A, necessary for vision, can delay loss of cone function in RP to preserve sight.[32,39]

Glaucoma

Glaucoma, a leading cause of blindness worldwide, is a progressive disease of the eye in which the nerve cells that send visual signals to the brain degenerate and gradually die. By the time this is noticed, it is usually too late to preserve sight. It is usually associated with high pressure inside the eyeball, which pinches the axons of the ganglion cells where they exit the eyeball. The pressure in the eye is created by fluid pumped into the eye from the bloodstream. The fluid pressure is drained by small canals around the edge of the iris. When the trabecular meshwork covering the canals gets blocked, the intraocular pressure increases and the optic nerves become damaged. Normal-tension glaucoma causes a similar type of damage to the optic nerve but is not associated with high pressure in the eyeball. It is thought to be caused by unusually fragile axons in the optic nerve, or restricted blood flow in the optic nerve.

In all types of glaucoma, damage to their axons causes the ganglion cells on the surface of the retina to progressively degenerate. Oxidative stress is thought to be a common component in the degeneration of ganglion cells in glaucoma.[7] Oxidative stress has been shown in the axons of animal models of glaucoma, and free radical scavengers can prevent retinal ganglion cell death.[40,41] The damage to the axons may be worsened when microcirculation of blood flow within the optic nerve is disrupted.[42] The ganglion cells are thought to die at different times during the disease because they receive differing secondary insults, including oxidative stress from light.[9]

The canals that normally regulate the intraocular pressure can be blocked by debris from degenerating eye tissue, especially the neurons of the retina, the iris, and lens due to oxidative damage from light absorption. The debris is carried to the canals where it can clog them and allow the pressure to build. The trabecular meshwork is also directly affected in glaucoma from oxidative stress, which damages the meshwork cells and their DNA.[40,43] This can be countered very effectively with antioxidants such as vitamins C and E, lutein, and glutathione.

The standard treatment for glaucoma is to lower the intraocular pressure. High levels of vitamin C (2,000–10,000 mg per day or higher) are very effective at reducing intraocular pressure, through its osmotic effect, and likely other mechanisms such as reducing lipid oxidation and increasing outflow through the trabecular mesh and canals that drain the eye.[44,45] In normal-tension glaucoma, supplemental magnesium may allow the blood vessels supplying the optic nerve to relax, increasing its blood supply. Increasing the neural energy supply is currently hypothesized to increase ganglion cell survival. One way to achieve this is with antioxidants that scavenge free radicals generated by light and oxidative stress.[41] To preserve ganglion cells under oxidative stress, oral supplements to enhance mitochondrial function such as lipoic acid, niacinamide (vitamin B3), and creatinine may prove useful.[42] In glaucoma, levels of vitamin C and other antioxidants such as glutathione are lower inside the eye, suggesting that they are protective against damage.[46] Although glaucoma is not considered to be a vitamin deficiency disease, vitamin E is known be an important regulator of the oxidative damage that causes glaucoma.[15] Vitamin E can delay the onset of glaucoma symptoms in retinal blood vessels.[5]

Diabetic Retinopathy

Diabetes is produced by an inability to utilize blood sugar (glucose), which causes damage to tissues throughout the body. Insulin secreted by the pancreas causes cells of most tissues to take up glucose from the bloodstream. Because the retina does not respond to insulin, it is particularly susceptible to diabetes and to damage caused by high blood sugar. Several nutrients, including alpha-lipoic acid, vitamins C and E, and magnesium and zinc, are thought to increase uptake of blood sugar and reduce blood pressure and are known to be helpful in preventing retinopathy.[47]

Cataracts

Cataracts are another leading cause of vision loss very common past age 60. During most of our life, the lens tissue can actively repair itself to keep the lens proteins intact. But with old age and damage due to oxidation from absorbing UV rays and ionizing radiation (the kind that has traditionally been considered most worrisome), the lens tissue cannot maintain itself in good condition,[6] and its crystalline protein becomes cloudy and absorbed water causes it to swell. Airline pilots have a higher rate of cataracts, thought to be caused by their exposure to radiation from outer space.[48] Although currently there is no treatment to cure cataracts, their onset can be delayed or prevented by antioxidants in the diet. The blood level of vitamin E is lower in patients with cataracts, suggesting the use of supplements to prevent cataract occurrence.[5,49,50] A combined supplement of vitamins C, E, and other antioxidants such as selenium and alpha-lipoic acid is helpful in reducing the occurrence of cataracts,[13,45,51] and this is thought to remove free radicals and enhance the activity of glutathione in the eye. Vitamin supplements are associated with reduced risk of cataracts if taken for 10 years or more.[45,52]

Need for Sufficient Doses

What are we to make of these tantalizing results and tentative conclusions? From test tube and animal studies, it is clear that to effectively neutralize free radicals the level of antioxidants must be sufficiently high. Indeed, large human studies using relatively low levels of supplemental nutrients have sometimes found little effect. For example, some randomized controlled trials (RCTs), widely considered to be the gold standard for testing the benefit of supplements, have not shown statistically significant health benefits for antioxidants. But when a benefit of supplements from an observational study on a specific at-risk group is backed up by a likely mechanism such as preventing oxidative stress, a negative result in a RCT cannot trump the positive result in the observational study.[53] The reason is that RCTs can be confounded by bias factors such as the complexities of diet and daily habits like smoking and related physiological and disease states. For example, some participants who take supplements are at risk because they have early indications of disease. Alternately, participants who take supplements may be health-conscious individuals without indications of disease. Both of these possibilities will introduce bias in a study about the benefits of supplements, which can confound the conclusion of the study.[53]

Thus, it seems likely that the equivocal results from some RCTs testing the benefits of antioxidants for prevention of eye disease are a consequence of the relatively low doses of supplements involved. For example, the amount of vitamin C typically taken in RCTs (often 500 mg or less) would not be expected to show a large effect.[3] The effects of low supplement levels on eye diseases are likely to be confounded by differences in diet correlated with other risk factors.[54] Further, many RCTs testing the effect of antioxidants on eye diseases have collected only short-term data (less than a few months) on antioxidant intake. Because oxidative damage in the eye is age-related, antioxidants are more likely to be beneficial when taken at relatively high doses over several decades.

Orthomolecular Doses

Although the minimum Recommended Dietary Allowance (RDA) for nutrients prevents the symptoms of acute deficiency, taking additional amounts of nutrients (i.e., orthomolecular doses) allows the body's metabolic reactions to proceed more fully, providing a greater health benefit.[55] An individual's need for nutrients such as vitamins C and E differs depending on his or her unique genetics, biochemistry, diet, and level of stress and disease.[3,51,56] Vitamin C cannot be synthesized by humans, primates, and guinea pigs, but most other animal species make 10,000–20,000 mg per day (relative to human body weight), and they make more when they are stressed physically or by disease. Typically, vitamin C is titrated to bowel tolerance, which for a healthy individual is an oral dose of 10,000–20,000 mg per day. However, when disease or oxidative stress affects the body, the gut absorbs more vitamin C according to the body's need, and then the individual's bowel tolerance can be tenfold greater.[3] Vitamin E to prevent oxidative stress and disease has been shown to be safe and effective at high doses (800–3,200 IU per day) for most people.[57] For these "megadoses," the benefit in reducing oxidative stress is likely to be more obvious. When taken in combination, a cocktail of nutrients including antioxidants dosed according to the individual's need will likely multiply the beneficial effects.

Common Benefit

Current knowledge about the risk of oxidative stress for eye diseases suggests the use of nutrient supplements because of the extensive literature over the past 70 years showing large benefits. Yet, because the necessary random controlled trials to test the optimal combinations and levels of supplements in eye disease have not been performed, the proper rationale depends on one's outlook; should one simply heed the standard conservative advice to wait until more is known before taking supplements?[53] From the evidence, it is apparent that many eye diseases have a common root in age-related oxidative stress, and that a common set of antioxidant supplements is likely to be helpful. What combinations and doses of supplements are optimal? The field of nutrition and age-related oxidative stress is moving quickly, and, as more trials of dietary and supplemental nutrients are published, we will surely learn much more about which combination is best. However, because the efficacy and safety of vitamins and nutrients is well known,[3,55] the rationale for picking the combination of nutrients seems clear. Individuals should take generous doses of those vitamins and nutrients known to be nontoxic, and a helpful guide is the orthomolecular literature.[55] Those with special conditions or needs should consult a nutrition-aware medical professional for precautions and to determine doses. Antioxidants are known to be synergistic, and it seems likely that a combination that maximally protects against age-related cataracts, for example, may also be effective in protecting against retinitis pigmentosa, macular degeneration, diabetic retinopathy, and glaucoma.

CONCLUSION

A combination of nutrients is most effective. A multitude of evidence shows that supplemental antioxidants and nutrients are effective at preventing eye disease, and when taken in combination is more effective than one or two taken alone. Thus, vitamins C and E, carotenoids (lutein/zeaxanthin), zinc, selenium, magnesium, and omega-3 fatty acids, when taken at the proper levels in combination with a well-balanced diet containing lots of fruits and vegetables over a decade or more, can do much to prevent oxidative damage to the eye and prevent or delay the onset of typical age-related eye diseases.[24,45,47] Zinc is found in relatively high concentrations in the retina and is necessary for several enzyme systems to preserve health.[24] Selenium in the proper amount is an important antioxidant and can help to prevent macular degeneration. Supplemental magnesium can correct a very common deficiency and helps to reduce blood pressure, maintain health of arteries, and prevent retinopathy. The carotenoids are helpful in preventing light from reaching the macular photoreceptors and are antioxidants that help to prevent oxidation caused by light. Vitamin E is helpful in reducing oxidation of fatty acids in cell membranes, which is very important for reducing damage to the retina and its photoreceptors. Vitamin C is helpful to prevent permeability and fragility of capillaries, and to neutralize free radicals, and it helps the body to regenerate vitamin E.

It is also helpful in reducing oxidation in all the tissues of the eye, and in reducing ocular pressure to prevent glaucoma. The omega-3 fatty acid docosahexaenoic acid (DHA) is concentrated in the retina; eicosapentaenoic acid (EPA) is used to make DHA. Low levels of DHA lead to degradation of the retina and loss of vision, and low levels may also contribute to diabetic retinopathy and macular degeneration.

Although proper nutrition is not a panacea, when taken together in a medically supervised program, these nutrients can do much to prevent diseases of the eye (and in the rest of the body). They are most effective taken at a sufficient level starting early in life.

REFERENCES

1. Rodieck RW. *The First Steps in Seeing.* Sunderland, MA: Sinauer, 1998.

2. Finkel T, Holbrook NJ. Oxidants, oxidative stress and the biology of ageing. *Nature* 2000; 408:239–247.

3. Hickey S, Saul, AW. *Vitamin C: The Real Story–The Remarkable and Controversial Healing Factor.* Laguna Beach, CA: Basic Health Publications, 2008, 91–102.

4. Azzi A. Molecular mechanism of alpha-tocopherol action. *Free Radic Biol Med* 2007;43:16–21.

5. Engin KN. Alpha-tocopherol: looking beyond an antioxidant. *Mol Vis* 2009;15:855–60.

6. Young RW. The family of sunlight-related eye diseases. *Optom Vis Sci* 1994;71:125–144.

7. Tezel G. Oxidative stress in glaucomatous neurodegeneration: mechanisms and consequences. *Prog Retin Eye Res* 2006;25: 490–513.

8. Skulachev VP, Anisimov VN, Antonenko YN, et al. An attempt to prevent senescence: a mitochondrial approach. *Biochim Biophys Acta* 2009;1787:437–461.

9. Osborne NN, Li GY, Ji D, et al. Light affects mitochondria to cause apoptosis to cultured cells: possible relevance to ganglion cell death in certain optic neuropathies. *J Neurochem* 2008; 105:2013–2028.

10. Young RW. The renewal of rod and cone outer segments in the rhesus monkey. *J Cell Biol* 1971;49:303–318.

11. Bouton SM Jr. Vitamin C and the aging eye: an experimental clinical study. *Arch Intern Med* 1939;63:930–945.

12. Gross RL. Collagen type I and III synthesis by Tenon's capsule fibroblasts in culture: individual patient characteristics and response to mitomycin C, 5-fluorouracil, and ascorbic acid. *Trans Am Ophthalmol Soc* 1999;97:513–543.

13. Rhone M, Basu A. Phytochemicals and age-related eye diseases. *Nutr Rev* 2008;66:465–472.

14. Terrasa AM, Guajardo MH, Marra CA, et al. Alpha-tocopherol protects against oxidative damage to lipids of the rod outer segments of the equine retina. *Vet J* 2009;182:463–468.

15. Veach J. Functional dichotomy: glutathione and vitamin E in homeostasis relevant to primary open-angle glaucoma. *Br J Nutr* 2004;91:809–829.

16. Skulachev VP. New data on biochemical mechanism of programmed senescence of organisms and antioxidant defense of mitochondria. *Biochemistry* (Mosc) 2009;74:1400–1403.

17. Jin HX, Randazzo J, Zhang P, et al. Multifunctional antioxidants for the treatment of age-related diseases. *J Med Chem* 2010;53:1117–1127.

18. Abouzeid H, Wolfensberger TJ. Macular recovery after retinal detachment. *Acta Ophthalmol Scand* 2006;84:597–605.

19. de Jong PT. Age-related macular degeneration. *N Engl J Med* 2006;355:1474–1485.

20. Bertram KM, Baglole CJ, Phipps RP, et al. Molecular regulation of cigarette smoke induced-oxidative stress in human retinal pigment epithelial cells: implications for age-related macular degeneration. *Am J Physiol Cell Physiol* 2009;297:C1200–1210.

21. Tan JS, Mitchell P, Kifley A, et al. Smoking and the long-term incidence of age-related macular degeneration: the Blue Mountains Eye Study. *Arch Ophthalmol* 2007;125:1089–1095.

22. Fletcher AE, Bentham GC, Agnew M, et al. Sunlight exposure, antioxidants, and age-related macular degeneration. *Arch Ophthalmol* 2008;126:1396–1403.

23. Age-Related Eye Disease Study Research Group. A randomized, placebo-controlled, clinical trial of high-dose supplementation with vitamins C and E, beta carotene, and zinc for age-related macular degeneration and vision loss: AREDS report no. 8. *Arch Ophthalmol* 2001;119:1417–1436.

24. Head KA. Natural therapies for ocular sisorders (part I): diseases of the retina. *Altern Med Rev* 1999;4:342–359.

25. van Leeuwen R, Boekhoorn S, Vingerling JR, et al. Dietary intake of antioxidants and risk of age-related macular degeneration. *JAMA* 2005;294:3101–3107.

26. Chiu CJ, Milton RC, Klein R, et al. Dietary compound score and risk of age-related macular degeneration in the age-related eye disease study. *Ophthalmology* 2009;116:939–946.

27. Tan JS, Wang JJ, Flood V, et al. Dietary antioxidants and the long-term incidence of age-related macular degeneration: the Blue Mountains Eye Study. *Ophthalmology* 2008;115:334–341.

28. Pemp B, Polska E, Karl K, et al. Effects of antioxidants (AREDS medication) on ocular blood flow and endothelial function in an endotoxin-induced model of oxidative stress in humans. *Invest Ophthalmol Vis Sci* 2010;51:2–6.

29. Christen WG, Glynn RJ, Chew EY, et al. Vitamin E and age-related macular degeneration in a randomized trial of women. *Ophthalmology* 2010;117(6):1163–1168.

30. Raniga A, Elder MJ. Dietary supplement use in the prevention of age-related macular degeneration progression. *NZ Med J* 2009;122:32–38.

31. Richer S, Stiles W, Thomas C. Molecular medicine in ophthalmic care. *Optometry* 2009;80:695–701.

32. Hamel C. Retinitis pigmentosa. *Orphanet J Rare Dis* 2006;1:40.

33. Tanito M, Kaidzu S, Anderson RE. Delayed loss of cone and remaining rod photoreceptor cells due to impairment of choroidal circulation after acute light exposure in rats. *Invest Ophthalmol Vis Sci* 2007;48:1864–1872.

34. Organisciak DT, Wang HM, Li ZY, et al. The protective effect of ascorbate in retinal light damage of rats. *Invest Ophthalmol Vis Sci* 1985;26:1580–1588.

35. Komeima K, Rogers BS, Lu L, et al. Antioxidants reduce cone cell death in a model of retinitis pigmentosa. *Proc Nat Acad Sci USA* 2006;103:11300–11305.

36. Usui S, Komeima K, Lee SY, et al. Increased expression of catalase and superoxide dismutase 2 reduces cone cell death in retinitis pigmentosa. *Mol Ther* 2009;17:778–786.

37. Kono S, Otsuji A, Hattori H, et al. Ataxia with vitamin E deficiency with a mutation in a phospholipid transfer protein gene. *J Neurol* 2009;256:1180–1181.

38. Neustadt J, Pieczenik SR. Medication-induced mitochondrial damage and disease. *Mol Nutr Food Res* 2008;52:780–788.

39. Berson EL. Long-term visual prognoses in patients with retinitis pigmentosa: the Ludwig von Sallmann lecture. *Exp Eye Res* 2008; 85:7–14.

40. Izzotti A, Bagnis A, Saccà SC. The role of oxidative stress in glaucoma. *Mutat Res* 2006; 612:105–114.

41. Schober MS, Chidlow G, Wood JP, et al. Bioenergetic-based neuroprotection and glaucoma. *Clin Experiment Ophthalmol* 2008;36:377–385.

42. Osborne NN. Pathogenesis of ganglion "cell death" in glaucoma and neuroprotection: focus on ganglion cell axonal mitochondria. *Prog Brain Res* 2008;173:339–352.

43. Saccà SC, Izzotti A. Oxidative stress and glaucoma: injury in the anterior segment of the eye. *Prog Brain Res* 2008;173: 385–407.

44. Linnér E. The pressure lowering effect of ascorbic acid in ocular hypertension. *Acta Ophthalmol* (Copenhagen) 1969;47: 685–689.

45. Head KA. Natural therapies for ocular disorders (part II): cataracts and glaucoma. *Altern Med Rev* 2001;6:141–166.

46. Ferreira SM, Lerner SF, Brunzini R, et al. Antioxidant status in the aqueous humour of patients with glaucoma associated with exfoliation syndrome. *Eye* (London) 2009;23:1691–1697.

47. Bartlett H, Eperjesi F. An ideal ocular nutritional supplement? *Ophthalmic Physiol Opt* 2004;24:339–349.

48. Rafnsson V, Olafsdottir E, Hrafnkelsson J, et al. Cosmic radiation increases the risk of nuclear cataract in airline pilots: a population-based case-control study. *Arch Ophthalmol* 2005; 123:1102–1105.

49. Rouhiainen P, Rouhiainen H, Salonen JT. Association between low plasma vitamin E concentration and progression of early cortical lens opacities. *Am J Epidemiol* 1996; 144:496–500.

50. Nourmohammadi I, Modarress M, Khanaki K, et al. Association of serum alpha-tocopherol, retinol and ascorbic acid with the risk of cataract development. *Ann Nutr Metab* 2008;52:296–298.

51. Packer L. Protective role of vitamin E in biological systems. *Am J Clin Nutr* 1991;53:1050S–1055S.

52. Jacques PF, Taylor A, Hankinson SE, et al. Long-term vitamin C supplement use and prevalence of early age-related opacities. *Am J Clin Nutr* 1997;66:911–916.

53. Fletcher AE. Controversy over "contradiction": should randomized trials always trump observational studies? *Am J Ophthalmol* 2009;147:384–386.

54. Millen AE, Gruber M, Klein R, et al. Relations of serum ascorbic acid and alpha-tocopherol to diabetic retinopathy in the Third National Health and Nutrition Examination Survey. *Am J Epidemiol* 2003;158:225–233.

55. Hoffer A, Saul AW. *Orthomolecular Medicine for Everyone: Megavitamin Therapeutics for Families and Physicians.* Laguna Beach, CA: Basic Health Publications, 2008.

56. Williams RJ, Deason G. Individuality in vitamin C needs. *Proc Nat Acad Sci USA* 1967;57:1638–1641.

57. Papas A. *The Vitamin E Factor: The Miraculous Antioxidant for the Prevention and Treatment of Heart Disease, Cancer, and Aging.* New York: HarperCollins, 1999.

PHYSICAN'S REPORT:
TREATMENT OF IRITIS AND HERPES ZOSTER WITH VITAMIN C

by Herschell H. Boyd, MD

A 56-year-old woman contacted me for treatment of her acute iritis (a painful inflammation of the eye), secondary glaucoma, and herpes zoster (an infection that increases risk of iritis). The patient was also suffering from frequent allergies and had had multiple episodes of iritis. Both cataracts had been removed. The patient lived in Butte, Montana, a mining town where pollution is so great that it caused vegetation to be denuded over a large radius. Hence, the patient needed to leave Montana with her family other than her husband who needed to work three more years before his retirement. The patient's daughter was diagnosed with chronic fatigue syndrome (CFS). The patient's husband and mother were suffering from multiple illnesses.

Treatment and Results

- **July 8, 1994, phone call:** Patient complained over the telephone of an iritis attack for several days. The symptoms were treated by another ophthalmologist but did not respond to dilation and cortisone. The patient was advised to take in addition to her cortisone and dilating drops 4,000 mg of vitamin C every 30 minutes.

- **July 9, 1994, phone call:** Patient called again. Iritis improved. No diarrhea. Patient was advised to increase her intake to 6,000 mg of vitamin C every 30 minutes.

- **July 11, 1994, office visit:** This was the first visit of this patient to the office. Iritis improving. The intraocular pressure was elevated to 23 mmHg in the eye affected by iritis. Cortisone drops were decreased to four times a day. Cycloplegic drops were discontinued.

- **July 13, 1994, office visit:** Iritis improved. No diarrhea yet. Patient was advised to increase intake to 8,000 mg of vitamin C every 30 minutes.

- **July 14, 1994, office visit:** No iritis. Intraocular pressure 22 mmHg. Patient developed a headache on right side of head. No diarrhea yet. Patient was advised to increase her intake to 12,000 mg of vitamin C every 30 minutes.

- **July 17, 1994, phone call from California:** Patient had traveled to California. The right side of her scalp was sore but no vesicles of zoster herpes visible. The 12,000 mg of vitamin C were continued.

- **July 20, 1994, phone call from California:** A physician was seen in California and diagnosed herpes zoster. A few vesicles developed on the scalp for three days, and the pain disappeared. Bowel dosage was reached. Patient slowly decreased her intake to 4,000 mg of vitamin C every hour in the following days.

- **August 8, 1994, office visit:** Patient returned from California. No iritis was present. Intraocular pressure was measured at 20 mmHg. Pain in her head had disappeared. Patient was advised to continue with 4,000 mg of vitamin C every hour since this seemed her bowel dosage at that time.

- **August 12, 1994, office visit:** No iritis. Interocular pressure 19 mmHg. No head pain. Patient was advised to continue with bowel dosage of vitamin C. Patient returned to Montana as she feels she may be able to stave off the ill effects of pollution with antioxidants. It may be of interest that this patient gave her 18-year-old daughter bowel dosage of vitamin C, in this case 120,000–150,000 mg per day, which achieved a marked improvement of CFS symptoms. Her husband's health improved as did her mother's. They all took vitamin C to the extent of bowel dosage.

- **October 13, 1994, letter:** Received letter from patient stating that "all the family was doing well and grateful for help and advice they have received."

Discussion

Irwin Stone,[1] in his book, *The Healing Factor, Vitamin C Against Disease* (1971) summarized the experience of using vitamin C with herpes zoster. It has been shown that vitamin C inactivates the herpes virus and clinical cases were treated in 1943 successfully with injections of vitamin C.

In 1953 it was reported that 327 cases of shingles were cured in three days of injections. In 1949 Dr. Kinnear injected eight shingle patients with ascorbic acid, and seven claimed cessation of pain within two hours after the first injection. Seven were said to have drying of the blisters within one day and clear of lesions in three days. Clearing of the lesions in three days was the same result in this patient treated orally with vitamin C.

Dr. Robert Cathcart[2] has stated in a letter of August 30, 1993, that he generally does not use intravenous (IV) ascorbic acid as it is expensive and time-consuming for the patient; however, at times if the patient is unable to tolerate the vitamin C because of burning in the stomach, IV vitamin C may be used for a few days, and following this the oral vitamin C is tolerated. Dr. Cathcart also uses oral vitamin C with the IV as this gives a double effect. He points out that one must stop giving oral vitamin C about 1 hour before the IV stops as diarrhea may occur upon cessation of the vitamin C. Then 30–60 minutes later oral vitamin C may be begun again.

It was suggested to this patient that she might do well with intravenous vitamin C, but she was only passing through town and felt that the large amounts of oral vitamin C were working well with no bowel problems except that she did complain of some gas as would be expected.

Along with the vitamin C, the patient was advised to take the following antioxidants and other substances three times daily: beta carotene (15 mg), vitamin E (400 IU), selenium (50 mg), vitamin B complex, multimineral, and L-lysine (500 mg).

Comments

1. Iritis was a manifestation of herpes zoster before herpes appeared.

2. Bowel dosage of vitamin C was approximately 500,000 mg per day to quench the free radicals of herpes zoster, plus whatever other toxic elements the patient's body may have accumulated by living in a polluted area. This is the largest amount of vitamin C ever prescribed to achieve bowel dosage by this author.

3. Treating the whole family in a toxic environment seemed logical and effective.

4. Treatment of iritis with cortisone and cycloplegic drops was not effective and could have led to a secondary glaucoma on a permanent basis.

5. My experience in treating herpes zoster with various drugs in the past has never been this effective in this short time span. Patients suffered from nine months to five years.

6. This is the most dramatic improvement in treating herpes zoster in my medical experience since graduating from medical school in 1952!

It is my feeling that the benign side effects of vitamin C both orally and intravenously far outweigh the toxic side effects of drugs that are not as effective for herpes zoster and certainly not for iritis. As physicians, we should consider vitamin C as the first weapon to use in these battles.

REFERENCES

1. Stone I. *The Healing Factor, Vitamin C Against Disease*. New York: Grosset & Dunlap, 1972, 74–75.
2. Cathcart RF. Personal letter, August 30, 1993.

From the *J Orthomolecular Med* 1995;10(2):97–99.

CATARACTS AND ORTHOMOLECULAR TREATMENT
by Abram Hoffer, MD, PhD

Free radicals and antioxidants are becoming increasingly popular and "establishment" in medicine. Damage caused by excessive oxidation and reversal of this damage or its prevention by antioxidants may be involved in cancer, mental illness (especially schizophrenia), and other degenerative diseases. Cataracts are also a byproduct of excessive oxidation. This is the price we pay for living in an atmosphere that is 20 percent oxygen and having to use it as a prime source of energy. But long before free radical theories were developed, a few physicians were using one antioxidant, ascorbic acid, to prevent and treat cataracts.

Dr. Irwin Stone's amazing book, *The Healing Factor: Vitamin C Against Disease*,[1] published in 1972, contains a brief review of the connection between ascorbic acid and cataracts. In 1939, workers in Argentina treated 60 patients (with a total of 113 cataracts) by daily injections of 50–100 milligrams (mg) of vitamin C twice a day for ten days. About 90 percent of the cataracts were benefited. That same year a Detroit physician gave patients 350 mg per day for four to eight weeks and found 60 percent had better vision. Improvement was noted in two weeks. He concluded, however, that vitamin C would not help established cataracts.

In 1952, D. T. Atkinson, an experienced ophthalmologist, gave 450 cases of incipient (very early) cataracts 1,000 mg of ascorbic acid per day and 20,000 international units (IU) of vitamin A. Other patients required surgery after about four years, but some after one year. From the treated group, only a small number required surgery. In some, the cataracts did not progress in up to 11 years.

In his discussion, Stone pointed out that the most striking change in lens-developing cataracts is a decrease in sulfhydryl groups (a sulfur and a hydrogen bonded to a hydrocarbon chain). These are destroyed by over-oxidation. They are also lower in vitamin C. The very high levels of ascorbic acid in the eye protect the lens protein from polymerizing (i.e., from becoming opaque). Anything that decreases vitamin levels will increase the tendency to develop cataracts.

Stone was concerned that these early studies had been consistently ignored. He wrote, "While some research shows that it is possible to slow down the cataractous process, no work could be found which would indicate that the proper use of ascorbic acid has been tried to reverse the cataractous process."

Other Therapeutic Nutrients

This oversight is being corrected. A report in *Canadian Family Physician* reviewed research at the University of Western Ontario.[2] Drs. James Robertson, Allan Donner, and J. Trevithick studied 175 senile cataract patients against 175 controls. The patients had undergone or were about to undergo cataract surgery. They were really surprised to find that people over age 55 who took daily supplements of vitamin E or vitamin C had a 44 percent and 30 percent chance, respectively, of developing senile (late-onset) cataracts. They also found that cataract-free patients drank five or more cups of tea per day. Tea contains tannic acid, a good source of pyrogallol, an antioxidant. Doses of vitamin E and vitamin C daily were 400 IU and 300–600 mg, respectively. This study is very important since about 15 percent of the population over age 55, especially women, will develop cataracts, and about 50 percent of all people over age 75 will have cataracts.

Other nutrients have been therapeutic for cataracts. Dr. Michael Lesser in *Nutrition and Vitamin Therapy* (1980)[3] reports on one case given 10,000 IU of vitamin A and 400 mg of riboflavin (vitamin B2) daily. The patient was developing cataracts and would soon need an operation. After several months on these vitamins her sight stabilized and then improved, and the cataracts began to recede.

From the *J Orthomolecular Med* 1998;3(2):61–62.

Dr. Richard A. Passwater in *Selenium as Food and Medicine* (1980)[4] further reviewed the biochemical pathology of cataracts. There is no doubt they result from excessive oxidation. Glutathione, a major antioxidant in the lens, increases the destruction of oxidizers; it contains the trace mineral selenium. Cataracts contain one-sixth the selenium content of normal lens tissue. In rats, selenium deficiency hastens development of cataracts.

I have discussed only a few of the nutrients essential in maintaining the integrity of lens tissue. It is likely many more are involved. Dr. Roger Williams has summarized it accurately in an issue of *Executive Health* when he wrote, "There is enough evidence now to indicate that faulty metabolism or metabolism inadequate for adapting to stresses is a major factor—and evidence too that not some panacea nutrient but rather a balanced team of nutrients has potential for preventing cataract formation and perhaps even for helping in the treatment of some existing, but not for advanced, cataracts."[5]

But nutrient therapy (especially antioxidant vitamins such as niacin, vitamin C, vitamin E, and minerals) may do more than slow down the rate of cataract formation. Some may be entirely reversed. In this report I will summarize two cases of cataracts responding to treatment in two of my patients. These two cases should stimulate others to treat their cataractous patients to determine what proportion will be resolved completely, and when are cataracts so well established that surgical treatment is the only solution.

Two Case Histories

C. W. developed some cloudiness of vision in 1984 at age 70. She had been taking vitamin C (1,500 mg), thiamine (100 mg), niacinamide (250 mg), and vitamin E (800 IU) daily. To this I recommended she add riboflavin (25 mg) and cod liver oil (3 capsules per day). One year later her lens was clear, and by August 1987 no further evidence of cataracts was evident on optometric examination. At no time did she take huge doses of vitamins.

The addition of riboflavin (vitamin B2) and cod liver oil, which is rich in vitamins A and D, was what she needed to halt and reverse the incipient cataracts developing in both eyes.

My second example, E. S., developed polycythemia vera in 1971. Her hemoglobin was 20 grams. Polycythemia vera is a blood disorder that causes the blood to be thicker than normal, which in turn slows the rate of blood flow through the veins to the small capillaries in the eyes. E. S. was treated with busulfan (Myleran) and continued to receive treatment with this drug now and then. By 1977 her hemoglobin was normal (14.1 grams), but by July 1981 she was anemic. She had entered a spent phase of extensive fibrosis and was diagnosed with myelofibrosis, a condition caused by the polycythemia. By December 1981 her hemoglobin was 7.2 grams. I first saw her in March 1982, at age 67. I started her on a comprehensive program but her hemoglobin continued to drop, reaching 6.2 in August 1982. I began to make adjustments in her multinutrient program and her hemoglobin began to increase, reaching 9.6 grams by December 1987. I will not detail what she was using as this is an example only of an improvement in cataracts. I was very pleased when she told me in October 1987 that she was able once more to read with her right eye. When seen last, December 8, 1987, her vision was even better.

These two examples of cataract reversal reinforce the evidence already discussed. It does not mean every cataract can be reversed, but it does mean that many cataracts, especially if caught early, can be reversed.

REFERENCES

1. Stone I. *The Healing Factor: Vitamin C Against Disease.* New York: Grosset & Dunlap, 1972.

2. Robertson J, Donner A, Trevithick J. *Canadian Family Physician* 1987;33:31.

3. Lesser M. *Nutrition and Vitamin Therapy.* New York: Grove Press, 1980.

4. Passwater RA. *Selenium as Food and Medicine.* New Canaan, CT: Keats Publishing, 1980.

5. Williams R. *Executive Health* 1976 (Dec);13.

CATARACTS AND VITAMINS: THE REAL STORY
by Damien Downing, MBBS, MSB, and Robert G. Smith, PhD

"Hidden danger of everyday supplements is revealed" blared the headline in the UK *Daily Mail*,[1] a newspaper that is well known for declaring that, for example, "coffee causes cancer" and "coffee reduces cancer risk" on different pages of the same issue. This time it is reporting on a study out of Sweden that appears to show that taking vitamin C or vitamin E supplements increases your risk of developing a cataract—by about 20 percent for C and 60 percent for E.[2] It makes a good headline, but does it make sense?

Is This Research?

No. They didn't give anybody anything, or do anything to them. This was just a computer exercise in which they reanalyzed postal questionnaires sent to the entire male population between the ages of 45 and 79 in an area of Sweden, and matched the responses to another database of cataract operations. Although the title says that it is "a population-based prospective cohort study," the term "prospective" would really mean that they followed the group of subjects (the cohort) closely over a period of time, without losing many of them. In fact, they simply had their computer go through some old electronic records. Nobody was interviewed, and no checks or validation exercises were carried out. No researcher met any of the men in the study, ever.

Is It Reliable?

No. The first really serious shortcoming of this paper (the gorilla in the room) is that half the men never replied in the first place, and then the authors deliberately excluded a lot more for reasons such as diabetes—one of the other main "outcomes" of the study and a big risk factor for cataracts. Finally, they omitted to account for another few thousand people, so that in the end they were only studying 27 percent of the original population. If they had randomly selected this sample of the population that would be fine, but in fact the subjects selected themselves by bothering to fill in and return the questionnaire, or not. What were their reasons? We know not. That means that already several types of selection bias have been introduced, and all the results are now meaningless.

There could even be what's known as "indication bias"—when cause and effect get mixed up. So, for instance, cataracts can take decades rather than years to develop, and people with early symptoms might be more likely to take supplements to ease their eyestrain. If the study goes on entirely in a computer, there's no way of telling.

Is It Scientifically Plausible?

No. The study contradicts many other studies that have shown either no effect or actual benefits of vitamins C and E for preventing cataracts and other eye diseases. Cataracts are common among older people, and it is well known that antioxidants can reduce the risk of developing them if taken long term. Smoking, obesity, and diabetes are well-known risk factors for cataracts,[3,4] and antioxidants are known to prevent the damage caused by these factors. In one study, vitamin C supplements taken over 10 years or more reduced the risk of cataracts by about 80 percent. This is a huge dose-related effect, strongly suggesting the benefit of antioxidants in preventing cataracts. The effect was not apparent for short-term use, suggesting that any shorter-term study may not identify the benefit.[5]

Studies should not be viewed in isolation because that leads to the "coffee causes cancer" and "coffee reduces cancer risk" absurdity. The effect of a discrepant study such as this is to marginally adjust the current information about risk. Let's say that based on previous studies, we thought there was an 80 percent probability that taking vitamins would help to prevent cataracts; after this one we might revise that to 75 percent. This is known as Bayesian probability (after an

From the *Orthomolecular News Service* March 5, 2013.

English minister 300 years ago) and makes a whole lot more sense than the supposedly black-and-white, 95 percent confidence-interval type of statistics used here. If a gambler isn't a Bayesian, he's an idiot; every hand, every throw, alters the odds. So does every study.

The conclusions here are also dodgy because there is no real data on the amounts of the vitamins taken—only a guesstimate from an earlier study of 248 men—and even occasional use was tabulated as use of supplements. For this to make a substantial difference to the health outcome isn't really plausible.

So, in Real Life?

To prevent age-related diseases of the eye including cataracts, the best current advice is to lower oxidative stress by stopping smoking, reducing excess weight (diabetes again), eating an excellent diet,[6,7] and taking a multivitamin supplement and additional supplements of vitamin C (3,000–6,000 milligrams [mg] per day in divided doses)[6,8] and vitamin E (400–1,200 IU of natural mixed tocopherols and tocotrienols).[9–12] This will greatly help prevent oxidation of the tissues of the eye. Artificial forms of vitamin E (dl-alpha-tocopherol) are only 50 percent as biologically active as the natural form (d-alpha-tocopherol). Taking alpha-tocopherol alone is thought to lower the effective uptake of the other beneficial forms of vitamin E, so it's important to take the natural form of mixed (alpha-, beta-, gamma-, delta-) tocopherols.

REFERENCES

1. Hagan P. How vitamin pills can raise risk of cataracts as hidden danger of everyday supplements is revealed. *Mail Online.* Feb 22, 2013. Available at www.dailymail.co.uk/health/article-2283178/How-vitamin-pills-raise-risk-cataracts-hidden-danger-everyday-supplements-revealed.html.

2. Selin JZ, Rautiainen S, Lindblad BE, et al. High-dose supplements of vitamins C and E, low-dose multivitamins, and the risk of age-related cataract: a population-based prospective cohort study of men. *Am J Epidemiol* 2013;177(6):548–555.

3. Mosad SM, Ghanem AA, El-Fallal HM, et al. Lens cadmium, lead, and serum vitamins C, E, and beta carotene in cataractous smoking patients. *Curr Eye Res* 2010;35(1):23–30.

4. Hiller R, Sperduto RD, Podgor MJ, et al. Cigarette smoking and the risk of development of lens opacities: the Framingham studies. *Arch Ophthalmol* 1997;115(9):1113–1118.

5. Jacques PF, Taylor A, Hankinson SE, et al. Long-term vitamin C supplement use and prevalence of early age-related lens opacities. *Am J Clin Nutr* 1997 Oct;66(4):911–916.

6. Mares JA, Voland R, Adler R, et al. and the CAREDS Group. Healthy diets and the subsequent prevalence of nuclear cataract in women. *Arch Ophthalmol* 2010 Jun;128(6):738–749.

7. Williams DL. Oxidation, antioxidants and cataract formation: a literature review. *Vet Ophthalmol* 2006;9(5):292–298.

8. Head KA. Natural therapies for ocular disorders, part two: cataracts and glaucoma. *Altern Med Rev* 2001 Apr;6(2):141–166.

9. Rouhiainen P, Rouhiainen H, Salonen JT. Association between low plasma vitamin E concentration and progression of early cortical lens opacities. *Am J Epidemiol* 1996 1;144(5):496–500.

10. Nourmohammadi I, Modarress M, Khanaki K, et al. Association of serum alpha-tocopherol, retinol and ascorbic acid with the risk of cataract development. *Ann Nutr Metab* 2008;52(4):296–298.

11. Seth RK, Kharb S. Protective function of alpha-tocopherol against the process of cataractogenesis in humans. *Ann Nutr Metab* 1999;43(5):286–289.

12. Engin KN. Alpha-tocopherol: looking beyond an antioxidant. *Mol Vis* 2009;15:855–60.

SUCCESSFUL REVERSAL OF RETINITIS PIGMENTOSA
by Merrill J. Allen, OD, PhD, and Raymond W. Lowry, OD

It is commonly taught that retinitis pigmentosa (RP) is a hereditary disease and that there is no cure. When young, the victim of RP usually has normal vision. This fact suggests that the primary cause of RP is a pathogen or a nutritional deficit and not inheritance. This idea is supported by the difficulty of doing RP research, and by our success with two patients treated with nutrients and with 200 microamperes (µA) of electricity. Neither of these unrelated patients have any known relatives with retinitis pigmentosa.

That researchers have had difficulty with the genetic concept of retinitis pigmentosa is summarized as follows:

> In order to pursue laboratory studies into inherited photoreceptor abnormalities, it is essential to have well-defined groups of patients with a common defect. This has rarely been achieved, the only sure way to ensure it until now being the investigation of persons with linked ancestry. Inheritance of RP can be autosomal recessive, autosomal dominant, or X-linked, and there is heterogeneity within the categories. In addition, spontaneous (simplex) cases occur without there being affected siblings or evidence of parental consanguinity. These may be inherited or acquired and meaningful studies will only be possible when the relationship to known diseases has been investigated.[1]

The nutritional factors began to come into focus when an epidemic of cat blindness similar to retinitis pigmentosa hit Australia in 1975.[2] As a result we now know that a critically essential nutrient for the retina is the amino acid taurine. Cats were receiving dog food that was labeled cat food, which did not contain taurine. The limited amount of taurine typical of human food can become unavailable if certain intestinal bacteria are present. Deficient diets as well as such a bacterial infection in members of a family can make RP seem to be inherited. Apparently these bacteria cause the kidneys to excrete taurine, so that supplementing with taurine may not provide the taurine needed by the eyes. If supplementation with taurine is not working, the specific antibiotic for treating these taurine-blocking pathogens is neomycin (Neo-Fradin).[3] Loss of dark adaptation is characteristic of retinitis pigmentosa. Studies have shown that dark adaptation is greatly improved by bilberries (European blueberries).

Regarding macular degeneration, which is also considered to be untreatable, Newsome[4] showed that zinc supplementation can slow but not stop vision loss. Michael and Allen's study[5,6] used nutrients and zinc the same as Newsome did, but they also applied 200 µA of electricity to closed eyelids. Acuity improved or was stabilized for 15 out of 25 macular degeneration patients, monitored for five years. Virtually all of Newsome's subjects, placebo and supplemented groups, lost vision in his two-year study, even though the supplemented subjects retained good acuity longer. Other studies have shown that the application of weak electrical currents to the eye has positive benefit in macular degeneration and other conditions.[7,8] There seem to be no known adverse effects from using microamperage electric current on the eyes. Our use of 200 µA on moist, closed eyelids produces only a sensation of flickering light.

An ocular supplement that contains antioxidants can stop the progression of age-related macular degeneration as shown by Richer.[9,10] Cheraskin[11] has shown that antioxidants are especially beneficial and that improved nutrition should be started earlier in life.

Retinitis Pigmentosa Study

With the above in mind, two RP patients have been monitored while they took a multiple vitamin plus mineral supplement, and 350 milligrams (mg) of bilberry, and 750 mg of taurine, three times daily, and received 200 µA of electricity applied to the eyelids during weekly and monthly office visits.

From the *J Orthomolecular Med* 1998;13(1):41–43.

Patient 1

Angela came for an eye examination at age 15, after the Mayo Clinic diagnosed her as having retinitis pigmentosa and recommended that she learn Braille. Two other ophthalmologists confirmed the diagnosis and advised that she would eventually go blind. For her first examination, Angela had to be led into the office. Her acuity was: left eye, $20/40^{-2}$; right eye, 20/200, and her visual fields were narrowed to less than 15 degrees.

Angela complained about clumsiness in walking and seeing floating spots. She had to give up the high school's marching band because of her inability to stay in line. After taking nutritional supplements and electrical treatments, starting in December 1992, Angela rapidly (in about one month) became an average, young lady able to move about and behave normally. She has continued the nutrients and electrical stimulation to the present time. Now she is happily married and has two children. Her last acuity check, December 14, 1997, was: OD, 20/20 and OS, $20/40^{+3}$. Her peripheral vision now is reasonably normal. She reports reasonably good night vision, and she has a standard driver's license. She reported that her vision now is fine. She continues with her daily multiple vitamins plus minerals, bilberry (300 mg), and taurine (750 mg). She had in-office electrical treatments for three years. Since June 1995 she has a 200-µA electrical stimulator at home. She uses it on her eyes about twice a day.

Patient 2

Barbara, age 37, was examined in September 1993. Records from four medical doctors diagnosed her as having RP. She had multiple, severe, visual field defects even though her acuity was: left eye, 20/30; right, 20/30. Her ability to drive and to walk, especially at night, was impaired as was her ability to read and to continue her work with learning disabled children. Barbara now drives 75 miles for her office visits. She could not do that before. Her visual fields are greatly improved. Her last check

in December 1997 was: left eye, 20/20, and right eye, 20/20. Regarding the success of her four years of nutritional supplements and electrical stimulation, she said: "Now I have no problems at all." Since June 1995, Barbara also has an electrical stimulator at home, which she uses on her eyes about twice daily.

■ CONCLUSIONS

For retinitis pigmentosa we have found a significant benefit from weak electrical currents applied to the eyes, and from using daily nutritional supplements. We have made remarkable visual and psychological improvements in two "incurable" retinitis pigmentosa patients. We recommend that all retinal problem patients including those with retinitis pigmentosa be provided, as a minimum, with proper nutritional supplements and microampere electrical stimulation.

REFERENCES

1. Voaden MJ. *Retinal Research.* New York: Pergamon Press, 1991, 294.

2. Hayes KC, et al. *Science* 1975;188:949.

3. Bradford RW, Allen HW. Taurine in health and disease. *J Adv Med* 1996;9:179–199.

4. Newsome DA, Swartz M, et al. Oral zinc in macular degeneration. *Arch Ophthal* 1988;106:192–198.

5. Michael, LD, Allen MJ. Nutritional supplementation, electrical stimulation and age-related macular degeneration. *J Orthomolecular Med* 1993;8:168–171.

6. Allen, MJ. Treating age-related macular degeneration. Letter. *Optom Vis Sci* 1994;71:293.

7. Kurtz JL. The principles and practice of ocular physical therapy for optometrists. *Am J Optom Publ* 1930.

8. Wallace L. The treatment of macular degeneration and other retinal diseases using bioelectromagnetic therapy. *J Optom Photother* 1997:3.

9. Richer S. Atrophic ARMD: a nutrition responsive disease. Guest editorial. *J Am Optomc Assoc* 1996;67:6–10.

10. Richer S. Multicenter ophthalmic and nutritional age-related macular degeneration study. Parts 1&2. *J Am Optomc Assoc* 1996;67:12–49.

11. Cheraskin E. Antioxidants in health and disease. *J Am Optomc Assoc* 1996;67:50–57.

EYE-PRESSURE LOWERING EFFECT OF VITAMIN C
by Herschell H. Boyd, MD

Vitamin C has been used since it was isolated in the early 1930s. Its use in lowering the pressure in glaucoma dates back to 1962 as reported in *Experimental Eye Research*.[1] Since then there have been many references in the foreign literature, but in the United States it has escaped the attention of the ophthalmologists. The purpose of this study was to document the pressure before the use of vitamin C and after the daily intake of maximum amounts of vitamin C, three times a day.

The study consisted of 50 consecutive patients who presented with intraocular (internal eye) pressure greater than 20 mmHg (the same pressure scale used for blood pressure readings), as measured by tonometery from August 1993 through March 1995. The highest pressure was 36 mmHg in the study. Out of 50 patients, 20 patients refused to take vitamin C and eye drops were used to lower the pressure in the standard manner. The age distribution of the patients ranged from 30–39 (1 patient), and 40–49 (6 patients), to 50–59 (5 patients), and 60–80 (18 patients). No visual field defects were found in any of the 50 patients. All 50 patients had open angles (the fluid drainage mechanism of the eye), and no angles were particularly closed as measured. (Debris from degenerating eye tissue is carried to the canals where it can block the drainage mechanism.)

Vitamin C Taken

The most vitamin C taken was 35,000 milligrams (mg) per day divided in three doses at mealtime. The least amount of vitamin C taken was 1,000 mg per day in two patients. The average intake for the 30 patients was 10,000 mg per day. It was suggested that patients take the vitamin until bowel intolerance and then back down, but this advice is almost always ignored by patients as they feel the idea is unreasonable and generally have this reinforced by friends and relatives who give statements of shock and dismay. But 20 out of 30 patients did take 10,000 mg or more per day so perhaps we should be pleased with this result.

The average drop in eye pressure was as follows:

- Right eye: 4.8 mmHg
- Left eye: 6.3 mmHg
- Both eyes: 5.6 mmHg

It is an interesting observation that individuals who take vitamin C regularly and have their intraocular pressure taken on a routine basis for their eye exam have pressures in the range of 10–13 mmHg commonly. It has been my experience that I have yet to find the first patient with a pressure over 20 mmHg who comes into the office and admits to taking any amount of vitamin C daily. It also seems to be generally true that those people who do have pressure elevated for the first time are those treating themselves with various toxic drugs, smoking, eating processed foods, and living a lifestyle saturated with free radicals. I assume the little amount of vitamin C they eat in a day is not enough to keep the eye pressure normal. Another interesting observation is that patients who already have taken intraocular pressure-reducing medication for years are generally unable to stop the medication and reverse the high pressure with vitamin C. This latter group is not unlike many diabetics, who finally are placed on insulin and cannot later usually get off the insulin, whereas before that the diabetes may be reversed.

One patient had the pressure decrease in one eye by 13 mmHg. Seven eyes dropped by 10–13 mmHg.

No side effects were encountered as vitamin C apparently has none. All drugs we use in glaucoma have multiple side effects including death.

Study Outcome and Application to Eye Disease

It is said that the aqueous fluid in the eye has 25 times the amount of vitamin C as in the blood. This may explain why the pressure decreased with the

From the *J Orthomolecular Med* 1995;10(3):165–168.

increased intake of vitamin C with an opening of the many canals, called Schlemm's canal, that regulate intraocular pressure. Any swelling in the area would be removed with the antihistamine effect of vitamin C. Further research could explain the possibility.

Another explanation of the pressure-lowering effect of vitamin C could be the ability of vitamin C to increase the number of T4 cells (immune cells that fight off infection foreign substances). Maybe debris is removed from the Schlemm's canal by T4 cells so iris pigment and inflammatory cells are unable to plug the outflow of the eye. Further studies could answer this question.

In 1969, Dr. Erich Linner explained that the fall in pressure in ocular hypertension was due to a reduction in the rate of aqueous flow and possibly by "bulk drainage by way of posterior uveoscleral routes,"[6] the drainage pathways at the back of the eye.

Since the patients in this study would not take amounts of vitamin C to bowel intolerance and then back down in dosage, the effects of vitamin C could be further improved from those obtained in this study. The reparative effects of vitamin C are certainly demonstrated and in my experience can be seen as well in other eye diseases.

Since vitamin C makes collagen needed to strengthen the blood vessel walls, those in the group who were diabetics quit bleeding in the retina (retinal hemorrhage) and elsewhere in the body. Diabetics have higher risk of developing glaucoma than non-

diabetics. This reduces the need for laser treatment to the retina and in many cases in the development of late glaucoma.[4]

It is generally agreed that macular degeneration occurs in 25 percent of the U.S. population over 55. This group can be helped enormously with antioxidants to improve what macula is left and protect the macular from worsening. People with glaucoma also become a major problem in management. In many cases my experience is that the vision may improve dramatically with vitamin C and other antioxidants. Here, too, it seems logical to affect lifestyle changes to eliminate free radicals.

Cataract removal represents the largest surgical expense in Medicare, and there are many patients in my practice who improve several lines of vision on the eye chart. One dramatic example was a woman with 20/40 eyesight, who achieved 20/20 vision in eight weeks with 12,000 mg of vitamin C each day. She was a smoker in her early 50s, and she has continued to smoke with good reason to cease.

The obvious savings financially for various payers is staggering. We may see the day when these people are told to take vitamin C by the insurers as they are totally cost-oriented and are unemotional in their thinking.

Functions of Vitamin C in the Eye

Ascorbic acid (vitamin C) has been reported to be of therapeutic benefit in numerous pathological

IN BRIEF

Results from this study may awaken ophthalmologists to the marvels of vitamin C in treating glaucoma. The study documented the pressure before the use of vitamin C and after the daily intake of maximum amounts of vitamin C, three times a day. Thirty patients (16 men, 14 women) were advised to take three divided doses of vitamin C in capsule form each day until loose stools occurred and then to back down slightly from this amount (bowel dosage) for a daily intake. The average daily intake for all patients was 10,000 milligrams per day. Twenty patients were forced to use eye drops to lower the pressure below 20 mmHg as they refused to take vitamin C. The findings were as follows: the greatest lowering of pressure was 13 mmHg; the least lowering of pressure was 1 mmHg; and the average for 30 patients was 10 mmHg. Thirty patients were controlled *only* with vitamin C—there was no occasion in which the pressure was not lowered with vitamin C. All drugs for glaucoma are seriously toxic, and vitamin C has no toxicity yet known. The patients also experienced many other good side effects from the vitamin C such as clearing of sinusitis and allergy symptoms, arthritis improvement, cholesterol lowering, laxative and diuretic effects, and other improvements associated with vitamin C intake of several thousand milligrams per day.

conditions, and researchers vary in their estimates of the daily requirement needed by humans. Animals, which are capable of synthesizing their own ascorbic acid, usually have tissue levels approaching saturation. Therefore, in man it would seem desirable to ensure the intake of ascorbic acid is sufficiently high for tissue saturation.[5]

This paper shows that in glaucoma, tissue saturation is needed to lower intraocular pressure. In a modern world of processed foods and excess free radicals, it is surprising that we have a relatively small group of glaucoma patients. Vitamin C concentrations have been shown to change in the body under various conditions of stress such as trauma, surgery, exposure to cold, after administration of cortisone or adrenocorticotropic hormone (ACTH), and during infection.[5] In ophthalmology we need to give vitamin C supplements for any of the glaucoma surgeries and for that matter with all our surgeries.

The lens in the eye is necessary for maintaining the normal level of ascorbic acid within the aqueous humor, vitreous body, and the cornea. The diminution of the intraocular ascorbic acid content does not take place when traces of lens fibers are present in the eye.[3] This could be an interesting study for glaucoma and cataract removal.

The structure of the vitreous body depends upon both the integrity of the meshwork of collagen fibers and on the maintenance of the polymeric state of the mucopolysaccharide hyaluronic acid, a major water-holding molecule in human and animal tissues. With a deficiency in vitamin C, abnormal mucopolysaccharide formation occurs. Disorganization of the vitreous body with the formation of vitreous bands is often associated with retinal detachment.[5] Here also the association of glaucoma with these people would be an interesting observation.

Michele Virno, MD, used 400–1,000 mg per kilogram (kg) of body weight of intravenous vitamin C to induce a "marked ocular hypotony [low intraocular pressure] in approximately 60 to 90 minutes." These good results instigated the idea to use vitamin C by mouth to lower intraocular pressure.[3]

Dr. Virno found in 1967 that 500 mg per kg of body weight of vitamin C in all patients with glaucoma resulted in a reduction of intraocular pressure. The vitamin C was given three to four times per day, and in some patients who could not be controlled with acetazolamide (Diamox) and 2 percent pilocarpine (Carpine)[1] it was possible to obtain almost normal pressures.

Erich Linner, MD, gave only 500 mg of vitamin C twice a day for four to six weeks and only decreased the pressure by 2–3 mmHg after two days of use. As Dr. Virno concluded, this was not enough but the idea was good in 1964.[2]

Irwin Stone, PhD, in his book *The Healing Factor: Vitamin C Against Disease* (1972), remarked: "Of all the disorders afflicting man, blindness causes the most widespread disability. Yet in spite of significant advances in eye research, the incidence of blindness is increasing. Megascorbic therapy might one day help to reverse this trend."

Dr. Stone reports that from 1965 to 1969 there were numerous papers reported on the prompt reduction of the intraocular pressure with two American journals in 1966 and 1967 reporting on the good results from Italian workers. There have been no American authors reporting on this exacting research or treatment of their patients.[7]

Dr. Stone made the very accurate observation that "research should be started immediately on population groups near 40 and older to determine the long-term effect of the inhibition of glaucoma by means of the continued daily intake of about 3,000–5,000 mg of vitamin C. This will help to determine if a simple and harmless ascorbic acid regimen can be worked out which will prevent blindness in our senior citizens." Cataracts and macular degeneration (eye diseases that are more common than glaucoma) would have immense benefit.

It is my experience that patients do not present with macular degeneration, cataracts, or glaucoma who have taken vitamins for years with vitamin C. One has to ask why it is that physicians in ophthalmology don't tell every patient to take the antioxidants with tissue saturation levels of vitamin C? The answer may be:

- It is not taught in medical school.

- Friends and associates don't use it.

- Medical literature does not have it currently.

523

- Standard of care does not include this treatment.

- Fear of being out of mainstream medicine.

- Fear of a lawyer charging that the "standard of care was not met."

- Double-blind studies have not been done recently.

- No office has a drug salesman selling vitamin C as there is not profit.

- Many patients cannot accept a treatment that does not involve drugs, as they always get from all other doctors.

- Fear of losing the confidence of a patient and his or her friends and family.

- Insurance payers will not reimburse the patient for treatment not on their toxic drug list.

- In glaucoma with even the best of drug therapy, an adverse result may occur with a resulting lawsuit and no help from the experts in glaucoma called upon to testify.

Why don't medical schools do research on vitamin C? As a past member of the advisory board at Vanderbilt University School of Medicine in Nashville, Tennessee, this same question was asked of the vice chancellor. The response was that at Vanderbilt Medical School the salaries of the workers there are paid by research grants from drug companies and from the National Institutes of Health in Washington, D.C. These two areas don't fund vitamin C. If a source of private money could be found, the medical school would be pleased to do studies as desired. A private foundation may be the salvation of glaucoma patients, and, of course, of the many other eye diseases we need to treat.

CONCLUSION

In this series of 30 patients there was no occasion in which the pressure was not lowered with vitamin C. The largest drop in pressure was 13 mmHg, and the average drop was 5.6 mmHg. All drugs for glaucoma are seriously toxic, and vitamin C has no toxicity yet known. The patients experienced many other good side effects from vitamin C not mentioned here such as clearing of sinusitis and allergy symptoms, arthritis improvement, cholesterol lowering, laxative effects, and other improvements associated with vitamin C intake of several thousand milligrams per day. Ophthalmologists may awaken to the marvels of vitamin C in treating glaucoma!

REFERENCES

1. Virno M, Bucci M. Oral treatment of glaucoma with vitamin C. *Eye, Ear, Nose and Throat Monthly* 1967;46:1502–1508.

2. Linner E. Intraocular pressure regulation and ascorbic acid. *Acta Soc Med Upsol* 1964;59:225.

3. Virno M, Bucci M, et al. Intravenous glycerol-vitamin C (sodium salt) as osmotic agents to reduce intraocular pressure. *Am J Ophthalmol* 1966;62(5):824–833.

4. Pope CN. *Diabetes* 1960;9:9.

5. Heath H. The distribution and possible functions of ascorbic acid in the eye. *Exp. Eye Res* 1962;1:362–367.

6. Linner E. The pressure-lowering effect of ascorbic acid in ocular hypertension. *ACTA Ophthalmologica* 1969;47:685–689.

7. Stone I. *The Healing Factor: Vitamin C Against Disease.* New York: Grosset & Dunlap, 1972, 126–132.

FATIGUE

A N EXPERIMENT WAS CONDUCTED BY James Lind in 1747 on the effect of citrus fruit on scurvy. During April and May while cruising on HMS *Salisbury* he conducted the first clinical controlled trial. He treated six pairs of sailors sick with scurvy. The first pair were given cider; the second pair, elixir of vitriol (sulfuric acid); a third pair, vinegar; a fourth pair, sea water; a fifth pair, each were given two oranges and one lemon for six days, at which time the supply of fruit ran out; and the last pair were given an electuary consisting of a mixture of seeds. By the time the fruit ran out the two lucky sailors who had received it were so much improved that they were nursing the remaining ten. Lind was convinced, but the British Admiralty was not.

Scurvy is extreme vitamin C deficiency. One of the key symptoms of scurvy is fatigue. Severe fatigue is also an acknowledged symptom of deficiency of vitamins, including vitamins B1 (thiamine), B2 (riboflavin), B3 (niacin) B6 (pyridoxine), B12 (cobalamin), biotin, folate (folic acid), and vitamins A, D, and E. Fatigue is also a recognized symptom of numerous mineral deficiencies, including iron, calcium, magnesium, chromium, and zinc.

Inadequate nutrient intake is the first thing that physicians should check for when they are presented with a chronically tired patient. It is usually the last. This section may help reinvigorate both the subject and the reader.

— ABRAM HOFFER, *JOM* 2004 (updated by A.W.S.)

TERMS OF FATIGUE

ANTIOXIDANTS. Vitamins, minerals, enzymes, or other compounds that help fight off the formation of free radicals and the damage caused by them.

CANDIDA ALBICANS. A yeast organism normally found in the body, an overgrowth of which causes the common yeast infection candidiasis.

CHRONIC FATIGUE SYNDROME (CFS). Extreme fatigue that generally can't be explained by any underlying medical condition. Other common symptoms include sleep difficulties, problems with concentration and short-term memory, flu-like symptoms, pain in the joints and muscles, tender lymph nodes, sore throat, and headaches.

HYPERINSULINISM. A disorder causing overproduction of insulin, which leads to low blood sugar, also known as hypoglycemia.

OXIDATIVE STRESS. An imbalance between the capacity of the body's antioxidant defense system and the level of free radicals. Oxidative stress increases when antioxidant defenses weaken or free radical levels rise.

STAGED MANAGEMENT FOR CHRONIC FATIGUE SYNDROME
by Erik T. Paterson, MD

I have no idea what chronic fatigue syndrome or whatever label may be used such as neuromyasthenia, myalgic encephalomyelitis, etc., is. However, despite attempts by some psychiatrists to claim it for their own, the evidence for its organicity is overwhelming.[1–10] That being the case, it is entirely within the province of most general practitioners or family doctors to manage.

The best explanation for chronic fatigue syndrome (CFS) that I have been able to distill is that it starts with a stressed organism, usually a person with a type A personality, a workaholic, someone who never refuses to take on new responsibilities—in other words a citizen, the kind of individual that no civilization can do without. On top of this comes stress from the various pollutants to which the individual is exposed, in the air, in the water, in the food consumed, and through other chemicals to which he or she becomes exposed. A virus infection, however one acquires it, is the final straw. No specific virus can be implicated, although the Epstein-Barr virus seems commonest in western North America.[11] In Europe it seems to be one of the enteroviruses.[12,13] The virus enters into a nondestructive relationship with either muscle cells,[14–16] or in the brain,[17] or both. In the body's attempts to attack the virus, it produces large amounts of cytokines (chemicals like interferon and interleukin 2) that help fight infection. It is the side effects of these agents that are responsible for most of the symptoms of the sufferers with CFS.[18]

Diagnostic Clues

Before treatment can be undertaken, a diagnosis must be made. Because CFS is a complex array of symptoms that may mimic other illnesses, its diagnosis is made by exclusion. The full clinical acumen of the practitioner must be brought to bear on the problem to make sure that no simpler, more easily treatable condition(s) is present.

The diagnostic list of what it could be includes depression, bipolar affective disorder, somatization disorders, the schizophrenias; multiple sclerosis, subacute combined degeneration of the cord (folic acid and vitamin B12 deficiencies), amyotrophic lateral sclerosis, neurosyphilis, parkinsonism; malingering (rare) chronic obstructive pulmonary disease; myocardial ischemia, cardiomyopathy, cardiac valvular disease; peptic ulcer disease, chronic hepatitis, chronic pancreatitis, ulcerative colitis, Crohn's disease, irritable bowel syndrome; gallbladder disease; giardiasis, chronic large bowel candidiasis; hypothyroidism, hyperthyroidism, Addison's disease; diabetes, reactive hyperinsulinism; acute and chronic urinary tract infections; myopathies, fibromyalgia (a condition often confused with CFS), food allergies or sensitivities; the anemias; arthritis; mineral disorders (calcium, magnesium, zinc, and copper), toxicity by iron, lead and mercury; and cancers of any body system. This list is not exhaustive. Often, though as one tries to exclude these, the tests are not diagnostic and one has to wait for further diagnostic clues.

There are, in fact, in the history two very common diagnostic clues. If the patient has suddenly become intolerant of all but small amounts of alcohol, then CFS is almost certainly the diagnosis. Similarly, if the patient is intolerant of regular doses of the tricyclic antidepressants (Aventyl, Norpramin, Tofranil, etc.), CFS is almost certainly the diagnosis. If both are present, then there is little doubt at all. And these almost entirely eliminate most psychiatric diagnoses. Probably the best policy of all is to maintain watchfulness over the patient's whole health with regular complete physical examinations and further diagnostic testing.

From the J Orthomolecular Med 1995;10(2):70–78.

Management Policies

Candida

Through bitter experience, I have learned that the very first measure I have to take after a thorough history and physical examination is to consider the issue of chronic bowel candidiasis (infection with the fungus *Candida albicans*). Diagnostic clues to this tend to be that the patient is female, is fertile, has taken oral contraceptives, has been subject to vaginal yeast infections, and has been exposed to many courses of antibiotics. Men can experience candidiasis too, especially if exposed to antibiotics or are partners of women prone to candidiasis. The only diagnostic test for this situation is a colonoscopy with multiple biopsies, which is expensive and has a high risk of serious complications. Stool cultures are useless.

By far the easiest way of making a diagnosis of candidiasis is to give a course of oral Nystatin, usually a dose of 1.5 million units three times per day for one week. This agent is not absorbed from the intestines and therefore cannot reach other places where chronic candida infection can occur. But it also means that no side effects are possible. If chronic bowel candidiasis is not involved, there is no response within the week. This does not mean that candida cannot become involved later.

If there is a mild to moderate infestation by candida, improvement starts to become apparent within two to three days. By the end of the week the patient is markedly better, but not well. A further month's course of Nystatin may restore the patient to full health. Avoidance of sugary/starchy foods with recolonization of the bowel by *Lactobacillus acidophilus* usually prevents recurrences. If full health is not achieved within the month, then the candida is only a contributory factor to the CFS and other measures must be taken. Even if full health is restored, recurrences can still occur, often from recolonization with candida from either a consort or spores from sites not reached by the Nystatin, such as the sinuses, middle ears, esophagus, bladder, prostate, and vagina. Other agents that do penetrate to these sites can be helpful such as ketoconazole (Nizoral) and fluconazole (Diflucan).

Where there is a severe infestation by candida, in two to three days there is a marked deterioration in the patient's condition. This situation is analogous to the Jarisch-Herxheimer reaction, which happens when large numbers of candida organisms, and some of the breakdown products, are absorbed causing the deterioration. In two to three days more, when most of the candida is dead, there is a rapid improvement. A further month's treatment, with the recurrence preventive measures as outlined above, can cure the patient. This is the situation that carries the best prognosis.

Further Diagnostic Testing

If candida is eliminated as a major player in the patient's condition, I proceed with complete bloodwork to determine if another underlying cause can be identified. Tests of function of T-cell subtypes, nuclear magnetic resonance (MRI) imaging, quantitative electroencephalograms, and positron emission tomography (PET) may also help determine if an underlying cause can be identified.

Basic CFS Treatment Protocol

Other conditions being ruled out, I then place the patient on a three- to four-month trial of the following basic protocol:

1. Limit activity to 75 percent of what you think you can do. This is the single most important measure without which nothing else can work. Some authorities go so far as to advocate limiting activities to 50 percent of the patient's tolerance. I emphasize that, if the patient becomes tired with any activity at all, then he or she has done far too

---

IN BRIEF

Chronic fatigue syndrome (CFS) is a multifactorial collection of illnesses that are very difficult to distinguish from each other but that have fatigue, muscle aches and pains, cognitive impairments, and often digestive disturbances in common. The diagnosis is by exclusion of other conditions. This leaves its management. There is, as yet, no single cure. But a staged approach frequently leads to major improvement, if not cure.

much. It seems that CFS patients must reserve at least 25 percent of their energy for getting better.

2. Reduce stress to a minimum. A real motherhood piece of advice that is often impossible to achieve.

3. Take vitamin C as per the instructions in the inset below.

4. Take a calcium/magnesium supplement equivalent to 1,000 mg of calcium per day for muscle pains and cramps.

5. Take eight capsules of evening primrose oil per day.[21]

6. Avoid junk foods.

Most patients will show some improvement on this line of management. In fact, if the duration of the illness has been less than two years, my experience is that a substantial majority of these patients will be cured by this line of management. Even if a cure does not occur, this does bring the patient onto a new plateau of health, and every other measure taken from this point on may bring the patient to a new plateau.

Other Therapies

Guided by the result of the investigations and other clues, I find that the following measures can improve matters for patients, bringing them stepwise to new plateaus of health.

A Hypoglycemic-Type Diet

Particularly, if the patient has an abnormal glucose tolerance test showing reactive hyperinsulinism; this is a slightly more rigorous form of the "junk-free diet" emphasizing a good breakfast and small, frequent snacks through the rest of the day, as opposed to three square gorges.[22]

A Therapeutic Fast and Provocative Food Test

Especially, if there is reason to believe that sensitivities to certain foods may be present,[23] a therapeutic fast may be suggested followed by a provocative food test.[24] For instructions on how to undertake a therapeutic fast, see the inset "Step 1: The Basics of Therapeutic Fasting" on the following page.

When you have successfully completed the fast, remember that it is only the first step. If you do nothing further, you will soon lose all the ground that

---

HOW TO TAKE VITAMIN C

Vitamin C is available in tablet or powder form.

- Vitamin C 1,000-mg tablets: It is best to take tablets with the strongest dose because they are the cheapest. If there are side effects from these, they are likely due to excipients (additives in the pills). Change brands without cornstarch, or use the pure crystalline powder, as below.

- Vitamin C crystals or powder: One-quarter teaspoon is roughly 1,000 mg. Take the ascorbic acid with a quarter teaspoonful of baking soda to neutralize it (if tablets cause acidity, use baking soda with them as well). Or try one-quarter teaspoon of calcium ascorbate or sodium ascorbate (nonacidic vitamin C salts). Use dissolved in unsweetened juice or water; like any excellent medicine, it does not taste good.

- Take vitamin C after food either three or four times per day, depending on your convenience and choice.

- Start with about 1,000 mg per dose.

- Every day increase the dose by 1,000 mg per dose. For example, on day 1, take 1,000 mg three or four times per day; on day 2, take 2,000 mg three or four times per day; and on day 3, take 3,000 mg three or four times per day, and so on.

- Continue, no matter how large the dose, until you get loose stool.

- Cut the dose down to the largest dose at which you do not get loose stool. The ideal result is to have two large, easy bowel motions per day.[20]

STEP 1: THE BASICS OF THERAPEUTIC FASTING

The following is the handout I provide to the patients to read and consider at length before they embark upon a therapeutic fast. It's important to know what to expect, especially because a person is apt to feel worse before feeling better.

When a person fasts, the individual starts feeling as if he or she is starving. This goes on for 48 hours, the person feeling worse and worse—and often wondering what they are doing and why. Then a chemical shift occurs in the body. It begins around the 48-hour mark. As it develops, the person feels better and better, and his or her mind becomes clearer and clearer. Usually between four and six days after the fast begins, the person feels better than ever before, free of any symptoms caused by (suspected) food allergies/sensitivities. Occasionally, it may take 10 days, or rarely, even longer. The maximum length of time I have taken a patient through a fast is 36 days, without harm.

Keep the following in mind:

1. Be determined. Decide that the fast is necessary, and that you need to stick with it through thick and thin, good and bad.

2. No food!

3. No drinks but water.

4. No candies or chocolates.

5. No cigarettes!

6. Drink plenty of spring or mountain water (if not available, then bottled), at least three liters (about 100 ounces) per day.

7. Get plenty of physical: a) if fasting at home, continue normal routine and take extra walks of at least two miles per day; b) if fasting in a hospital, walk around as much as possible and make frequent use of the exercise equipment in the physiotherapy room.

8. Twice daily showers or baths.

9. Expect that the first 48 hours will be the worst, and increasingly severe before there is any improvement.

you have so courageously gained through the fast. Unless you go on to testing yourself, it was pointless to do the fast. The next step is a provocative food testing. For instructions, see the inset "Step 2: The Basics of Provocative Food Testing" at right.

Sleep

Lack of effective sleep is among the most distressing symptoms of CFS. The usual hypnotics are usually ineffective or poorly tolerated. As noted above, most of the tricyclic antidepressants are poorly tolerated, almost diagnostic of CFS. But small doses of such antidepressants may help sleep quite well. The best-tolerated drug of this group seems to be trazodone (Desyrel); zopiclone (Imovane), not an antidepressant, also seems well tolerated and effective for sleep. Clonazepam (Klonopin), alone of the anti-anxiety benzodiazepine drugs, also seems helpful.

Antidepressants

While CFS is not depression, depression often logically occurs in CFS and makes it the potentially lethal condition with the risk of suicide. Serotonin reuptake inhibitors such as doxepin (Sinequan), clomipramine (Anafranil), and trazodone boost serotonin levels in the brain and in small doses are often effective and tolerated. (Serotonin is one of the brain's principal brain chemicals responsible for improving mood.) Some of the selective serotonin reuptake inhibitors are even more effective, but they take between one and four months to begin to show their effectiveness. Often gastrointestinal disturbances occur early on with them, but usually these settle down again quite soon. Fluoxetine (Prozac) I have not found useful. But many patients have benefited from sertraline (Zoloft). Since these agents work best if given in the morning after breakfast, they may be used in combination with the drugs used to help sleep. Phenelzine, a monoamine oxidase inhibitor that prevents the substance monoamine oxidase from breaking down serotonin, has helped one of my patients.

Thyroid Hormone

Even if thyroid function testing seems normal, if the patient's basal temperature is below 96.8°F (36°C), a trial of thyroid hormone might improve

STEP 2: THE BASICS OF PROVOCATIVE FOOD TESTING

This list is designed to be used only after the patient has successfully passed through a therapeutic fast and is free of *all* symptoms. The testing is carried out by exposing the patient to only *one* new food substance at a time, either by eating or drinking it, the time being most conveniently mealtimes.

If there is a reaction, this will be felt as a return of any, or all, or any combination of the patient's symptoms, or a rise in pulse rate, between 20 and 30 minutes after trying the food, of greater than 10 beats per minute over the rate at the time the food was taken—where there is no other explanation of that rise. Very rarely, reactions may be delayed for up to 60 to 90 minutes.

No reaction will last for more than an hour or so.

From these reactions (or lack of) two lists are built up. The first list consists of those foods to which a reaction took place and that should be avoided whenever possible thereafter. The second list consists of those foods to which no reaction occurred, and that can be safely taken at any of all of the following meals. All mealtimes following a fast should be considered testing sessions. (Numbers refer to notes below.)

Milk[1]	Coffee	Tomato
Bread[2]	Tea	Carrot
Corn[3]	Sugar	Celery
Eggs	Salt	Broccoli
Bacon[4]	Pepper	Cucumber
Apricots	Pineapple	Raspberries
Cheeses[5]	Peanuts	Cauliflower
Beef	Peas	Zucchini
Chicken	Rice	Apple
Turkey	Potato	Pear
Fish[6]	Lettuce	Orange
Cherries	Peach	Strawberries

The actual order should be varied according to circumstances and convenience.

Foods not on the list that are particularly liked, and taken often, or disliked, and taken rarely, should be added to this list because there is a strong possibility that these are the most likely offending foods.

Care should be taken that only one new food is added at each mealtime so there is no confusion at all over which is the substance that might be causing the trouble.

The list is only preliminary and just forms the basis for detailed and life-long testing.

This is not a scientific exercise, but a tool for long-term change in lifestyle. Like real life it is a matter of trial and error.

If you start deteriorating again, something has been missed. There is no problem about fasting again until you become well again. Then you can backtrack on the testing until you have found what was missed.

Foods may occur in combination. It is vital to become knowledgeable about what is actually in what you eat. The unsuspected ingredient is what may be making you ill. Where you are in any doubt, leave it alone.

What makes this horribly difficult is that you may be reacting to other environmental factors as well. These include pollution from nearby industry, such as pulp-mills, fumes from floor cleaning chemicals or paint, scents in cosmetics worn by visitors, contaminants in the water supply, molds, spores, pollens, animal dander, and infections (candida being especially important). Too much artificial light can be harmful, or too little sunlight. Most important of all is cigarette smoke.

If too many foods are found to cause reactions for avoidance to be possible or practicable, or something(s) is being consistently missed, then referral to a knowledgeable dietitian who has experience with "rotation diets" can be made.

This is not a list of all possible foods. It is a general guide to further testing, and other foods should be added to it as they are encouraged.

NOTES:

1. One glass of milk is representative of all dairy products, and anything to which dairy products have been added.

2. Two slices of bread, representative of all wheat products, and anything to which wheat has been added.

3. Corn is added to many processed foods. Read the labels.

4. Ham can be used instead; neither should be sugar cured.

5. Even though you test against dairy products and do not react, you cannot assume that you do not react to cheese. Each of the cheeses should be tested individually.

6. Each kind of fish, shellfish especially (allergies to these can be severe), should be tested individually.

the energy levels of the patient. But this should be monitored with frequent thyroid-stimulating hormone (TSH) tests to prevent hyperthyroidism (too much thyroid hormonal activity), which can be very exhausting and dangerous.

Vitamins

• *Vitamin B12:* Even if blood vitamin B12 (cobalamin) levels are normal, injections of vitamin B12 have helped a lot of my patients. Vitamin B12 is an excellent anti-anxiety, antidepressant, and anti-fatigue vitamin. I am not at all impressed with oral therapy with this vitamin. The dose and frequency of injections are highly individual. The color of the injection solution is the natural color of the vitamin, not that of any additive, since it is self-preserving. The best dose is that which just tinges the urine some time over the next six hours or so after an injection, ranging from 1,000 to 25,000 micrograms (mcg) per dose. And the benefits of each injection, if an effective dose is given, are apparent within one to two days. How long each injection is effective is also highly variable. Some patients need an injection every day, every second day, or so, up to every one to two months. If the dose of the vitamin B12 has to be reduced or given less frequently, as shown by increased spillage of color into the urine, this is an indication that the patient's condition is improving. A similar effect happens with vitamin C, a return of diarrhea forcing reduction of dosage indicating an improvement of the illness.

• *Coenzyme Q10 (CoQ10):* This solid, waxlike substance is derived from cholesterol and is critical in the cellular energy-generating system called oxidative phosphorylation. CoQ10 is often helpful in improving patients' energy levels to a greater or lesser extent—rather like vitamin B12. From 150 to 300 mg per day seems the best doses range.

• *Niacin:* The famous niacin flush is very exhausting to patients with CFS. This limits vitamin B3's usefulness. But if it can be tolerated in the dose of 3,000 mg per day, it does seem to help with both the depression and the poor energy. The procedure I use to introduce it is as follows: Start with 100 mg

tablets. Take one-half tablet three times per day after meals for one week. Then, take 1 tablet three times per day after meals until finished. Next, switch to the 500-mg tablets. Take one-half tablet three times per day after meals for one week. Then, take 1 tablet three times per day after meals for one week. Then, take 2 tablets three times per day after meals for the rest of your life.

• *Pyridoxine:* Vitamin B6 does help in CFS in a dose of 500 mg per day. The reported neuropathy, which has scared many patients from taking it, only happens if no other vitamins are being used and is very rare. It is particularly useful in women if the CFS is complicated by premenstrual syndrome when the dose is doubled from the time of ovulation to the onset of menses. The effect is partially, at least, due to the inhibition of prolactin from the pituitary.

• *Thiamine:* Vitamin B1 helps in a fashion similar to vitamin B6, but I know of no corresponding endocrine effect.

• *Other Vitamins:* On an individual basis, combinations of other water-soluble and fat-soluble vitamins have also helped some patients. I know of no way of predicting who will respond to what, except by trial and error.

Activity

Increasing activity can be a good thing, but it must be restricted to the limits of the patients' energy levels. Otherwise they get worse not better.

Pain Relief

Non-steroidal anti-inflammatory drugs (NSAIDs) are almost universally unhelpful in patients with CFS. The one exception seems to be ketorolac (Toradol), which is helpful with the muscle pains. As the muscle pains improve with the general improvement in the patient's condition, the pains tend to become localized into discrete trigger points. These respond, just as in fibromyalgia, to local injections of local anesthetics within seconds. Such injections are not curative however, but the need for them, that is the number of trigger points, becomes less with time.

Psychotherapy

The only psychotherapy of any value to CFS patients is explanation of the condition and education about its nature and management. There have been numerous attempts by psychiatrists to rationalize this condition as being in some ways psychogenic[25-27] and to make it their exclusive arena of management. But their arguments have been subject to close critical study and found lacking in any factual basis.[28,29] Other measures that do help include relaxation techniques such as deep, slow breathing, balanced relaxation (especially helpful with headaches), focused relaxation (especially helpful when there are stress effects from the unconscious, more effective than formal psychotherapy, and cheaper), relaxation tapes (but can be a stress to a CFS patient in their own right), and meditation.

■ CONCLUSION

None of these measures are curative, but, when they, or any combination of these therapies, are added to the basic protocol, the combination may bring the patient as close to a cure as can be expected. I must emphasize that when a treatment has been tried and has shown no benefit over three to four months, it ought to be abandoned. I also have to grant that a substantial portion of patients become well again in time. These treatments, it might be argued, may be of purely placebo effect. But no one has shown that CFS is a placebo-responsive illness. Nor do placebos take months or years to take effect. No curative therapy for CFS is yet available, except, in some instances, when treatment can be begun in less than two years from the onset of the illness. But in a staged manner, considerable improvement can be achieved in a majority of patients.

REFERENCES

1. Buchwald D, et al. A chronic illness characterized by fatigue, neurologic and immunologic disorders, and active human herpes virus type 6 infection. *Ann Intern Med* 1992;116:103–113.

2. Behan WMH, et al. Mitochondrial abnormalities in the post viral fatigue syndrome. *Acta Neuropathologica* 1991;83:61–65.

3. Demitrack MA, et al. Evidence for impaired activation of the Hypothalamic-pituitary adrenal axis in patients with chronic fatigue syndrome. *J Clin. Endocrin & Metab* 1991;73(6):1224–1234.

4. Bakheit AMO, et al. Possible up regulation of hypothalamic 5-hydroxytryptamine receptors in patients with post viral fatigue syndrome. *BMJ* 1992;304:1010–1012.

5. Archard LC, et al. Post-viral fatigue syndrome: persistence of enterovirus RNA in muscle and elevated creatine kinase. *J R Soc Med* 1988;81:326–329.

6. Gow JW, et al. Enteroviral sequences detected by polymerase chain reaction in muscle biopsies of patients with the post viral fatigue syndrome. *BMJ* 1991;302:692–696.

7. Behan PO, et al. The post viral fatigue syndrome: an analysis of the findings in 50 cases. *J Infect* 1985;10:211–222.

8. Gow JW, Behan WMH. Amplification and identification of enteroviral sequences in the post viral fatigue syndrome. *Br Med Bull* 1991;47:872–885.

9. Jamal GA, Hansen S. Post-viral fatigue syndrome: evidence of underlying organic disturbance in the muscle fibre. *Eur Neurol* 1989;29:272–276.

10. Arnold DL, et al. Excessive intracellular acidosis of skeletal muscle on exercise in a patient with a postviral exhaustion/fatigue syndrome: a P31 nuclear magnetic resonance study. *Lancet* 1984;i:1367–1369.

11. Jones J. Possible role for Epstein-Barr Virus (EBV) in the chronic fatigue syndrome. In: *The Clinical and Scientific Basis of Myalgic Encephalomyelitis–Chronic Fatigue Syndrome* edited by JA Goldstein. Ottawa, ON: Nightingale Research Foundation, 1992, 269–277.

12. Dowsett EG, et al. Myalgic encephalomyelitis (M.E.): a persistent enteroviral infection? In: *The Clinical and Scientific Basis of Myalgic Encephalomyelitis–Chronic Fatigue Syndrome* edited by JA Goldstein. Ottawa, ON: Nightingale Research Foundation, 1992, 269–277, 285–291.

13. Yousef GE, et al. Chronic enterovirus infection in patients with postviral fatigue syndrome, *Lancet* 1988;i:146–150.

14. Archard LC, Cunningham L. Molecular virology of muscle disease: persistent virus infection of muscle in patients with postviral fatigue syndrome. In: *The Clinical and Scientific Basis of Myalgic Encephalomyelitis–Chronic Fatigue Syndrome* edited by JA Goldstein. Ottawa, ON: Nightingale Research Foundation, 1992, 343–347.

15. Warner CL, et al. Neuromuscular abnormalities in patients with chronic fatigue syndrome. In: *The Clinical and Scientific Basis of Myalgic Encephalomyelitis–Chronic Fatigue Syndrome*, edited by JA Goldstein. Ottawa, ON: Nightingale Research Foundation, 1992, 348–351.

16. Doyle D. An account of 100 muscle biopsies in epidemic myalgic encephalomyelitis (EME). In: *The Clinical and Scientific Basis of Myalgic Encephalomyelitis–Chronic Fatigue Syndrome* edited by JA Goldstein. Ottawa, ON: Nightingale Research Foundation, 1992, 352–356..

17. Hyde B, et al. Magnetic resonance in the diagnosis of M.E./CFS: a review. In: *The Clinical and Scientific Basis of Myalgic Encephalomyelitis–Chronic Fatigue Syndrome* edited by JA Goldstein. Ottawa, ON: Nightingale Research Foundation, 1992, 425–431.

18. Mowbray JF, Yousef GE. Immunology of postviral fatigue syndrome. *British Medical Bulletin*, 1991:Al A:886–894.

19. Paterson ET. Aspects of hypoglycemia. *J Orthomolecular Pysch* 1982;11:151–155.

20. Cathcart RC. *Proceedings Orthomolecular medical society.* 2nd Annual Meeting, San Francisco, Feb. 1977.

21. Behan PO, et al. The use of EFAs in chronic fatigue syndrome. *Acta Neurol Scand* 1990;82:209–216.

22. Jenkins DJA, et al. Nibbling versus gorging: metabolic advantages of increased meal frequency. *NEJM* 1989;321(14):929–934.

23. Loblay RH, Swain AR. The role of food intolerance in chronic fatigue syndrome. In: *The Clinical and Scientific Basis of Myalgic Encephalomyelitis–Chronic Fatigue Syndrome* edited by JA Goldstein. Ottawa, ON: Nightingale Research Foundation, 1992, 521–538.

24. Cott A. Controlled fasting treatment for schizophrenia. *J Orthomolecular Pysch* 1974;3(4):301–311.

25. Woods TO, Goldberg DP. Psychiatric perspectives: an overview, post-viral fatigue syndrome. *British Medical Bulletin* 1991:908–918.

26. Sharpe M. Psychiatric management of PVFS: post-viral fatigue syndrome. *British Medical Bulletin* 1991:989–1005.

27. Davis H. CFS: fact or fiction? *BCMJ* 1993:35(8):582–584.

28. Dutton DG. Depression/somatization explanations for the chronic fatigue syndrome: a critical review. In: *The Clinical and Scientific Basis of Myalgic Encephalomyelitis–Chronic Fatigue Syndrome* edited by JA Goldstein. Ottawa, ON: Nightingale Research Foundation, 1992, 491–508.

29. Hickie I. The psychiatric status of patients with the chronic fatigue syndrome. In: *The Clinical and Scientific Basis of Myalgic Encephalomyelitis–Chronic Fatigue Syndrome* edited by JA Goldstein. Ottawa, ON: Nightingale Research Foundation, 1992, 509–518.

VITAMIN C AND FATIGUE

by Emanuel Cheraskin, MD, DMD

What is the connection between vitamin C and fatigue? The correlations are abundant, beginning with the earliest medical writings and still appearing in the most recent professional literature.

A Look Back into the Future

There is the old adage, variously described that, those who have not read history are destined to repeat it. At the end of the Middle Ages, sailors began to make ever more daring voyages out from western Europe. We know that Portuguese sailors began to explore Africa in the 1400s, finally rounding the Cape in 1487. It soon became obvious, though, that on such voyages the men at sea became quite ill. Their hands and feet swelled and their gums grew over their teeth, which made eating difficult if not impossible. One of the earliest, most impressive and relevant findings was inordinate tiredness. As a matter of fact, many a sailor was punished because the captain accused him of malingering. The truth of the matter was the poor soul was too tired to perform his duties.

For our purposes, we can skip the subsequent experiences with the French, English, and the Dutch. There is ample documentation that their navies suffered the same fate. Back to the Portuguese, who quite by accident encountered the Moors, who were carrying oranges, which seemed to provide a magical cure.

One naval surgeon who became particularly interested in the devastation of scurvy at sea was James Lind, now the most celebrated name in the history of this subject. It was during one such outbreak of scurvy that this British physician carried out his now famous experiment, probably the first controlled trial in clinical nutrition, or even in any branch of clinical science. He studied a group of sailors all with scurvy under what today would be viewed as an acceptable double-blind experience. This terrible syndrome responded almost magically to the consumption of oranges and lemons.

The Now and New Scurvy

As we have just learned, the vitamin C connection was established with the recognition that, an absence of what later became known as vitamin C, led to a fatal disease identified as scurvy.

When the correlation was finally and firmly established, the scientific community rested with the happy thought that here was a specific substance associated with a specific syndrome.

From this time on until the middle of the 1900s, not much occurred clinically. True, there were some isolated brilliant discoveries like the 1928 identification of vitamin C by Albert Szent Györgyi. However, from a practical clinical standpoint, the two centuries from 1750 to the early 1900s could be viewed as the dark ages.

In October 1939, John Crandon,[1] a resident surgeon attached to Harvard Medical School placed himself on a diet of bread, crackers, eggs, cheese, beer, pure chocolate, and sugar with supplements of yeast and all the then known vitamins other than C. At the beginning of the trial, chemical analysis of his blood plasma for ascorbic acid gave a value of 1.0 milligrams (mg) percent. Crandon had continued his surgical work all this time. And most important to point out, before he demonstrated any physical signs, there was an obvious feeling of tiredness. After 26 weeks, Crandon was given a fatigue test. He could run at seven miles per hour for only 16 seconds and showed rapid exhaustion in other measurements. One gram (1,000 mg) of C was given intravenously each day for a week. A subjective improvement was noticed in the first 24 hours.

Five investigators from Zagreb, in the former Republic of Yugoslavia,[2] looked beyond this traditional concept. They sought the acme (the ultimate in well-being) through a continuing series of vitamin studies extending over a number of years. One phase emphasized the effect of ascorbic acid supplementation on physical working capacity in adolescent boys. After daily administration for two months of 70 mg ascorbic acid, the mean plasma vitamin C in the 49 subjects in the experimental group rose four and one-half fold. There was a bonus of improved oxygen utilization. Conversely, no convincing changes in biochemical state or in oxygen consumption could be shown in the 42 placebo-supplemented children. Hence, according to Suboticanec-Buzina and his Yugoslavian colleagues from the Department of Nutrition at the Institute of Public Health, it is clear that overall performance can be heightened even in seemingly healthy kids.

There is much more to the story. One vitamin C expert (Dr. C. A. B. Clemetson, author of a monumental three-volume review of the subject[3]) best described the picture: clearly about half the boys in the supplemented group showed a very marked increase in working capacity, such as would likely make the difference between losing and winning their next soccer game. Moreover, their improved ascorbate status could lift their spirits and would most probably improve their resistance to infection.

More Vitamin C, Less Fatigue

We here at the University of Alabama Medical Center have also looked at this connection.[4] The vitamin C intake of 411 dentists and their spouses was determined from data on daily vitamin C consumption in a food-frequency questionnaire. The mean number of fatigue symptoms listed in answers to the seven questions comprising Section I of the Cornell Medical Index Health Questionnaire (CMI) was designated the fatigability score. The relationship between the two variables was determined by calculating the tiredness grade for different levels of vitamin C intake.

The 81 subjects who consumed less than 100 mg of ascorbic acid per day reported a fatigability mark averaging 0.81. Conversely, the 330 participants ingesting more than 400 mg of the ascorbates per day reported an exhaustion index of only 0.41. Those taking the RDA for vitamin C reported approximately twice the fatigue symptomatology as those taking about seven times the RDA.

Quite apart, it is well known that, with advancing age, there is increasing weariness. Old people get more tired than young folks. With that in mind, these same data were reexamined in terms of the aging process.[5] With time, there is a rise in fatigability in those individuals consuming approximately 41 mg of C. In contrast, people ingesting an average of 318 mg of the ascorbates do not display this increment. What is particularly noteworthy is that the average 57-year-old utilizing about seven times the RDA showed a mean score (0.4), which is less than the average 33-year-old (0.7) demonstrating the RDA for vitamin C.

REFERENCES

1. Crandon JH. *N Engl J Med* 1940;223(10):353–369.

2. Suboticanec-Buzina K. *International Journal for Vitamin and Nutrition Research* 1984;54(1):55–60.

3. Clemetson CAB. *Vitamin C*. Boca Raton, FL: CRC Press, 1989.

4. Cheraskin E. *J Am Geriatr Soc* 1976;24(3): 136–137.

5. Cheraskin E. Unpublished data.

From the *J Orthomolecular Med* 1994;9(1):39–45.

CHANGES IN WORKER FATIGUE AFTER VITAMIN C ADMINISTRATION

by Hang-Hwan Yeom, MD, PhD, Gyou Chul Jung, MD, Sang Woo Shin, MD,

Sun Hyun Kim, MD, PhD, Jong Soon Choi, MD, Whang Jae Lee, MD, PhD,

Jae S Kang, MD, PhD, Keun Jeong Song, MD, PhD

Fatigue is extremely common in patients. Everybody experiences this symptom during life, even in the absence of any disease. However, doctors, as well as the general population, tend to neglect symptoms of fatigue, attributing it not to illness but to a normal response to the exertions of life.

The relevant rates of fatigue prevalence vary considerably, depending on whether the fatigue being examined is characterized by tiredness, weakness, or exhaustion. The phenomenon of fatigue is usually divided into fatigue, chronic fatigue, and chronic fatigue syndrome. The boundary between fatigue, chronic fatigue, and chronic fatigue syndrome is also fairly arbitrary, as these are obviously subjective terms.[1] According to many researchers, the prevalence of fatigue was more than 27 percent, whereas chronic fatigue had a prevalence of 1–10 percent and chronic fatigue syndrome evidenced a prevalence of 0.2–0.7 percent in the general population.[2–6] In our home country of Korea, Kim and others reported that the prevalence of chronic fatigue was 8.4 percent and that chronic fatigue syndrome occurred in 0.6 percent of the general population.[7]

The prevalence and severity of fatigue in workers is substantially higher than in the general population due to the stress inherent to the modern work environment. Also, many workers have many diseases or risk factors of many diseases. If workers don't take early steps to reduce their fatigue, they may experience serious difficulty and reduced work efficiency.

Despite considerable worldwide efforts, no single cause has been discovered to explain fatigue symptoms. It appears likely that multiple factors promote its development, sometimes with the same factors both causing and being caused by fatigue. A great number of recent studies have demonstrated that oxidative stress may be involved in its development. The role of oxidative stress in fatigue is an important area for current and future research, as it suggests the use of antioxidants in the treatment of fatigue. Specifically, the dietary supplements glutathione, N-acetyl cysteine, alpha-lipoic acid, oligomeric proanthocyanidins, ginkgo biloba, vitamin C, and *Vaccinium myrtillus* (bilberry) may exert beneficial effects.[8,9]

Vitamin C is a powerful antioxidant, and exists in a variety of fruits and vegetables.

Fatigue is the initial symptom of experimental scurvy, and a marginal vitamin C deficiency may induce fatigue, lassitude, and depression—all of which have been shown to respond to supplementation.[10–13] Although some early reports have failed to find any evidence of decreased serum levels of vitamin C in chronic fatigue syndrome (CFS) patients, no current assay technique for the measurement of ascorbic acid is entirely satisfactory; therefore, this single report of serum vitamin C levels arguably does not eliminate the possibility that a subset of CFS patients may be vitamin C deficient.[14,15]

The principal objective of this study was to evaluate changes in fatigue in workers after vitamin C administration.

Materials and Methods

We consecutively examined 44 workers who work regularly from 9:00 A.M. to 6:00 P.M. The exclusion criteria included the following: pregnancy, cancer, cardiovascular diseases, and infection.

Written consent was obtained from all study subjects. They were orally administered 6,000 milligrams (mg) of vitamin C daily for two weeks. We then investigated the demographic data and assessed any changes in the patients' fatigue scale and blood tests. The demographic data included the sex, age, and exercise status of the patients. The

From the *J Orthomolecular Med* 2008;23(4):205–209.

fatigue scales used included both a fatigue severity scale (FSS) and a visual analogue scale (VAS).[16] The blood tests conducted included vitamin C; hemoglobin A1C (HgA1C), C-reactive protein (CRP), aspartate aminotranferase (AST), alanine aminotranferase (ALT), r-GTP, and cortisol. The fatigue scale and blood test levels prior to and after vitamin C administration were compared.

Results

The subjects included 27 males (67.5 percent) and 13 females (32.5 percent). The patients' ages ranged from 34 to 39. No patients were excluded due to side effects of vitamin C.

Fatigue Severity Scale

The FSS is a 9-item scale that measures the severity of fatigue and how much it affects the person's activities and lifestyle, with scores ranging from 1 to 7. Patients are asked to respond to each statement (e.g., "I am easily fatigued," "Exercise brings on my fatigue," etc.) on a scale of 1 to 7, with 1 indicating "strongly disagree" and 7 indicating "strongly agree." A higher score indicates higher fatigue levels. The VAS, the other fatigue scale used, consists of 18 items relating to the subjective experience of fatigue. Each item asks patients to place an "X," representing how they currently feel, along a visual analogue line that extends between two extremes (e.g., from "not at all tired" to "extremely tired"). In fatigue, both FSS and VAS improved after vitamin C administration. VAS scores improved on average from 5.5–7.5 to 4.5–6.5 after vitamin C administration. Also, FSS improved from 5.0–6.5 to 3.5–4.5 after vitamin C administration.

Blood Tests

The blood tests prior to and after vitamin C administration were reduced. The vitamin C level in the blood increased from 43–55.0 to 69.0–95.0 micromoles per liter (µmol/L) after vitamin C administration. In liver function tests, the subjects reported significantly lower levels of AST, ALT, and r-GTP following vitamin C administration. The cortisol levels in the blood, an indicator of adrenal stress, were reduced from 12.0–15.5 to 9.0–11.6 micrograms per deciliter (µg/dL), and CRP levels, a sign of inflammation, were reduced from 0.1–0.3 to .05–.07 milligrams per liter (mg/L) after vitamin C administration. Also, HgA1C levels, a marker of blood glucose (sugar) levels, were reduced from 6.0 to 5.0 percent after vitamin C administration.

Discussion

Fatigue is a common experience, and most people experience feelings of fatigue during their regular lives. Thus, fatigue is a property both of normal experience and of certain diseases. We believe that fatigue should be considered a symptom or disease in cases in which the fatigued person perceives him- or herself to be ill. If an individual experiences fatigue symptoms for an extended period, that individual may be suffering from a disease of which fatigue is a symptom. Particularly in workers, the prevalence of fatigue symptoms is now growing at a rapid rate, due principally to the heavy stress inherent to the modern work environment.

The cause or causes of fatigue remain unclear, however, a number of recent studies have demonstrated that oxidative stress may be involved in its development.[17] The role of oxidative stress in

IN BRIEF

In recent research, the role of oxidative stress has been an important factor in fatigue. The principal objective of this study was to evaluate changes in fatigue in workers after vitamin C administration. We consecutively examined 44 workers who work regularly. They were orally administered 6,000 milligrams of vitamin C daily for two weeks. We then investigated the demographic data and assessed any changes in the patients' fatigue scale (VAS, FSS) and blood tests (vitamin C, HgA1C, CRP, AST, ALT, r-GTP, cortisol). In fatigue, both VAS and FSS improved after vitamin C administration. In blood tests, AST, ALT, r-GTP, HgA1c, CRP, and cortisol were reduced after vitamin C administration. From this study we can conclude that vitamin C administration reduced fatigue symptoms and improved blood tests with fatigue in workers.

fatigue is an important area for current and future research, as it suggests that antioxidants might prove useful in the management of fatigue.[18]

In this study, the subjects reported significant improvements in fatigue following vitamin C administration. Vitamin C is a powerful antioxidant and an essential cofactor in the formation of carnitine, an amino acid important for producing energy.[19] Also, according to reports, approximately 15 percent of American adults are deficient in vitamin C.[20] Twenty-five years ago, this percentage was far lower, at approximately 3–5 percent of American adults.[21] Thus, modern people appear to have an unfulfilled vitamin C requirement.

In this study, subjects evidenced improvements in some blood levels (AST, ALT, r-GTP, cortisol, CRP, HgA1C) after vitamin C administration.

AST, ALT, and r-GTP, which are associated with liver function and cortisol, are all hormone-related. Reduced blood levels of these compounds on these tests were associated with improvements in the subjects' fatigue.

C-reactive protein (CRP) is secreted by the liver in response to inflammatory hormones called cytokines. It was identified recently as a stronger predictor of cardiovascular events than LDL cholesterol.[22] Recently, a meta-analysis indicated that individuals in the top third of CRP plasma concentrations (2.4 mg/L) were two times as likely to have coronary heart disease as compared to those in the lowest third of CRP concentrations (1.0 mg/L).[23] In our study, the blood levels of the subjects' CRP decreased after vitamin C administration. This result was reminiscent of several other studies showing that the antioxidant components in fruit and vegetables like carotenoids, vitamins C and E, and flavonoids may contribute to this anti-inflammatory effect.[24,25] The consumption of a diet low in antioxidants was shown to result in inflammation, whereas antioxidant supplementation has been shown to ameliorate inflammation.[26]

HgA1C is an integrated measure of plasma glucose and is intended to represent glucose concentrations in blood averaged over a two- to -three month period. In 1987, Cerami and others summarized the interaction of glucose with protein and its associa-

tion with human aging and diabetic disorders.[27] Additionally, a reduction in glycation (sugar molecules bonding to proteins or fats) has been suggested to prevent diabetic disorder and to retard the aging process. Although the duration of this study was only two weeks, the blood level of HgA1C was decreased by 0.58 percent. These results were reminiscent of those of other studies.[28,29] In the report of Khaw and others, a lowering of 0.2 in hemoglobin glycation in the population would reduce total mortality by 10 percent.[30]

CONCLUSION

In workers, fatigue is a very important problem. If workers can resolve this problem at an early time, they can help prevent fatigue-associated diseases and increase their work efficiency. After reviewing the relevant results, we believe that antioxidants such as vitamin C may serve to reduce fatigue in workers.

REFERENCES

1. Ranjith G. Epidemiology of chronic fatigue syndrome. *Occupat Med* 2005;55:13–19.

2. Meltzer H, Grill D, Petticrew M, et al. The prevalence of psychiatric morbidity amongst adults living in private households. London: *HMSO*, 1995.

3. Lloyd AR, Hickie I, Boughton CR, et al. Prevalence of chronic fatigue syndrome in an Australian population. *Med J Aust* 1990;153:522–528.

4. Bates DW, Schmitt W, Buchwald D, et al. Prevalence of fatigue and chronic fatigue syndrome in a primary care practice. *Arch Intern Med* 1993;153(24):2759–2765.

5. Kroenke K, Wood DR, Mangelsdorff AD, et al. Chronic fatigue in primary care. Prevalence, patient characteristics, and outcome. *JAMA* 1988;260(7):929–934.

6. Hickie IB, Hooker AW, Hadzi-Pavlovic D, et al. Fatigue in selected primary care settings: sociodemographic and psychiatric correlates. *Med J Aust* 1996;164(10):585–588.

7. Kim CH, Shin HC, Won CW. Prevalence of chronic fatigue and chronic fatigue syndrome in Korea: community-based primary care study. *J Korean Med Sci* 2005;20(4):529–534.

8. Jung GC, Yeom CH, Cho BC, et al. The effect of intravenous vitamin C in people with fatigue. *J Korean Acad Fam Med* 2006;27(5):391–395.

9. Grant JE, Veldee MS, Buchwald D. Analysis of dietary intake and selected nutrient concentrations in patients with chronic fatigue syndrome. *J Am Diet Assoc* 1996;96:383–386.

10. Hodges RE, Hood J, Canham JE, et al. Clinical manifestations of ascorbic acid deficiency in man. *Am J Clin Nutr* 1971;24:432–443.

11. Kinsman RA, Hood J. Some behavioral effects of ascorbic acid deficiency. *Am J Clin Nutr* 1971;24:455–464.

12. Heseker H, Kubler W, Pudel V, et al. Psychological disorders as early symptoms of a mild-to-moderate vitamin deficiency. *Ann NY Acad Sci* 1992;669:352–357.

13. Gerster H. The role of vitamin C in athletic performance. *J Am Coll Nutr* 1989;8:636–643.

14. Grant JE, Veldee MS, Buchwald D. Analysis of dietary intake and selected nutrient concentrations in patients with chronic fatigue syndrome. *J Am Diet Assoc* 1996;96(4):383–386.

15. Lee W, Davis KA, Rettmer RL, et al. Ascorbic acid status: biochemical and clinical considerations. *Am J Clin Nutr* 1988;48:286–290.

16. Krupp LB, LaRocca NG, Muir-Nash J. The Fatigue Severity Scale: Application to patients with multiple sclerosis and systemic lupus erythematosus. *Arch Neurol* 1989;46:1121–1123.

17. Logan AC, Wong C. Chronic fatigue syndrome: oxidative stress and dietary modifications. *Altern Med Rev* 2001;6(5):450–459.

18. Werbach MR. Nutritional strategies for treating chronic fatigue syndrome. *Altern Med Rev* 2000;5(2):93–108.

19. Reda E, D'Iddio S, Nicolai R, et al. The carnitine system and body composition. *Act Diabetol* 2003;40:S106–113.

20. Hampl JS, Taylor CA, Johnston CS. Vitamin C deficiency and depletion in the United States: The Third National Health and Nutrition Examination Survey, 1988–1994. *Am J Pub Health* 2004;94:870–875.

21. U.S. Department of Health and Human Services. Hematological and nutritional biochemistry reference data for persons 6 months–74 years of age: United States, 1976–1980. In: *Advance Data from Vital and Health Statistics, No. 83–1682.* Hyattsville, MD: National Center for Health Statistics, 1982, 124–139.

22. Ridker PM, Rifai N, Rose L, et al. Comparison of C-reactive protein and low-density lipoprotein cholesterol levels in the prediction of first cardiovascular events. *N Engl J Med* 2001;347:1557–1565.

23. Danesh J, Whincup P, Walker M, et al. Low-grade inflammation and coronary heart disease: prospective study and updated meta-analyses. *BMJ* 2000;321:199–204.

24. Calfee-Mason KG, Spear BT, Glauert HP. Vitamin E inhibits hepatic NF-B activation in rats administered the hepatic tumor promoter, phenobarbital. *J Nutr* 2002;132:3178–3185.

25. Meydani, SN, Wu D, Santos, MS, et al. Antioxidants and immune response in aged persons: overview of present evidence. *Am J Clin Nutr* 1995;62:1462S–76S.

26. Sanchez-Moreno C, Cano MP, de Ancos B, et al. High-pressurized orange juice consumption affects plasma vitamin C, antioxidative status and inflammatory markers in healthy humans. *J Nutr* 2003;133(7):2204–2209.

27. Cerami A, Vlassare H, Brownlee M. Glucose and aging. *Sci Am* 1987;256(5):90–96.

28. Krone CA, Ely JTA. Ascorbic acid, glycation, glycohemoglobin, and aging. *Med Hypoth* 2004;62:275–279.

29. Sargeant LA, Warham NJ, et al. Vitamin C and hyperglycemia in the European prospective investigation in cancer, Norfolk (EPIC-Norfolk) study. *Diabetes Care* 2000;23(6):726–732.

30. Khaw KT, Wareham N, et al. Glycated haemoglobin, diabetes, and mortality in men in Norfolk cohort of European Prospective Investigation of Cancer and Nutrition (EPIC Norfolk). *BMJ* 2001;322:1–6.

HIV/AIDS

IMAGINE: A 50 PERCENT REDUCTION IN AIDS cases just from vitamins. That is counterintuitive, yet demonstrated. It's been known since 1993 that nutrition stops AIDS better than any pharmaceutical drug. Over 20 years ago, a Johns Hopkins study (Tang, *Am J Epidemiol* 1993) demonstrated that supplements slow AIDS and even help halt it. The seven-year-long study of 281 HIV-positive men showed that those taking vitamins had only about one half as many new AIDS outbreaks as those not taking supplements.

The real wonder is that the dosages used were so small: only 715 milligrams of vitamin C a day, and about five times the U.S. RDA of the B vitamins and beta-carotene. Larger, orthomolecular amounts would almost certainly save still more lives. Even so, Dr. Tang and his coworkers concluded that "the highest levels of total intake (from food and supplements) of vitamins C and B1 and niacin were associated with a significantly decreased progression rate to AIDS (as were) vitamin A, niacin, and zinc."

Then, eleven years later, a Harvard study once again showed that the use of supplements slowed progression from HIV-positive to AIDS by the same astonishing 50 percent (Fawzi, *N Engl J Med* 2004). Furthermore, this newer study also reported a 27 percent decrease in deaths among AIDS patients taking vitamin supplements. Many health professionals have never heard about this study, and most of the public did not see it reported in the news media. This section documents success with perhaps the most controversial use of nutrient therapy for one of the most controversial of diseases.

Most of this chapter is new to the public and professions as well. It is very important material that previously had not seen the light of day beyond the *Journal of Orthomolecular Medicine*.

— A.W.S.

TERMS OF HIV/AIDS

AIDS. Also called acquired immune deficiency syndrome; an immune system disorder in which the body's ability to defend itself is greatly diminished.

CD4 CELL. Immune system cells that fight infection. The CD4 cell is a type of white blood (immune) cell that has molecules called CD4 on its surface; CD4 cells start the immune response that protects the body from infectious invaders such as viruses and bacteria.

CD4 CELL COUNT. A measurement of how many CD4 immune cells are circulating in the patient's blood.

DRUG COCKTAIL. No single drug has been effective in stopping the HIV virus, and thus HIV medications are taken in combination in order to be more effective. These combinations are known as HAART (highly active antiretroviral therapy) and are widely referred to as a drug cocktail.

HIV. Human immunodeficiency virus invades key white blood (immune) cells called T lymphocytes and multiplies; it causes a breakdown in the body's immune system, eventually leading to overwhelming infection and/or cancer. It belongs to a group of viruses called retroviruses.

HIV ANTIBODY TESTING. A positive result on a confirmed HIV antibody test means that HIV antibodies are present and the individual is infected (HIV-positive) with the virus; a negative result means that most likely the individual is not infected (HIV-negative) with HIV, although it can take three to six weeks, and sometimes up to three months before HIV antibodies show up.

KARNOFSKY PERFORMANCE SCALE. An assessment tool used to gauge a patient's functional status and ability to carry out activities of daily living.

LYMPHOCYTE. A type of white blood cell (also called T-cells or T-lymphocytes) that helps the body to fight infection.

SELENOENZYME GLUTATHIONE PERIOXIDASE. An enzyme made from the mineral selenium, and the amino acids cysteine, glutamine, and tryptophan, that appears to protect against viral infection and to be a prime target of the HIV virus.

VIRAL LOAD. A measurement of the amount of HIV in the blood.

ZIDOVUDINE (also known as AZT). The primary drug used to treat HIV infection.

HIV/AIDS: A NUTRIENT DEFICIENCY DISEASE?
by Harold Foster, PhD

HIV/AIDS is a very serious disease and is occurring or will be occurring everywhere . . . except in some areas where the soils are very rich in selenium such as in Senegal. This is the view of medical geographer and researcher Harold D. Foster, PhD. Dr. Foster is not only trying to persuade the scientific world of the real cause of HIV/AIDS but also how to deal with it. His following papers are very important for they point out the direction we must go.

The four essential nutrients used in Dr. Foster's African studies are non-toxic: selenium and the three amino acids, glutamine, tryptophan, and cysteine. They will do no harm, unlike AIDS drugs, which produce profound changes in lipid and lipoprotein metabolism and an increased risk of coronary artery disease. The HIV by itself impairs reverse cholesterol transport from macrophages. There is no evidence that these nutrients have any pathological impact on cholesterol metabolism. As a rule, xenobiotic (toximolecular) drugs are characterized by the large number of pages required to describe their side effects and toxic qualities. In sharp contrast orthomolecular nutrients are not toxic and any side effects are minor, rare and never life threatening. The costs of treating HIV/AIDS will be enormously reduced if these simple and effective nutrients are used.

I treated three patients with AIDS about 15 years ago and they all recovered with the use of the nutrients I normally use, including selenium. The preliminary therapeutic trials and pilot trials reported by Foster support his hypothesis that this disease is caused by a deficiency of the components of glutathione peroxidase, of which selenium is a very important one. In Africa the diet is so poor that amino acid deficiency is common. In other countries like North America this deficiency is not as marked but selenium deficiency is a significant problem.

There will be a major catastrophe if Foster's hypothesis is submerged by the antiretroviral idea and is not examined as quickly and fully as possible.

—ABRAM HOFFER

As described in many of my published papers and my book *What Really Causes AIDS* (2006), because HIV (human immunodeficiency virus) and humans both encode for the selenoenzyme glutathione peroxidase, the virus competes with its host for the four nutrients required to produce this antiviral enzyme, namely: selenium, cysteine, tryptophan, and glutamine. I have argued that this means the symptoms of AIDS can be prevented by supplementation with this trace element and three amino acids. What follows is supporting evidence for this hypothesis.

Here is a report from the girlfriend of a former drug addict who, in the spring of 2002, became the first AIDS patient to use this nutritional approach. He was infected by hepatitis A, B, and C and, of course, HIV.

My partner began taking the cocktail while still using cocaine, heroin, and other drugs, as well as drinking his face off. The alcoholism at first got worse as he sought to replace harder drugs with beer. During this time he had full-blown AIDS and it seemed certain he would be dead soon despite the HAART [highly active antiretroviral therapy] cocktail prescription. After talking to you and reading your book together [*What Really Causes AIDS*], we focused on nutrition, specifically getting the selenium into him, and also me as an extra protection against exposure to the viruses.

We also understood better the relationship between the drugs and alcohol and the progression of his diseases. Even after the HIV seemed to be under control, his hep C was bothering him. As he learned to take better care of himself nutritionally, and eventually managed to quit all substances with the help of NA [Narcotics Anonymous], he seemed to be on the road to health. Within a few months his viral load was

From the *J Orthomolecular Med* 2005;20(2):67–69.

undetectable. When he went travelling and was unable to access either the cocktail or the nutrients, he quickly became ill again. By the time he came home he was once again quite sick, full-blown AIDS. However, after returning home and once again taking the selenium and other nutrients you suggested, as well as returning to the cocktail, he quickly got better. This time the improvement happened over a period of weeks.

"People's minds are changed through observation and not through argument."
—WILL ROGERS

Open Clinical Trials in Africa

As of November 2004, this former dying hepatitis A-, B-, and C-AIDS patient is symptom free and working on a construction site doing heavy labor. About a year ago, I set up HD Foster Research Inc. to produce a product containing selenium, cysteine, tryptophan, and glutamine in a single capsule. I then began giving this product away to African hospices, hospitals, and clinics where HIV/AIDS patients were being treated. Open trials began in an AIDS hospice in South Africa, where five out of six AIDS patients greatly improved. We discovered in South Africa that problem cases had extreme diarrhea, developed secondary deficiencies, and could not absorb adequate nutrients. Future trials will probably provide the nutrients in powder form to such patients. The other initial

small trial took place in a Kenyan clinic. The patients there were weak and passing into AIDS. They soon recovered their energy and are now in much better health. None of the patients in either of these trials had ever taken antiretroviral drugs.

Encouraged by these results, two larger open trials were set up. The first, in a Ugandan hospital, involved 40 HIV/AIDS patients. After one month, 77 percent reported a noticeable improvement in their health. These results were better than they seemed at first glance because seven of these patients also had tuberculosis and four also suffered from syphilis. Improvement continued with the passage of time. As a student helping to conduct this open, quality-of-life trial wrote: "One of our patients, who was on home care, walked into the clinic on Monday, which was exciting for us. There was also a man we hadn't met before, who had been a homecare patient of [two earlier medical students involved in the trial], and he had been bedridden for four years. He also walked into the clinic on Monday!"

In Zambia, the nutritional supplements were provided to a childcare and adoption society. The initial report from this organization was on 15 orphans and guardians who were HIV/AIDS patients; several also had tuberculosis. Here is a direct quotation:

> The general impressions [of the use of the nutrients] from our target group were positive and encouraging. Most people given, improved within the first two weeks of taking these food supplements (i.e., a noticeable improvement started between second to third week of taking

IN BRIEF

AIDS is a deficiency disease caused by HIV. HIV-1 contains a gene that is virtually identical to that which allows humans to produce the enzyme, glutathione peroxidase. As the virus is replicated, it begins to seriously compete with its host for the four nutrients needed to make this enzyme, specifically the trace element selenium and the three amino acids, glutamine, cysteine, and tryptophan. As infection increases, serious deficiencies of these nutrients develop. Inadequate selenium causes the immune system to collapse, the thyroid to malfunction, and depression to develop. Glutamine deficiency leads to muscle wasting and diarrhea. Shortages of cysteine result in skin problems such as psoriasis and greater susceptibility to infection. A lack of tryptophan causes diarrhea, dermatitis, dementia, and ultimately death. It becomes easy for other pathogens to infect the patient, and the infected person has developed the disorder we call AIDS. The treatment of HIV/AIDS, therefore, should always include diets elevated in these four nutrients to reverse such deficiencies.

the supplements). For instance most people given had their complexions improve, hair texture, and general outlook of their bodies improved. The supplements also made them to have enough energy to even move around, others have gained weight, and some of those who were bedridden have even started walking on their own.

Additional Confirmations and Observations

Beyond such open clinical trials, I have been receiving e-mails from HIV/AIDS patients who have read *What Really Causes AIDS* and have followed the protocol that was suggested in this book. Here is the most recent example, received November 5, 2004.

> I am an HIV-positive patient. Since I started following your (selenium, cysteine, tryptophan, and glutamine) remedy I have remarkably recovered. I came across your article in a magazine *Nexus* by chance and that's when I started the remedy. To be honest, I was nearly dying and I would like to take this opportunity to thank you for your help and advice you are giving to the HIV sufferers. My HIV tests are now alternating from positive (+) to negative (-), well I reckon soon I will stay on the negative for good.

At a recent workshop, at which I lectured on HIV/AIDS and other diseases, a doctor informed me that prior to my book's publication, he usually had about 30 HIV/AIDS patients. Today, he routinely refers them to *What Really Causes AIDS* and he now has none sick enough to need his attention.

A publication that supports the nutritional treatment of HIV/AIDS is definitely worth mentioning here. Roland Kupka, Sc.D., and colleagues have published a paper on the relationship between death from AIDS and plasma selenium levels in pregnant women, in Tanzania.[1] In summary, blood was collected from 949 pregnant women and saved for 5.7 years, by which time 306 of them had died. Statistical analyses showed that the lower her original plasma selenium level, the more likely the woman was to have died of AIDS. This selenium-death relationship was statistically significant. This link, of course, has been obvious for years and is the key to at least slowing the diffusion of HIV. It's unfortunate that 306 women had to die to prove the obvious, as the previously described open trials have shown, HIV/AIDS patients need extra selenium.

■ CONCLUSION

In closing, I would like to make a few additional observations. There can be little doubt that AIDS is a nutritional disease, caused by a virus. However, AIDS patients with severe diarrhea also develop secondary nutritional deficiencies that, in and by themselves, can, if neglected, prove fatal. As a result, my next batch of nutritional supplements includes a well-balanced vitamin/mineral mixture, designed to address that problem, in addition to the key nutrients, selenium, cysteine, tryptophan, and glutamine. Patients taking antiretrovirals as well as the four key nutrients seem to progress very well, showing that there is no antagonism between the conventional treatment and my own suggested protocol. However, HAART, no doubt, still carries its normal side effects. What is needed now is a large (200 patient) scientific study that cannot be ignored so easily.

REFERENCES

1. Kupka R, Msamanga GI, Spiegelman D, et al. Selenium status is associated with accelerated HIV disease progression among HIV-1-infected pregnant women in Tanzania. *J Nutr* 2004;134(10):2556–2560.

THE FAILURE OF MEDICAL SCIENCE TO PREVENT AND TO ADEQUATELY TREAT HIV/AIDS: AN ORTHOMOLECULAR OPPORTUNITY

by Harold D. Foster, PhD

The chaos surrounding the medical science of HIV/AIDS provides orthomolecular medicine with an opportunity to provide society with simple but essential strategies to prevent and treat this deadly disease. In a recent issue of this journal, an orthomolecular model was put forward to explain how HIV replication caused AIDS by removing the nutrients required to produce glutathione peroxidase.[2] This publication also proved that the conventional model of how this virus causes AIDS is incorrect. Since this is the case, it is hardly surprising that treatment protocols, based on this model, are also faulty.

Treatment: Measuring Disease Progression Conventional Predictions

In 1996, Mellors and colleagues[4] published a paper in *Science* claiming that the numbers produced by the viral load test could be used to accurately predict the progression of HIV-positive patients into AIDS. Viral load numbers were soon used by doctors and research scientists as a method of persuading healthy HIV-positive patients with high numbers to "hit early and hard with the newly approved drugs [highly toxic protease inhibitors], while AIDS doctors throughout the world started using viral load for everything from diagnosing illness to confirming HIV infection."[5]

The truth is that viral loads are a very poor tool to predict anything. In the *Journal of the American Medical Association,* a national team of orthodox AIDS researchers, led by Rodriguez and Lederman[6] of Case Western Reserve University in Cleveland, Ohio, presented the results from studying 2,800 untreated HIV-positive patients. They concluded that viral load measures failed in over 90 percent of cases to either predict or explain immune status.

In short, the viral load test is worthless. To cite Rodriguez and colleagues[6] "HIV RNA [ribonucleic acid] level predicts the rate of CD4 cell decline only minimally in untreated persons. Other factors, as yet undefined, are likely to drive CD4 cell losses in HIV infection."

Orthomolecular Predictions

The orthomolecular model, put forward by Foster,[1,2] stresses that, as HIV-positive patients' progress into AIDS, the virus depletes their bodies of selenium and the amino acids glutamine, cysteine, and tryptophan, so causing a decline of levels of glutathione peroxidase.

If this is the case, then declines in such nutrients would be useful predictors of disease progression. This is indeed the case. Numerous studies have shown selenium deficiency in the plasma of individuals with HIV/AIDS.[7–9] The worse the AIDS symptoms become, the more depressed the plasma selenium levels. Indeed, Baum and coworkers[7] have demonstrated that in both HIV-1-positive drug-using males and females, depressed selenium plasma levels are a far more accurate predictor of mortality than falling CD4 T-cell counts. This also was found to be true of HIV-infected children.[10] Baum and coworkers'[7] longitudinal study, for example, collected data on CD4 T-lymphocyte count, antiretroviral treatment, and plasma levels of vitamins A, E, B6, and B12, and selenium and zinc. A total of 21 of the 125 participants, adult drug users, died of HIV-related causes during this 3.5-year study. Only CD4 T-lymphocyte counts over time and selenium deficiency were significantly associated with mortality, with a lack of selenium being by far the most superior indicator of who was the most likely to die of AIDS. This was true also of selenium levels in infants.[10]

That adults and children who quickly died of AIDS had both depressed CD4 T-lymphocyte counts and very depleted plasma selenium stores[7,10] is no coincidence. Rather, it seems much

From the *J Orthomolecular Med* 2008;23(1):6–12.

more likely that this viral decline provides evidence of a positive feedback system in which a fall in selenium causes a reduction of CD4 T-cells because this trace element is essential for the production of T lymphocytes.[12] Such a drop in the efficiency of the immune system can also be documented by measuring the levels of glutathione peroxidase, the selenoenzyme that appears to protect against viral infection and to be a prime target of HIV. These declines in the efficiency of the immune system, caused by selenium inadequacy, then allows infection by other pathogens, resulting in a further decline in selenium. The "selenium-CD4 cell tailspin" is beginning its downward spiral.[11] It is clear, therefore, that the way to predict the future health of HIV-positive patients is not through measuring viral loads but by assessing levels of selenium and/or glutathione peroxidase. This is exactly what was done in the Mengo Nutritional Trial, recently conducted in Kampala, Uganda.[12] This clinical trial found that as glutathione peroxidase levels rose, so too did CD4 cell counts, Karnofsky scores (measuring the patient's quality of life), and body weights.

In summary, patient selenium and glutathione peroxidase levels are far better methods of predicting future health, or lack of it, than are the measurement of viral loads. To illustrate, at the beginning of the Mengo trial, the 160 HIV-positive patients in Group A had a median CD4 cell count of 347 per cubic millimeter (mm^3) and a median glutathione peroxidase level of 3,628 units per liter (L). One year later, after taking 37 nutrients daily, the median CD4 cell count of this group had risen to 388 cells per mm^3 and their median glutathione peroxidase levels had more than doubled to 8,573 units/L. Improvements in weight and Karnofsky scores were also highly statistically significant.[12] The levels of the selenoenzyme glutathione peroxidase appear to be the optimum indicator of future immune function and survival rates in HIV-positive individuals.

Conventional Side Effects

There is no doubt that antiretroviral drugs, often given as the HAART cocktail, can prolong life in patients who are receiving no other form of treatment. From the time of entering HIV care, the projected life expectancy for a patient is 24.2 years.[13]

The question arises, however, "what is the quality of this life?" To quote from *Science*'s News Focus,[14] "Confronting the Limits of Success" six years ago, new cocktails of anti-HIV drugs transformed prospects for infected people in industrialized countries. Now, serious limitations have become apparent. Indeed, two years after the *Journal of Orthomolecular Medicine* (2008) introduction of HAART, new side effects began to appear in treated patients. These included nausea and anemia, and odd distributions of fat known as lipodystrophy. Other metabolic abnormalities have since developed that lead to diabetes-like problems, heart disease, and brittle bones.

Research has appeared proving that a common mainstay of HAART, the drug AZT, is likely to be carcinogenetic.[15] A European study also has shown that deaths from liver-related disease among HIV-positive patients with similar CD4 cell counts has increased since the introduction of HAART.[16] So too has HIV-associated renal disease.[17] Similarly, the use of combined antiretroviral therapy is a strong independent risk factor for subclinical carotid atherosclerosis in drug-treated HIV patients, clearly showing its cardiovascular toxicity.[18]

In addition to the physical decline associated with antiretrovirals, mental disorders also are unusually common among HIV-patients treated with them.[19] One reason for this is that these drugs tend to be large molecules that cannot pass the blood-brain barrier. As a result, the brain acts as a sanctuary for HIV.[20] For example, 3D scans reveal tissue damage in the brains of many AIDS patients. In color-coded images, researchers have shown that there may be as high as 15 percent tissue losses in the centers of the brain that regulate movement and coordination. Thinning also is seen in the reasoning and language centers.[21] In addition to these brain scans, the National Institute of Mental Health are funding a long-term brain function study of HIV-positive patients that hopes to enroll about 1,600 drug-treated individuals. Initial findings already suggest that about 50 percent of such patients have subnormal performance. To quote Clifford,[20] "They might be slower on computer keyboards, working crossword puzzles, or have difficulty keeping track of what's been said in a conversation. They may even begin to move more slowly."

In summary, antiretrovirals are keeping HIV-infected patients alive longer. However, as a consequence of the properties and side effects of these drugs, patients are developing lipodystrophy, diabetes, liver and kidney problems, carotid atherosclerosis, and brain thinning and associated subnormal performance. It is also likely that they are increasing their risk of subsequently developing cancer.

Orthomolecular Side Effects

The orthomolecular treatment of HIV/AIDS involves diets that are high in specific nutrients that are essential for all human survival. Nutritional intake must specifically provide elevated levels of those nutrients, selenium, cysteine, glutamine, and tryptophan, that HIV replications remove from the body.[1,2,12] There is no evidence that these nutrients, especially if provided in foods such as Brazil nuts, spirulina, desiccated liver, or yogurt cause any adverse side effects. Naturally, they should not be ingested at abnormally high levels.

The author has published several articles, describing open and closed trials, that have established that such nutrients can reverse the downward HIV/AIDS spiral, even when AIDS patients are very close to death.[24] Indeed, many of the orthomolecularly treated HIV/AIDS patients claim to be healthier than at any previous time in their lives. Selenium, of course, is known to extend life span and reduce the risk of death from cancer[25] and cardiovascular disease.[26]

Conventional Expenses

According to Schackman and coworkers,[27] from the time of entering HIV care, the average patient life expectancy is an additional 24.2 years. Such a patient's medical care lifetime-discounted costs, are $385,200. Undiscounted cost is $618,900 for adults who begin antiretroviral treatment with CD4 cell counts less than 350/muL. Seventy-three percent of these predicted costs are to pay for antiretroviral medications, 13 percent for inpatient care, 9 percent for outpatient care, and 5 percent for other HIV-related medications and laboratory

costs. If antiretroviral treatment begins in a patient with a CD4 cell count of less than 200/muL, projected survival time is 22.5 years, with a discounted lifetime cost of $354,100 and an undiscounted cost of $567,000.

Orthomolecular Expenses

It is not yet possible to provide similar data for orthomolecular treatment. However, in South African, Ugandan, and Zambian trials with HIV/AIDS, patients have been successfully treated for a year or longer with nutrients costing between $60 and $300 annually.[23,24] These patients have, in many cases, proved so healthy after a few months that it is possible that over a lifetime their treatment cost will be effectively negative. That is, they will require less medical treatment than they would have received had they not been HIV-positive and, therefore, not receiving nutritional supplements. Since they are generally well enough to quickly return to work, the addition of their wages to the economic equation would certainly result in negative costs for the orthomolecular treatment of HIV/AIDS in such third world patients.

Conventional Prevention Strategies

In April 1984, Health and Human Services secretary Margaret Heckler held a press conference to announce that Dr. Robert Gallo of the National Cancer Institute had discovered the cause of AIDS, the retrovirus HTLV-III (later called HIV). She expressed hope that a vaccine against this virus would be produced within two years.[28] Heckler was no Nostradamus, more than 23 years later there is no vaccine for HIV. To quote Horton[29] writing in 2004:

> But contrary to the predictions and promises of most AIDS experts, the signs are that a vaccine to prevent HIV infection will not be found for, at the very least, several decades to come—if at all. Those responsible for carrying on the global fight against AIDS do not accept this grim outlook, at least publicly. Yet it is a conclusion, based on all the evidence gathered so far, which increasingly defies rebuttal. Until the gravity of this scientific failure is openly acknowledged, a serious debate about how to end HIV's lethal grip on some of the poorest

and most vulnerable human populations in the world cannot take place.

Of course, this criticism by Horton is not new. In 1992, Dr. Albert Sabin, developer of the oral polio vaccine, claimed: "The available data provides no basis for testing any experimental vaccine in human beings or for expecting that any HIV vaccine could be effective in human beings."[30] Nevertheless, the search goes on. In 2004, for example, world expenditure on AIDS vaccine research was between $600 and $700 million, $582 million being provided by the United States.[31]

What has medical science to show for the billions of dollars spent in AIDS vaccine research? Well, in 2007, the cream of the crop vaccine, being tested in the "STEP Study" failed spectacularly. Not only did the vaccine not prevent HIV infection, but those receiving it proved more likely to be infected with the virus than those volunteers receiving the placebo.[32] This study included 3,000 males and females, ages 18 to 45 who, because of their lifestyles, were considered at high risk of HIV infection.

One hundred of these volunteers were from Seattle, the rest were drawn from 15 other U.S. cities and from Peru, Brazil, Canada, Australia, Jamaica, Haiti, Puerto Rico, and the Dominican Republic.

Orthomolecular Strategies: Soil Remineralization

What are the reasons for the timing of the first AIDS pandemic, and indeed for the increased ability of viruses to cross the species barrier from animals to humans?[33,34] There seems to be a minimum daily dietary selenium intake above which, as seen in Senegal[6] and Finland,[35] HIV cannot be easily transmitted. This appears to be because the body's antioxidant defense system, especially the selenoenzyme glutathione peroxidase, acts as an internal defense against viral infection, preceding the formation of antibodies. For this reason, HIV is having its greatest difficulty in

NUTRIENTS BOOST NATURAL ANTIRETROVIRAL ENZYME IN HIV-INFECTED PATIENTS

A double-blind, randomized, clinical trial has shown that HIV-positive patients given supplemental nutrients can stop their decline into AIDS. The study, conducted at Mengo Hospital, Kampala, Uganda, was designed to test the impacts of two nutrient mixtures on the body's ability to produce glutathione peroxidase and to monitor any effects of such changes on levels of CD4 T-lymphocytes, body weight and quality of life.

For the study, 310 patients were randomly divided into two groups, both receiving nutritional supplements for a year, one group receiving an additional seven nutrients. In both groups, serum glutathione peroxidase levels increased by 250 percent. This enzyme normally declines as HIV/AIDS progresses. CD4 cell counts, indicative of an improving immune system, also rose in both treatment groups. In addition, quality of life, as measured using the Karnofsky scale also increased over the year. Patients' gains in glutathione peroxidase, CD4 cell counts, weight, and quality of life were all highly sta-

tistically significant. Both males and females benefited to the same degree from the two nutrient combinations.

These results are consistent with those of smaller open nutritional supplement trials that have been conducted elsewhere in Sub-Saharan Africa.[1] It seems clear that inadequate nutrition plays an extremely important role in the progression into AIDS of HIV-infected patients. These results also are consistent with Foster's model[2-3] of the development of AIDS, which suggests that deficiencies of glutathione peroxidase play a key role in the process, which can be reversed with nutritional supplementation.

REFERENCES

1. Bradfield M. *J Orthomolecular Med* 2006;21(4):193–196.
2. Foster HD. *What Really Causes AIDS*. Victoria, BC: Trafford Publishing, 2002.
3. Foster HD. *Med Hypotheses* 2004; 62(4):549–553.

Excerpted from the *Orthomolecular Medicine News Service*, October 25, 2013.

infecting those with diets elevated, either naturally or by design, in the trace element selenium and in the amino acids cysteine, glutamine, and tryptophan. Together these nutrients stimulate the body's production of glutathione peroxidase.[36–37]

As Foster wrote in the *Well Being Journal*,[34] "If this is correct, any drop in selenium in the food chain would naturally encourage the diffusion of HIV and indeed many other viruses. In the second half of the twentieth century, coal combustion more than doubled, oil consumption increased by a factor of almost 8 and natural gas was used as a fuel at a rate of roughly 11 times that of 1950. Simultaneously, large parts of the earth were deforested and much of the wood burned." The resulting high levels of sulfur and nitrogen, emitted into the atmosphere, were largely converted into sulfuric and nitric acids, increasing the acidity of associated precipitation. Acid rain altered soil pH and so reduced selenium's bioavailability.

Similarly, potassium, nitrogen, and phosphorus in commercial fertilizers are further depressing the uptake of selenium in crops. These processes reduce the dietary intake of selenium by humans, animals, and insects, triggering viral mutation and promoting associated pandemics.

Naturally, the effects of decreased selenium bioavailability have been most obvious in those unfortunate regions, like sub-Saharan Africa, where levels of this trace element are naturally depressed in the food chain. This is the fundamental reason why sub-Saharan Africa is so badly affected by the HIV/AIDS pandemic.

Field trials in China have shown that the addition of selenium to fertilizers, table salt, and/or animal fodder can greatly reduce Keshan disease (a cardiomyopathy) by slowing the diffusion of Coxsackie virus B.[38] This is also true of the hepatitis B and C viruses and liver cancer.[39,40] The addition of selenium to fertilizers in Finland, mandated nationally in 1984, has apparently also significantly reduced the incidence of HIV infection.[38]

It seems that, for a fraction of the money spent with no return on HIV vaccine research, the AIDS and other viral pandemics could be halted by increasing the global dietary intake of selenium. Such a strategy would be particularly effective if combined with efforts to increase protein consumption worldwide.

CONCLUSION

As William A. Hasteltine[41] pointed out in a 1992 lecture to the French Academy of Sciences, "The future of AIDS is the future of humanity." Hasteltine, then chief retrovirologist at Harvard's Dana-Farber Cancer Institute, went on to add that "unless the epidemic of AIDS is controlled, there is no predictable future for our species." Soon afterward he testified to a U.S. Senate hearing,[42] pointing out that by the year 2000 we might see 50 million people who had been infected by HIV.

In his opinion, by 2015 the total number dead or dying from this cause could reach 1 billion, that is, about one-sixth of the current global population. Hasteltine may have been a little optimistic: the AIDS pandemic has not been controlled and by the end of 2000, 57.9 million people had been infected with HIV, 21.8 million of whom were already dead.[43] We are at, or near, the tipping point.[44] If the orthomolecular strategies described in this article are not applied globally, very soon there will be, as Hasteltine suggested, no predictable future for our species.

REFERENCES

1. Foster HD. *What Really Causes AIDS*. Victoria: Trafford Publishing, 2002.

2. Foster HD: How HIV replication causes AIDS: an orthomolecular model. *J Orthomolecular Med* 2007; 22(3):123–128.

3. Ho DD. Viral counts in HIV infection. *Science* 1996;272 (5265):1124–1125.

4. Mellors JW, Rinaldo CR Jr., Gupta P, et al. Prognosis in HIV-1 infection predicted by the quantity of virus in plasma. *Science* 1996;272(5265):1167–1170.

5. Alive and Well AIDS Alternatives. The failure of viral load tests: *JAMA* study shakes AIDS science, angers HIV advocates. Retrieved from www.aliveandwell.org.

6. Rodriguez B, Sethi AK, Cheruvu VK, et al. Predictive value of plasma HIV RNA level on rate of CD4 T-cell decline in untreated HIV infection. *JAMA* 2006; 296(12):1498–1506.

7. Baum MK, Shor-Posner G, Lai S, et al. High risk of HIV-related mortality is associated with selenium deficiency. *J Acquir Immun Defic Syndr and Hum Retrovirol* 1997;15(5):370–374.

8. Dworkin BM. Selenium deficiency in HIV infection and the acquired immunodeficiency syndrome (AIDS). *Chemico-Biological Interactions* 1994;91(2–3):181–186.

9. Schrauzer GN, Sacher J. Selenium in the maintenance and therapy of HIV-infected patients. *Chemico-Biological Interactions* 1994;91(2–3):199–205.

10. Campa A, Shor-Posner G, Indacochea F, et al. High risk of HIV-related mortality is associated with selenium deficiency. *J Acquir Immun Defic Syndr and Hum Retrovirol* 1997;15(5):508–513.

11. Foster HD. AIDS and the "selenium CD4 T-cell tailspin": the geography of a pandemic. *Townsend Lett Doctors Patients* 2000:290:94–99.

12. Namulemia E, Sparling J, Foster HD. Nutritional supplements can delay the progression of AIDS in HIV-infected patients: results from a double-blind, clinical trial at Mengo Hospital, Kampala, Uganda. *J Orthomolecular Med* 2007;22(3):129–136.

13. Schackman BR, Gebo KA, Walensky RP, et al. The lifetime cost of current human immunodeficiency virus care in the United States. *Med Care* 2006;44(11):990–997.

14. Cohen J. Confronting the limits of success. *Science* 2002;296(5577):2320–2324.

15. National Toxicology Program. NTP toxicology and carcinogenesis studies of AZT (CAS No. 30516-87-1) and AZT/alpha-interferon A/D B6C3F1 mice (Gavage Studies). *Natl Toxicol Program Tech Rep Ser* 1999;469:1–361.

16. Harding A. European HIV study finds rise in liver-related deaths. *Reuters* January 2002. Retrived from www.medscape.com/viewarticle.

17. Röling J, Schmid H, Fischereder M, et al. HIV-associated renal diseases in highly active antiretroviral therapy-induced nephropathy. *Clin Infect Dis* 2006;42(10):1488–1495.

18. Jerico C, Knobel H, Calvo N, et al. Subclinical carotid atherosclerosis in HIV-infected patients: role of combination antiretroviral therapy. *Stroke* 2006;37(3):812–817.

19. Pence BW, Miller WC, Gaynew BN, et al. Psychiatric illness and virologic response in patients in initiating highly active antiretroviral therapy. *J Acquir Immune Defic Syndr* 2007;44(2):159–166.

20. Brink S. Brain escapes benefits of antiretrovirals. *Guardian Weekly* Nov 25–Dec 1, 2005:5.

21. Thompson PM, Dutton RA, Hayashi KM, et al. 3D mapping of ventricular and corpus callosum abnormalities in HIV/AIDS. *Neuroimage* 2006;31(1):12–23.

22. Clifford cited by Brink op.cit.

23. Foster HD. HIV/AIDS: a nutritional deficiency disease. *J Orthomolecular Med* 2005;20(2):67–69.

24. Bradfield M, Foster HD. The successful orthomolecular treatment of AIDS: accumulating evidence from Africa. *J Orthomolecular Med* 2006;21(4):193–196.

25. Foster HD: The geography of disease family trees: the case of selenium. In Bobrowsky PT, ed. *Geoenvironmental Mapping: Methods, Theory and Practice*. Rotterdam: Balkema Publishers 2001, 497–529.

26. Foster HD. Coxsackie B virus and myocardial infarction. *Lancet* 2002;359(9308):804.

27. Schackman BR, Gebo KA, Walensky RP, et al. The lifetime cost of current human immunodeficiency virus care in the United States. *Med Care* 2006;44(11):990–997.

28. In their own words . . . NIH researchers recall the early year of aids: timeline, 1981–1988. Retrived from http://72.14.253.104 /search?q=cache:Ko8kWXqcaQQJ:aidshistory.nih.gov/timeline/in dex.html+vaccine+ALOS+prediction+historyy&hl=en&ct =clnk&cd=2&gl=ca.

29. Horton R. AIDS: the elusive vaccine. *New York Review of Books* 2004;51(14):1–7.

30. Sabin A. Cited in Miller SK. HIV strategy will fail says vaccine veteran. *New Scientist* September 1992:8.

31. Associated Press. Foxnews.com. AIDS vaccine funding shrinking. Retrieved from www. foxnews.com/story/0,2933, 148281,00.html.

32. Song KM, Ostrom CM. Failure of AIDS vaccine punctures soaring hopes. *Seattle Times,* November 8, 2007.

33. Henderson M. Deadly viruses mutating to infect humans at rates never seen before. *Times on Line.* August 15, 2006. Retrieved from www.timesonline.co.uk/article/0,3–2049697.html.

34. Foster HD. A nutritional solution to AIDS and other viral pandemics. *Well Being Journal* November/December 2006; 15(6):1–10.

35. Foster HD. AIDS in Finland. *J Orthomolecular Med* 2005; 20(3):221–222.

36. Foster HD. The role of the antioxidant defense system in preventing the transmission of HIV. *Med Hypoth* 2007; 69(6):1277–1280.

37. Foster HD. Host-pathogen evolution: implications for the prevention and treatment of malaria, myocardial infarction and AIDS. *Med Hypoth* 2008;70(1):21–25.

38. Cheng YY. Selenium and Keshan disease in Sechuan Province, China. In: Combs GF Jr, Spallholz JE, Levander OA, Oldfield JE (eds). *Selenium in Biology and Medicine*. New York: Van Nostrand Reinhold, 1987: 877–891.

39. Yu SY, Li WG, Zhu YJ, et al. Chemoprevention trials of human hepatitis with selenium supplementation in China. *Biol Trace Elem Res* 1989;20:15–22.

40. Yu SY, Hu YJ, Li WG, et al. A preliminary report on the intervention trials of primary liver cancer in high-risk populations with nutritional supplementation of selenium in China. *Biol Trace Elem Res* 1991;29:289–294.

41. Hasteltine WA. cited in More cases, same old question. *Philadelphia Inquirer* June 6, 1993. Review and Opinion D1.

42. Hasteltine WA. cited in Large AIDS increases predicted by early 2005. *Vancouver Sun* Dec 15, 1992, A12.

43. Worldwatch Institute. *Vital Signs 2001: The Trends That Are Shaping Our Future.* New York: WW Norton, 2001.

44. Gladwell M. *The Tipping Point: How Little Things Can Make a Big Difference.* New York: Little, Brown & Company, 2002.

VITAMINS AND MINERALS REDUCE AIDS MORTALITY: IGNORING SUPPLEMENTS MEANS UNNECESSARY DEATHS

by Andrew W. Saul, PhD

Twenty-six years ago, I worked with a client (a woman in her late 20s) who was HIV positive. She was a heavy drinker and drug user, a smoker, and had a terrible diet and a series of bad personal relationships. Her health was deteriorating. Desperate, she decreased her drug and alcohol use. She still smoked, ate a poor diet, and was under great stress. She took multivitamin/multimineral supplements irregularly. But she took a lot of vitamin C very regularly, for over two decades.

• Twenty-six years later, doctors cannot detect HIV in her system. They now say that she never had it. She did. She probably still does. But they cannot find it. She has no symptoms.

• Robert Cathcart, MD, in California, treated AIDS patients with up to 200,000 milligrams of vitamin C a day. He found that, with very large intakes of vitamin C, even advanced AIDS patients lived significantly longer and had far fewer symptoms. His findings appeared in the August 1984 issue of *Medical Hypotheses*.[1]

Note that publication date: 1984, some 30 years ago. This clinical finding is very important. So important that it is hard to believe that the entire Wikipedia entry for Dr. Cathcart was deleted. His work was arbitrarily judged "too unsubstantial to provide notability" (see http://en.wikipedia.org/wiki/Wikipedia%3AArticles_for_deletion%2FRobert_Cathcart).

Perhaps even Wikipedia might find it difficult to ignore this research:

• A 1993 study at Johns Hopkins demonstrated that larger than RDA-dosages of multivitamin supplements slow AIDS and even help halt it. The seven-year-long study of 281 HIV-positive men showed that those taking vitamins had only about one half as many new AIDS outbreaks as those not taking supplements.[2]

• In 2004, a Harvard study by Fawzi and others found that vitamins cut AIDS deaths by 27 percent and slow the progression to AIDS by 50 percent. The study authors said, "Multivitamins also resulted in signifi-cantly higher CD4+ and CD8+ cell counts and significantly lower viral loads . . . Multivitamin supplements delay the progression of HIV disease."[3]

Here you have something truly interesting: in 1984, 1993, and 2004, studies showed that HIV patients taking vitamins are 50 percent less likely to develop full-blown AIDS, and that vitamin-taking AIDS patients live considerably longer, with far fewer symptoms. Have you heard anything about this on TV, or in a newspaper or magazine? Or a college course? Or from your health-care provider?

And now, in 2013, a new study in the *Journal of the American Medical Association (JAMA)* confirms it yet again. In HIV-infected adults, "supplementation with a single supplement containing multivitamins and selenium was safe and significantly reduced the risk of immune decline and morbidity."[4]

Yes, that was with a *single* multivitamin supplement with added selenium.

Harold D. Foster, PhD, advocated the use of selenium and amino acids, plus antioxidants, for HIV/AIDS a decade ago.[5-7] But the new *JAMA* study does not appear to mention his work at all. Yet the public *has* been told, for months and years and decades, that they do not need multivitamins or other dietary supplements; told that supplements do no good; told that supplements are harmful; and told that supplements even increase death rates.

In short, the public has been lied to—for decades. How many lives have been lost that could have been saved?

REFERENCES

1. Cathcart RF. *Med Hypotheses* 1984;14(4):423–433.
2. Tang AM. *Am J Epidemiol* 1993;138(11):937–991.
3. Fawzi WW. *N Engl J Med* 2004;351(1):23–32.
4. Baum MK. *JAMA.* 2013;310(20):2154–2163.
5. Foster HD. *Med Hypotheses* 2003;60(4):611–614.
6. Foster HD. *Med Hypotheses* 2004;62(4):549–553.
7. Foster HD. *Med Hypotheses* 2007;69(6):1277–1280.

Excerpted from the *Orthomolecular Medicine News Service*, December 17, 2013.

NUTRITIONAL SUPPLEMENTS CAN DELAY THE PROGRESSION OF AIDS IN HIV-INFECTED PATIENTS: RESULTS FROM A DOUBLE-BLIND CLINICAL TRIAL AT MENGO HOSPITAL, KAMPALA, UGANDA

by Edith Namulemia, MSc Epid, James Sparling, MD, and Harold D. Foster, PhD

There is clearly a relationship between the global diffusion of HIV/AIDS and the nature of local diets.[1] In HIV infection, for example, deficiencies of specific nutrients have been shown to be associated with more frequent opportunistic infections, faster progression of the disease, and higher AIDS mortality.[2-4] Furthermore, Fawzi and coworkers[5] have reported an increase in CD4 cell count in HIV-infected patients receiving micronutrients.

The mineral selenium appears to play a key role in this relationship. Ogunro and colleagues,[6] for example, have shown that as HIV/AIDS progresses, both selenium levels and mean glutathione peroxidase activity declines. Consequently, they suggest that selenium supplementation would be of immense benefit to HIV-1/AIDS infected patients. Kaiser and coworkers[7] also have recently demonstrated that micronutrient supplements, including selenium, N-acetyl cysteine, and L-glutamine significantly increased CD4 cell count in HIV-infected patients receiving highly active antiretroviral therapy (HAART). Indeed, Foster[8] has argued that the major symptoms seen in AIDS are due to extreme deficiencies of selenium and the three amino acids, cysteine, glutamine, and tryptophan, caused by production of a variant of glutathione peroxidase by HIV.

The major objectives of this clinical trial were to establish whether nutritional supplementation could slow the decline of HIV-positive patients to AIDS and improve their CD4 cell counts and quality of life, as shown by Karnofsky scores. If so, the study sought to determine whether such improvements were associated with increases in serum glutathione peroxidase levels.

Method: Study Design

This was a prospective, randomized, double-blind clinical trial designed to determine the affects of two nutritional supplement mixtures on HIV-1 disease progression, in HIV-infected patients who were not receiving any antiretroviral treatment. These mixtures were designed to increase the body's production of glutathione peroxidase to determine whether elevated levels of this selenoenzyme changed the natural history of HIV infection. All the study participants were outpatients of the Mengo Hospital in Kampala, Uganda. The trial lasted one year.

Study Subjects and Site

Enrollment began in June 2005 and concluded in October of the same year. This individual recruitment process took 2 weeks and so, although patients were involved with the trial for 54 weeks, they actually received the assigned supplements for 52 weeks. By the end of enrollment in October, 310 HIV-positive patients had been recruited. Of the enrolled patients, 249 were female and 61 male. In women, the median age at the trial's start was 36.0 years (25 percentile 30.0 years, 75 percentile 40.0 years). In men, the median age was 39.0 years (25 percentile 33.7 years, 75 percentile 45.5 years).

Participants were given one of two nutrient supplement combinations identified as A or B, to be taken three times daily with meals, for 52 weeks (Table 1). Patients who were pregnant, had a baseline CD4 T-lymphocyte count of 200 or less, or who were receiving antiretroviral treatment were excluded from trial participation. However, patients who suffered from other additional illnesses, such as tuberculosis, were accepted for enrollment. All clinical staff and student assistants were unaware of the patient group treatment assignments. All trial participants agreed to return, at six weekly intervals, to Mengo Hospital to receive nutritional supplements and for measurement of CD4 cell counts, serum glutathione peroxidase, weight, and quality-of-life assessments as required.

From the *J Orthomolecular Med* 2007;22(3):129–136.

Study Medications

Two nutritional combinations were designed and encapsulated specifically for use in this trial. The medications given to patients in Group B consisted of 30 nutrients with a filler of organic sugar (Table 1). This combination of nutrients had been found, in small open trials, to stimulate appetites in HIV-positive patients.[9] The logic behind this approach was to establish whether greater appetite was sufficient to encourage HIV-positive individuals to increase their consumption of local foods to a point at which enough selenium and amino acids were digested to normalize glutathione peroxidase levels. Serious loss of appetite is a common symptom of HIV/AIDS.[10]

The capsules taken by Group A patients contained the same 30 appetite-stimulating supplements but also included the additional seven nutrients shown in Table 1. The latter nutrients were designed to directly promote the body's production of glutathione peroxidase and, in addition to amino-acid rich desiccated beef liver, included L-selenomethionine, N-acetyl cysteine, L-glutamine, hydroxytryptophan, alpha-lipoic acid, and ascorbic acid. Patients receiving this mixture of supplements did not have to rely on their own diet to provide the selenium, cysteine, tryptophan, and glutamine thought necessary to boost body glutathione peroxidase levels.[11]

Capsule sizes and dosages were identical and their appearances were extremely similar. Both nutrient supplements were taken three times daily (six capsules in total) with food.

TABLE 1. NUTRITIONAL COMBINATIONS USED IN MENGO HOSPITAL HIV-POSITIVE OUTPATIENT TRIAL (GROUPS A AND B)		
AMOUNT PER SERVING	GROUP A	GROUP B
Calcium	23 mg	23 mg
Magnesium	23 mg	23 mg
Boron	0.2 mg	0.2 mg
Zinc	1.1 mg	1.1 mg
Vanadium	2 mcg	2 mcg
Copper	100 mcg	100 mcg
Chromium	8 mcg	8 mcg
Manganese	620 mcg	620 mcg
Silica	770 mcg	770 mcg
AEP iron (2-amino ethanol phosphate)	600 mcg	600 mcg
Iodine	2.9 mcg	2.9 mcg
Strontium	25.7 mcg	25.7 mcg
Molybdenum	0.3 mcg	0.3 mcg
Vitamin A	390 IU	390 IU
Provitamin A	390 IU	390 IU
Vitamin D3	31 IU	31 IU
Vitamin B1	1.9 mg	1.9 mg
Vitamin B2	1.9 mg	1.9 mg
Vitamin B3	7.8 mg	7.8 mg
D-calcium pantothenate	7.8 mg	7.8 mg
Vitamin B6	1.9 mg	1.9 mg
Vitamin B12	8 mcg	8 mcg
Vitamin C (calcium ascorbate)	23 mg	23 mg
Vitamin E (d-alpha tocopherol)	5 IU	5 IU
Vitamin K (phytonadione)	23 mcg	23 mcg
Biotin	8 mcg	8 mcg
Folic acid	31 mcg	31 mcg
Choline	4 mg	4 mg
Inositol	4 mg	4 mg
PABA (para-aminobenzoic acid)	2 mg	Nil
Dessicated beef liver	400 mg	Nil
L-glutamine	180 mg	Nil
Hydroxytryptophan (5-HTP)	180 mg	Nil
N-acetyl cysteine	180 mg	Nil
Alpha-lipoic acid	30 mg	Nil
Ascorbic acid	40 mg	Nil
L-selenomethionine	200 mcg	Nil
Organic sugar as a filler	Nil	Yes

Mg = milligram; mcg = microgram; IU = international units

Clinical and Laboratory Evaluations

Potential study patients underwent an initial screening at Mengo Hospital. This involved collection of demographic data, medication history and a laboratory testing of CD4T cell levels. Eligible participants then returned to this hospital for baseline and follow-up visits on a six-weekly basis for 52 weeks. Glutathione peroxidase levels were measured at baseline on entering the trial, after 30 weeks and at the end of the trial, as were CD4T cell counts. Patients were also weighed during each of their hospital visits. Karnofsky quality-of-life scores were taken at baseline and at 30 and 52 weeks.

Results

The trial began with 310 patients, 160 of whom were randomly assigned to Group A and 150 to Group B. During its 52-week duration, 47 patients exited the program, 29 from Group A and 18 from Group B. This represented a loss to follow-up of some 15.2 percent. In Group A, 3 left because of pregnancy, 14 were lost to follow-up, 4 withdrew consent, 2 died from tuberculosis, and 1 from esophageal cancer. Two further patients died from unknown causes and another from severe anemia. In Group B, over the course of the trial, 1 patient left because of pregnancy, 6 were lost to follow-up, one withdrew consent, 4 died of tuberculosis, 2 from cancer, and 4 of undiagnosed illnesses. As a consequence, 81.9 percent of patients in Group A and 88.0 percent of those from Group B completed the yearlong trial. The statistical analyses that follow refer to these patients. Beyond simple measures of central tendency, the Sign Test and the Wilcoxon Signed-Rank Test (two

common testing methods for comparing data) were used to establish whether the obtained results were statistically significant.

Immunological, Biochemical Parameters

From baseline over the one-year period of follow-up, 92 patients in Group A experienced an increased in the CD4 counts, while the remaining 39 showed a decrease (Table 2). Nevertheless, the mean/median CD4 count for Group A as a whole rose from 400/347 to 446/388 cells per mm3, increases that were statistically significant. Similarly, from base measurement to week 52, 89 patients in Group B showed an increase in their CD4 counts, while the remaining 41 displayed a decrease. The mean/median CD4 count for Group B rose from 400/335 to 446/394 over the year. Again, the Wilcoxon Signed-Rank Test and the Sign Test both established these gains to be of statistical significance.

At the beginning and end of the 52-week trial, glutathione peroxidase levels were measured in 92 patients from Group A. Of these patients, 77 had experienced an increase in the levels of this selenoenzyme, while the remaining 15 showed decreases. As a whole, 92 patients in Group A, for whom glutathione peroxidase levels were measured, showed mean/median increases from 3,825/3,628 units per liter (L) at the beginning of the 52-weeklong trial to 8,894/8,573 units/L at its end. Similarly, glutathione peroxidase levels were measured in 92 members of Group B at the start

TABLE 2. CHANGES (INCREASES/DECREASES/NO CHANGE) IN CD4 CELL COUNTS, SERUM GLUTATHIONE PEROXIDASE, WEIGHT AND KARNOFSKY SCORES FROM BASELINE MEASUREMENT TO 52 WEEKS

GROUP A	CD4 CELL COUNT	GLUTATHIONE PEROXIDASE	WEIGHT	KARNOFSKY SCORES
Increase	92	77	69	68
No change	0	0	17	27
Decrease	39	15	41	34
GROUP B				
Increase	89	81	76	71
No change	0	0	8	27
Decrease	41	11	42	31

and endpoint of the trial. Of these, 81 had experienced an increase and 11 a decrease in levels of this selenoenzyme. This group, as a whole, showed rises in mean/median glutathione peroxidase levels from 3,862/3,602 units/L to 9,839/9,203 units/L over the 52-week trial. These increases were considered statistically significant.

Clinical Parameters

Over the 52 weeks, 67.7 percent of the patients in Group A either increased or remained the same in weight. Mean weight increased from 60.1 kg to 61.1 kg (132 to 134 lbs)—a statistically significant gain. Similarly, 66.7 percent of the patients in Group B either increased or remained the same in weight over the yearlong trial. Mean weight for Group B rose from 62.0 kg to 63.4 kg (136 to 139 lbs), during the 52 weeks. Again, a weight gain that was of statistical significance.

Quality of life, as measured by the Karnofsky scores[13] also had risen during the duration of the trial in both groups. In Group A, for example, these scores rose or remained the same in 73.6 percent of patients, while the mean of this measure increased from 81 to 85. In Group B scores rose or remained unchanged in 76.0 percent of patients, while the mean rose from 82 to 86.

Comparison of Groups A and B and of Males and Females

Four analysis models were used to compare changes in CD4 cell counts, serum glutathione peroxidases, weight, and Karnofsky scores, over 52 weeks, using two factors: nutritional supplements and gender. Neither of these two factors was considered significant. That is, during this trial, there were no statistically significant gender differences in the results obtained, nor were there any statistically significant differences in changes in CD4 cell count, serum glutathione peroxidase, weight, or Karnofsky scores between Group A and B patients. In summary, both genders showed similar immunologic, biochemical, and clinical improvements, regardless of which of the two nutritional combinations they were taking.

Discussion

The major objective of this clinical trial was to determine whether either, or both, of the nutritional supplement mixtures, described in Table 1, could slow or reverse the progression to AIDS of HIV-infected patients who were not taking antiretroviral drugs. When the trial ended, the majority of patients from both Groups A and B felt that this goal had been achieved. Many patients, for example, described significant appetite increases, together with the return of their ability to walk long distances. Most also reported being happier. The quantitative data supported these claims. It has been long established that selenium and associated glutathione peroxidases are essential components of the human immune system.[14] In the trial described here, two related, but distinct, nutritional treatments were both able to increase serum glutathione peroxidase levels in HIV-infected outpatients by roughly a factor of 2.5, over a 52-week period. Such increases would be very unexpected in HIV-positive patients who are not receiving antiretroviral drugs since serum selenium and glutathione peroxidase levels both normally decline as HIV/AIDS progresses.[15–16]

Simultaneously, the CD4 cell counts, indicative of an improving immune system, rose in both treatment groups. Such improvements are also atypical of HIV-positive patients not taking antiretroviral drugs. To illustrate, a healthy CD4 cell count is somewhere between 500 and 1500 cells per cubic millimeter of blood. Normally, as observed at Mengo Hospital and confirmed elsewhere,[17] in HIV-positive patients not receiving antiretroviral, the count decreases on average about 50 to 100 cells each year. If this is the case, one might have expected CD4 cell counts (mean/median) to have fallen to some 325/272 in patients in Group A and 325/260 in Group B after the completion of the 52-week trial. In fact, these measures of central tendency were, as described, 446/338 and 446/394 at trial's end. That is, both nutrient groups had mean and median CD4 cell counts that were roughly 120 cells per cubic millimeter of blood higher than expected in HIV-positive patients not receiving antiretroviral treatment. Increases in weight and

Karnofsky score were also indicative of a general clinical improvement in health of both treatment groups. While these relationships do not prove that increasing glutathione peroxidase levels cause improvements in CD4 cell counts, weight gains, and higher personal evaluation of health, they are certainly consistent with this hypothesis. These analyses strongly support providing nutritional supplements for all HIV-1/AIDS patients, although it is clear that further clinical trials are required to establish optimum dosages and nutrient combinations.

CONCLUSION

This trial shows that both nutrient combinations (Table 1), taken for 52 weeks by HIV-positive patients who were receiving no antiretroviral drugs, can significantly slow their decline into AIDS. The associated improvement is associated with increases in glutathione peroxidase levels, CD4 cell counts, body weights, and improvements in quality of life scores. These results are consistent with those of smaller open trials using nutritional supplement that have been conducted elsewhere in sub-Saharan Africa.[18] It seems clear that inadequate nutrition plays an extremely important role in the progression into AIDS of HIV-infected patients. These results also are consistent with Foster's model[19] of the development of AIDS, which suggests that deficiencies of glutathione peroxidase play a key role in the process.

REFERENCES

1. Foster, HD. Halting the AIDS pandemic. In Janelle DG, Warf B, Hansen K, eds. *WorldMinds: Geographical Perspectives on 100 Problems.* Dordrecht, Netherlands: Kluwer Academic, 2004:69–73.

2. Semba RD, Tang AM. Micronutrients and the pathogenesis of human immunodeficiency virus infection. *Br J Nutr* 1999;81:181–189.

3. Tang AM, Graham NM, Saah AJ. Effects of micronutrient intake on survival in human immunodeficiency virus type 1 infection. *Am J Epidemiol* 1996;143:1244–1256.

4. Friis H, Goma E, Michaelson KF. Micronutrient interventions and HIV pandemic. In Friis H, ed. *Micronutrients and HIV Infection.* Boca Raton, FL: CRC Press, 2002:219–246.

5. Fawzi WW, Msamanga GI, Spiegelman D, et al. A randomized trial of multivitamin supplements and HIV disease progression and mortality. *NEJM* 2004;351:23–32.

6. Ogunro PS, Ogungbamigbe TO, Elemie PO, et al. Plasma selenium concentration and glutathione peroxidase activity in HIV-1/AIDS infected patients: a correlation with the disease progression. *Niger Postgrad Med J* 2006;13(1):1–5.

7. Kaiser JD, Campa AM, Ondercin JP, et al. Micronutrient supplementation increases CD4 count in HIV-infected individuals on highly active antiretroviral therapy: a prospective, double-blind, placebo-controlled trial. *J Acquir Immune Defic Syndr* 2006;42(5):523–528.

8. Foster HD. *What Really Causes AIDS.* Victoria, BC: Trafford Publishing, 2002.

9. Bradfield M, Foster HD. The successful orthomolecular treatment of AIDS: accumulating evidence from Africa. *J Orthomolecular Med* 2006;21(4):193–196.

10. Shabert JK, Winslow C, Lacey JM, et al. Glutamine-antioxidant supplementation increases body cell mass in AIDS patients with weight loss: a randomized double-blind control trial. *Nutrition* 1999;15(11–12):860–864.

11. Moriorino M, Aumann KD, Brigelius-Flohe R, et al. Probing the presumed catalytic triad of a selenium-containing peroxidase by mutational analysis. *Z Ernahrungswiss* 1998;37(Supp. 1):118–121.

12. SPSS Inc. *SPSS base 15.0 Use's Guide.* Chicago: SPSS Inc., 2006.

13. The Measurement Group.com. Definition: Karnofsky Severity Rating. Retrieved from www.themeasurementgroup.com /Definitions/Karnofsky.html.

14. Dworkin BM, Rosenthal WS, Wormser GP, et al. Abnormalities of blood selenium and glutathione peroxidase activity in patients with acquired immunodeficiency syndrome and AIDS-related complex. *Biol Trace Elem Res* 1988;15:167–177.

15. Dworkin BM. Selenium deficiency in HIV infection and the acquired immunodeficiency syndrome (AIDS). *Chem Biol Interact* 1994;91(2–3):181–186.

16. Look MP, Rockstroh JK, Rao GS, et al. Serum selenium, plasma glutathione (GSH) and erythrocyte glutathione peroxidase (GSH-PX) levels in asymptomatic versus symptomatic human immunodeficiency virus-1 (HIV-1) infection. *Eur J Clin Nutr* 1997;51(4):266–272.

17. AIDS Meds. Com T-cell Test. Retrieved from www.aidsmeds.com/articles/TCellTest_4727.shtml.

18. Foster HD. HIV/AIDS: A nutrient deficiency disease. *J Orthomolecular Med* 2005;20(2):67–69.

19. Foster HD. How HIV-1 causes AIDS: implications for prevention and treatment. *Med Hypotheses* 2004;62(4):549–553.

HIGHLY BENEFICIAL RESULTS IN THE TREATMENT OF AIDS

by Joan C. Priestley, MD

AIDS is truly the scourge of America. At this point, the very word "AIDS" is certainly as charged as the word "cancer" ever was. This disease is a very traumatic experience for anyone who has been exposed to the AIDS virus, especially with all the media hype that abounds today. The dominant thought is that everyone who has been exposed to the virus is going to die, soon, of the virus. I believe that's totally untrue. AIDS is a chronically manageable infection and will prove to be a curable disease. It's just a matter of time.

In America, we've been dealing with AIDS for 10 years now. After 10 years of virtually ignoring this disease, we're at the point now where 88 cases of AIDS are reported to the CDC every day. Right now, it is estimated that there are over a million and a half carriers of the virus in our country, many of whom don't know that they've been exposed to the AIDS virus. After a person is diagnosed with AIDS, their average life span is only about 15 months. Not my clients, but this is true for the average AIDS patient.

In Western medicine, we tend to believe that pharmaceutical drugs are the salvation of the world, and we tend to wait expectantly for some "magic bullet" to cure this disease. I don't think AIDS can ever be treated effectively in this somewhat myopic fashion. It's too complicated a disease and has too many other factors involved.

Five-Point Empowerment Program

Is there any other way to approach this disease? I certainly think that there is. To date, I have seen over 600 HIV-positive clients. I first developed my protocol in 1986 in Key West, Florida. I also developed a largely gay clientele. I was known somewhat as a vitamin lady. I was the only woman M.D. south of Miami, and I was the only one who was even remotely interested in nutrients in all of Florida, it seemed. My gay clients came to me and said, "We don't have enough money to take AZT," because none of them had insurance. "Figure out something. There has to be something else that we can do. Are there any principles you can teach us? Is there any way we can help strengthen our general bodies and our general immune system?"

Starting in 1986, I began investigating the idea of whether diet has anything to do with disease. But at the time it was a mystery to me. So I read medical literature and flew to other doctors' offices around the country (the few holistic doctors who are taking care of AIDS clients). I gradually developed a protocol of my own independently for the treatment of HIV disease called the Five-Point Empowerment Program. Now note, I did not say the cure of HIV, but the treatment of HIV. The program, I discovered, was extremely similar to the protocols used by the other major holistic AIDS doctors.

Point 1: Stress Reduction

The first point of the Empowerment Program is stress reduction. I tell all my clients that if they can reduce their stress—or more accurately, their experience of stress—they will enhance their response to the AIDS virus, as well as their response to life in general.

Stress reduction, as I define it, includes lifestyle changes. I ask all my clients if they smoke, drink alcohol, do any recreational drugs, and whether it would be an issue for them to stop using these substances. If my clients will not stop drinking and not stop smoking, I won't see them again. I approach that issue by simply telling them, "I'm always here for you, and I'd be happy to see you again when you've been clean and sober for 30 days."

If they are willing to make these changes, that's wonderful. If they're not, I give them a protocol handout and usher them out the door. There have been some studies, finally, that have indicated that cocaine and marijuana and cigarettes definitely accelerate the AIDS virus and also depress the immune system.

From the *J Orthomolecular Med* 1991;6(3&4):174–180.

Point 2: Dietary Changes

The second point of the Five-Point Empowerment Program is dietary changes. These clients really need to clean up their diet. In general, people with the AIDS virus need more protein and higher quality calories. They also need to get the sugar out of their diet and keep the yeast under control. Although yeast lives in all of us normally, in the presence of HIV, yeast becomes a cofactor that seems to accelerate the progress of the AIDS virus. Keeping the yeast under control is a major part of AIDS treatment.

I want my patients to eat a largely vegetarian diet, with all the salads, vegetables, grains, and legumes they can stuff down comfortably every day. In addition, I want them to eat more chicken, fish, eggs, and soybean products such as tofu and soy milk. I also ask my patients to simply stop eating all animal meats and cow milk products like butter and cheese. I also ask them to consume mostly fresh, whole, unprocessed, and uncanned foods.

Point 3: Supplement Use

The third point in the Empowerment Program is the use of nutrients. I love using nutrients instead of drugs. I use nutrients in two ways with people with HIV disease. The first method involves the use of nutrients as "replacement therapy."

People who have been exposed to the AIDS virus have definite nutritional deficits secondary to malabsorption. That's been proven time and again, mainly by Dr. Donald Kotler, a gastroenterologist who works at St. Luke's–Roosevelt Hospital in New York. He has actually convinced his clients to let him stick tubes down their throats and do intestinal biopsies.

People who have the virus in their body have difficulty absorbing a multitude of nutrients for several reasons. The AIDS virus inactivates intestinal cells through cell mechanisms. The AIDS virus also stimulates the person's own white blood cells to create autoimmune intestinal disease. These patients develop sprue, more commonly known as celiac disease. They have a sensitivity to gluten (a component of wheat, rye, oats, barley,

and related grain hybrids) and often develop lactase deficiency (the inability to digest lactose, or milk sugar) too. Their dietary needs are different and their absorption is impaired also. So, I use nutrients as replacement therapy. Because these people have deficits, I have to use larger doses available only as supplements. Vitamin and other supplements are necessary to get these patients to absorb the minimum from those larger doses just equal what the normal population could absorb solely from food, for instance.

Let's talk about the nutrients that people with AIDS seem to benefit from taking. Well, first and foremost, of course, is vitamin C. It really is the foundation, a cornerstone of an AIDS management–AIDS prevention program. I always use vitamin C in what I proudly refer to as "Linus Pauling doses," since it was Dr. Pauling's excellent research publications that were very influential in my decisions to use really high megadoses of vitamin C.

How much is enough? Well, most of my clients seem to get loose stools at about 15,000–18,000 mg of vitamin C per day. The scientific name for this is the "diarrhea dose" of vitamin C. In addition, I have my clients do an intravenous immune drip at least once a month. And that shuttles in another 25,000 mg of C intravenously.

Every so often I'll run across someone who obviously has some kind of smoldering infection that they're just keeping at bay with their extra-high doses of vitamin C. The house record is 240,000 mg of vitamin C, per day, by mouth, with no diarrhea. When people already have diarrhea, I ask them to take vitamin C anyway. My experience has been that a lot of time they'll take a certain amount of vitamin C and their diarrhea will stop. Why? Because they're finally taking enough vitamin C to kill all the bugs causing their diarrhea. Then they'll go up, up, up on their vitamin C dose and they'll get diarrhea again. That's their true "diarrhea dose" of vitamin C. So, as long as vitamin C doesn't aggravate someone's diarrhea, I have no hesitation in suggesting that he or she take these phenomenal doses.

AIDS must be one of those diseases that involve free radicals (unstable molecules that can damage cells) because most of my core program nutrients are antioxidants and free-radical quenchers. The premiere one, of course, is vitamin C, followed right along next in importance by vitamin A (in the form of beta-carotene, 25,000 IU), vitamin E (400–800 IU), and N-acetyl cysteine (at least 1,200 mg). This last compound becomes the antioxidant glutathione in our own bodies. I'm investigating intravenous glutathione as a way of bypassing NAC, but it's very expensive.

Remember that antioxidants, such as vitamin C, glutathione, and vitamin E, help neutralize the free-radical cascade and prevent cellular damage, so it's important to give all four of these major antioxidants, as well as the major minerals.

AIDS patients have also been found to be lacking in most minerals, such as calcium, magnesium, selenium, molybdenum, iron, and zinc. Not all these deficiencies are seen in one person, of course, but people with AIDS have been studied by various

SELENIUM AND IMPAIRED ABSORPTION IN AIDS' PATIENT

"Research has shown that there may be problems in nutrient absorption even in asymptomatic HIV-positive individuals. HIV patients need to take larger amounts of vitamins than uninfected individuals to attain the same blood levels. With selenium, a dose of 400 micrograms (mcg) seems reasonable for HIV-infected individuals, if they have impaired absorption. (The U.S. RDA is 55 mcg.) For an AIDS patient who is demonstrably deficient in selenium, an even higher daily dose (up to 800 mcg) for a brief period of time (several weeks) to get his or her blood levels up, followed by a decrease to 400 mcg, is an effective strategy. This question of dose level naturally arouses concerns because in the past so much has been made of the potential toxicity of selenium. I believe that the danger of serious toxicity with selenium supplementation has been exaggerated. The signs of chronic selenium toxicity—garlic odor of breath and sweat, metallic taste in mouth, brittle hair, and fingernails—are distinctive, and easily reversed by lowering the dose."

E.W. Taylor. *J Orthomolecular Med* 1997;12(4):227–239.

institutions, and they tend to be deficient in vitamin C, vitamin A, vitamin E, and/or all these other minerals. Why? I think because they also lack the ability to make enough stomach acid to properly absorb nutrients, and they also seem to have pancreatic problems. They can't make enough of the pancreatic enzymes needed for digestion. So, I correct that too. I give betaine hydrochloride and also use pancreatic enzymes as replacement therapies.

Quercetin is the jewel of the program. Quercetin is a bioflavonoid found in orange rinds, and it is known to synergize vitamin C. Quercetin is also the only natural substance I've found that blocks the AIDS virus, the same way AZT blocks the AIDS virus. AZT is the only drug we've come up with, after a billion dollars of research in ten years. Quercetin costs less than $20 a month, and has none of the side effects of AZT.

Some other things I give my clients are more controversial. I give them oral peroxide (food-grade hydrogen peroxide) because I think there's value in oxygenators as well as antioxidants. I also use a lot of super-saturated potassium iodide (a form of iodine), called SSKI. Iodine has some anti-HIV activity. So, all my patients get 8 drops of SSKI. It's a good thyroid tonic, also. CoQ10, another antioxidant and oxygenator, evening primrose oil, and fish oils decrease inflammatory prostaglandins and increase the anti-inflammatory prostaglandins. I also developed a B vitamin shot that has all the B vitamins in it, a lot of B12 and every other B vitamin that exists. All my clients get a B shot once a week.

It's my professional opinion that some of the anemia seen with AIDS, and a lot of the dementia (called AIDS dementia complexes), actually are not due to the AIDS virus; these problems are due to B vitamin deficiencies that accumulate gradually in people who have been exposed to the AIDS virus. These deficiencies are unrecognized by most Western-trained physicians. We just blame everything on the AIDS virus. I've helped my patients prevent dementia by giving them high doses of B vitamins. They don't have any mental deterioration.

Last, but not least, I give garlic to all my patients. Garlic is a superb antibiotic and is used for treating fevers and many infections. Think of it as nature's sulfur drug. Any way they can get it down—garlic suppositories, garlic liquid, garlic in their ears for ear infections. I have also read several articles on intravenous garlic extract, which has been used successfully to treat cryptococcal meningitis (usually a fatal disease in the presence of HIV infection).

Point 4: Use of Medications When Necessary

The fourth part of the Five-Point Empowerment Program is appropriate use of drugs. Drugs do have a place to play in the treatment of AIDS, but I think it's a minor one. Where Western medicine really shines, I feel, is in acute care and trauma management. If I get hit by a truck, get me to an emergency room in a Western-based hospital. But, when it comes to the treatment of cancer and other slowly developing degenerative disease, Western medicine has, by and large, just fallen flat on its face. We really have to look further or elsewhere.

Point 5: Mind Food

The fifth point of the protocol is what I call "nutrition for the mind." I ask my clients to do a number of other therapies that may include visualizations, affirmations, forgiveness exercises, massage classes, deep breathing, or simply taking a stick to a tree and just beating out their internal feelings. I also ask them to get involved in other equally important issues of our planet, whether it's animal rights or the homeless mess or doing something to promote environmental issues; there are any number of other causes that these people especially could contribute to. People with AIDS still have tremendous talent. A lot of them are on disability, and these service groups take their minds off thinking about the virus for 24 hours a day.

Future Treatment of AIDS

We are going to see holistic, alternative, and nutritional treatments become much more prominent in the management of HIV disease; this is a new phenomenon. It's why I feel to some extent that AIDS is the greatest thing that's happened to holistic medicine. With cancer, the argument is always raised that we're just taking people away from traditional treatments and giving them this alternative mumbo jumbo, and that we're cheating people from receiving effective treatments. Which, of course, isn't true, but that's the argument that is used. Well, there is no effective, traditional treatment for AIDS. These people have nothing else to use.

What kind of results have I had? I've seen 600 clients at least once. About 200 of them are doing the program on a quasi-regular basis, and about 100 people are doing it devotedly. In general, it's rare that my clients get sick. I ask them to always call the office and let us know when they have to go into the hospital. By and large, they just don't get sick. They certainly don't die. In the last two years, I have only seen about 20 deaths out of those 100 who have been on my protocol with devotion.

Many of the patients who died were not well when they first came to my office. They had lymphoma or Kaposi's sarcoma (a cancer associated with HIV infection), or they had had several episodes of other infections and their life expectancy was statistically very short, anyway. But even at that, many had hospital admissions where they just kind of bounced in and bounced out again. For the most part, they just seem to coast along without complications. They do extremely well. In fact, my patients have very good statistics where disease progression and mortality are concerned. They are, on the whole, above the national average of those who have pursued pharmaceutical protocols.

THE SUCCESSFUL ORTHOMOLECULAR TREATMENT OF AIDS: ACCUMULATING EVIDENCE FROM AFRICA

by Marnie Bradfield, MA, and Harold D. Foster, PhD

As HIV replicates, it deprives HIV-positive individuals of the selenoenzyme glutathione peroxidase and its four key components, namely, selenium, cysteine, glutamine, and tryptophan.[1-3] Slowly but surely, this depletion process causes severe deficiencies of all these nutrients. Their lack, in turn, is behind the major symptoms of AIDS, including the collapse of the immune system and an increased susceptibility to cancer, myocardial infarction, depression, muscle wasting, diarrhea, psychosis, and dementia. As these nutrient deficiencies cause failure of the immune system, associated pathogenic cofactors become responsible for their own unique symptoms, such as tuberculosis, *pneumocystis carinii* pneumonia, and toxoplasmosis.[4] Any successful treatment for HIV/AIDS must therefore, include normalization of the body's levels of glutathione, glutathione peroxidase, selenium, cysteine, glutamine, and tryptophan.

Clinical Trials

Initially, an attempt was made to test this hypothesis in the cheapest way possible, by developing a simple nutrient mixture of selenomethionine and beef liver. This, for example, was used in open trials in a South African hospice where five of six AIDS patients greatly improved when provided with it.[5] Another small trial took place in a Kenyan clinic. Here the patients were weak and passing into AIDS. They soon recovered their energy and regained their health when given selenium and desiccated beef liver.

Encouraged by such results two further larger open trials were set up. In Zambia, the nutritional supplements were given to a childcare and adoption society.[5,15] Orphans and guardians who were HIV/AIDS patients experienced dramatic improvement when given this selenium-amino acid-enriched nutrient mixture. Most showed noticeable improvement in the second to third weeks after receiving these supplements. In Uganda, at the Mengo Hospital in Kampala where

a 40-HIV/AIDS-patient open trial also was set up, after one month 77 percent of these patients reported noticeable health improvement.

The success of these open trials encouraged the researchers to conduct a 318-patient, double-blind clinical trial, also in Uganda at the Mengo Hospital. As of this time, the study is almost completed, and the results will be available early in 2007. [Editor's note: For study results, see the article "Nutritional Supplements Can Delay the Progression of AIDS in HIV-Infected Patients" earlier in this chapter.] Since the Ugandan authorities would not allow the use of a placebo, one of the researchers Dr. Harold Foster developed a nutrient mixture that was thought likely to be an optimum treatment for HIV/AIDS. Designed to stimulate the immune system and to correct all AIDS-associated nutritional deficiencies, this mixture contained desiccated beef liver, selenomethionine, L-glutamine, hydroxytryptophan (5-HTP), N-acetyl cysteine, and cofactors of glutathione peroxidase such as alpha-lipoic acid and ascorbic acid. In addition, the supplement included 30 other nutrients, designed to replace losses due to diarrhea. Half of the patients in the Mengo trial received the nutritional supplement. The other 50 percent of patients were given 30 nutrients, which did not include either selenium or desiccated beef liver.

Soon after the start of the double-blind hospital trial in Uganda, the authors of this article met for the first time and Marnie Bradfield took samples of this multinutrient supplement to Africa. Bradfield, a public health nurse whose family has business interests in South Africa, has traveled to and throughout sub-Saharan Africa since 1970. Her mission in Africa was to give the multinutrient supplement to dying AIDS patients who were not receiving other forms of medication. What follows is her description of the results of this project.

From the *J Orthomolecular Med* 2006;21(4):193–196.

Sibongile's Story

"In 2003, Gilbert, an employee of our small company in South Africa, asked to go home to Zimbabwe to bury his brother saying, 'They said my brother has died of HIV/AIDS.' When Gilbert returned to Johannesburg, he was distraught and reported that his sister-in-law, Sibongile, had been 'unable to go to the grave.' She too had AIDS and was 'lying on the floor dying.' As a result, Gilbert was about to become the guardian of the three minor children in Sibongile's family.

"I had read Dr. Foster's book *What Really Causes AIDS* (2006) and felt sure that the orthomolecular approach he suggested could cause no harm to the people I was meeting in South Africa, where in some regions the level of soil selenium is among the lowest in the world. When Gilbert came to me in great consternation and distress about the state of Sibongile and her family, I asked him if she wanted to take some of Dr. Foster's *muti* (a generic term for medicine among Ngune-speaking people). He agreed and we found a way to quickly send a bottle of the supplement to Zimbabwe. Within a few weeks we heard from other relatives that this woman, who had been moribund, seemed to be improving.

"Over the next several weeks Sibongile continued to get better. Soon she was able to move to her own room, where she began to look after her children, cooking for them and taking them to school. Sibongile took the multinutrient for one month and then continued to receive 400 mcg of selenium each day. Her recovery is viewed by her African neighbors and friends as nothing short of a miracle. As far as is known, Sibongile is celibate. In 2004, she began to feel unwell but she quickly recovered when given a further monthly course of the multinutrient supplement. This was followed by a resumption of 400 mcg of selenium daily."

Gerson's Story

"In November 2004, Gerson, a 44-year-old painter employed by my family's business, became ill and almost certainly was suffering from AIDS. Later he would recall in his own words, 'I was weak, weak . . . like a feather, the wind could blow me over. I was slowly dying.' I spoke to Gerson and started him on the first series of multinutrient trials. By the time he began he was seriously ill, unable to eat, very thin, and lying on the floor. If he could not manage to take three tablets a day, he would take two, or what was possible. I told Gerson that I needed to know each day how many capsules he had taken, at what time, and how he felt, and I gave him a calendar on which to note this information. He faithfully did this and much to his amazement later told me that he knew within four or five days that he was 'getting better.' As he said on a filmed interview, 'I said these pills . . . they work . . . they very good.'

"Gerson took a one-month course of the supplement and then began to receive 400 mcg of selenium each day. However, after a few months, he appeared to be increasingly less well and was given a second series of the multinutrient supplement. Since that time he has been on 400 micrograms of selenium daily and, as of August 29, 2006, he was healthy and back at work. However, a note from another African woman in October tells me that Gerson sometimes 'forgets to take his muti' and only remembers when he does not feel well. Such may be the nature of compliance in chronic disease."

Victor's Story

"In January 2005, a 19-year-old employee, Victor, failed to return to work after the long Christmas holiday. His brother, who was also an employee and who had gone home on holiday on December 5, 2004, announced that Victor had tuberculosis but that something else was wrong because he was losing a lot of weight and had no strength. Our company could not get anyone up to see Victor for three months, as he lived five hours up the Great North Road near the Zimbabwe border. Finally, Gilbert (previously mentioned and Sibongile's brother-in-law) was able to go. When he returned from bringing the supplement, food, and other provisions to Victor, he had very sad news. Gilbert said he was sure Victor would die. He was living with his mother, who was spoon-feeding him. Victor 'had no flesh on his body . . . he could not stand . . . he could not even sit on the chair.' On June 22, 2005, Gilbert and my husband and I went to visit Victor.

"Victor, who did not know we were coming, was sitting out in the sunshine and got up to walk to meet us at our car, using a walker that we had sent him. Victor said he was much better, although he 'was having an upset stomach' from taking the supplement. (Hence, I developed a simple protocol for muti ingestion whereby the patient eats some food, takes the supplement, and then more food, in addition to marking the calendar notations.)

"This may seem very simple, but life in the developing world is fraught with challenges that oftentimes deter someone from following even basic routines. Victor has severe foot drop in his left foot and thus far this has not been corrected. However, he was well enough to undertake the five-hour journey to Johannesburg in June and was then walking with one stick only. It is possible that Victor may have received some antiretrovirals on a visit to the hospital to treat his tuberculosis but, if so, they were not given to him outside the institution. The great bulk of his improvement in health appears to have been caused by the multinutrient and the subsequent use of selenium."

John's Story

"In addition, John, a hardworking 28-year-old, took to staying in his bed about every third day. He simply could not get up and, if he did, he was too weak to work. He had a deep rasping cough and was rapidly becoming skeletal in appearance. In October 2005, I went to talk to him about his health. He agreed that 'I am not good . . . and I have my children, they will have no one if I die.' I suggested to John that he start a nutritional supplement. He took the orthomolecular nutrient mixture for one month. Within a week, John had improved dramatically and was able to get out of bed and come to work even in the extreme heat of the sub-Saharan summer. John received a one-month course of multinutrients and, thereafter, received 400 mcg of selenium daily. He is still in good health and working."

Prince's Story

Shortly after John began to recover, in early November 2005, I noticed that Prince, a conscientious and excellent employee, began to show symptoms of AIDS. He dramatically lost weight and rapidly became exhausted early in the day, and often had to go home to bed. I went to talk to him about his health and asked him if he would take the muti and try it. He did so for one month, and then came back to me, as he knew there was something else he needed to take. I gave him his first bottle of selenium and now he takes 400 mcg daily. As of October 12, 2006 he is alive, well, and working."

Albert's Story

"Albert, John's brother, was also a family employee. In December 2006, he was working nearby and I realized that he had lost a lot of weight . . . and was moving slowly. He had continued to come to work, but I could see that he was rapidly deteriorating. The muscles on Albert's arms were very thin and he was actually very frail. When I asked about his health, he told me "I can't eat . . . food not taste good . . . I feel bad . . . weak.' Then he asked if he could have some 'muti like you gave John.' We agreed that he should start. He did so for one month and then subsequently went onto the selenium maintenance dose. One morning in early January, I asked him how he was feeling. His face lit up in a huge smile . . . and he said 'Great . . . great . . . can eat lots . . . can work lots.' As of my last update on Albert, in October 2006, he was doing well, working, and taking his daily selenium supplements."

■ CONCLUSION

Several conclusions appear obvious from the African nutritional trials being used to test the efficacy of selenium and amino acids as a treatment for HIV/AIDS. Firstly, it is possible to reverse all the symptoms of AIDS in dying patients using nutrition alone. Secondly, this requires selenium and the amino acids cysteine, tryptophan, and glutamine. Thirdly, while selenium alone can slow HIV replication, eventually HIV/AIDS patients also need amino acid supplements. These can be given temporarily until deficiencies are corrected. The patients can then return to selenium supplementation alone for several months, until the more complex nutritional mixture is again required for another month. There appear to be no adverse side effects from these nutritional treatments and patients are delighted with their greatly improved health status.

REFERENCES

1. Taylor EW. Selenium and viral diseases: facts and hypotheses. *J Orthomolecular Med* 1997;12(4):247–239.

2. Foster HD. *What Really Causes AIDS*. Victoria, BC: Trafford Publishing, 2002.

3. Foster HD. How HIV-1 causes AIDS: implications for prevention and treatment. *Med Hypotheses* 2004;62:549–553.

4. Foster HD. AIDS and the "selenium-CD4T cell tailspin": the geography of a pandemic. *Townsend Lett* 2000;209:94–99.

5. Foster HD. HIV/AIDS–A nutritional deficiency disease? *J Orthomolecular Med* 2005;20(2):67–69.

AIDS: A TREATABLE COMBINATION OF NUTRITIONAL DEFICIENCIES

New clinical reports from Zambia, Uganda, and South Africa indicate that AIDS may be stopped by nutritional supplementation. A number of members of the medical profession have observed that high doses of the trace element selenium, and of the amino acids cysteine, tryptophan, and glutamine can together rapidly reverse the symptoms of AIDS, as predicted by Dr. Harold D. Foster's nutritional hypothesis.[1] These nutrients are necessary for the human body to produce the enzyme glutathione peroxidase. This enzyme is strongly anti-retroviral and can greatly reduce HIV replication. Unfortunately, HIV has developed the ability to compete with the body for these four nutrients because shortages of them allow its more effective replication. Specifically, HIV has a gene that allows it to produce an analogue of glutathione peroxidase.

Diets high in selenium, cysteine, tryptophan, and glutamine seem to have two major benefits for AIDS patients:

1. They replace these four nutrients in the body, correcting the deficiencies HIV has caused. AIDS is what we call these combined deficiency symptoms.

2. High levels of these four key nutrients push up the body's glutathione peroxidase levels, making it much more difficult for HIV to replicate. This enzyme also beneficially interferes with the replication of hepatitis B and C. Nutritionally treated patients are still HIV-positive but seem to generally remain in good health unless they start to eat a diet that once again is poor in one or more of these nutrients. If this occurs, glutathione peroxidase levels fall, HIV begins to be replicated and the AIDS cycle begins again.

Some countries or regions, like Senegal and Bolivia, have been very fortunate. Their bedrock is naturally elevated in selenium and their diets are normally high in the three amino acids. As a result, they are rarely infected by HIV. Others, like Finland, have wisely mandated the addition of selenium to their fertilizers, with similar results. In contrast, some regions like Kwazulu-Natal, South Africa, have bedrock and soils that contain little selenium and diets are poor in one or more of the key nutrients. For example, corn (maize) is low in both selenium and tryptophan. As a result, populations eating a great deal of corn are easy to infect with HIV and die very quickly of its associated nutritional deficiencies (AIDS).

To halt AIDS, to stop HIV from replicating, the needed nutrient levels are high. Selenium, for example, is taken at several times the commonly recommended daily allowance for the first month. Dosage is considered in more detail in *What Really Causes AIDS*.[2]

REFERENCES

1. Foster HD. *Med Hypotheses* 2004;62(4):549–553.

2. Foster HD. *What Really Causes AIDS*. Victoria, BC: Trafford, 2002.

Excerpted from the *Orthomolecular Medicine News Service*, April 26, 2006.

HYPERACTIVITY AND OTHER LEARNING AND BEHAVIORAL DISORDERS

CRITICISMS AND LAWSUITS over the hazards of tranquilizers, methylphenidate (Ritalin), and related pharmaceuticals are on the rise. But neither court nor controversy can cure a child. "Battered parents" (Dr. Abram Hoffer's term) need to know what to do, and now. Saying "no to drugs" also requires saying "yes" to something else. That something else is nutrition, properly employed.

Over his 55-year practice, Dr. Hoffer successfully treated a large number of behaviorally impaired children with supplemental vitamins. He would also provide an instruction directly to the child, leaning over and saying, "No junk!" Dr. Hoffer said that he never saw any child that failed to grasp what he meant. But many adults ask, "If this approach is so good, how come my doctor doesn't already use it?" The answer may have more to do with medical politics than with medical science. Consider Hoffer's views on attention-deficit hyperactivity disorder (ADHD): "The DSM system (the standard of the American Psychiatric Association) has little or no relevance to diagnosis. It has no relevance to treatment, either, because no matter which terms are used to classify these children, they are all recommended for treatment with drug therapy" combined, sometimes, with other non-megavitamin approaches. "If the entire diagnostic scheme were scrapped today, it would make almost no difference to the way these children were treated, or to the outcome of treatment. Nor would their patients feel any better or worse." Statements like these do not exactly endear one to the medical community.

For those who say there is insufficient scientific evidence to support nutrition-based therapy for learning disabilities like ADHD and other children's behavior disorders, this section will demonstrate that they haven't been looking hard enough.

—A.W.S.

567

TERMS OF LEARNING AND BEHAVIORAL DISORDERS

ANTIPSYCHOTICS. Medications such as aripiprazole (Abilify), risperidone (Risperdal), and quetiapine (Seroquel) that are increasingly being prescribed to treat attention-deficit hyperactivity disorder and other behavior problems.

CONNERS' RATING SCALE. A widely used diagnostic tool written by C. Keith Conners, PhD, which is considered the accepted rating scale of attention-deficit hyperactivity disorder. It has a rating scale for parents, teachers, children. The higher the score (0–40), the more severe is considered to be the problem.

DIAGNOSTIC AND STATISTICAL MANUAL OF MENTAL HEALTH DISORDERS (DSM). The standard classification system used by practitioners to diagnose disorders, including attention-deficit hyperactivity disorder.

MUTAGEN. A substance that can produce changes (mutations) in DNA, which can prevent a gene from functioning properly.

NEUROTOXIN. A substance that can alter and eventually disrupt or kill neurons (nerve cells) that transmit and process signals in the brain and other parts of the nervous system.

NEUROTRANSMITTER. A chemical made from amino acids that is used to carry messages throughout the brain's network of cells.

PSYCHOSTIMULANTS. Medications such as methylphenidate (Ritalin), dextroamphetamine (Dexedrine), or dextroamphetamine-amphetamine (Adderall), which are stimulants that decrease impulsivity and hyperactivity, and increase attention.

SALICYLATE. A chemical found naturally in many fruits and vegetables that is also a major ingredient of aspirin and other pain-relieving medications.

TERATOGEN. A substance that can cause malformation of an embryo.

CHILD PSYCHIATRY: DOES MODERN PSYCHIATRY TREAT OR ABUSE?
by Abram A. Hoffer, MD, PhD

Jay, six years old, was forced into the modern psychiatric system from which he was rescued three years later by Marty McKay, PhD, a clinical psychologist, and from Child Welfare by a court order. By then he had seen 60 physicians and had been diagnosed with dozens of diagnoses, including mental retardation, attention-deficit hyperactivity disorder (ADHD), Tourette's syndrome, oppositional-defiant disorder, obsessive-compulsive disorder, conduct disorder, and the then current favorite childhood-onset bipolar mood disorder. He was treated with combinations of toxic drugs with no evidence they were therapeutic. Toward the end of his treatment program he was on methylphenidate (Ritalin), divalproic acid (Depakote), and quetiapine fumarate (Seroquel). He was saved by the relentless effort of Dr. McKay, who insisted that the University of Toronto's Hospital for Sick Children take him under care away from his psychiatrist. It took ten months to get him off the drugs. He had stopped growing. Since then he has regained his health. The long-term effect of this massive long-term toxic drugging is not known.

Rebecca Riley was not so lucky. She died from an overdose of two of the drugs prescribed for Jay. This tragic event was featured on the CBS *60 Minutes* report "What Killed Rebecca Riley," on September 30, 2007. Rebecca was the youngest child in a dysfunctional family living in Hull, Massachusetts. Her two older siblings were already on massive drug medication. At two and a half, she was diagnosed with ADHD and bipolar disorder. She was prescribed Seroquel, a favorite antipsychotic for adult schizophrenic patients; Depakote, an anticonvulsant for adults; and clonidine (Catapres), a drug for lowering blood pressure. On December 13, 2006, she was found dead, lying on the floor near her mother's bed from an overdose of drugs. Her parents are charged with murder and are in jail waiting trial. On December 12, Rebecca appeared to have a cold. Her mother gave her some acetaminophen (Tylenol) and some more clonidine because she did not go to sleep. Then she laid her down beside her on the floor and fell asleep. When her mother woke up, Rebecca was dead.

The publicity given to Rebecca's death spurred Massachusetts into the beginning of regulatory action. A *Boston Globe* journalist[1] reported "Although cases like the overdose of Rebecca Riley are rare, the prescription of psychiatric drugs to young children is not. Doctors last year prescribed clonidine—a drug sometimes used to treat hyperactivity that was found in lethal quantities in the girl's bloodstream—to 955 children under age seven in MassHealth (a public assistance health insurance program). Doctors also prescribed antipsychotic drugs, which raise the risk of diabetes and obesity, to 536 children under age seven. The largest provider of mental health services for MassHealth, Massachusetts Behavioral Health, identified 35 preschoolers in the first three months of the system who were taking three psychiatric medications or one antipsychotic drug." [Editor's note: In January 2011, Tufts Medical Center, which insured the doctor who prescribed the psychiatric drugs for Rebecca Riley, awarded her estate $2.5 million.]

The Psychiatric Diagnosis

The official diagnostic standard of the American Psychiatric Association (APA) is the *Diagnostic and Statistical Manual* (DSM) *of Mental Disorders* [now in its fifth edition, May 2013]. This system of diagnosing is not as popular in other areas of the world, and doubts are developing about its usefulness even in North America.[2] It is not reliable in that several independent psychiatrists examining the same individual will come to several different diagnostic conclusions.

Prescientific medicine faced similar problems. It had to be descriptive since there were no laboratory tests or other accurate diagnostic methods available. Pain in the chest, worse on inhalation and exhalation, and fever suggested that something may be

From the *J Orthomolecular Med* 2008;23(3):139–152.

wrong in the lungs. Pneumonia was a high-risk-of-death disease and before antibiotics became available one of the standard treatments was mustard plaster (a poultice of mustard seed powder). Today, we know that there are many causes of pneumonia. Tests help us to determine the real cause and then appropriate treatment is given.

Modern psychiatry is in the mustard-plaster stage of scientific diagnosis. This is understandable if the tests are not available but it is unforgivable when available tests are not used. Psychiatrists over 100 years ago did use tests when they became available. Around 1900 a textbook of psychiatry discussed differential diagnosis of psychosis, which included pellagra (vitamin B3 deficiency), scurvy (vitamin C deficiency), syphilis of the brain, and dementia praecox. The two vitamin deficiency syndromes were removed eventually from psychiatry and came under proper care by public health professionals and other doctors. The addition of small amounts of niacin (vitamin B3) to flour almost eradicated pellagra. (This was one of the greatest public mental health measures ever and did more to decrease the incidence and prevalence of psychosis than all of psychiatry has done.) General paresis of the insane (syphilis) was diagnosed by a blood test and disappeared from psychiatry. Dementia praecox also disappeared by being renamed schizophrenia.

There was little further progress in psychiatric diagnoses until orthomolecular psychiatry developed. In 1960 my research group in Saskatchewan, Canada, discovered a substance in the urine of psychiatric patients called the "mauve factor," as it stained the paper chromatograms mauve. We used this as a way of characterizing a condition we called malvaria (later renamed pyroluria by Carl Pfeiffer, MD),[4] a metabolic condition caused by excessive levels of pyrroles in the body. These patients came from several diagnostic groups, including schizophrenics, who excreted too much of this factor into their urine. Dr. Pfeiffer eventually described a large number of different syndromes of schizophrenia. Each requires a rather different program. For if the disease is present due to a deficiency or a need for a lot of niacin, it will not respond to any other vitamin or treatment. Drugs are not specific; they swamp the whole bio-chemical machinery of the body and affect everything. They cannot be expected to be curative in the way that discovering the cause and treating it is.

Of the 40 or more different attention-deficit hyperactivity disorders in children, the main treatment is Ritalin no matter which of the 40 labels is attached to the child. A child may be seen by 10 different psychiatrists and be given 10 different diagnoses and numerical classifications, and yet leave the office with the same prescription.

Conflicts of Interest and Diagnosis of Attention-Deficit Hyperactivity Disorders

Colleen Clements, PhD, associate professor of psychiatry at the University of Rochester in New York, is a medical ethicist who writes a column for the *Medical Post*.[5] She is very concerned about the pervasive use of Ritalin and other stimulants for the treatment of children diagnosed with one of the ADHD disorders. She points out that 1) ADHD is a classification with dubious scientific basis; 2) there are no well-established norms against which to judge the behavior of these children; 3) long-term treatment with these drugs interferes with normal development and society appears to benefit more than the child does from this treatment, and; 4) the condition that a serious deviation must be present before treatment is started is ignored. Children are put in an illness category, which is degrading of their normality and worth. In a following issue she makes her points more dramatically: drug prescriptions to children and adolescents increased from 275 per 100,000 in 1995 to 1,438 per 100,000 in 2002. This is a fivefold increase; 40 percent were on another drug as well.

Between 1950, when I first became interested in psychiatry, and 1965, the older diagnoses were used. Various degrees of retardation were diagnosed based primarily on the IQ test. Down's syndrome was diagnosed on physical appearance. A few schizophrenic children were recognized using adult criteria. Autism had only been recently described and was so rare most doctors never saw any cases. A few hyperactive children were recognized. They were called minimally brain damaged. But this was very unpopular with their parents who heard only the word "brain damage" and not the word "minimally." Eventually, the term was dropped and replaced by hyperactivity. From 1965 to today, there has been an explosion of diagnostic categories. The DSM-IV introduced the attention-deficit system listing about 40 different categories each with its own diagnostic number. Yet, all the diagnoses are descriptive. None has any real meaning.

The problem is, psychiatric diagnosis contrary to all diagnosis in medicine is not scientific. It is descriptive, legal, and moral. There are many variations in the way people behave and think and there is no limit to the number of descriptive diagnostic categories. I fully expect that one day the DSM will be thicker than the telephone books of large cities.

There must be a reason and one is conflict of interest. A flagrant example of conflict of interest is reported by Cosgrove et al.[6] She and her colleagues examined the financial relationship between DSM-IV panel members and Big Pharma. Out of 170 panel members, 56 percent had one or more financial associations with Big Pharma. All the members of the panel on Mood Disorder and Schizophrenia had these ties. If a company has a drug released for treatment of schizophrenia, it will profit them handsomely if the criteria for this condition are so relaxed, so altered, that many patients not previously diagnosed schizophrenia will become so under the new guidelines. If diagnosis were scientific, this would play little role but since the diagnosis is more psychological and political, it does play a major role.

Psychiatry knows that this is a profitable semantic game.[7] It is not stupid. Thus, Dr. Michael First, director of the project that reviewed DSM-IV, expects fewer new categories will be added because "they're hard to get rid of. It's disruptive to eliminate a disorder people have been using." This statement gives the game away. Because real diseases cannot be gotten rid of so easily simply by deleting them from the diagnoses manuals. If they can be added and later deleted simply by a popular vote or by popular pressure, are they really disorders? Or are they sophisticated ways of describing behavior that might better be used in novels and public discourse and not tied to diseases where they do harm to victims of these diag-

noses? But there is a glimmer of hope. Dr. First indicates that in the new DSM-V some laboratory tests may be included in the diagnosis.[8]

The Effects of Psychiatric Drugs on Children

The latest mass trend is to diagnose children as bipolar. Today, in the United States, there are 1 million children on toxic adult drugs for their bipolar disorder. They are diagnosed as early as age three. Anne Duffy, MD,[9] in a review concludes that as currently diagnosed, bipolar disorder does not manifest as such typically until at least adolescence. The title of her paper is a question "Does Bipolar Disorder Exist in Children? A Selected Review." After reviewing 41 published reports, she concludes that it does not. She writes, "Chronic fluctuating abnormalities of mood, over activity and cognition and conduct disturbances have been described in very young children. Whether this syndrome represents an early variant of bipolar disorder or some other psychiatric disturbance is at this time unknown and requires further research."

A report by Madsen et al[10] found a significant association between the amount of tranquilizers (sedatives) taken over years in grams and cerebral cortex atrophy. The estimated risk of atrophy increases by 6.4 percent for each additional 10,000 milligrams (mg) of tranquilizer drug. Gur et al[11] reported that tranquilizers increased sub-cortical volumes in schizophrenic patients. These changes were not present in patients not on this medication. They suggested these changes were in response to receptor blockade and could decrease the effect of treatment. In other words, these drugs damage the brain and decrease the odds these patients can ever recover.

At age two children's brains start to develop rapidly and reach adult weight by age five. Between ages two and five, the brain triples in weight and this is the period when children are more impulse than control. They have to learn ways of dealing with others and with aggression so that they will become good members of society. How can the developing brain deal with these if inhibited with toxic drugs? It is well known that children are much more sensitive to drugs, even to the additives that are present in our food.

571

Forty years ago Dr. Ben Feingold, a well-known and respected allergist, reported that these additives made some children develop these problems. His work was totally rejected except by parents of the children who found their children became better when these additives were removed. A panel of the U.S. National Institutes of Health (NIH) determined in 1982 that there was no scientific evidence to support these claims. The majority of clinical studies done at that time including some that were controlled, all showed that Feingold was wrong. The paradigm at that time opposed his conclusions. The paradigm is now changing and the recent studies, also controlled, show that Feingold was right.[12] As the paradigm changes it becomes easier to insinuate these out-of-the box studies and to get them accepted. Most people do not realize that to the medical profession, the term "scientific" means it has been accepted by the paradigm. If it is outside the paradigm, it is not scientific.

Allowing these children to be diagnosed bipolar on vague behavioral changes that are simply a learning process is like giving a license to kill, if not the child, then his or her mental growth and development.

ADHD and Stimulant Drugs

As the diagnostic term hyperactivity became more popular, the use of stimulant drugs also increased beginning with the amphetamines (speed), and later with Ritalin, which has evolved into different names and different formulations for the same drug. These stimulants had what was called a paradoxical effect on these active children. It relaxed them. (Given to adults they were stimulants and were used to treat conditions with excessive sleepiness and to control excess sedation of the anticonvulsants.) They were very effective and needed no double-blind studies to show that they did something. Children who were out of control would quickly settle down. This was great for schools who could not deal with too many hyperactive children in the classes. The drugs would be given in the morning, which would keep them more or less down, until they went home when the effect of the drug was gone and their hyperactivity once more exerted itself. Teachers appreciated these

drugs more than did their parents. (Adults taking these drugs were given barbiturates to help them sleep and amphetamines in the morning to waken them up.) They were widely abused. One of my patients became addicted to amphetamines given to him when young to keep his weight down and later became schizophrenic. A few children not liking the side effects of these drugs would not swallow them and would sell them (aka "kiddie coke") to their older school chums. But over the past two decades they have been replaced by Ritalin. Diagnosing children with one or more of the 40 diagnostic categories for attention deficit gave the doctor permission to give them any combination of Ritalin and other drugs.

Health Canada, the department responsible for the country's public health, warns that ADHD drugs can be deadly, even for youngsters (*Times Colonist*, Victoria, BC, May 27, 2006). It should have said especially for youngsters whose lives may be destroyed by these drugs, which include Adderall, Attenade, Biphentin Concerta, Dexedrine, Ritalin and Ritalin SR, and Strattera. The potential market is immense and explains why so many different names are used for almost the same drugs for these children. Health Canada warns that they may cause heart disease and even death but does not mention many other very serious side effects such as loss of appetite, suppression of growth, and the consequences on personality by long-term drug use, and later addictions, but some doctors are not convinced as they see more benefit than risk. This is a logical point of view if one does not know that there are much better alternatives to these drugs, which are effective and do not cause any of the side effects listed.

The Ritalin advocates have new ammunition in their major attempt to retain this drug for the treatment of children, the National Institute of Mental Health, which sponsored what it calls "the first long-term, large-scale study designed to determine the safety and effectiveness of treating preschoolers who have attention-deficit hyperactivity disorder with methylphenidate (Ritalin)." Not surprisingly, they found it safe and effective when used in low doses for preschoolers, ages three to five. The study found that children in this age range are more sensitive than older children to the medication's side effects and therefore should be closely monitored.

Let's tease out the relevant data from this carefully worded document designed to support their conclusions:

1. The study ran for 70 weeks. This may be a long time in contrast to the usual few months drug studies but is very short term in respect to these children growing into their mid teens. Malnutrition may not show its worst toxic side effects for up to 20 years. To call this a long-term study is surely a major stretch. They also called it a large scale study but only 303 children were included. The term "large scale" is unwarranted even if that sample size was probably adequate. The description "long term" and "large scale" are used to soothe the public.

2. Safety. Adverse effects are worse than with older children.

3. The medication slowed the children's growth rates. Over the 70 weeks of the study, they grew one-half inch less than the expected rates. Suppose we estimate what would happen if these children remained on trial for ten years, into their teens, which is not that uncommon. This is difficult as growth is not linear with respect to age but we can estimate that on the average they would be 5 inches shorter and weigh 30 pounds less. How many teenagers would appreciate having their height and weight cut down that much? Height has economic and competitive advantages for both men and women. I know of no teenagers who would be happy if they knew that was going to occur.

4. Eleven percent had to drop out of the study as a result of intolerable side effects. For example, while some children lost weight, weight loss of 10 percent or more of the child's baseline weight was considered a severe enough side effect for the investigators to discontinue the medication. Other side effects included insomnia, loss of appetite, mood disturbances such as feeling nervous or worried, and skin-picking behaviors. Can a treatment which makes one out of ten worse really be considered safe and effective?

Children and Antipsychotics

I consider psychiatric drugs essential evils with major emphasis on the word "evil." They are essential for many patients but evil when used in large doses and forever. They are less evil when used in much smaller doses and for shorter periods, and if combined with orthomolecular psychiatric methods. They should be used like crutches and thrown away when they are no longer needed. Much more attention must given to the toxic side effects of antipsychotics. One of the major toxic long-term side effects is that it is almost impossible to ever fully get well when on the medication. The natural recovery rate when patients with mental disorders are given proper shelter, good food, and are treated with civility and respect is around 40 percent. When treated by modern psychiatry, it drops down to about 10 percent.

A SIGNATURE CASE HISTORY

In 1960, a physician called me from the United States. He was crying as he told me about his son, age 12, who was in hospital. He had just been advised that there was no treatment, no hope, and that he should lock him up in a California state mental hospital and forget about him. That was very common advice. I advised his father that he should obtain some niacin and take it to the hospital to discuss with his son's psychiatrist. I did not think that any knowledgeable doctor would be afraid of a vitamin. This was a failure as the psychiatrist became very angry, denounced the use of niacin saying that they had tested it and that it would fry his brains. Both statements were equally not true. I have been on niacin for over 50 years and so far my brain appears not to have been fried. Father then began to visit his son daily and while there, he fed him jam sandwiches made up of a slice of bread, a layer of jam, niacin powder, another layer of jam and a slice of bread. Three months later he wanted to go home. He completed Grade 12 in the top 5 percent of high school students in the country. Later, he studied medicine, obtained his MD degree, and became a research psychiatrist. He spent one summer working in Linus Pauling's laboratory.

In Sweden, government legislation enforces the "substitution principle"[12] This means that, if a safer alternative is available for any toxic chemical added to the environment, food, and so on, there is a legal obligation to use the safer compound. This is a very enlightened policy, not used in the North America. It should be enforced in all forms of chemotherapy including antipsychotic medication to replace drugs that are dangerous and for which there are safer alternatives. I consider treating with psychiatric drugs palliative chemotherapy for psychiatric conditions, and about as effective as is chemotherapy for cancer. And in the same way that chemotherapy for cancer leaves patients very sick, so treatment with antipsychotics causes the tranquilizer psychosis that is often confused with the original psychosis.

Side effects, usually involuntary movements, can be permanent and are hence evidence of brain damage. A report in 1985 in the *Mental and Physical Disability Law Reporter* indicates courts in the United States have finally begun to consider involuntary administration of the so-called major tranquilizer/antipsychotic/neuroleptic drugs to involve First Amendment rights because antipsychotic drugs have the capacity to severely and even permanently affect an individual's ability to think and communicate. In *Molecules of the Mind: The Brave New Science of Molecular Psychology* (1987), Professor Jon Franklin[14] observed: "This era coincided with an increasing awareness that the neuroleptics not only did not cure schizophrenia, they actually caused damage to the brain. In severe cases, brain damage from neuroleptic drugs is evidenced by abnormal body movements called tardive dyskinesia. However, tardive dyskinesia is only the tip of the iceberg of neuroleptic-caused brain damage. Higher mental functions are more vulnerable and are impaired before the elementary functions of the brain such as motor control."

Orthomolecular Treatment: Why Is Not Every Child Getting the Benefit?

By 1960, I had been using large doses of vitamin B3 (niacin or niacinamide) for seven years for treating schizophrenia, lowering cholesterol, and decreasing the ravages of senility and other conditions.[15] But I had very little experience with its beneficial effects in helping children with learning and behavioral disorders. (These are usually correlated as it is rare that a child will suffer from one set of these symptoms and not the other.) That year, however, I began using this vitamin to help children.

In 1999,[17] I described 110 brief case histories of children under the age of 14 whom I had treated with orthomolecular methods. It is obvious that many of them, if seen by a child psychiatrist, would be diagnosed with one or more of the attention-deficit disorders and bipolar. They would have been treated with antipsychotic drugs and none would have recovered. The first three children I treated in 1960 recovered. No double-blind studies were needed. Today, I have treated well over 2,000 patients under the age of 14.[17] There were very few failures.

My conclusions have since been recorded in dozens of publications and in several books, and there has been massive corroboration by physicians who used the treatment I had described.[16] If this treatment is as good as I have seen and described, why is not every child getting the benefit? Why is psychiatry loading these children with heavy doses of Ritalin and atypical antipsychotic drugs? Why did Jay and his family have to suffer so much? Why did it take the intense dedication of Dr. McKay to save Jay's life and allow him to become a functioning human being?

The orthomolecular treatment theory and practice is based on the modern paradigm about the use of vitamins as treatment and not only to prevent a few deficiency disease such as pellagra, scurvy, rickets. The treatment is more complex than just handing out a few vitamin pills. That is how it started, but it became clear that the whole field of nutrition is involved. That is why in my books on children I give so much space to nutrition.

The first element is to correct the diet of the child. Too many consume huge amounts of food artifacts such as the sugars, harmful fats, and products made from refined flour. Just as important is to eliminate foods to which the child is allergic. This has been totally ignored by medicine except by a few clinical ecologists who are also ignored. If the child is sick because she is eating large amounts of milk to which she is allergic, the child will not recover until that has been corrected. The child can eat all good foods.

After the child and his parents are instructed with respect to what to eat and when (i.e., to have three meals each day), he is started on the appropriate vitamins. For a child with behavioral and/or learning disorders, the two B vitamins—niacin (B3) and pyridoxine (B6)—are the most important. When I first began to treat with vitamins I used only vitamin B3, but later it became clear that vitamin B6 also played a role especially for autistic children. Vitamin C is needed as no one ever gets enough from food. Vitamin D is needed especially in northern countries where ultraviolet light is rare most of the year. And since it is rare for any person to have only one deficiency, it is good to add a multi B-complex preparation. The most important minerals are zinc and selenium.

Perhaps a more detailed description may be more persuasive. Ben was my first child to receive orthomolecular treatment. Being the first he, his family, and his response remain fresh in my mind. If a picture is worth a thousand words perhaps one good anecdote is worth dozens of brief case histories.

The Case of Ben

One evening, early in 1962, my friend George called to say he was very worried bout his youngest son, Ben. Nine years old, Ben had become a behavioral problem with a learning disability. Today, he would be diagnosed as suffering from ADHD or one of its many variants. Progress at school was so slow his teachers began to prepare his parents to have him go to a school for slow learners, perhaps even to a school for the mentally retarded. But before anyone was aware that Ben had such a problem, he had tested 120 on an IQ (intelligence quotient) test. To his father, a public administrator, and his mother, a teacher, this was not only perplexing but very disturbing. I asked George to bring Ben to my office on the fifth floor of the University Hospital, now the Royal University Hospital, in Saskatoon. At the time, I was director of psychiatric research, and associate professor of psychiatry at the medical school.

"The DSM system (the standard of the American Psychiatric Association) has little or no relevance to diagnosis. It has no relevance to treatment, either. No matter which terms are used to classify these children, they are all recommended for treatment with drug therapy. If the entire diagnostic scheme were scrapped today, it would make almost no difference to the way these children were treated, or to the outcome of treatment. Nor would their patients feel any better or worse."

— ABRAM HOFFER

I was not very keen on seeing Ben since I had little experience in treating children. The few children I had seen in the previous ten years were all considered either slow learners or had various degrees of severe retardation and no treatment was available for them. The modern type of hyperactive learning-disordered child was extremely rare in 1960. But George was so disturbed I set aside my worry about making a proper assessment of Ben.

Ben came into my office with his father. He was a good-looking boy, appeared healthy, with none of the physical stigmata of the seriously retarded children seen in old psychiatric textbooks. He did not know why he had been brought to see me, and he denied having any problems or symptoms. His father gave me his developmental history. He was walking by 14 months and speaking by 20 months. Both parents considered him an ideal child until he entered Grade 1 when he was seven years old. By the end of 1960, his mother noticed a change in behavior. He became more anxious, could not fall asleep at night, and, if he did sleep, he woke up frequently during the night. School became harder for Ben. When the family moved to a different part of the city and he was moved to a different school, he had even more problems. His teachers were worried about his erratic performance at school and told his parents he was in a "shell." Reading and spelling were very poor. He finished Grade 3 with a D average in spite of extensive tutoring and drilling at home by his mother.

In July 1961, he was examined by a mental health clinic specializing in treating children. Ben's mother told them he had a very poor memory, reversed letters, and had no knowledge of phonics. His eyes skipped back and forth so much she tried to keep him focused by using a ruler under the lines. His teachers reported he was not working up to his best ability, spent a lot of time day-dreaming, wasting time, and therefore falling behind. His marks were very low. He did not complete his assignments and did not bother to write his exams, nor could he be motivated. At home Ben was negative to his father, missed a lot of school, and often would come home after school hours not having gone to school that day. The clinic blamed the move to a new school and sibling rivalry with his brother, a year and a half older. They recommended remedial reading, which proved to be ineffective.

After my examination, I was puzzled. Nothing appeared that could explain the deterioration of this child to his present state. I arranged to analyze his urine for the kryptopyrroles (originally called "mauve factor"). This was the substance, which I previously mentioned, that my research group had discovered in the urine of a majority of schizophrenic patients we treated, but it was also found in a smaller number of patients with other diagnoses. Over the previous few years, I had found that any patient with this substance in their urine more closely resembled schizophrenia than they did other diagnostic groups and that they responded very well to large doses of vitamin B3.

The next day we found large quantities of kryptopyrrole in Ben's urine. I started Ben on niacinamide (3,000 mg) three times each day after meals. His parents continued this regimen for several months. George called me again that fall and told me that Ben was normal. He had been given remedial reading for two months by the clinic, who then pronounced him well, but he had shown no progress whatever before starting on the vitamin. He had spent the summer happily getting caught up with his reading.

One of his teachers prepared a report on Ben which she sent to me in 1973. George had advised her that Ben had done so badly in previous classes that he was called "stupid" in school and had responded by not answering any questions during class. But to her surprise she found him active in group discussions and volunteering answers. Here is what she wrote: "The first thing that his parents noticed in Ben's improvement after he showed an improvement in his health was his desire to go to school. Ben started to do his assignments, but at first he found the excuse of hunting for his books and pencils in his desk to delay him in starting his assignments promptly." The teacher started keeping his books on her desk for some time, but midway through the term Ben took the initiative to get his books out promptly and began his assignments. Previous to vitamin therapy, Ben had no desire to take down all the notes given in the allotted time. When anything was dictated, Ben would have a hard time keeping up. Then he would become very tense and, so to speak, "fold up." This would happen in some exams, especially in Spelling and Arithmetic, which he was slow doing, and then he would run out of time.

These problems soon began to disappear. Many other improvements were noted physically, socially, emotionally, and educationally. Ben at the beginning of the term would pride himself with the fact his mother was also a teacher. Later on in the term, Ben also started to mention his father and brother. "Ben is no longer shy," his teacher reported. "He is a sparkling personality; not afraid to speak up. He has started to take an interest in sports, in which he excels and which should be encouraged. He now gets along well with the children at school and at camp. He will assume leadership and organization duties. Ben now can read with eye-reversal not noticeable in reading and seldom in writing. Ben would go up on the stage to sing, say a speech, and read the morning scripture to the whole student body and the staff. All of these things he did well with little nervousness and tension noticeable. Ben also reads books without being told and enjoys reading them."

In 1966, Ben had completed Grade 7 with a low A average. In Grade 9 he went to a track meet, participated in extracurricular activities, and worked as stage manager for a school play. He was so busy he finished his scholastic year with a C average. Nevertheless, his parents were delighted with his state of normality.

In 1970, his mother wanted me to see him again. Ben had not taken niacinamide for two years, and she was worried that he might relapse. Ben had forgotten he had ever seen me and did not understand why he should take vitamin pills. I explained the situation to him, and he agreed he would start again and keep taking the vitamins and niacinamide until age 18. Later Ben married. He is raising a family and has a responsible permanent job. He meets my criteria for recovery: he is free of symptoms and signs of illness, he gets on well with his family and with the community, and he is employed and pays taxes.

Although Ben was one of the first children I tested for kryptopyrrole and advised to take large doses of niacinamide, he is an excellent example of what can be done for these children with so-called learning disabilities and behavioral disorders if they are examined, diagnosed, and treated with the correct, orthomolecular approach. Ben's treatment and response to a vitamin in large doses is a prototype of what can be achieved through diet and nutrient supplements, not only for "ill" children like Ben, but also for "healthy" children.

Discussion

I still marvel at the fact that a disease, which was very seldom diagnosed in children a few years ago, is found in millions of children down to the age of two to such a degree that they are given antipsychotic drugs. This may be due to the "cascade phenomenon." *New York Times* science reporter John Tierney[18] writes, "Cascades are especially common in medicine." This phenomenon leads to widespread errors and mistaken consensus agreements. Tierney continues, "Doctors take their cues from others, leading them to overdiagnose some faddish ailment (called bandwagon diseases) and overprescribe certain treatment (like the tonsillectomies once popular for children). Unable to keep up with the volume of research, doctors look for guidance from an expert—or at least someone who sounds confident."

The idea that bipolar is so common originated at Harvard University with Joseph Biederman, MD, chief of child psychopharmacology at Massachusetts General Hospital. In a CBS program he defined the disorder more broadly so that more children could be diagnosed. He was very confident. Here we have the needed elements for a "cascade" to start—the opinion by a respected scientist attached to Harvard. How many psychiatrists would stand up against a scientist from a distinguished university? The idea was also very attractive and helpful to Big Pharma, which found an enormous new market for these drugs. I also find it bizarre that a diagnostic system such as the DSM that has never been validated and that is useless and harmful, can have been accepted so quickly by the profession and that a treatment, for which there is no evidence that it works for children and has not been released for this purpose, can have become so popular in a very few years, whereas orthomolecular treatment—which has been developing over decades and which has been corroborated every time it has been used—is hardly known. Of course, the massive sweep of bad ideas is not unique to psychiatry.

■ CONCLUSION

Psychiatric diagnosis as described in DSM-IV is not scientific, nor useful, either for treatment or prognosis, and should be abandoned. It should be replaced by etiologic diagnosis, such as allergies, and vitamin and mineral deficiency and dependency. Present diagnosis is harmful to children. It is a license to kill. Palliative toxic psychiatric chemotherapy should follow the "substitution principle" mandated in Sweden for toxic environmental chemicals.

The adoption of these two policies would eliminate a large number of harmful conditions including brain damage, suicide, diabetes, abnormal blood lipid levels, and associated cardiovascular disease. On a social level, it would eliminate much pain, hardship, family disruption, and chronic invalidism.

REFERENCES

1. Allen S. Tracks children on psychiatric drugs: prescriptions eyed after overdose. *Boston Globe,* Oct 7, 2007.

2. Parker G. Through a glass darkly: the disutility of the DSM nosology of depressive disorders. *Can J Psychiatry* 2006;51:879–886.

3. Goldney RD. The utility of the DSM nosology of depressive disorders. *Can J Psychiatry* 2006;51:874–878.

4. Hoffer A, Osmond H. Malvaria: a new psychiatric disease. *Acta Psychiat Scand* 1963;39:335–366.

5. Clements C. ADHD: America: the drugged. *Medical Post* (Toronto) May 2, 2005, 12–13.

6. Cosgrove L, Krinsky S, Vijayaraqhavan M, et al. Financial ties between DSM-IV panel members and the pharmaceutical industry. *Psychotherapy and Psychosomatics* 1996;75:154–160.

7. Gerstel J. Road rager, mad spouse: ill or nasty? Psychiatric labels cast wide net on human foibles. *Toronto Star,* June 16, 2006.

8. First MB. Including laboratory tests in DSMIV diagnostic criteria. *Am J Psychiat* 2006;163:2041–2042.

9. Duffy A. Does bipolar disorder exist in children? A selected review. *Can J Psychiat* 2007;52:400–415.

10. Madsen A, Keiding N, Karle A, et al. Neuroleptics in progressive structural abnormalities in psychiatric illness. *Lancet* 1998;352:784.

11. Gur RE, Manny V, Mozley PD, et al. Subcortical MRI volumes in neuroleptic-naive and treated patients with schizophrenia. *Am J Psychiat* 1998;155;1711–1717.

12. Schab DW, Trinh, NH. Do artificial food colors promote hyperactivity in children with hyperactive syndromes? A meta-analysis of double blind placebo controlled trials. *J Dev Behav Pediatr* 2004;25(6):423–434.

13. Luymes G. Chemicals are quiet killers: report. *Times Colonist* (Victoria), Oct 7, 2007.

14. Franklin J. *Molecules of the Mind: The Brave New Science of Molecular Psychology.* New York: Atheneum, 1987.

15. Hoffer A, Foster HD. *Feel Better, Live Longer with Vitamin B3.* Toronto ON: CCNM Press, 2007.

16. Hoffer A. *Hoffer's ABC of Natural Nutrition for Children.* Kingston, ON: Quarry Press, 1999.

17. Hoffer A. *Healing Children's Attention and Behavior Disorders.* Kingston, ON: Quarry Press, 2005.

18. Tierney J. Diet and fat: a severe case of mistaken consensus. *New York Times,* Oct 9, 2007.

BIPOLAR KIDS NEED NUTRITION,
NOT JUNK FOOD AND MORE DRUGS

by Andrew W. Saul, PhD

The *New York Times* magazine cover story, "The Bipolar Kid" (September 14, 2008), is a very bleak article. While emphasizing the miseries of living with such a child, Jennifer Egan's article offers little hope except for ever-increasing doses of lithium. Long on discussions of definitions and diagnoses, it is remarkably short on treatment alternatives. Not a word about diet. Not a word about vitamins. Indeed, in this 9,500-word feature, describing the daily life of an out-of-control, beyond-ADHD boy, the word "nutrition" is not mentioned at all. Neither are the words "sugar" or "caffeine."

What astounding omissions. Pediatrician Lendon H. Smith nationally famous as "The Children's Doctor," was very plain in stating that sugar causes profound mood disorders.[1] He specifically advised parents to give their children a "sugarless diet without processed foods." It is not easy. The Center for Science in the Public Interest has reported that children between the ages of six and eleven drink nearly a pint of soda a day. Twenty percent of toddlers drink soda, nearly a cup daily.[2] And, of the seven best-selling soft drinks, six have caffeine in them. In sensitive people, caffeine can cause psychotic behavior.[3]

Not a Word About Food Chemicals

Food colorings and benzoate preservatives increase childhood hyperactivity, according to research published in *Archives of Disease in Childhood* (June 2004).[4] The study, involving 277 preschool children, also demonstrated that withdrawing these chemical additives decreased hyperactivity. When additives were reintroduced, there was once again an increase in hyperactivity. "Additives do have an effect on overactive behavior independent of baseline allergic and behavioral status," said lead author Dr. J. O. Warner. So many parents, and any of us who have taught school the day after Halloween, can verify this.

It is possible that the children profiled in the *New York Times* story are unusual in that they do not consume any sugar, or any artificial food colorings, or any benzoate preservatives, or any caffeine-laced soft drinks. But it is much more likely that they do. The article ignored these important factors even though health professionals are increasingly aware that the normal functioning of the brain and nervous system is nutrient-dependent and additive sensitive. Dr. Ian Brighthope says, "What is going on in the mind can be influenced by the nutrients and chemicals going into it. You can't get anywhere with a patient with psychiatric symptomatology if their brain is hungry, starved, or poisoned."[5]

Yet in the entire *Times* article, the words "allergy" and "junk food" are not mentioned, not even once. Children's learning and behavior problems often begin in their parents' grocery carts. Allergist Benjamin Feingold was convinced of the negative effect of food chemicals on children's behavior and the role of good nutrition in treatment.[6] Says the Feingold Association: "Numerous studies show that certain synthetic food additives can have serious learning, behavior, and/or health effects for sensitive people."[7]

Not a Word About Vitamins

Another word totally absent from the *Times* article is "vitamin." Psychiatrist Abram Hoffer has had decades of experience and considerable success treating children's behavioral disorders with vitamins. High doses of vitamin B3 (niacin or niacinamide) were first used by Hoffer and colleague Dr. Humphry Osmond in the early 1950s. The trials were double-blind and placebo-controlled. Over half a century later, vitamin therapy has still been largely ignored by the psychiatric profession and, evidently, by some newspapers.

What a loss to patients and their families. I know and personally observed a preadolescent who was having serious behavioral problems in school and at home. Interestingly enough, the child had already been taking physician-prescribed little bits of niacin, though totaling less than 150 milligrams (mg) per day, but evidently it wasn't enough to be effective. When tried, drugs (especially Adderall) actually made him worse: far more angry and dangerously confrontational. I was present when his parents had to hold him down while he screamed death threats at them. In desperation, his mother finally tried giving him 500 mg of niacin, three times daily (1,500 mg total). There was some improvement. With about 500 mg every two hours (an astounding 6,000–8,000 mg/day), the boy was a new person. He was now a cheerful, cooperative, affectionate youngster. Adding vitamins C and B6 to his regimen helped even more. His school performance soared, the teachers loved him, and they repeatedly said so. At age 15, his maintenance dose was about 3,000 mg per day. He has since graduated from high school and is successfully employed. This is exactly in line with what Dr. Hoffer has repeatedly demonstrated for over 50 years.[8]

Two Sides to a Story

People often ask, "If this treatment is so good, how come my doctor doesn't know about it? How come it is not in the newspaper?" Those are good questions. The *New York Times* should know that reporting one side is not good reporting. To tell the whole story, we need nutrition. So do bipolar children.

REFERENCES

1. Smith L. *Foods for Healthy Kids*. New York: McGraw-Hill, July 1981.

2. Jacobson MF. Available at www.cspinet.org/sodapop /liquid_candy.htm. Accessed Sept 18, 2008.

3. Whalen R. *Welcome to the Dance: Caffeine Allergy, a Masked Cerebral Allergy and Progressive Toxic Dementia*. Victoria, BC: Trafford Publishing, 2005.

4. Bateman B. *Arch Dis Child* 2004;89(6):506–511.

5. Interview. *Food Matters*. Thornleigh, AU: Permacology Productions, 2008.

6. Feingold BF. *Why Your Child Is Hyperactive*. New York: Random House, 1985.

7. www.feingold.org/pg-research.html and www.feingold.org /pg-news.html.

8. Hoffer A. *Healing Children's Attention & Behavior Disorders: Complementary Nutritional and Psychological Treatments*. Toronto, ON: CCNM Press, 2004.

Excerpted from *Orthomolecular Medicine News Service*, October 16, 2008.

THE BENEFITS OF GOING BEYOND CONVENTIONAL THERAPIES FOR ADHD
by Gary Null, PhD, and Martin Feldman, MD

Attention-deficit hyperactivity disorder (ADHD) has the distinction of being the most thoroughly studied of all the behavioral/emotional disorders of childhood.[1] But despite the continuing focus on this disorder, experts in the topic acknowledge that many aspects of ADHD—from its etiology to the best form of treatment—continue to be poorly understood or controversial.[2,3]

Two such controversies stem from the ADHD protocols of conventional medicine, which use subjective methods of diagnosis and mind-altering pharmaceuticals such as Ritalin and Adderall. Although these drugs are central nervous system stimulants, in the case of ADHD they have the paradoxical effect of calming the patient. Unfortunately, they also put the growing number of children and adolescents who are diagnosed with ADHD at risk of the adverse effects associated with these drugs, particularly methylphenidate (Ritalin, Concerta, Metadate, Focalin, Methylin). The negative effects range from insomnia and decreased appetite to movement disorders such as tics and the stunting of children's growth. An analysis of orthodox medicine's approach to diagnosing and treating ADHD will reveal the benefits of using more natural methods of treating the collection of symptoms now grouped under the ADHD label.

Problems of Diagnosis

ADHD has become the most commonly diagnosed behavioral disorder of childhood, characterized by the core symptoms of inattention, impulsivity, and hyperactivity. Data on its prevalence vary. The American Psychiatric Association (APA) reports that 3 to 5 percent of school-age children have ADHD[4]; the American Academy of Pediatrics reports 4 to 12 percent.[5] The most stringent estimate in a recent study by the Mayo Clinic puts the figure at 7.4 percent of children by age 19.[6] In a controversial development, the diagnosis of ADHD and use of stimulant medications have been increasing among adults.[7] According to one

expert, the literature suggests that "ADHD is best conceptualized as a lifelong disability rather than as a childhood disorder."[8]

However, the diagnosis of ADHD and its treatment with pharmaceuticals have been largely concentrated in the United States,[9,10] making ADHD an American phenomenon and raising questions about whether it is a true disorder. It is of interest that the use of methylphenidate for ADHD has increased sharply in many other countries—mostly European ones—as well, according to the International Narcotics Control Board. Consumption in countries such as Belgium, Germany, Iceland, and the Netherlands increased by 150 percent to 350 percent in a recent five-year period. Consumption in Australia and Canada, formerly main consumer countries of methylphenidate, has leveled off or declined, although they are the only countries besides the United States to report significant use of amphetamines for the treatment of ADHD.[11]

In diagnosing ADHD, physicians and psychiatrists use a variety of assessment tools and rating scales, such as the Conners'/Clinical Assessment of Depression (CAD) scales and the diagnostic criteria presented in the APA's *Diagnostic and Statistical Manual of Mental Disorders*. DSM-IV (1994) defines three major subtypes of the diagnosis of attention-deficit hyperactivity disorder (ADHD): predominantly inattentive, predominantly hyperactive-impulsive, and a combined type. (This condition also is referred to as attention-deficit disorder, ADD. The APA replaced its former diagnosis of ADD—with or without hyperactivity—with the unidimensional ADHD diagnosis in 1987, then specified the three subtypes in 1994.)[12, 13]

Children with ADHD may have one, two, or all three of the core symptoms of inattention, hyperactivity, and impulsivity. Thus, a child may be diagnosed with ADHD even if he or she is not hyperactive. Girls, for example, often fall into the

From the *J Orthomolecular Med* 2005;20(2):75–88.

inattentive subtype.[14] However, a 2000 review of the diagnosis of ADHD points out that the DSM-IV criteria for this disorder are phenomenologic rather than etiologic and are much more relevant for children than for adolescents and adults.[15]

An easy-to-see problem with this approach to diagnosis is that the assessments are not definitive. The National Institutes of Health (NIH) believes the diagnosis of ADHD can be made reliably using diagnostic interview methods, but it also said in its 1998 Consensus Statement on ADHD that "there is no independent valid test for ADHD."[16] Although new testing methods are being developed, the diagnosis of ADHD remains far less objective than that of other abnormalities, where specific tools such as blood tests, x-rays, and sonograms are used to determine the presence of the disorder.

Furthermore, the answers provided by parents and teachers on behavior rating scales—to questions such as how much a child fidgets or whether he/she is easily distracted—are subjective. What one person views as distractibility, another may view as natural inquisitiveness. Some of the questions also are based on questionable values or assumptions. For example, the Conners' Parent Rating Scale[17] asks whether the child "actively defies or refuses to comply with adults' requests." In some life situations, though, disobedience is a virtue.

Another problem with the ADHD diagnosis is that it may apply a medical label to behaviors that fall at one end of a spectrum of normal patterns. The NIH says in its Consensus Statement: "Clinicians who diagnose this disorder have been criticized for merely taking a percentage of the normal population who have the most evidence of inattention and continuous activity and labeling them as having a disease. In fact, it is unclear whether the signs of ADHD represent a bimodal distribution in the population or one end of a continuum of characteristics." The NIH observes that one of the problems of diagnosis is to "determine the appropriate boundary between the normal population and those with ADHD."[18]

The APA states itself that the diagnosis of ADHD is not an easy one to make. The symptoms are similar to those of many other childhood disorders.[19] Psychiatrist Abram Hoffer has stated: "You can take this same difficult child to ten psychiatrists and come back with ten different diagnoses. But no matter what the diagnosis is, they all put him on Ritalin."[20] To add to the complexity, approximately 65 percent of patients with ADHD may have one or more coexisting disorders, such as anxiety, communication, mood, conduct, oppositional defiant and learning disorders, and Tourette's syndrome.[21]

One researcher suggests that more exact diagnostic guidelines may emerge from ADHD-related tests of executive functioning, neuroimaging, and genetics that have been developed in recent years.[22] But any such diagnostic methods are likely to be controversial as well. According to a 2004 article, while the current evidence on the genetics of ADHD will provide important clues to its etiology, it is not sufficient to justify the use of genetic screening tests. The authors add that "genetic information on susceptibility to ADHD has the potential to be abused and to stigmatize individuals."[23]

Also open to controversy are the results of neuroimaging studies that have identified supposed abnormalities in structural and functional aspects of the brains of ADHD patients.[24] Researchers have interpreted these findings to mean that the disorder may have a biological basis. For example, a 2003 study in the *Lancet* found reduced regional brain sizes and gray-matter abnormalities in cortical components of attentional systems that may help account for ADHD symptoms.[25]

Research associating ADHD with brain abnormalities does not withstand a critical analysis, however. A review of neuroimaging studies published in *Clinical Neuropharmacology* in 2001 states that, while the results of such studies are often used to support a biological basis for ADHD, "inconsistencies among the studies raise questions about the reliability of the findings." At the time of publication, the researchers found that "no specific abnormality in brain structure or function has been convincingly demonstrated by neuroimaging studies." They concluded that the neuroimaging literature "provides little support for a neurobiologic etiology of ADHD."[26]

Some doctors are already using brain-scanning technologies in the assessment of ADHD, according to a *Wall Street Journal* article. One such method even exposes the patient's brain to a small amount of radioactive material, which is used to illuminate brain activity. However, most researchers believe the use of brain-scanning techniques to diagnose ADHD is premature and impractical, given the expense of the tests and the lack of standard guidelines for interpreting the scans.[27]

Another more objective test of ADHD is available. The Developmental Biopsychiatry Research Program at Harvard's McLean Hospital has developed a diagnostic tool called the McLean Motion and Attention Test (M-MAT) that monitors fine body movements during a computerized task to measure hyperactivity, impulsivity, and attention. Because a child can be retested after taking a dose of medication, the test helps determine whether the drug will be effective for him or her. The researchers believe this test will address the concerns of many physicians that the diagnosis of ADHD is "too subjective, often pathologizes normal childhood behavior, and masks the detection of other important problems, such as a learning disorder."[28]

Conventional Treatment of ADHD

Psychostimulants have become the primary treatment for those diagnosed with ADHD, fueling what the NIH has called one of the major controversies regarding this disorder. The agency noted in 1998 that the growing prescription of these drugs for the short- and long-term treatment of ADHD has led to intensified concerns about their potential overuse and abuse.[29]

The stimulants used to treat ADHD include methylphenidate, mixed salts of amphetamine (Adderall), dextroamphetamine sulfate (Dexedrine, Dextrostat), and, to a much lesser extent, pemoline (Cylert). The methylphenidates and amphetamines are available in short- and long-acting versions. In late 2002, Eli Lilly introduced the first nonstimulant medication approved by the Food and Drug Administration (FDA) for the treatment of ADHD. This drug, atomoxetine (Strattera), is a selective norepinephrine reuptake inhibitor. It had the strongest launch ever for an ADHD drug and was the first such medication approved for the treatment of adults as well as children and adolescents.[30,31]

Stimulant-type drugs still lead this market, however, and numerous studies document their growing prescription during the 1990s.[32–36] One study found that the use of psychotropic medications among young people had reached nearly adult utilization rates in 1996, with stimulants ranked first in the three groups examined.[37] Another study reported sizable increases in the use of stimulants and other medications among even two to four year olds.[38]

Perhaps most disconcerting is a four-year analysis of the use of stimulants in an area of North Carolina that found that the majority of nine- to sixteen-year-old children who took these medications had never had any impairing ADHD symptoms reported by their parents. They did have symptoms and behaviors that were classified as ADHD, but "these typically fell far below the threshold for a DSM-III-R diagnosis of ADHD," say the researchers.[39]

One study finding evidence of overdiagnosis was conducted in southeastern Virginia, where the incidence of grade-school children receiving ADHD medications was two to three times as high as the expected rate of the disorder. By fifth grade, 18 to 20 percent of Caucasian boys were taking ADHD drugs.[40] Meanwhile, a study of the prevalence of stimulant prescriptions in 1999 found wide variations among states, ranging from a high of 6.5 percent in Louisiana to a low of 1.6 percent in the District of Columbia. The authors suggest that areas of both overuse and underuse may exist.[41]

The use of stimulant-type drugs to treat ADHD has grown despite a lack of understanding of their therapeutic action. Methylphenidate and amphetamines are stimulants of the central nervous system (10 milligrams of Ritalin are equivalent to 5 milligrams of amphetamine), yet in patients with ADHD the drugs have a paradoxical effect and reduce the symptoms of inattention, hyperactivity, and impulsive behavior.

Researchers acknowledge that stimulants' method of action in treating ADHD is not well understood.[42–44] According to the *Journal of the American Medical Association*, Nora Volkow, MD, a leading researcher in the imaging of drug effects in the brain, said of methylphenidate in 2001: "As a psychiatrist, sometimes I feel embarrassed about the lack of knowledge because this is, by far, the drug we prescribe most frequently to children."[45]

A 2001 study by Dr. Volkow and colleagues provided direct evidence, for the first time, that therapeutic doses of methylphenidate significantly increase extracellular dopamine in the human brain by blocking dopamine transporters. The researchers postulate that the drug's amplification of weak dopamine signals in ADHD patients enhances task-specific signaling, improving attention and reducing distractibility.[46]

Other research in this area includes a 2003 study that measured regional cerebral blood flow in ADHD patients while they were on and off methylphenidate. The results suggested that Ritalin reduces ADHD symptoms by modulating regions of the brain associated with motor function.[47] A study from Harvard Medical School found evidence that methylphenidate alters activity and attentiveness in children with ADHD in a rate-dependent manner. There was a clear inverse association between the severity of symptoms and the degree of therapeutic response.[48]

Some recent evidence about the dosages of stimulants prescribed to young people is of interest: While the common practice is to increase a child's dosage as he or she grows, this may not be necessary for all patients.[49] In one clinical trial, 40 percent of children who took half the dose of methylphenidate that had kept their symptoms stable, along with a placebo, had equally good ADHD control and fewer side effects.[50] Another study found that the greatest benefit in academic performance and classroom behavior came with the lowest dose studied,[51] while a third reported that "adolescents with ADHD may not necessarily require more medication than younger children to achieve a similar therapeutic effect."[52]

Questions Regarding ADHD Drugs

In addition to uncertainties about the diagnosis of ADHD and the method of action of ADHD drugs, questions remain about the quality of studies of stimulant medications, the safety of these drugs, and the implications of long-term use in young patients with developing brains.

In 2001, pharmacologist Howard Schachter and colleagues published a meta-analysis of 62 randomized trials of the efficacy and safety of short-acting methylphenidate. The trials involved 2,897 participants under age 18 diagnosed with attention-deficit disorder. Their treatment lasted 3 weeks on average and 28 weeks at most. The meta-analysis found a significant effect of methylphenidate for each primary outcome. However, it also found that the collection of trials "exhibited low quality" based on scores from two separate indices. The analysis concluded that the drug's "apparent beneficial effects are tempered by a strong indication of publication bias and the lack of robustness of the findings, especially those involving core ADD features."[53]

An earlier meta-analysis of 77 randomized controlled trials of both pharmacological and non-pharmacological interventions for ADHD also found that studies of this disorder "have low reporting quality, methodological flaws, and heterogeneity across outcome measures and tests." This analysis makes a noteworthy point about efficacy: It found that methylphenidate may reduce behavioral disturbance in children with ADHD, but that "academic performance does not appear to be improved with stimulants."[54] Likewise, the NIH consensus statement on ADHD refers to the "consistent findings that despite the improvement in core symptoms, there is little improvement in academic or social skills."[55]

Research on the long-term effects and safety of ADHD medications has been especially lacking. Schachter's meta-analysis notes that while short-acting methylphenidate has a statistically significant clinical effect in the short-term treatment of ADHD, the "extension of this placebo-controlled effect beyond four weeks of treatment has not been demonstrated."[56] In fact, the prescribing information for Adderall XR and Concerta state that the effectiveness of the drug beyond three weeks and four weeks, respectively, has not been systematically evaluated in controlled trials. Even so, the average number of years children are being treated for ADHD is increasing.[57] And according to a study of psychotropic drugs (such as stimulants, sedatives, and antidepressants) used with preschoolers, earlier ages of initiation and longer

"What use do you make of your physician?" said the king to Molière one day. "We chat together, sire; he gives me his prescriptions; I never follow them, and so I get well."

—JULES-ANTOINE TASCHEREAU, author of *Histoire de la Vie et Des Ouvrages de Molière*, 1825

durations of treatment mean that "the possibility of adverse effects on the developing brain cannot be ruled out."[58]

One often cited study of longer-term ADHD treatments, the Multimodal Treatment Study of Children with ADHD, lasted 14 months. In this clinical trial, 64 percent of children, ages 7 to 9.9 years, were reported to have side effects from ADHD medications (mild side effects for 49.8 percent; moderate for 11.4 percent; severe for 2.9 percent). Interestingly, the authors say that 6 of the 11 severe side effects—such as depression, worrying, and irritability—"could have been due to nonmedication factors."[59] But as psychiatrist and author Peter Breggin, MD, points out, double-blind placebo-controlled clinical trials have shown that the three side effects mentioned above are common adverse reactions to stimulants.[60]

A clearer picture of the long-term consequences of stimulant use is beginning to emerge from animal studies conducted in the past few years. These studies have found, for example, that Ritalin has the potential to cause long-lasting changes in brain cell structure and function[61]; that a repeated, clinically relevant dose of methylphenidate markedly inhibits immediate-early gene expression in the brain[62]; that chronic exposure to methylphenidate during pre- and periadolescent development made the animals significantly less responsive to natural rewards than control animals and significantly more sensitive to stressful situations, with an increase in anxiety-like behaviors,[63] and that early exposure to methylphenidate causes behavioral changes that last into adulthood, including some changes that may be beneficial (less sensitivity to cocaine reward) and others that may be detrimental (increases in depressive-like signs).[64]

The lack of information on long-term effects isn't the only worrisome factor in the treatment of ADHD. Young people also are increasingly being prescribed multiple medications at the same time. For example, a child prescribed methylphenidate for ADHD may also take a selective serotonin reuptake inhibitor (SSRI) antidepressant.[65] A review by researchers at Johns Hopkins medical institutions found that the data supporting the use of concomitant psychotropic medication are based almost entirely on case reports and small-scale, non-blind assessments.[66] Other studies also document the simultaneous use of multiple psychoactive drugs by children.[67,68] The Johns Hopkins review concludes: "Substantive systematic evidence is needed to clarify this increasingly common, inadequately researched child psychopharmacologic practice."[69]

Another shortcoming in the research on pediatric drug use may undermine safety data as well: There is no common method used to elicit and report data on adverse events in clinical studies, according to a 2003 review of 196 pediatric psychopharmacology articles published over the past 22 years. The inconsistency in the ascertainment of safety data "is a major limitation that likely impairs the ability to promptly and accurately identify drug-induced adverse events," state the reviewers. "Research on how best to standardize safety methods should be considered a priority in pediatric psychopharmacology."[70]

Adverse Effects

Stimulant-type drugs generally are described as a safe treatment for ADHD, causing relatively mild side effects that may be related to dose and may decrease with time.[71,72] Yet as a review published in 2002 notes, there is a substantial amount of variation both in response to these drugs and in adverse drug reactions.[73] Although 75 to 90 percent of ADHD patients respond well to amphetamine and methylphenidate, says another review, there is a subset of patients who either do not respond to the drugs or who experience side effects that preclude their use. These side effects include tics, a severe loss of appetite, and marked insomnia.[74]

In their analysis of 62 randomized trials, Schachter and colleagues conclude that methylphenidate "has an adverse event profile that requires consideration." For almost all of the adverse events reported, patients taking methylphenidate had a higher percentage of the effects than did those taking the placebo. According to data derived from parent/self-reported adverse effects, the number of study participants required for five prominent adverse events to be identified were as follows: 4 patients for a decreased appetite, 7 for insomnia, 9 for all stomachache events, 10 for all drowsiness events, and 11 for all dizziness events.[75]

According to a 2002 review, side effects of methylphenidate such as nervousness, headache, insomnia, anorexia, and tachycardia (rapid heartbeat) increase linearly with dose, while overdoses can cause agitation, hallucinations, psychosis, lethargy, seizures, tachycardia, dysrhythmias (heart rhythm problems), hypertension, and hyperthermia.[76] A study of long-acting methylphenidate published in 2003 found that only two side effects, insomnia and decreased appetite, were more common at higher doses. In this group of 5 to 16 year olds, younger and smaller children were more likely to experience sleep problems and a diminished appetite at higher dosages.[77]

A study of even younger children, ages 4.0 to 5.11 years, raises serious questions about the growing use of stimulants in preschoolers. In this study of 11 young children with developmental disabilities and ADHD, 5 who took methylphenidate experienced significant adverse effects, such as severe social withdrawal, increased crying, and irritability, especially at the higher dose of 0.6 milligrams per kilogram (mg/kg) of body weight. The researchers state that "this population appears to be especially susceptible to adverse drug side effects."[78]

Another medication, Cylert, can cause acute and sometimes fatal hepatic failure. Its black box warning in the United States was revised in 1999, stating that Cylert should not ordinarily be considered a first-line drug treatment for ADHD.[79] [This drug was removed from the U.S. market in 2005.] The drug also has been withdrawn from the United Kingdom and Canadian markets (it is available with restrictions through a special access program in Canada).[80,81] What follows is a discussion of some of the side effects associated with stimulant-type drugs used to treat ADHD, particularly methylphenidate.

Mental Effects

Stimulants can cause a variety of negative effects on mental functioning. In his book *Talking Back to Ritalin* (1998), Peter Breggin, MD, discusses some of the adverse experience reports for Ritalin submitted to the FDA's Spontaneous Reporting System from 1985 through 1997. Among these data, which represent only a small fraction of the total adverse events experienced by a drug's users, were reports of depression (48 reports for depression, 11 for psychotic depression); personality disorders (89); agitation (55); hostility (50); abnormal thinking (44); hallucinations (43); psychosis (38); and emotional instability (33), along with reports of amnesia, anxiety, confusion, nervousness, neurosis, stupor, paranoid reactions, and, in a few cases, manic reactions.[82]

Dr. Breggin points out that stimulants impair the function of the basal ganglia in the brain, and this dysfunction can impede higher mental functions and cause obsessions, compulsions, and abnormal movements. In two studies of stimulants, the rate of obsessive-compulsive disorder (OCD) symptoms was 51 and 25 percent, respectively.[83,84] Another study found that 42 percent of children experienced obsessive overfocusing.[85] Parents and teachers may mistakenly see these OCD symptoms as an improvement, says Dr. Breggin, but drug-induced OCD is in fact a severe type of brain dysfunction.[86] Case reports also document stimulant-induced obsessive compulsiveness.[87,88]

The potential for psychotic behavior in Ritalin users is included in the drug's packaging information. A 1999 chart review of children with ADHD treated in an outpatient clinic found a 6 percent rate of psychotic behavior among stimulant users. Six of the 98 children who took a stimulant (they were followed an average of 21 months) developed psychotic or mood-congruent psychotic symptoms during treatment.[89]

As for mania, a study of 34 adolescents hospitalized for this disorder found that patients who had used stimulants in the past had an earlier age at onset for bipolar disorder than those without prior stimulant exposure. In fact, those who had used at least two stimulants developed bipolar disorder at a younger age than those who had been treated with one such drug.[90] The authors of a 2004 article also hypothesize that the earlier age of onset for bipolar disorder in the United States than in the Netherlands (where the prevalence among adults and adolescents, but not prepubertal children, is similar to that of the United States) may be related to the greater use of antidepressants and stimulants for depression or ADHD by American children.[91]

Movement Disorders

Children taking methylphenidate may develop involuntary muscle contractions and limb movements. A 2003 review reports that the increased use of stimulants, antipsychotic agents, and antidepressants in children has inevitably led to more young patients experiencing side effects such as movement disorders. Those associated with these drugs include acute dystonic reaction and tardive dyskinesia. The reviewer states: "Unlike the isolated abnormal involuntary movements associated with drugs prescribed for epilepsy or asthma, movement syndromes . . . associated with psychotropic drugs are complex, difficult to recognize, and potentially seriously disabling."[92]

In a retrospective chart review involving 555 subjects, a total of 7.8 percent of those treated with stimulants developed tics (8.3 percent of methylphenidate users; 6.3 percent of dextroamphetamine users; 7.7 percent of pemoline users). The children who developed tics were significantly younger than those who did not.[93] Another cross-sectional analysis and chart review of 122 children with ADHD treated with stimulants found that approximately 9 percent developed tics or dyskinesia. One child developed Tourette's syndrome (a condition involving motor and/or vocal tics).[94] Other studies and case reports bear out the association between stimulants and abnormal movements.[95–97]

Growth Effects

Another disturbing side effect of stimulants is the stunting of growth that occurs in some children who take moderate to high doses over a period of years. This stunting occurs not only because stimulants can diminish a child's appetite but also because they may alter the body's natural balance of growth hormones.[98]

A study conducted at Yale University School of Medicine, published in 2003, examined the growth of 84 patients with ADHD who took stimulants and compared their height standard deviation (SD) scores with those of untreated biological siblings. The researchers found significant differences in mean height SD scores between treated children and siblings after two years of treatment. These findings "suggest that the prevalence of growth-suppressive effects of methylphenidate is greater than previously suspected."[99]

Another 2003 study in Australia tracked 51 children treated with dexamphetamine (dextroamphetamine in the United States) or methylphenidate for six to 42 months. In the first six months, 86 percent of the patients had a height velocity below the age-corrected mean and 76 percent lost weight. The children's height and weight standard deviation score (SDS) showed a progressive decline that was statistically significant after 6 and 18 months. During the first 30 months, height velocity was significantly attenuated (with a mean height deficit of approximately 1 centimeter (about half an inch) per year in the first two years).[100]

Cardiovascular Effects

Several recent studies have documented changes in cardiovascular functioning that can occur when children take stimulants. In a study of 17 boys taking methylphenidate or Adderall, diastolic blood pressure load increased significantly while the subjects were on Adderall. Systolic blood pressure and heart rate also differed between on and off medication.[101] A study of 14 healthy subjects found that intravenous doses of methylphenidate significantly increased heart rate, systolic and diastolic blood pressures, and epinephrine (adrenaline) concentration in plasma. The blood pressure changes were significantly correlated with increases of dopamine in striatum and of plasma epinephrine levels caused by the drug, supporting the hypothesis that methylphenidate-induced blood pressure increases are due in part to the drug's central dopaminergic effects.[102]

The cardiovascular effects of methylphenidate can be deadly. According to FDA adverse reaction reports—which are notoriously incomplete—there were 160 Ritalin-related deaths between 1990 and 1997, most of them related to cardiovascular functioning. Dr. L. Dragovic, Oakland County, Michigan, medical examiner, explains that drugs such as methylphenidate stimulate the body's adrenergic system when used repetitively, affecting everything that has as its chemical pathway mediators and transmitters such as adrenaline, noradrenaline, and dopamine. The enhancement of the adrenergic system over many months or years will produce changes in small blood vessels. Some cells will be lost, and scarring will occur as the body tries to repair the area. The blood vessels will narrow. "The changes that we're seeing in kids who have been on Ritalin for about eight years are basically the same as the changes in someone that has been abusing cocaine regularly over a period of years," says Dr. Dragovic.[103]

Potential for Drug Abuse

According to the U.S. Drug Enforcement Administration (DEA), of all the psychoactive drugs prescribed to young children in the United States, only two substances that are widely used to treat children are subject to the Controlled Substances Act (CSA): methylphenidate and amphetamine. The DEA identifies these drugs as "powerful stimulants" and places them in Schedule II of the CSA, which contains substances that have the highest abuse potential and dependence profile of all drugs with medical utility.[104]

In testimony before Congress in 2000, a DEA official reported that extensive research "unequivocally indicates that both methylphenidate and amphetamine have high abuse liabilities." The data show that animals and humans cannot tell the difference between cocaine, amphetamine, and methylphenidate when they are taken in the same way at comparable doses. "In short, they produce effects that are nearly identical," he said. Improper use of methylphenidate (tablets can be abused orally, crushed and snorted, or dissolved in water

and injected) poses significant risks, with high doses producing agitation, tremors, euphoria, palpitations, and other problems. Abuse of this drug also has been associated with psychotic episodes, paranoid delusions, and hallucinations.[105]

Natural Therapies for ADHD

Given the risks that children face in taking stimulant-type drugs, it stands to reason that parents may want to use more natural methods of treating ADHD symptoms. A 2003 review of nutrition in the treatment of ADHD found that nutritional factors such as food additives, refined sugars, food sensitivities/allergies, and deficiencies of fatty acids have been associated with this disorder. The authors say there is growing evidence that "many children with behavioral problems are sensitive to one or more food components that can negatively impact their behavior." One study proving this statement found that 19 of 26 children who met the criteria for ADHD responded favorably to a multiple-item elimination diet. In an open challenge, all 19 reacted to many foods, dyes and/or preservatives. Sixteen of them completed a double-blind placebo-controlled food challenge, which found a significant improvement on placebo days compared with challenge days. The researchers state that "dietary factors may play a significant role in the etiology of the majority of children with ADHD."[106]

The value of nutritional therapies in addressing ADHD was demonstrated in a recent study comparing the effects of Ritalin with those of food supplements. In this study, 10 children with ADHD took the drug and 10 took dietary supplements. Subjects in both groups showed significant gains on the outcome measures used, such as the Intermediate Visual and Auditory/Continuous Performance Test. The supplements used in the study included a mix of vitamins, minerals, phytonutrients, amino acids, essential fatty acids, phospholipids, and probiotics that attempted to address the biochemical risk factors of ADHD. The researchers concluded: "These findings support the effectiveness of food supplement treatment in improving attention and self-control in children with ADHD and suggest food supplement

587

treatment of ADHD may be of equal efficacy to Ritalin treatment."[107]

Natural therapies for ADHD, such as those discussed here, target the symptoms of this disorder without posing the risks of conventional treatment. Considering the many controversies surrounding ADHD—an unidentified cause, a subjective diagnosis, and exposure to potentially harmful medications—there is clearly room for treatment options that avoid those considerable risks.

REFERENCES

1. Jensen PS, Achenbach TM, Rowland AS. Epidemiologic research on ADHD: what we know and what we need to learn. From the conference, Attention-Deficit Hyperactivity Disorder: A Public Health Perspective, sponsored by CDC, National Center for Environmental Health, and the Department of Education, Office of Special Education Programs, Atlanta, GA, Sept 23–24, 1999.

2. Diagnosis and treatment of attention-deficit hyperactivity disorder (ADHD). National Institutes of Health Consensus Statement 1998;16(2):1–37.

3. Jensen, op. cit.

4. American Psychiatric Association. Fact sheet: attention deficit/hyperactivity disorder, May 2001.

5. American Academy of Pediatrics. AAP releases new guidelines for treatment of attention-deficit/hyperactivity disorder. News release. Oct 1, 2001.

6. Barbaresi WJ, Katusic SK, Colligan RC, et al. How common is attention-deficit/hyperactivity disorder? Incidence in a population-based birth cohort in Rochester, Minn. Arch Pediatr Adolesc Med 2002;156(3):217–224.

7. Stemstein A. Not just for kids: adults deal with ADHD in work place. ABCNEWS.go.com, Dec 2, 2003.

8. Rowland AS. Epidemiologic research on ADHD: what we know and what we need to learn. From the conference, Attention-Deficit Hyperactivity Disorder: A Public Health Perspective, sponsored by CDC, National Center for Environmental Health, and the Department of Education, Office of Special Education Programs, Atlanta, GA, Sept 23–24, 1999.

9. DeGrandpre R. Ritalin Nation. New York: W.W. Norton, 1999, 160.

10. UN narcotics czar warns of overconsumption of mind-altering drugs. Psychiatry Today Annual meeting, June 24–27, 2002.

11. Report of the International Narcotics Control Board for 2003. From www.incb.org/e/ind_ar. htm.

12. Crystal DS, Ostrander R, Chen RS, et al. Multi-method assessment of psychopathology among DSM-IV subtypes of children with attention-deficit/hyperactivity disorder: self, parent, and teacher reports. J Abnormal Child Psychol 2001;29(3)189–205.

13. Diagnosing ADHD: guidelines for diagnosis. From www.adhdinfo.com, Novartis Pharmaceuticals Corp.

14. Ibid.

15. Hechtman L. Assessment and diagnosis of attention-deficit/hyperactivity disorder. Child Adolesc Psychiatr Clin N Am 2000;9(3):481–498.

16. Diagnosis and treatment of attention-deficit hyperactivity disorder (ADHD), op. cit., p. 7.

17. Conners CK. "Conners' Parent Rating Scale–Revised (S)," Multi-Health Systems Inc., North Tonawanda, NY.

18. Ibid, p. 7–8.

19. American Psychiatric Association, op. cit.

20. Sahley BJ. Stop ADD Naturally: Cutting-Edge Information on Amino Acids, Brain Function and ADD Behavior. San Antonio, TX: Pain & Stress Publications, 2003, 9.

21. Treatment of attention-deficit/hyperactivity disorder. Summary: Evidence Report/Technology Assessment, No.11. AHCPR Publication No. 99-E017, Dec 1999. Rockville, MD: Agency for Health Care Policy and Research.

22. Hechtman, op. cit.

23. Yeh M, Morley KI, Hall WD. The policy and ethical implications of genetic research on attention-deficit hyperactivity disorder. Aust N Z J Psychiatry 2004;38(1–2):10–19.

24. Krause KH, Dresel SH, Krause J, et al. The dopamine transporter and neuroimaging in attention-deficit hyperactivity disorder. Neurosci Biobehav Rev 2003;27(7):605–613.

25. Sowell ER, Thompson PM, Welcome SE, et al. Cortical abnormalities in children and adolescents with attention-deficit hyperactivity disorder. Lancet 2003 Nov 22;362(9397):1699–1707.

26. Baumeister AA, Hawkins MF. Incoherence of neuroimaging studies of attention deficit/hyperactivity disorder. Clin Neuropharmacol 2001;24(1):2–10.

27. Parker-Pope T. New ADHD tests claim more objective diagnoses. Wall Street Journal Dec 10, 2002. Posted at www.southcoasttoday.com/pnk/p051o131.htm.

28. McLean Hospital. Teicher lab develops ADHD diagnostic tool. McLean Hospital Research Community: News. Updated Jan 8, 2003. Available at: http://research.mclean.org/news/news2003018mmat.html.

29. Diagnosis and treatment of attention-deficit hyperactivity disorder (ADHD), op. cit., p. 5, 20.

30. Eli Lilly and Co.. About Strattera. From www.strattera.com, 2003.

31. Rosack J. Med check: regulatory and legal briefs. Psychiatric News 2003;38(23):22.

32. Zito JM, Safer DJ, DosReis S, et al. Psychotropic practice patterns for youth: a 10-year perspective. Arch Pediatr Adolesc Med 2003;157(1):17–25.

33. Shatin D, Drinkard CR. Ambulatory use of psychotropics by employer-insured children and adolescents in a national managed care organization. Ambul Pediatr 2002;2(2):111–119.

34. Olfson M, Gameroff MJ, Marcus SC, et al. National trends in the treatment of attention deficit hyperactivity disorder. Am J Psychiatry 2003;160(6):1071–1077.

35. Robison LM, Sclar DA, Skaer TL, et al. National trends in the prevalence of attention-deficit/hyperactivity disorder and the prescribing of methylphenidate among school-age children: 1990–1995. *Clin Pediatr* (Phila) 1999;38(4):209–217.

36. Rushton JL, Whitmire JT. Pediatric stimulant and selective serotonin reuptake inhibitor prescription trends: 1992 to 1998. *Arch Pediatr Adolesc Med* 2001;155(5):560–565.

37. Zito, op. cit.

38. Zito JM, Safer DJ, dosReis S, et al. Trends in the prescribing of psychotropic medications to preschoolers. JAMA, 2000 Feb 23;283(8):1025–1030.

39. Angold A, Erkanli A, Egger HL, et al. Stimulant treatment for children: a community perspective. *J Am Acad Child Adolesc Psychiatry* 2000;39(8):975–984.

40. LeFever GB, Dawson KV, Morrow AL. The extent of drug therapy for attention deficit-hyperactivity disorder among children in public schools. *Am J Public Health* 1999;89(9):1359–1364.

41. Cox ER, Motheral BR, Henderson RR, et al. Geographic variation in the prevalence of stimulant medication use among children 5 to 14 years old: results from a commercially insured US sample. *Pediatrics* 2003;111(2):237–243.

42. Volkow ND, Wang G, Fowler JS, et al. Therapeutic doses of oral methylphenidate significantly increase extracellular dopamine in the human brain. *J Neurosci* 2001 Jan 15;21(2):RC121.

43. Teicher MH, Polcari A, Anderson CM, et al. Rate dependency revisited: understanding the effects of methylphenidate in children with attention-deficit hyperactivity disorder. *J Child Adolesc Psychopharmacol* 2003;13(1):41–51.

44. Langleben DD, Acton PD, Austin G, et al. Effects of methylphenidate discontinuation on cerebral blood flow in prepubescent boys with attention-deficit hyperactivity disorder. *J Nucl Med* 2002;43(12):1624–1629.

45. Vastag B. Pay attention: Ritalin acts much like cocaine. *JAMA* 2001 Aug 22/29;286(8).

46. Volkow, op. cit.

47. Schweitzer JB, Lee DO, Hanford RB, et al. A positron emission tomography study of methylphenidate in adults with ADHD: alterations in resting blood flow and predicting treatment response. *Neuropsychopharmacol* 2003;28(5):967–973.

48. Teicher, op. cit.

49. Mendenhall D. Behavior therapy with Ritalin pushed for teens with ADHD. Post-gazette.com, June 4, 2001.

50. Placebo study indicates lower doses may effectively treat ADHD. Sciencedaily.com, May 6, 2003. Study by Dr. Adrian Sandler and Dr. James W. Bodfish presented at the Pediatric Academic Societies Annual Meeting, May 3, 2003.

51. Evans SW, Pelham WE, Smith BH, et al. Dose response effects of methylphenidate on ecologically valid measures of academic performance and classroom behavior in adolescents with ADHD. *Exp Clin Psychopharmacol* 2001;9(2):163–175.

52. Findling RL, Short EJ, Manos MJ. Developmental aspects of psychostimulant treatment in children and adults with attention-deficit/hyperactivity disorder. *J Am Acad Child Adolesc Psychiatry* 2001;40(12):1441–1447.

53. Schachter HM, Pham B, King J, et al. How efficacious and safe is short-acting methylphenidate for the treatment of attention-deficit disorder in children and adolescents? A meta-analysis. *CMAJ* 2001 Nov 27;165(11):1475–1488.

54. Jadad AR, Boyle M, Cunningham C, et al. Treatment of attention-deficit/hyperactivity disorder. *Evid Rep Technol Assess* (Summ) 1999;11:i–viii,1–341.

55. Diagnosis and Treatment of Attention-Deficit Hyperactivity Disorder (ADHD). NIH Consensus Statement, 1998 Nov 16–18;16(2):10.

56. Schachter, op cit.

57. Rowland, op. cit.

58. Prescriptions for stimulants, antidepressant on the rise for preschoolers. *JAMA/Medscape Wire,* Feb 22, 2000. From www.childadvocate.net/meds.htm.

59. The MTA Cooperative Group. A 14-month randomized clinical trial of treatment strategies for attention-deficit/hyperactivity disorder. *Arch Gen Psychiat* 1999;56:1073–1086.

60. Breggin PR. A critical analysis of the NIMH Multimodal Treatment Study for attention deficit/hyperactivity disorder (The MTA Study). From www.breggin.com/mta.html.

61. Baker L. Scientists study effects of Ritalin. *University at Buffalo Reporter* Nov 8, 2001. Results of study presented at the Society for Neuroscience Annual Meeting, Nov 11, 2001.

62. Chase TD, Brown RE, Carrey N, et al. Daily methylphenidate administration attenuates c-fos expression in the striatum of prepubertal rats. *Neuroreport* 2003;14(5):769–772.

63. Bolanos CA, Barrot M, Berton O. Methylphenidate treatment during pre- and periadolescence alters behavioral responses to emotional stimuli at adulthood. *Biol Psychiat* 2003;54 (12):1317–1329.

64. Carlezon WA, Mague SD, Andersen SL. Enduring behavioral effects of early exposure to methylphenidate in rats. *Biol Psychiat* 2003;54(12):1330–1337.

65. Newswise.com. Ritalin and Prozac: more kids using both drugs. University of Michigan study by Jerry Rushton, et al., presentation to the annual meeting of the Pediatric Academic Societies and the American Academy of Pediatrics, May 13, 2000.

66. Safer DJ, Zito JM, Dos Reis S. Concomitant psychotropic medication for youths. *Am J Psychiat* 2003;160(3):438–449.

67. Harel EH, Brown WD. Attention deficit hyperactivity disorder in elementary school children in Rhode Island: associated psychosocial factors and medications used. *Clin Pediatr* (Phila) 2003;42(6):497–503.

68. Martin A, Van Hoof T, Stubbe D, et al. Multiple psychotropic pharmacotherapy among child and adolescent enrollees in Connecticut Medicaid managed care. *Psychiatr Serv* 2003;54 (1):72–77.

69. Safer, op. cit.

70. Greenhill LL, Vitiello B, Riddle MA, et al. Review of safety assessment methods used in pediatric psychopharmacology. *J Am Acad Child Adolesc Psychiat* 2003;42(6):627–633.

71. Treatment of attention-deficit/hyperactivity disorder. Summary, Evidence Report/Technology Assessment: No 11. AHCPR Pub No. 99-E017. Rockville, MD: Agency for Health Care Policy and Research, 1999.

72. Diagnosis and treatment of attention-deficit hyperactivity disorder (ADHD), op. cit., p. 13.

73. Masellis M, Basile VS, Muglia P, et al. Psychiatric pharmacogenetics: personalizing psycho stimulant therapy in attention-deficit/hyperactivity disorder. *Behav Brain Res* 2002;130(12): 85–90.

74. Pliszka SR. Non-stimulant treatment of attention-deficit/hyperactivity disorder. *CNS Spectr* 2003;8(4):253–258.

75. Schachter, op. cit.

76. Klein-Schwartz W: Abuse and toxicity of methylphenidate. *Curr Opin Pediatr* 2002;14(2):219–223.

77. Stein MA, Sarampote CS, Waldman ID, et al. A dose-response study of OROS methylphenidate in children with attention-deficit/hyperactivity disorder. *Pediatrics* 2003;112 (5):e404.

78. Handen BL, Feldman HM, Lurier A, et al. Efficacy of methylphenidate among preschool children with developmental disabilities and ADHD. *J Am Acad Child Adolesc Psychiat* 1999;38(7):805–812.

79. Abbott Laboratories. "Dear Health Care Professional" letter. Posted on U.S. FDA website.

80. Advisory: liver complications result in withdrawal of attention deficithyperactivity disorder drug Cylert. *Health Canada Online* Sept 22, 1999.

81. Current problems in pharmacovigilance: Volatil (pemoline) has been withdrawn. Medicines Control Agency, Committee on Safety of Medicines, Sept 1997.

82. Breggin PR. *Talking Back to Ritalin.* Cambridge, MA: Perseus Publishing, 2001;43–44.

83. Borcherding BV, Keysor CS, Rapoport JL, et al. Motor/vocal tics and compulsive behaviors on stimulant drugs: is there a common vulnerability. *Psychiatric Research* 1990;33:83–94 (cited in Breggin).

84. Castellanos FX, Giedd JN, Elia J, et al. Controlled stimulant treatment of ADHD and comorbid Tourette's syndrome: effects of stimulant and dose. *J Am Acad Child Adolesc Psychiat* 1997;36:589–596 (cited in Breggin).

85. Solanto MV, Wender EH. Does methylphenidate constrict cognitive functioning? *J Am Acad Child Adolesc Psychiat* 1989;28:897–902 (cited in Breggin).

86. Breggin, op. cit;37.

87. Kotsopoulos S, Spivak M. Obsessive-compulsive symptoms secondary to methylphenidate treatment. *Can J Psychiat* 2001;46(1):89.

88. Kouris S. Methylphenidate-induced obsessive-compulsiveness. *J Am Acad Child Adolesc Psychiat* 1998;37(2):135.

89. Cherland E, Fitzpatrick R. Psychotic side effects of psychostimulants: a 5-year review. *Can J Psychiat* 1999;44(8):811–813.

90. DelBollo MP, Soutullo CA, Hendricks W. Prior stimulant treatment in adolescents with bipolar disorder: association with age at onset. *Bipolar Disord* 2001;3(2):53–57.

91. Reichart CG, Nolen WA. Earlier onset of bipolar disorder in children by antidepressants or stimulants? An hypothesis. *J Affect Disord* 2004;78(1):81–84.

92. Rodnitzky RL. Drug-induced movement disorders in children. *Semin Pediatr Neurol* 2003;10(1):80–87.

93. Varley CK, Vincent J, Varley P, et al. Emergence of tics in children with attention-deficit hyperactivity disorder treated with stimulant medications. *Compr Psychiat* 2001;42(3):228–233.

94. Lipkin PH, Goldstein IJ, Adesman AR. Tics and dyskinesias associated with stimulant treatment in attention-deficit hyperactivity disorder. *Arch Pediatr Adolesc Med* 1994;148(8):859–861.

95. Borcherding, op. cit.

96. Bower B. Study of stimulant therapy raises concerns. *Science News Online* 2000;158(5).

97. Senecky Y, Lobel D, Diamond GW, et al. Isolated orofacial dyskinesia: a methylphenidate-induced movement disorder. *Pediatr Neurol* 2002;27(3):224–226.

98. Sears W, Thompson L. *The AD Book: New Understandings, New Approaches to Parenting Your Child.* New York: Little, Brown & Co. 1998;235.

99. Lisska MC, Rivkees SA. Daily methylphenidate use slows the growth of children: a community based study. *J Pediatr Endocrinol Metab* 2003;16(5):711–718.

100. Poulton A, Cowell CT. Slowing of growth in height and weight on stimulants: a characteristic pattern. *J Paediatr Child Health* 2003;39(3):180–185.

101. Stowe CD, Gardner SF, Gist CC, et al. 24-hour ambulatory blood pressure monitoring in male children receiving stimulant therapy. *Ann Pharmacother* 2002;36(7–8):1142–1149.

102. Volkow ND, Wang GJ, Fowler JS, et al. Cardiovascular effects of methylphenidate in humans are associated with increases of dopamine in brain and of epinephrine in plasma. *Psychopharmacol* (Berl) 2003;166(3):264–270.

103. Gary Null interview with Dr. Dragovic, Feb 13, 2001.

104. Woodworth T. U.S. Drug Enforcement Administration Congressional Testimony before the Committee on Education and the Workforce: Subcommittee on Early Childhood, Youth and Families, May 16, 2000.

105. Ibid.

106. Boris M, Mandel FS. Foods and additives are common causes of the attention deficit hyperactive disorder in children. *Ann Allergy* 1994;72(5):462–468.

107. Harding, op. cit.

TREATMENT OF LEARNING DISABILITIES
by Allan Cott, MD

Learning disabilities constitute one of the most prevalent and urgent medical problems afflicting children not only in the United States but in most countries of the world. Evidence is accumulating that learning disabilities are frequently of genetic origin and may be related to genetic vitamin dependency. This article presents for consideration a most important variable in the learning process: the biochemical disorders that interfere with learning and a new adjunct to treatment, which involves the use of massive doses of vitamins and the maintenance of proper nutrition to create the optimum molecular environment for the brain.

There are effective alternatives to drug treatment or effective treatments for that one-third to one-half of the many millions of children who are not helped by drugs. In my experience treating the hyperactive learning-disabled child with orthomolecular interventions, better than 50 percent are helped. These statistics achieve greater significance because the children treated have failed to improve with the use of methylphenidate (Ritalin) or amphetamines (Adderall and Dexedrine).

Parents Who Refuse to Accept the Cliches

Many parents were searching for an alternative to drug therapy because their children were experiencing the side effects of insomnia, loss of appetite with concomitant weight loss, or a reaction of fatigue and sedation when the drug was given in doses large enough to control the hyperactivity. Many children had been tried on a regime of various psychotropic (tranquilizer) medications that failed because they produced the paradoxical effect of overstimulation and increased the hyperactivity and disturbed behavior. Many parents had read of the orthomolecular approach or had spoken to other parents whose children were achieving notable improvement on the regime and sought this as the primary treatment. Since the orthomolecular approach is compatible with all other substances used in drug intervention and since the megavitamins potentiate the action of most drugs, the treatments can be combined. This is frequently done early in treatment while the vitamin doses are gradually being raised to the optimal maintenance level and more rapid control of the hyperactivity is required. At times, tranquilizer medication is added at the request or insistence of the school authorities to bring the hyperactive, disruptive behavior under more rapid control.

The large majority of children treated by the orthomolecular approach improve without the use of drugs. Fortunately, very few parents accept the cliches with which their concerns about their child's development *are* met by many of their pediatricians and family physicians. They are not satisfied with "boys are slower than girls," "you're an anxious mother, your baby is fine," "lots of healthy children do not speak until they are four years old," or "there's nothing to worry about if your baby creeps backwards or sideways." It has been my experience that the mothers most often are first in noticing their child's problems, while in a very low percentage of cases it is the pediatrician who first makes the diagnosis. Many parents, after reading about the orthomolecular approach, instituted the recommended dietary changes and found these changes alone brought about a dramatic reduction in hyperactivity. Other parents purchased vitamins and reported improvement when their child was given several of the vitamins used in the treatment.

During the treatment of several hundred psychotic children, I noted and reported that in most cases in which parents persisted in the proper administration of the vitamins and diet, significant improvement in many areas of functioning was achieved. The most significant and earliest sign of improvement reported by parents was a decrease in hyperactivity, which led to improved concentration and attention span with a resultant improved capacity for learning. Trials were then begun with

From the *J Orthomolecular Psych* 1974;3(4):343–355.

the orthomolecular treatment in children exhibiting specific learning disabilities, the child diagnosed as hyperactive or with minimal brain dysfunction, the child described as being of near- or above-average intelligence with certain learning or behavioral disabilities ranging from mild to severe, which are associated with deviations of function of the central nervous system. Until these studies were begun, most remedial specialists stressed the more peripheral aspects of a handicapped child's performance and ignored the biochemical basis of his or her disturbed behavior and impaired ability to learn. Improvement under the orthomolecular treatment is directing the attention of the scientific community to the central processes and closer scrutiny of the biochemical processes of the learning-disabled child. In this means of intervention, remedial efforts are directed toward both brain function and body chemistry. In addition to the employment of perceptual-motor techniques and pharmacotherapy, attempts should be made to improve the child's biochemical balance through the use of orthomolecular techniques.

Improving Brain Function

Orthomolecular treatment has been described previously, but its definition bears repetition. Dr. Linus Pauling, in his classical paper on orthomolecular psychiatry in 1968, defined this approach as the treatment of illness by the provision of the optimum molecular composition of the brain, especially the optimum concentration of substances normally present in the human body. The implications for much needed research in the more universal application of orthomolecular treatment are clear. There is rapidly accumulating evidence that a child's ability to learn can be improved by the use of large doses of certain vitamin and mineral supplements, and by improvement of his general nutritional status through removal of junk foods from his daily diet.

With orthomolecular treatment, results are frequently quick in starting and the reduction in hyperactivity often dramatic, but in most instances several months elapse before significant changes are seen. The child exhibits a willingness to cooperate with his parents and teachers. These changes are seen in the majority of children who failed to improve with the use of the stimulant drugs or tranquilizer medications. The majority of the children I see have been exposed to every form of treatment and every known tranquilizer and sedative with little or no success even in controlling the hyperactivity. Concentration and attention span increases, and the child is able to work productively for increasingly larger periods of time. He ceases to be an irritant to his teacher and classmates. Early intervention is of the utmost importance not only for the child but for the entire family, since the child suffering from minimal brain dysfunction is such a devastating influence on the family constellation. He is the matrix of emotional storms, which envelop every member of the household and disrupt both their relationship to him and to each other.

Based on empirical data, the application of orthomolecular principles can be successful in helping many learning-disabled children. Positive results have been obtained when the treatment regimen consisted of the following vitamins: niacinamide or niacin (1,000–2,000 milligrams [mg]) daily depending upon body weight, ascorbic acid (1,000–2,000 mg) daily; pyridoxine (200–400 mg) daily, calcium pantothenate (200–600 mgs) daily. The vitamins are generally administered in divided doses twice daily. Magnesium oxide powder is frequently used for its calming effect on the hyperactivity. One-half teaspoon of the powder is added to the vitamin intake twice daily along with 1 tablet of calcium gluconate or calcium lactate twice daily.

These are starting doses of the vitamins for children weighing 35 pounds or more. If a child weighs less than 35 pounds, 1,000 mg daily of niacinamide and ascorbic acid are used in 500-mg doses administered twice daily. If the child shows no signs of intolerance after two weeks, the dose is increased to 1,000 mg twice daily. In the smaller child the pyridoxine and calcium pantothenate are started at 100 mgs twice daily and gradually increased to twice the amount. In a child weighing 45 pounds or more, an optimum daily maintenance level of approximately 3,000 mg grams of niacinamide and 3,000 mg of ascorbic acid is reached. Frequently, vitamin B12 (cobalamin), vitamin E, riboflavin (vitamin B2), thiamine (vitamin B1), folic acid, and L-glutamine can be valuable additions to the treatment. No serious side effects have resulted in any of the hundreds of children treated with these substances. The side effects, which occur infrequently (nausea, vomiting, increased frequency of urination or bowel movements), are dose-related and subside with reduction of the dose.

It has been shown that proper brain function requires adequate tissue respiration, and Dr. O. Warburg (1966), Nobel laureate in biochemistry, described the importance of vitamins B3 and C in the respiration of all body tissues in the maintenance of health and proper function.

It is my belief that those children and adults in all diagnostic categories who benefit from the massive doses of vitamins are not always suffering from vitamin deficiencies but rather from a genetic vitamin dependency.

Improving Body Chemistry

Back in 1970, Dr. L. E. Rosenberg of the Department of Genetic Research at Yale University reported that of the dozen known disorders involving genetic vitamin dependency, pyridoxine (vitamin B6) is involved in five. Genetic dependency is described as a condition in which normal levels of vitamins are insufficient for the body and can be treated successfully only by massive doses of vitamins.

Rosenberg found that in many instances up to 1,000 times the usual vitamin requirements are needed to prevent the disease from expressing itself. Laboratory findings with animals have shown a direct relationship between vitamin intake and learning enhancement. It has been found by some researchers that injections of vitamin B12 markedly enhanced learning in rats.

Control of the child's diet is an integral part of the total treatment and failure to improve the child's nutritional status can be responsible for achieving minimal results. Greater concern must be shown for the quality of the child's internal environment in which his cells and tissues function if we are to help him attain optimal performance. The removal of offending foods from the diet of

disturbed or learning-disabled children can result in dramatic improvement in behavior, attention span, and concentration.

Since many disturbed and learning-disabled children are found to have either hypoglycemia (low blood sugar), hyperinsulinism (high blood insulin), or dysinsulinism, sugar and rapidly absorbed carbohydrate foods should be eliminated from their diets. It has been the universal observation of those investigators who assess children's nutritional status that they eat a diet that is richest in sugar, candy, sweets, and in foods made with sugar. The removal of these foods results in a dramatic decrease in hyperactivity. Most children do not drink milk unless it is sweetened with chocolate syrup or some other syrupy additive. All the beverages that they consume every day are spiked with sugar—soda, caffeinated cola drinks, highly sweetened "fruit juices," and other concoctions— which are sold to them on TV commercials. The child who drinks any water at all is indeed rare.

The appalling fact about the constant consumption of these junk foods is the parents' belief that these foods are good for their children. Parents must realize that they litter their children's bodies by making these unnatural junk foods available to them and incorporating them in their daily diet. Children will not voluntarily exclude these foods from their diet, they must be helped to accomplish this. These foods should not be brought into the house. The child must learn the principles of proper nutrition and proper eating from his parents. The dissemination of this knowledge is far too important to entrust it to the writers of TV commercials whose aim is to sell rather than educate.

The author has taken many dietary histories, which revealed that the usual "nutritious" breakfast for some children consists of a glass of soda or "coke" and a portion of chocolate layer cake! For the child with hypoglycemia, such food assures a drop in blood sugar level for several hours, during which time that child's brain function is impaired so that she cannot learn well even if she does not suffer from learning disabilities. At best, the breakfast menu of the majority of learning-disabled children is poorly balanced and varies from the above extreme by the substitution of sugar-frosted cereals. The glucose in the bloodstream is one of the most important nutrients for the proper functioning of the brain, and the maintenance of a proper glucose level is essential in the creation of an optimum molecular environment for the mind.

No Valid Reason for Delay

Orthomolecular treatment has many advantages that make it especially suitable for large numbers of children. Treatment can be directed by parents and paraprofessionals, reducing to a minimum the occasions upon which the child must be brought to a specialist for therapy. It is inexpensive, as it does not depend on complex machinery or equipment, or on the long-term use of psychotropic drugs. Of great importance is the role it could serve as a preventive as well as a therapeutic measure because it could easily be included in prenatal and infant care programs everywhere. These are important considerations in view of the evidence that neurologically based and biochemically based learning disabilities are especially frequent among children from low-income areas.

The relationship of severe malnutrition to infant mortality, disease, and retardation in physical development are all well documented. In recent years evidence has accumulated that malnutrition has adverse effects on mental development and learning as well.

Because research cannot at this time give an unequivocal or full answer to the question of what effect malnutrition or malnourishment has on intellectual development is not a valid reason to delay programs for improving the nutritional status and eating practices of mothers and infants. Information demonstrating the benefits of good nutrition in improved health, physical growth, and improved learning already justifies such efforts.

We cannot afford the luxury of waiting until causes can be unquestionably established by techniques yet to be developed. We cannot postpone managing as effectively and honestly as possible the millions of children who desperately need help now.

REFERENCES

Bronfenbrenner U. Dampening the unemployability explosion. *Saturday Review* Jan 4, 1969.

Cott A. Orthomolecular approach to the treatment of learning disabilities. *Schizophrenia* 1971;3(2):95–105.

Cott A. Megavitamins: the orthomolecular approach to behavioral disorders and learning disabilities. *Academic Therapy* 1972;7(3).

Hoffman MS. Early indications of learning problems. *Academic Therapy* 1972;7(1).

Mayer J. World Wide Report. *Medical Tribune* Jan 19, 1970.

Michaelson AI, Sauderhoff MW. Lead poisoning. *Medical World News* Sept 7, 1973.

Montagu A. *Life Before Birth.* New American Library, 1964. Office of Child Development and the Office of the Assistant Secretary for Health and Scientific Affairs, Dept. of HEW: "Report of the Conference on the Use of Stimulant Drugs in the Treatment of Behaviorally Disturbed Young School Children," 1971.

Pasamanick B, Rogers ME, Lillienfeld AM. Pregnancy experience and the development of behavior disorder in children. *Am J Psychiatry* 1956;613–618.

Silbergeld EK, Goldberg AM. *Medical World News* Sept 7, 1973, 7.

Warburg, O. The Prime Cause and Prevention of Cancer. Lindau Lecture1966.

Wendle WF. Developmental behaviors delayed appearance in monkeys asphyxiated at birth. *Science* 1971;171(3976):1173–1175.

Williams RJ. The nutritive value of single foods. Paper presented to the National Academy of Sciences, Apr 28, 1971.

Wunderlich R. *Kids, Brains and Learning.* St. Petersburg, FL: Johnny Reads Inc, 1970.

VITAMIN TREATMENT OF HYPERACTIVITY IN CHILDREN AND YOUTH: REVIEW OF THE LITERATURE AND PRACTICAL TREATMENT RECOMMENDATIONS

by Jonathan E. Prousky, ND

Attention-deficit hyperactivity disorder (ADHD) involves symptoms such as hyperactivity, inattention, and impulsivity, leading to impairments in daily functioning, scholastic performance, and relationships with peers. Stimulant medication has been used to treat problems associated with ADHD for more than 50 years. Approximately 3–5 percent of children receive a diagnosis of ADHD.[1] Some 2.8 percent of United States youth (ages 5–18) received stimulant medication in mid-1995.[2] In a more recent publication, the prevalence of stimulant use among youth under 19 was reported to be about 2.9 percent, amounting to some 2.2 million youth.[3] The data is fairly consistent, demonstrating that nearly 3 percent of all youth are diagnosed with ADHD and prescribed stimulant medication.

While the rationale for stimulant medication is to reduce the symptoms associated with ADHD, critics have argued that Ritalin (methylphenidate) and similar stimulant medications are overly prescribed and inherently dangerous.[4] Results from double-blind placebo-controlled clinical trials and animal laboratory research suggest that stimulant medication itself can contribute to abnormal behaviors by causing adverse drug effects on the central nervous system of the child.[5] It is unfortunate that options other than stimulant medication are not typically provided to patients and their families. Promoting stimulant medication implies that ADHD is a homogenous medical disorder and that stimulant medication is the only effective treatment. However, the etiology of ADHD is not homogeneous.

Numerous possible contributory factors may include sensitivities to food additives, intolerances to foods, nutrient deficiencies and imbalances, heavy metal intoxication, toxic pollutant burden, or abnormal thyroid activity.[6] Given the heterogeneous nature of this disorder, treatments other than stimulant medication might be better suited to some youth with ADHD.

The vitamin approach, a plausible alternative treatment, has been dismissed as ineffective and potentially dangerous.[7] After reviewing several publications on vitamin therapy for the treatment of childhood hyperactivity, I will demonstrate that vitamin therapy deserves to be taken seriously since there are compelling single-blind studies showing benefits from high-doses of single B vitamins with an acceptable risk-to-benefit (i.e., safety) profile. The results from double-blind studies are equivocal due to methodological flaws. Therefore, those reports cannot be used to support or dismiss the merits of combining high doses of several B vitamins and ascorbic acid for the treatment of childhood hyperactivity.

Review of Double-Blind Studies

Orthomolecular pioneer Dr. Allan Cott was probably the leading proponent of using the vitamin approach for treating childhood learning disabilities.[8,9] He treated 500 children with vitamins and reported that vitamin therapy was more effective than any other treatment available. Dr. Cott's program involved the following vitamins taken orally—in pill, capsule, or liquid form—in daily doses: niacin or niacinamide (1,000–2,000 milligrams [mg]), increasing to 3,000 mg if the child weighs more than 45 pounds; ascorbic acid (1,000–2,000 mg); vitamin B5 as calcium pantothenate (400–600 mg); and vitamin B6 (200–400 mg).

Cott noted that vitamin therapy decreased hyperactivity and improved concentration and attention span, yielding a greater capacity for learning. The program sometimes afforded dramatic results in a very short time, but normally three to six months of treatment was needed to produce significant changes. With respect to safety, Cott found no negative effects, except for brief

From the *J of Orthomolecular Med* 2011;26(3):119–126.

flushing when starting niacin and nausea when taking too much niacinamide.

Following Cott's reports and reports by other clinicians,[10–13] three double-blind, placebo-controlled trials were conducted to assess the vitamin approach for children with hyperactivity.

Double-Blind Trial #1

In this study, children (ages 5–12) with a diagnosis of minimal brain dysfunction (MBD) were given either a placebo or the megavitamin regimen.[14] MBD, an older term for ADHD, was diagnosed when children displayed a combination of symptoms, such as hyperactivity, distractibility, short attention span, incorrigibility, labile explosiveness, incoordination, and perceptual motor problems. Of the children, 16 were given the placebo, while 15 were given the vitamin treatment program which was comprised of vitamin B3 (2,000 mg as niacin), of ascorbic acid (2,000 mg), vitamin B5 (400 mg as calcium pantothenate), vitamin B6 (200 mg as pyridoxine), and glutamic acid (1,000 mg) taken orally in twice daily divided doses. The length of the trial was two weeks. The differences between the placebo and vitamin groups, as determined by several different rating scales, were not statistically significant. The authors recommended against the vitamin approach unless dietary history, specific symptoms, or biochemical findings suggest a specific vitamin deficiency.

When reviewing the data more closely, there were greater improvements in the ratings of children in the vitamin group compared to children in the placebo group. This suggests that either the patient number was too small for statistical significance, or that the trial duration was insufficient to demonstrate a therapeutic effect. Since Cott observed that three to six months of treatment are usually required before benefits can be obtained, the results of this two-week controlled clinical trial should not be used to dismiss the possible benefits that vitamin therapy might confer upon hyperactive children.

Double-Blind Trial #2

This six-month trial included 20 youth (ages 7–14), comprising 17 boys and 3 girls.[15] Even though the diagnoses of the participants were heterogeneous, each one had been diagnosed as hyperactive, or as having MBD, or both. Participants taking psychostimulant medication were withdrawn from their medication at least three months before the controlled clinical trial. Eight boys and two girls were randomly assigned to the vitamin group, whereas nine boys and one girl were assigned to the placebo group. Each participant in the vitamin group received daily dosages (according to weight) of vitamin C (1,000–3,000 mg), vitamin B3 as niacinamide (1,000–3,000 mg), vitamin B5 (200–600 mg), and vitamin B6 (500–750 mg).

All participants, regardless of treatment, followed a high-protein, low-carbohydrate, sugar-free diet. On one day during each weekend, participants were allowed a "junk food" day to

IN BRIEF

Approximately 3–5 percent of children receive a diagnosis of attention-deficit hyperactivity disorder (ADHD). Some 3 percent of all youth (less than 19 years old) diagnosed with ADHD in the United States take stimulant medication. It is unfortunate that options other than stimulant medication are not typically provided to patients and their families. The vitamin approach, a plausible alternative treatment, has been dismissed as ineffective and potentially dangerous in spite of the fact that numerous publications on vitamin therapy for the treatment of childhood hyperactivity suggest that this approach deserves to be taken seriously. Several compelling single-blind studies show benefits from high-doses of single B vitamins and indicate an acceptable risk-to-benefit (i.e., safety) profile. The results from three double-blind studies are equivocal due to methodological flaws so these cannot be used to support or refute the safety or conclude about the merits of treating childhood hyperactivity with high doses of several B vitamins and ascorbic acid. It may be preferable to treat hyperactive children and youth with a simplified vitamin regimen, since a complicated ortho-molecular regimen involving numerous daily interventions can prove too cumbersome and onerous for the majority of parents and their children to follow. The reviewer proposes an algorithmic approach using single B vitamins.

ensure compliance and manageability for the parents. Most of the participants did not need the "junk food" day after they acclimated to the diet. Numerous rating scales were administered before and following the trial. In addition, urine testing for the mauve factor (i.e., urinary excretion of kryptopyrrole, a marker for overactive oxidation) was done to see if elevated levels of the mauve factor predicted a better response from the vitamin treatment. The results demonstrated no significant differences between the vitamin and placebo groups on the rating scales administered before and after the trial. There were also no significant differences in how participants responded to megavitamin treatment even if it was determined at trial entry that they had abnormal mauve factor test results.

A closer examination of the trial data revealed that both groups had significant improvements in their behavior. For example, the total behavior checklist score prior to trial was 79.2 in the vitamin-treated group and 67.2 in the placebo group. Following the trial, these scores decreased to a 52.6 and 48.6 in the vitamin and placebo groups, respectively. This might mean that the diet employed, rather than the vitamin or placebo treatments, was responsible for the behavioral gains seen in this trial. Since this trial was not designed to assess the therapeutic effects of dietary control upon behavior, it cannot be assumed that these results arose from adherence to a healthier diet. The Hawthorne effect (a result of the parents' enthusiasm and high expectations) may have influenced the outcome. Additionally, the fact that each participant was six months older, and presumably more mature at trial conclusion, could have contributed to the gains seen in both groups.

Double-Blind Trial #3

This trial was comprised of 41 children with a diagnosis of ADHD.[16] There were 6 girls and 35 boys in the vitamin group, and 39 girls and 36 boys in the control group. The design of this trial was complex, in that, there was a 3-month open clinical period (denoted as Stage 1), followed by a double-blind crossover trial (denoted as Stage 2) for children that had a positive therapeutic response

during Stage 1. All children were administered intelligence and achievement tests, given physical and neurological examinations, and had extensive blood work (at baseline and at the end of Stages 1 and 2) assessing nutrient levels and testing elements by blood chemistry analysis (e.g., fasting glucose, creatinine, calcium, phosphorus, and alkaline phosphatase). Behavioral assessments were done throughout the trial. All medications or programs used to treat ADHD were discontinued one week before study entry.

During Stage 1, the daily vitamin regimen was gradually increased, depending on tolerability, from 1,000 mg of vitamin B3 (as niacinamide), 1,000 mg of vitamin C, 400 mg of vitamin B5, and 200 mg of vitamin B6 to 3,000 mg of vitamin B3, 3,000 mg of vitamin C, 1,200 mg of vitamin B5, and 600 mg of vitamin B6. A washout period of six weeks separated Stages 1 and 2. Stage 2 was comprised of four trial periods, each six weeks in duration. During Stage 2, the assignment of treatment was done randomly in two possible arrangements: 1) drug (vitamin)-placebo-drug-placebo; or 2) placebo-drug-placebo-drug. No specific dietary plan was prescribed or recorded during Stages 1 and 2, except that parents were instructed to provide well-balanced and wholesome meals.

Twelve children (29 percent) showed behavioral improvements during Stage 1 and were given the opportunity to participate in Stage 2 of the trial. Only seven children participated in Stage 2 of the trial. Five of the 12 children did not enter Stage 2 due to a variety of somatic complaints resulting from the vitamin regimen, including nausea, anorexia, gagging, and abdominal pain. All seven children in Stage 2 of the trial were boys with a mean age of 8.9 years. One child was removed during Stage 2 as a result of unacceptable behavior. The overall results demonstrated that during Stage 2 there were no statistically significant differences in the rating scales between the vitamin and placebo treatments. In some cases, teachers and mothers noted declines in behavior problems (e.g., improved conduct, better learning, and less hyperactivity) resulting from the vitamin regimen compared to the placebo. No statistically significant differences were found in serum vitamin C or vitamin B6 levels of the treatment or the control participants. During vitamin treatment, 17 of the 41 participants (42 percent) had significant elevations of serum transaminase levels that exceeded the upper limits of normal. (These elevations, common in niacin therapy, indicate higher liver activity.) In some cases these levels required four to six weeks to return to baseline values. The investigators of this study concluded that the vitamin approach had no benefits and was possibly dangerous due to hepatic enzyme abnormalities resulting from quantities of vitamins exceeding Recommended Dietary Allowance (RDA) ranges.

From my analysis, conclusions different from those of the study investigators can be drawn. In Stage 1 of the trial, 12 children (29 percent) had significant therapeutic responses to the vitamin regimen. The duration of treatment during Stage 1 was three months, a sufficient period of time to observe potential therapeutic benefits from the vitamin regimen. Seven children participated in Stage 2 but were taken off their vitamin regimen for six weeks, and were then provided either an alternating placebo or the vitamin regimen in six-week intervals for a total of 24 weeks or six months. The six-week intervals might not have been sufficient to observe therapeutic responses from the vitamin regimen, especially since the duration of time given during Stage 1 of the trial was 12 weeks. It might have been destabilizing for the vitamin responders to be placed on and then off treatment in six-week intervals during Stage 2 of the trial. This could have negatively influenced the results. As for the vitamin approach being potentially harmful to the liver, none of the children developed clinical jaundice, hepatomegaly, or sustained weight loss during the trial. Increased transaminase levels require clinical vigilance but are not normally a clinical concern unless the values are markedly elevated in conjunction with relevant patient symptomatology.[16a]

Review of Single-Blind Studies

Orthomolecular pioneer Dr. William Kaufman published a report in 1953 describing how therapeutic doses of niacinamide (900–4,000 mg in divided daily doses) alleviated agitated hyperactivity and depression in elderly patients as long as they remained on the vitamin.[17] None of Kaufman's patients had classic pellagra. To my knowledge, Kaufman's report was one of the first to establish a relationship between vitamin B3 and hyperactivity.

Single-Blind Trial #1

Almost two decades later, Dr. Abram Hoffer published a single-blind placebo-controlled trial design that assessed the therapeutic effects of administering niacin or niacinamide to children under 13 years of age exhibiting disturbing behavior.[18] The diagnoses of these children varied, but they were all ill. Some were very disturbed; most had hyperactivity. Thirty-eight children entered the study in 1967, but six could not complete the required three-year study period.

All children were given 1,500 to 6,000 mg a day of niacinamide, or rarely niacin if there was no response to the niacinamide. Each child also took 3,000 mg of vitamin C daily, and rarely very small doses of tranquilizers or antidepressants.

After the child recovered, even if it took three months or two years, vitamin B3 was discontinued and the child continued with an equivalent dose of a placebo, along with ascorbic acid and very small doses of tranquilizers or antidepressants (if previously prescribed). Each child was kept on the placebo until he or she relapsed, at which point the parents resumed the vitamin B3 treatment. The vitamin C and drug therapies were unaltered during the entire study period. Of the 32 children in the study, 24 went through the treatment-placebo-treatment cycle. Only Hoffer and the children's parents were privy to the exact treatment, but the children were blinded. In all 24 cases, the children recovered while taking vitamin B3, then relapsed within one month of taking the placebo, and recovered again when resuming vitamin B3.

Dr. Hoffer noted that the recovery from vitamin B3 was slower following the placebo. The remaining eight patients in this study were almost recovered and had yet to be placed on the placebo.

In a later publication, Hoffer reported additional findings from this study.[19] At the conclusion of the trial in 1974, he had a cohort of 37 children to report on. Out of 37 children in total, 19 were normal and 6 were much improved. Of the remaining 12 children, 3 were not improved and the results for 9 were not known. Thus, 25 out of 37 children (68 percent) were normal or much improved by the addition of niacinamide or niacin. Hoffer reported that the chief reason for failure was the inability of the child to remain on the vitamins prescribed. These results, according to Hoffer, confirmed a vitamin B3 dependency syndrome in some children.

He concluded that children should be given a therapeutic trial of vitamin B3 if they exhibit three of four specific features: 1) hyperactivity, 2) deteriorating school performance, 3) perceptual changes, and/or 4) an inability to acquire or maintain social relationships.

Single-Blind Trial #2

In 1982, Dr. Arnold Brenner reported on his experiences with 100 youth (ages 4–15) given brief therapeutic trials with single doses of specific B-complex vitamins.[20] He hypothesized that subgroups of youth with hyperactivity might respond to pharmacologic doses of specific B-complex vitamins. The majority of youth had a diagnosis of MBD with hyperactivity, attention span deficit, distractibility, impulsivity, emotional instability, and learning deficits. Six youth with hyperactivity were also phobic, neurotic, or borderline schizophrenic. The majority of youth were on stimulant medication (i.e., d-amphetamine or methylphenidate), which was discontinued prior to clinical trials with specific B-complex vitamins. Dr. Brenner conducted two complex single-blinded controlled trials with these 100 youth. In all cases, the parents and youth were blinded, but not Brenner.

In Trial 1, patients were given four coded envelopes with specific instructions: 1) 100 mg of vitamin B1 four times daily for three days; 2) one lactose (placebo) pill given twice daily for three days; 3) 218 mg of vitamin B5 twice daily for three days; and 4) 100 mg of vitamin B6 three times daily for three days. In most cases, the tablets were crushed and ingested with applesauce. The interval or time between envelopes was usually one day and not the recommended three to four days. If there was no benefit or if an adverse reaction resulted, the treatment was discontinued and then therapeutic trials with other treatments (i.e., other envelopes) were attempted. Table 1 describes the results from Trial 1.

TABLE 1. RESULTS FROM TRIAL 1: THERAPEUTIC RESPONSES TO SPECIFIC B VITAMINS AND PLACEBO			
THERAPEUTIC AGENT	IMPROVED	WORSENED	NO CHANGE
Vitamin B1 (thiamine)	26	22	52
Lactose (placebo)	6	19	75
Vitamin B5 (calcium pantothenate)	23	9	68
Vitamin B6 (pyridoxine)	18	16	66
No change with any therapeutic agent	N/A	N/A	38

Once there was a noted benefit from one of the particular treatments, the youth was entered into Trial 2. In Trial 2, youth were maintained for an additional seven-day period on the specific treatments (vitamins or placebo) that they responded to in Trial 1. Following this additional seven-day period, youth that responded were placed on a placebo to assess for relapses, while youth that did not respond were put back on medication and/or received behavior therapy. If relapses resulted when on the placebo, youth were then placed on the specific vitamins they had previously responded to—or placebo if they did not relapse—for long-term treatment with frequent follow-up. The long-term treatment and follow-up extended to four years, and the daily doses of the vitamins or the placebo were periodically reduced or discontinued to assess their ongoing therapeutic value. In addition, two-thirds of youth that did not respond in a robust manner during Trial 2 were provided with niacinamide, various B-complex vitamins, minerals, or elimination diets to further assess the value of these treatment combinations. A full response was deemed to be equal to or better than stimulant medication. Table 2 describes the results from Trial 2.

TABLE 2. RESULTS FROM TRIAL 2: SEVEN-DAY TRIALS AND LONG-TERM FOLLOW-UP OF YOUTHS TAKING SPECIFIC B VITAMINS AND PLACEBO

THERAPEUTIC AGENT	NUMBER OF PATIENTS	FULL RESPONDERS
Vitamin B1 (thiamine)	21	11
Lactose (placebo)	6	1
Vitamin B5	15	4
Vitamin B6 (pyridoxine)	18	9

Given the heterogeneous nature of the hyperactivity syndrome, Brenner concluded that some youth with the hyperactivity syndrome might benefit from a program of B-complex vitamins. He noted that vitamin responsiveness was likely dependent on such physiological factors as decreased ingestion, intestinal absorption, impaired utilization, increased metabolic requirements, increased excretion, or degradation of the vitamin. He also noted that some youth required only short-term administration of specific vitamins, which likely meant that treatment corrected a specific deficiency. On the other hand, other youth required long-term administration, which was suggestive of biochemical dependencies.

Discussion

Only one of three controlled trials (i.e., Double-Blind Trial #2) raised some doubts as to the merits of a vitamin regimen using several B vitamins and vitamin C for the treatment of childhood hyperactivity. The remaining two controlled trials (i.e., Double-Blind Trials #1 and #3) had methodological problems meaning that their conclusions refuting the vitamin approach should be questioned until better designed studies are completed. Hoffer asserted that the double-blind approach is flawed since only the vitamin-dependent children would adequately respond to treatment.[12] Until investigators can prove their groups of youth to be homogenous with respect to etiology, Hoffer argues that double-blind studies evaluating the vitamin approach will yield inconclusive results.

As for the single-blind studies, the results are promising. The pooled data from Brenner's study demonstrated that 20 out of 60 youth (33 percent) had sustained clinical responses from the long-term use of individual B vitamins, sometimes in

TABLE 3. AN ALGORITHMIC APPROACH USING SINGLE B VITAMINS TO TREAT PATIENTS WITH HYPERACTIVITY AND ASSOCIATED PROBLEMS

TREATMENT	DAILY DOSE	DURATION	CLINICAL RESPONSE
Niacinamide	1,500 mg (increasing to 12 weeks with comparable amounts of vitamin C)	12 weeks	If sufficient, patient to remain on treatment with regular monitoring (i.e., transaminases); if insufficient, proceed to 2
Vitamin B6 (pyridoxine)	300 mg (consider adding 2 mg folic acid and 50 mg elemental zinc)	12 weeks	If sufficient, patient to remain on treatment with regular monitoring; if insufficient, proceed to 3
Vitamin B6	Increase dose to 1,000 mg	12 weeks	If sufficient, patient to remain on treatment with regular monitoring (i.e., peripheral neuropathy and central nervous system toxicity); if insufficient, proceed to 4
Vitamin B1 (thiamine)	400 mg	12 weeks	If sufficient, patient to remain on treatment with regular monitoring (i.e., urticaria or other dermatoses); if insufficient, proceed to 5
Vitamin B5 (calcium pantothenate)	500 mg	12 weeks	If sufficient, patient to remain on treatment with regular monitoring; if insufficient, reassess patient and provide other treatments

combination with other nutrients (i.e., folic acid, niacinamide, and zinc), for up to four years. Hoffer's single-blind results showed an astounding 68 percent response rate from the long-term use of niacinamide (and rarely niacin) among hyperactive youth when followed for up to seven years.

Using single doses of a specific B vitamin does appear to be a viable option, especially if stimulant medication is to be avoided or if the clinical response from stimulant medication becomes undesirable for a variety of reasons (e.g., weight loss, anorexia, and lack of clinical improvement). Having each patient complete therapeutic trials of one B vitamin at a time seems preferable to using a daily program consisting of several B vitamins, vitamin C, and minerals, since compliance issues would be less likely to result from this approach. I have developed an algorithmic approach based on efficacy (i.e., from the cited data). This approach simplifies treatment when a single nutrient dependency is implicated in a patient's hyperactivity and associated problems (see Table 3).

It is appropriate to consider vitamin dependencies in the differential diagnosis of hyperactivity. The 16th edition of *The Merck Manual of Diagnosis and Therapy* defines a vitamin dependency as that which relates to "coenzyme function and results from an apoenzyme abnormality that can be overcome by administration of doses of the appropriate vitamin that are many times the Recommended Dietary Allowance (RDA)."[21] In the 17th edition of this prestigious medical text, the definition of a vitamin dependency was slightly modified as resulting "from a genetic defect in the metabolism of the vitamin or in the binding of the vitamin-related coenzyme to its apoenzyme."[22] The authors note that to correct the altered metabolic pathway, vitamin doses of 1,000 times the RDA are sometimes necessary. Thus, a vitamin dependency is only correctable by increasing the intake of a particular vitamin to levels greater than could be achieved from dietary sources alone.

An enzyme-catalyzed reaction could be corrected by increasing doses of vital micronutrients. A 2002 report validated the concept of vitamin dependencies for the treatment of 50 common genetic diseases. In this report, the need for doses of vitamins far in excess of RDA amounts were deemed necessary as a means of increasing coenzyme concentrations and correcting defective enzymatic activity.[23]

CONCLUSION

Due to methodologically flawed studies, the results of double-blind studies cannot be used to endorse or to dismiss the vitamin approach for the treatment of hyperactivity. The results of single-blind studies are promising. These studies provide evidence that vitamins can ameliorate hyperactivity in vitamin-dependent children and youth.

REFERENCES

1. Woodard R. The diagnosis and medical treatment of ADHD in children and adolescents in primary care: a practical guide. *Pediatr Nurs* 2006;32:363–370.

2. Safer DJ, Zito JM, Fine EM. Increased methylphenidate usage for attention-deficit disorder inthe 1990s. *Pediatr* 1996;98(6 Pt 1):1084–1088.

3. Zuvekas SH, Vitiello B, Norquist GS. Recent trends in stimulant medication use among U.S. children. *Am J Psychiatr* 2006; 163:579–585.

4. Safer DJ. Are stimulants overprescribed for youth with ADHD? *Ann Clin Psychiatr* 2000;12:55–62.

5. Breggin PR. What psychologists and psychotherapists need to know about ADHD and stimulants. Changes: *Int J Psychol Psychother* 2000;18:13–23.

6. Kidd PM. Attention-deficit /hyperactivity disorder(ADHD) in children: rationale for its integrative management. *Altern Med Rev* 2000;5:402–428.

7. Baumgaertel A. Alternative and controversial treatments for attention-deficit/hyperactivity disorder. *Pediatr Clin North Am* 1999;46:977–992.

8. Cott A. Orthomolecular approach to the treatment of learning disabilities. *Schizophrenia*, 1971;3:95–105.

9. Cott A. Treatment of learning disabilities. *Orthomolecular Psychiatr* 1974;3:343–355.

10. Hoffer A. Treatment of hyperkinetic children with nicotinamide and pyridoxine. *Can Med Assoc J* 1972;107:111–112.

11. Rees EL. Clinical observations on the treatment of schizophrenic and hyperactive children with megavitamins. *J Orthomolecular Psych* 1973;2:93–103.

12. Hoffer A. Letter: hyperactivity, allergy and megavitamins. *Can Med Assoc J* 1974;111:905, 907.

13. Silverman LB. Orthomolecular treatment in disturbances involving brain function. *J Orthomolecular Psych* 1975;4:71–84.

14. Arnold LE, Christopher J, Huestis RD, et al. Megavitamins for minimal brain dysfunction. *JAMA* 1978;240:2642–2643.

15. Kershner J, Hawke W. Megavitamins and learning disorders: a controlled double-blind experiment. *J Nutr* 1979;109:819–826.

16. Haslam RHA, Dalby T, Rademaker AW. Effects of megavitamin therapy on children with attention-deficit disorders. *Pediatrics* 1984;74:103–111.

16a. Parson, William B. *Cholesterol Control without Diet.* 2nd ed. Lilac Press, 2000.

17. Kaufman W. The use of vitamin therapy to reverse certain concomitants of aging. *J Am Geriatr Soc* 1955;3:927–936.

18. Hoffer A. Vitamin B3 dependent child. *Schizophrenia* 1971;3:107–113.

19. Hoffer A. *Healing Children's Attention & Behavior Disorders.* Toronto, ON: CCNM Press Inc., 2004;208–211.

20. Brenner A. The effects of megadoses of selected B complex vitamins on children with hyperkinesis: controlled studies with long-term follow-up. *J Learn Disabil* 1982;15:258–264.

21. *The Merck Manual of Diagnosis and Therapy.* 16th ed. Rathway, NJ: Merck Research Laboratories.1992;959.

22. *The Merck Manual of Diagnosis and Therapy.* 17th ed. Whitehouse Station, NJ: Merck Research Laboratories. 1999;33.

23. Pauling L. *Orthomolecular psychiatry.* Varying the concentrations of substances normally present in the human body may control mental disease. *Science* 1968;160:265–271.

23. Ames BN, Elson-Schwab I, Silver EA. High-dose vitamin therapy stimulates variant enzymes with decreased coenzyme binding (increased Km): relevance to genetic diseases and polymorphisms. *AmJ Clin Nutr* 2002;75:616–658.

TREATING ADHD WITH VITAMIN B3

by Andrew W. Saul, PhD

ADHD is not caused by a drug deficiency. But it may indeed be caused by a profound nutrient deficiency, more accurately termed nutrient dependency. Although all nutrients are important, the one that an ADHD child is most likely in greatest need of is vitamin B3 (niacin or niacinamide). Over 60 years ago, niacinamide therapy pioneer Dr. William Kaufman wrote:

Some patients have a response to niacinamide therapy which seems to be the clinical equivalent of "decreased running" observed in experimental animals. When these animals are deprived experimentally of certain essential nutriments, they display "excessive running," or hyperkinesis. When these deficient animals receive the essential nutriments in sufficient amounts for a sufficient period of time, there is exhibited a marked "decrease in running."

The benefit is so profound, said Kaufman, that a person receiving niacinamide treatment

may wonder whether or not his vitamin medications contain a sedative . . . Analysis of his history indicates that prior to niacinamide therapy he suffered from a type of compulsive impatience, starting many projects, which he left unfinished as a new interest distracted him, returning perhaps after a lapse of time to complete the original project. Without realizing it, he was often careless and inefficient in his work, but was "busy all the time."

This report appeared, almost as a side note, on page 73 of Kaufman's 1949 book, *The Common Form of Joint Dysfunction*. So accurately does it describe the problems of ADHD children that it is difficult to believe that vitamin B3 has been so thoroughly ignored for so long.

Dr. Kaufman continues:

With vitamin therapy, such a patient becomes unaccustomedly calm, working more efficiently, finishing what he starts, and he loses the feeling that he is constantly driving himself. He has leisure time that he does not know how to use. When he feels tired, he is able to rest, and does not feel impelled to carry on in spite of fatigue . . . If such a patient can be persuaded to continue with niacinamide therapy, in time he comes to enjoy a sense of well-being, realizing in retrospect that what he thought in the past was a super-abundance of energy and vitality was in reality an abnormal "wound-up" feeling, which was an expression of aniacinamidosis (niacin deficiency).

Dr. Kaufman's observation that niacinamide is an effective remedy for hyperactivity and lack of mental focus is very important. With ADHD, orthodox medicine seems unwilling even to admit nutrient deficiency as a causal factor, let alone a curative one. Such nutritional information as does make news generally stays far from the headlines, unless, of course, it is critical of vitamins. The most widely publicized vitamin therapy trials tend to be low-dose, worthless, negative, or all three. Mass media attention to a given nutritional research study appears to be inversely proportional to its curative value.

Therefore, the public and many physicians remain unaware of the power of simple and safe natural methods due to contradictory, inadequate, or just plain biased media reporting. When the press touts the supposed "dangers" of vitamins while simultaneously overlooking the very real dangers of having kids on long-term drug maintenance, it strains at a gnat and swallows a camel. Whereas drug side effects fill the *Physician's Desk Reference (PDR)* to bursting, the chief side effect of niacinamide is failure to take enough of it. The quantity of a nutrient that cures an illness indicates the patient's degree of need for the nutrient. This amount may be quite high. A dry sponge holds more milk.

Dr. Kaufman advocated relatively modest quantities of niacinamide (250 milligrams) per dose but stressed the importance of the frequency (six or eight times a day) of those doses. Frequently divided doses are maximally effective. The precise amount of niacinamide that an ADHD child requires needs to be thoughtfully considered by parent and physician alike.

To learn more about Dr. William Kaufman's observations about ADHD clinical success with high-dose vitamin therapy:

* Vitamin deficiency, megadoses, and some supplemental history. A letter by William Kaufman, MD, PhD, April 7, 1992. is available at www.doctoryourself.com/kaufman2.html.

* *The Common Form of Joint Dysfunction* (1949) is long out of print, but the full text has been posted online for free reading at www.doctoryourself.com/kaufman6.html.

* In 2002, Dr. Kaufman's papers were acquired by the University of Michigan, Special Collections Library, 7th Floor, Harlan Hatcher Graduate Library, Ann Arbor, MI 48109. Email at special.collections@umich.edu.

* A bibliography of Dr. Kaufman's work will be found at www.doctoryourself.com/biblio_kaufman.html.

From the *J Orthomolecular Med* 2003;18:29–32.

THE ADVERSE EFFECTS OF FOOD ADDITIVES ON HEALTH: A REVIEW OF THE LITERATURE WITH SPECIAL EMPHASIS ON CHILDHOOD HYPERACTIVITY

by Tuula E. Tuormaa

A food additive is any substance not commonly regarded or used as food, which is added to, or used in or on, food at any stage to affect its keeping quality, texture, consistency, taste, color, or alkaline/acid balance, or to serve any other technological function in relation to food, and includes processing aids in so far as they are added to or used in or on food.[1,2] Food additives in use today can be divided roughly into three main types: cosmetics (to enhance appearance), preservatives (to extend shelf-life), and processing aids (to facilitate food preparation).[3] The growth in the use of food additives has increased enormously in the past 30 years, totaling now over 200,000 tons per year.[4,5] Therefore, it has been estimated that today about 75 percent of the Western diet is made up of various processed foods, with each person now consuming an average 8–10 pounds of food additives per year, and some possibly eating considerably more.[5–7] With the great increase in the use of food additives, there also has emerged considerable scientific data linking food additive intolerance with various physical and mental disorders, particularly with childhood hyperactivity.[8–31]

The Feingold Hypothesis

Allergist Benjamin F. Feingold was one of the first physicians to speak out against food additives. Dr. Feingold and his team, when working under a National Institutes of Health grant, discovered in 1964 that low-molecular weight compounds, like artificial food dyes, can produce behavioral disorders in susceptible individuals.[8–13,44–46] After collecting evidence based on over 1,200 cases, they found that hyperactivity, including other neurophysiological disturbances, can be induced in some children when they consume certain chemicals such as food additives, as well as some naturally occurring salicylates. He arrived at this conclusion by observing that certain children, who

seem to react neurophysiologically to aspirin (acetylsalicylic acid), reacted also in a similar manner to natural foods containing salicylates. This led him to study further the effect of other low molecular compounds, such as artificial food additives, on children's health and behavior, finding similar results. He also observed that as the affected individuals seem to react negatively to allergy skin tests, the reaction involved could not be based on an allergic/immunological mechanism, but rather on some pharmacological/toxic mechanism.[13]

Using clinical observations and parental testimony, Feingold found that in approximately 30–50 percent of hyperactive children, the adverse behavior pattern displayed could simply be a direct manifestation of an elevated sensitivity to certain low-molecular weight compounds, such as synthetic food additives as well as to foods containing natural salicylates. He observed further that the children, whose hyperactive behavior was a direct manifestation of this elevated sensitivity, can be treated effectively by simply removing from their diet all foods containing artificial food additives as well as foods containing natural salicylates.[13] Using a similar dietary regimen, he also claimed success in helping children suffering from a variety of learning disabilities.[10]

Feingold's claims originated primarily from anecdotal reports; however, there have been since several subsequent scientific evaluations to test his hypothesis, some supportive,[14–22] some unsupportive,[47–51] and some finding only a very limited support (i.e., that only the very youngest of the children responded).[20,51–53] It has been speculated, however, that this wide discrepancy between different observations may have been due to the differentiation between the levels of food colors used in the test conditions.[19–25] This may have been indeed the case.

From the *J Orthomolecular Med* 1994;9(4):225–243.

For example, Drs. C. Keith Conners[51] and J. Preston Harley[53] employed in their challenge procedure 26 milligrams (mg) of artificial food colors daily; Dr. B. Weiss used 35 mg[20]; and a study by Dr. James Swanson, which incidentally found a clear supportive evidence to Feingold's hypothesis, used a daily challenge dose of 100–150 mg.[19] In fact, it has been found that this highest daily challenge dose of 100–150 mg of food additives is the most realistic amount to be employed in any test procedure.

This became apparent when the Food and Drug Administration (FDA) studied 5,000 randomly selected children between the ages of 5 and 12 and determined that the 90th percentile for daily consumption of artificial food dyes within this age group was 150 mg. For the population as a whole, the FDA found an average daily mean to be 57.5 mg, while the 90th percentile range was between 100 and 300 mg per day.

Food Additives and Side Effects

The following are some of the most commonly used additives as well as their common side effects.

Common Food Dyes

• *Tartrazine* (E102) is primarily used by the candy, soft drink, and baked good industries. It is one of the colors most frequently implicated in food intolerance studies.[2,5,16,31,33,35,54–62] Adverse reactions to tartrazine seem to occur most commonly in subjects who are also sensitive to acetylsalicylic acid, a finding which was also observed by Feingold and his team. Depending on the test protocol followed, it has been found that between 10–40 percent of aspirin-sensitive patients are indeed usually also affected by tartrazine,[101] the reactions including asthma,[2,55,61–64] urticaria,[2,59,61–65] rhinitis,[62–64] and, as previously mentioned, childhood hyperactivity.[9–13]

A major breakthrough in the understanding of the mechanisms involved in acetylsalicylic-acid intolerance came also with discovery that aspirin, including other non-steroidal anti-inflammatory drugs, inhibit the synthesis of prostaglandins (substances that mediate regulation of inflammation), by selectively blocking the cyclooxygenase path-

way, resulting in an enhanced production of leukotrienes.[67–69] Excessive leukotriene production in turn leads to vascular permeability, causing edema and inflammation, which is directly associated with various airway constriction disorders, including asthma.[2,70,71]

One study found that an oral administration of 50 mg of tartrazine to 122 patients suffering from allergy-related disorders evoked the following reactions: feeling of suffocation, weakness, heat sensation, palpitations, blurred vision, rhinitis (chronic sneezing and/or a congested, drippy nose), pruritus (itchy skin), and urticaria (hives and/or raised itchy welts). Even though 50 mg could be considered a substantial dose, such a quantity of tartrazine could easily be consumed by an individual drinking only a few bottles of soft drinks per day.[56]

Another carefully conducted double-blind placebo-controlled trial on 76 children diagnosed as hyperactive showed that tartrazine and benzoates (a chemically similar substance) provoked abnormal behavior patterns in 79 percent of them.[29] In addition, a double-blind placebo-controlled trial on 10 hyperactive children when compared to controls found that tartrazine increases urinary zinc secretion and decreases serum and salivary zinc concentrations in hyperactive children, with a corresponding deterioration in their behavior. This phenomena was not found among the controls. It was suggested therefore that tartrazine seems to act as a zinc-chelating agent in susceptible individuals. Furthermore, that zinc depletion may also be one of the potential causes of childhood hyperactivity.[60]

Although tartrazine seems to be most frequently associated with adverse reactions,[72] there are also other coloring agents that are known to cause mental and/or physical ill-effects.[33,73]

• *Caramel coloring* (E150), of which over 100 different formulations are currently in use, is widely used by the cola drinks industry, as well as the beer and alcohol industries. It is also used as a coloring agent in baked goods, potato chips, soy and Worcestershire sauces, chocolate-flavored products, gravy browning, and a variety of other foods. The main recurring problem about the safety of caramels concerns the presence of an impurity called 4-methylimidazole, produced by processes using ammonia, which leads to convulsions when fed to rats, mice, and chicks. It has been also found that ammoniated caramels can affect adversely the levels of white blood cells and lymphocytes in laboratory animals. Furthermore, a study on rabbits provided evidence that even small doses of ammoniated caramels seem to inhibit the absorption of vitamin B6 (pyridoxine).[33]

• *Carmoisine* (E122) is used mainly in candy, baked goods, cake icing, jams, preserves, and chewing gum. It was found by the U.S. Certified Color Manufacturers Association to be unavoidably contaminated with low levels of beta-napthylamine, which is a well-known carcinogen;[33] it has also been found to be mutagenic in animal studies.[5] It is now banned in the United States.

• *Erythrosine* (E127) is a red dye used in baked goods, candy, and candied cherries. It has been found to act as a potent neurocompetitive-dopamine inhibitor of dopamine uptake by nerve endings when exposed in vitro on a rat brain.[74] Other studies have shown that erythrosine can have an inhibitory action also on other neurotransmitters, resulting in an increased concentration of neurotransmitters near the receptors, thus functionally augmenting the synaptic neurotransmission.[75,76] There is now some evidence that a reduced dopamine turnover may lead to childhood hyperactivity.[77] Similar findings have been linked with a reduction of noradrenaline.[78] Erythrosine also has been found to have a possible carcinogenic action when tested on animals.[5]

• *Sunset Yellow* (E110), used in beverages, candy, baked goods, has been found to damage kidneys and adrenals when fed to laboratory rats.[33] It has also been found to be carcinogenic when fed to animals.[5]

Common Preservatives

• *Benzoates* (E210-E219) are preservative used mainly in marinated fish, fruit-based fillings, jam, salad dressings, soft drinks, and beer, and have been found to provoke urticaria, angioedema (swelling most often around the lips and eyes), and asthma.[2-33,79] Furthermore, they have also been directly linked with childhood hyperactivity.[29]

• *Butylated hydroxyanisole* (BHA/E320) are used to retard rancidity in cereals, chewing gum, potato chips, vegetable oil, soup mixes, and cheese spread. It has been found to be tumor-producing when fed to rats.[83] In human studies, BHA has been linked with urticaria, angioedema, and asthma.[84,85]

• *Monosodium glutamate* (MSG/E621) is used as a flavor enhancer in soups, , salad dressings, chips, frozen entrees, luncheon meats, and many restaurant foods. It has been associated with a conjunction of symptoms in susceptible individuals, such as severe chest and/or facial pressure and overall burning sensations, not unlike a feeling that the victim is experiencing a heart attack.[48] MSG has been also found to precipitate a severe headache and/or asthma in susceptible individuals.[86,87] In susceptible children MSG has been linked with epilepsy-type "shudder" attacks.[88] In animal studies it has been found to damage the brains of young rodents.[35]

• *Nitrates and nitrites* (E249-E252) are used as preservatives, and coloring and flavoring agents in bacon, ham, luncheon and cured meats, hot dogs, smoked fish, corned beef, and some cheeses. They have been found to cause headaches in susceptible individuals.[81] In addition, these chemicals have been linked with cancer both in animal[5-33] and human studies.[82] They have also been found to be mutagenic when fed to mammals.[5]

• *Sulfites* (E220-E227) prevent discoloration and are used mainly in dried fruits, fruit juices and syrups, fruit-based dairy desserts, biscuit dough, cider, beer, and wine. They have been linked with pruritus, urticaria, angioedema, and asthma.[2,31,33,80,81] When fed to animals, sulfites have also been found to have a mutagenic action.[5]

Common Sweeteners

• *Saccharin*, known as Sweet N' Low, is an artificial sweetener that is widely used by the soft drink and diet industry as a sugar substitute. It has been shown to produce cancer when tested on animals.[68,89–91] Saccharin has also been found to be mutagenic[68,92,93] and growth inhibiting,[94] as well as to cause congenital malformations in animal studies.[95] The fact that any substance that has been found to be carcinogenic also seems to have a mutagenic action was established by testing 300 different carcinogenic chemicals for mutagenicity. The results showed that of the 300 carcinogenic chemicals tested, 90 percent were also found to have a mutagenic action.[96]

• *Aspartame* (E951), more popularly known as Equal and NutraSweet, of which the key ingredient is the amino acid phenylalanine, is also widely used by the soft drink and sweet food industry. When fed to rats, aspartame was found to double the level of phenylalanine in their brains, which re-doubled when other carbohydrates were consumed at the same time. This combination was found to give a great rise in brain tyrosine, followed by a considerable reduction in brain tryptophan levels.[97,98] Low tryptophan levels have been directly linked with both aggressive and violent behavior.[99–105] Furthermore, as dietary tryptophan acts as a precursor for serotonin, reduced tryptophan levels will also result in a reduction of brain serotonin levels, which has been directly linked with both hyperactive and aggressive behavior.[106–111]

• *Sucrose* (table sugar), which is a simple molecular substance artificially refined from complex carbohydrates, thus called a refined carbohydrate, can be found in most of our foods. An excessive refined carbohydrate consumption has been directly associated with a high incidence of both criminal and antisocial behavior.[28,34]

Stephen Schoenthaler, PhD, and his team conducted several double-blind studies among thousands of incarcerated juvenile offenders, finding a clear correlation between high sugar/junk food intake and the incidence of antisocial behavior. In all studies, the primary dietary revision to reduce sugar consumption was organized by simply replacing sugary drinks and junk food snacks with fruit juices and nutritious snacks such as nuts and fresh fruits. After implementing this simple dietary policy with 276 incarcerated offenders, informal disciplinary actions were lowered 48 percent, when contrasting the 12 months before and after nutritional revision. Assault and battery was lowered 82 percent, theft 77 percent, horseplay 65 percent, and refusal-to-obey-an-order 55 percent.[112,113] When similar diet policy was designed for 1,382 offenders confined in three different juvenile institutions, there was a clear 25 percent reduction in rule violations. All 1,382 juveniles served as their own controls and the length of the pre- and post-intervention period lasted for three months each.[158]

Similar findings were observed when the behavior of 2,005 incarcerated offenders was analyzed for 24 months. In the second half of the experiment (after 12 months of the initial observation period), the offenders were no longer allowed foods/drinks containing added sugar or artificial additives; instead they were offered nuts, fruit, and fruit juices. After implementing the low-sugar diet policy the incidence of rule violations fell 21 percent; assaults and fights, 25 percent; and general disruptions, 42 percent.[115] The consumption of sucrose/additive-rich foods was not only seen to worsen the behavior of young offenders, but, when given to children diagnosed as hyperactive, these foods seemed greatly to increase their restless and destructive behavior.[116,117] Similar results were established among a group of normal preschool children, as sucrose was found significantly to correlate with their "inappropriate behavior" pattern.[118]

Allergy or Intolerance?

Allergic intolerance in susceptible individuals can be caused by a variety of substances. However, in the majority of cases, cross-sensitivity and the possibility that several nutritionally related factors are working together should not be overlooked.

The most convincing evidence that this is indeed so, comes from a well-conducted double-blind placebo-controlled crossover trial by Dr. J. Egger and his team when studying 76 hyperactive children to find out whether diet can contribute to behavioral disorders. The results showed that 79 percent of the children tested reacted adversely to artificial food colorants and preservatives, primarily to tartrazine and benzoic acid. These produced a marked deterioration in their behavior.

However, no child reacted to them alone. In fact, 48 different foods were found to produce symptoms among the group of children tested. For example, 64 percent reacted to cow's milk, 59 percent to chocolate, 49 percent to wheat, 45 percent to oranges, 39 percent to eggs, 32 percent to peanuts, and 16 percent to sugar. Interestingly, it was not only that the children's behavior improved after the individual dietary modification, but most of the associated symptoms also improved considerably, such as headaches, fits, abdominal discomfort, chronic rhinitis, aches in limbs, skin rashes, and mouth ulcers.[29]

Another similar double-blind controlled food trial by Egger and his team was conducted on 88 children suffering from frequent migraines. As before, most children reacted to several foods/chemicals. However, the following foods/chemicals were found to be most prevalent: cow's milk provoked symptoms in 27 children, egg in 24, chocolate in 22, both orange and wheat in 21, benzoic acid in 14, and tartrazine in 12. Yet again, interestingly, after dietary modification, not only migraine improved but also associated symptoms such as abdominal pain, aches in limbs, fits, rhinitis, recurrent mouth ulcers, asthma, eczema, as well as various behavioral disorders.[178]

These two studies are a prime example of how problems created by adverse dietary factors are typically polysymptomatic and multisystem in type. In order to create a reaction in susceptible individuals, probably a whole range of mechanisms coexist.

It has been already established that a reaction to low molecular compounds, such as artificial food additives, do not appear to be immunological but rather pharmacological or toxic in type. Also, it has been suggested that low molecular compounds, such as food additives, may simply act as haptens (partial antigens) and, after attaching themselves to macromolecules, can become antigenic, thus producing an allergenic reaction in susceptible individuals.[66,134] Even Feingold was careful not to talk about allergy in its true sense in connection with food additives but rather preferred the term "elevated sensitivity."

Who Is Affected?

Young children seem to serve always as the first sentinels of any environmental contamination because of their immaturity of enzymatic detoxifying mechanism, incomplete function of excretory organs, low levels of plasma protein capable of binding toxic chemicals, and incomplete development of physiological barriers such as the blood-brain barrier.[135] The young, developing nervous system seems to be particularly vulnerable. For example, results of some research studies, which incidentally were rather critical of Feingold's claims, found that only the very youngest of the children tested reacted adversely to artificial food additives.[20,48,51–53]

It should be stressed, however, that the period of organ formation and development stretches long before the moment of birth. Fetal alcohol syndrome is a useful example, which arises with fetal exposure to neurotoxic agents such as alcohol.[36–38] Similar adverse effects have been attached to maternal smoking,[36,37,39] to lead contamination,[36,37,40–43] and now, more recently, to food additives.[35,36,37,135] Using animal experiments, it has been found that the fetus may be more susceptible to tumor development than an adult animal.

Evidence is also accumulating that non-carcinogenic substances may cause a variety of biochemical changes, including alterations in the fetal enzyme development at levels at which the mother is asymptomatic.[135]

One class of compounds dangerous to the fetus, often in very low concentration, are the mutagens, which are able to react with and injure chromosomes and genes carrying the genetic code. Furthermore, it has been found that mutagens not only cause mutations but are also capable of damaging and killing living cells, thus inflicting the greatest damage very early in pregnancy or during the weeks before conception.[36] Mutagens are reported to differ from other poisons in that the human or animal body does not seem to have a metabolic space within which they could be metabolized and rendered harmless (i.e., there appears to be no satisfactory evidence of "no effect" doses or "threshold doses" at which they would not inflict genetic chromosomal damage).[36]

The mutagenicity of mutagenic substances varies widely, depending on the dose consumed. As previously mentioned, most substances that have been found to be mutagenic also seem to have a carcinogenic action.[96] Out of the food additives mentioned in this paper, the following have been found in animal studies to have either mutagenic or carcinogenic action: BHA, carmoisine, erythrosine, nitrates/nitrites, saccharin, and sulfites. Furthermore, the following food additives have been found to be teratogenic when tested on animals: aspartame, BHA, MSG, and saccharin.[5] However, it has been argued that these toxicological food additive tests on animals for the assessment for human safety levels are really a waste of time. First of all, experiments on animals are conducted on healthy species fed on a nutritious diet, not on the malnourished, elderly, or sick. Secondly, only one agent is tested at a time, whereas humans are known to consume an elaborate cocktail of 12 to 60 different additives in the course of a single meal.[5] This may also be a reason why we still remain ignorant of the number of people really affected by the consumption of food additives.

Surveys on food intolerance per se have shown that as many as 2 in 10 people believe that they react badly to certain foods or to their constituents, whereas less than 2 in every 100 has been considered to be the official figure. This finding is based on the fact that only the latter statistical results can be measured using presently acceptable diagnostic techniques.[136] However, a recently published report indicates that small children are much more likely to react to certain foods. Although the exact numbers are not known, surveys suggest that 1 child in 10 may be affected in some way.[137]

Nutritional and Toxic Chemical Influences on Behavior

Dietary and toxicological factors in behavioral disorders have been sadly neglected by mainstream psychiatry, even though it is known that brain function itself involves subtle chemical and electrical processes, which can be easily altered and modified with the use of various psychoactive drugs. Therefore, it is difficult to comprehend why the role of nutritional influences on behavior has been completely ignored, even though the precursors of neurotransmitter molecules, essential for the brain function, are only found in foods. Furthermore, that they cannot be synthesized nor stored by the brain, unless introduced by appropriate dietary substances.

When the availability of these dietary precursors are reduced, the neurotransmitter synthesis will become impaired, with the consequent changes in both thinking process and behavior. When this happens, learning and memory tasks may become impaired or disturbed, intellectual development inhibited, and overt behaviors disordered, depending upon which dietary precursor is deficient or missing. In addition, various neurotoxins such as alcohol, heroin, LSD, nicotine, lead, organic solvents, individual food intolerances, and some food additives can modify neurotransmitter release, resulting in subtle or exaggerated behavioral changes.[34,98,155,156]

Food Additives and Malnutrition

Another form of risk posed by additives is the loss of the nutritional value of a food, which can result in inappropriate diets and subclinical malnutrition. The common factor in most foods containing additives is their high sugar and fat content. Pure sucrose, by definition, contains literally no nutrients, only calories; fat, on the other hand, contains few nutrients and is very high in calories. In addition, foods containing additives are mainly processed foods that have lost a substantial proportion of their nutritional value through the processing procedure. Even though some vitamins and/or minerals are sometimes added to some foods after processing, the ratio of essential nutrients to calories is usually still quite inadequate, resulting in a high calorie, but a low nutritional, intake. This type of diet, because of the high calorie and low nutritional content, can result in less than optimum nutrition and therefore subclinical and/or marginal malnutrition.

A study examining the nutritional status of 65 inner city schoolchildren showed that 63 percent of the children obtained more than 35 percent of their calorie intake from foods as fat and 88 percent of the children consumed more than 11 percent of their calories from added sugar. A third of the children had nothing to eat for breakfast before going to school and the remainder consumed only confectionery (sweet, refined, processed foods) and/or potato chips. Forty percent of the girls and 34 percent of the boys ate no fresh fruit during the week they kept the diary. For the majority of children, the mean intake of essential nutrients such as calcium, magnesium, iron, zinc, vitamin A, riboflavin (vitamin B2), and folate was found to be considerably below the lowest recommended nutrient intake.

In addition, iron deficiency is directly associated with attention-deficit disorders, irritability, and with poor scholastic achievement;[138,139] zinc deficiency with irritable, tearful, sullen, and possibly also hyperactive behavior;[60,140] calcium deficiency with anxiety neurosis;[34] and magnesium deficiency with fidgeting, anxious restlessness, as well as with learning disabilities.[141] Furthermore, the lack of an adequate high-protein breakfast in schoolchildren has been linked with a poor academic performance.[142–144]

Finally, an excessive sugar-rich food consumption without the presence of an adequate amount of protein can lead to reactive hypoglycemia, with its most disturbing antisocial and behavioral consequences.[28,119–132] Also, the diets on which the schoolchildren existed seem to be so low in essential nutrients, vitamins, and minerals that it may not be inappropriate to suggest that most of these children were also suffering from a subclinical malnutrition, which in turn has been directly linked with behavioral disorders and scholastic failures, as well as with antisocial and criminal behaviour.[47,145–152]

Discussion and Recommendations

The use of food additives has increased enormously in the last few decades. As the result, it has been estimated that today about 75 percent of the Western diet is made up of various processed foods, each person consuming an average 8–10 pounds of food additives per year, with some possibly eating even more.

The following adverse effects have been attributed to the consumption of food additives: eczema, urticaria, angioedema, exfoliative dermatitis, irritable bowel syndrome, nausea, vomiting, diarrhea, rhinitis, bronchospasm, migraine, anaphylaxis, hyperactivity, and other behavioral disorders.[31]

There is also now clear evidence that the health of the nation in the United Kingdom has deteriorated considerably during the last few decades. This was found by Dr. Michael Wadsworth, when he compared the health records of over 5,000 people born in 1946 to their first-born children a generation later. The survey found among the new generation a substantial increase in hospital admissions of children up to the age of four, a tripling of instances of asthma, a sixfold increase in both eczema and juvenile diabetes, as well as a double increase in obesity.[158]

The number of children admitted to psychiatric hospitals has also risen sharply. The latest official figures have shown between 1985 and 1990 a 42 percent rise in the number of under 10-year-olds seen by the psychiatric services and a 65 percent increase in children aged between 10 to 14, whilst the admissions of 15- to 19-year-old juveniles to psychiatric hospitals had increased 21 percent. Even some children as young as five years of age are ending up in psychiatric wards.[159,160]

Crime is also presently on top of the political agenda. In fact, the present rising trend of the criminal statistics and violence resembles today more of an epidemic disease, with symptoms including mental disarrangement combined with a complete lack of any behavioral or emotional control.[201] Whilst the crime statistics relentlessly rise, the government and the media are trying to put the blame on varied sociopolitical influences such as TV and film violence, poverty, lack of parental guidance, alleged child abuse, frustration, lack of motivation, lack of appropriate prisons or institutions, the police, and so on. In fact, the blame has been pointed at most things, but never on faulty nutrition. Yet, as this paper has shown, an inappropriate nutrition can modify brain function resulting, in susceptible individuals, in a severe mental dysfunction, including manifestations of criminal and violent behavior.

When this happens, several nutritional factors might be working together; however, the following fundamental dietary factors must be taken into consideration when confronting anyone displaying an inappropriate behavior pattern: Is the person concerned living on a high-sugar, high-food additive diet that lacks an appropriate amount of good protein? Is the diet completely lacking in foods high in vitamin and mineral content such as fresh fruits and/or salads? Could the person have an allergic intolerance to any foods he or she is consuming regularly? Could the person suffer from a toxicological burden of heavy metal contamination, such as lead, cadmium and/or aluminum, or a deficiency of an essential trace element?[157]

■ CONCLUSION

It must be stressed that this paper is most definitely not trying to insinuate that all negative behavior manifestations are nutritional in origin, as sociopolitical influences certainly do play a part. However, it must be always remembered that a healthy and non-toxic brain can usually receive information and process it in an intelligent and positive manner, as opposed to a malnourished and toxic brain that simply does not possess the same capability.

As seen from the above, inadequate nutrition and subclinical malnutrition seem to be two of the basic reasons for a myriad of physical and mental health problems of today. This could be easily rectified by reducing the wide use of non-essential food additives, which in turn would simply restrict the amount of non-nutritious foods presently on sale, resulting in a wider uptake of more nutritionally dense foods.

The main excuse of the food manufacturers and the government officials for the importance of the use of preservatives is that without them foods would soon spoil. This argument is indeed quite realistic. However, it is interesting to note that of the nearly 4,000 different additives currently in use, over 3,640 are used purely for cosmetic reasons and as coloring agents, the preservatives accounting for less than 2 percent of all additives when counted by number or by weight.[161]

The other continued reason for the approval of the use of additives is based on the argument that they are present in foods on such a minute scale that they must be therefore completely harmless. This argument may be almost acceptable regarding additives with a reversible toxicological action. However, with additives that have been found to be both mutagenic and carcinogenic, neither the human nor animal body is able to detoxify. There-

fore even very minute doses of these additives, when consumed continuously, will eventually result in an irreversible toxic burden, resulting finally in cancer formation and/or in chromosomal and fetal damage. This is quite unacceptable, particularly as the majority of these dangerous agents belong to the food coloring group.

In order to improve the present situation, the following recommendations are made:

• All non-essential food additives should be banned, particularly all cosmetic agents such as food colorants.

• All foods that include additives with carcinogenic, mutagenic, and teratogenic properties should be clearly labeled with the appropriate warning.

• All food additives should be banned from foods that may be consumed by infants and young children.

• The amount of TV advertising that encourages children to buy and eat unhealthy junk food should be vigorously cut down as children are presently surrounded by images promoting extremely unhealthy eating habits.

• All foods that have little or no nutritional value should be discouraged from all promotions.

• All foods, drinks, or medications currently exempt from declaring additives must in future be required to do so. Adverse reactions to undisclosed excipients should be always suspected whenever patients present with recurrent, unexplained symptoms, particularly allergies.[31]

• Finally, all young children diagnosed as hyperactive, including children currently seen by psychiatric services, should always be screened first for evidence of a possible food/chemical intolerance as even the simplest dietary changes such as avoiding foods containing food additives like colored candy or carbonated and sugary drinks can bring about a remarkable improvement in their health and behavior.[162]

I think it would be appropriate to suggest that we must now finally insist that the government must pass a law refusing permission for the food industries to add continuously into our everyday foods and beverages demonstrably toxic agents for cosmetic purposes only.

REFERENCES

1. The Food Labeling Regulations (S.I. 1980, No:1849), 1980.

2. Food intolerance and food aversion: a joint report of the royal college of physicians and the British Nutrition Foundation. *J Royal College of Physicians of London* 1984;18(2).

3. *The London Food Commission: Food Adulteration and How to Heat It.* London: Unwin Paperbacks, 1988.

4. Based on information from Industrial Aids Ltd Depth Study of the food additives industry, London 1980, updated by discussions with market researchers, and Key Note Food Flavourings and Ingredients, London, 1985.

5. Miller M. *Danger! Additives at Work.* London Food Commission, London 1985.

6. Taylor RJ. *Food Additives.* Chichester: John Wiley & Sons, 1980.

7. ACARD. The Food Industry and Technology, Cabinet Office, Advisory Council for Applied Research and Development, HMSO, London, 1982.

8. Feingold BF. Food additives and child development. *Hospital Practice* 1973;21:11–12,17–18.

9. Feingold BF. Adverse Reactions to Hyperkinesis and Learning Disabilities (H-LD) Congressional Record, S-1973, 39–42,1973.

10. Feingold BF. Hyperkinesis and learning disabilities linked to artificial food flavors and colors. *Am J Nutr* 1975;75:797–803.

11. Feingold BF. *Why Your Child Is Hyperactive.* New York: Random House, 1975.

12. Feingold BF. Hyperkinesis and learning disabilities linked to the ingestion of artificial food colors and flavors. *J Learn Disabilities* 1976;9:19–27.

13. Feingold BF. Dietary management of behavior and learning disabilities. In: *Nutrition & Behavior* edited by SA Miller. Philadelphia, PA: Franklin Institute Press, 1981.

14. Cook PS, Woodhill JM. The Feingold dietary treatment of the hyperkinetic syndrome. *Med J Austr* 1976;2:85–90.

15. Brenner AA. A study of the efficacy of the Feingold diet on hyperkinetic children. *Clin Pediatr* 1977;16:652–656.

16. Levy F, Dumbrell S, Hobbes G, et al. Hyperkinesis and diet: a double-blind crossover trial with a tartrazine challenge. *Med J Austr* 1978;1:61–64.

17. Williams JI, Cram DM. Diet in the management of hyperkinesis: a review of the tests of Feingold hypotheses. *Canadian Psych Assoc J* 1978;23:241–248.

18. Margen S, Weiss B, William HH. Report on phase II-FDA contract 223-76-2040: a dietary challenge study of artificial food colors in children 1–7 years old with behavioral disturbances. Dec 15, 1978.

19. Swanson JM,Kinsbourne M. Food dyes impair performance of hyperactive children on laboratory learning tests. *Science* 1980;207:1485–1487.

20. Weiss B, Williams JH, Margen S, et al. Behavioral responses to artificial food colors. *Science* 1980;207:1487–1489.

21. O'Banion DR. *An Ecological and Nutritional Approach to Behavioral Medicine.* Springfield, IL: Charles C. Thomas, 1981.

22. O'Shea JA, Porter SF. Double-blind study of children with hyperkinetic syndrome treated with multi-allergen extract subclinically. *J Learning Dis* 1981;14(4):189–237.

23. Silbergeld EK, Anderson SM. Artificial food colors and childhood behavior disorders. *Bull New York Acad Med* (2nd series) 1982;58(3):275–295.

24. Weiss B. Food additives and environmental chemicals as sources of childhood behavior disorders. *J Am Acad Child Psvch* 1982;21(2):144–152.

25. Rippere V. Food additives and hyperactive children: a critique of Conners. *Br J Clin Psych* 1983;22:19–23.

26. King DS. Psychological and behavioral effects of food and chemical exposure in sensitive individuals. *Nutrition and Health* 1984;3:137–151.

27. Menzies IC. Disturbed children: the role of food and chemical sensitivities. *Nutrition and Health* 1984;3:39–54.

28. Schauss AG. Nutrition and behavior: complex interdisciplinary research. *Nutrition and Health* 1984;3:9–37.

29. Egger J, Carter CM, Graham PJ, et al. Controlled trial of oligoantigenic treatment in the hyperkinetic syndrome. *Lancet* 1985 Mar 9:540–545.

30. Schoenthaler SJ, Doraz WE, Wakefield JA. The impact of a low food additive and sucrose diet on academic performance in 803 New York City public schools. *Int J Biosocial Res* 1986;8(2):185–195.

31. Smith JM. Adverse reactions to food and drug additives. *European J Clin Nutr* 1991;45(Supp. I):17–21.

32. Dickerson JWT. Diet and Hyperactivity. *J Human Nutr* 1980;34:167–174.

33. Miller M, Millstone E. *Food Additives Campaign Team: Report on Color Additives.* London: FACT, 1987. 34. Bryce-Smith D. Environmental and chemical influences on behaviour and mentation. *Chem Soc Rev* 1986;15:93–123.

35. Weiss B. *Food Additive Safety and Evaluation: The Link to Behavioral Disorders in Children.* New York: Plenum Publishing, 1984, 221–250.

36. Wynn M, Wynn A. *The Prevention of Handicap or Early Pregnancy Origin: Some Evidence for the Value of Good Health Before Conception.* London: Foundation for Education and Research in Childbearing, 1981.

37. Barnes B and Bradley SG. *Planning for a Healthy Baby.* London: Ebury Press, 1990.

38. Tuormaa TE. Adverse effects of alcohol on reproduction: literary review. *International Journal of Biosocial & Medical Research* 1994:14(2).

39. Tuormaa TE. Adverse effects of tobacco smoking on reproduction and health: literary review. *Journal of Nutrition and Health* 1995;10:105–120.

40. Bryce-Smith D. Lead and brain function. In: *Food and Health Science Technology* edited by GG Birch and KJ Parker. London: Applied Science Publishers, 1980.

41. Bryce-Smith D. Lead induced disorders and mentation in children. *Nutrition and Health* 1983;1:179–194.

42. Davies S. Lead and disease. *Nutrition and Health* 1983;2(3/4):135–145.

43. Tuormaa TE. The Adverse Effects of Lead. *J Nutr Med* 1994;4(4):449–461.

44. Freeman EH, Feingold BF, Schlesigner K. Psychological variables in allergic disorders: a review. *Psychosomatic Medicine* 1964;26:543.

45. Feingold BF, Singer MT, Freeman EH. Variables in allergic disease: a critical appraisal of methodology. *J of Allergy* 1966;38:143.

46. Feingold BF. Recognition of food additives as a cause of symptoms of allergy *Ann. of Allergy* 1968;26:309.

47. Lipton MA, Nemeroff CB, Mailman RB. Hyperkinesis and food additives. In: *Nutrition and Brain* edited by RJ Wurtman and JJ Wurtman. New York: Raven Press, 1979.

48. Stare FJ, Whelan EM, Sheridan M. Diet and hyperactivity: is there a relationship? *Pediatrics* 1980;66:521–525.

49. Kavale KA, Forness SR. Hyperactivity and diet treatment: a meta-analysis of the Feingold hypothesis. *J of Learning Dis* 1983;16:324–330.

50. Mattes JA. The Feingold diet: A current reappraisal. *J of Learning Dis* 1983;16:319–323.

51. Conners CK, Goyette CH, Southwick MA, Lees JM, et al. Food additives and hyperkinesis: A double-blind experiment. *Pediatrics* 1976;58:154–166.

52. Goyette CH, Conners CK, Petti TA, et al. Effects of artificial food colors on hyperkinetic children: A double-blind challenge study. *Psychopharmacology Bull* 1978;14:39–40.

53. Harley J, Ray R, Tomasi L, et al. Hyperkinesis and food additives: testing the Feingold hypothesis. *Pediatrics* 1978;61:818–828.

54. Lockey SD. Allergic reactions due to FD&C yellow no. tartazine, an aniline dye used as coloring agent and identifying agent in various steroids. *Ann Allergy* 1959;17:719–721.

55. Freedman BJ. Asthma induced by sulphur dioxide, benzoate and tartazine contained in orange drinks. *Clin Allergy* 1977;7:407–415.

56. Neuman I, Elian R, Nahum H, et al. The danger of "yellow dyes" (tartazine) to allergic subjects. *Clin Allergy* 1978;8:65–68.

57. Peterson MA, Biggs DF, Aaron TH. Comparison of the effects of aspirin, indomethacin and tartazine on dynamic pulmonary compliance and flow resistance in the guinea pig. Proc Western Pharmacology Society (Seattle), 1980;23:121–124.

58. Weliky N, Heiner DC. Hypersensitivity to chemicals: correlation to tartazine hypersensitivity with characteristic serum IgD and IgE immune response pattern. *Clin Allergy* 1980;10:375–394.

59. Juhlin L. Recurrent urticaria: clinical investigation of 330 patients. *Br J Dermatology* 1981;104:369–381.

60. Ward NI, Soulsbury KA, Zeittel VH, et al. The influence of the chemical additive tartazine on the zinc status of hyperactive children: a double-blind placebo-controlled study. *J Nutr Med* 1990;1:51–57.

61. Juhlin L, Michaelson G, Zetterstrom O. Urticaria and asthma induced by food and drug additives in patients with aspirin sensitivity. *J Allergy and Clin Immunol* 1972;50:92–98.

62. Vendanthan PK, Menon MM, Bell TD, et al. Aspirin and tartrazine oral challenge: incidence of adverse response in chronic childhood asthma. *J Allergy and Clin Immunol* 1977;60:8–13.

63. Stenius BSM and Lemola M. Hypersensitivity to acetylsalicylic acid (ASA) and tartrazine in patients with asthma. *Clin Allergy* 1976;6:119–129.

64. Settipane GA, Chafee FH, Postman IM, et al. Significance of tartrazine sensitivity in chronic urticaria of unknown aetiology. *J Allergy and Clin Immunol* 1976;57:541–546.

65. Noid HE, Schulze TW, Winkelman RK. Diet plan for patients with salicylate-induced urticaria. *Arch Dermatology* 1974;109:866–868.

66. Johnson HM, Peeler JT, Smith BG. Tartrazine: quantitative passive hemagglutination. Studies on a food-borne allergen of small molecular weight. *Immunochemistry* 1971;8:281–287.

67. Vane JR. Inhibition of prostaglandin synthesis as a mechanism of action for aspirin-like drugs. *Nature (New Biol)* 1971;231:232–235.

68. McIntyre BA, Philip RB. Effect of three non-steroid agents on prostaglandin synthesis in vitro. *Throm Res* 1977;12:67.

69. Regtop H. Nutrition leukotrienes and inflammatory disorders. *Yearbook of Nutritional Medicine, 1984/85.* New Canaan, CT: Keats Publishing, 55–70.

70. Dahlen S, Samuelsson B. Leukotrienes are potent constrictors of human bronchi. *Nature* 1980;288:484.

71. Weiss JW, Drazen JM et al. Airway constriction in humans produced by inhalation of leukotriene. *JAMA* 1977;249:2814.

72. Anon N. Tartrazine: a yellow hazard. *Drug Ther Bull* 1980;15:53–55.

73. Anon N. E-numbers, doctors and patients: food for thought. *Drug Ther Bull* 1984;22:41–42.

74. Lafferman JA, Silbergeld EK. Erythrosin B inhibits dopamine transport in rat caudate synaptosomes. *Science* 1979;205:410–412.

75. Logan WJ, Swanson JM. Erythrosin B inhibition of neurotransmitter accumulation by rat brain homogenates. *Science* 1979;206:363–364.

76. Snyder SH. Putative neurotransmitters in the brain: selective neuronal uptake, subcellular localization, and interactions with centrally active drugs. *Biol Psychiatry* 1970;2:367–389.

77. Shaywitz BA, Cohn DJ, Bowers MB. CSF monoamine metabolites in children with minimal brain dysfunction: evidence for alterations of brain dopamine: a preliminary report. *J Pediatr* 1977;90:67–71.

78. Shekim WO, DeKirmeryian H, Chapel JL. Urinary catecholamine metabolites in hyperkinetic boys treated with d-amphetamine. *Am J Psychiatry* 1977;134:1276–1279.

79. Michaelsson G and Juhlin L. Urticaria induced by preservatives and dye additives in foods and drugs. *Br J Dermatology* 1973;88:525–532.

80. Stevenson DD, Simon RA. Sensitivity to ingested metabisulphites in asthmatic subjects. *J Allergy Clin Immunol* 1981;68:26–32.

81. Henderson WR, Raskin NH. Hot dog headache: individual susceptibility to nitrite. *Lancet* 1972;1:1162–1163.

82. Taylor G. Nitrates, nitrites, nitrosamines and cancer. *Nutrition and Health* 1983;2:1.

83. Ehrlichman J. Why the scandal of BHA leaves a nasty taste in the mouth. *Guardian*, May, 22, 1987.

84. Thune P, Grandholt A. Provocation tests with antiphlogistica and food additives in recurrent urticaria. *Dermatologica* 1975;151:360–367.

85. Juhlin L. Incidence of intolerance to food additives. *Int J Dermatology* 1980;19:548–551.

86. Collins-Williams C. Intolerance to additives. *Ann Allergy* 1983;51:315–316.

87. Allen DH and Baker GJ. Chinese restaurant asthma. *New Engl J Med* 1981;305:1154–1155.

88. Reif-Lehrer L. Possible significance of adverse reactions to glutamate in humans. *Federation Proceedings* 1976;35:2205–2211.

89. Bryan GT, Erturk E, Yoshida O. Production of urinary bladder carcinomas in mice by sodium saccharin. *Science* 1970;168:1238.

90. Ashby J, Styles JA, Anderson D, Paton D. Saccharin: an epigenetic carcinogen/mutagen. *Food Cosmet Toxicol* 1978;16:95–103.

91. Reuber MD. Carcinogenicity of saccharin. *Envir Health Perspect* 1978;25:173–200.

92. Masubuchi M, et al. The mutagenicity of sodium saccharin: dominant lethal test; II cytogenic studies. *Mutat Res* 1978;54:218–219.

93. Moore CW, Schmick A. Recombino-genicity and mutagenicity of saccharin in saccharomyces. *Mutat Res* 1979;67:215–219.

94. Batzinger RP, Ou SYL, Bueding E. Saccharin and other sweeteners: mutagenic properties. *Science* 1977;198:944–946.

95. Lederer J, Pottier-Arnauld AM. Influence de la saccharine sur de developpement de l'embryon chez la rate gestante [in French]. *La Diabete* 1973;21:13.

96. Claxton LD, Barry PZ. Chemical mutagenesis: an emerging issue for public health. *Am J Public Health* 1977;67:1037–1042.

97. Weiner MA. *Maximum Immunity*. Bath, UK: Gateway Books, 1986, 73–74.

98. Wurtman RJ. *Nutrition and the Brain*. New York: Raven Press, 1977.

99. Werbach MR. *Nutritional Influences on Mental Illness*. Tarzana, CA: Third Line Press, 1991, 11–13.

100. Mawson AT, Jacobs KW. Corn consumption, tryptophan, and cross-national homicide rates. *J Orthomol Psychiatry* 1978;7:227–230.

101. Morand C, Young SN, Ervin FR. Clinical response of aggressive schizophrenics to oral tryptophan. *Biol Psychiatry* 1983;18:575–578.

102. Young SN, Chouinard G, Annable L.et al. The therapeutic action of tryptophan in depression, mania and aggression. In: *Progress in Tryptophan and Serotonin Research* edited by HG Schlossberger et al. New York: Walter de Gruyter, 1984.

103. Kitahara M. Dietary tryptophan ratio and homicide in Western and Southern Europe. *J Orthomolecular Med* 1986;1(1):13–16.

104. Young SN and Teff KL. Tryptophan availability, 5HT synthesis and 5HT function. *Prog Neuropsychopharmacol Biol Psychiatrv* 1989;13(3–4):373–379.

105. Volavka J, et al. Tryptophan treatment of aggressive psychiatric in-patients. *Biol Psychiatrv* 1990;28(8):728–732.

106. Brown GL, Ebert MH, Goyer PF, et al. Aggression, suicide and seretonin: relationship to CSF amine metabolites. *Am J Psychiatry* 1982;139:741–746.

107. Iversen LL. Introduction, neurotransmitters and CNS disease. *Lancet Review* Oct. 23–Dec 18, 1982.

108. Linnoila M, Virkkunen M, Scheinin M, et al. Low cerebrospinal fluid 5-hydroxyindo-leacetic acid concentrations differentiates impulsive from non-impulsive violent behaviour. *Life Sci* 1983;33:2609–2614.

109. Virkkunen M. Aivojen seretooni ja aggres-siivisuus. *Duodecim* 1986;102:850–852.

110. Roy A, et al. Monoamines, glucose metabolism, aggression towards self and others. *Int J Neurosci* 1988;41(3–4):261–264.

111. Van Praag HM. Affective disorders and aggression disorders: evidence of common biochemical metabolism. *Suicide Life Theat Behav* 1986;16(2):103–132.

112. Schoenthaler S. Diet and crime: an empirical examination of the value of nutrition in the control and treatment of incarcerated juvenile offenders. *Int J Biosocial Res* 1983;4(l):25–39.

113. Schoenthaler S, Doraz W. Types of offences which can be reduced in an institutional setting using nutritional intervention: a preliminary empirical evaluation. *Int J Biosocial Res* 1983;4(2):74–84.

114. Schoenthaler S. The Los Angeles probation department diet-behavior program: an empirical evaluation of six institutions. Int *J Biosocial Res* 1983;5(2):88–98.

115. Schoenthaler S. The Northern California diet-behavior program: an empirical examination of 3000 incarcerated juveniles in Stanislaus Country juvenile hall. *Int J Biosocial Res* 1983;5(2):99–106.

116. Prinz RJ, Roberts, Hantman E. Dietary correlates of hyperactive behavior in children. *J Consult Clin Psychol* 1980;48(6):760–769.

117. Crook WG. Food additives and hyperactivity. *Lancet* May 15, 1982:1128.

118. Goldman JA, et al. Behavioral effects of sucrose in preschool children. *J Abnorm Child Psychol* 1986;14(4):565–577.

119. Fishbein D. The contribution of refined carbohydrate consumption to maladaptive behaviors. *J Orthomolecular Psychiatry* 1982;ll(l):1–4.

120. A case of functional hypoglycaemia: a medicolegal problem. *Br J Psychiatry* 1973;123:353–358.

121. Bolton R. Hostility in fantasy: a further test of the hypoglycaemia-aggression hypothesis. *Aggressive Beh* 1976;2:257–274

122. Bolton R. The hypoglycaemia-aggression hypothesis; an overview of research. In: *Biosocial Bases of Antisocial Behavior* edited by SA Mednick. New York: Cambridge University Press, 1985.

123. Buckley RE. Hypoglycaemia, temporal lobe disturbances in aggressive behavior. *J Orthomolecular Psych* 1979;8(3):188–192.

124. Mozer K. *Physiology of Hostility.* Chicago, IL: Markham Publishing Co, 1971.

125. Neziroglu FA. Behavioral and organic aspects of aggression. In: *Biological Psychiatry Today* edited by J Obiols, et al. Amsterdam: Elsevier Publishing, 1979, 1215–1222.

126. Yarura-Tobias JA, Netziroglu FA. Violent behavior, brain dysrhythmia and glucose dysfunction: a new syndrome. *J Orthomolecular Psych* 1975;4:128–188.

127. Yarura-Tobias JA, Neziroglu FA. Aggressive behavior, clinical interfaces. In: *Saint Vincent; Edizioni Centro Culturale & Congressi* edited by I Vazelli and I Morgese, 1981.

128. Virkkunen M. Reactive hypoglycaemic tendency among habitually violent offenders; a further study by means of the glucose tolerance test. *Neuropsyhobiology* 1982;8:35–40.

129. Virkkunen M, Huttunen MO. Evidence of abnormal glucose tolerance test among violent offenders. *Neuropsychobiology* 1982;8:30–34.

130. Virkkunen M. Insulin secretion during glucose tolerance test in antisocial personality. *Br J Psychiatry* 1983;142:598–604.

131. Virkkunen M. Reactive hypoglycaemic tendency among habitually violent offenders. *Nutr Review* 1986;(Suppl):94–103.

132. Tuormaa TE. *An Alternative to Psychiatry.* Book Guild Ltd, 1991, 132–161.

133. Egger J, Carter CM, Wilson J, et al. Is migraine a food allergy? A double-blind controlled trial of oligoantigenic diet treatment. *Lancet* 1983:865–869

134. McGovern JJ, Gardner RW, Brenneman LD. The role of naturally occurring haptens in allergy. *Ann Allergy* 1981;47:123.

135. Joint Expert Committee on Food Additives of the United Nations Food and Agriculture Organisation and the World Health Organisation. *Environmental Health Criteria* 1987;70:46–65.

136. Young E, et al. A population study of food intolerance. *Lancet* 1994;343:1127–1129.

137. Adverse Reactions to Food, Topical Update 2. National Dairy Council Publication, 5/7 John Princes Street, London W1M OAP, 1994.

138. Webb T, Oski F. Behavioral status of young adolescents with iron deficiency anemia. *J Spec Education* 1974;8(2):153–156.

139. Lozoff B and Brittenham GH. Behavioral aspects of iron deficiency. *Prog Hematol* 1986;14:23–53.

140. Moynahan EJ. Zinc deficiency and disturbances of mood and visual behavior. *Lancet* 1976;1:91.

141. Durlach J. Clinical aspects of chronic magnesium deficiency. In: *Magnesium in Health* edited by MS Seeling. New York: Spectrum Publications, 1980.

142. Pollitt E, et al. Fasting and cognitive function. *J Psychiatr Res* 1983;17:169–174.

143. Pollitt E, et al. Brief fasting, stress, and cognition in children. *Am J Clin Nutr* 1981;34:1526–1533.

144. Connors CK, Blouin AG. Nutritional effects on behavior of children. *J Psychiatr Res* 1983;17:193–201.

145. Latham MC and Cobos F. The effects of malnutrition on intellectual development and learning. *Am J Public Health* 1971;61:1307–1324.

146. Hoffer A. Relation of crime to nutrition. *Humanist in Canada* 1975;9(3):2–9.

147. Schauss A. *Diet, Crime and Delinquency.* New York: Parker House, 1981.

148. Reed B. Food, *Teens and Behavior.* Natural Press, 1983.

149. Galler JR. Malnutrition: a neglected cause of learning failure. *Postgrad Med* 1986;80:225–230.

150. Schoenthaler S J. Doraz WE, Wakefield JA. The impact of a low additive and sucrose diet in academic performance in 803 New York City public schools. *Int J Biosocial Res* 1986;8(2):138–148.

151. Eysenck HJ and Eysenck SBG, eds. *Improvement of I.Q. and Behavior as a Function of Dietary Supplementation: A Symposium.* Oxford, UK: Pergamon Press, 1991.

152. Bryce-Smith D. The Third Leg. Lecture in the Power of Prevention Conference, 24th June, Oxford, UK, 1994.

153. The Gardner Merchant School Meals Survey "What Are Our Children Eating?" Gardner Merchant. Educational Services, Kenley House, 1994.

154. Doyle W, et al. Maternal nutrient intake and birthweight. *J Human Nutr and Dietetics* 1989;2:415–422.

155. Wynn SW, et al. The association of maternal social class with maternal diet and the dimensions of babies in the population of London women. *Nutrition and Health* 1994;9:303–315.

156. Smithells RW, et al. Possible prevention of neural tube defects by preconceptional vitamin supplementation. *Lancet* 1980;ii:339–340.

157. Laker M. On determining trace element levels in man: to uses of blood and hair. *The Lancet* 1978;2:260–262.

158. Wadsworth M. Intergenerational differences in child health. Report to British Society for Population Studies Conference, August 1985.

159. Thompson D, Pudney M. Mental Illness: The Fundamental Facts. *Mental Health Foundation Publication,* 1990.

160. Gorman J. Mental Health Statistics, MIND Information Unit, Dec 1993.

161. London Food Commission; *Food Adulteration and How to Beat It.* London: Unwin Paperbacks, 1988.

162. Bunday S, Colquhoun V. Why the lack of treatment for hyperactive children? *J Nutr Med* 1990;1:361–363.

RAISING STUDENT ACHIEVEMENT THROUGH BETTER NUTRITION
by Helen F. Saul, MSEd

It seems only natural that, by now, people would be well aware of the importance of eating healthy foods. However, if you were to take a field trip through your average school cafeteria, you might notice that the foods on the students' trays don't reflect that thinking. In the school's defense, are fruits, vegetables, and whole grains offered? Yes. Are they fresh, appetizing, unprocessed, and low in salt and sugar? Not exactly. In the popular documentary *Super Size Me,* the field representative of Sodexho, a company that services over 400 K-12 schools nationwide, stated: "We are hoping through nutrition education the students will learn to make the right food choices without restricting what they can purchase."[1] However, it is rare that I see a student taking a large helping of the gray-green canned peas, rubbery canned fruit, or a large helping of lettuce and tomatoes on their meat taco. (I like vegetables, and even I don't eat those.)

Between a slice of pizza or a tiny sorry-looking salad, what would the average kid choose? By not offering appetizing healthy foods, are we setting the kids up to make bad choices? In a school district like mine where over 40 percent of the students are on free and reduced lunch programs, they are far less likely to come in with a (more expensive) healthy bagged lunch. As for the bagged lunches, they seem to come in an array of colors, few if any of which belong to fruit or vegetables.

Adopting a better nutrition program in schools will not only affect positive changes in behavior, attendance, and overall health, it will also improve students' ability to learn and thus raise their levels of achievement. Reduce problem behaviors and referrals, increase student learning, raise test scores, and lower dropout rates? It is an administrator's dream. The dream however can become a reality, and schools have done just that by providing healthier food choices for students.

Background

In June of 1946, President Harry S. Truman signed the National School Lunch Act. "The federally assisted meal program was established as 'a measure of national security, to safeguard the health and well-being of the Nation's children and to encourage the domestic consumption of nutritious agricultural commodities.'" Additionally, in 1966, President Lyndon B. Johnson signed the Child Nutrition Act and remarked, "good nutrition is essential to good learning."[2] Yet, to this day we are struggling in our schools to get kids to attend, behave, and achieve. "The one place where the impact of our fast food world has become more and more evident is in our nation's schools."[1]

The Nutritional Resource Foundation, created by nutritionist Barbara Stitt, PhD, and her husband Paul Stitt who holds a MS degree in biochemistry, is dedicated to helping students and adults alike eat more healthy diets. They point out the humbling statistic that "less than one in three children and adolescents meet dietary recommendations for limiting intake of saturated fat, less than one in five eats enough fruits and vegetables." Additionally, "meals served at school are often more deficient in produce than those at home. Fast foods have overtaken school cafeteria food and soft-drink machines have displaced real fruit juices as well as milk. When vegetables are offered, they are typically the steam-table variety, overcooked, and unappetizing."[3] While originally schools began providing students with food to help improve their health, especially those from families that could not feed them adequately, now schools are the ones creating health problems for children.

Defining the Problem

Test scores are low, and programs such as No Child Left Behind have shown little improvement. The *Washington Post* reports: "Most troubling for educators are the sluggish reading skills among middle-school students, which have remained virtually unchanged for 15 years, according to the National

From the *J Orthomolecular Med* 2006;21(2):80–84.

Assessment of Educational Progress."[4] Administrators cringe at decreases in test scores, and remaining stagnant is not much of an accomplishment.

Schools have adopted breakfast programs, says Julie Skolmowski MPH, RD, because they know

> that well-nourished students that skip breakfast perform worse on tests and have poor concentration.[6] Nutrients play a major role in learning abilities. If children's bodies are left deficient day after day, as are most in America, their brains will not function properly and they will be under performing . . . Research suggests that skipping breakfast can affect children's intellectual performance, and even moderate under-nutrition can have lasting effects on cognitive development. Children who are hungry are more likely to have behavioral, emotional, and academic problems at school.[3]

So, how many schools give students breakfast? But what kind of breakfast are they eating? While we might maintain that we have come a long way and we have nutrition guidelines in our schools that must be followed, we still have children who are undernourished and underachieving, and our test scores are not where we want them. According to Abram Hoffer, a medical doctor who also holds a PhD in nutrition,

> Over 75 percent of our current diet consists of processed food. This diet is deficient in fiber, too rich in processed fats, too rich in simple sugars, and deficient in vitamins, minerals, and essential fatty acids . . . It is also too rich in additives . . . Food additives decrease the nutritional quality of foods.[7]

Jane Hersey, National Director of the Feingold Association of the United States, a group dedicated to helping children and adults apply scientifically proven dietary techniques for better behavior, learning, and health for over 30 years, further emphasizes that "typically, the reaction [to food additives] will be one of these: a change in behavior, a change in the ability to focus and learn."[8] Why would we want to detract from the very skills and behaviors students need in order to be successful?

For some kids, the meal at school may be the only one they get that day. But we should be reminded that all children, regardless of socioeconomic status, are at risk for poor nutrition. As the number of parents in the workforce increases, children are left to fend for themselves when preparing meals at home. Therefore, it is our responsibility to make the meals they eat at school of the highest quality. This benefits not only the child but also the entire climate, culture, and success of the building.

A parent should be tuned into whether or not their child is getting the proper nutrition. Lendon Smith, MD, known nationally as the "Children's Doctor," asked parents to tune into statements like these during a school conference: "I know he knows the work, but he won't put it on paper"; "He won't work up to his ability"; "Some days he has it; the next day it's gone." These comments suggest "nutritional factors are a part of the explanation. The off-and-on phenomenon is the clue to fluctuating blood sugar . . . nutrition is the key factor in helping this particular child."[9]

The School Nutrition Association (SNA) is recognized as the authority on school nutrition and has been "advancing the availability, quality, and acceptance of school nutrition programs as an integral part of education since 1946."[5] Reading through their 2005 report, "School Nutrition Market Trends: Environmental Scan Update," I found that pizza was named the top entrée during the 2003–2004 school year. In the same report it was indicated that "poor nutrition and physical inactivity are shown to cost schools academic achievement and significant amount of funding."[10] Perhaps they have considered that the two may be related.

How Do We Fix It?

If good food is available, children will eat it. Dr. Smith insisted that what is needed is for somebody to do something about the avalanche of junk food, which increasingly displaces nutritious food in the diets of these kids and disposes them to rampage.[9] If we want to increase the success of a nutrition program, we need to remove the junk, and then add the nutrients. "There is rapidly accumulating evidence that a child's ability to learn can be improved by . . .the improvement in general nutritional status through removing junk foods from his daily diet," says Dr. Hoffer.[7] This starts with setting standards: What foods will we serve in our schools?

In an alternative charter school in Appleton, Wisconsin, they have adopted a nutrition program that goes above and beyond the requirements. These are their goals:

• Get everyone eating five servings of fresh fruit, fresh vegetables, and whole grains every day.

• Promote and serve more fresh fruits and vegetables.

• Eliminate food with artificial coloring, artificial flavoring, and sweeteners.

• Encourage parents and kids to pack healthy lunches.

• Teach basic nutrition concepts.

• Reduce children's intake of hydrogenated fat, saturated fat, sugar, and caffeine.

The above will, among other benefits, increase attendance in school and work, and improve the behavior and learning ability of students.[3]

Not only do you feed them right, you tell them why they are being fed this way and how to make their own healthy food choices as well. "Several studies have shown that when schoolchildren are introduced to a new food in school, become familiar with it, and learn about its origins and food value, they are more likely to eat it in the lunchroom and encourage their parents to serve it."[3] Ultimately, we want children to learn how to make good food choices on their own, as they won't always have the school to rely on.

Good Outcomes

Is this goal being met? In this day and age even "computers are now helping school foodservice workers ensure that the meals offered in schools comply with nutrition standards," and yet "it is another challenge altogether to ensure that students consume the nutritious foods provided."[11] However, if there are no unhealthy choices available, it will be difficult for a student to eat a meal that is not nutritionally beneficial to them.

RAISING STUDENT ACHIEVEMENT

Here is a sample of the foods now available for students in the breakfast and lunch programs[3] in the Appleton Central Alternative Charter School.

The breakfast menu includes:

• Bottled water, 100 percent juice, milk, and blended energy drinks.

• Whole-grain foods free of additives, dyes, artificial preservatives, and saturated fats.

• Granola, peanut butter, almond butter, natural fruit preserves, and fresh fruits.

The lunch menu includes:

• Bottled water, 100 percent juice, milk, and blended energy drinks.

• Whole-grain foods free of additives, dyes, artificial preservatives, and saturated fats.

• A salad bar filled with dark green lettuce, tomatoes, carrots, cucumber, mushrooms, olives, peanuts, sunflower seeds, broccoli and cauliflower, boiled eggs, whole-grain croutons, home-made applesauce, cabbage, peach and pear slices, pineapple, and fruity salad.

• Meats including lean pork, chicken, turkey, and fish.

• A variety of spices, soymilk products, and tofu are used as natural flavor enhancers.

Meals are cooked on site, and no frying is allowed in a grease product.

According to the Nutritional Resource Foundation, outcomes of this Wellness and Nutrition Program included "increased ability to concentrate in the school setting, more on task-behavior; increased cognitive development; ability to think more clearly, objectively, and rationally; and dropouts and expulsions may be dramatically reduced." A teacher commented, "We noticed a change from the get-go. All teachers reported that students were able to concentrate for longer periods in class."[3] Teachers and principals have observed that "grades are up, truancy is no longer a problem, arguments are rare, and teachers are able to spend their time teaching." Superintendent Dr. Thomas Scullen noted that the kids are coming to school, expulsions are rare, the drop-out rate is almost nil, and, although he expected a healthy diet would improve behavior, he was surprised that it had such an impact on academic performance.[12]

The Whitefish Central School in Montana has also adopted this program. Over the past three years, "teachers report that they have gained between 10 and 15 percent additional teaching time since the children have calmed down and are more alert and able to focus. This is reflected in the fact that the school now ranks academically in the 76th percentile in the state." They also found that "there has been another change in the cafeteria: the amount of food wasted has been cut in half, from 85 to 100 pounds per day, to about 45 pounds."[13]

Other schools with similar desired outcomes are also showing success.

A recently released study by WestEd, a non-profit research, development and service agency, found that California schools with students who routinely engaged in healthy eating and physical activity had larger subsequent gains in test scores than other schools. "These studies show what we have known—that healthy school meals play a critical and positive role in students development and learning process," said Donna Wittrock, president of the American School Food Service Association.[14]

What Does It Cost?

Adopting a program like the one in the Appleton School District "costs about the same as any other school lunch program."[1] Perhaps the question we should be asking though is not what does it cost, but what will it cost if we do not adopt a strong nutrition and wellness program in our schools?

Action for Healthy Kids (AFHK) recently released a report titled *The Learning Connection*[15] that summarizes evidence demonstrating the negative impact poor nutrition, inactivity, and weight problems can have on student achievement. According to former U.S. Surgeon General Dr. David Satcher,

The Learning Connection examines the impact of the root causes of childhood overweight and reveals a strong link between children's health and academic success. This report provides insight on possible costs to schools as the result of poor nutrition, inactivity, and weight problems, and makes the case for additional research to find more definitive data.

Dietician Julie Skolmowski writes,

The consequences *The Learning Connection* presents for the learning process as well as to school budgets are striking. The report also quantifies dollars that schools lose when children are absent from school—small amounts for individual students but this can add up. Particularly, the report demonstrates that, "Even an average school with a high absence rate based on poor nutrition and physical inactivity would lose from $95,000 to $160,000 per year in state aid."[6]

Our students are not the only ones that cost the district money when they are not healthy; sick teachers cost money too. "The Appleton, Wisconsin, Alternative High School serves fresh, homemade foods that the students and faculty enjoy. The full cost for this transformation was only about $20,000 per year—a fraction of what schools now spend to address the learning and behavior problems that are being caused, in part, by junk foods."[3] Principal LuAnn Coenen said, "I can't buy the argument that it is too costly for schools to provide good nutrition for their students. I found that one cost will reduce another. I don't have the vandalism. I don't have the litter. I don't have the need for high security."[16] One teacher noted that, "We're concerned about new band uniforms. We're concerned about the football team. We're concerned about textbooks. Why not be concerned about nutrition? Nutrition should be part of the general operating budget."[12] A member of the Board of Education in the Los Angeles Unified School

---

"One grandmother is worth two MDs."

— ROBERT MENDELSOHN

district observed, "It's not about money; it's not about economics; it's about health."[1]

Support

In order for any change to be accepted, people need to be shown the advantages of doing it. If your district is not ready for a full-blown nutrition program, there are ways to gradually introduce healthy eating habits. Here are some steps to consider:

• Use soy yogurt for dressings and tartar sauce.

• Use reduced fat mayonnaise.

• Use whole grain flour; have fresh fruit available.

• Try lower fat cheeses.

• Reduce amount of butter used in cooking.

• Offer vegetarian toppings on pizzas.

• Use lean meat.

• Eliminate the deep fryer.

• Limit the choice of hot dogs or foods high in salt, bad fat, and coloring to no more than once monthly.

• Remove salt shakers.

• Offer low-in-sugar breakfast items.

• Clearly define the limits of fat and sodium that you expect in the foods served.[17]

As with any change, "it starts with leadership. You have to believe that what you're going to do is going to work, and then you have to have the teachers on board. Once you are able to convince them, it is pretty simple to get the kids to follow."[18] Schools around the country are trying to get kids more interested in school lunches. Some examples cited by the School Nutrition Association:

• In National City, California, the School Board passed a resolution proclaiming the week National School Lunch Week. Legislators, board members, and parent groups have been invited to "do" lunch with the district's students. Materials include posters, bookmarks, and a parent newsletter.

• In Adams County, Colorado, every day has a themed menu with items such as "Rift Valley Baked Chicken" and "Call of the Wild Carrot Sticks." The district also will have special giveaways for parents and children and Take Your Family to Lunch Day.

• In Polk County, Florida, the Discovery Academy will become wild: tiki huts will cover each terminal at the end of the lunch line, vines and animals of every description will adorn the walls, a homemade full-sized Jeep will be on hand, and special surprises will be given away to students. Child nutrition staff will be sporting animal aprons and headdresses. A skit on the importance of good nutrition will be presented, and students will walk under a life-sized giraffe to receive their lunch.[14]

Now we just have to make sure that all the foods that are offered to kids in school are extremely nutritious. If we are going to get them excited about food, we had better make sure it is the right kind of food.

The information is out there. There is research to back it up. We must do what our students need and give them the competitive edge. Higher test scores, better attendance, and reduction of behavioral problems: it's not just an administrator's dream; it can be an administrative reality.

REFERENCES

1. *Super Size Me* [DVD]. 2004. New York: Kathbur Pictures, Inc.

2. School Nutrition Association. Program history and data. Retrieved Jan 2006, from www.schoolnutrition.org/Index.aspx?id=71.

3. Nutritional Resource Foundation. Roadmap to Healthy Foods in Schools. Manitowoc, WI, 2004.

4. Romano L. Improvement appears slight since No Child Left Behind. *Washington Post*, Oct 20, 2005. Retrieved Jan 2006, from www.nutritionalresourcefoundation. org/articles/school/ ?p=3#more-3.

5. School Nutrition Association. SNA overview. Retrieved Jan 2006 from www. schoolnutrition.org/Index.aspx?id=1307.

6. Skolmowski J. AFHK reports show link between nutrition and academic achievement. Nov 4, 2004. www.schoolnutrition .org/Index.aspx?id=883 Retrieved Nov 2005.

7. Hoffer A. *Dr. Hoffer's ABC of Natural Nutrition for Children.* Ontario, Canada: Quarry Press, 1999, 89.

8. Hersey J. *Healthier Food for Busy People: 20 Little Rules to Help You Navigate the Supermarket.* Alexandria, VA: Pear Tree Press, undated.

9. Smith L. *Feed Your Kids Right: Dr. Smith's Program for Your Child's Total Health.* New York: Mc-Graw Hill, 1979, 222, 227.

10. SNA releases new report on school nutrition market trends. Retrieved November 2005, from http://www.schoolnutrition.org /Index. aspx?id=931.

11. Kretsch M. Helping school kids reach nutritional excellence. 2005. Retrieved Jan 2006, from www.ars.usda.gov/is /AR/archive/oct05/form1005.pdf.

12. Feingold Association of the United States. *Behavior, Learning and Health: The Dietary Connection.* Atlanta, GA, 2003.

13. Anderson K. Montana school cleans up the playground, then the food. Pure Facts, Sept 2004, 2.

14. School Nutrition Association. School lunch: Something to get wild about. Retrieved Jan 2006, from www.schoolnutrition.org /Index.aspx?id=944.

15. Action for Healthy Kids. The learning connection: the value of improving nutrition and physical activity in our schools. Sept 23, 2004. Retrieved from www.actionforhealthykids. org/pdf/LC _Color_120204_final.pdf.

16. *Impact of Fresh, Healthy Foods on Learning and Behavior* [DVD]. Manitowoc, WI: Natural Ovens Bakery, 2004.

17. Evers C. *How to Teach Nutrition to Kids.* Portland, OR: Carrot Press, 1995.

18. *Eat, Exercise, Excel.* [VHS] Wichita, KS: The Center for the Improvement of Human Functioning, 2004.

TREATING CHILDREN WITH HYPERACTIVE SYNDROME: A MEMOIR

by M. C. Giammatteo PhD, EdD

I had a joint practice with offices in Oregon and Washington during the late '60s and early '70s. Our treatment for alcoholics was a simple use of all B-complex vitamins and ascorbic acid (vitamin C). We noticed that patients reacted within weeks in a more positive manner and were focused on problem solving rather than problem blaming, fixing situations rather than fixing blame. We began to teach others the protocol as well as to broaden the scope to self-destructive behaviors and techniques for cures.

The Alcoholics Anonymous (AA) people did not seem to feel we were on the right track, but the Oregon Council on Alcohol and Drug Treatment did. They wrote one complete newsletter about our theories in their 1967 mental health newsletter, and asked my partner and me to give a series of continuing education workshops on "Self-Defeating and Self-Destructive Behaviors" to physicians, psychologists, social workers, and registered nurses. The workshops were taught in major hospitals in Oregon, Alaska, Washington, California, and Hawaii for about six or seven years. A number of participants asked if we worked with children of alcoholics and we responded indicating we were using the same techniques slightly modified for our third- through sixth-grade clients. We also worked with a family treatment model.

Treatment Model

Our model for children was simple and easy to use. The children were administered 1,500–3,000 milligrams (mg) of vitamin B3 (niacin) daily for 90 days along with about 5,000 mg of ascorbic acid (vitamin C) daily, along with one clove of garlic in the vegetable meal recommended per day.

We went by weight and feedback from the child and the parents to adjust the dosage of the vitamin B3 and vitamin C. Usually the flushing experience (from the niacin) and the slight potential for diarrhea (form the vitamin C) were the only problems our patients reported. We also had the parents give a cup of coffee to the child before their first visit. We suggested a Saturday morning and asked them to notice the behavior of the child. When parents reported that the child seemed to calm down and was more focused, we knew we had a child that was having problems with hyperactivity behaviors. This protocol worked up to about age 12 for boys.

The children were asked also to start on an exercise program with a small trampoline and perceptual training skills.

The parents were given eating behavior handouts, which asked the child to discuss the color, size, and smell of the food being eaten, and to place their fork and spoon down after each bite before chewing. Green leafy vegetables and fruits were recommended and added sugars were to be cut from their diets for the next three months. Yogurt, kale, and spinach, along with bran cereals, were recommended for their food sources and were also to be recorded in their food diary kept with the parents.

The children were asked to list and talk out the things that caused them stress. They also kept a journal with words and pictures telling about their self-reported changes. They shared these journal entries with me once every week for month one, every other week for month two, and one last time about three weeks before their last or next to last visit depending on feedback and progress. The program took about 90 days and included seven to nine visits.

Each visit took place in my 20-by-22-foot office, which had three mirrors lining one wall. One mirror was placed at the far right, one centered, and one to the far left. The child was asked to face mirror one (far right) and tell what he or she wished to change about their behavior, thinking, and feeling . . . then with each of the six or seven steps over to mirror two, the child would tell one small change required to meet with the desired change. With

From the J Orthomolecular Med 2006;21(3):170–173.

each of the remaining six steps over to the third mirror (far left), the child focused on the positive feelings resulting from the changed attitude and behavior. Our motto was, Do that which is justified rather than justifying that which you do.

The children were asked to have a parent call me every month or so for any signs or concerns. The parents were sent to local colleges to take courses in parenting if we thought it was a major part of the problem. We also asked the child or parent to tell us of any new stressors that developed, which we and would then discuss during our visits. These included:

• Physical stressors: Living conditions, broken bones, etc.

• Nutritional stressors: Poor eating habits and a high sugar intake.

• Social stressors: Challenges and losses such as healthy child to sick, smart kid to slowest, a geographical move to a new district, school, or state; parental divorce; value losses; belief losses; organizational/environmental stressors in the classroom (type of lighting, noise level, structured seating vs. open seating arrangements, etc).

• Self-talk stressors: Negative thoughts and self-talk.

Case Study: Robert

After a psychiatrist met with seven-year-old Robert, his parents were told the child would require institutionalization. The special education people where he resided were making no headway with the child. His younger brother manifested none of the behavioral and learning problems that Robert exhibited. The parents had tried several forms of treatment in the time between Robert's fourth and seventh birthdays. A graduate student in psychology working in the district had been made aware of the treatment format I used at the clinic. She met with the parents explaining some of my techniques.

Robert's parents scheduled an appointment. On his first visit, Robert oriented almost immediately to what we were doing and when I placed my hands under his, looked him in the eyes, and asked, Are you ready? he nodded. We threw him a beanbag and he said his name. This was done each time as he caught the beanbag. We then had him spell each letter of his name timed to the catching of the beanbag. By the end of the first session, Robert was taken to the other room where his parents were being given the nutritional and food information required. Robert asked the nurse if he could spell his name. We used the beanbag technique and, when he spelled his name, the mother was excited. The father, an engineer, saw the demonstration as a weird non-scientific approach, and when he was told about the vitamin therapy along with the food intake concepts he balked at additional treatment. The mother said he had filed for divorce two months prior to our first visit with Robert. Nevertheless, Robert began the vitamin therapy under our control the first visit. We started him out with 1,500 mg of vitamin B3 and 5,000 mg of vitamin C, while a staff member watched him for the next half of an hour. During that time a staff member also made suggestions for exercise, home activities, and meals to both parents. The clients were told the child could call me at home if they felt uncertain or had treatment questions. Robert responded with "neat."

Each visit thereafter we would introduce more stress into his activities until he was doing many things approaching the low end of the normal range. His visual acuity changed so that his myopia was now also opening up and we used near- and far-point accommodation exercises, which are more or less standard in developmental optometry.

On Robert's second visit, he reported that he felt like he could jump out of his skin and that he wanted to say so much . . . would we listen? He was then given 2,000 mg of vitamin B3 daily, along with the same dosage of vitamin C and the one clove of garlic per day at mealtime. He had a sense of humor and wanted to know if he would turn green from all that green stuff. We had several sessions with the mother and began to wonder why such a diagnosis was given to their child. She reported that her son was always upset at mealtimes and was fearful of not being perfect, and that he started to get clumsy by age three to such an extent that the father thought he was retarded. It seemed obvious that by association Robert had learned to be a behavior "problem." He did, however, present all the signs of the hyperactive child: he was unable to really focus on tasks or to socialize; he was disruptive in class and often would get up and move quickly from the front of the room to the back. When put in a special education classroom, his behavior continued to be disruptive. The district wanted the consulting psychiatrist to do a final analysis since the educators and the father had reached their wits' end.

On our third meeting, Robert was reporting as was the special education department that he was calming down and participating in the discussions with the other children. The nurse got Robert's mother to begin volunteering with children with similar presenting problems, and she became an advocate for this type of program. When her divorce was final, she also volunteered in another district.

By the remaining sessions, all outside sources reported the outstanding turnaround that Robert had made. After a year of educative and skills-training sessions without the vitamin approach, Robert's mother relocated to Hawaii. Nine years later, we found that Robert had entered the University of Hawaii and was majoring in biology. A number of years later, while in Hawaii for a seminar, a phone call to my room brought me up to date on Robert: he was completing his requirements for a medical degree.

CONCLUSION

As in Robert's case, at the end of 90 days using the above protocol, we had children who were able to give up medications they had been taking formerly. Teacher reports were indicative of positive observable behavior changes. Parents also were advised to maintain the vitamin portion of treatment after a 30-day waiting period because my colleague and I felt that it played an important role in bringing about the positive and observable changes.

The majority of the physicians and medical support in our community understood what we were attempting to do and would ask questions about the treatment model from time to time. The medical personnel at a local level included one orthomolecular psychiatrist and several family practice clinics. They were all supportive and referred children patients and alcoholic patients to us at a rate that kept our offices fully booked. Overall, we had positive results in our local community. When the concepts were presented at our medical association meeting in Oregon, the people enjoyed the input but most found reasons why that protocol would not work in their setting. They felt people wanted a "pill" approach or a prescription.

RADIATION SICKNESS

LARGE AREAS OF THE WORLD are becoming exposed to radioactive pollution from nuclear reactors, plutonium disposal, and uranium mining. Contamination by catastrophic nuclear accidents at Chernobyl in 1986 and Fukushima in 2011 is of worldwide concern. However, there is good news.

Workers with severe radiation exposure at the Fukushima nuclear plant had major reduction in cancer risk when supplemented with vitamin C and other antioxidative nutrients. Sixteen men, ages 32 to 59, worked five to six weeks in a radiation contaminated area, collecting contaminated water, measuring radiation levels, operating heavy machinery, and removing debris. Blood samples were obtained to measure whole blood counts and blood chemistry, plasma levels of free DNA, and 47 cancer related gene expressions. Four workers who took intravenous vitamin C (25,000 mg) therapy before they went in, and continuously took antioxidative supplements during the working period, had no significant change in both free DNA and overall cancer risk. Three workers who did not have preventive intravenous vitamin C had an increase in calculated cancer risk. After two months of intervention with intravenous vitamin C and oral antioxidative nutritional supplements, free DNA returned to normal level and cancer risk score was significantly decreased (Yanagisawa, www.doctor yourself.com/Radiation_VitC.pptx.pdf).

This important clinical demonstration confirms research done nearly 20 years ago showing that pretreatment with vitamin C, by oral intake or injection, increased sperm head survival after the injection of radioactive iodine-131 in mice (Narra, *J Nucl Med* 1993). Oral intake of alpha-lipoic acid and vitamin E reduced urinary radioactivity and oxidative stress in irradiated children in Chernobyl (Korkina, *Biochem Soc Trans* 1993). Furthermore, there have been numerous scientific studies about the radioprotective effects of other vitamins, minerals, and antioxidative nutrients, as discussed in this chapter.

—ATSUO YANAGISAWA

TERMS OF RADIATION SICKNESS

ANTIOXIDANT. A molecule that donates electrons to render free radicals harmless.

APOPTOSIS. Cell death.

BIOLOGICAL HALF-LIFE. Time required for one-half of a given amount of a radioactive substance to disintegrate.

DEOXYRIBONUCLEIC ACID (DNA). A complex protein within cells that carries genetic information.

EXTERNAL RADIATION. Exposure to radiation that stops when you are no longer near the source.

FREE RADICAL. An unstable molecule that is damaging to the organs and tissues of the body.

GRAY. A measure of radiation exposure. Specifically, the absorption of one joule of ionizing radiation by one kilogram of matter.

INTERNAL RADIATION. Radionuclide particles that get deposited in the body by inhalation, ingestion, or skin contact.

IODINE-131. A cancer-causing radioactive form of iodine and a principal element released from nuclear reactor accidents.

IONIZING RADIATION. A form of radiation made up of highly unstable atoms that release an energy that is strong enough to dislodge electrons in cells of living tissue and to damage or kill that tissue.

RADIATION SICKNESS. Symptoms and illness resulting from excessive exposure to ionizing radiation. Severity of symptoms may range from nausea, bleeding, and vomiting to delayed medical problems such as cancer and genetic mutations; the bone marrow, gastrointestinal tract, and reproductive tract are especially sensitive to radiation injury.

RADIONUCLIDE. A radioactive particle of an unstable atom that gives off energy.

FUKUSHIMA RADIATION RELEASE IS WORSE THAN YOU HAVE BEEN TOLD: WHAT YOU CAN DO TO PROTECT YOURSELF

by Steve Hickey, PhD, Atsuo Yanagisawa, MD, PhD, Andrew W. Saul, PhD, Gert E. Schuitemaker, PhD, and Damien Downing, MBBS, MSB

In the fall of 2011, the Japanese College of Intravenous Therapy (JCIT) presented a study that Fukushima workers had abnormality gene expression, which may be avoided using dietary antioxidants, especially vitamin C. The data was presented in Japan, Taiwan, and Korea. The JCIT sent letters to the government urging the government to tell the people how they may protect themselves from radiation. To date, the recommendation has been ignored by the Japanese government and the Tokyo Electric Power Company (TEPCO).

Linus Pauling gained the Nobel Peace Prize in part based on his calculations of the number of deaths from nuclear weapons fallout.[1] He was supported by physicist and father of the Soviet bomb Andrei Sakharov, who also later received the Nobel Prize for Peace.[2] These and other scientists estimated that there would be an extra 10,000 deaths worldwide for each megaton nuclear test in the atmosphere. A nuclear reactor can contain much more radioactive material than a nuclear weapon. Fukushima had six reactors, plus stored additional radioactive material and nuclear waste.

How Radiation Damages Cells

Ionizing radiation acts to damage living tissue by forming free radicals. Essentially, electrons are ripped from molecules. Removing an electron from an atom or molecule turns it into an ion, hence the term *ionizing radiation*. X-rays, gamma rays, and alpha and beta radiation are all ionizing. Most of the damage occurs from ionizing radiation generating free radicals in water, as water molecules are by far the most abundant in the body. While avoiding unnecessary exposure to ionizing radiation is clearly preferable, people affected by Fukushima do not have the luxury of avoiding contamination.

Antioxidants: Free-Radical Scavengers

Free-radical scavengers, as the name suggests, mop up the damaging radicals produced by radiation. The more common term for free radical scavenger is antioxidant. Antioxidants replace the electrons stripped from molecules by ionizing radiation. Antioxidants have long been used in the treatment of radiation poisoning.[3–7] Most of the harm from ionizing radiation occurs from free radical damage that may be quenched by the free electrons antioxidants provide. Fortunately, safe antioxidants are widely available as nutritional supplements. Vitamin C is the prime example.

Why Vitamin C?

Vitamin C is of particular importance and should be included at high intakes for anyone trying to minimize radiation poisoning. High dose vitamin C provides continual antioxidant flow through the body. It is absorbed from the gut and helps to replenish the other antioxidants. When it is used up, it is excreted in the urine. Importantly, it can chelate (grab onto) radioactive heavy metal atoms and help eliminate them from the body. Large dynamic flow doses of vitamin C (about 3,000 milligrams [mg], taken four times a day, for a total of 12,000 mg) would exemplify antioxidant treatment. Higher doses have been used by Dr. Atsuo Yanagisawa and colleagues.[8,9]

Shortly after the disaster, Dr. Damien Downing described how supplements can help protect against radioactive fallout.[10] The *Orthomolecular Medicine News Service* issued an update on the response to Fukushima in Japan.[11] Recently, Dr. Gert Schuitemaker has provided a review of vitamin C as a radio-protectant for Fukushima contamination.[12] [Editor's note: These articles are among those that follow.]

People living in the areas affected by radioactive contamination can take antioxidant supplements, especially high doses of vitamin C, to counteract the negative consequences of long-term low dose radiation exposure, as well as to protect the health of coming generations.[12,13] People who have a possible internal or external radiation exposure should take antioxidant supplements to maintain an optimal antioxidant reserve. Because of the enormous size and oceanic spread of Fukushima contamination, this literally applies to everyone.

REFERENCES

1. The Nobel Foundation. Linus Pauling–facts: Nobel Peace Prize 1962, biography. Available at: www.nobelprize.org/nobel _prizes/peace/laureates/1962/pauling-facts.html.

2. The Nobel Foundation. Andrei Sakharov–facts: Nobel Peace Prize 1975, biography. Available at: www.nobelprize.org/nobel _prizes/peace/laureates/1975/sakharov-facts.html.

3. Brown SL, Kolozsvary A, Liu J, et al. Antioxidant diet supplementation starting 24 hours after exposure reduces radiation lethality. *Radiat Res* 2010;173:462–468.

4. Zueva NA, Metelitsa LA, Kovalenko AN, et al. Immunomodulating effect of berlithione in clean-up workers of the Chernobyl nuclear plant accident [Article in Russian]. *Lik Sprava* 2002;1:24–26.

5. Yamamoto T, Kinoshita M, et al. Pretreatment with ascorbic acid prevents lethal gastrointestinal syndrome in mice receiving a massive amount of radiation. *J Radiat Res* (Tokyo) 2010;51(2):145–156.

6. Gaby A. Intravenous nutrient therapy: the "Myers' Cocktail." *Alt Med Rev* 2002;7(5):389,403.

7. Narra VR, Howell RW, Sastry KS, et al. Vitamin C as a radioprotector against iodine-131 in vivo. *J Nucl Med* 1993;34(4):637–640.

8. Yanagisawa A. Orthomolecular approaches against radiation exposure. Presentation Orthomolecular Medicine Today Conference, Toronto, 2011. Available at: www.doctoryourself .com/Radiation_VitC.pptx.pdf.

9. Green MH, Lowe JE, et al. Effect of diet and vitamin C on DNA strand breakage in freshly-isolated human white blood cells. *Mutat Res* 1994;316(2):91–102.

10. Downing D. Radioactive fallout: can nutritional supplements help? A personal viewpoint. *OMNS*, May 10, 2011. Available at: www.orthomolecular.org/resources/omns/v07n04.shtml.

11. Saul AW (ed.). Vitamin C prevents radiation damage, nutritional medicine in Japan. *OMNS*, Feb 1, 2012. Available at: http://orthomolecular.org/resources/omns/v08n06.shtml.

12. Schuitemaker GE. Vitamin C as protection against radiation exposure. *J Orthomolecular Med* 2011;26(3):141–145.

13. Yanagisawa A, Uwabu M, Burkson BE, et al. Environmental radioactivity and health. Official JCIT Statement, March 29, 2011. Available at: http://media.iv-therapy.jp/wp-content/uploads /2012/05/Statement.pdf.

VITAMIN C IS SCIENTIFICALLY PROVEN TO PROTECT FUKUSHIMA VICTIMS FROM RADIATION EFFECTS

People have been misinformed about the tragedy at Fukushima and its consequences. There is a continuing cover-up, the reactors have not been stabilized, and radiation continues to be released. The Japanese College of Intravenous Therapy (JCIT) has recently released a video for people wishing to learn more about how to protect themselves from contamination by taking large doses of vitamin C.

- Part 1: www.youtube.com/watch?v=Rbm_MH3nSdM

- Part 2: www.youtube.com/watch?v=j4cyzts3lMo

- Part 3: www.youtube.com/watch?v=ZYiRo2Oucfo

- Part 4: www.youtube.com/watch?v=51Ie8FuuYJw

All four parts of the video are also available here http://firstlaw.wordpress.com. Readers may link to, embed in their web pages, and make copies of the video for free distribution.

Steven Carter, director of the International Society for Orthomolecular Medicine, writes, "The International Society for Orthomolecular Medicine is pleased to have participated in the making of this important DVD on the protective effects of intravenous vitamin C on radiation exposure from the Fukushima nuclear plant in March 2011. We are in full support of the valuable work of Dr. Yanagisawa and his colleagues, and we very much appreciate the commitment of Mr. Daisuke Shibata, who has made it possible for the free distribution of the video around the world. May this orthomolecular message raise awareness and foster improvement in the treatment of radiation exposure."

Excerpted from the *Orthomolecular Medicine News Service*, May 14, 2012.

VITAMIN C CAN PREVENT RADIATION DAMAGE: RESULTS FROM FUKUSHIMA NUCLEAR POWER PLANT WORKERS

by Atsuo Yanagisawa, MD, PhD

On March 11, 2011, there was a terrible earthquake and tsunami in Japan. The earthquake and tsunami killed more than 15,000 people and nearly 3,000 people are still missing. One unfortunate consequence of these events has been the environmental disaster caused by the release of radiation from the Fukushima nuclear power plant. This has deeply troubled people around the world. We have to consider the effects of this radiation exposure on our air, water, and contaminated food chain. From the experiences of Chernobyl disaster, radiation exposure affects our health and causes many diseases including cancer, heart disease, neurological disorders, birth defects, allergic disorders, and other serious health problems.

Damage from External Sources of Radiation

The DNA in our cells is injured by radioactivity through two routes: a direct route and an indirect route. Radiation can strike the DNA molecule directly and damage it; this is the direct route. Most people believe that the direct route is the only cause of radiation damage on DNA. No! The direct route causes only 20 percent of all injury from radiation. So, what is the other 80 percent caused by? The other 80 percent of radiation injury is caused by the indirect route. Radiation hits and ionizes water molecules, producing free radicals that react and damage DNA molecules. This is a key point and very important part: indirect radiation injury via free radicals is the main cause of DNA damage, and this is the 80 percent. These mechanisms are widely known and are even written about in the textbook of medical radiology and medical physics as a common knowledge. So now, you can imagine that why radiation-induced free radicals can be neutralized by antioxidative nutrients including vitamin C.

There are many scientific studies demonstrating the protective effects of vitamin C on radiation-induced cellular injury. The paper, "Pretreatment with ascorbic acid prevents lethal gastrointestinal syndrome in mice receiving a massive amount of radiation" was published March 2010, one year before the Fukushima accident, and was written by the National Defense Medical College and Ground Self-Defense Force in Japan. Ten years earlier, in 1999, a nuclear power plant accident occurred in Japan. Nuclear power plant workers who were exposed to high doses of radiation developed severe bone marrow failure and thereafter underwent stem cell transplantation. However, they developed severe gastrointestinal damage with diarrhea and bleeding (known as gastrointestinal syndrome, or GIS), and eventually died from multiple organ failure. The authors thought that, if a radiation accident unfortunately occurred, prevention of radiation-induced damage, in particular GIS, is of vital importance to the rescue team.

Mice could survive less than 8 gray (Gy) whole body irradiation (WBI). However, mice receiving 8 Gy or more all died at 10 to 24 days, because of radiation-induced severe GIS. Bone marrow transplantation (BMT) 24 hours after radiation can rescue mice receiving 12 Gy or less. However, no mice receiving 14 Gy survived.

Then, 150 milligrams (mg) of vitamin C per kilogram (kg) of body weight daily was orally administered for 3 days, and then the mice received 14 Gy of irradiation. This dose of vitamin C is equivalent to giving 9,000 mg of vitamin C to a man weighing 60 kg (132 lbs). Pretreatment with vitamin C markedly improved radiation-induced gastrointestinal damage, thereby rescuing mice receiving 14 Gy in combination with BMT.

The authors from the National Defense Medical College and Ground Self-Defense Force in Japan commented in this article: "When we undertake the rescue of victims from a radiation-contaminated

---

Lecture presented at the Algerian Society for Nutrition and Orthomolecular Medicine, Algiers, Algeria, January 26, 2013.

area just after a radiation accident or terrorism, it is important for the rescue team to promptly take vitamin C orally." On March 13, 2011, the rescue team of National Self-Defense Force took vitamin C when they were in the Fukushima nuclear power plant. However, the government and the Tokyo Electric Power Company (TEPCO) never gave vitamin C to the people working in the Fukushima nuclear power plant until today.

Damage from Internal Sources of Radiation

We need to also consider internal radiation. Internal radiation is caused by aspiration or ingestion of radionuclide particles via air or food contamination. In 1993, Narra and others showed the effect of vitamin C on internal radiation injury in the animal experiment. Intratesticular injection of iodine-131 (radioactive isotopes of iodine) decreased sperm survival in mice and is known as a model of internal radiation injury. Pretreatment of intratesticular injection of vitamin C or oral intake of vitamin C increased sperm survival after the injection of iodine-131 in mice. Thus, vitamin C is a radio-protector when radionuclides are incorporated in the body and the dose is delivered frequently soon after exposure.

In 1994, Green and colleagues investigated the effect of vitamin C on radiation damage using human blood. Blood samples were taken before and one hour after breakfast with oral ingestion of 35 mg of vitamin C per kg of body weight. This dose is equivalent to a 132-pound man taking only 2,000 mg of vitamin C. Samples were immediately irradiated using a cobalt-60 hotspot, and DNA damage was measured using the comet assay (a standard technique for evaluating DNA damage and repair). As a result, vitamin C ingestion showed a significant reduction in DNA damage due to irradiation and its peak effect was four hours after ingestion. Thus, oral intake of vitamin C can prevent radiation-induced DNA damage in humans. According to the numerous scientific research papers, radiation injury can be protected by not only vitamin C but other antioxidative nutrition as well.

Protective Supplement Protocol

On March 29, 2011, 17 days after the accident, seven physicians and I from the Japanese College of Intravenous Therapy (JCIT), an international consortium of 420 physicians, 22 dentists, and 12 veterinarians, formed a working group and issued an official statement on "Environmental Radioactivity and Health." In it we state,

It is our strongest recommendation that those living in the affected areas regularly take antioxidant supplements such as vitamin C to counteract the negative consequences of long-term low dose radiation exposure as well as to pro-

IN BRIEF

Yamamoto T, et al. Pretreatment with ascorbic acid prevents lethal gastrointestinal syndrome in mice receiving a massive amount of radiation (*J Radiation Res* 2010;51(2):145–156). While bone marrow or stem cell transplantation can rescue bone marrow aplasia [when the bone marrow doesn't make enough new blood cells] in patients accidentally exposed to a lethal radiation dose, radiation-induced irreversible gastrointestinal damage (GI syndrome) is fatal. We investigated the effects of ascorbic acid on radiation-induced GI syndrome in mice. Ascorbic acid (150 mg/kg/day) was orally administered to mice for three days, and then the mice underwent whole body irradiation (WBI). Bone marrow transplantation (BMT) 24 hours after irradiation rescued mice receiving a WBI dose of less than 12 gray (Gy). No mice receiving 14 Gy-WBI survived, because of radiation-induced GI syndrome, even if they received BMT. However, pretreatment with ascorbic acid significantly suppressed radiation-induced DNA damage in the crypt cells and prevented denudation of intestinal mucosa; therefore, ascorbic acid in combination with BMT rescued mice after 14 Gy-WBI. DNA microarray analysis demonstrated that irradiation up-regulated [increased] expressions of apoptosis-related genes in the small intestine, including those related to the caspase-9-mediated intrinsic pathway as well as the caspase-8-mediated extrinsic pathway, and down-regulated [decreased] expressions of these genes in ascorbic acid-pretreated mice. Thus, pretreatment with ascorbic acid may effectively prevent radiation-induced GI syndrome.

tect the health of coming generations. It is further recommended that those working in environments that require exposure to high concentrations of radiation should immediately undergo high dose intravenous vitamin C therapy along with a vigorous antioxidant supplementation program.

Our recommendations were as follows:

Recommendation #1

If environmental radioactivity becomes twofold higher than usual, women of childbearing age should take antioxidant supplements to keep *optimal* antioxidative reserve.

- Vitamin C: 1,000–2,000 mg, 3–4 times daily, or liposomal vitamin C (highly absorbable vitamin C) 1,000 mg, 2 times daily
- Alpha-lipoic acid: 100–200 mg, 2 times daily
- Selenium: 50–200 micrograms (mcg), 2 times daily
- Vitamin E: 100–200 mg, 2 times daily
- Other essential vitamins and minerals

Recommendation #2

If environmental radioactivity levels becomes more than fivefold higher than usual, people of all ages should take antioxidant supplements to keep *maximum* antioxidative reserve.

- Vitamin C: 2,000–3,000 mg, 3–4 times daily, or liposomal vitamin C 1,000 mg, 2 times daily
- Alpha-lipoic acid: 300 mg, 2 times daily
- Selenium: 200 mcg, 2 times daily
- Vitamin E: 200 mg, 2 times daily
- Other essential vitamins and minerals

Recommendation #3

The following is our recommendation for people who work at radiation-contaminated areas in the Fukushima nuclear plant. It consists of intravenous (IV) vitamin C to be taken before and after work along with daily oral antioxidant supplements.

- Intravenous vitamin C: 25,000 mg as part of a Myers' cocktail (a magnesium, calcium, and B-vitamin mixture), administered before and after exposure

- Liposomal vitamin C: 2,000 mg, 3 times daily
- Alpha-lipoic acid: 300 mg, 2 times daily
- Selenium: 200 mcg, 2 times daily
- Vitamin E: 200 mg, 2 times daily
- Other essential vitamins and minerals

We sent this statement and its recommendations to the government, TEPCO, congressmen, and media of TV news, journals, magazines, and newspapers. However, they did not respond. Not a word. Nothing! The statement was ignored. I regret to say that I am deeply disappointed in our government.

Effect of Vitamin C in Fukushima Nuclear Plant Workers: A Pilot Study

In 2011, we examined cancer-related gene expression in 16 men who had worked at severe radiation environment at Fukushima nuclear plant. We also confirmed the improvement of cancer risk score by the supplementation of vitamin C and other antioxidant nutrition. This study was not supported by the government nor by TEPCO.

The study was approved by the ethical committee of the JCIT. Study subjects were 16 men, ranging in age from 32 to 59, who worked five to six weeks at the radiation-contaminated area of Fukushima nuclear power plant after March 12, 2011. All subjects were temporary workers of a sub-subcontractor company of TEPCO. Work operations at the contaminated area were collecting contaminated water, measuring radiation level in the plant area, removing debris, and operating heavy machinery.

Blood samples were obtained every few days after the end of the working period. In four workers, blood was obtained before and after the working period. We measured 1) whole blood counts and blood chemistry, 2) plasma levels of free DNA, 3) 47 cancer-related gene expressions, and 4) then calculated the worker's cancer risk score. An increase in plasma levels of free DNA suggests frequent cellular damage or apoptosis. Cancer patients tend to show an increase in free DNA and we defined 25 nanograms per milliliter (ng/mL) as a cutoff value of normal. The cancer risk score was calculated using an equation formed by the logistic analysis from the value of 47 cancer-related gene expressions. The score tends to increase in cancer patients and we defined the score of 38 as a cutoff value of normal.

The results: Plasma-free DNA was increased in two of twelve workers, and cancer risk score was increased in three of twelve workers. So, five of twelve workers showed abnormal values after the two to three months working period at the nuclear power plant. We proceeded to intervene in those five workers. Our interventions included 25,000 mg of intravenous (IV) vitamin C and the oral supplements listed in Recommendation #3 above. The five workers were treated with IV vitamin C twice a month and oral antioxidant supplements for two months. After which free DNA was decreased to normal levels after two months of intervention. Surprisingly, cancer risk scores of all five workers were significantly decreased. The number was small but significant.

In general, such scores never change during such short period, even in cancer patients and normal healthy subjects. In one worker, the value of cancer risk score did not returned to the normal value. Why? This worker returned to Fukushima and worked again during that two-month period. So this may be the reason why his cancer risk score did not return to normal levels. Finally, his score returned to normal after four months of intervention.

In four workers, we studied the effect of IV vitamin C and antioxidant nutrition before and after five to six weeks of nuclear plant work at Fukushima. The workers were given a one-time IV of vitamin C (25,000 mg) therapy before they went to Fukushima and continuously took oral antioxidant supplements during the working period. No significant change was seen in both values of free DNA and cancer risk score. The number was small but they did not show any risk of cancer on DNA.

To recap:

1. We evaluated the effects of radiation exposure on cancer-related gene expression in 16 men who worked five to six weeks at the radiation contaminated area of Fukushima nuclear power plant.

2. After working, plasma free DNA was increased in two of twelve workers, and cancer risk score was increased in three. After the two-month intervention with intravenous vitamin C and oral antioxidant supplements, free DNA returned to normal level and cancer risk score was significantly decreased.

3. No significant change was seen in four workers who took IV vitamin C before working and continuous intake of antioxidant supplements during the working period.

4. Increase in cancer risk by radiation exposure can be protected by antioxidant nutritional intervention. Fukushima workers in the radiation-contaminated area should take antioxidant nutrition therapy immediately.

CONCLUSION

The JCIT Working Group had concluded that "Only vitamin C and other nutritious antioxidant supplements can save the people's lives from radiation injury."

The biggest concern today is the impact of radioactivity on people's health on planet Earth, especially, the health of women and children, and the next generations. Orthomolecular nutritional medicine is the way to protect our health from radiation.

Let us make this world a safer and more peaceful place.

VITAMIN C AS PROTECTION AGAINST RADIATION EXPOSURE
by Gert E. Schuitemaker, PhD

In 2011, a 9.0-magnitude earthquake and a subsequent 30-foot high tsunami wave struck Japan. It led to a serious nuclear accident at the Fukushima nuclear power plant (NPP) with the release of a substantial amount of radiation. Of primary concern was the protection against radioactive contamination of the population, of the rescue workers, and of the people trying to control the nuclear disaster in locales and in areas surrounding the nuclear power plant.

The mechanistic measures taken by the authorities included evacuation of the population, decontamination showers of clothing, and the use of protective clothing for workers at the nuclear site. All of these measures are aimed to minimize contamination. Except for potassium iodide tablets that protect the thyroid gland against radioactive isotopes of iodine (i.e., iodine-131), there has been little implementation of orthomolecular protection methods by the Japanese authorities.

This article highlights the opinions of Dr. Atsuo Yanagisawa that were presented at the 40th Orthomolecular Medicine Today Conference in Toronto, April 29, 2011, to support the use of oral and/or intravenous vitamin C (ascorbic acid), as well as other antioxidants, as internal protectants against radiation exposure.

Published Evidence

Studies with vitamin C, financed partially by the Japanese Ministry of Defense under the Special Research Program, demonstrate that vitamin C can limit the adverse effects of radiation exposure in mice.[1] In the main part of the study, mice were pretreated with 150 milligrams (mg) of vitamin C per kilogram (kg) of body weight daily for three days and then were exposed to 14 gray (Gy) of whole body radiation, followed by bone marrow transplant (BMT) at 24 hours post-radiation. There was a 42 percent survival in the mice pretreated with vitamin C prior to radiation compared to no survival if only provided with vitamin C post-radiation. Of note, when mice were pretreated with vitamin C, but not given BMT, none survived. The best results were obtained when vitamin C was given before radiation exposure and was then combined with BMT.

The results of this animal study suggest that patients and rescue workers should consider supplementing with vitamin C since accidental exposures to a lethal dose of radiation might be mitigated when combined with bone marrow or stem cell transplants. Vitamin C can significantly decrease DNA damage in the cells of the intestinal crypt (a gland located in the lining of the small intestine and colon), preventing damage to the intestinal mucosa. Radiation in the small intestine leads to the expression of genes involved in cell death (apoptosis), which is reduced by supplemental vitamin C.

The Japanese government became involved in this research due to a nuclear accident in 1999. People exposed to high doses of radiation developed severe bone marrow aplasia and required stem cell transplantation. These people developed severe intestinal damage with diarrhea and bleeding and subsequently died from multiple organ failure despite intensive supportive therapy. This severe gastrointestinal condition resulting from high doses of radiation is known as fatal gastrointestinal syndrome (GIS). It is also an unfortunate complication of abdominal radiation therapy in cancer patients.

There are currently no effective therapies against GIS due to extensive radiation exposure. Vitamin C might help to prevent or limit severe gastrointestinal damage, thereby preventing fatal GIS. Unfortunately, the rescue team members of the National Self-Defense Force did not get intravenous vitamin C or even vitamin C supplements when they were in the Fukushima nuclear power plant.[2]

From the *J Orthomolecular Med* 2011;26(3):144–145.

Additional Vitamin C Experiments

Dr. Venkat R. Narra and others demonstrated that vitamin C mitigates radiation-induced damage from tissue-incorporated radionuclide (i.e., iodine-131).[3] In this study, an experimental model of sperm cell development in mice was used since it closely resembles that of humans.[3] The experiment showed that vitamin C protected mice sperm cells that were previously injected with radioactive iodine. As a result of vitamin C, the 37 percent sperm survival dose (D37) increased by a factor of 2.2 compared with the D37 in animals receiving only the radionuclide. In a separate experiment, mice were placed on a vitamin C-enriched (1 percent by weight) diet five days prior to the administration of the radionuclide. The vitamin C-enriched diet was continued for seven days post-radionuclide. The vitamin C–enriched diet was found to have a similar therapeutic effect to that of injected vitamin C, which led the researchers to conclude that vitamin C may play an important role as a radio-protector against accidental or medical radiation exposures, especially when radionuclides are chronically incorporated in the body.

In another study, nucleated cells from freshly isolated whole blood taken from normal human subjects before and one hour after they had eaten a meal in combination with approximately 35 mg of vitamin C per kg of body weight were subjected to ionizing radiation (i.e., radioactive cobalt).[4] The addition of vitamin C led to significant reductions in DNA damage, with its therapeutic effects peaking four hours post-ingestion.

The vitamin C studies presented here suggest that it should be used to mitigate radiation damage following acute exposures, chronic exposures, and as prophylaxis against potential radiation exposures.

OFFICIAL STATEMENT TO THE JAPANESE GOVERNMENT

At the request of Dr. Yanagisawa, the Japanese College of Intravenous Therapy issued an official statement on March 29, 2011, directed toward the Japanese government: "It is our strongest recommendation that those living in the affected areas regularly take antioxidant supplements such as vitamin C to counteract the negative consequences of long-term low dose radiation exposure as well as to protect the health of coming generations. It is further recommended that those working in environments that require exposure to high-concentrations of radiation should immediately undergo high-dose intravenous vitamin C therapy along with a vigorous antioxidant supplementation program."

Key Role of Antioxidants

Radiation can damage DNA in two ways: 1) by directly ionizing (breaking) DNA molecules; and 2) indirectly by ionizing water in body cells, where free radicals are formed, which in turn damages DNA. There are scientific reports documenting the benefits of using a complement of several radio-protective antioxidant orthomolecules, which presumably mitigate DNA damage.

In one study, a combination of antioxidants (i.e., alpha-lipoic acid, vitamins C and E, selenium, N-

IN BRIEF

The nuclear accident in Fukushima, Japan, in March 2011, led to drastic mechanistic measures (e.g., evacuation, decontamination showers of clothing, and use of protective clothing by rescue workers) to protect the population against imminent and future radiation exposure. Besides mechanistic measures, no orthomolecular protection measures other than iodine supplementation were taken, although scientists from Japan's Ministry of Defense had demonstrated that oral vitamin C in mice protects against radiation injury. This article highlights the opinions of Dr. Atsuo Yanagisawa that were presented at the 40th Orthomolecular Medicine Today Conference in Toronto (April 29, 2011) to support the use of oral and/or intravenous vitamin C (ascorbic acid), as well as other antioxidants, as internal protectants against radiation exposure.

acetyl cysteine, and coenzyme Q10) improved the survival of mice following total-body irradiation.[5] The mice not given antioxidants were dead by day 16, but four of fourteen mice that were given antioxidants immediately after total-body irradiation were alive on day 16. When antioxidants were delayed by 24 hours post-exposure, there was a marked increase in survival, which resulted in fourteen of eighteen mice surviving at 30 days compared to none surviving when given a diet supplemented with antioxidants immediately after total-body irradiation. When administered 24 hours post-radiation, the antioxidant combination improved bone marrow cell survival and moderated lethality, yielding a radiation protection factor of approximately 1.18.

In another study, 600 mg per day of alpha-lipoic acid was taken orally by nine individuals who had been involved in the clean-up of the Chernobyl nuclear accident.[6] These individuals were given the alpha-lipoic acid 11 to 12 years following their exposure and only took the antioxidant daily for two months. The results demonstrated normalization of various immune parameters such as neutrophil phagocytic activity (a measure of white blood cells that fight disease), complement titer (a measure of antibody strength), and reaction of autorosette formation (a measure of immune responsiveness and adaptation).

CONCLUSION

An optimal antioxidant reserve, therefore, plays a key role in the protection against radiation-induced injury. The general population in locales and in areas surrounding nuclear power plants should protect themselves with daily antioxidant supplementation. Potassium iodide should also be included to saturate the thyroid. This will ensure that the thyroid absorbs less radioactive isotopes of iodine in cases of a radioactive disaster. Potassium iodide tablets during or immediately after a disaster is especially useful if an individual is iodine deficient.

See Appendix 4 "Radiation-Injury Protocol" for Dr. Yanagisawa's supplement recommendations for protecting against radiation-induced injury.

REFERENCES

1. Yamamoto T, Kinoshita M, Shinomiya N, et al. Pretreatment with ascorbic acid prevents lethal gastrointestinal syndrome in mice receiving a massive amount of radiation. *J Radiat Res* 2010; 51:145–156.

2. Yanagisawa A. Orthomolecular approaches against radiation exposure. 40th Orthomolecular Medicine Today Conference. Toronto, Ontario. April 29, 2011.

3. Narra VR, Howell RW, Sastry KSR, et al. Vitamin C as a radio-protector against iodine-131 invivo. *J Nucl Med* 1993;34:637–640.

4. Green MH, Lowe JE, Waugh AP, et al. Effect of diet and vitamin C on DNA strand breakage in freshly-isolated human white blood cells. *Mutat Res* 1994;316:91–102.

5. Brown SL, Kolozsvary A, Liu J, et al. Antioxidant diet supplementation starting 24 hours after exposure reduces radiation lethality. *Radiat Res* 2010;173:462–468.

6. Zueva NA, Metelitsa LA, Kovalenko AN, et al. Immunomodulating effect of berlithione in clean-up workers of the Chernobyl nuclear plant accident [in Russian]. *Lik Sprava* 2002;(1):24–26.

7. Gaby AR. Intravenous nutrient therapy: the "Myers' cocktail." *Altern Med Rev* 2002;7:389–403.

RADIOACTIVE FALLOUT: CAN NUTRITIONAL SUPPLEMENTS HELP?
by Damien Downing, MBBS, MSB

The Fukushima nuclear accident has already been described as "the largest accidental release of radiation we have ever seen,"[1] and it's not over yet. Already, radioactive plutonium, strontium, and iodine have reached the continental United States.

Should We Worry?

When the earthquake and tsunami hit northeast Japan on March 11, 2011, it disabled all the multiple safety mechanisms at the Fukushima nuclear power plant. Fires started in three of the six reactors, and 24 hours later a large hydrogen explosion caused the collapse of part of the structure. From then on, radioactive material would have been released to the atmosphere. This is reasonable to assume, despite the usual assurances from the operators, the Tokyo Electric Power Company (TEPCO), and the Japan Atomic Energy Agency. Six days later, after all, traces of radioactive material were detected in Washington State[2] and then right down to California. This material can only have reached the United States by the airborne route.

Fukushima is now off the media map, replaced by dramatic political events. Contrast this with the coverage that was given to the Chernobyl disaster. Perhaps at that time there was a sense that the destruction of a nuclear power plant in the Ukraine was a metaphor for the failure of the Soviet Union. But Fukushima is, or will eventually prove to be, a far worse disaster. It is one that will be underplayed. The world is committed to nuclear power, and we will not be shown its true dangers. Do not expect to be told the whole truth when reading reassuring statements from industry or governments. Fukushima is affecting us all.

Radioactive elements released from Fukushima include plutonium, strontium, cesium, and iodine. Ten days after the tsunami, Japanese scientists reported increased radioactive cesium and iodine (radioactive particles) in seawater offshore of Fukushima, and they rapidly reached levels "more than 1 million times higher than previously existed."[3] More serious radiation levels are likely in the United States when this polluted seawater reaches the west coast, which is estimated to take from 18 months to 3 years.

More Serious? Why? Because . . .

- There will be radioactive elements that are ingested or absorbed by people, animals, and plants.

- They will biomagnify, concentrating up the food chain, as do all pollutants.

- They won't go away; once inside us they will stay there.

There are two different kinds of radiation: external, when you are exposed to radiation sources around you (the Fukushima clean-up workers are currently getting a lot of that), but that stops when you are no longer near the source; and internal, when a source of radiation gets into your body and stays there. This is much more serious because you are constantly exposed for much longer. Former Russian agent Alexander Litvinenko was killed in London that way in 2006—by being given, probably swallowing in a beverage, some highly radioactive polonium. Traces of the same polonium were found on some airline seats, but nobody seems to have been harmed by sitting in them.

You may already have been exposed to (mostly) depleted uranium back in 2003. Despite official denials, it does seem to be true that increases in uranium were detected in Berkshire, England, nine days after the start of Shock and Awe (U.S. invasion of Iraq using an attack strategy to intimidate the enemy into surrender based on striking specific targets rather than all-out bombing).[4] To get there it must have traveled across the whole of the United States.

Excerpted from the *Orthomolecular Medicine News Service*, May 11, 2011.

By the time it reaches the continental United States the radiation from Fukushima will be very spread out, so individual doses will be very small. But they will be on top of the radiation to which we are all exposed already: from x-rays, from flying at 30,000 feet, from radon in the ground, and on top of all other exposures.

Epidemiologist Dr. Steven Wing makes the useful point that whether a dose of radiation is spread thickly across just a few thousand people, or much more thinly across tens of millions, around the same number of cancers will result. So although the increase in individual risk from Fukushima is likely to be tiny for any individual in the United States, it will still amount to a major public health problem. Case in point:

• The Chernobyl nuclear disaster certainly caused thousands of premature deaths in a sweep across northern Europe and may have caused more than a million deaths.[5] But Fukushima is worse in several ways.

• At Chernobyl there were only 180 tons of nuclear fuel on-site, whereas at Fukushima there are thousands of tons.

• Chernobyl is 250 miles from the nearest sea, but Fukushima is on the coast. Already the radiation released to sea from there is 10 to 100 times worse than Chernobyl.

• Chernobyl was sealed into a "sarcophagus," although too late to prevent some airborne release. Fukushima is and will likely continue releasing radiation into the sea for some time. Best case scenarios (from the nuclear industry, of course) are saying it will take nine months to shut the reactors down and seal them. Skeptics say that you truly cannot "seal" a reactor with concrete because the radioactive material will then go downward, into the soil and the water table, and end up in the sea anyway.

You may say, "Surely the government has this all in hand?" Well, the strange thing is that the Environmental Protection Agency (EPA) is set to revise its Protective Action Guides— the levels of radiation that it deems safe for us to be exposed to, from food, water, air, or soil. Some of the upper limits are rising more than 1,000-fold, into the "will

definitely give cancer to some people" zone. You can read more about this at www.collapsenet.com,[6] which also gives useful email addresses in case you want to express your views to the EPA. I know it looks like another one of "those" websites, but this is corroborated many times over elsewhere.

The European Union (EU) moved quickly to respond. On March 25, EU Regulation 297/2011[7] came into force. Although this looks like a sensible precaution, requiring testing of foods from affected areas of Japan for radioactivity, it in fact introduces upper limits for radioactivity that are significantly *higher* than previous ones.

What Can You Do?

For each radionuclide there is a different risk and a different set of measures. The U.S. Department of Homeland Security funded a guidelines paper in 2006 that among others addressed the following radioactive elements.[8]

Radioactive Iodine-131

For this threat, we take regular iodine, to minimize the amount of radioactive iodine that gets taken up by the thyroid. Various forms, such as potassium iodide, do work, but only if given before or within 12 hours of exposure. And, since iodine-131 has a half-life of eight days, by the time it gets from Fukushima to the United States there won't be much radioactivity left.

Uranium

Uranium (half-life: thousands of years) is there in Fukushima in large quantities in the fuel rods. No reports of it being found in the environment yet, but there's plenty of time. And even depleted (non-radioactive) uranium is a highly toxic heavy metal, and one to which anybody who served in the first or second Gulf War, or in Bosnia or Kosovo, has probably been exposed. So a Fukushima exposure would just add to that toxicity. For uranium there are protocols worked out by the U.S. military. Large doses of sodium bicarbonate (baking soda, in the orange box) minimize the damage caused by uranium and encourage its excretion in the kidneys. You can buy bicarbonate in bulk for less than a dollar per pound. It is certainly worth stocking up on. You can absorb it through the skin, so a good fistful in a warm bath, which you sit in for 15–20 minutes, is the simplest way to take it in.

Cesium-137

This has a half-life of 30 years and like uranium is still a toxic metal even when not radioactive. The U.S. government stockpiles the chemical Prussian blue for removing cesium.[9] Prussian blue is ferric ferrocyanide—Fe7(CN)18 plus a load of water. It is not absorbed from the gut; it can only trap cesium (and also thallium) as it is recycled through the bile to gut to blood again. It works by cutting the biological half-life (time to get rid of half the total body burden) from about 80 days to 25. But that would still take three months to bring the level below 10 percent of starting, which is plenty of time to do harm. Prussian blue was used in photography before we went digital, so there might be some left in your garage. Leave it there and *do not* try this at home. Prussian blue contains cyanide, a strong poison.

Plutonium

When uranium is used in a reactor it converts to plutonium, which is a big worry. Plutonium is extremely dangerous. It is estimated that 1,000 mg could kill 10 million people. This is what the Centers for Disease Control (CDC) and Prevention has to say:

> Because it emits alpha particles, plutonium is most dangerous when inhaled. When plutonium particles are inhaled, they lodge in the lung tissue. The alpha particles can kill lung cells, which causes scarring of the lungs, leading to further lung disease and cancer. Plutonium can enter the blood stream from the lungs and travel to the kidneys, meaning that the blood and the kidneys will be exposed to alpha particles. Once plutonium circulates through the body, it concentrates in the bones, liver, and spleen, exposing these organs to alpha particles. Plutonium that is ingested from contaminated food or water does not pose a serious threat to humans because the stomach does not absorb plutonium easily and so it passes out of the body in the feces.[10]

What can you do about it? There are no grounds for thinking iodine or bicarbonate will work. The medical recommendation at present is diethylenetriaminepentaacetate acid (DTPA), which is a version of ethylenediaminetetraacetic acid (EDTA)—a chelating (detoxifying) agent, specific to transuranic elements.

In each of the above exposures, of course, you should get to a doctor, fast, and get the appropriate treatment. But an exposure coming from Fukushima is likely to be a dirty mix of any or all of these, so we need some universal measures. There are three worthwhile ones, all of which you can do for yourself.

Antioxidant Vitamins

It's easy to get down to the health store and buy some bottles of these, and in these circumstances an overdose is the last thing to worry about. While the shelves are full of nutritional and herbal products that might help, my personal advice would be to take:

• Vitamin C (water-soluble antioxidant): 3,000–5,000 milligrams (mg), three times daily; option to combine water-soluble and oil-based forms.

• Vitamin E (fat-soluble antioxidant) mixed tocopherols and tocotrienols: About 400 international units (IU), once daily.

• Alpha-lipoic acid (operates in both water and lipid compartments, spares both vitamins C and E): 100 mg or more, three times daily.

Glutathione

This amino acid is known to chelate certain minerals, but there's no evidence that it works on radioactive ones. Some experts say nothing does. However, it's a crucial antioxidant, which will protect against radiation damage and help to mop up the toxic molecules produced. Take loads: say 1,000 mg, three times daily. And because it can be tricky to absorb, consider using the oil-based version that you rub into your skin.

Phosphatidylcholine

If you turned up in the ER in an Eastern bloc country with acute radiation exposure, they would give you a IV shot of phosphatidylcholine. It is found in egg yolk, organ meats, and lecithin supplements and is easily absorbed into our membranes as a phospholipid. There are no human experiments I know of, thankfully, but this is backed up by some doctors: ionizing radiation first disturbs the phospholipid metabolism, then provokes severe inflammatory reactions, and finally leads to death . . . The survival of rats exposed to lethal doses of radiation was clearly prolonged with phospholipid supplementation.[11] You can get phosphatidylcholine in liquid or capsule form: take at least a tablespoon or equivalent daily, with food.

If you've got the time, it's wise to build all of these up slowly, or they may give you loose bowels for a few days. If you haven't got the time, you have bigger things to worry about.

REFERENCES

1. Buesseler K. Japan's irradiated waters: how worried should we be? CNN Opinion, Apr 26, 2011. Available at: www.cnn.com/2011/OPINION/04/26/buesseler.fukushima.radiation/index.html?_s=PM:OPINIO.

2. Environmental Protection Agency. Japanese nuclear emergency: EPA's radiation monitoring. EPA website, Mar 11, 2011. Available at: www.epa.gov/japan2011.

3. Shinbun Y. Fukushima I nuke plant: radioactive iodine and cesium in seawater detected. EXSKF, Mar 22, 2011. Available at: http://ex-skf.blogspot.com/2011/03/fukushima-i-nuke-plant-radioactive.html.

4. Sircus M. No danger no concern no sanity. Dr. Sircus.com, Mar 19, 2011. Available at: http://blog.imva.info/medicine/danger-concern-sanity.

5. Yablokov AV. Mortality after the Chernobyl catastrophe. *Ann N Y Acad Sci* 2009;1181:192–216.

6. Kane M. Fallout. Collapse Network, Mar 24, 2011. Available at: www.collapsenet.com/free-resources/collapsenet-public-access/item/723-fallout.

7. European Commission. Commission implementing regulation (EU) No. 297/2011, Mar 26, 2011. Available at: http://eurlex.europa.eu/LexUriServ/LexUriServ.do?uri=OJ:L:2011:080:0005:0008:EN:PDF.

8. Marcus C, et al. Medical management of internally radiocontaminated patients. Report for Dept. of Homeland Security, June 2006. Available at: www.acnmonline.org/docs/MMRSManualCarol_Marcus.pdf.

9. Dept. of Health and Human Services. Prussian blue, insoluble (radiogardase). Rediation Emergency Medical Management, Aug 30, 2013. Available at: www.remm.nlm.gov/prussianblue.htm.

10. Centers for Disease Control and Prevention. Radioisotope brief: plutonium. Emergency Preparedness and Response, May 10, 2006. Available at: http://emergency.cdc.gov/radiation/isotopes/plutonium.asp.

11. Gundermann KJ. The "essential" phospholipids as a membrane therapeutic. Institute of Pharmacology and Toxicology, Szczecin, Poland, 1993.

SCHIZOPHRENIA AND PSYCHOSIS

SCHIZOPHRENIA IS ONE OF the most important chronic diseases. It does not kill as many people as cancer or heart disease, but in another sense it does terminate the life every person is entitled to—a life that is relatively free from pain and is normally productive. The person with schizophrenia should be able to achieve whatever he or she could as if they had never been ill once they have recovered from their acute illness. But this does not happen. The natural recovery rate is probably less than 25 percent, and the addition of any or all of the tranquilizers when used alone does not yield any better results. In 1850, Dr. John Conolly reported a 50 percent recovery rate. He used decent, humane care, good food, and shelter. I have yet to meet a schizophrenic who recovered from drugs alone who is practicing medicine, law, piloting a commercial jet, running a bank, or doing any of the many skilled jobs upon which our society must depend.

For this reason, the stigma of mental disease has remained strong in spite of best efforts to convince the public that it is a disease like others. In my opinion, the stigma will dissipate only when the results of treatment are as predictable and as effective as are the treatments for the majority of other chronic conditions. We are ready for this now, but it has been impossible to persuade the psychiatric profession. We should be working on behalf of our patients, and not on behalf of the drug companies persuaded by the massive drug advertising campaigns, the major post-graduate trainers. We should use what is known, while at the same time trying to perfect and to develop new treatments. Governments should demand from their public health departments that they seek out and use the best possible treatment as a way of reducing disease costs. What is the value of searching for the perfect drug? So far in the vast field of medicine, there are no xenobiotics that do more than alleviate a few symptoms and often at a major price to the patient. Diseases are caused by nutrient deficiencies, by nutrient *dependencies,* by toxicities, by biochemical abnormalities. They are not caused by a drug deficiency. Schizophrenia is not due to a deficiency of Haldol or any other tranquilizer.

The latest trend in medicine is to talk about "evidence-based" medicine, meaning using the treatment that is the most effective at the least cost. If this new principle were applied to the treatment of schizophrenia, there would be no doubt whatever that orthomolecular treatment would be the treatment of choice. The cost of using any other treatment is $2 million per lifetime for every schizophrenic because they do not become well, while the cost of orthomolecular treatment is infinitesimally small compared to this since the majority of acute patients will become well.

The *Journal of Orthomolecular Medicine* was founded over 25 years ago to provide a forum for the discussion of schizophrenia since no other journals would carry this type of information. I have dedicated my professional career toward this cause. I will continue to publish clinical data to demonstrate that schizophrenic patients can get well, and to prove that they deserve a chance to achieve this objective.

—ABRAM HOFFER, *JOM* 1995

TERMS OF SCHIZOPHRENIA AND PSYCHOSIS

ACIDOSIS. A condition in which body chemistry becomes imbalanced and overly acidic, and that if left unbalanced can interrupt all cellular activities and functions.

ADRENOCHROME. Oxidization product of adrenaline (also known as "pink adrenaline"); a neurotoxic hallucinogen.

AXON. The fiberlike extension of a neuron by which it sends information to target cells.

CATECHOLAMINE. Neurotransmitters known as dopamine, epinephrine, and norepinephrine that are active in both the brain and the central nervous system.

DENDRITE. A treelike extension of a neuron and the primary site for receiving and integrating information from other neurons.

HOD TEST. Hoffer-Osmond Diagnostic Test. A simple card-sort test developed by Drs. Abram Hoffer and Humphry Osmond in 1961 for assisting in the diagnosis of schizophrenia.

METHYLATION. A process, central to mood control, among other functions, in which a molecule donates one of its methyl groups to another substance in the body.

NEURON. The basic working unit of the brain, a cell specialized for the transmission of information and characterized by long, fibrous projections called axons, and shorter, branchlike projections called dendrites.

NEUROTRANSMITTER. A chemical released by neurons at a synapse for the purpose of relaying information to other neurons via receptors.

PELLAGRA. Niacin deficiency disease; symptoms include hallucinations, depression, anxiety, confusion, memory loss, anorexia, fatigue, and psychosis very much like schizophrenia.

PHENOTHIAZINES. Antipsychotics that include chlorpromazine (Thorazine), haloperidol (Haldol), and perphenazine (Phenothiazine), which are used to treat schizophrenia and other psychotic disorders by controlling symptoms by affecting the brain neurotransmitters dopamine and serotonin.

POLYPHARMACY. The use of multiple drugs simultaneously; a "drug cocktail" would be an example. Disadvantages include difficulty in telling which medicine is working and which is or are not; increased side effects due to drug-drug interactions.

PORPHYRIA. A group of inherited and acquired disorders in which an important part of hemoglobin, called heme, is not made properly; the resulting buildup of abnormal amounts of porphyrins can manifest with neurological complications.

PSYCHOSIS. A severe symptom of psychiatric disorders characterized by an inability to perceive reality.

PYROLURIA. Originally known as malvaria, pyroluria is a genetic abnormality in hemoglobin synthesis resulting in a deficiency of zinc and vitamin B6 (pyridoxine) and the buildup of kryptopyrroles in the body.

SYNAPSE. A physical gap between two neurons that functions as the site of information transfer from one neuron to another.

TARDIVE DYSKINESIA. A disorder that involves involuntary movements, especially of the lower face, and a serious side effect that occurs from antipsychotic medications.

WILSON'S DISEASE. A rare inherited disorder of copper metabolism in which excessive amounts of copper accumulate in the body. The buildup of copper leads to damage in the liver, brain, and eyes.

ORTHOMOLECULAR TREATMENT OF SCHIZOPHRENIA
by Abram Hoffer, MD, PhD

In 1968, Dr. Linus Pauling stated, "I have reached the conclusion, through arguments summarized in the following paragraphs, that another general method of treatment, which may be called ortho-molecular therapy, may be found to be of great value and may turn out to be the best method of treatment for many patients." Immediately following this, Professor Pauling defined orthomolecular psychiatric therapy as "the treatment of mental disease by the provision of the optimum molecular environment for the mind, especially the optimum concentrations of substances normally present in the body."

In 1968, the Committee on Therapy of the American Schizophrenia Association, consisting of around a dozen physicians all practicing what was then called megavitamin therapy for schizophrenia and other diseases, felt the need for a unifying concept. Dr. Linus Pauling's concept of orthomolecular psychiatry seemed most appropriate at that time and still does because we all realized that we were, in fact, practicing a form of orthomolecular medicine.

Evolution of the Concept

The historical roots of orthomolecular psychiatry go back many years. One of the major roots began with the vitamin pioneers like Dr. Casimir Funk who first coined the term "vitamine." He was followed by a long line of distinguished vitaminologists and nutritionists. But a few have a special interest for us because they introduced the use of megavitamins into psychiatry. These are men like Goldberger, Sydenstricker, and Joliffe and many others who did much of their work in mental hospitals. It includes psychiatrists like Cleckly, Medlicott, Sherill, Washburne, Thompson, and Proctor. Gould completed very valuable work in England nearly 20 years ago.

Adrenochrome Hypothesis of Schizophrenia

Another major root arose from the work that was started in Saskatchewan, Canada. With Osmond who recently arrived from England, I began to develop what was called the adrenochrome hypothesis of schizophrenia. Adrenochrome, an oxidized derivative of adrenaline, is made in the body and rapidly converted into adrenolutin; both of these compounds are hallucinogens. We realized that the establishment of the adrenochrome hypothesis would require many decades, and we were not prepared to wait patiently for this great day before developing a therapeutic program. In 1952, there were no specific therapies for schizophrenia. We, therefore, made the assumption that our adrenochrome hypothesis might be correct and began to develop therapeutics that could be used to counteract the production of these endogenous hallucinogens.

Water-Soluble Vitamins

An examination of the chemistry involved suggested to us that the water-soluble vitamins might be the most important factors in the treatment of schizophrenia. Of these, ascorbic acid (vitamin C), thiamine (vitamin B1), riboflavin (vitamin B2), and niacin (niacinamide or vitamin B3) seemed most relevant. The one that seemed the most promising was niacin. This was based upon the fact that a number of mental illnesses had already yielded to treatment with small doses of niacin. We also knew that pellagra, which had, at one time, been endemic around the Mediterranean Basin and southern United States, was remarkably like schizophrenia.

Megadoses of Niacin

It also arose from observations that niacin in larger dosages had been used for the treatment of bromidism (neurologic and dermatologic effects caused by excessive or prolonged use of sedative

This paper was presented at the joint meeting of the American Schizophrenia Association, the Canadian Schizophrenia Association, and the Schizophrenia Association of Great Britain; London, England, September 28–30, 1971, and subsequently published in the *J Orthomolecular Psych* 1972;1(1)46–55.

bromides). We began to use megadoses because we were aware that, if 1,000 or 2,000 milligrams (mg) a day of niacin had worked on chronic schizophrenics, this certainly would have been reported. We did not realize that due to error in philosophy, psychiatrists had prevented examination of the use of large dosages of vitamin B3 for the treatment of chronic schizophrenia. When schizophrenic patients were given 1,000 mg of niacin per day and recovered, they were promptly rediagnosed with pellegra. This prevented proper examination of these dosages for chronic schizophrenics.

In addition, up until 1950 when most of this work was done, niacin was very expensive and the idea of giving dosages of up to 30,000 mg a day could not have arisen, as it would have depleted most of the research budgets of these men.

We, therefore, decided to begin with at least 3,000 mg of niacin per day and to go up to 30,000 mg, if necessary, in a carefully controlled research program. It was our hope that the use of this vitamin would effectively cut down the production of adrenochrome and in this way would allow the normal, reparative processes of the body to become more effective.

Vitamin C

Another root of orthomolecular psychiatry comes from the work of Dr. Irwin Stone who has been gathering the literature on vitamin C or, as he prefers to call it, ascorbic acid. It is Dr. Stone's thesis that over the course of millions of years certain essential nutrients that were manufactured within the body can no longer be made and species have become dependent upon external sources. Without ascorbic acid, man is one of the few species who will develop scurvy. Every person, therefore, suffers from a condition called hypoascorbemia (chronically low blood vitamin C levels), which is kept in control only as long as that person is able to maintain his exogenous supplies of ascorbic acid.

Biochemical Individuality

Another major root was the work of Professor Roger Williams, who has shown with remarkable clarity the marked individuality of people. It is clear that there is sufficient biochemical individuality so that one day a proper examination of a person's enzymes would be enough to identify him.

Orthomolecular Medicine

Finally, a major historical root was the work of Professor Linus Pauling, who established a basis for the term orthomolecular medicine with his pioneering work on sickle cell anemia and its relationship to hemoglobin (the pigment in blood that carries oxygen). Dr. Pauling, having examined all of these roots, developed his present concept of orthomolecular medicine and showed how it would be possible for species of animals to drop certain enzymes and become more dependent upon external sources of nutrients.

Dr. Pauling concluded,

The functioning of the brain is affected by the molecular concentrations of many substances which are normally present in the brain. The optimum concentrations of these substances for a person may differ greatly from the concentration provided by his normal diet and genetic machinery. Biochemical and genetic arguments support the idea that orthomolecular therapy, the provision for the individual person of the optimum concentration of important, normal constituents of the brain, may be the preferred treatment for many mentally ill patients.

Then he goes on to say,

It is suggested that the genes responsible for abnormalities (deficiencies) in the concentration of vital substances in the brain may be responsible for increased penetrants of the postulated gene for schizophrenia and that the so-called gene for schizophrenia may itself be a gene that leads to a localized cerebral deficiency in one or more vital substances.

A Megavitamin Approach to Schizophrenia

The present orthomolecular program for treating schizophrenia was developed chiefly by members of the Committee on Therapy of the American Schizophrenia Association. Each physician uses essentially the same program although there are minor variations in dosages and in the adjunctive therapies that are used. The program is based on our philosophy that schizophrenia is a chronic condition that is more comparable as a model to diabetes, which requires the continuous use of insulin and diet, than it is to pneumonia, which will respond to one series of treatments of antibiotics.

In the orthomolecular approach, we apply the simplest treatment first, then depending on the response, apply more difficult and varied treatments until the patient has achieved either a full or near recovery. The program cannot be defined in terms of months or years. No trial is completed until at least five years have lapsed from the beginning of the treatment. Several patients have become well after seven years.

Treatment

Patients are started on 3,000–4,000 mg of vitamin B3 per day. Vitamin B3 is used to cover both niacin, the form that produces a flush the first few times it is taken, and nicotinamide, which is not a vasodilator. I start with nicotinamide with all patients under the age of 21 simply because young people have a much harder time with the flush. With male patients over 21, I start with niacin because of the positive side effects, such as the lowering of cholesterol levels and the decrease in the incidence of coronary disease as well as a decrease in the incidence of senility. With women who are concerned about the cosmetic effect of the flush, I start with nicotinamide but otherwise will begin with niacin.

Chronic patients tend to do better with niacin, the reason being that it is possible to increase the dose to higher levels. There is a maximum dose beyond which one cannot go, not because it will produce any serious toxicity, but because it produces physiological reactions such as nausea and vomiting, which severely limits further intake. As a rule, it is seldom possible to go beyond 6,000 or 9,000 mg a day of nicotinamide, but it is quite possible to go up to 25,000 or 30,000 mg a day of niacin without developing nausea and vomiting.

In addition to the vitamin B3, patients are also given ascorbic acid from 1,000 to 3,000 mg per day and other water-soluble vitamins. I use vitamin B1 (thiamine) if there is a good deal of depression and vitamin B6 (pyridoxine) if there is a good deal of muscular hyperactivity, for example, in the hyperkinetic child or in the epileptic. For fatigue, I use vitamin B12 (cobalamin).

In addition to adjusting the vitamins, patients are placed on a nutritious diet, which means reducing the intake of refined foods such as flour and sugar, increasing the frequency of feeding, and, of course, increasing the proportion of protein.

Attention must also be given to the use of minerals such as zinc, calcium, magnesium, and iodine.

Many early cases of schizophrenia will not require anything more than this nutritional approach. I have a series of several hundred who have never received any other chemotherapies commonly used in psychiatry. However, if the patient is severely disturbed or severely depressed, it may be essential to temporarily use sedatives and other drugs. I use moderate quantities of tranquilizers on outpatients because the vitamin approach tends to improve the efficiency of these substances. Patients admitted to the hospitals where I work are treated with heavy dosages of tranquilizers because it is important to bring them under control within 48 hours.

At the initial interview, the patients are given perceptual tests. The one that I commonly use is the Hoffer-Osmond Diagnostic (HOD) Test, which has proven to be a very efficient diagnostic aid, not only for diagnosing, but also for monitoring treatment. It also has great value in determining when relapse is occurring. Another test is the Experimental World Inventory (EWI) test developed by Dr. El Meligi and Dr. Osmond, which is a much more sophisticated test.

After the patient has been on this program for a reasonable period of time, say about a month, he is reevaluated. If he is much improved, he is continued on the same program until he has made a complete recovery. By recovery, I mean that this patient, if examined by the most objective psychiatrist, would not show any evidence of residual disability.

The dosages of vitamin B3 may have to be varied in order to achieve this state; between 3,000 and 30,000 mg a day for niacin and usually between 3,000 and 9,000 mg a day for nicotinamide. However, once the patient has recovered, the dosages are slowly reduced until a proper maintenance is obtained. This is usually well under 9,000 mg per day although a few cases have been higher. Tranquilizers and any other sedatives are slowly removed from the program.

If patients do not respond in a reasonable period of time, I will continue to work with them trying out various forms of drugs and sometimes adding to the therapeutic program penicillamine, known commercially as Cuprimine, up to 1,000 mg per day. Penicillamine is a copper-chelating agent that picks up extra quantities of copper from the body.

For nonresponders, a five-year program is laid down that might include bringing the patients back into the hospital every six to twelve months for the application of various medications and megavitamins, which might be of some help to them. I will also use injectable vitamins. These are special research cases. I do not give up unless the patient is taken away from me either by his own wish or by going to one of the local mental hospitals, which will usually immediately discontinue the megavitamin program that they had been following.

Expected Results

One can expect the following results. If one were to start with a cohort of schizophrenic patients, who were ill for one year or less, but who have not been injured by residing in a chronic mental hospital, one would expect over a two-year period to achieve over 90 percent recovery rate. The other 10 percent will be better and none will have been made worse.

If, however, one started with a cohort of patients who have been sick between one and ten years but who have not been injured by residing in a chronic mental hospital, one would expect perhaps 70 percent recovery or better.

If one were to start with a chronic population who have been treated in chronic mental hospitals for anywhere from one to twenty or more years, the recovery results are very much less and I would be surprised if one could get more than 25 percent recovery. However, even with these chronic cases, most of them will be vastly improved and will be able to function in the community to a limited degree.

I have for the past five years been following about 25 chronic schizophrenics whose average duration of stay in hospitals had been around 25 years. They have been on the megavitamin approach. I have been astonished at the remarkable improvement in some of them although none will ever be considered well. I am positive that had these unfortunate schizophrenics been started on the program 20 years ago most of them today would be well.

Evidence the Megavitamin Approach Works

It is the fashion today to depend upon double-blind control experiments to establish new treatments in psychiatry. I really cannot complain about this because Dr. Osmond and I directed the first double-blind control experiment in the history of psychiatry in 1951 in Saskatchewan. The first experiment was a controlled study of the effect of certain yeast nucleotides. The second double-blind experiment was a study comparing the efficacy of niacin, nicotinamide, and a placebo in each case using 3,000 mg per day.

Double-Blind Study of 30 Acute Schizophrenic Patients

This study was started at the General Hospital in Regina, Sackatchewan. Thirty acute schizophrenic patients admitted to this hospital and diagnosed by their own clinicians were randomized using random numbers into three groups of roughly 10 each. All of the 30 patients received the usual psychotherapy given at this unit, which was very dynamic and gave each patient about three hours per week of psychotherapy. Tranquilizers had not yet been introduced. In addition, each therapist gave his patient electroconvulsive therapy (ECT) if this was indicated. Ten of the patients received 3,000 mg of niacin per day. This group would be betrayed by the flush due to the nicotine acid and, therefore, could not be considered a proper control group. However, a second group was given nicotinamide, which does not produce any flush, while the third group received the placebo.

The clinical and nursing staff were informed that there would only be two medications in this trial—a placebo and the niacin. They would assume that all of the patients who flushed were receiving niacin and that the others were on the placebo. In fact, half of the non-flushers were on nicotinamide. The patients were all evaluated before the treatment by a team of psychologists and clinicians. The study ran 33 days at the end of which time the medication was discontinued and the patients were reevaluated.

One Year Follow-Up

We decided not to use discharge criteria alone because it had become obvious that whether or not a patient was discharged did not depend primarily upon his own clinical state. It depended much more upon what the psychiatrist felt about him. The patients were followed up for one year by a trained worker who did not know which treatment they had had in the hospital. Patients were recalled at three-month intervals. At the end of 12 months, after the last patient had been treated, the code was broken and the results were evaluated.

Evaluation of the Study

It turned out that of the 10 or so patients receiving niacin, 7 had remained well over that year. Of the 10 or so nicotinamide patients, 7 or 8 had remained well, while of the 10-placebo patients only 3 had remained well. Around 75 percent of the patients receiving vitamins had remained well, whereas only one-third of the patients receiving the placebo had remained well. It is important to remember that about two-thirds of all the patients had also received ECT so that this was a study of the combination of ECT plus megavitamins.

Double-Blind Study of 82 Schizophrenic Patients

The results of the study were relatively clear-cut, but it seemed very important to us not to report this until we repeated the study on a larger scale, to make sure there had been no hidden errors. We, therefore, started the second double-blind clinical experiment using the same design except that this time we did use niacin and a placebo while informing the staff that we were going to follow the previous design. With our second study, we were able to treat 82 patients. The results were very similar.

Additional Studies with Schizophrenic Patients

In the meantime, I encouraged a psychiatrist working on our staff to run a study on a group of chronic schizophrenic patients using 3,000 mg per day. We proved to our own satisfaction that this dose was inadequate for this group of patients since none of them got well.

Additional evidence is based from the combined experience of the Committee on Therapy, which has a total experience of 15,000 schizophrenic patients or more. We have compared notes every year for the past five years. There is no doubt that we are all obtaining similar results.

Schizophrenic Twins

Recently, I reviewed a series of 11 identical schizophrenic twins. Of these 11 identical twins, every twin treated with the megavitamin B3 approach recovered, whereas, every twin treated by the standard, that is, tranquilizer approach, was still ill. The most striking pair are a couple of women who were so identical at birth that their parents could not tell them apart and who were able to confuse their teachers and their boyfriends for a long time.

They both became psychotic about 25 years ago, and over the next 20 years each one suffered frequent relapses. They went into a mental hospital at least once a year for between one and three months and between their admissions to hospital were barely able to function. About five years ago, one of these twins consulted her family physician for backache. He diagnosed her schizophrenic, started her on the megavitamin B3, and she recovered. Her identical twin had a similar history except that she was not permitted to start on the megavitamin by her psychiatrist. The control twin, therefore, not receiving therapy but receiving expensive psychotherapy and tranquilizer therapy, has in the past three years been readmitted to a psychiatric ward at least a dozen times.

Evidence Is Conclusive

Looking over the evidence, I have concluded that every physician who has used the orthomolecular approach, as described, with care, skill, and industry, has gotten identical results. On the other hand, every physician who has not used the program, as described, has been disappointed in its results. This should not be very surprising.

A few papers have appeared recently with claims that the results of the megavitamin approach have not been obtained. When these papers are examined carefully, it is obvious that they have not followed the orthomolecular approach because of ineffective low doses and without the other nutrients.

Expansion of Orthomolecular Concept

One of the greatest but perhaps least well-known psychiatrists was Dr. John Conolly who worked in England at Hanwell Hospital over 130 years ago. Dr. Conolly had a modern conception of psychosis, which he described as a perceptual disease. I am at a loss to understand how this brilliant work by Dr. Conolly has been so totally submerged in British psychiatry and only now is beginning to emerge. It is ironic that the first hospital to be called the John Conolly Hospital is now being built in New Jersey by Dr. Jack Ward and his associates.

Dr. Jack Ward, many years ago, became aware that a large number of patients (not schizophrenic but with many perceptual changes and high scores on the HOD test) responded very quickly to megavitamin B3. His concept was taken up by Dr. Bella Kowalson, who wrote a brief paper describing a disease she called metabolic disperception (that is, problems of metabolism bringing about disperceptions). Most of her patients were schizophrenic, but she felt that her term was not only more accurate but was much safer for her to use since as a general practitioner she did not want to argue with her psychiatric colleagues about her right to diagnose schizophrenia. In any event, we are now aware of a large number of patients who do suffer major perceptual changes that can be diagnosed by the clinical interview but that can be done more economically by the use of the HOD and EWI Tests. They do respond very well on the megavitamin or orthomolecular approach.

Schizophrenia—An Orthomolecular Disease

I have concluded after reviewing all of this material that schizophrenia is one of the orthomolecular diseases. If a person consumes a diet too low in vitamin B3 and if his average requirements are normal, he will develop pellagra. This is a condition that is so like schizophrenia that they are easily confused. If, however, the person has an average diet containing average quantities of vitamin B3 but due to some defect in his chemistry requires quantities of vitamin B3 that are not provided by the diet, he will suffer from exactly the same deficiency, but he is said now to have a dependency condition since the error is in his body and not in the diet. It is my contention that schizophrenia is a vitamin B3–dependency condition. It is also my contention that this vitamin B3–dependency condition can strike at any time from infancy to senility. If it strikes or becomes apparent before puberty, then it will take on any of the forms of learning and other behavioral disabilities.

Study of 30 Children with Learning or Behavioral Disorders

I am completing a study on about 30 children who were all either learning or behavioral disorders. I was not concerned about their diagnosis but merely about the fact that they were not doing well at home or at school and had been referred to me by their family physician. They were all placed upon orthomolecular treatment and, in every case where this was followed, recovered. There were a very small number where treatment could not be continued due to factors beyond my control. After these young patients had recovered, they were given placebo instead of nicotinamide and, in every case, within one month had relapsed to their previous condition. When they were again placed upon nicotinamide, they once more recovered but in many cases it took a much longer period of time thereafter, as if one major relapse had had a gravely pathological effect on their need for vitamins thereafter.

In my opinion, the majority of childhood illnesses of this nature, where there are perceptual and behavioral changes that can be measured using perceptual tests or behavioral tests, are instances of vitamin B3 dependency. During adolescence this takes the form of rebellion, hostility, excessive use of drugs like LSD, marijuana, and, more recently, heroin and methadone. These young children also suffer from a variety of perceptual disturbances that, by and large, are ignored by psychiatrists who deal with them and who are not aware that these are there.

Adulthood Schizophrenia

If the condition should express itself during adulthood, then, of course, we have the more typical cases of adulthood schizophrenia. We, however, run into the difficulty of diagnoses in that various countries use different diagnostic criteria and people who are considered schizophrenic in Canada and the United States might be considered not to have schizophrenia in England. These discrepancies in diagnosis will disappear as soon as all of the psychiatrists begin to use proper perceptual tests to aid them in their diagnosis.

If the condition should strike after the age of 60, these patients may be diagnosed senility. I have a fair number of so-called senile patients who have been treated with the orthomolecular approach and who are now normal.

Many Need More Essential Nutrients

Finally, there is a most important expansion of this program to include most people. According to Dr. Linus Pauling, there are at least 40 to 50 essential nutrients and perhaps 50,000 enzymes in the body. It is quite obvious that we are all different and it makes sense to believe that a large number of people may require extra quantities of one or more of these essential nutrients. At the moment, there is no scientific way of determining which of these nutrients are lacking, although a beginning has been made in this area. Dr. Arthur Robinson, working with Dr. Linus Pauling, has shown that schizophrenic patients tend to retain more ascorbic acid, niacin, and pyridoxine then do normal controls. When they are given a test dose of these vitamins, much less appears in their urine than it does in normal people. Their theory is that a body that requires these vitamins will tend to excrete less. This technique might one day be developed to determine which of these nutrients any one of us might lack. There is, however, a practical way, which is for each one of us to run experiments on ourselves with the essential nutrients, none of which are toxic. By trying out these nutrients, one after the other and measuring our own response, we could soon discover whether or not we do suffer from these orthomolecular or perhaps, minor diseases.

■ CONCLUSION

I have outlined the evolution of the orthomolecular approach where various historical streams of research have come together and have been combined into a major stream that we call orthomolecular psychiatry. Orthomolecular therapy in psychiatry has been proven more effective for treating schizophrenia than standard therapy. It is coming into use very rapidly for treating learning and behavioral problems in children, for alcoholics, and for other patients with many perceptual difficulties.

ORTHOMOLECULAR TREATMENT FOR SCHIZOPHRENIA: A REVIEW
by Raymond J. Pataracchia, ND

Various segments of the schizophrenic population fall into subgroups of distinct biochemical imbalance. We often see subgroups of essential fatty acid deficiency, inadequate nutriture, dysglycemia (unstable blood sugar), food intolerance, digestive compromise, malabsorption, undermethylation, niacin (vitamin B3) deficiency, vitamin C deficiency, heavy metal toxicity, pyridoxine (vitamin B6) deficiency, zinc deficiency, brain hypothyroidism, and adrenal insufficiency. Complementary and alternative medicine (CAM) has a key role in the treatment of schizophrenia. The goal of optimal complementary treatment is to correct the biochemical imbalance. In schizophrenia, we can assess cases with lab tests and target our treatment accordingly. CAM treatment involves the use of nutritional supplements, nutraceuticals (food components with medicinal qualities), amino acids, and botanicals.

Biochemical Imbalances: Part 1

Dietary changes are also implemented in treatment. In Part 1 of this review we will cover the research on essential fatty acid deficiency, inadequate nutriture, dysglycemia, food intolerance, digestive compromise, malabsorption, undermethylation, vitamin B3 deficiency, and vitamin C deficiency.

The EFA-Deficient Schizophrenic

Chronic schizophrenics have increased phospholipid neuron membrane breakdown (oxidative stress) that concentrates in the frontal cortex and other brain areas.[1,2] Pro-inflammatory cytokine involvement in development may set the stage for oxidative stress from early development onward.[3,4] Omega-3 fats have a neuroprotective and anti-inflammatory role. Sixty percent of the dry weight of the brain is fat. Essential fatty acids (EFAs), including omega-3 and omega-6, are good fats, not saturated with hydrogen, and, unfortunately, not readily provided in the North American diet. Investigators note an integral need for omega-3 supplementation for schizophrenia, mood, and behavior disorders.[3,5] EFAs are important components of nerve cell walls, and they are involved in neurotransmitter electrical activity.

Eicosapentaenoic acid (EPA) is an omega-3 fat that is slightly more unsaturated than an omega-6 fat. Brain membrane structure is compromised in chronic schizophrenia, and EPA has demonstrated some potential in keeping brain neuron degeneration at bay and in reducing psychotic symptoms.[6–12] Omega-3 EFAs may eventually gain notice as "a safe and efficacious treatment for psychiatric disorders in pregnancy and in breast-feeding [moms]."[6,13] Fish have high amounts of omega-3s and high-EPA supplements are derived from fish. The higher the EPA content, the more useful it is for schizophrenics.[7]

A balanced essential fatty acid profile may also be mediated by vitamin B3, but more research is needed to identify the role of vitamin B3 on the EFA profile of schizophrenics.

The Schizophrenic with Inadequate Nutriture

Neurotransmitter production is dependant on amino-acid protein building blocks (phenylalanine, tyrosine, tryptophan, etc.) supplied from the diet. The catecholamines dopamine, norepinephrine, and epinephrine are derived from the amino acids phenylalanine and tyrosine. Catecholamines (a type of neurotransmitter) are involved in executive functions and motivation. Serotonin, the " feel good" neurotransmitter, is derived from the amino acid tryptophan. Protein nutriture is very important for schizophrenia and for general mental well-being. I have seen many schizophrenics respond when they start increasing their protein intake with each meal. A diet that has 40 percent protein,

From the *J Orthomolecular Med* Part 1, 2008;23(1):21–28 and Part 2, 2008;23(2):95–105.

40 percent carbohydrate, and 20 percent fat is ideal for most schizophrenics.

Many schizophrenics do not eat three meals a day and their diet is invariably carbohydrate dominant. Carbohydrate-dominant North American diets release glucose (blood sugar) to the bloodstream quickly. Most schizophrenics require a dietary change that incorporates complex carbohydrates. They also do well to avoid high-glycemicload foods including junk food, white sugar, white rice, and white bread. If they have a poor appetite, this can lead to inadequate nutriture. Poor appetite may be associated with zinc or iron loss.

Fat nutriture is important in schizophrenia. Cold-water fish with teeth have a fat profile suitable for schizophrenics. Salmon, tuna, mackerel, herring, cod, and trout provide the highest omega-3 profile. Other high EFA sources include scallops, shrimp, flaxseeds, walnuts, winter squash, and kidney beans.

Inadequate nutriture can also occur with gastrointestinal compromise, malabsorption, and low thyroid function.

The Dysglycemic Schizophrenic

The brain's demand for glucose is so immense that about 20 percent of the total blood volume circulates to the brain, an organ that represents only 2 percent of body weight. The brain demands a substantial amount of glucose to maintain its high metabolic rate. Gluco-sensing neurons regulate glucose availability in the brain as a fail-safe mechanism to ensure homeostasis (equilibrium of body functions) of brain glucose levels.[15]

In schizophrenia, it seems likely that glucose transporters are compromised with consequent intraneuronal glucose deficits.[15] McDermott and de Silva mention that this hypoglycemic state has the potential to cause "acute symptoms of misperceptions, misinterpretations, anxiety and irritability— the usual features of prodromal [early] and first-onset schizophrenia." Epidemiological investigations show us that schizophrenics are at increased risk for dysglycemia.[17] Psychiatric meds also have some potential to induce hyperglycemic or insulin-resistant states and this can be addressed, at least in part, with a nutritional adjunct.[18]

The hypoglycemic state involves a sharp rise of simple sugars in the blood followed by a sharp decline that robs the neurons of their main energy source; the sharper the decline, the greater the effect on brain cells. Typical hypoglycemic symptoms include irritability, poor memory, late afternoon blues, poor concentration, tiredness, cold hands, muscle cramping, and "feeling better when arguing."

Schizophrenics with hyperglycemia, much like diabetics, present with hypoglycemic mental symptoms because the glucose doesn't get into brain neurons. Brain neurons starved for energy behave differently and mental function declines.[19,20] It is not clear if dysglycemia has a causative role in schizophrenia but it can be deemed an aggravating factor.

It is said that hypoglycemia is 100 percent treatable in compliant patients. This emphasizes the need to address diet. The dysglycemic schizophrenic requires three solid meals (of 40 percent protein) a day and sometimes additional protein-containing snacks. Many schizophrenics need to be educated on complex versus simple carbohydrates and the avoidance of junk food and sugar. When schizophrenics increase their protein intake, they release glucose to the brain at a steady rate and sugar cravings lessen. Chromium and zinc are useful for sugar balance and botanical medicine is useful in advanced hypoglycemia.

The Food-Intolerant Schizophrenic

Schizophrenics, just like the general population, have the potential to exhibit mild or severe food intolerance symptoms.[21–25] The digestive tract reacts to food allergens by eliciting an immune response. Undigested food byproducts can be toxic (e.g., peptides with opiate-like properties), pass through the gut wall, enter the bloodstream, and reach the brain with subsequent brain function compromise.[23,26–28] I have several clients who have an increased severity and frequency of hallucinations, delusions, depression, anxiety, irritability, and insomnia when they eat an intolerant food. We see schizophrenics that experience a wide range of food-related physical symptoms such as headaches, skin eruptions, palpitations, weakness, painful digestion, constipation, diarrhea, and arthritis. In schizophrenia, gluten, dairy, and eggs are commonly not tolerated.[22,23,29] Other common food intolerances include tree nuts, citrus, fish, legumes, and crustaceans.

It is helpful to survey patient responses with a seven-day diet diary. Often schizophrenics are tired, weak, irritated, and moody after eating intolerant foods. Typically, they either hate the intolerant food or crave it, and this may be due to the toxic effects of opioid-eliciting peptides. It is not uncommon to see patients that have fasted in the past and report that they feel better. This is a good indication that they have a food intolerance. An elimination diet followed by provocation is helpful to assess cases clinically. Elaborate lab testing may not need to be implemented but IgG Elisa testing can be quite useful to assess food intolerances that are less obvious.[21,30] IgG responses are provoked when there is a delayed response. IgG tests report the severity of the delayed reaction and also provide a rotation diet schedule. Many investigators have noted improvements with dietary restriction of food intolerants. In our clinic, a small but significant portion of schizophrenics experience profound improvements after removing intolerant foods.

Some researchers estimate 10 percent of schizophrenics having severe food intolerances.[31] More research is needed to understand the pathophysiology, epidemiology, and clinical presentation of the food-sensitive subset of schizophrenics.[32]

The Schizophrenic with Digestive Compromise and Malabsorption

I constantly see gastrointestinal problems in schizophrenia including constipation, spastic obstipation (neuromuscular disturbance of the colon), bloating, cramping, abdominal discomfort, irritable bowel syndrome (IBS), and gastroesophageal reflux disease (GERD). Compromised gastrointestinal function leads to malabsorption of nutrients. These patients often require higher doses of nutrients and medications. Lack of stomach acid can reduce intrinsic factor (key to extracting B12 from foods) and diminish vitamin B12 utilization, which is essential for methylation and neurotransmitter formation. Poor bowel transit locks in toxins

and they build up, tax the immune system, and reduce the absorptive surface area. Poor bowel transit may be due to lack of peristalsis, low thyroid function, or magnesium deficiency. Adequate water intake is about 8 cups per day for the average adult. This is essential to keep toxins moving out and bowel contents hydrated. CAM treatment for digestive dysfunction and low thyroid function helps to alleviate digestive symptoms and also reduces the need for high nutrient dosing. Intact gastrointestinal health is a prerequisite for improved outcome in schizophrenia.

The Undermethylated Schizophrenic

Schizophrenic researchers are well aware that certain brain tracts are overstimulated while others are understimulated (hypofrontality). If we can methylate efficiently, we have the machinery to form neurotransmitters in areas of the brain that are understimulated and neurotransmitter deficient. In our clinic, we see a good portion of schizophrenics with methylation compromise as indicated by elevated fasting homocysteine levels. Elevated homocysteine levels and methylation compromise are common in schizophrenia.[33–41] Elevated homocysteine levels have also been correlated with an increased severity of symptoms.[42]

Nutritional treatment with vitamin B12, folic acid, and other methylators can restore methylation status. In schizophrenia, investigators have found disrupted folic acid pathways.[43,44] These schizophrenics have a greater need for folic acid supplementation.[42] Investigators suspect a causal link between elevated homocysteine and methylenetetrahydrofolate reductase (MTHFR).[45] Many schizophrenics have adequate dietary intake of vitamin B12 and folate yet their homocysteine levels are high.[46] These studies support the hypothesis that schizophrenic pathogenesis may be inherent.

The Vitamins B3- and C-Deficient Schizophrenic

Schizophrenics are poor at filtering the influx of sensory information and this causes perceptual dysfunction (hallucinations, illusions). Overstimulated brain pathways have an excess of neurotransmitters and symptoms are, in part,

653

caused by neurotransmitter overstimulation of the prefrontal cortex. Many neurotransmitter pathways are involved; some overstimulated, others understimulated. In a schizophrenic brain, vitamin B3 and vitamin C together have the potential to intervene and limit the production and oxidation of excess catecholamines in the brain.

Vitamin B3 is one of the few methyl acceptors in the body. As a methyl acceptor, vitamin B3 can limit, in a regulated fashion, neurotransmitter production.[49] When under stress, vitamin B3 can also limit adrenal gland conversion of noradrenaline to adrenaline (excitatory neurotransmitters). Peripherally, this acts as a fail-safe mechanism to prevent excessive adrenaline production and consequent readily autoxidizable catecholamine end products.

A catecholamine-rich cerebral environment is prone to oxidization, and oxidized metabolites are neurotoxic and hallucinogenic to humans.[50-54] In the healthy brain, oxidized catecholamines convert back to a stable form (neuromelanin), a process that has the effect of "neutralizing" or "storing" unwanted toxins.[53,54] Smythies proposes that neuromelanin neutralization is compromised in schizophrenia and it may play a causative role.[52,53] Both vitamins B3 and C have the potential to reduce oxidized catecholamine intermediates.[55] In the adrenal gland, vitamin C is found in high concentrations to keep oxidation at bay.[49]

As a separate mechanism of action, vitamin B3 and vitamin C are physiologically antagonistic to copper. They can help to limit dopamine overproduction that overstimulates the prefrontal cortex and disturbs executive functions. Excess copper is very common in schizophrenia and copper is a cofactor in dopamine production. When dopamine pathways are overstimulated, serotonin (the opposing feel-good master neurotransmitter system) can become downregulated. This may in part account for some of the negative symptoms of schizophrenia.

Vitamin B3 can be found in several supplemental forms such as niacin, niacinamide, and inositol hexaniacinate. Niacin and inositol hexaniacinate are dosed safely in the gram (thousands of milligram) range in the treatment of intermittent claudication, hypercholesterolemia, and Raynaud's disease. Sufficient doses of vitamin B3 for schizophrenia are also in the gram range. Niacinamide and inositol hexaniacinate are flush-free. Pure niacin causes flushing due to the release of peripheral histamine stores. When dosed in the gram range, pure niacin causes a head down flushing response during day one and two of dosing. This subsides with subsequent gram-range dosings. The inositol hexaniacinate form of vitamin B3 is well tolerated and has a great safety profile. Numerous investigators report the use of inositol hexaniacinate in the 4 gram (4,000 mg) daily range without a single adverse reaction.[56-58] Inositol hexaniacinate and pure niacin also promote brain blood flow that can be important in schizophrenic hypofrontality. Vitamin B3 has an interesting side-effect of longevity. The Mayo Clinic found significant reductions in mortality in subjects with high baseline cholesterol who used niacin alone.[59,60]

The B3-deficient state is typified in the disease pellagra, the rarely seen vitamin B3-dependent disease state. Classic symptoms of pellagra include psychosis, hallucinations, depression, anxiety, confusion, memory loss, anorexia, and fatigue.[61,62] Pellagrins and schizophrenics respond well to vitamin B3.

The positive results of B3 treatment have been noted in six double-blind trials on schizophrenic cohorts and an optimal dosing strategy is indicated.[63-80]

Vitamins B3 and C are anti-stress vitamins. Practitioners who treat schizophrenics with vitamin B3 and vitamin C continue to report positive responses.[63,81-83]

Biochemical Imbalances: Part 2

This two-part review on schizophrenia describes various segments of the schizophrenic population that fall into subgroups of distinct biochemical imbalance. To recap, these subgroups include essential fatty acid deficiency, inadequate nutriture, unstable blood sugar (dysglycemia), food intolerance, digestive compromise, malabsorption, undermethylation, vitamin B3 deficiency, B6 deficiency, vitamin C deficiency, zinc deficiency, heavy metal toxicity, brain hypothyroidism, and hypoadrenia. In Part 2 of this review, we discuss heavy metal toxicity, vitamin B6 deficiency, zinc deficiency, brain hypothyroidism, and hypoadrenia.

Heavy Metal Toxicity in Schizophrenia

Most heavy metals are free radicals that induce oxidative stress (lipid peroxidation) and have an affinity for brain tissue.[1,2] Free radical-mediated neurotoxicity and oxidative stress are implicated as a causative factor in schizophrenia.[3,4] These free radicals have the ability to compromise and/or destroy brain tissue and, in so doing, decrease the availability of viable brain tissue. Note that other mechanisms of brain tissue compromise are involved in schizophrenia, so the added burden of toxic metals is to be avoided.

Elevated heavy metal levels are associated with schizophrenic pathology.[4–8] It is not uncommon to see toxic levels of copper, lead, mercury, aluminum, arsenic, and cadmium in schizophrenics. We find some of the most advanced schizophrenic cases having three or more heavy metals. Heavy metal toxicity is also associated with attention-deficit hyperactivity disorder (ADHD), anxiety, obsessive-compulsive disorder (OCD), depression, bipolar disorder, and dementia.

Heavy metals are excreted by using the body's metal-removing protein, metallothionein.[2,9] In the process of ridding the body of heavy metals, this protein loses zinc.[10] Zinc loss in schizophrenia in turn compromises the ability to transcribe proteins and make neurotransmitters. Investigators recognize compromised brain protein transcription pathways in schizophrenia.[3,11] Zinc deficiency is associated with schizophrenia and other psychiatric pathologies including mood dysfunction and dementia.[9]

Lead disrupts mental function.[12] Toxic lead levels are associated with psychosis.[13] Lead toxicity is also associated with behavior disturbance, mood disorder, learning disabilities, insomnia, immune compromise, brain damage, and delayed infant development. Lead has been found to disrupt the carriage of thyroid hormone (T4) into the brain.[14,15] If you are a city dweller, you are exposed to lead and the risk of lead toxicity rises with age. With widespread pesticide use, lead accumulates in the food chain. Lead is found in paints, print color, glass, batteries, rust protectants, alloys, and old water pipes and bathtubs.[16]

Mercury is toxic and has no therapeutic use; in fact, it disrupts dopamine and norepinephrine metabolism.[17] It is not uncommon to find elevated mercury in patients with schizophrenia. Mercury is found in fluorescent lights, vaccines, thermometers, and fish, animals, and plants exposed to toxic environments. Dental fillings contain on average about 40 percent mercury, which has the potential to leach with electrolytic decay. Mercury often causes headaches, nervous irritability, memory decline, depression, rapid fatigue, nausea, stomachaches, and allergic susceptibilities.[16] Mercury has a strong affinity for the brain but also sequesters in the liver, kidney, and spleen.

Aluminum can be toxic in patients with schizophrenia, mood disorders, Alzheimer's disease, and digestive system pathologies. Aluminum disrupts enzyme function and is well-documented to disrupt cognition, learning, and memory. Environmental sources of aluminum include aluminum cookware (especially from heating and deglazing with an acid such as vinegar or wine), drinking boxes, processed cheese, deodorants, and drinking water (aluminum is more soluble in our acidic magnesium deficient drinking water).[18]

In excessive concentrations, copper has a toxic effect and, in schizophrenia, contributes to excess catecholamine oxidation, the end products of which are unstable toxic hallucinogens.[6,19] We have found copper toxicity to be the most common heavy metal pattern in schizophrenia. It is also associated with ADHD, autism, depression, anxiety, bipolar disorder, and paranoia. With copper toxicity we see clinical zinc deficiency.[20] Copper is abundant in food and water as it is found in soil, pesticides, and animal feed. Since World War II we have been exposed to

---

"Niacin and niacinamide are equally effective for schizophrenia, but higher doses of niacin can be tolerated without nausea. Inositol hexaniacinate (a no-flush form of niacin) works, too, but not quite as well. Only niacin or inositol hexaniacinate can lower cholesterol; niacinamide does not."

— ABRAM HOFFER

---

greater levels of copper due to copper piping in modern homes and the widespread use of birth control pills (estrogen-based). Estrogen dominance is associated with higher circulating copper levels and copper is thought to transfer via placenta from generation to generation.[20] Other copper sources include copper tea pots, copper sulfate treated Jacuzzis or swimming pools, drinking water, dental fillings, prenatal vitamins, and copper intrauterine devices (IUDs). Neuroleptics (antipsychotics), antibiotics, antacids, cortisone, cimetidine (Tagamet), ranitidine (Zantac), and diuretics often encourage copper-dominant biochemistry.

The liver produces the copper-regulating proteins metallothionein and ceruloplasmin, and with low thyroid function, their hepatic protein synthesis is diminished. The body attempts to remove excess copper by excreting it out of the liver via gallbladder excretion to the bowel. Vitamin B3, vitamin C, and zinc are helpful clinically because of their physiological antagonism to copper.

Schizophrenics relapse when thyroid function is low.[21] Poor thyroid function encourages heavy metal retention. Conversely, heavy metals seem to play a major role in blocking peripheral enzyme conversion of thyroxine (T4) to triiodothyronine (T3).[22–25] Heavy metal removal involves mobilizing and eliminating the metal and this is often best done after thyroid function has been optimized. The organs involved in the elimination of the metal tend to function more efficiently when thyroid metabolism is intact. It is also essential to avoid environmental exposures to heavy metals.

Zinc and B6 Deficiency in Schizophrenia

Zinc and iron are the most concentrated metals in the human brain. Zinc is important to several biochemical pathways as over 200 enzymes are zinc dependant. Zinc deficiency is very common in schizophrenia.[7–9] Insufficient levels of zinc are also associated with depression, dementia, mental retardation, learning disability, lethargy, and apathy.[26] Zinc is essential for the synthesis of serotonin and melatonin.[20] It is crucial to brain development because it plays a major role in protein synthesis.[20,26] In the brain, zinc lowers excitability by moderating N-methyl-D-aspartate (NMDA) receptor

release of excitatory glutamate. Zinc is involved in the synthesis of inhibitory gamma-aminobutyric acid (GABA) by the modulation of glutamate decarboxylase activity. Among the zinc-dependant proteins are metallothionein, which is essential for heavy metal regulation and zinc bioavailability. The synthesis of metallothionein and the enzyme copper-zinc superoxide dismutase are essential in preventing oxidative damage.[20] Zinc protects against fatty-acid peroxidation, which destroys neuron structure and function. Zinc is involved in neuronal membrane structure and functioning and may play a key role in blood-brain-barrier integrity.[27] Zinc is involved in storing biogenic amines in small packages called synaptic vesicles and in their transport and release from the axon.

The biogenic amine histamine regulates nucleus accumbens activity, which is responsible for filtering sensory information and communicating with the amygdala, ventral tegmentum, and hypothalamus (structures in the limbic area that control emotional responses). In the limbic system, zinc is involved in the biochemistry of emotional regulation. In the pituitary gland and hypothalamus, zinc is involved in hormonal metabolism.

Vitamin B6 (pyridoxine) is involved in the breakdown of the amino acids tyrosine, tryptophan, and histidine into the neurotransmitters norepinephrine, serotonin, and histamine, respectively.[28] B6 deficiencies are associated with schizophrenia, depression, and behavior disorders. It is a cofactor in homocysteine remethylation.[29] Vitamin B6 has been found useful in memory acquisition, with just a 20-milligram (mg) dose.[30] It has demonstrated usefulness in controlling neuroleptic-induced akathisia (psychomotor restlessness) and drug-induced movement disorders.[31–33] B6 is essential for the synthesis of antioxidants such as metallothionein, glutathione, and CoQ10, which help prevent neuronal oxidative stress. Vitamin B6 (and zinc) are involved in the synthesis of glutamic acid decarboxylase (GAD), which blocks excitotoxicity with eventual secondary oxidative damage. Vitamin B6 is also essential for glutathione peroxidase and glutathione reductase, which are helpful in preventing decay of the mitochondria (parts of cells where energy is produced).

The major neurotransmitters of the brain are derived from protein building blocks and precisely assembled according to messenger RNA (mRNA) transcription of neuronal DNA templates. Brain tissue samples of schizophrenics have been assessed with high-dimensional biology and found to be compromised in basic mRNA transcription and protein synthesis.[3]

These perturbations influence an array of neuronal changes in the schizophrenic brain among which are neurotransmitter synthesis and mitochondrial functioning. Oxidative stress can cause these perturbations and the ensuing changes in neuronal structure and function may be integral in understanding schizophrenic pathophysiology.

It is interesting to note here that zinc and vitamin B6 together are needed by the body as cofactors for neurotransmitter synthesis; zinc is needed for transcription and B6 is needed for transamination. Previous investigators have described vitamin B6 and zinc depletion in the context of pyroluria. In this metabolic syndrome (where high amounts of kryptopyrroles circulate in the blood and manifest themselves as behavioral abnoralities), vitamin B6 and zinc interact with 2,4-dimethyl-3-ethylpyrrole and are readily excreted.[34–42]

Hypoadrenia in Schizophrenia

Thyroid and adrenal function are compromised in many schizophrenics.[21,43] The thyroid and adrenal are pivotal endocrine glands. Many symptoms common to adrenal dysfunction are seen in thyroid dysfunction and vice versa. The adrenal works in concert with the thyroid gland and often both glands need to be supported together.[44,45]

Hypothalamic-pituitary-adrenal axis dysregulation is integrally associated with schizophrenia.[21,43] The adrenal glands are involved in stress response, sugar metabolism, electrolyte balance, peripheral epinephrine synthesis, blood pressure regulation, and sex hormone metabolism. Many schizophrenics who are heavy coffee drinkers have low adrenal function. Low adrenal symptoms include sluggishness on waking, stress intolerance, lack of enjoyment, post-traumatic stress, addiction, dizziness, low blood pressure, fluctuant body temperature, insomnia at 4:00 A.M., immune compro-

mise, hypoglycemia, dermatitis, PMS, phobia, and poor libido. Schizophrenics can be warm at times and at other times cold with trouble adapting to daily temperature extremes. Fluctuant body temperatures and heat intolerance are a sign of low adrenal function, which often accompanies low thyroid function.[46] Adrenal symptoms are a good indicator of adrenal status. In some cases, saliva testing is useful to assess the adrenal hormones dehydroepiandrosterone (DHEA) and cortisol. Cortisol is part of the stress response but elevated cortisol disturbs mental function. Cortisol levels are commonly elevated in schizophrenics and depressives.[47,48] Adaptogens and supplements can be used effectively to support adrenal function without elevating cortisol.

Hypothyroidism in Schizophrenia

Active thyroid hormones are responsible for enabling cells at the DNA level to maintain their metabolic rate. Thyroid hormones also maintain oxygen availability in the brain and elsewhere. With healthy thyroid hormone function, our cells produce energy and complete their tasks efficiently. When tissue cells including neurons have energy, they work efficiently. When thyroid function is low, cells remain in a state of hypofunction. Hypofunctioning cells work slowly and produce minimal energy. Consequently, fewer enzymatic reactions occur, cells don't give off heat, and core body temperature decreases. Intolerance to cold is a typical complaint in low thyroid function.[21] When body temperature is insufficient, enzymatic reactions do not occur as readily, yet these reactions are needed throughout the body for, among other things, neurotransmitter synthesis. It is not uncommon to have schizophrenics report that they feel warm despite having low average body temperature.

Low thyroid symptoms are seen often in psychosis.[21,49–51] In treatment-resistant depression, psychiatric thyroid-augmentation treatment is frequently applied.[52,53] The most obvious low thyroid symptoms include impaired cognition, easy weight gain, fatigue, pain, headache, irritability, anxiety, panic, PMS, depression, poor memory, poor concentration, insomnia, constipation, indigestion, hair loss, high cholesterol, and frequent infection.[21,52,54,55]

The digestive tract of a low thyroid patient has poor motility and slow stool transit, which results in constipation and inefficient nutrient absorption.[56] In low thyroid patients, core body temperatures are often so low that digestive enzymes do not reach their reaction threshold. Patients with varied non-specific complaints often have low thyroid function.

Classic hypothyroidism, occurring in a small percentage of schizophrenics, is a problem with the inability to produce adequate thyroid hormone. In classic "conventional" hypothyroidism, blood tests show low output of thyroid hormone T4 with elevated thyroid-stimulating hormone (TSH) levels. Immune involvement as in Hashimoto's thyroiditis is usually seen in 80 percent of classic hypothyroid cases. In one study Othman and others assessed a sample of 249 chronic schizophrenics and reported a prevalence of thyroid antibodies in 20 percent of cases.[57] Many blood thyroid imbalances are found to correlate with the degree of symptom presentation, as for example, in acute psychotic episodes.[58]

The reliance on thyroid blood tests in schizophrenia leads practitioners astray because a large portion of schizophrenics show "normal" blood test measures but, paradoxically, have a low core body temperature and low thyroid symptoms (fatigue, psychosis, depression, etc). There is no accepted diagnostic agreement on this physiological state, however, Wilson's temperature syndrome (WTS) has emerged as a condition that meets this criteria. WTS factors in the possibility of inefficient conversion of T4 to active T3 despite having adequate circulating thyroid hormone T4.[52,53,59] In classic hypothyroidism and WTS, we can implement desiccated thyroid, sustained-release T3, and botanical medicine.

Brain Hypothyroidism

The brain is highly dependent on thyroid hormone for the regulation of dopamine, norepinephrine, and serotonin pathways.[50,60,61] Brain hypothyroidism has been described by Hatterer and others as a state that occurs when systemic T4 does not readily cross into the brain.[62] Active-thyroid hormone T3 is synthesized in the brain by brain type II 5'-deiodinase conversion of T4 to T3.[53,63] Brain neurons therefore depend on a ready supply of T4. The choroid plexus of the brain produces transthyretin (TTR), a transport protein that binds T4 and transports it across the blood-cerebral spinal fluid barrier to the brain.[63] Transthyretin is significantly decreased in the cerebral spinal fluid (CSF) of schizophrenics versus healthy controls.[64] This suggests that schizophrenics lack adequate amounts of T4 in the brain. Without adequate T4, brain cells remain hypometabolic and this may, among other things, reduce neurotransmitter synthesis and disrupt the regulation of dopamine, norepinephrine, and serotonin.

Huang and others suggest that low CSF transthyretin may prove useful as a biomarker for early diagnosis of schizophrenia.[65] Also of interest is the fact that lead has been linked to the reduction of CSF transthyretin in humans.[14,15] Reduced CSF transthyretin is also seen in depression and suicidal propensity.[66,67] Many schizophrenics and depressives relapse when thyroid function drops.[21]

Blood thyroid levels can be normal in the context of brain hypothyroidism. T4 to T3 conversion by brain type II 5'-deiodinase can be inhibited by cortisol.[68,69] This is important because cortisol levels are commonly elevated in schizophrenics, especially during stress. Cortisol is an adrenal stress hormone and, during stressful periods, we tend to conserve energy by shutting down thyroid hormone production.

Antithyroidal Adrenochrome

Adrenochrome is a quinone and many molecules in this class are antithyroidal. In schizophrenia, a ready supply of oxidized adrenaline may account for thyroid compromise. Adrenochrome has the ability to induce oxidative stress and functional changes in thyroid tissue and peripheral metabolism.[70–78] It is not known to what degree adrenochrome damages the thyroid gland. Skoliarova suggests that functional changes can be inferred from the structural "deterioration" of the thyroid and pituitary gland of chronic schizophrenics autopsied 20 minutes to five hours post-mortem.[79]

Thyroid Treatment

There are some remarkable studies reporting the outstanding efficacy of thyroid therapy in acute and chronic schizophrenia. A study by Danziger reported in 1958, showed that 100 days of optimally dosed desiccated thyroid or thyroxine with vitamin B complex lead to the full recovery of 54 (45 percent) of 80 schizophrenics.[80] Twenty of the 80 patients were given thyroid therapy alone while 60 of the 80 patients were given thyroid plus electroconvulsive therapy (ECT). Fifteen (75 percent) of the 20 patients given thyroid therapy recovered fully, and 39 (65 percent) of the 60 patients given thyroid therapy plus ECT recovered fully. Of the 15 patients, 2 were sick for 60 or more months, 2 were sick for 24–60 months, 5 were sick for 12–24 months, and 6 were sick less than 6 months. Of the 39 patients, 6 were sick for 60 or more months, 5 were sick for 24–60 months, 11 were sick for 12–24 months, and 17 were sick less than six months. After discharge, the incidence of relapse was very small with a maintenance treatment that kept the basal metabolic rate (BMR) in check. Full recovery was defined appropriately; that is, being "symptom-free, returning to a former place in society/occupation and accepted as well by family, friends and co-workers." The prognosis of the 80 patients at the onset of the study was "generally unpromising" as they were treatment resistant to ECT, psychoanalysis, and psychotherapy (none had taken antipsychotic medications before).

Many of the 80 schizophrenic patients reported by Danziger required high doses of natural desiccated thyroid (128–1,280 mg) or synthetic thyroxine (1–9 mg). Of the 54 patients that recovered with thyroid therapy or thyroid plus ECT, only four required 640 mg or more of desiccated thyroid, and only two required up to 4 mg of thyroxine. Such doses were probably required to combat adrenochrome's antithyroid effects and to make up for the lack of T4 transport from the CSF to the brain ("brain hypothyroidism"). Hoskins and others report on the tolerance of schizophrenics for even higher doses of desiccated thyroid than those used by Danziger.[81,82] To enable good treatment outcome, the BMR is raised to a level that likely improves the function and production of respiratory enzymes in the cerebrum.[83] In Danziger's study, first-episode cases had the best response,

however, one third of the chronic cases (five plus years post-onset) experienced full recovery as well.

A double-blind efficacy study reported by Lochner and others in 1963 used T3 (triiodothyronine) treatment in a six-week trial on 30 chronic male schizophrenics eight plus years post-onset.[84] Typical tranquilizers prescribed at the time were discontinued several weeks prior to treatment. Patients were included if they tolerated withdrawal without exhibiting aggressive behavior. Fifteen subjects were randomly assigned to the thyroid group and another 15 subjects to the placebo control group. Red blood cell uptake of iodine 131-T3 was normal for all subjects at baseline; they were euthyroid according to blood tests. The treatment group received 50 micrograms (mcg) of T3 two times a day for one week, then 100 mcg two times a day (200 mcg per day) for six weeks.

In this short treatment period, 7 of the 15 patients treated with T3 responded very well. They had improved motor activity, work performance, spontaneity, sociability, and logical/relevant thinking. Some reported they were "more lively" and could "think better." Mood improved and they showed interest in their environment. They showed improvements in executive functioning; some voiced "plans for the future" and wanted to visit relatives, return to work, and resume family relationships outside of the hospital. Five of the 15 patients had some worsening. Two of these five patients were responsive and cooperative with generally better mood but exhibited hallucinations and delusions that had been repressed and were tense, restless, and loquacious. Another two of these five patients became non-conversive and tense with reduced facial expression and motor retardation. The last of these five patients became incoherent, irritable, and explosive with increased hallucinations, delusions, and activity. The remaining 3 of the 15 experienced no change.

All schizophrenics returned to their previous state shortly after discontinuation of treatment. Lochner's study was reproduced by Scheuing and Flach with the same cohort, and a consensus of results was determined.[85] The results with T3 are impressive when you consider the short treatment duration, the long duration of the cohorts' illness, and the failure to implement optimal dosing strategy. Doses of 200 mcg of T3 may have been too high for those patients that aggravated in the given six-week time frame of the study. Conversely, 200 mcg may not have been a high enough dose for those schizophrenics that did not respond. To my knowledge, the use of T3 in first-episode schizophrenia has not been fully investigated.

Hoffer also reports on 12 schizophrenic patients treated with niacin and optimally dosed desiccated thyroid.[71] Of the 11 patients that completed the treatment, 9 had benefited. Six of the 9 were moving toward rapid recovery and had very much improved. The remaining 3 were improving consistent with increasing doses of desiccated thyroid. The average maintenance dose of desiccated thyroid was 300 mg per day.

As adrenochrome-reducing nutrients, vitamin B3 and C play a key role in reducing the oxidative stress on the thyroid gland. This thyroid link may explain in part, why vitamins B3 and C yield such good success in treatment. As a final note on thyroid function, blood testing can help rule out the hyperfunctioning state typical of Grave's disease.[58]

■ CONCLUSION

To summarize, the key causative factors of schizophrenia include essential fatty acid deficiency (oxidative stress), inadequate nutriture, hypoglycemia, food intolerance, digestive dysfunction, malabsorption, undermethylation (neurotransmitter deficiency), vitamin B3 deficiency, B6 deficiency, vitamin C deficiency, zinc deficiency, heavy metal toxicity, and thyroid and adrenal dysfunction. Modern research continually confirms that these factors are important to schizophrenic pathophysiology. This is why, in support of Dr. Hoffer's original

work, we now see downregulated niacin receptors in parts of the limbic system of schizophrenics.[86]

The list of assessments and treatments described herein is not exhaustive but represents the core considerations of optimal complementary treatment for schizophrenia. Orthomolecular treatment can be implemented safely as an adjunct to conventional psychiatric therapy. Schizophrenics treated with orthomolecular medicine experience positive changes. Response is based on the degree of severity and the duration of illness. We see schizophrenics who have been sick for a year or two who start responding within weeks. Schizophrenics sick over five years are less responsive initially but improve with long-term care. The pathological deterioration of brain tissue in schizophrenia should impel us to use orthomolecular treatment to keep oxidative stress at bay. The necessity of early screening and early intervention is important for both orthomolecular and conventional psychiatric treatment. In first-episode cases, a cocktail of desiccated thyroid (or sustained-release T3), vitamin B3, and vitamin C may be the best early detection-intervention program ever developed. Complementary treatments for schizophrenia have been in the workings since the 1930s. A large outcome study is needed to compare the efficacy of orthomolecular treatment versus psychiatric medication.

Orthomolecular treatment should play a key role in mainstream mental health care and schizophrenic patients/families constantly express their desire to see that happen.[87,88] Conventional mental health costs are exorbitant in comparison to orthomolecular treatment costs and the potential for improved quality of life should empower practitioners to be steadfast in addressing core underlying biochemistry.[89]

660

REFERENCES: PART 1

1. Fendri C, Mechri A, Khiari G, et al. Oxidative stress involvement in schizophrenia pathophysiology: a review. *Encephale* 2006;32(2 Pt 1):244–252.

2. Gattaz WF, Schmitt A, Maras A. Increased platelet phospholipase A2 activity in schizophrenia. *Schizophr Res* 1995;16(1): 1–6.

3. Song C, Zhao S. Omega-3 fatty acid eicosapentaenoic acid. A new treatment for psychiatric and neurodegenerative diseases: a review of clinical investigations. *Expert Opin Investig Drugs* 2007;16(10):1627–1638.

4. Das UN. Can perinatal supplementation of long-chain polyunsaturated fatty acids prevents schizophrenia in adult life? *Med Sci Monit* 2004;10(12):HY33-HY37.

5. Greenwood CE, Young SN. Dietary fat intake and the brain: a developing frontier in biological psychiatry. *J Psychiatry Neurosci* 2001;26(3):182–184.

6. Freeman MP. Omega-3 fatty acids in psychiatry: a review. *Ann Clin Psychiatry* 2000;12(3):159–165.

7. Horrobin DF. Treatment of schizophrenia with eicosapentaenoic acid (EPA). Nutritional Medicine Today 29th Annual Conference. Vancouver, BC, Apr 8, 2000.

8. Bennett CN, Horrobin DF. Gene targets related to phospholipid and fatty acid metabolism in schizophrenia and other psychiatric disorders: an update. *Prostaglandins Leukot Essent Fatty Acids* 2000;63(1–2):47–59.

9. Richardson AJ, Easton T, Puri BK. Red cell and plasma fatty acid changes accompanying symptom remission in a patient with schizophrenia treated with eicosapentaenoic acid. *Eur Neuropsychopharmacol* 2000;10(3):189–193.

10. Puri BK, Richardson AJ, Horrobin DF, et al. Eicosapentaenoic acid treatment in schizophrenia associated with symptom remission, normalisation of blood fatty acids, reduced neuronal membrane phospholipid turnover and structural brain changes. *Int J Clin Pract* 2000; 54(1):57–63.

11. Horrobin DF. The membrane phospholipid hypothesis as a biochemical basis for the neurodevelopmental concept of schizophrenia. *Schizophr Res* 1998;30(3):193–208.

12. Puri BK, Easton T, Richardson AJ. Normalisation of positive and negative symptoms of schizophrenia following dietary supplementation with essential fatty acids: a case study. *Biol Psychiat* 1997;42:189S.

13. Koletzko B, Agostoni C, Carlson SE, et al. Long-chain polyunsaturated fatty acids (LC-PUFA) and perinatal development. *Acta Paediatr* 2001;90(4):460–464.

14. Smesny S, Rosburg T, Riemann S, et al. Impaired niacin sensitivity in acute first-episode but not in multi-episode schizophrenia. *Prostaglandins Leukot Essent Fatty Acids* 2005;72(6): 393–402.

15. Rao J, Oz G, Seaquist ER. Regulation of cerebral glucose metabolism. *Minerva Endocrinol* 2006;31(2):149–158.

16. McDermott E, de Silva P. Impaired neuronal glucose uptake in pathogenesis of schizophrenia–can GLUT 1 and GLUT 3 deficits explain imaging, post-mortem and pharmacological findings? *Med Hypotheses* 2005;65(6):1076–1081.

17. Voruganti LP, Punthakee Z, Van Lieshout RJ, et al. Dysglycemia in a community sample of people treated for schizophrenia: the Diabetes in Schizophrenia in Central-South Ontario (DiSCO) study. *Schizophr Res* 2007;96(1–3):215–222.

18. Bergman RN, Ader M. Atypical antipsychotics and glucose homeostasis. *J Clin Psychiatry* 2005;66(4):504–514.

19. Cox D, Gonder-Frederick L, McCall A, et al. The effects of glucose fluctuation on cognitive function and QOL: the functional costs of hypoglycaemia and hyperglycaemia among adults with type 1 or type 2 diabetes. *Int J Clin Pract Suppl* 2002;129:20–26.

20. Mitrakou A, Ryan C, Veneman T, et al. Hierarchy of glycemic thresholds for counter regulatory hormone secretion, symptoms, and cerebral dysfunction. *Am J Physiol* 1991;260(1 Pt 1): E67–E74.

21. Hardman G, Hart G. Dietary advice based on food-specific IgG results. *Nutrition & Food Science* 2007;37(1):16–23.

22. Jackson JA, Neathery S, Kirby R. Hidden food sensitivities: a common cause of many illnesses. *J Orthomolecular Med* 2007;22(1):27–30.

23. Cade R, et al. Autism and schizophrenia: intestinal disorders. *Nutritional Neuroscience* 2000.

24. Crowe SE, Perdue MH. Gastrointestinal food hypersensitivity: basic mechanisms of pathophysiology. *Gastroenterology* 1992;103(3):1075–1095.

25. Hall K. Allergy of the nervous system: a review. *Annals of Allergy* 1976;36(1):49–64.

26. Takahashi M, Fukunaga H, Kaneto H, et al. Behavioral and pharmacological studies on gluten exorphin A5, a newly isolated bioactive food protein fragment, in mice. *Jpn J Pharmacol* 2000; 84(3):259–265.

27. Dohan FC. Genetic hypothesis of idiopathic schizophrenia: its exorphin connection. *Schizophr Bull* 1988;14(4):489–494.

28. King DS. Psychological and behavioral effects of food and chemical exposure in sensitive individuals. *Nutr Health* 1984;3(3):137–151.

29. Ross-Smith P, Jenner FA. Diet (gluten) and schizophrenia. *J Hum Nutr* 1980;34(2):107–112.

30. Atkinson W, Sheldon TA, Shaath N, et al. Food elimination based on IgG antibodies in irritable bowel syndrome: a randomised controlled trial. *Gut* 2004;53(10):1459–1464.

31. Edelman E. *Natural Healing for Schizophrenia: A Compendium of Nutritional Methods.* Eugene, OR: Borage Books, 1996.

32. Kalaydjian AE, Eaton W, Cascella N, et al. The gluten connection: the association between schizophrenia and celiac disease. *Acta Psychiatr Scand* 2006;113(2):82–90.

33. Haidemenos A, Kontis D, Gazi A, et al. Plasma homocysteine, folate and B12 in chronic schizophrenia. *Prog Neuropsychopharmacol Biol Psychiatry* 2007;31(6):1289–1296.

34. Herrmann W, Obeid R. Review: biomarkers of folate and vitamin B(12) status in cerebrospinal fluid. *Clin Chem Lab Med* 2007;45(12):1614–1620.

35. Herrmann W, Lorenzl S, Obeid R. Review of the role of hyperhomocysteinemia and B-vitamin deficiency in neurological and psychiatric disorders–current evidence and preliminary recommendations. *Fortschr Neurol Psychiatr* 2007;75(9):515–527.

36. Zammit S, Lewis S, Gunnell D, et al. Schizophrenia and neural tube defects: comparisons from an epidemiological perspective. *Schizophr Bull* 2007 Jul;33(4):853–858.

37. Regland B. Schizophrenia and single-carbon metabolism. *Prog Neuropsychopharmacol Biol Psychiatry* 2005;29(7):1124–1132.

38. Neeman G, Blanaru M, Bloch B, et al. Relation of plasma glycine, serine, and homocysteine levels to schizophrenia symptoms and medication type. *Am J Psychiatry* 2005;162(9): 1738–1740.

39. Regland B, Germgård T, Gottfries CG, et al. Homozygous thermolabilemethylenetetrahydrofolate reductase in schizophrenia-like psychosis. *J Neural Transm* 1997;104(8–9):931–941.

40. Regland B, Johansson BV, Gottfries CG. Homocysteinemia and schizophrenia as a case of methylation deficiency. *J Neural Transm Gen Sect* 1994;98(2):143–152.

41. Freeman JM, Finkelstein JD, Mudd SH. Folateresponsive homocystinuria and "schizophrenia." A defect in methylation due to deficient 5,10-methylenetetrahydrofolate reductase activity. *N Engl J Med* 1975;292(10):491–496.

42. Goff DC, Bottiglieri T, Arning E, et al. Folate, homocysteine, and negative symptoms in schizophrenia. *Am J Psychiatry* 2004;161(9):1705–1708.

43. Gilbody S, Lewis S, Lightfoot T. Methylenetetrahydrofolate reductase (MTHFR) genetic polymorphisms and psychiatric disorders: a HuGE review. *Am J Epidemiol* 2007;165(1):1–13.

44. Roffman JL, Weiss AP, Purcell S, et al. Contribution of methylenetetrahydrofolate reductase (MTHFR) polymorphisms to negative symptoms in schizophrenia. *Biol Psychiatry* 2008;63 (1):42–48.

45. Casas JP, Bautista LE, Smeeth L, et al. Homocysteine and stroke: evidence on a causal link from mendelian randomisation. *Lancet* 2005;365(9455):224–232.

46. Regland B, Johansson BV, Grenfeldt B, et al. Homocysteinemia is a common feature of schizophrenia. *J Neural Transm Gen Sect* 1995;100(2):165–169.

47. Parnetti L, Bottiglieri T, Lowenthal D. Role of homocysteine in age-related vascular and non-vascular diseases. *Aging* (Milan, Italy) 1997;9(4):241–257.

48. Zaremba S, Hogue-Angeletti R. NADH: (acceptor) oxidoreductase from bovine adrenal medulla chromaffin granules. *Arch Biochem Biophys* 1982;219(2):297–305.

49. Wakefield LM, Cass AE, Radda GK. Functional coupling between enzymes of the chromaffin granule membrane. *J Biol Chem* 1986;261(21):9739–9745.

50. Paris I, Cardenas S, Lozano J, et al. Amino-chrome as a preclinical experimental model to study degeneration of dopaminergic neurons in Parkinson's disease. *Neurotox Res* 2007; 12(2):125–134.

51. Graumann R, Paris I, Martinez-Alvarado P, et al. Oxidation of dopamine to aminochrome as a mechanism for neurodegeneration of dopaminergic systems in Parkinson's disease. Possible neuroprotective role of DT-diaphorase. *Pol J Pharmacol* 2002;54(6):573–579.

52. Smythies JR. Oxidative reactions and schizophrenia: a review-discussion. *Schizophr Res* 1997;24(3):357–364.

53. Smythies J. On the function of neuromelanin. *Proc Biol Sci* 1996;263(1369):487–489.

54. Smythies J. Redox aspects of signaling by catecholamines and their metabolites. *Antioxid Redox Signal* 2000;2(3): 575–583.

55. Siraki AG, O'Brien PJ. Prooxidant activity of free radicals derived from phenol-containing neurotransmitters. *Toxicology* 2002;177(1):81–90.

56. Sunderland GT, Belch JJ, Sturrock RD, et al. A double-blind randomized placebo controlled trial of Hexopal in primary Raynaud's disease. *Clin Rheumatol* 1988;7(1):46–49.

57. Ring EFJ, Porto LO, Bacon PA. Quantitative thermal imaging to assess inositol nicotinate treatment for Raynaud's syndrome. *J Int Med Res* 1981;9:393–400.

58. Holti G. An experimentally controlled evaluation of the effect of inositol nicotinate upon the digital blood flow in patients with Raynaud's phenomenon. *J Int Med Res* 1979;7:473–483.

59. Berge KG, Canner PL. Coronary drug project: experience with niacin. Coronary Drug Project Research Group. *Eur J Clin Pharmacol* 1991;40(Suppl1):S49–S51.

60. Pauling L. *How to Live Longer and Feel Better*. New York: W.H. Freeman & Co, 1986.

61. Pitche PT. Service de dermatologie. *Sante* 2005;15(3): 205–208.

62. Hoffer A. Vitamin B3 dependency: chronic pellagra. *Townsend Lett for Doctors & Patients* 2000;207:66–73.

63. Hoffer A. *Orthomolecular Treatment For Schizophrenia: Megavitamin Supplements and Nutritional Strategies for Healing and Recovery*. Los Angeles: Keats Publishing, 1999.

64. Hoffer A. Orthomolecular treatment for schizophrenia. *Natural Med J* 1999;2(3):12–13.

65. Hoffer A. *Vitamin B-3 and Schizophrenia: Discovery, Recovery, Controversy*. Kingston, ON: Quarry Press, 1998.

66. Hoffer A. Correspondence: follow-up reports on chronic schizophrenic patients. *J Orthomolecular Med* 1994;121–123.

67. Hoffer A. Chronic schizophrenia patients treated ten years or more. *J Orthomolecular Med* 1994;9(1):7–37.

68. Hoffer A. Orthomolecular Medicine. In: *Molecules in Natural Science and Medicine: An Encomium for Linus Pauling* edited by ZB Maksic and M Eckert-Maksic. Chichester, England: Ellis Horwood Ltd, 1991.

69. Hoffer A. *Orthomolecular Medicine for Physicians*. New Canaan, CT: Keats Publishing, 1989.

70. Hoffer A. *Common Questions on Schizophrenia and Their Answers*. New Canaan, CT: Keats Publishing, 1987:129–146.

71. Hoffer A. The adrenochrome hypothesis of schizophrenia revisited. *Orthomol Psychiat* 1981;10(2):98–118.

72. Hoffer A, Osmond H. Schizophrenia: another long term follow-up in Canada. *Orthomol Psychiat* 1980;9(2):107–115.

73. Hoffer A, Osmond H. In reply to the American Psychiatric Association Task Force Report on Megavitamins and Orthomolecular Therapy in Psychiatry. Burnaby, BC: Canadian Schizophrenia Foundation, 1976.

74. Hoffer A. Natural history and treatment of thirteen pairs of identical twins, schizophrenic and schizophrenic-spectrum conditions. *Orthomol Psychiat* 1976;5:101–122.

75. Hoffer A. Mechanism of action of nicotinic acid and nicotinamide in the treatment of schizophrenia. In: *Orthomolecular Psychiatry* edited by D Hawkins and L Pauling. San Francisco: W.H. Freeman & Co, 1973.

76. Hoffer A. Treatment of schizophrenia with a therapeutic program based upon nicotinic acid as the main variable. Vol 2. In: *Molecular Basis of Some Aspects of Mental Activity* edited by O Walaas. New York: Academic Press, 1967.

77. Hoffer A. Five California schizophrenics. *J Schizophren* 1967;1:209–220.

78. Hoffer A, Osmond H. *How to Live With Schizophrenia.* Rev. ed. New York: University Books, 1997.

79. Hoffer A, Osmond H. *The Chemical Basis of Clinical Psychiatry.* Springfield, IL: C.C. Thomas, 1960.

80. Hoffer A, Osmond H, Callbeck MJ, et al. Treatment of schizophrenia with nicotinic acid and nicotinamide. *J Clin Exper Psychopathol & Quart Rev Psychiat Neurol* 1957;18(2):131–158.

81. Dardanelli L, Del Pilar Garcia AM. Successful recoveries with orthomolecular treatment. *J Orthomolecular Med* 2001;16(1):52–58.

82. Wenzel KG. Orthomolecular treatment for mental health: the roles of hypoglycemia, pyrroluria and histamine disturbances, 2000. Nutritional Medicine Today 29th Annual Conference, Vancouver, BC, Apr 8, 2000.

83. Walsh WJ. *Biochemical Treatment of Mental Illness and Behavior Disorders.* Naperville, IL: Health Research Institute, 1997.

REFERENCES: PART 2

1. Kelly G. Peripheral metabolism of thyroid hormones: a review. *Altern Med Rev* 2000;5(4):306–333.

2. Aschner M, Cherian MG, Klaassen CD, et al. Metallothioneins in brain: the role in physiology and pathology. *Toxicol Appl Pharmacol* 1997;142(2):229–242.

3. Prabakaran S, Swatton JE, Ryan MM, et al. Mitochondrial dysfunction in schizophrenia: evidence for compromised brain metabolism and oxidative stress. *Molec Psychiat* 2004;9(7):684–697, 643.

4. Yao JK, Reddy RD, van Kammen DP. Oxidative damage and schizophrenia: an overview of the evidence and its therapeutic implications. *CNS Drugs* 2001;15(4):287–310.

5. Kunert HJ, Norra C, Hoff P. Theories of delusional disorders. An update and review. *Psychopathology* 2007;40(3):191–202.

6. Wolf TL, Kotun J, Meador-Woodruff JH. Plasma copper, iron, ceruloplasmin and ferroxidase activity in schizophrenia. *Schizophr Res* 2006;86(1–3):167–171.

7. Stanley PC, Wakwe VC. Toxic trace metals in the mentally ill patients. *Niger Postgrad Med J* 2002;9(4):199–204.

8. Wallwork JC. Zinc and the central nervous system. *Prog Food Nutr Sci* 1987;11(2):203247.

9. Ebadi M, Iversen PL, Hao R, et al. Expression and regulation of brain metallothionein. *Neurochem Int* 1995;27(1):1–22.

10. Chimienti F, Jourdan E, Favier A, et al. Zinc resistance impairs sensitivity to oxidative stress in HeLa cells: protection through metallothioneins expression. *Free Radic Biol Med* 2001;31(10):1179–1190.

11. Aschner M. The functional significance of brain metallothioneins. *FASEB J* 1996;10(10):1129–1136.

12. Goyer RA. Nutrition and metal toxicity. *Am J Clin Nutr* 1995;61(3 Suppl):646S–650S.

13. Bahiga LM, Kotb NA, El-Dessoukey EA. Neurological syndromes produced by some toxic metals encountered industrially or environmentally. *Z Ernahrungswiss* 1978;17(2):84–88.

14. Zheng W, Lu YM, Lu GY, et al. Transthyretin, thyroxine, and retinol-binding protein in human cerebrospinal fluid: effect of lead exposure. *Toxicol Sci* 2001;61(1):107–114.

15. Zheng W, Blaner WS, Zhao Q. Inhibition by lead of production and secretion of transthyretin in the choroid plexus: its relation to thyroxine transport at blood-CSF barrier. *Toxicol Appl Pharmacol* 1999;155(1):24–31.

16. Wenzel KG, Pataracchia RJ. *The Earth's Gift to Medicine: Minerals in Health and Disease.* Alton, ON: KOS Publishing, 2005.

17. Rajanna B, Hobson M. Influence of mercury on uptake of [3H]dopamine and [3H]norepinephrine by rat brain synaptosomes. *Toxicol Lett* 1985;27(1–3):7–14.

18. Foster HD. What Really Causes Alzheimer's Disease? 2004. Avaliable at: www.hdfoster.com.

19. Rigobello MP, Scutari G, Boscolo R, et al. Oxidation of adrenaline and its derivatives by S-nitrosoglutathione. *Nitric Oxide* 2001;5(1):39–46.

20. Johnson S. Micronutrient accumulation and depletion in schizophrenia, epilepsy, autism and Parkinson's disease? *Med Hypothesis* 2001;56(5):641–645.

21. Heinrich TW, Grahm G. Hypothyroidism Presenting as Psychosis: Myxedema Madness Revisited. Prim Care Companion. *J Clin Psychiat* 2003;5(6):260–266.

22. Gupta P, Kar A. Cadmium induced thyroid dysfunction in chicken: hepatic type I iodothyronine 5'-monodeiodinase activity and role of lipid peroxidation. *Comp Biochem Physiol C Pharmacol Toxicol Endocrinol* 1999;123(1):39–44.

23. Gupta P, Kar A. Role of ascorbic acid in cadmium-induced thyroid dysfunction and lipid peroxidation. *J Appl Toxicol* 1998;18(5):317–320.

24. Chaurasia SS, Kar A. Protective effects of vitamin E against lead-induced deterioration of membrane associated type-I iodothyronine 5'-monodeiodinase (5'D-I) activity in male mice. *Toxicology* 1997;124(3):203–209.

25. Barregård L, Lindstedt G, Schütz A, et al. Endocrine function in mercury exposed chloralkali workers. *Occup Environ Med* 1994;51(8):536–540.

26. Pfeiffer CC, Braverman ER. Zinc, the brain and behaviour. *Biol Psychiat* 1982;17(4):513–532.

27. Noseworthy MD, Bray TM. Zinc deficiency exacerbates loss in blood-brain barrier integrity induced by hyperoxia measured by dynamic MRI. *Proc Soc Exp Biol Med* 2000;223(2):175–182.

28. Marz RB. *Medical Nutrition from Marz*. Portland, OR: Omni-Press, 1997.

29. Levine J, Stahl Z, Sela BA, et al. Homocysteine-reducing strategies improve symptoms in chronic schizophrenic patients with hyperhomocysteinemia. *Biol Psychiat* 2006;60(3): 265–269.

30. Deijen JB, van der Beek EJ, Orlebeke JF, et al. Vitamin B6 supplementation in elderly men: effects on mood, memory, performance and mental effort. *Psychopharmacology* (Berl), 1992;109(4):489–496.

31. Lerner V, Bergman J, Statsenko N, et al. Vitamin B6 treatment in acute neuroleptic-induced akathisia: a randomized, double-blind, placebo-controlled study. *J Clin Psychiat* 2004;65(11): 1550–1554.

32. Lerner V, Kaptsan A, Miodownik C, et al. Vitamin B6 in treatment of tardive dyskinesia: a preliminary case series study. *Clin Neuropharmacol* 1999;22(4):241–243.

33. Sandyk R, Pardeshi R. Pyridoxine improves drug-induced parkinsonism and psychosis in a schizophrenic patient. *Int J Neurosci* 1990;52(3–4):225–232.

34. Wenzel KG. Orthomolecular Treatment for Mental Health: The Roles of Hypoglycemia, Pyrroluria and Histamine Disturbances. Nutritional Medicine Today 29th Annual Conference. Vancouver, BC, Apr 8, 2000.

35. Jackson JA, Riordan HD, Neathery S, et al. Case from the center: urinary pyrrole in health and disease. *J Orthomolecular Med* 1997;12(2):96–98.

36. Edelman E. *Natural Healing for Schizophrenia: A Compendium of Nutritional Methods*. Eugene, OR: Borage Books. 1996.

37. Hoffer A. Schizophrenia: an evolutionary defense against severe stress. *J Orthomolecular Med* 1994;9(4):205–221.

38. Pfeiffer CC. *Mental and Elemental Nutrients*. New Canaan, CT: Keats Publishing, 1975.

39. Sohler A, Holsztynska E, Pfeiffer CC. A Rapid Screening Test for Pyroluria;Useful in Distinguishing a Schizophrenic Subpopulation. *J Orthomolecular Psych* 1974;3:273–279.

40. Pfeiffer CC, Iliev V. Pyrroluria, urinary mauve factor, causes double deficiency of B6 and zinc in schizophrenics. *Fed Proc* 1973;32:276.

41. Sohler A, Beck R, Noval JJ. Mauve factor re-identified as 2,4-dimethyl-3-ethylpyrrole and its sedative effect on the CNS. *Nature* 1970;228(278):1318–1320.

42. McGinnis WR, Audhya T, Walsh WJ, et al. Discerning the mauve factor. Part 1. *Altern Ther* 2008(Mar/Apr);14(2):40–50.

43. Mello AA, Mello MF, Carpenter LL, et al. Update on stress and depression: the role of the hypothalamic-pituitary-adrenal (HPA) axis. *Rev Bras Psiquiatr* 2003;25(4):231–238.

44. Abdullatif HD, Ashraf AP. Reversible subclinical hypothyroidism in the presence of adrenal insufficiency. *Endocr Pract* 2006;12(5):572.

45. Candrina R, Giustina G. Addison's disease and corticosteroid-reversible hypothyroidism. *J Endocrinol Invest* 1987;10(5):523–526.

46. Michel V, Peinnequin A, Alonso A, et al. Decreased heat tolerance is associated with hypothalamo-pituitary-adrenocortical axis impairment. *Neurosci* 2007;147(2):522–531.

47. Ritsner M, Maayan R, Gibel A, et al. Elevation of the cortisol/dehydroepiandrosterone ratio in schizophrenia patients. *Eur Neuropsychopharmacol* 2004;14(4):267–273.

48. Swigar ME, Kolakowska T, Quinlan DM. Plasma cortisol levels in depression and other psychiatric disorders: a study of newly admitted psychiatric patients. *Psychol Med* 1979;9(3):449–455.

49. Contreras F, Menchon JM, Urretavizcaya M, et al. Hormonal differences between psychotic and non-psychotic melancholic depression. *J Affect Disord* 2007;100(1–3):65–73.

50. Bauer M, London ED, Silverman DH, et al. Thyroid, brain and mood modulation in affective disorder: insights from molecular research and functional brain imaging. *Pharmacopsychiat* 2003;36 Suppl 3:S215–S221.

51. McGaffee J, Barnes MA, Lippmann S. Psychiatric presentations of hypothyroidism. *Am Fam Physician* 1981;23(5):129–133.

52. Jackson IM. The thyroid axis and depression. *Thyroid* 1998;8(10):951–956.

53. Oppenheimer JH, Braverman LE, Toft A, et al. A therapeutic controversy. Thyroid hormone treatment: when and what? *J Clin Endocrinol Metab* 1995;80(10):2873–2883.

54. Westphal SA. Unusual presentations of hypothyroidism. *Am J Med Sci* 1997;314(5):333–337.

55. Heitman B, Irizarry A. Hypothyroidism: common complaints, perplexing diagnosis. *Nurse Pract* 1995;20(3):54–60.

56. Shafer RB, Prentiss RA, Bond JH. Gastrointestinal transit in thyroid disease. *Gastroenterol* 1984;86(5 Pt 1):852–855.

57. Othman SS, Kadir KA, Hassan J, et al. High prevalence of thyroid function test abnormalities in chronic schizophrenia. *Australian and NZ J Psychiat* 1994;28:620–624.

58. Roca RP, Blackman MR, Ackerley SM, et al. Thyroid hormone elevations during acute psychiatric illness: relationship to severity and distinction from hyperthyroidism. *Endocrine Res* 1990;16(4):415–447.

59. Lum SM, Nicoloff JT, Spencer CA, et al. Peripheral tissue mechanism for maintenance of serum triiodothyronine values in a thyroxine-deficient state in man. *J Clin Invest* 1984;73(2): 570–575.

60. Haddow JE, Palomaki GE, Allan WC, et al. Maternal thyroid deficiency during pregnancy and subsequent neuropsychological development of the child. *N Engl J Med* 1999;341(8):549–555.

61. Brouwer A, Morse DC, Lans MC, et al. Interactions of persistent environmental organohalogens with the thyroid hormone system: mechanisms and possible consequences for animal and human health. *Toxicol Ind Health* 1998;14(1–2):59–84.

62. Hatterer JA, Herbert J, Hidaka C, et al. CSF transthyretin in patients with depression. *Am J Psychiat* 1993;150(5):813–815.

63. Schreiber G. The evolutionary and integrative roles of transthyretin in thyroid hormone homeostasis. *J Endocrinol* 2002;175(1):61–73.

64. Wan C, Yang Y, Li H, et al. Dysregulation of retinoid transporters expression in body fluids of schizophrenia patients. *J Proteome Res* 2006;5(11):3213–3216.

65. Huang JT, Leweke FM, Oxley D, et al. Disease biomarkers in cerebrospinal fluid of patients with first-onset psychosis. *PLoS Med* 2006;3(11):e428.

66. Sullivan GM, Mann JJ, Oquendo MA, et al. Low cerebrospinal fluid transthyretin levels in depression: correlations with suicidal ideation and low serotonin function. *Biol Psychiat* 2006;60(5):500–506.

67. Sullivan GM, Hatterer JA, Herbert J, et al. Low levels of transthyretin in the CSF of depressed patients. *Am J Psychiat* 1999;156(5):710–715.

68. Hidal JT, Kaplan MM. Inhibition of thyroxine 5'-deiodination type II in cultured human placental cells by cortisol, insulin, 3',5'-cyclic adenosine monophosphate, and butyrate. *Metabolism* 1988;37(7):664–668.

69. Visser TJ, Leonard JL, Kaplan MM, et al. Kinetic evidence suggesting two mechanisms for iodothyronine 5'-deiodination in rat cerebral cortex. *Proc Natl Acad Sci, USA* 1982;79(16):5080–5084.

70. Foster HD. What really causes schizophrenia? 2003. Available at: www.hdfoster.com.

71. Hoffer A. Thyroid and schizophrenia. *J Orthomolecular Med* 2001;16(4):205–212.

72. Langer P, Földes O. Effect of adrenaline on biliary excretion of triiodothyronines in rats mediated by alpha 1-adrenoceptors and related to the inhibition of 5'-monodeiodination in liver. *J Endocrinol Invest* 1988;11(7):471–476.

73. Nauman A, Kamin ski T, Herbaczyn ska-Cedro K. In vivo and in vitro effects of adrenaline on conversion of thyroxine to triiodothyronine and to reverse-triiodothyronine in dog liver and heart. *Eur J Clin Invest* 1980(Jun);10(3):189–192.

74. Ceremuzyn ski L, Herbaczyn ska-Cedro K, Broniszewska-Ardelt B, et al. Evidence for the detrimental effect of adrenaline infused to healthy dogs in doses imitating spontaneous secretion after coronary occlusion. *Cardiovasc Res* 1978;12(3):179–189.

75. Maayan ML, Ingbar SH. Effects of epinephrine on iodine and intermediary metabolism in isolated thyroid cells. *Endocrinology*, 1970;87(3):588–595.

76. Hoffer A, Osmond H. *The Hallucinogens*. Academic Press, New York, 1967.

77. Hupka S, Dumont JE. In vitro effect of adrenaline and other amines on glucose metabolism in sheep thyroid, heart, liver, kidney and testicular slices. *Biochem Pharmacol* 1963;12:1023–1035.

78. Pastan I, Herring B, Johnson P, et al. Studies on the mechanism by which epinephrine stimulates glucose oxidation in the thyroid. *J Biol Chem* 1962;237(2):287–290.

79. Skoliarova NA. Morphology of the endocrine system in schizophrenia according to early autopsy findings (the hypophyseal-thyroid system). *Zh Nevropatol Psikhiatr Im S S Korsakova* 1975;75(7):1045–53.

80. Danziger L. Thyroid therapy of schizophrenia. *Dis Nerv Syst* 1958;19(9):373–378.

81. Hoskins RG, Sleeper FH. The thyroid factor in dementia praecox. *Am J Psychiat* 1930;87:411–432.

82. Hoskins RG, Walsh A. Oxygen consumption ("Basal Metabolic rate") in schizophrenia: II. Distribution in 214 cases. *AMA Arch Neurol Psychiat* 1932;28:1346–1364.

83. Danziger L, Kindwall JA. Thyroid therapy in some mental disorders. *Dis Nerv Syst* 1953;14(1):3–13.

84. Lochner KH, Scheuing MR, Flach FF. The effect of L-triiodothyronine on chronic schizophrenic patients. *Acta Psychiatr Scand* 1963;39:413–26.

85. Scheuing MR, Flach FF. The effect of L-triiodothyronine on chronic schizophrenic patients. *Am J Psychiat* 1964;121:594–595.

86. Miller CL, Dulay JR. The high-affinity niacin receptor HM74A is decreased in the anterior cingulate cortex of individuals with schizophrenia. *Brain Res Bull* 2008;77(1):33–41.

87. Zammit S, Lewis S, Gunnell D, et al. Schizophrenia and neural tube defects: comparisons from an epidemiological perspective. *Schizophr Bull* 2007;33(4):853–858.

88. Regland B. Schizophrenia and single-carbon metabolism. *Prog Neuropsychopharmacol Biol Psychiatry* 2005;29(7):1124–1132.

89. Rössler W, Salize HJ, van Os J, et al. Size of burden of schizophrenia and psychotic disorders. *Eur Neuropsychopharmacol* 2005;15(4):399–409.

CHRONIC SCHIZOPHRENIC PATIENTS TREATED 10 YEARS OR MORE
by Abram Hoffer, MD, PhD

Dr. Humphry Osmond and I began to use niacin (vitamin B3) and ascorbic acid (vitamin C) in large doses for treating acute schizophrenics in 1951. Based on the results obtained from pilot studies, we began the first double-blind therapeutic trials in the history of psychiatry in 1953. By then we knew that these vitamins were safe even in multigram doses, that they could be taken for long periods of time, and that the side effects were minimal and easily dealt with. Our first two double-blind experiments showed that patients who were given vitamin B3 in doses of at least 3,000 millgrams (mg) per day had a much better prognosis compared to those who received a placebo. We concluded that the addition of this vitamin to the standard treatment of that day doubled the two-year recovery rate of acute schizophrenics. Our second conclusion was that chronic patients did not respond to this vitamin, even with large doses. This was based upon a large number of patients we had treated at University Hospital in Saskatchewan, and upon a study completed by Dr. O'Reilly in 1955. O'Reilly was a research psychiatrist associated with our research group. He found that there was slight therapeutic activity, but we did not think it was adequate to alter our conclusion.

These two main conclusions are very important in view of the controversy that erupted following our reports of the therapeutic efficacy of vitamin B3 because the investigators who tried to repeat our work did so by not repeating it. That is, they used chronic patients without acknowledging that their patients were different from the type we had used and on whom we had based our original claims. When they did their studies with chronic patients, they found as we had, that there was no response. The only investigator who tried to corroborate our conclusions was Dr. Wittenberg,[58,59] who published two studies. In the first, he found no significant improvement over the placebo. In the second, he found that the acute members of their group responded exactly the same as had our acute patients. Two-thirds of his group were chronic and they had not responded. Wittenberg

thus completely confirmed our claims. However, the critics have since then refused to refer to his second paper, while giving full publicity to his first paper. I had been placing almost all the patients under my care on vitamin B3, whether acute or chronic, and eventually I began to accumulate evidence that it did have substantial activity but that it took a long time for it to become manifest, and it required the use of other nutrients and medication as well.[8,9,37,41,46]

Since 1965 I have treated a very large number of chronic patients using the entire orthomolecular approach. The results have been much superior to those seen when only drugs are used. I concluded long ago that for these patients the best treatment must include everything that is available. The results are not as good as they are for acute patients, but a major proportion of the patients can be returned to a life that falls into a range normal for our diverse society.

Follow-Up Results from First Double-Blind Studies

Antipsychotic drugs were introduced with great fanfare once the initial resistance from the National Institutes of Mental Health in Washington was overcome. The initial skepticism of psychiatrists was replaced by an overly enthusiastic evaluation that these drugs would rapidly restore patients to health. In our report in 1964, Dr. Osmond and I summarized the results of a 10-year follow-up of patients treated in two psychiatric wards in Saskatchewan. From that report,[37] we showed that patients treated with naicin plus other treatments responded much better than had patients treated by drugs alone. The first study included the first few patients given this vitamin in 1952 before tranquilizers came into general use. By the end of that 10-year follow-up period, tranquilizers had become the main treatment. The latter, the second

From the *J Orthomolecular Med* 1994:9:7–37.

study group, was treated at University Hospital group between 1956 and 1962. After orthomolecular treatment the amount of time the first group spent in the hospital decreased to 40 percent of the time they had spent in hospital before treatment. In sharp contrast, the tranquilizer-treated group was in the hospital eight and half times longer.

Another way of showing the effect of niacin is in decreasing the need for further admissions. With niacin, 16 patients had only 3 readmissions in a 10-year period. Of 27 patients not on niacin, over the same time period, there were 72 readmissions; these patients were treated before the tranquilizers were introduced. The second study group was treated at University Hospital at the onset of the drug era. They were mostly treated by other psychiatrists who had no interest in research, but who were persuaded by residents to try it out. There was very little input from me. This follow-up data showed that those patients who had received niacin were less likely to be readmitted to the hospital, and those that were had shorter stays.

We also examined the number of suicides. There were five from the untreated group (on tranquilizers and/or ECT only), and none from the niacin group. The suicide rate was 1.47 per 100 patients over the seven-year period. This was in agreement with an earlier study when we found four patients killed themselves from a group of 98, and none from a vitamin group of 73. Putting this data together we found that the suicide rate for the non-vitamin group was 0.22 suicides per 100 per year, or 220 per 100,000. It was a rate 22 times as great as the prevalent rates then for any normal population. Johnstone and others[44] reported that out of 532 patients there were two suicides over the decade for women, 13 times the expected rate from a normal population, and five suicides for men, or about 19 times the normal rate. This is very close to the Saskatchewan suicide rate of tranquilizer-treated patients compared to no suicides for the vitamin-treated patients. The English group were treated with tranquilizers. Placing schizophrenic patients on tranquilizers only thus exposes them to a suicide rate 22 times normal. We wrote, "We believe any drug which produced this high a mortality would soon be removed unless of course no other drugs were

The suicide rate of patients with schizophrenia is about 20 times that of healthy people of the same age. The cost of saving those lives with niacin therapy would be about 25 cents per patient per day.
—HUMPHRY OSMOND and ABRAM HOFFER

available to treat the conditions, which untreated produced a much higher risk of death."

The results reported completely corroborate the 1952 results. The studies were conducted in two different hospitals in different cities, and separated about five years from each other. The therapists were different also. Finally, the second set of data was obtained during the tranquilizer era of psychiatry. Yet both sets of data were very similar. It is apparent tranquilizers have not decreased readmissions very much, if at all. Niacin, on the other hand, has made a great difference to the natural history of schizophrenia. There can be few who can still doubt that every schizophrenic patient should be given niacin therapy. It is clear we greatly underestimated the ability of psychiatrists to be doubtful.

We concluded that

There can be no a priori reason why massive [amounts of] niacin should not alter the outcome of schizophrenia. Apart from deep prejudice or sheer inertia, it is worth trying because it meets one of the major requirements of any treatment, that of "doing the sick no harm." Two-thirds of those who develop schizophrenia are more or less crippled by it and return to hospital for periods ranging from a few weeks to several years. Our studies suggest that at least half of the crippled two-thirds will be well if given nacin, and some of the others will be helped. We think that these young people, who are doomed to be in and out of mental hospitals for most of their lives, have a right to be given niacin even if medical people are skeptical. Nothing can be lost and as we have shown, belief or skepticism seems to have very little bearing upon the effects of this treatment.

Follow-Up Studies

Eleven years later Bockoven and Solomon[1] also found that tranquilizers did not improve the long-term prognosis of schizophrenic patients. They compared the outcome of two five-year follow-up studies on patients treated at their hospital between 1947 and 1952, and between 1967 and 1972. The first group could not have gotten any tranquilizers while the second group was given the full benefit of this treatment. They concluded that the outcome was almost the same with one possible exception, the tranquilizer group fared worse and required much more social supports for them to keep going. Almost every thorough study published since then has shown the same results. The last one was reported by Dr. James D. Hegarty of McLean Hospital in Belmont, Massachusetts. *Science News* described his findings as follows:

Many psychiatrists regard the introduction of antipsychotic medication in the 1950s as a boon for the long-term adjustment of people with schizophrenia, a devastating disturbance of thought and emotion. But an analysis of research conducted over the past century indicates that psychiatric definitions of schizophrenia, rather than new treatment, primarily account for observed improvements or decline in the condition of schizophrenics over time. James D. Hegarty and his colleagues identified 359 studies from the United States, Europe, Russia, and China in which scientists used specific criteria to diagnose schizophrenia in 15 or more individuals and then tracked the patients progress for at least one year. At least 15 percent of the schizophrenics studied from 1900 to 1930 showed significant improvement, Hegarty's team contends. That figure rises to 30 percent between 1930 and 1970, and then declines to about 15 percent again in research covering the past 20 years, they say. Studies in the first and last time periods generally used narrow definitions of schizophrenia, often requiring continuous signs of disturbance for at least six months. Projects in the middle period relied on broader definitions with no minimum time limits on symptoms. In studies for 1930 to 1970, more patients got better because they had milder

problems to begin with Hegarty maintains. The poorer outcome for schizophrenics studied after 1970 may also reflect the discharge of many patients from state mental hospitals and the lack of community mental health care for people with severe psychiatric disorders, he adds.[7]

E. C. Johnstone and colleagues[44] reported their results of a follow-up study of 532 schizophrenic patients treated over a 10-year period beginning in January 1975. It is one of the most thorough studies of this kind. They had a mean of 1.68 admissions before entering this cohort with a range zero to 22 admissions. The total number of admissions was 5.37 with a range of one to 40 admissions. During the decade study they averaged 3.69 admissions. The group averaged 1.68 admissions before entering the study and this increased to 3.69 admissions on the average during the study. This again is comparable to the data obtained in Saskatchewan, where it was found that tranquilized patients had to be admitted much more often. It is difficult to compare these patients outcome with mine since they used different criteria. Of major interest is their determination that only two patients were in the best occupational level, and 25 in the next best (that is, only 27 out of 532, about 5 percent, were in the best two occupational levels). Fewer than 20 percent were employed but there was no breakdown to illustrate the type of employment they had. Over 50 percent of their sample still suffered from morbid symptoms. They also compared a five-year cohort beginning in 1970 and found that they were almost identical with the latter group in outcome, even though the latter group had much more contact with social and medical agencies. From the latter group over 90 percent were in good contact with the agencies, whereas from the earlier group only 60 percent were in contact. The authors wrote,

More than 90 percent of patients received medical and/or social support, and 45 percent were supervised by a consultant psychiatrist. This was much closer supervision than had been provided for schizophrenic patients from the same service ten years previously . . . Few patients are now out of touch with the medical services and many more are receiving specialist supervision, and yet they are no better in these terms. The findings do raise the question of whether there is anything to be gained by the increased level of care given to the later sample.

Orthomolecular: The Optimum Approach for Schizophrenia

Over the past month I have seen a large number of my chronic schizophrenic patients who have been under treatment with me for at least ten years. I was impressed with their great improvement over what they had been like the first few years after they started on this treatment. I also thought how sad it is that psychiatrists have refused to look at this treatment and thereby have deprived their patients of their chance for an equivalent recovery and themselves of the opportunity to see schizophrenic patients who are getting well. They are not simply putting in time being heavily tranquilized.

It is possible that psychiatry, the least physiological of all the medical specialties, may one day catch up and realize that it will have to come into the newer medicine, which is examining with great interest a large number of nutrients and their potential benefit to patients. These include niacin, which lowers cholesterol levels and elevates high-density lipoprotein ("good") cholesterol, and the antioxidant vitamins such as beta-carotene, and vitamins C and E, which have been shown to prevent the development of arteriosclerosis,[47,52,53–55] and to extend life.[5] These and other vitamins used in optimum doses—meaning, in much larger than those needed to prevent the vitamin deficiency diseases such as scurvy and pellagra—are for the first time in 50 years beginning to receive some attention as therapeutic compounds with a vast potential for helping patients. I hope that by publishing these case histories (to follow) and reporting exactly what their present state is, this might increase the level of interest among psychiatrists.

Research physicians publish rather brief papers for two main reasons: 1) There is a keen demand for space, and journals like to publish as many authors as they can in one issue without cutting in too heavily into the pages devoted to advertising (up to 50 percent of the pages). 2) Case histories have disappeared from journal articles, as if living patients no longer existed or counted for very much. Instead, authors describe their methods, describe what criteria they used in selecting their groups of patients that were used in their prospective double-blind controlled studies, and provide ample charts and statistics. I have read many papers where it is impossible to get any feeling for a single patient. In my opinion the object of a medical report is to report honestly what one has seen and in such a way that other physicians and readers will understand what was done, what the results were and what kind of patients were treated, and what was the outcome. This paper represents the type of paper that was common 40 years ago. By and large readers find these papers much more interesting. This is why letters to the editor are so much more interesting. They have not been vetted to death by skeptical reviewers as have been almost all the papers published.

A treatment that started out simply by using one or two vitamins and adding them to the current treatment program has become much more complex as newer findings have been incorporated into the program. Today, orthomeocular treatment includes the following main elements.

Diet

This has been one of the major stumbling blocks for orthodox psychiatrists who have never been able to understand that food plays an enormous role not only in physical disease. There are two basic changes that must be made. The first is to remove as much as possible the many additives that are placed in modern prepared or processed foods. One simple rule will remove a major proportion of these: it is the *no sugar rule*. I advise my patients to avoid all foods to which anyone has added sugar, such as pastry, candy, soda, ice cream, cakes, and so on. Any examinations of processed and packaged foods shows the intimate association between sugar and other additives. The second rule is to avoid any foods to which the patient is allergic or that cause any physical or mental discomfort. Elimination diets may be needed to determine these. In many cases a simple allergy history will locate them.[28,31]

Vitamins

The main vitamins used in orthomolecular psychiatry are vitamin B3, vitamin B6, vitamin C, and to a much lesser degree vitamin B12 and folic acid.

- Vitamin B3: This term includes niacin, also known as niacinamide. I prefer niacinamide for young people and for all patients who might not like the cosmetic effect of flushing after they have taken niacin. However, niacin is the best one for elderly patients and for lowering cholesterol levels. The dose varies from 1,000 milligrams (mg) to many more thousands of milligrams per day. Niacin is best given three times per day since it is water soluble and easily excreted. The usual starting dose for adults is 1,000 mg, three times a day. Patients advised to start on niacin must be warned about the flush and how to deal with it. If any dose level causes nausea and later vomiting, it must be lowered to below this nauseant level. If this level is too low for either one, a combination of both can be used. For a detailed discussion of the properties of vitamin B3, see Hoffer,[8–11,14–27] and Hoffer and Osmond.[36,41]

- Vitamin B6 (pyridoxine): There is one main indication for using this vitamin for schizophrenics. It is the condition know as pyroluria. The condition is diagnosed by a urine test, which measures for the presence of kryptopyrrole (also known as mauve factor).[12,13,35,38,40] If a urine test is not available, it can be suspected by a few clear physical signs such as white areas in the finger nails, stretch marks on the body, or premenstrual tension. The dose is usually under 1,000 mg daily. I start with 250 mg and occasionally have to increase it to 500 or 750 mg. It is best given in association with one of the zinc salts such as zinc gluconate or citrate or sulfate.

- Vitamin C (ascorbic acid): I consider this a most important nutrient for everyone, especially when they are sick. It is a good antistress vitamin. It does not decrease the stress but certainly increases the ability of the person to cope with it. It prevents the development of arteriosclerosis and also increases longevity. The books by Stone,[56] Pauling,[47] Cathcart,[2] Cheraskin,[3] and Cheraskin, Ringsdorf, and Sisley[4] must be considered essential reading for anyone interested in using vitamin C. Dr. Pauling effectively disposes of the myth that vitamin C causes kidney stones, see also Hoffer.[29] For a discussion of vitamin C and the prolongation of life for cancer patients, see Hoffer and Pauling.[43]

Minerals

All the minerals are essential but a few play a particularly important role in the treatment of the mentally ill. Zinc and manganese are important, especially in combination with vitamin B6 since the double dependency exists so frequently,[49–51] particularly in areas where the drinking water is high in copper leached from copper plumbing, and deficient in manganese.

- Zinc: The dose is between 50 and 100 mg per day, which is safe for this water-soluble mineral. Any of the salts can be used. I use either zinc gluconate or zinc citrate available in 50 mg tablets. The indications are described by Pfeiffer,[49] Pfeiffer, Mailloux, and Forsythe,[50] and Pfeiffer, Ward El Melegi, and Cott.[51]

- Manganese: Kunin[45] discovered that tardive dyskinesia is caused by a deficiency of manganese, which is bound by and excreted with the tranquilizers used over a long period of time. When the manganese is restored, in most cases combined with vitamin B3, the condition is removed within a matter of days or weeks. I have seen how effective it can be. Hawkins[6] surveyed psychiatrists who had treated, all together, over 58,000 patients. They could not recall a single case of tardive dyskinesia. The dose is anywhere between 15 and 50 mg daily and may be combined in a solution with zinc.

Drugs

The major psychiatric drugs are used following the usual indications. When combined with the dietary, nutrient program, eventually much lower doses are adequate. This has the major advantage that patients are less handicapped by the tranquilizers and there is much less chance of getting the usual tranquilizer side effects and toxic reactions. Orthomolecular doctors have never been opposed to the use of drugs as part of the overall program. They are opposed to the use of drugs only because they are not helping patients become well when used this way.

Psychiatrists are faced with what I have called the tranquilizer dilemma. It is the same kind of blindness to fact, the same kind of denial that dogged psychiatry for years after these drugs first came into general use. For a long time they could not believe that these drugs could cause tardive dyskinesia. The psychiatric literature contained many articles denying that this could happen and attacking the psychiatrist who first brought this to public attention and insisted it was a real phenomenon. The dilemma follows from two true propositions: 1) That tranquilizers are helpful in reducing and eliminating symptoms and signs from schizophrenic patients. 2) That they are equally effective in making normal people sick. The first proposition will never be denied by any physician who has used them. The second proposition is based on what happens to normal subjects when they take these drugs by accident and upon the outcome of giving these drugs to normal people.

The object of giving drugs to patients is to start the process of recovery. At first this is exactly what they do. They rather quickly decrease the intensity of the symptoms and signs presented by the schizophrenic patients. But as the patient begins this process and their symptoms decrease in intensity and frequency, their physiology, which must also become more and more normal, begins to respond to the drugs as if they were well, that is, the drugs make them sick. They produce the tranquilizer psychosis. The tranquilizer psychosis is iatrogenic, induced by the doctor who has prescribed the drug. It causes both mental and physical symptoms.

The physical symptoms are lethargy, uncoordination, tremor, fatigue, excessive sleepiness, impotence, dry mouth, difficulty in urination, increased sensitivity to sun, and excessive weight gain. These symptoms provide some of the main reasons why patients refuse to take these drugs after most of their psychosis has come under control. But the mental symptoms are even worse. They include difficulty in concentration, decrease in memory, disinterest, apathy, depression, and irresponsibility.

Tranquilizers convert one psychosis to another. This was first pointed out by Professor Meyer-Gross, shortly after these drugs were introduced from France into England and the United States. He said, "Tranquilizers convert one psychosis into another." The tranquilizer psychosis prevents the unfortunate patient from becoming a normal member of society because with these symptoms no one can function at jobs or occupations where these symptoms and signs are a handicap, such as practicing law or medicine, or being a normal cook or architect or worker on the farms or in the factories. Would you allow your surgeon to operate on you if you knew she was taking 300 mg of chlorpromazine (Thorazine) daily?

Psychiatrists have tried to deal with this dilemma in only one way—by decreasing the dose, by searching for newer drugs that are less apt to cause severe side effects such as clozapine (Clozaril), and in the extreme by placing the patient on a drug-free program. This would be great if the original psychosis did not start to come back as it does in the vast majority of cases. The unfortunate patient is caught between these two psychoses and like a swing oscillates back and forth. Visualize two mountain ranges separated by a valley. One mountain range represents the original schizophrenic psychosis. The other represents the tranquilizer psychosis. Both are equally undesirable with a major difference. Psychiatrists seem to be more content to have their patients permanently on the tranquilizer mountain range while patients try desperately to escape into the valley that represents normality. As soon as the drugs are started they begin to work and after a few weeks or months both patients and their families are happy since the major symptoms are moderated and the patient appears to be getting well. Later on with the continued treatment as the patient becomes more normal, the tranquilizer psychosis begins to appear. Eventually, the entire schizophrenic psychosis has been replaced by the tranquilizer psychosis. The major difference is that society is much more tolerant of the latter psychosis than it is of the first. The major difference for the patient is that the psychosis has been changed from a "hot" to a "cool" psychosis.

Hot signs and symptoms are those that families and society find most intolerable and that are the reasons why these patients are admitted to a hospital or, if the mental hospitals refuse to accept them, into prison. By the latter, I mean that many psychiatric wards and hospitals will refuse to accept patients if they do not want them for a variety of reasons and the easiest way to keep them out is to find them not mentally ill, as was the case with one of the patients I will describe later.

These are the symptoms that most normal people will find intolerable. They include:

• Perceptual disorder: Visions, especially if the patient talks about them; voices, especially if the patients act upon them (e.g., by setting fires); other senses, if the patient responds with inappropriate behavior.

• Thought disorder: These changes may lead to inappropriate behavior such as wandering nude downtown, accusing someone of poisoning them, etc.

• Mood disorder: Manic behavior or suicidal depression.

• Behavioral disorder: Any abnormal persistent activity, such as hopping on one foot all day, or rocking all day, or any inappropriate social activity.

Cool signs and symptoms are the same as the hot signs and symptoms listed above, only decreased or eliminated so that the overall behavior is now much more tolerable to families and to society. They are much more tolerable in an acute sense but in the long run will become just as intolerable. It is one of the main factors in making it impossible for families to look after their chronic tranquilized children and forces them into group homes or other sheltered homes like those of the Salvation Army. Tranquilizers produce a variety of cool symptoms that comprise part of the tranquilizer psychosis.

Tranquilizers cool the hot symptoms and add a few more to the unfortunate patient. The tranquilizer psychosis is a combination of cool symptoms originally present in the patient combined with the new symptoms induced by the drugs. The dilemma is that, while tranquilizers cool the hot symptoms, they do not remove them and they add their own form of toxic reactions. (This does not apply to the antidepressants that in most cases are much more benign and do not restrict patients activities and behavior to the same degree. It is

possible to be normal while on antidepressant drugs.) Of course this is also possible when the amount of drug needed to cool or eliminate symptoms is so low the tranquilizer psychosis symptoms are not generated. This is the case with many of the chronic patients I will describe further on. The optimum dose of drugs must be used at all stages of the treatment process. They must be decreased as soon as possible, the objective always being to eliminate them.

Tranquilizers work very quickly compared to the much slower action of the nutrients. Here is a comparison of the two major treatment modalities:

• Tranquilizers act rapidly, decrease intensity of signs and symptoms, and cause pyschosis

• Nutrients act slowly, remove signs and symptoms, and are nontoxic.

The solution to the tranquilizer dilemma is to combine both treatments as is done by orthomolecular psychiatrists. By combining these two treatments, one takes advantage of the rapidity of the drugs with the much better final effect of the vitamins and minerals. At the beginning of treatment, patients, if they have hot symptoms, are placed on the appropriate drugs and at the same time the nutrient program is started. As soon as the patient begins to respond, the dose of drugs is slowly and carefully decreased, waiting weeks or even months before any major reduction is made.

Eventually, with most acute patients, the drug is lowered to such a low dose it can no longer produce the tranquilizer psychosis or is eliminated. As the patient recovers, the nutrients gradually take over and once the patient is well they will in most cases keep them well. If they do relapse, it is not nearly as severe and usually they respond much more quickly the second time around. The revolving door syndrome whereby patients are rotated in and out of hospitals is eventually effectively removed. I have seen patients who had 30 admissions when they were started on this program and who eventually did not need any more admissions. The HOD Test is very helpful in following patients and will warn about an impending relapse long before it becomes apparent to the patient or to the physician.[34,39,40]

Other Factors

The other factors are the hospital, or nursing home (i.e., the place where the patient is housed and sheltered, the ancillary services such as social work, occupational therapy, and the psychology division). The nursing service is the most important in the hospital setting since they know the patient and their progress much better than any one else in the institution. All are important, but in my opinion the most important is the treatment program. In the same way, the most ideal hospital dealing with the diabetic will not get very far if it ignores the use of diet and insulin or other antidiabetic drugs.

Community Support Services

These are vital, especially for the chronic patients, many of whom do not need to be rehabilitated but habilitated. They have never been normal and when they recover they will need a total educational program to make them fit for social activity, for work, and so on.

When Is a Patient Well?

Institutions prepare annual reports for the governments who provide the funds with which they operate. When I worked for the Department of Public Health in Saskatchewan, I read each report put out by the institutions with a great deal of interest. They provided information such as the number of staff in various categories; the number of patients admitted, discharged, still in hospital; and the number of tests given. But nowhere did I ever see a breakdown that would tell me how many were treated successfully. I would have liked to see this statistic. When I would talk to my colleagues in psychiatry and psychology about evaluating patients after treatment, they were all very loathe even to get involved. Their usual answer was that it was very difficult to determine when patients were better and that it would require large research grants to work out methods for making these measures. I understood why they were so reluctant. It simply indicated that changes in patients after treatment were so subtle that only carefully worked out subtle tests could make these determinations. On one occasion at one of the morning clinical conferences at the University of Saskatchewan where I was one of the professors, I suggested to the meeting that we should hold a type of psychiatric post mortem whenever a patient who had been in hospital and discharged had to be returned. I suggested that these returnees should be conferenced and we would discuss why they had failed to stay in the community. There was a cold, dead silence and nothing more was said about this. I pointed out that surgeons were not reluctant to have pathologists do post-mortem examinations on their post-surgical patients and that they learned a good deal from this.

Since most people can tell when a person is psychotic or bizarre and this is known to members of the family, it must be relatively easy to conclude whether or not a person has something the matter with him or not. The solution was therefore to use common-sense criteria that any person could understand. It would be of no value to try to judge the degree of thought disorder that was present, the quantity of depression, or the intensity of the hallucinations. One would merely disregard most of these subjective findings and look at those variables that determine whether a person can function in the community. I, therefore, selected four measures of recovery or of wellness:

1. Freedom from symptoms and signs: 1 point.

2. Ability to get on reasonably well with family: 1 point.

3. Ability to get on reasonably well with the community: 1 point.

4. Able to work at a job or to be active in the same way as was the case before the illness struck. If the patient never had been engaged in this kind of activity, they would be judged by the ability to perform any useful work: 1 point. The ability to pay income tax is an important measure of recovery.

With these criteria I used the following scale: well (4 points); much improved (3 points); improved (2 points); not improved (1 point).

Clinical Descriptions of 27 Schizophrenic Patients

1) K. G., Born 1945

As a youngster K. G. was shy and sensitive and occasionally had to be given tranquilizers. At age 18 he had Asian flu with a fever, up to 105°F. He was admitted to the hospital with hallucinations. Following that he required several admissions, including one to hospital in Vancouver, B.C., where he was started on a vitamin program with marked improvement. Later he relapsed and was admitted to an institute in Victoria, for a series of ECT. Then he went to an institute in Vancouver, for six months, had two more ECT series receiving 30 treatments. After discharge he lived in a boarding house for a year. When I saw him he was confused, his speech was garbled, it was impossible to communicate with him, and he was very inappropriate. He was depressed. He required Thorazine (400 mg) to keep some kind of control.

He was admitted February 27–March 13, 1978, and again August 4, 1978 because of obstructive jaundice caused by the tranquilizer. In 1978 he was no better and he was switched to Haldol and eventually to long-acting Haldol by injection. He needed several more admissions as follows: October 17–27, 1984, October 1–December 1, 1986, and January 28–February 10, 1988. By then he was much better. When I saw him recently he came alone, was well dressed, told me about his activities in the group home and at a rehabilitation workshop. It was quite easy to engage him in conversation. He is on long-acting Haldol by injection (200 mg every four weeks), plus Haldol (90 mg/day), and Kemadrin (5 mg/3x per day). His vitamins include nicotinamide (500 mg/3x per day) and folic acid (5 mg/day). He was seen the following number of times: 1977–78 (21 times); 1979–80 (15 times); 1981–82 (12 times); 1983–84 (11 times); 1985–86 (6 times); 1987–88 (8 times); 1989–90 (1 time); and 1991–92 (7 times). I classified him as improved.

2) L. T., Born 1955

When first seen in 1979, L. T. complained she had been depressed since 1972. It started in high school. She left home at age 16 because she could not stand her stepfather. She married at age 17 and divorced soon after. She felt no emotion during the separation but later was depressed. She did not respond to antidepressants, which made her feel like a vegetable. When I saw her she was unreal, had out of body experiences, and heard her own thoughts. She was paranoid when depressed and was at this time depressed. I started her on the orthomolecular program and she began to respond.

She was very depressed again and was admitted to the hospital March 7 for one month. She was then well and released until November 13, 1986, when she was admitted again. She has remained well since. She is on the following program, nicotinamide (1,000 mg/3x per day), vitamin C (12,000 mg/day), pyridoxine (250 mg/day), zinc citrate (50 mg/day), Ludiomil (100 mg/day), Prozac (40 mg/day), and Thorazine (200 mg/day). She married and has two normal children. She has been seen the following number of times: 1979–80 (13 times); 1981–82 (10 times); 1983–84 (7 times); 1985–86 (14 times); 1987–88 (8 times); 1989–90 (3 times); and 1991–92 (6 times).

Only a person who has come through the schizophrenic experience can really relate what it was like. Here is her account of her illness and recovery.

When I was 15, in 1970, my mother, youngest brother, and myself moved into some low-income housing on our own. My two older brothers had fled by then. It was at this time when I acutely began to feel the difference between myself and the other kids at school. I felt superior to them. I never had to study and felt a slight contempt for those who did. I felt crazy. I remember spending classes engraving my eraser with my compass to produce a rubber stamp which said insane. It became my trademark. It was also about this time that I decided to go on the pill and, although I had not yet menstruated, my doctor prescribed them for me. When I spoke to this same doctor about my confusion and depression, he assured me these were normal teenage feelings. I figured the fault lay within myself.

I maintained the same inadequate diet, which I believe had paramount consequences and included lots of cola drinks, pizzas, hot dogs, chips, cheezies, cakes, and candies. I started drinking anything alcohol; I began smoking tobacco and pot, and doing street drugs. I stopped short of taking heroin. Part of this shift was due to living in a large metropolis, where peer pressure is difficult to avoid. Part was also due to being 16 and 17 years old during the hippie era. LSD was in. Most of it was an escape from the increasingly difficult reality of my life.

I tried school counselors. They told me I was having normal adolescent anxieties. I moved into a boarding home. I went to doctors, another general practitioner, then a psychiatrist. Both prescribed Valium. This really did wonders for my depression.

I tried suicide twice. Then I went to live in the streets. I began to think that if I didn't do something, I would really go crazy. So I ended up marrying one of my street friends and leaving for British Columbia. After two years the marriage collapsed, and I found myself alone and back where I had been born, in Victoria.

Shortly after my arrival in Victoria I met someone very special. I knew that when I met him, but never realized just how special he was until it was all over and there he was still loving me. We were living together when things really began getting worse. I started having the hallmark auditory hallucinations; whispery, demeaning voices; mild visual hallucinations; delusions; and sometimes very vivid illusions involved in schizophrenia. My thoughts did not make sense—I had too many thoughts—violent and hateful thoughts. I went from being extroverted to extremely withdrawn. I would sit in one place for hours at a time. I was afraid to look in the mirror. I became extremely agitated by sound, wouldn't answer the telephone, refused to see anyone. I hated eating. I became very superstitious. I began experiencing anxiety attacks, where the earth fell away or I was pulled up out of my skin. I lost all feeling. Time slowed down. I would bang my head and pull my hair to try and stop the noise, the pain in my soul. I would circle around and around upon waking, trying to figure out what I should do. Should I wash my face, brush my teeth first. What should I do?

Finally my common law husband came home one day and said he'd heard about some old fellow in town who might help me. He was a naturopath. For about a year I visited this marvelous little man (who is over 90). He taught me about diet, and why. He told me to eat whole, raw foods, and to stay away from stimulants and why. He also piqued my interest in vitamins. When it was clear that he could help me no further, he told me about a specialist who would really know what to do. A referral from a general practitioner was necessary, but I thought this would pose no problem. But the doctor I had been seeing for four years refused to refer me. He told me I would do better coming to his group therapy sessions than in going to that "quack." That quack you may have guessed was Dr. Hoffer.

It took two more doctors before finally finding one, albeit a reluctant one, to get my referral. My first visit to Dr. Hoffer hallmarked the turning point of my life. He gave me the Hoffer-Osmond Diagnostic (HOD) Test, which confirmed I was schizophrenic. Then, he told me all about schizophrenia, explaining carefully what I could do to overcome it. He prescribed vitamins, minerals, and medication and firmly spoke to me about proper nutrition.

I remember about three weeks into the program feeling very despondent. I just didn't feel any better. Dr. Hoffer suggested I do the HOD test again. Much to my amazement, there was a 30 point difference in scores. This, along with some encouragement and adjustments in medication and supplements, kept me going for another three months, when the bottom fell out of my world. I think because I had begun to get better, this particularly bad slip seemed to me, worse than ever before. I went into the hospital. I had a series of ECT. About two months after getting out of the hospital, I began to notice a climbing of mood. Over the next few months, many other signs became apparent. Separately, they did not seem like much, but, collectively, they really pointed at recovery. My menses became more regular, my muscles stopped aching, my perceptions straightened out. I noticed I could remember things better and retain more and more information. Even now, and I spoke to Dr. Hoffer about this recently, my brain actually feels as though it is regenerating. I told him if this keeps up, I'll actually be a genius by 1990.

Having reached my goal of becoming well, in 1980, at the age of 25, I felt a need to test out my health. Perhaps I could go back to work? Having failed several times at holding a job for any length of time in the past, I found myself fairly shaky about the idea. I decided to start with part-time work. When that went all right, it gave me the confidence I needed to move on to bigger and better things. In May of 1981 I married the man I mentioned as being so special earlier on. They say you marry for better or worse. Certainly he and I had already experienced the worst before we got married.

In April of 1983, after three years of successful part-time work and two years of a successful marriage, I completed a normal pregnancy with the birth of a beautiful baby boy. I maintained my vitamin program throughout the pregnancy, having managed with doctors' guidance to wean off all medications in the year prior to becoming pregnant. I have been medication free ever since a total of four years, keeping on with the diet, vitamins, and lifestyle.

I found a job in a small office and shortly thereafter found myself becoming involved as a volunteer in the Friends of Schizophrenics Society. I had discovered the group after attending a lecture series on schizophrenia that was put on by the local hospital and mental health centers. They were looking to establish a chapter in Victoria, so I jumped in with both feet. This was the chance I had been waiting for. Ever since I'd become well, I had been trying to figure out a way to help other schizophrenics. Surely what had worked for me would work for some of them as well. This is where I began to make my being schizophrenic into a positive force.

For the future I would like to see a pooling of all the accumulated knowledge, a cooperative effort in research, and, ultimately, because of these efforts an end to schizophrenia. I believe schizophrenics can act as a powerful force in ensuring this end. We must keep reminding those who are working for us, that they are working for us, that there is no time for political quibbling and controversy. So that all of us together can one day say, Our minds used to think without us.

This wish expressed by this patient arose from the controversy that was generated in the group when she told them that a major part of her recovery arose from the use of the vitamin program. Other patients were interested but the professional people were not. They had indoctrinated Friends of Schizophrenics into pursuing their only main objective, which was to provide support to the friends of the patients. They were convinced that tranquilizers were all that one could offer and that taking vitamins was a waste of time.

3) E. P., Born 1954

I saw E. P. in 1980 when she had been suffering since 1969. She had been admitted to a psychiatric hospital in Winnipeg for six months and there received nine ECT. She had almost total amnesia about that admission but she was told that she was very paranoid. In 1975 she began to suffer from chronic fatigue. She started on a vitamin program that she followed until 1974 and during this time was much better. When she discontinued her vitamins, she became depressed and tired. When I saw her she complained that people were watching her. She had seen visions in the past. She was paranoid with a lot of blocking, and she was tired and depressed. I admitted her to the hospital December 1–7, 1981 and again February 18–March 21, 1982. Since then she has been improving steadily with fewer swings into depression. In 1958 she moved into her own apartment. It had taken her about two years to feel ready to leave her parents home. She is now well on the following program: Fluanxol (4.5–9 mg/day), niacin (2,500 mg/day), vitamin C (12,000 mg/day), Eskalith (300 mg/3x per day), and Cogentin (1 mg/day). She was seen the following times: 1979–80 (5 times); 1981–82 (14 times); 1983–84 (11 times); 1985–86 (14 times); 1987–88 (14 times); 1989–90 (9 times); and 1991–92 (7 times). I consider her well.

4) E. B., Born 1953

In 1974 E. B. became very paranoid and withdrawn. She believed people were laughing at her. Several months later she was well. When I saw her she heard voices and heard a tape recorder in her apartment, as she had earlier. She was again very paranoid believing people were gossiping about her, and had been plotting against her in the past. This included arranging for her to have a car accident. She also felt bugged. Depression and fatigue were present. She was admitted on three occasions: June 18–22, 1981, December 11–19, 1981, and September 4–January 8, 1982. Early in 1985 she still saw visions, and black-robed people walking through her apartment. By midyear they were gone. The voices continued to bother her for several years. But for the past three years she has been free of them. She is on Thorazine (500 mg/day), nicotinamide (4,000 mg/day), and vitamin C (3,000 mg/day). She was seen the following times: 1979–80 (5 times); 1981–82 (14 times); 1983–84 (11 times); 1985–86 (14 times); 1987–88 (14 times); 1989–90 (9 times); and 1991–92 (7 times). I classed her as much improved since she is still not able to work.

5) S. D., Born 1953

During her midteens she became epileptic with grand mal and petit mal seizures. She was well controlled with anticonvulsant medication but from that time on she remained depressed. She was admitted on seven occasions to psychiatric hospitals, receiving ECT during some of these. Then she went to Hollywood Hospital, Vancouver, and was given more ECT in combination with a vitamin program. Following that she was much better. When I saw her in 1979, she still suffered from visions and from voices that ordered her to hurt herself. This she would often do by holding a burning cigarette to her skin until she had punched through the skin. She was very paranoid, depressed, and nervous. She was admitted January 15–March 4, 1980. She married in October 1984 to a very difficult, unsympathetic man who worked very hard at two jobs. She was admitted again July 7–13, 1986. During the summer of 1989 she went off all her program largely because of her husband, who did not approve of any of it, and she suffered a serious relapse. Her family physician restarted the program and she improved and is now well. She is on Modecate (50 mg intramuscularly every two weeks), Anafranil (50 mg before bed), niacin (2,000 mg/3x per day), vitamin C (4,000 mg/day), folic acid (5 mg/day), and zinc gluconate (100 mg/day). She has been seen the following times: 1979–80 (10 times); 1981–82 (6 times); 1983–84 (13 times); 1985–86 (15 times); 1987–88 (8 times); 1989–90 (2 times); and 1991–92 (3 times).

6) J. L., Born 1949

During the first visit, in 1976, it was impossible to get any information from J. L. He walked in with his mother and promptly turned his back to me and spent the next five minutes or more looking over the books on my wall bookcase. His mother had to persuade him to sit down and face me. She told me he had been uncoordinated as a child and later had a learning problem. He did learn to read and later became an avid reader. At age 18, he read about LSD and then told his mother he had been seeing visions as long as he could remember. In 1968 he was admitted and spent two months in the hospital receiving ECT, which was continued afterward as an outpatient. He received about 100 treatments in all. In 1974 he was readmitted for three months to Hollywood Hospital and there given Thorazine (1,600 mg/day). He had been started on a vitamin program two years before. On examination he reported visions, voices to which he responded, and hearing his own thoughts. In his thoughts he was paranoid, blocked a lot, had a poor memory, and was not able to engage in any intelligent discussion. He also had violent mood swings. Since then he has continued to improve and is now improved.

I saw J. L. again in June 1992. His present state is so good it is difficult to realize how sick and deteriorated he was when I saw him first. We had a long discussion and reviewed his earlier presenting symptoms. He remembered his voices and visions, which have been gone for many years. He was helpful in the group home where he lived and took on more responsible tasks. He was much more sociable both in the home and at a center for schizophrenic patients that he attends. He laughed and had a good sense of humor. Whereas at one time he would walk 8 to 10 miles daily, he had greatly reduced this since he had so many more useful activities to do. He maintained close contact with his family and his non-identical twin brother. He could be classed as much improved but has lost so much out of his life from his chronic illness that he will probably never be able to work and be self-supporting. It is possible to talk to him reasonably intelligently, he had no more outbursts, creates no problems at the group home, continues to read, and is in good physical condition. He is on the following program: nicotinamide (2,000 mg/3x per day), vitamin C (1,000 mg/3x per day), pyridoxine (250 mg/3x per day), vitamin E (400 IU/day), zinc sulfate (220 mg/2x per day), Anafranil (75 mg before bed), Trilafon (12 mg before bed), and Valium (10 mg/2x per day). He was seen the following number of times: 1979–80 (10 times); 1981–82 (6 times); 1983–84 (13 times); 1987–88 (8 times); 1989–90 (2 times); and 1991–92 (3 times).

7) G. H., Born 1963

I saw this young girl for the first time as a result of a strange series of events. In 1981 I received a phone call from both parents who were very disturbed about their daughter because she was in prison. None of the psychiatric wards on the lower mainland of British Columbia would admit her to their hospital and the judge had ordered her to be held in prison. They wanted to know if I would admit her to a hospital in Victoria. I replied that I could not do so since I had not seen her and that I would have to evaluate her myself before deciding. They then appeared before the judge and told him that I would admit her believing that once I saw her I would really agree that this was essential.

A few days later they all arrived and I was able to examine her. Her mother told me she had always been a nervous child from age three when she became hyperactive with a learning disorder. When 14 she went to a private school but had to drop out because she began to binge on junk food and became disoriented. She gained 20 pounds in a short time and later became bulemic, and lost a lot of weight. When she came home she was referred to a health center at the University of British Columbia for four months and later to a center for delinquent and other behaviorally disturbed teenagers for one and a half years. At age 17 she was made a ward of the government. In November 1980, she was found to be unmanageable in the group home and she was again admitted to a hospital for two months. She left against advice to go home. In January 1981, she set fire to her mattress because she was angry at the world. She was admitted again, then followed up as

an outpatient at a health center. During this period she made three serious suicide overdose attempts. Her behavior remained hyperactive and bizarre. For a while she was in and out of institutions, where they found her to be mentally normal and discharged her home. Again she set a fire to her curtains. The police were called and she was arrested and taken to a nearby prison because the judge could not find a single unit that would admit her. She had been blackballed since she had been found "mentally normal" and had no right to be admitted to a psychiatric unit. She was released to her parents' care by the judge on condition they see me. The judge believed I had promised to admit her.

She told me about the visual hallucinations present from age 15. She saw people with knives and had told her mother about this. She heard voices that ordered her to do bad things like setting fires. She felt weird and heard her own thoughts. She was also very paranoid, believing people were plotting against her, watching her. She blocked a lot and could not concentrate. On top of all these symptoms, she was very depressed. I had no choice but to admit her. Not to have done so would have been, in my opinion, not only very bad psychiatry but malpractice.

She was in the hospital September 11–October 11, 1981, and again April 9– July 18, 1983. Her final admission was February 25–April 16, 1986, because the voices had come back and were ordering her to set fires, which she would not do. Since then she has been improving steadily and has been well for the past four years. On her birthday, June 1, 1992, she called me to tell me she felt great and that she was hoping she would soon get a job for which she had applied. She has been taken care of by a general practitioner in Vancouver familiar with the orthomolecular treatment program. She is on the following program: Nozinan (100 mg/day), Lithium (300 mg/3x per day), thyroid medication (60 mg/day), niacin (1,000 mg/3x per day), vitamin C (1,000 mg/3x per day), Kemadrin (5 mg/2x per day), and Modecate (50 mg intramuscularly every 7 days). I consider her well. She was seen the following number of times: 1981–82 (12 times); 1983–84 (11 times); 1985–86 (7 times); 1987–88 (3 times); 1989–90 (4 times); and 1991–92 (1 time).

8) D. P., Born 1961

D. P. became very restless and disturbed after a period of hectic activity in preparing for going to college. Her mind ran out of control and she began to hear Satan. At night in her home when she heard the house creak she knew this was Satan. One night she heard him knock three times and she knew this meant he was coming to get her so that she could not go with Christ. The next day she smashed a record she had been listening to the previous day. I saw her later that year when she described her auditory hallucinations, her paranoid ideas about being watched, and her severe anxiety. I admitted her September 16–25, 1980. Later she was able to trace the onset of symptoms to 1977. By March 1981, she was well and working. She was admitted again February 15–27, 1984, because the voices came back but by the end of that year she was well.

I saw her again in the summer of 1981. She had been told by her coworkers about her powerful body odor. She was so embarrassed that she quit. They had considered her dirty, which she was not. She had a typical schizophrenic body odor. I reassured here and advised to drink one glass of cranberry juice each morning. (One of my patients had discovered this and since then I have found it to be very effective.) Soon after she got another job and has remained well since. She is on nicotinamide (1,000 mg/3x per day), vitamin C (3,000 mg/day), vitamin B6 (250 mg/day), zinc gluconate (50 mg/day), Anafranil (75 mg before bed), and Nozinan (50–100 mg/day). She was seen the following number of times: 1979–80 (3 times); 1981–82 (13 times); 1983–84 (15 times); 1985–86 (3 times); 1987–88 (2 times); 1989–90 (3 times); and 1991–92 (3 times). I class her as well.

9) D. M., Born 1954

D. M. was admitted April 1977 because of manic-like behavior with great overexcitement. She had been working aboard a ship where she became very delusional and developed hallucinations. She saw Christ and God in people's eyes and heard Christ's voice in an attitude of prayer. She heard herself think and felt unreal. She showed thought disorder with confusion, paranoid ideas about plots against her, and blocked a lot. With these she was also deeply depressed. She was admitted again May 19–August 2, 1977. By 1978 she was well and has remained free of schizophrenia since then. I have seen her often merely to monitor her treatment and response. She has been well for many years, since 1978. In the meantime she completed her master's degree and married, and is getting along well. She is on nicotinamide (1,000 mg/3x per day) and vitamin C (1,000 mg/3x per day) most of the time. She was seen the following number of times: 1977–78–11; 1979–80 (10 times); 1981–82 (17 times); 1983–84 (16 times); 1985–86 (8 times); 1987–88 (5 times); 1989–90 (3 times); and 1991–92 (3 times).

10) J. K., Born 1921

Seen in 1977 she told me that she had her first breakdown in 1962. She suddenly became psychotic and was diagnosed schizophrenic. She began to feel peculiar and because of severe pain in her stomach was afraid to eat. Her behavior became bizarre; for example, she began to burn her objects in her house, practiced yoga in the street, and urinated on the street. She heard voices. Recently, she once more described how frightened she had been with these phenomena. She was admitted to hospital and was given one ECT. She then persuaded her family to take her home and she was discharged against advice. Since then she had remained very tired to the point she did not feel human.

When I examined her she had no perceptual symptoms, she blocked a lot and had a poor memory and poor concentration, her head felt dull, and she found it hard to follow conversation. She is the type of schizophrenic who would be counted as having responded to treatment simply because she no longer appeared in the mental health system even though she had never recovered but was able to function in the community. Her daughter is a chronic schizophrenic patient still in a mental hospital. I started her on the vitamin program. By the end of 1980 she was well. She is on niacin (2,000 mg/day), vitamin C (2,000 mg/day), pyridoxine (250 mg/day), and zinc gluconate (50 mg/day) combined with Serentil (20 mg/day), Librium (10 mg/day), and thyroid medication (60 mg/day). She was seen the following number of times: 1977–78 (8 times); 1979–80 (18 times); 1981–82 (6 times); 1983–

84 (6 times); 1985–86 (8 times); 1987–88 (5 times); 1989–90 (3 times); and 1991–92 (3 times).

11) L. K., Born 1954

L. K. became ill in 1978 when she was very nervous. I saw her the following year when she complained she could hear her own thoughts, was paranoid, and blocked a lot, and she was very anxious. I diagnosed her anxiety state and started her on a vitamin program. In 1980 I rediagnosed her schizophrenic after she told me about her visions of people in the pictures on walls and hearing voices. She was admitted September 2–29, 1980, July 14–22, 1982, and for the last time July 15– Aug 3, 1985. Early in 1983 her child was born. For a while the department of human resources threatened to take away her baby but her parents took on that responsibility and eventually took charge. She has been doing a fairly good job since then with the help of her parents. Her parents at one point did not accept that her unusual behavior resulted from an illness and had considered her as bad and lost to the family. Once they understood what was happening, they changed their attitude toward her. She is now a single mother living in her own apartment and looking after her child. She is on the following program and follows it very carefully: nicotinamide (3,000 mg/day), vitamin C (1,500 mg), folic acid (5 mg), vitamin B complex (50 mg), Nozinan (210 mg before bed), Elavil (50 mg before bed), and Kemadrin (5 mg/day). She has been seen the following number of times: 1979–80 (6 times); 1981–82 (14 times); 1983–84 (9 times); 1985–86 (19 times); 1987–88 (13 times); 1989–90 (10 times); and 1991–92 (4 times). I class her as well.

12) J. P., Born 1945

J. P. had developed very slowly and was considered retarded. Speech began when she was 9 months, and then stopped until age two and a half. She went to a special school but did not learn much. Three years in a convent taught her more than all her years at the special schools. She learned to read and write. At age 16, she was admitted to a hospital, near Calgary, and many times after until age 20. She was then started on a vitamin program by Dr. Max Vogel and thereafter was a lot better. She and her

mother moved to British Columbia in 1977. When I saw her she felt unreal and was paranoid believing people were talking about her. She was depressed. She had visual illusions and spoke to the Beatles when she saw pictures of them. She had physical evidence of a pyridoxine-zinc deficiency. I started her on a revised vitamin program but could not see her very often as she was living in Vancouver. After many months of agitation, she was moved to a group home in Victoria and was started on Loxitane (60 mg/day). Since then I have been seeing her more regularly. There has been a striking improvement and she is now much improved. She got on well at the group home, is taking rehabilitation courses, and was looking forward to her mother moving to retire to Victoria so that they could both live together again. The change in her in a few months has been dramatic. She is on nicotinamide (3,000 mg/day), vitamin C (3,000 mg/day), pyridoxine (500 mg/day), and a vitamin B complex daily.

13) A. B., Born 1962

I first saw A. B. in 1978 after he had been ill for one year. He had been admitted to hospital for one month. After discharge he was unable to go to school and took a correspondence course at home. He was started on vitamins four months before I saw him. During that first examination he told me about feeling watched, about the visions and voices he had in the past, and about his paranoid ideas about people out to get him and having plotted against him in the past. He was also depressed. I admitted him on October 27–28, 1980, but he was discharged at the request of his mother after one day because his father was seriously ill at home. In 1987 his mother took him to a nearby hospital, where he came under the care of Dr. Moke Williams for 20 days. Since then there has been substantial steady improvement year by year and he is now much improved. He is on nicotinamide (3,000 mg/day), vitamin C (3,000 mg/day), Ativan (1 mg before bed), and Anafranil (50 mg before bed). He came in for his annual check June 10, 1992. He told me that he was well except that he had been slightly depressed for the past two weeks. His major problem now was that he had gained 20 pounds over the past year. His mother agreed that he was well. He was seen the following number of times: 1979–80 (4 times); 1981–82 (0 times); 1983–84 (1 time); 1985–86 (2 times); 1987–88 (1 time); 1989–90 (1 time); and 1991–92 (2 times).

14) S. M., Born 1951

S. M. was always hyperactive according to her husband. In 1980 she suffered a miscarriage giving birth to a dead fetus. She delivered again in 1981 by caesarian section. For the next three weeks she was hyperactive. Because she was overweight she was placed on medication to suppress her appetite. She became psychotic seven days before admission August 4–11, 1982. She denied having any perceptual symptoms, yet was delusional (e.g., she was convinced she was the sister of Terry Fox, a man who ran across Canada to bring attention to the cancer problem), and her behavior had been bizarre. She fled into the street nude. She had two more admissions: September 20–October 8, 1982 and October 29–November 15, 1982. In January 1983 she separated. Since then she has been stable and well having worked at her previous profession as a hairdresser most of the time. She has had several relationships since and had dealt with them in a normal manner. She is now on the following program: Lithium (300 mg), nicotinamide (3,000 mg), vitamin C (1,500 mg), pyridoxine (500 mg), Valium (30 mg), Trilafon (16 mg), and Elavil (560 mg), all daily. She was seen the following number of times: 1981–82 (4 times); 1983–84 (14 times); 1985–86 (12 times); 1987–88 (10 times); 1989–90 (9 times); and 1991–92 (6 times).

15) J. W., Born 1950

J. W. came to see me in 1979 when he told me he had been sick since 1963. At puberty he went "crazy," developed a fear of being seen, and hid as much as he could for the next five years. He also rubbed his eyes incessantly until, he believed, he had damaged them. By age 17 he was in hospital in North Bay, Ontario, for three months. He was admitted again when he was 28 in Terrace, British Columbia. In between he married. This turned out well. When I saw him he believed people were watching him. He told me about the visions and voices he had experienced in 1978, and he still felt unreal occasionally. In his thinking he was paranoid, confused, his memory was poor, there was blocking, and ideas were running through his head. He was also very depressed. At that time he was on 400 mg of Thorazine per day. I admitted him in December 1979 for 17 days. In February 1980 he was nearly well. But he needed another admission in May 1980 for 18 days. In June 1981 he completed his diploma at a community college. Since then he has been working full time. He is now on nicotinamide (500 mg/3x per day), vitamin C (4,000 mg/day), and Valium (15–20 mg/day). I classify him as well.

16) R. B., Born 1950

In 1968 R. B. developed a serious prolonged tremor. The following year he was admitted to the hospital for 10 days and later to the closest mental hospital for eight months. By 1972 he had been in a hospital in Vancouver several times. He was then given a series of ECT and started on a vitamin program. This he had been following when I saw him in 1976. He then told me about his voices to which he would talk or shout back, about feeling unreal, about believing people were watching him. He was paranoid, blocked a lot, and was depressed. I continued him on the vitamins. In 1977 he developed infectious hepatitis. By April 1992 he was improved. His program consisted of niacin (500 mg/3x per day), vitamin C (1,500 mg/3x per day), nicotinamide (1,000 mg/3x per day), Haldol (2 mg before bed), Tofranil (25 mg in the morning), and Anafranil (25 mg before bed). He was seen the following number of times: 1977–78 (8 times); 1979–80 (12 times); 1981–82 (6 times); 1983–84 (5 times); 1985–86 (3 times); 1987–88 (2 times); 1989–90 (1 time); and 1991–92 (2 times).

17) B. W., Born 1965

Seen in 1979 B. W. complained that it all started in 1965 when he was working with heavy equipment that was very noisy. He stated that it "blew his mind." I have never been able to figure out exactly what this meant to him but it has been a very disturbing symptom since then. He was able to work until 1973. Then he was in a car accident and was in the hospital for 14 days. He was then treated at a mental health facility in 1978 for three months. When I saw him he complained of people watching him, hearing voices and distorted sounds so that he could not hear music properly, and having feelings of unreality. He was blocked, his concentration was down, and he was depressed. Subsequently, he was admitted to the hospital on December 5, 1979, for six days, January 28, 1980, for seven weeks, and June 17, 1981, for six weeks. He was in again from August 22 to October 23, 1991. He is on the following program: niacin (1,500 mg/3x per day), vitamin C (1,000 mg/3x per day), Haldol (75 mg/day), Cogentin (6 mg/day), and Ativan (4 mg before bed). I class him as improved.

18) B. A., Born 1956

In 1977 B. A. dropped out of university to join a religious cult. Several years later he came back home still suffering from euphoria and expressing similar religious convictions. When I saw him he complained of voices and visions and was convinced he was getting messages from God. He was paranoid and blocked and suffered from depression. On February 24, 1983, he was admitted for three weeks still complaining of the same symptoms. After that he continued to improve. He has been fully employed for the past eight years. He is on Tofranil (25 mg in the morning), Anafranil (50 mg at bed), Elavil (59 mg at bed), nicotinamide (1,000 mg/3x per day), ascorbic acid (1,000 mg/3x per day), pyridoxine (250 mg/day), zinc sulfate (220 mg/day), and Nozinan (125 mg/day). I have him classed as well.

19) C. C., Born 1949

This patient was very nervous in his teens and was first admitted in 1972 for two months. After discharge he moved to a farm and separated from his wife. In 1973 he was admitted again for two months. After this discharge he ran out of money, stopped all medication, and relapsed requiring his third admission in 1974. Until 1977 he remained on Moditen but this left his mind in a fog and he was changed to Haldol. When I saw him he was having visual and auditory hallucinations and believed people were looking at him all the time. He was

paranoid, delusional, and his memory and concentration were poor. He had continued to suffer episodes of depression. He told me he had taken LSD over a period of time about 60 times and also had drank too much alcohol. By 1979 he began to improve but was still disorganized, depressed, and found it hard to express himself. In April 1979, I doubled his nicotinic acid to 6,000 mg daily. In 1990 I saw him at a supermarket when he told me that he had just completed his B.A. at the university and was looking for summer employment.

He was interviewed by a reporter from the *Times Colonist* in Victoria. This is what he wrote:

C. C. was diagnosed as schizophrenic in 1979. By that time he had been sick for eight years and hospitalized four or five times. After sailing through high school, he entered university and began working toward a degree in engineering. But he soon began to feel unaccountably depressed and anxious. "I used to start crying in class because I was overcome by feelings of not being in control. I started sleeping long hours. I would fall asleep in the hallways at the university. His trouble stayed nameless for a long time. The big problem was I didn't know what was wrong with me. I was never told the word schizophrenic; it was never applied to me." His wife to whom he complained of hearing voices left him. His behavior drove her away. "People abandoned me and I have forgiven them because I was impossible," said C. C, who is articulate and speaks in measured tones.

After he first began to get symptoms, rather than becoming quickly psychotic, he began getting progressively more ill. His hallucinations got worse. When he sat on a chair, he felt it whirling him around the room. When he looked at his arms, he saw pictures but no flesh. Gradually, his life fell apart. Friends fled and the material props of existence slipped out from under him. "I was left all alone in a house with no furniture. When they finally came to get me, they found me curled up behind the refrigerator in the fetal position." His arms were covered with burns. In an attempt to drive the illness out, he had branded himself repeatedly with a fireplace poker. He was taken to hospital in a straitjacket.

In 1978 he moved to Victoria, wanting to make a fresh start in a place that had a reputation for being more spiritually and culturally evolved. He went to see Dr. Hoffer and was relieved when the psychiatrist told him he was sick and could be helped. Until then all he had heard was, "You're weird. You're crazy. You're possessed." Today, he takes a maintenance dose of an antipsychotic drug and doesn't think of going off it. Having lost nearly two decades of his life, he is back at school studying for a bachelors degree in biochemistry.

He is on niacin (2,000 mg/3x per day), vitamin C (1,000 mg/day), vitamin B6 (250 mg/day), zinc sulfate (110 mg/day), and Valium (5 mg/day). I consider him well.

20) C. P., Born 1955

I saw C. P. first in 1978. Her first symptoms started six years earlier while she was attending first-year university. Three years later she took the year off because she suffered from marked mood swings. She moved around a lot and received counseling. Finally, she felt weird, began to hallucinate, and believed that poison had been put into her food. She was admitted to a hospital for three months receiving six ECT and medication. She was then advised that she would never be well. When I saw her she described how she had believed people were watching her, had voices and visions, and felt unreal. She was less paranoid than she been before but still believed there was a plot against her. She blocked a lot and complained that ideas were racing in her mind and that her memory and concentration were poor. With that she was depressed. She was admitted to the hospital July 1981 for three months. By October 1981 she was well. But she was admitted again on February 27, 1982 until March 20, 1982, on two certificates. She was suffering severe hallucinations. I admitted her again on July 1, 1983, but on July 30 she discharged me refusing to follow the program any more.

Many years later she reestablished contact with me by writing me long detailed letters about her progress. In April 1991 she told me she had married, was getting on well, and was operating a store with her husband. In January 1992, she reported she was on a gluten-free diet that she found helpful. In April 1992, she once more wrote to tell me she had been in the hospital for three months and had received another ECT series. Again the voices had been very severe. She was started on Clozaril. She had been on nutrients as well, including nicotinamide (2,000 mg/day), vitamin C (500 mg/3x per day), zinc gluconate (50 mg/day), pyridoxine (100 mg/day), and a vitamin B complex once daily. She said that she had gone off this entire program July 1991 for about two months but then went back onto it. I have classed her as well, even though she had a brief resurgence that responded rapidly to treatment. She was seen two times in 1979–1980, 13 times in 1981–1982, three times in 1983–1984, and once in 1991–1992.

21) R. W., Born 1940

R. W. became psychotic in his early teens. He was then treated in some of the top psychiatric institutions in the United States, including one and a half years at the Menninger Clinic in Houston, Texas, one year at the Institute of Living in Hartford, Connecticut, and in a large number of other hospitals ranging from Florida to New York State. Early in 1971 his father, a New York industrialist, called and asked whether I would be willing to take his son on for treatment. By then he had been sick with no improvement for more than half of his life. By then he had spent about $500,000 on treatment.

At the time I was conducting an experiment to determine what was the most important element in any treatment program for psychiatric patients. I was then at the University Hospital, in Saskatoon, a professor of psychiatry, and director of psychiatric research for the province. The university hospital cost $80 per day and provided ideal ratios of staff to patients. I believe there was at least one staff per patient, perhaps more. At the same time the closest mental hospital treated the same type of patients and their daily cost was around $20 per day. In those heady years when mental hospitals were improving so fast it was commonly believed by psychiatrists and by superintendents of hospitals that one could produce much better treatment results by increasing the ratio of staff to patients. They believed there was almost a direct correlation between this ratio and outcome. I became quite skeptical about this when I found out from research carried out in my division that the results obtained in treating schizophrenic patients were as good at the mental hospital at $20 per day as they were at the university hospital at $80 per day. We should have seen an outcome from the latter up to four times as good.

The major elements in any treatment program are the treating staff, the site of treatment (such as the hospital, clinic, home, the streets, etc.), and the treatment process (i.e., psychotherapy, medication, nutrition, nutrients, etc.). The university hospital and the mental hospital used the same treatment programs, provided the same quality of food, and differed only in the staff to patient ratios. That study suggested that staff to patient ratio was a minor factor. To further test these conclusions, I arranged with the proprietor of a new nursing home in Saskatoon to admit chronic patients under my care. They were coming from the rest of Canada and from the United States. The nursing home would charge the families $20 per day. It would provide nursing supervision, a single room, and I would be responsible for the treatment program. I had agreed to have no more than two patients there at one time. They had none of the usual facilities available to the patients at the university hospital (i.e., no psychologists, no social workers, no occupational therapists, no physiotherapists, and no residents, nor medical students).

My first objective was to find out whether the nursing home could manage these psychotic patients. Everyone was a treatment failure from mental hospitals elsewhere. Within a month it was clear that we were not having any unusual difficulties. The patients did not run away any more than they would have from the hospitals. In fact, the elderly patients in these homes enjoyed having young men and women schizophrenic patients around because they added some life to the setting. Most of the patients offered to help with looking after the seniles and others. I treated over 60 patients in this nursing home over a period of several years. An analysis of the follow-up data showed that the results I was getting with these very chronic sick patients was the same as the results I obtained with similar patients at the university hospital. This reinforced my conclusion that the treatment is the most important single variable. The results I was getting were much superior to the results obtained by using ECT alone or tranquilizers alone. Of course, there must be adequate psychiatric and nursing supervision. But more money should be put into the treatment program than into the facilities and other aspects of treatment if one is to conserve money and get the same good results.

I explained this to the patient's father and I agreed to take his son into the nursing home. By then he had been treated by Dr. Moke Williams in Florida, who had to give him a series of ECT, and later he was treated by Dr. David Hawkins in New York, who also had to give him another series of ECT. He was brought to Saskatoon accompanied by a nurse and he was installed in the nursing home. Very slowly he began to improve. Eventually, I found a family in Saskatoon who took him and when I moved to Victoria another fine family took him in as a member. He now lives in Victoria in his own area, which includes his living room, bedroom, private bathroom, and the run of the house. He eats with the family. He is almost a member of the family. I see him every two weeks. If I were to introduce him to any psychiatrist and not tell them anything about his history, I doubt they would diagnose him as schizophrenic this time, not unless they spent a lot of time with him. He is still paranoid at times but most of the time he is pleasant, cooperative, and well dressed. He spends a lot of time reading books and magazines. He goes with the family on outings. He is as happy as he will ever be. But he still must remain on a very extensive nutrient program with heavy doses of tranquilizers and Anafranil (75 mg per day). He has not needed any more ECT nor has he been admitted to any hospital since coming under my care.

For the first few months after he started on the orthomolecular treatment in Saskatoon, he was totally confused. One time I saw him sitting alongside a woman who was so deteriorated mentally she did not know where she was or what she was doing. Yet R. W. sat patiently beside her trying to teach her how to play checkers. He was completely unaware that she was in an entirely different world. I have classed him improved because he still suffers from symptoms and he is still unemployable.

In 1975 a colleague examined him and wrote the following report:

He has a flat, inexpressive face although at time he appears to be grimacing. His speech is confused and rambling. His affect is basically flat but at times inappropriate. He describes his moods as being very high or very low. He feels that he enjoys life and that life is worth living. He denies suicidal ideas. His thought content showed some rather vague paranoid-delusional ideas concerning religion. However, there appears to be no systematized delusional system. He denies having had any hallucinations at any time. His thought processes show thought blocking, circumstantial thinking, and tangential thinking. At times he also showed punning and clang associations (words based on double meanings and similar sounds rather than coherent meaning). He tried to be abstract in his thinking but tended toward concreteness. There is no confusion, however both his recent and remote memory are very poor. His general knowledge was very good and his intelligence seems to be in the high-normal range. Diagnosis: Chronic hebephrenic schizophrenia.

He is improved.

22) G. J., Born 1951

I saw G. J. in 1971 after he had been sick for two years. He had become very nervous, could not concentrate, and had to drop out of school. He was admitted to Winnipeg General Hospital for three months, where he was given 20 ECT. After that he continued to feel unreal, numb, and frozen. In 1970 he was admitted again for 10 days, followed by three months at the Manitoba Hospital in Brandon. He was discharged in April 1970 but was back in December for four days. When I saw him he suffered from visual illusions, saw his face change in the mirror, heard voices, felt unreal, and heard his own thoughts. He was paranoid, believing everyone was watching him and he could not concentrate. His mood was flat, he felt half dead.

In April 1972 I admitted him to Extendicare, the nursing home that was admitting my patients (described in previous case history). He was started on the vitamin program. He had to be admitted again in Winnipeg, April 14, 1975, for another six ECT. He came under my care again in September 1975 and I admitted him to City Hospital, Saskatoon, for three weeks for treatment of his jaundice. By October that year he was better but still very ill. He was admitted in Kelowna for a few weeks, but since the hospital refused to give him his vitamins he stopped going there.

In March 1977, his aunt who was being very helpful wrote:

It has been nearly two years since I have been in touch with you. G. J. is feeling so well and hasn't had a real setback since you last saw him in the hospital in Saskatoon when you treated him for jaundice.

In April 1987, I wrote to his doctor who had referred him,

I saw this patient in November 1983 at which time he was getting along fairly well. He had done reasonably well until last winter when he began to feel sick, especially around Christmas. His Modecate had to be increased and now he is taking 25 mg every seven days. He is somewhat better now but still not as good as he was. At times he tends to be very paranoid, and he is still preoccupied with thoughts which he finds extremely unpleasant. He is also taking Lithium (750 mg per day) compared to the smaller quantity he was taking before, but I think this is a good idea. I have started him on Anafranil (100 mg before bed) to replace the other antidepressant he was on.

In April 1991, I wrote:

G. J. pointed out that the last summer had been difficult for him because he was much more paranoid than he had been, and it required some readjustment of his medication. By fall, however, he was better. This past winter has been better than the previous winter, and since coming back to British Columbia he has been feeling good. He discussed some of his delusional ideas, which he is trying hard to control. Over the past four days his sense of taste has returned. It first deserted him in 1978 when he became ill. He also reported how lights appeared to be exaggerated last year but they are better now. I think he is continuing to make slow subtle progress.

His program consisted of niacin (1,500 mg/3x per day), vitamin C (2,000 mg/3x per day), pyridoxine (800 mg/day), manganese (50 mg/day), selenium (200 micrograms/ day), Lithium (750 mg/day), zinc gluconate (50 mg/ day), and a few other vitamins. I have classed him much improved.

23) T. D., Born 1961

T. D. became a behavioral problem in 1975. But for the previous two years her work at school deteriorated. She became irresponsible, sexually active, and began to have temper outbursts. She began to suffer blackouts, experienced visual hallucinations and illusions, and her behavior became strange. She had taken LSD several times. When I saw her she told me about her visions and voices, her feelings of unreality (e.g., her legs did not feel attached to her body). Her concentration was poor, and she was very paranoid and very depressed. I started her on a treatment program but for several years she refused to take even vitamins because she was convinced they were poisonous. Eventually, she trusted me enough and began to follow the vitamin program carefully but she remained very suspicious of drugs. Her baby was born October 1980. I admitted her to the hospital in November 1982 for four days. She had her last admission in May 1986 for 10 days. She has been well for the past three years and has been active in the movement to help schizophrenic patients. She is currently taking niacin (1,500 mg/3x per day), vitamin C (1,000 mg/3x per day), Elavil (225 mg before bed), and Thorazine (25 mg before bed). She was seen the following number of times: 1977–78 (1 time); 1979–80 (0 times); 1981–82 (3 times); 1983–84 (8 times); 1985–86 (26 times); 1987–88 (17 times); 1989–90 (11 times); and 1991–92 (0 times).

24) J. J., Born 1946

J. J. is an example of a chronic patient who was treated very intensively for many months but who did not remain on the program after he went home.

He is a good example of the type of response usually obtained with chronic patients taking only tranquilizers. I saw him for the first time in 1971 after he was admitted to the nursing home I have already described. He came with his mother who filled in the details of his history. He told me he had been depressed for four years. One year after onset he was treated at an institue in Toronto, for four months receiving eight ECT. He was slightly better. But there was evidence of trouble long before. As a child he had been very nervous and as a youth he suffered from a learning disorder. After discharge from the hospital, he tried several jobs but could not carry on with any of them. In 1970 he suddenly stopped the Thorazine he was taking. Two weeks later he was catatonic. It was necessary to place him back on the high doses he was on before. When I saw him he reported that people were watching him, told me about his visions of various people and his voices and scenery, and how he heard his own thoughts and felt unreal. He was paranoid, spoke with a peculiar phraseology, and his concentration was poor. Both parents were involved in a plot against him. He was in a nursing home August 31–November 25, 1971. Then he returned home but would not stay with the program. He continued to drink too much and would not follow a sugar-free diet. He came back again July 28–September 5, 1973. I was then told that he had refused to take the vitamins because he had trouble swallowing pills and had to chew them or grind them up. I got him back on the program. He then returned home somewhat better but within a few weeks at home he once more became noncompliant and would not follow the program. His mother tried her best to keep him on the program but his father was very skeptical all along about it and he made little effort to support his wife. Recently, I was informed that he is still ill, not doing well at all, and is in an institution.

Another young man was in the nursing home at the same time. He too received the vitamin program. He went back home. Today, 28 years later, I received a phone call from his mother who was visiting friends in Victoria. She called to bring me up to date. I had forgotten about him and have not been able to locate his file. She told me he was doing well. He had not needed to go back to any hospital. After his treatment in Saskatoon he had done remarkably well and was working five hours each day in one of the supermarkets. He was living in a group home and still followed his vitamin program with the support of his psychiatrist. He again illustrates the beneficial effects of the orthomolecular program if it is maintained. J. J. illustrates what happens when it is not followed.

25) J. M., Born 1968

J. M.'s mother wrote to me in June 1971. Following that discussion she brought him to Saskatoon and I saw him July 2, 1971. I found that he had been treated at a hospital in Toronto in 1968 for two weeks. He was clearly psychotic, hearing voices with a series of paranoid delusions. He believed that the world was going to end, and that he somehow was influencing events outside, including the weather and the world international situation. He was inappropriate, agitated. The conditions had settled in after a few weeks. He was started on medication and responded but remained apathetic, without drive, and always worried and nervous. He showed the early manifestations of tranquilizer psychosis. He had to be readmitted shortly after discharge to readjust his medication, which had been causing severe side effects. When I examined him he spoke to me about his feeling that people were watching him, about being very self-conscious and unreal, and about his deep depression.

He responded very rapidly to the vitamin program but in December 1973 became jaundiced. The doctors immediately concluded he has developed a vitamin B3 jaundice but it turned out to be obstructive and cleared, and when he went back on the vitamins it has not recurred. He still continued to suffer from anxiety and episodes of depression. In May 1974, he did a four-day water fast to determine which foods he might be allergic too. On the fourth day he was well. Thereafter, he avoided certain foods. In 1979 his mother told me he had completed first-year nursing and was well. He had married and had a daughter. In 1986 I was informed that he was well. In 1991 he is still well and now has two children. He has been working at his profession since he graduated about 10 years ago.

As a professional watcher of my colleagues, I am interested in their reaction to patients who tell them they have gotten better on vitamins when they have failed to respond to tranquilizers. This family ran into the usual number of roadblocks in their attempt to get their son well. For example, one psychiatrist, who had never tried out any of the program, told them when they came to see him, "You Hoffer people do have your believers" sarcastically. He suggested by this, that only their faith in me had made him well. This is curious since no double-blind experiment has ever shown that faith alone will help schizophrenics get well, even though faith is an important ingredient in any program and should accompany the use of tranquilizers as well. Another psychiatrist told the family in 1974, "Vitamin therapy is pure crap." He interpreted the disease in their son as arising from family hostility. He told the family, "J. M. was like a fluffy little bird in the nest and that not just his mother, but the whole family was not willing to release him to anyone else." This is very poetic but neither scientific nor medically correct. Shortly after that he was transferred to a different hospital where the attitude to them was more sympathetic and helpful, and less tainted by Freudian jargon. I have classed him as well.

26) G. L., Born 1954

G. L. became sick in 1974 following the taking of LSD on three occasions. She became very depressed and suicidal and was admitted for two days. In 1975 she practiced Transcendental Meditation, went to first-year university, and drank heavily. Following her second suicide attempt, she was admitted to the University of British Columbia's Health Sciences Center, for one month, where she was diagnosed with schizophrenia. After discharge she became more obsessional, felt she was falling apart, and again was admitted for another month. In November 1975, she was in again for two months and again in 1976. Later she was admitted to an institute in Victoria and readmitted on July 5, 1977 when I saw her for the first time. By then she believed people were watching her. The feeling was so strong she was afraid to ride in buses or to go out. She saw walls falling in on her and once saw a suit hanging in her closet become a person of whom she was very fearful. She also heard voices. She was very paranoid, believing people were talking about her, running her down. Her concentration was poor. On top of all that she was very depressed, tense, and suicidal. She then told me she had taken a 10-day fast in 1975 and toward the end had felt marvelous. I started her on the orthomolecular program. She recovered and remained well until 1980 when she began to drink wine heavily. In August 1983, she was depressed but by mid-1986 she was well again and still on her vitamin program. In December that year she made another suicide attempt by setting fire to her apartment. She was in a group home for a while. In 1991 she married but later they separated. She had remained well, had one child, and had developed her own business, which required 10 employees. In May 1992 she was again pregnant, but then it was discovered she had thyroid cancer and this was resected. She was placed on a different vitamin program, including a lot more ascorbic acid. Two weeks after surgery she told me she felt great and was back administering her business. I class her as well.

27) R. S., Born 1958

I first saw R. S. during his third admission to the hospital. He described his visions of God and of love, and his voices that were of two types: the good and the bad. He also believed people were watching him. He was paranoid, believing that someone was going to kill him, and his mood was inappropriate. He was in the hospital May 20–June 16, 1979. I then started him on the orthomolecular program. By July that year he was much better. Early in 1980 he began to show signs of tardive dyskinesia, which cleared in one month when he was started on manganese. In March 1980, he made a suicide attempt by overdosing, was seen in the emergency room, but did not have to be admitted. He was admitted again December 25–January 2, 1980. I saw him in 1984 when he reported that he had not taken his vitamins but had remained on medication. He appeared well and was able to hold two jobs. But after going off all the medication for one month, he relapsed and was readmitted from June 19 to June 30, 1988. He then had been

off his vitamins for seven years. I placed him back on this program again. He has been compliant since then and has been well many years, on Haldol (3 mg/day) plus niacin and vitamin C. He is still fully employed and gets on well with his employer. He was seen the following number of times: 1979–80 (17 times); 1981–82 (3 times); 1983–84 (1 time); 1985–86 (0 times); 1987–88 (4 times); 1989–90 (12 times); and 1991–92 (11 times).

The patient told me he had stopped taking his niacin for one month because he wanted to re-experience his hallucinations again. Within a few days his voices came back and they were the same as they had been before. He became paranoid again. He felt his judgment was affected. For example, he began to believe everything he read. He then resumed the niacin and within four days the hallucinations were gone again.

Discussion

This series of 27 schizophrenic patients is not a randomly selected sample from a larger population of schizophrenics. They were selected using the following criteria: 1) They have been under treatment at least 10 years. 2) With a couple of exceptions, they have been ill an average of seven years before they came for treatment; their average age was 40. 3) They had not been responsive to any previous treatment. From this group of 27, excluding the one chronic patient who did not follow the program, 11 are working, two are married and looking after their family and home, two are single mothers looking after one child, and three are managing their own business. One received a MA, another received a BSc, and a third received a diploma from a community college.

The mean number of times the patients were seen over two-year intervals beginning with the years 1977–78 and ending with the years 1991–92 steadily decreased. The range averaged from a maximum of 9.6 times seen in the earlier intervals with a steady decrease in this statistic until in the last two years it was around four. Number of times seen is one of the criteria I use in determining how patients are getting along. The sicker they are the more frequently are they seen. This is a joint decision since in most cases once they have started to improve I ask them to decide whether they should be seen at intervals of one month, or two, or three, or when they think they would like to come back again. If it is left open, they are told they may call to set up another appointment whenever they feel there is a need to do so. The nurse in charge of group homes decides when patients should be seen again, for the two patients living in these homes. In my opinion chronic patients who are still taking tranquilizers should be seen once or twice each year to monitor progress and to detect side effects. I have found over the past 40 years that patients are more compliant when they are in steady contact with their physician. This means that even when well the mean number of times seen per two-year period will be between two and four.

Chronic patients respond very slowly to treatment and in this series there was little change in the first half of the follow-up period. Only in the past five to seven years has there been a steady and enduring improvement. This cannot be ascribed to the use of new and improved tranquilizers since with these drugs alone this is not the usual response. However, it is possible that combined with the nutrients the newer tranquilizers may have become more effective. Another factor might have been the use of antidepressants, especially clomipramine (Anafranil). I have found this to be very useful in reducing and eliminating paranoid ideas. I consider recurrent paranoid ideas equivalent to obsessive-compulsive ideas. I began to use it when I realized I had never seen cheerful paranoids. It occurred to me that if I could remove their depression it might be easier to let go of their paranoid ideas.

This slow response is a major disadvantage since few psychiatrists in private practice are willing to work that long with their patients, and too often in mental hospitals patients who are discharged are not followed long enough by the same psychiatrist. In my opinion follow-up must be done by physicians who can change the medications and nutrients as needed.

There undoubtedly is some bias in this chronic population. They were willing to stay compliant for this period of time. The patients who would not follow the program would not appear in this kind of follow-up. In my opinion compliance is much less of a problem when orthomolecular treatment is used

since the dose of tranquilizers is much less and there is less incentive for patients to go off the program.

Because of these factors one cannot generalize beyond the parameters of this study. But it does show that chronic patients, who are compliant over enough years, do improve substantially. To deprive them of this chance for recovery and for improvement is to me the height of irresponsibility. Double-blind purists will dismiss this conclusion because it is not a prospective double-blind controlled study. However, such a study, even if I thought it scientifically valid, would be impossible to carry out. I cannot visualize any substantial body of schizophrenic patients taking a placebo for this length of time, nor would it be ethical to expose them to such a charade. Those who demand double blinds are simply using this as a weapon against the use of this particular treatment. There is of course a way of rebutting this data. That is, for any skeptical psychiatrist to select from their caseload a similar group of patients who have been only on tranquilizers and to show that they have done equally well. I would be delighted to see such a series since in my clinical experience going back from the time tranquilizers first were introduced in 1955 I have not been able to find such patients and such responses with the use of these drugs only.

Recently Waring, Lefcoe, Carver, and others reported the course and outcome of 34 early schizophrenic patients. They had had one episode or one admission and were classed as early (acute) patients. According to their description, they were the best group to treat from a prognostic point of view because they had had only one episode, and they came from intact nuclear biologic families who were informed about their diagnosis. They were followed for five years. Sixty percent were still living at home and 82 percent were involved in follow-up. Only one was not on medication of whom half were on antipsychotic drugs. Forty-five percent who had been working at the onset were still working but work time was often reduced to part-time for extended periods of time.

Thus, with the best possible group of patients, given good and dedicated care by professionals and warm and supporting parents, only 40 percent were able to work part- or full-time. With these kind of patients, orthomolecular treatment over two years would have yielded at least 90 percent full recovery. With the use of the best possible ancillary treatment including only drugs, this group has not done as well as the chronic group described in this report. Nor is it likely that the early group will do much better over the next five years, since as I have shown, it is not possible to get well on tranquilizers alone. The authors ended their report as follows "only time will tell whether this cohort is able to work and love in their adult years."

■ CONCLUSION

From this group of 27 patients treated over 10 years, 18 are now well, 3 are much improved, 5 are improved, and 1 is the same as he was at the beginning of this study. The one not improved did not remain on the program after returning to his home in Ontario. None are worse. I have described the criteria I have used earlier in this report. This does not mean that they will be able to escape from seeing psychiatrists at regular intervals. If they are on medication, it is mandatory that they be followed to ensure they come to no harm from the drugs. In addition, problems arise now and then as they do with any group of patients who have a chronic disease, such as diabetes mellitus for example. The second major conclusion is that orthomolecular treatment is safe even when used for over 10 years. The third conclusion is that no major side effects are caused by the smallish doses of tranquilizers that many of these patients still require. The program does not produce tranquilizer psychosis. The tranquilizer dilemma is solved.

The final conclusion is that schizophrenic patients find the program palatable and will remain compliant. They are able to look forward to continuing improvement. I expect that if I could do another follow-up in 10 more years with the same group, the follow-up results would be even better. The onus is now on orthodox psychiatry to demonstrate by research of their own that there is a major fault in these conclusions. It is not good enough to assume that this is all due to a series of unproven assumptions such as a placebo effect, faith, or even some monstrous conspiracy to show

something works when in fact it does not. Or will the profession adopt the stance of a California psychiatrist who recently testified for 15 minutes before a judge that one of the patients was psychotic since she believed that vitamins had been helpful to her?

REFERENCES

1. Bockoven JS, Solomon HC. Comparison of two five-year follow-up studies: 1947–1953 and 1967–1972. *Am Jl Psychiatry* 1975;132:796–801.

2. Cathcart RF. Vitamin C: the non toxic , non rate limited antioxidant free radical scavenger. *Med Hypotheses* 1985;18:61–77.

3. Cheraskin E. *The Vitamin C Controversy; Questions and Answers.* Wichita, KS: Bio-communications Press, 1988.

4. Cheraskin E, Ringsdorf, WM, Sisley EL. *The Vitamin C Connection.* New York: Harper & Row, 1983.

5. Cowley G. Live longer with vitamin C. *Newsweek,* May 18, 1992.

6. Hawkins DR. The prevention of tardive dyskinesia with high dosage vitamins: a study of 58,000 patients. *J Orthomolecular Med* 1986;1:24–26.

7. Hegarty JD. Summarized in *Science News,* May 16, 1992.

8. Hoffer A. Nicotinic acid: an adjunct in the treatment of schizophrenia. *Am J Psychiatry* 1963;120:171–173.

9. Hoffer A. *Niacin Therapy in Psychiatry.* Springfield, IL: C.C. Thomas, 1962.

10. Hoffer A. Treatment of organic psychosis with nicotinic acid (a single case). *DisNerv Syst* 1965;26:358–360.

11. Hoffer A. The effect of nicotinic acid on the frequency and duration of re-hospitalization of schizophrenic patients: a controlled comparison study. *Int J Neuropsychiatry* 1966;2:234–240.

12. Hoffer A. A comparison of psychiatric inpatients and outpatients and malvaria. *Inter J Neuropsychiatry* 1965;1:430–432.

13. Hoffer A. Malvaria and the law. *Psychosomatics* 1966;7:303–310.

14. Hoffer A. Five California schizophrenics. *J Schizophrenia* 1967;1:209–220.

15. Hoffer A. Biochemistry of nicotinic acid and nicotinamide. *Psychosomatics* 1967;8:95–100.

16. Hoffer A. Safety, Side Effects and Relative Lack of Toxicity of Nicotinic acid and Nicotinamide. *Schizophrenia* 1969;1:78–87.

17. Hoffer A. Pellagra and schizophrenia. Academy of Psychosomatic Medicine, Buenos Aires, Jan. 12–18, 1970. *Psychosomatic* II, 1979:522–525.

18. Hoffer A. A vitamin B-3 dependent family. *Schizophrenia* 1971;3:41–46.

19. Hoffer A. Vitamin B-3 dependent child. *Schizophrenia* 1971;3:107–113.

20. Hoffer A. Megavitamin B-3 therapy for schizophrenia. *Can Psychiatric Ass J* 1971;16:499–504.

21. Hoffer A. Orthomolecular treatment of schizophrenia. *Orthomolecular Psych* 1972:46–55.

22. Hoffer A. Treatment of hyperkinetic children with nicotinamide and pyridoxine. *Can Med Ass J* 1972;107:111–112.

23. Hoffer A. Mechanism of action of nicotinic acid and nicotinamide in the treatment of schizophrenia. In: *Orthomolecular Psychiatry* edited by DR Hawkins and L Pauling. San Francisco: W.H. Freeman, 1973.

24. Hoffer A. Hong Kong veterans study. *J Orthomolecular Psych* 1974;3:34–36.

25. Hoffer A. Natural history and treatment of thirteen pairs of identical twins, schizophrenic and schizophrenic-spectrum conditions. *J Orthomolecular Psych* 1976;5:101–122.

26. Hoffer A. Megavitamin Therapy for Different Cases. *J Orthomolecular Psych* 1976;5:169–182.

27. Hoffer A. To the Editor. Tardive dyskinesia treated with manganese. *Can Med Ass J* 1977;117:859.

28. Hoffer A. Orthomolecular nutrition at the zoo. *J Orthomolecular Psych* 1983;12:116–128.

29. Hoffer A. Ascorbic acid and kidney stones. *Can Med Ass J* 1985;132:320.

30. Hoffer A. Niacin, coronary disease and longevity. *J Orthomolecular Med* 1989;4:211–220.

31. Hoffer A. *Orthomolecular Medicine for Physicians.* New Canaan, CT: Keats Pub, 1989.

32. Hoffer A. *Vitamin B-3 (Niacin) Update.* New Canaan, CT: Keats Pub, 1990.

33. Hoffer A, Osmond H, Callbeck MJ, et al. Treatment of schizophrenia with nicotinic acid and nicotinamide. *J Clin Exper Psycho-pathol* 1957;18:131–158.

34. Hoffer A, Kelm H, Osmond H. *The Hoffer-Osmond Diagnostic Test.* Huntington, NY: RE Krieger Pub Co, 1975.

35. Hoffer A, Mahon M. The presence of unidentified substances in the urine of psychiatric patients. *J Neuropsychiatr* 1961;2:331–362.

36. Hoffer A, Osmond H. *The Chemical Basis of Clinical Psychiatry.* Springfield, IL: CC Thomas, 1960.

37. Hoffer A, Osmond H. Treatment of schizophrenia with nicotinic acid: a ten year follow-up. *Acta Psychiat Scand* 1964;40:171–189.

38. Hoffer A, Osmond H. The relationship between an unknown factor (us) in the urine of subjects and hod test results. *J Neuropsychiatry* 1961;2:363–368.

39. Hoffer A, Osmond H. People are watching me. *Psychiatric Quart* 1963;37:7–18.

40. Hoffer A, Osmond H. Malvaria: a new psychiatric disease. *Acta Psychiat Scand* 1963;39:335–366.

41. Hoffer A, Osmond H. Some psychological consequences of perceptual disorder and schizophrenia. *Int J Neuropsychiatry* 1966;2:1–19.

42. Hoffer A, Osmond H. *How to Live with Schizophrenia.* New York: Citadel Press, 1974, revised 1992.

43. Hoffer A, Pauling L. Hardin Jones biostatistical analysis of mortality data for cohorts of cancer patients with a large fraction surviving at the termination of the study and a comparison of survival times of cancer patients receiving large regular oral doses of vitamin C and other nutrients with similar patients not receiving those doses. *J Orthomolecular Med* 1990;5:143–154.

44. Johnstone EC, et al. Disabilities and circumstances of schizophrenic patients: a follow-up study. *Brit J Psychiatry* 1991;159 (Supp 13):33.

45. Kunin RA. Manganese and niacin in the treatment of drug-induced dyskinesias. *J Orthomolecular Psych* 1976;5:4–27.

46. Osmond H, Hoffer A. Massive niacin treatment in schizophrenia: review of a nine-year study. *Lancet* 1963;1:316–320.

47. Pauling, L. *How to Live Longer and Feel Better.* New York: W.H. Freeman & Co, 1986.

48. Pauling L, Rath M. An orthomolecular theory of human health and disease. *J Orthomolecular Med* 1991;6:135–138.

49. Pfeiffer CC. *Mental and Elemental Nutrients.* New Canaan, CT: Keats Pub, 1975.

50. Pfeiffer CC, Maillous R, Forsythe L. *The Schizophrenias: Ours to Conquer.* Wichita, KS: Bio-Communications Press, 1988.

51. Pfeiffer CC, Ward J, El-Melegi M, et al. *The Schizophrenias: Yours and Mine.* New York: Pyramid Books, 1970.

52. Rath M, Pauling, L. Solution to the puzzle of human cardiovascular disease: its primary cause is ascorbate deficiency leading to the deposition of lipoprotein(a) and fibrinogen/ fibrin in the vascular wall. *J Orthomolecular Med* 1991;6:125–134.

53. Rath M, Pauling L. Apoprotein(a) is an adhesive rotein. *J Orthomolecular Med* 1991;6:139–143.

54. Rath M, Pauling L. A unified theory of human cardiovascular disease leading the way to the abolition of this disease as a cause for human mortality. *J Orthomolecular Med* 1992;7:5–15.

55. Rath M, Pauling L. Plasmin-induced proteolysis and the role of Apoprotein(a), Lysine and Synthetic Lysine analogues. *J Orthomolecular Med* 1992;7:17–23.

56. Stone, I. *The Healing Factor: Vitamin C Against Disease.* New York: Grosset & Dunlap, 1972.

57. Waring EM, Lefcoe DH, Carver C, et al. The course and outcome of early schizophrenia. psychiatric. *J University of Ottawa* 1988;13:194–197.

58. Wittenborn JR. A search for responders to niacin supplementation. *Archives General Psychiatry* 1974;31:547–552.

59. Wittenborn JR, Weber ESP, Brown M. Niacin in the Long-Term Treatment of Schizophrenia. *Arch Gen Psychiatry* 1973;28:308–315.

BACKGROUND TO NIACIN TREATMENT

by Humphry Osmond, MD

Fifteen years ago Dr. Abram Hoffer and I began the first double-blind trial of niacin and niacinamide in Saskatchewan, Canada. It was also, so far as we knew, the second double-blind study undertaken in North America, for we had, ourselves, recently completed the first some months earlier.[1]

In those days the double-blind trial, which has become over the years something of a sacred cow, was an innovation, foisted upon clinicians by statisticians and methodologists, and viewed with suspicion by most clinicians. It was accorded none of the reverence that it now receives. Methodologists and statisticians were, however, loud in their praises for the new device even though they had at that time very little evidence with which to support their belief. Today, when such trials are two a penny, sophisticated statisticians and methodologists are less enchanted, and sometimes highly critical.[2,3]

We had already striking clinical evidence that our treatment helped in the treatment of schizophrenia. A recent follow-up of our first eight patients given niacin over 15 years ago shows that our original impressions were not ill founded since all eight are well today. Eight cases is not many; however, James Lind's 1753 classic study of scurvy employed only 12 men, and, when the two who had been given citrus fruit got well, he judged correctly that he had a remedy for scurvy.[4] Joseph Lister's 1867 famous paper on compound fractures described 11 cases of whom one died, one had to be amputated, and the other nine recovered. We have no evidence that more would have been learned using the most modern experimental designs.

The Days of Phenothiazines

One feature of our studies in the treatment of schizophrenia with niacin and other methods is that we sometimes underestimated these niacin studies with what would now be regarded as exemplary caution. Unluckily, we picked one of the worst possible times for such scientific reserve. Those who were marketing the phenothiazines, having doubtless compared the safety of their sub-stances with the barbiturates and similar compounds, promoted and advertised them with resolve. Millions of dollars were spent on developing new ones, testing those already found, and informing medical men about those considered to be valuable. To be more acceptable in the climate of the 1950s, phenothiazines were frequently and rather ingenuously described as being mere adjuncts to psychotherapy. There was at that time no evidence whatever that schizophrenia was benefited by psychotherapy; indeed, Freud, Federn, Jung, and many others had at various times expressed doubts as to whether this ever happened. In a very recent survey of the phenothiazines after 14 years use Kinrose-Wright noted, "There is no convincing evidence that intensive psychotherapy with or without inadequate atarac-tic (tranquilizing) medication can benefit the majority of psychotic patients. There is ample evidence that adequate phenothiazine treatment without psychotherapy can benefit them. There is also evidence that if these patients are maintained and supervised on adequate doses of phenothiazines for indefinite periods they may be kept out of the hospital and remain in the community. Unfortunately, there is also evidence that unless they are actively rehabilitated into a productive life, the majority of chlorpromazine-maintained patients will exist to become chronically disabled citizens."[6] There is little doubt that the effect upon psychiatric morale of these useful substances encouraged those who worked in mental hospitals to insist upon reforms that were long overdue. The operation, staffing, equipping, and general design of mental hospitals have all been benefically affected by the breathing space given by the phenothiazines. It would be both churlish, untruthful, and lacking in gratitude to Henri Laborit, whose ingenuity and perceptiveness played so large a part in furthering their great value.

From the *Journal of Schizophrenia* 1967;1(1):126–131.

However, once the first five years had elapsed, many of us were curious to know whether the long-term outcome of schizophrenia had changed for the better. During those heady days, little notice was taken of niacin and we simply continued our studies on the prairies. It took about a decade for psychiatrists to grasp what Dr. J. D. W. Pearce of St. Mary's Hospital, London, has wittily described in these words: "In the old days we had the closed door, then the open door, and now we have the revolving door." Shortly before this, Enid Mills in a compassionate but rather depressing book called *Living with Mental Illness* (1962) had shown that even when good policies were used in a well-run hospital, many people left the hospital to live very miserable lives outside it in spite of phenothiazine treatment.[7]

An Old Orphan Treatment

As the years passed and we studied our niacin data, we found more and more evidence that those who took the vitamin in addition to other treatments did better than those who did not do so. It was natural that we should become increasingly interested in these findings as the shortcomings of the valuable phenothiazines became clearer. Our double-blind experiments[8,9] and a later one by Denson[10] all suggested that particularly in early schizophrenia the outcome could be altered for the better by the rather humdrum means of giving large doses of a well-known vitamin. We had, however, great difficulty in getting anyone else to try our treatment, even though we were advocating one of the cheapest, safest, and easiest of treatments ever suggested in psychiatry. Cynically, perhaps, we have sometimes felt that this was its main disadvantage. In addition ours was an orphan treatment. No great pharmacological house was prepared to spend a small fortune on testing and promoting a non-proprietary substance. It would have been unreasonable to expect them to do so. This resulted in very few psychiatrists ever hearing about niacin and those who did were suspicious. One asked why more people did not use it, if it was as good as we claimed.

Five- and 10-year follow-up studies continued to show benefits that no one had been able to claim for the phenothiazines alone. It was clear that niacin did not work as quickly as the newer substances but luckily they were compatible and possibly synergistic with it. We published repeatedly, but, in 1963, after the monograph on niacin therapy that had stirred very little interest was completed,[11] we decided to write a popular book. For a decade we had informed our colleagues about our findings in the accepted professional manner without exciting even the mildest curiosity. Those findings showed that, if careful observation and follow-up of several hundred cases, combined with a variety of statistical evaluations and the use of a chemical and psychological test, both of an objective kind, meant anything, then we had evidence that we could improve the long-term outcome of schizophrenia—by very simple means. In the course of the years, we had developed a concept of schizophrenia very different from that put forward by Kraepelin, Bleuler, or Freud and his disciples. This would have been no surprise in other branches of medicine, but, to at least some psychiatrists, concepts developed in the late 19th or early 20th centuries are considered sacrosanct. Psychiatrists almost alone in medicine today still parade old ideas as if they were icons rather than guideposts along the way.

Due to this curious series of accidents, many of our colleagues first learnt about our niacin treatment from their patients who had read our only non-professional book, *How to Live with Schizophrenia* (1966). This book led some kind people in the press, radio, and TV to hail the use of niacin as a new discovery. But this is not true. It is an old discovery! Some psychiatrists, indignant it seems at being told something by their patients of which they were unaware, have spoken angrily about this new discovery being made available to the lay public before being told to the profession. Had this been a new discovery and had the profession been so uninformed, we would have been the first to deplore such a gaffe. However, since this is no new discovery and since professional articles and books have referred to our clinical research work repeatedly, there is no need to apologize. We are not responsible for the combination of information explosion and the ethical advertising implosion, which hid the use of niacin from the profession. It has, however, been gratifying to find that some of our colleagues who have read our papers and have been courteous enough to give this treatment a fair trial appear to have achieved results very similar to our own. They are not often dramatic but they work.

Innovation Rarely Welcome

We had thought that university and mental hospital psychiatrists would be among the first to use our treatment. We reasoned that the former, who had more time for research, reading, and reflection, would be curious about our discovery; while the latter, working in hospitals often swamped by enormous numbers of readmissions and seeing the dismal consequences of long-established schizophrenia, would be most anxious to explore anything that might reduce chronicity if employed early. Since niacin is so inexpensive and safe, we assumed that directors of mental hospitals would be keen to try a treatment that might save money and reduce laboratory work. It seemed to us that private practitioners would be too busy to study such new methods, might be discouraged because niacin is often rather slow to act, and await the decision of the leaders of the profession before trying anything new. We have been wholly mistaken. It seems that it is in the offices of private practitioners that the shortcomings of current treatments are seen in the most vivid, immediate, and striking manner. In addition, private practitioners see patients who are bold and articulate enough to complain about the discomfort of taking tranquilizers, which, useful as they undoubtedly are, often produce side effects.

All this would make one think that great and sustained efforts would have been made to enquire carefully into any treatment, however unlikely, that might offer some prospect of changing the long-term outlook of schizophrenia. Yet, to expect this would be to ignore not only the history of medicine but also that of science. Medical men are, generally speaking, like every one else—they do not enjoy innovation and tend to do what

is customary. Failure to be convinced by well-planned experiments is not by any means unique to medicine. An article on learning in planarians (flat worms) puts the matter clearly: "When is a replication not a replication? Answer: When nobody has read the original study and did not believe it anyhow." After quoting some discouraging experiences in which repeated replication did not convince, he continues, "What good does it do to publish replications over and over again if no one reads them? On the other hand, what good does it do to replicate an experiment if no one believes you?"[12] Yet, it is far easier to assess results in an elegant laboratory study of learning in flat worms than it is in clinical psychiatry where human beings are so much more difficult to control and live so much longer. To assess the result of the psychiatric treatment adequately, experiments must often last for months, years, or even decades.

Innovation is rarely welcome. For as the English poet John Milton observed sourly, "Truth never comes into the world, but like a bastard, to the ignominy of him that brought her forth." However, there have been many happy and successful bastards, love-children worthy of the name. Our views about unconventional children and unconventional ideas are determined largely by our set, our customary posture when meeting the unexpected or the unknown. There have been times when bastardy was no slur, indeed, it was thought to confer greater vigor. The niacin treatment is, we hope and believe, robust enough to survive the scorn and disregard of the orthodox, it may even come to thrive on it.

It is one of the very few treatments in psychiatry that comes close to meeting Claude Bernard's requirements for human experiments, where he said, "Those that can only harm are forbidden. Those that involve no foreseeable harm to the patient are innocent and therefore permissible. Those that may do good are obligatory." Of how many other treatments for schizophrenia could this be said?

694

REFERENCES

1. Clancy J. et al. Design and planning in psychiatric research: illustrated by the Weyburn Nucleotide Project. *Menninger Clinic Bulletin* 1954;18:147–153.

2. Chassan JB. *Research Design in Clinical Psychology and Psychiatry.* New York: Appleton Century Crofts, 1967.

3. Hogben L. *Statistical Theory.* New York: Norton, 1957.

4. Lind J. *Treatise on Scurvy.* London, 1753.

5. Lister J. Antiseptic principle in the practice of surgery. *British Med Journal* 1867;2:246.

6. Kinross-Wright J. The current status of the phenothiazines. *JAMA* 1967;200:461–464.

7. Mills E. *Living with Mental Illness.* London: Routledge & Kegan Paul, 1962.

8. Hoffer A. et al. Treatment of schizophrenia with nicotinic acid and nicotinamide. *Journal of Clinical and Experimental Psychopathology* 1957;18:131–158.

9. Hoffer A, Osmond, H. A card-sorting test helpful in making psychiatric diagnosis. *Journal of Neuropsychiatry* 1961;2:6.

10. Denson, R. Nicotinamide in the treatment of schizophrenia. *Diseases of the Nervous System,* 1962;23:167–172.

11. Hoffer A. *Niacin Therapy in Psychiatry.* Springfield, Illinois: Charles Thomas, 1962.

12. McConnell JV. Worms (and things). *Journal of Biological Psychology* 1967;9:1–4.

PHYSICIAN'S REPORT: ALLAN'S SECOND CHANCE

by Abram Hoffer, MD, PhD

Allan consulted me when he was 34 years old. He had been hyperactive his entire life. About eight years before I saw him, he had become depressed and paranoid. His paranoid delusions got worse until he was committed to a mental hospital for six months. Treatment included a series of electroconvulsive therapy (ECT). He improved slowly. By 1972 he was able to work at a day-care center but again became hyperexcitable and paranoid. He was discharged from his job. He was then started on orthomolecular treatment. During the summer of 1973 he stopped all the vitamins and began to drink excessively. His psychosis recurred, leading to his second admission to the same mental hospital, subsequently transferring to a private hospital for one year. During this year he received 20 ECT combined with moderate amounts of B vitamins. He improved slowly. When I saw him, he stated he had been free of psychosis for over one year. His diagnosis had been schizophrenia on remission.

At this point, each reader of this brief anecdote should try to predict Allan's future course. Did he remain sick thereafter, with frequent readmissions, on social assistance, lonely, unemployed, and unemployable? Did he remain stable but unable to work because he was suffering from the tranquilizer psychosis (fatigue, apathy, disinterest, tremor), or was he able to overcome his illness and become a normally productive and responsible person? After you make your prediction based on what I have written, read on.

I added niacin 3,000 milligrams per day to his program. He was normal three months later. He married in October 1978. In November 1989 he reported he had been employed full time for ten years in a job he liked. Both he and his wife were very pleased. On February 14, 1995, he called me to thank me for his good health. He added that he felt better than he ever could remember, was very cheerful and upbeat, and was still faithful to his vitamin regime.

I consider Allan well because: 1) he is free of symptoms; 2) he gets on well with his family; 3) he gets on well in the community; and 4) he is employed full time and pays taxes. Before he was started on vitamins he had spent nearly two years in hospital. He had had several jobs but could not cope with his day-care job. After treatment with niacin was started, he was able to work within three months.

From the *J Orthomolecular Med* 1995;10(2):68–89.

ZINC AND MANGANESE IN THE SCHIZOPHRENIAS

by Carl C. Pfeiffer, MD, PhD, and Scott LaMola

The essential trace elements zinc and manganese have been noted as factors in brain disease since the 1920s. The first suggestion that a trace element deficiency might be a factor in mental disease was that of Derrien and Benoit[19] who found a high level of urinary zinc (Zn) in a dying porphyric female patient showing abnormal psychiatric symptoms. Pyroluria is a familial disorder that occurs with stress. The first use of a trace element as treatment for schizophrenia was that of Reiter, [61] who found intravenous manganese (Mn) to be effective. He found that 23 to 50 patients improved after the injections. Schrijver[67] gave manganese chloride intravenously to 23 patients with good improvement in 3 patients, and possible improvement in 7. Helweg[29] treated 95 chronic schizophrenics with negative results. Tindinge[73] used either oral or intravenous Mn in 75 patients and found only one dramatic improvement. Reed[60] used a control schizophrenic group of 30 patients and found that 18 percent of the controls were discharged from the hospital in one year, while 37 percent of the Mn-treated schizophrenic patients (30 patients) were discharged. Reed used a Mn solution intravenously twice weekly over a period of 15 weeks, followed by manganese chloride twice daily by mouth.

Manganese

W. M. English[21] studied many schizophrenics but had the best results with Mn in those who had been psychotic only two weeks to three years. Of 38 such patients, an increase in body weight, physical improvement, and mental improvement occurred in 22 patients. Some of the chronic patients also improved. R. G. Hoskins[33] used manganese dioxide intramuscularly in 30 patients with only 2 improved, 2 worse, and 26 unchanged. Although Hoskins failed to follow the experimental procedure and design of the successful investigators, his study triumphed and manganese hydrochloride intravenously was no longer used. We found in 1968[81] that oral Mn produced a three-fold increase in excretion of copper (Cu) in schizophrenic patients and that the combination of Zn and Mn was even more effective in promoting urinary-Cu excretion.

In 1965 Professor Roger Williams called our attention to the paper of Kimura and Kumura,[42] who found the brains of schizophrenics at autopsy to have only 50 percent of the Zn content of control brains. This low level of Zn held constant for the frontal, occipital, and hippocampal portions (three of the four different sections) of the brains studied. We know that Zn is essential in the hippocampal portion of the brain, where histamine is stored in histaminergic nerve endings. We, therefore, purchased an atomic absorption spectrophotometer for measuring concentrations of elements analyzed in body tissues and juices. We have seen over 15,000 outpatients and each outpatient has had blood serum and hair analyzed for both the trace and toxic elements.

From 1966 to 1971, we observed lasting clinical benefit with zinc-manganese combination drops in many patients who had high-hair or high-serum Cu levels and low serum Zn levels. By 1977 we had perfected the method for whole-blood Mn determination, so we now encounter schizophrenics who initially are high in serum Cu and low in both serum Zn and whole-blood Mn. These biochemical abnormalities revert to normal, as the patient improves mentally and physically. In our opinion, the use of Mn and Zn to reduce the Cu burden of the body and restoration of Zn in the hippocampus allows for a reduction in the need for major tranquilizers in the schizophrenic. In some cases this Cu excess with Zn and Mn deficiency is the only biochemical imbalance.

By 1971 we had objective data showing that mauve-positive schizophrenic patients (identified by measuring kryptopyrroles in the urine)[37] actually excreted almost twice as much Zn as did schizophrenic patients who were not mauve positive.

From the *J Orthomolecular Psych* 1983;12(3): 215–234.

Kryptopyrrole is an avid aldehyde reacting agent that we have shown to combine irreversibly with pyridoxal phosphate (the active form of vitamin B6). The new molecule then chelates Zn with the combined product appearing in the urine. The whole syndrome is stress induced so the susceptible patient when stressed, quickly becomes vitamin B6 and Zn deficient. Armed with this knowledge we can effectively treat the pyroluric patient and we have written several papers on the signs, symptoms, and treatment of pyroluria.[51,52]

By 1977 our method for whole-blood Mn was applied to all outpatients, both new and old. This revealed that many patients who had been treated with Zn alone had become Mn deficient. With new patients, the diagnostic categories with the lowest Mn levels were the epileptics, hypoglycemics, pylorurics, and schizophrenics. Zinc is easily and rapidly absorbed from the gut but Mn is poorly absorbed and we don't know at present how to increase the whole-blood Mn other than by the administration of large doses of Mn gluconate daily over a long period of time. We have tried all of the presently marketed oral preparations of Mn. We have not tried parenteral or intravenous Mn as a supplement.

Practical Aspects of Manganese Supplements

In the 1977–1979 period, we noted low blood Mn levels in many of our schizophrenic patients and, therefore, increased the dose of oral Mn, using either 10 milligrams (mg) elemental or 50 mg of Mn gluconate. To our surprise, the blood Mn level in many instances continued to be low or go to a lower level. Most of these patients were receiving 30 mg of Zn gluconate morning and night, which in retrospect is a large dose since the body needs only 10–15 mg a day. Patients with normal eating habits would require less supplementation since 5–8 mg is obtained from a good diet. When the Zn supplement is reduced to 15 mg a day, the blood Mn level will usually rise with a daily dose of 10–20 mg of Mn. (Note: that this dose is two to four times the recommended daily intake.)

We are at present studying the factors that may increase the absorption of Mn from the intestinal tract. When normal subjects in the fasting state take 150 mg of Mn as the gluconate (or amino acid chelate) this dose does not cause a significant rise in the serum Mn level over a period of four hours. The eating of a breakfast high in manganese content does not significantly elevate the serum Mn levels. Ninety percent of the blood Mn is contained in the red blood cells or erythrocyte, which has a life of 120 days. The determination of whole blood Mn is useful in our clinic since patients are seen every three to six months. Patients with a blood Mn below 8 nanograms per gram (ng/g or ppb) slowly develop macrocytosis (high cell volume and elevated cell hemoglobin). These patients have normal serum folate and vitamin B12 levels and the macrocytosis responds to a dietary supplement of Mn with the Zn supplement reduced to a maximum of 15 mg per day.

With Zn alone and sometimes supplemented with a combination of zinc, manganese, and vitamin C, morning and evening, the patient's whole blood Mn will decrease over a treatment period of

---

IN BRIEF

The essential trace elements zinc and manganese have been noted as factors in brain disease since the 1920s. The combined use of zinc and manganese in schizophrenia is based on: 1) increased urinary excretion of copper when both zinc and manganese are given orally, 2) zinc alone causes a decrease in blood manganese, and 3) the double deficiency of zinc and manganese frequently is found in patients with excess copper. The mauve factor (kryptopyrrole) is known to increase the excretion of zinc and pyridoxine (vitamin B6). In children insufficient levels of zinc and manganese have been associated with lowered learning ability, apathy, lethargy, and mental retardation. Hyperactive children may be deficient in zinc, manganese, and vitamin B6 and have an excess of lead and copper. Alcoholism, schizophrenia, Wilson's disease, and Pick's disease are brain disorders dynamically related to zinc and manganese levels. Zinc has been employed with success to treat Wilson's disease, acrodermatitis enteropathica (abnormal fatty acid metabolism), and specific types of schizophrenia.

4–12 months. These low Mn levels can result in depression, intolerance to oral Zn, possible increase in autoimmune reactions and the afore-mentioned macrocytosis. The finding of a lowered Mn blood level with prolonged Zn supplementa-tion has occurred in psychiatric, arthritic, senile, and cardiac patients. Thus, all diagnostic cate-gories can be harmed by large prolonged doses of Zn without Mn.

With this new concept we have treated prob-lem patients with large oral doses of Mn. In one severely allergic male, age 45, whom we had treated for 15 years, we suggested 50 mg of Mn morning and night. He felt somewhat better with this dose, so he cautiously increased the dose to 100 mg, three times per day. Before starting this dose his blood Mn was 6 ng/g. After three months of the large dose, his blood Mn was 11 ng/g. One month later the level was 8.5 ng/g, and a year and a half later it was 10.5 ng/g. Normal is 10–20 ng/g. Physical examination, blood pressure, pulse, and chem screen showed no abnormalities. During the period of 300 mg of Mn orally per day, he gained 11 needed pounds in body weight and was able to tolerate foods that normally caused severe depres-sive reactions. With the higher blood levels of Mn, this patient now can tolerate small doses of Zn, which previously caused severe depression.

Manganese Levels in the Hair of Schizophrenics

Other than the therapeutic trials of Mn in schizo-phrenics by Reiter in 1929,[61] the first demonstra-tion of a possible deficiency of Mn was reported in our survey in 1974. We found Mn to be low in the hair of schizophrenics, and in males (but not in females) Mn decreased with age. Barlow[3] found Mn to be significantly lower in the hair of schizo-phrenics compared to a control population. Bowen[8] found the Mn in hair of Indonesian chil-dren to be normal but protein-deficient Indonesian children had a level five times higher. The hair copper level in these same children was two times higher. Perhaps the continuous ingestion of tropi-cal fruits (high in Mn) with a low-protein diet might account for the very high Mn level of the protein-deficient Indonesian children. Ryan and

others[64] reported Mn hair levels of both male and female patients diagnosed with multiple sclerosis to be one-half that of a normal population. The hair Zn levels of the MS patients were not lower than the controls.

Manganese and Tardive Dyskinesia

Excesses of the metal ions of manganese, mercury, copper, cadmium, and lead all appear to cause mal-functions of the central nervous system in animals and man. Manganese is unusual among these ions since neurological abnormalities have been associ-ated with both a deficiency and an excess of Mn.

Neuroleptic (antipsychotic) drugs are known to cause tardive dyskinesia in which the patient exhibits involuntary, rhythmic movements of the tongue, lips, and facial muscles; sometimes exhibit-ing abnormal trunk movements or twisting and writing (choreoathetoid) movements of the extremi-ties. This condition is usually reversible but in the long run may become irreversible in some patients.

In his earlier work with psychiatric patients who developed tardive dyskinesia on neuroleptic drugs, Kunin[43] tried antiparkinson agents and *Rauwolfia serpentina* (a plant containing reserpine, an alkaloid substance with powerful sedative effects) to no avail. He then recalled the work of Borg and Cotzias,[4] who reported that phenoth-iazines form free radicals with manganic (triva-lent) ions in vitro. Manganese is found in high concentrations in the extrapyramidal system (the network of nerves that help regulate motion). He reasoned that phenothiazines might chelate Mn, thus binding it electrochemically, and that this might make it unavailable for some presumed function as an enzyme activator. It seemed plausi-ble that by providing extra dietary Mn the defi-ciency would be corrected and the dyskinesia might thereby improve.

Kunin[43] found in 15 cases of tardive dyskinesia treated with Mn, 7 were completely relieved; 3 cases were much improved; 4 were improved, and only 1 was unimproved. Good results followed Mn doses of at least 15 mg and up to 60 mg a day. Niacin, at doses of 100–500 mg, was of significant benefit in treating dyskinesia in 3 of the 15 cases. Mean content of Mn in the hair of a psychiatric patient population averaged 0.8 parts per million (ppm). The tardive dyskinesia patients averaged 0.46 ppm. It is concluded that Mn appears to be of value in treating many cases of tardive dyskinesia and it may also be of value in preventing the occurrence of dyskinesias.

Manganese and Seizures

Mn deficiency also affects cerebral motor function. Hurley and others[35] demonstrated a relationship between seizure activity and Mn deficiency in rats. The seizure threshold was found to be significantly lower in Mn-deficient animals. Tanaka[71] has presented a preliminary report on low blood Mn levels in epileptic patients.

Sohler and others[68] compared blood Mn levels in a group of patients with seizure activity to a control group. Blood Mn levels from control subjects had a mean of 14.8 ng/g while the blood Mn levels were significantly lower in the patients with seizure activity, at 9.9 ng/g. The clinical significance of the low blood Mn levels remains to be evaluated. In uncontrolled trials we find that Mn is helpful in controlling seizures of both minor and major types.

Both Mn and choline deficiencies are believed to interfere with membrane stability and this could be responsible for facilitating the propagation of seizure activity. We suggest these findings warrant the use of dietary supplements of Mn for the control of seizure activity. The remission of seizures is frequently dramatic.

Apparently, the essential trace element Mn is a basic, direct legacy from vegetable life to animal life. Tropical fruits are naturally high in Mn with tea leaves the highest. Plants cannot convert the sun's energy without Mn (photosynthesis) and man cannot live without Mn since at least six important enzymes require Mn for normal function. Compared to Zn, Mn is poorly absorbed and both Mn and Zn are rapidly excreted. The absorption of Mn and Cu are equally slow but Cu is sequestered in the absence of Zn and Mn and may cause harmful effects. Because of the slow absorption of Mn, the beneficial effects of Mn in man may not be evident for weeks and months. Except for the occasional elevation of blood pressure, oral Mn is without serious side effects.

Manganese and the "Empty" Basophil

The blood histamine level correlates with the absolute basophil count since most of the blood histamine is contained in the basophils, a white blood cell.[56] On all patients we perform both determinations and expect the histamine to be near the mean of 48 nanograms per millilter (ng/mL) and the basophil count at about 35 cells per cubic mL. When the patient is Mn deficient, some may have a high basophil count (i.e., 75, with a normal or low-blood histamine). We call this the "empty" basophil syndrome. The patient responds clinically to an oral Mn supplement and has a rise in the blood histamine level to correlate with the high basophil count.

Summary—Manganese

Although often ignored by nutrition-conscious individuals, Mn is an essential trace metal frequently deficient in our diet. A component of at least six known enzymes, Mn is required for efficient sugar metabolism, for the production of cartilage (a vital structural component of our bodies) and for the manufacture of cyclic AMP (a cellular second messenger).

Low Mn levels have been associated with epilepsy and schizophrenia. Studies dating back to 1929 indicate that schizophrenics improve with supplementary Mn and our experience with Mn-deficient schizophrenics at the Princeton Brain Bio Center supports this. We have also discovered that Mn-deficient patients may suffer depression, which clears up when Mn is included in the treatment program. Seizure patients may respond dramatically to Mn.

Unfortunately, most diets, even the best planned, tend to be deficient in this important trace metal. Our Mn-deficient farmlands often produce fruits and vegetables lacking adequate levels. And, many of our frequently eaten foods contain little Mn. For example, meat, even liver, provides little Mn. Foods rich in Mn include nuts, whole grains, spices, legumes, and tea leaves. Tropical fruits such as pineapple, banana, papaya, and mango are particularly good sources.

However, patients with low Mn blood or hair Mn levels will need supplementary Mn in addition to a good diet. Fortunately, Mn is well tolerated, even at high doses (up to 300 mg per day). However, occasionally in patients over 40, Mn can raise blood pressure and produce tension headaches. If this occurs, the Mn dose should be stopped until the blood pressure normalizes and the headaches disappear. Dried or fresh tropical fruits and tea can then be used as a source of Mn.

Low Zinc and High Copper in Some Schizophrenics

In 1966, when we found that some schizophrenic patients had low levels of blood histamine, we turned to a study of their Zn and Cu levels as possible factors in the storage and destruction of body histamine. (Histamine triggers inflammatory response.) Those patients registering low in histamine were also low in zinc and serum folate and high in serum Cu.[56]

Occasionally a high Cu level was accompanied by a high-serum creatine phosphokinase (CPK) level. Meltzer and others[45] have studied serum CPK extensively. In sheep poisoned with Cu, the CPK levels are tremendously high,[72] so that a high-serum Cu level plus increased motor activity may cause a rise in CPK in the occasional schizophrenic. Over a 10-year period, we have used folic acid and vitamin B12 to treat patients with low-serum histamine levels and high-serum Cu levels. These two vitamins reduce the need for the large doses of niacin used in megavitamin therapy; the use of folate and vitamin B12 in histapenic patients makes reasonable doses of niacin effective. With these nutrients, plus Zn and Mn, the Cu burden of the patient decreased over a three-month period, and the blood histamine level usually rises to a normal level.

Experience in the diagnosis and treatment of large numbers of schizophrenic patients has led us to separate three main biotypes: 50 percent are histapenic (low-blood histamine, high-serum Cu, low folate), 20 percent are histadelic (high-blood histamine, low- or normal-serum Cu), and 30 percent are normal in Cu and histamine but excrete large quantities of kryptopyrrole in their urine, depleting them of vitamin B6 and Zn.[53]

The low-histamine (histapenic) biotype of schizophrenia is frequently an environmentally produced copper overload with a resultant nutrient imbalance. Patients may be deficient in folic acid, vitamin B12, niacin, Zn, and Mn. Behavioral symptoms in high-copper histapenia include paranoia and hallucinations in younger patients, but depression may predominate in older patients. The patient is usually classified as having chronic or process schizophrenia.

Others have found that the administration of folic acid will correct severe psychosis caused by folate deficiency. A 15-year-old girl was found to suffer homocysteinuria (genetic disorder of metabolism of the amino acid methionine) and symptoms of schizophrenia. Folate and pyridoxine greatly improved the patient's condition.[2] There have been many well-documented reports of other folate-responsive behavioral disorders.[5–7,14]

Folic Acid in Low-Histamine, High-Copper Patients

We have used folic acid plus vitamin B12 for over 12 years to treat histapenic high-copper patients, who have hallucinations or paranoia in the early years of life or depression in later years. This is effective therapy that augments the effects of zinc, niacin, and vitamin C. With this therapy the serum Cu level is reduced, and the blood histamine rises to the normal range of 40 to 70 ng/ml after five to six months of therapy. The psychiatric symptoms decrease as the biochemical values approach more nearly normal levels.[56]

Folic Acid in High-Blood Histamine, Normal-Copper Patients

Histadelic (high-blood histamine) patients are characterized by fast oxidation, little fat, long fingers and toes, severe depression, compulsions, and phobias. These patients respond to mild antifolate drugs such as phenytoin (Dilantin) and agents that decrease histamine such as calcium salts and methionine in doses of 1,000–2000 mg per day. Folic acid makes histadelic patients worse, and even the folic acid in food may cause seasonal depression, which we have termed "salad bowl depression." A reducing diet composed mainly of spinach or lettuce has caused depression in some histadelic patients. These examples are obviously dietary extremes, but the patient who is depressed each summer in the salad season may be histadelic. Even the 0.4-mg dose of folic acid in many multivitamins is enough to produce increased depression in the histadelic patient. When a mildly depressed histadelic patient is given 1 mg of folic acid per day, a severe agitated depression may result. Therefore, we do not use folic acid in any schizophrenic patient until we know the absolute basophil count or the blood histamine level. Since the blood histamine is contained primarily in the basophils, the absolute basophil count may frequently serve to differentiate histapenic (low-blood histamine) and histadelic patients.

Therapy with niacin, folic acid, zinc, and manganese can change a low-blood histamine patient into a high-blood histamine depressed patient.[25] This has occurred many times in our experience and is corrected by a reduction in the dose of folic acid or the elimination of folic acid for a week and thereafter the use of a smaller dosage. Our usual 1–2 mg per day dose of folic acid is sufficient for the histapenic high-copper patient.

Some of the florid symptoms in the high-copper histapenic patient will respond promptly to therapy with folic acid, niacin, vitamin C, zinc, and manganese. The drippy palm syndrome, which forces the patient to carry a wad of tissues in each hand to absorb the sweat, responds within one to four weeks to this vitamin-mineral regime. The hypomania (a moderate form of mania), hallucinations, and mind racing are subdued within three to four weeks. In other patients, insomnia may be rectified in the same period. The degree of paranoia decreased very slowly, so that full remission may take 12–15 months. Relief of paranoia parallels the attainment of a normal Cu level in the blood serum.

The simple histapenia-histadelia concept allows a therapeutic trial of "running for the other goal line." If a patient worsens with folic acid and niacin, this therapy is stopped. Then the history and laboratory data are reviewed, and the patient may be tried on methionine, calcium, and phenytoin therapy to see if this provides improvement. Many allergic patients do not store histamine in their basophils because of antigen-antibody interaction. Thus, our allergic patient may have an abnormally low-blood histamine.

Excess copper is the primary imbalance of histapenics. The Cu comes from the drinking water, food, and inappropriately formulated vitamins plus minerals, which are overloaded with 2 mg of copper. Phenytoin (diphenylhydantoin) elevates copper levels.[77] High Cu levels antagonize folic acid through a complex web of trace metal interactions. Pregnant women and young women on the birth control pill will have abnormally low-blood histamine levels because of the high-estrogen levels. Copper levels also rise with the increase in estrogens. High copper levels increase the activity of histaminase (diamine oxidase), a copper-containing enzyme that oxidizes histamine.[38,39,74] Vitamin C-deficient guinea pigs show progressive rises in serum copper levels.

People with pellagra have elevated serum, hair, and urinary copper levels; skin histidine is low.[62,76] These return to normal with niacin treatment. Reduced availability of nictotinamide adenine dinucleotide (NADH), important in supplying energy to cells, has been reported in folate deficiency. The skin of pantothenic acid-deficient rats has a fivefold increase in copper level, as compared with controls. It has been reported that a single large dose of pantothenic acid (vitamin B5) effectively lowers the high serum Cu level for a one week period.

Plasma concentrations of Zn decrease during pregnancy, whereas Cu levels increase. Zinc and Cu are antagonistic in the human body and probably compete for the same sites on the protein carrier, metallothionine. Histamine is stored in the mast cells and basophils in a zinc-heparin-histamine complex.[40,41]

Zinc

Zinc is an essential nutrient in the development of neurons (nerve cells) of the normal brain. Rats Zn deficient in prenatal and early postnatal periods develop abnormal brains. In adults rendered Zn deficient only postnatally, abnormal behavior is manifest without demonstrable abnormal structure. Both hippocampal and cerebellar development in rats occur postnatally with the cerebellar cortex (the outer surface of the cerebral hemispheres) acquiring nearly all its cellular constituents and the hippocampus acquiring 85 percent of its neurons during the first three weeks of life.[36] Zinc is involved in the maturation and function of the mossy fiber pathway (excitatory pathways). Histochemical observations indicated increasing levels of Zn in the hippocampal mossy fiber layer after 20 days of age. Between 18 and 22 days hippocampal Zn increased by 35 percent to reach adult levels.

Zinc deficiency during the critical period for brain growth permanently affects brain function. When this deficiency is imposed throughout the latter third of pregnancy, brain size is decreased; there is a reduced total brain cell count and the cytoplasmic nuclear ratio is increased, implying an impairment of cell division in the brain during the critical period of neuronal proliferation.[36] In adult life, male rats so treated display impaired shock avoidance and female rats are significantly more aggressive at a high level of shock than adult females whose mothers were Zn sufficient during pregnancy.[28,75] Zinc deficient animals are more susceptible to a standard stress.

Zinc deficiency has been shown to impair DNA, RNA, and protein synthesis in the brains of suckling rats.[26] Zinc deficiency results in impaired incorporation of thymidine into brain DNA. Incorporation of sulfur into protein is also decreased. Zinc deficiency also decreases the concentration of total lipid in brain while phospholipids and fatty acids are not affected.

Rat pups suckled for 21 days by their mothers fed a zinc-deficient diet demonstrated impaired body growth and smaller cerebella and hemispheres compared to pups given adequate zinc.[26] A smaller hippocampus is also associated with zinc deficiency.[11] A deficiency of dietary Zn during the suckling period of the rat results in the pups having smaller forebrains, reduced cell numbers, and decreased RNA and DNA.[26] Buell and others[11] found that postnatal Zn deficiency in rats results in fewer brain neurons with a decrease in the total amount of DNA. The hippocampus showed similar deficits.

A deficiency of nerve growth factor may occur with Zn deficiency. One nerve growth factor is a small basic protein with three distinct types of subunits.[78] Two molecules of Zn are present in the complex and Zn participates in holding the structure together.[20,47] In the absence of Zn, the subunits separate. Nerve growth factor is required for the survival and development of certain sympathetic and sensory neurons. It is equally clear that nerve growth factor affects a wide variety of other cells as well. Nerve growth factors are present on the plasma membrane and almost certainly at the synaptic ending as well.[20] Nerve growth factor action increased dendritic attachments that require elevated levels of RNA synthesis, which is Zn dependant.

Zinc and Amino Acids

Zinc deficiency greatly alters amino acid metabolism and balance. Some amino acids have important neurotransmitter functions in the brain. Hsu[34] studied the effects of Zn deprivation on the levels of free amino acid in plasma, urine, and skin extracts of rats. He found significantly higher concentrations of threonine, leucine, and isoleucine both in the urine and plasma of Zn-deficient animals. Higher concentrations of taurine, glutamic acid, valine, and lysine as well as urea were also observed in the Zn-deficient urine. Zinc deficiency causes a significant increase in the brain catecholamines, norepinephrine, and dopamine.[80] Total plasma amino acids are increased.[79] Histidine was especially elevated while plasma glutamic acid was depressed. Histamine from histidine, glutamic acid directly, acetylcholine from choline, serotonin from tryptophan, and catecholamines from tyrosine are neurotransmitters affected by dietary control. Changes in amino acid levels in Zn deficiency were affected by abnormalities in amino acid utilization and excretion.[79]

Zinc and Behavior

Zinc deficiency in humans is associated with apathy, lethargy, amnesia, and mental retardation, often with considerable irritability, depression, and paranoia.[59] Caldwell and others[13] have shown that the rats born to mildly Zn-deficient mothers are mentally retarded and do not learn as well as rats from Zn-supplemented mothers. Prior to the above studies, Caldwell and coworkers observed a significantly inferior learning ability in the surviving offspring of mildly Zn-deficient mothers, compared to similar rats from Zn-supplemented mothers. These effects of Zn deficiency were subsequently confirmed and extended.[28,65,66,75] Colleagues visiting Iran and Egypt are told that 30 percent of the young children are slow learners. It may not be a coincidence that these areas of the world, which have been farmed for centuries, no longer have much available Zn in the soil.[58]

Hesse and others[31] have found that adult rats chronically deprived of dietary Zn do not behave as hippocampal-intact animals; the evidence suggests that the deficiency alters the electrophysiological properties of normally Zn-rich hippocampal mossy fibers.[31] The behavioral characteristics of these animals differed from controls and were substantially parallel to those reported for animals with excess glucocorticoids (stress hormones).[31] Zinc-deficient rats show latency in the platform box test, cul de sac and retrace errors, and open field errors.[13,65,66] Zinc-deficient rats[9] show significant differences in stereotypic behavior (grooming, licking) and motor function (rapid changes in position, backward locomotion, and rapid jerky movements). These behavioral abnormalities correlated with high levels of the catecholamines.

Disperception can occur during deficiency states and Zn has been useful in otology.[63] Henkin and others[30] have noted that one of syndromes of acute Zn loss is cerebellar dysfunction. Zinc supplementation following Zn deficiency reverses excessive emotionality.[53]

Each of three major phenothiazines increases the total brain zinc uptake in all animals tested, more in rats than in mice.[17] The following regional changes were detected in rat brains. Occipitotemporal cortex, thalamus, and hippocampus became more zincophilic (zinc-absorbing), the thalamus especially under chloropromazine (Thorazine) and the hippocampus under perphenazine (Trilafon) treatment. Zinc deficiency clearly alters behavior through both primary and secondary metabolic pathways.

Brain Content of Zinc and Disease

McLardy[44] observed a 30 percent deficit of Zn brain content in early onset schizophrenics and chronic alcoholics. Other researchers have observed a decrease in hippocampal Zn in schizophrenics.[42] Zinc deficiency elevates catecholamines in rat brain.[9,80]

Lead displaces Zn from the hippocampal mossy fiber system.[12,46] Rabbits exposed to copper, iron, and Zn are significantly decreased in these regions. The decrease in Zn was most significant in the interior hippocampus. Staton and others[70] have also described Zn deficiency-Cu excess presenting as schizophrenia. In Wilson's disease patients (a genetic disorder resulting in excessive copper accumulation in the liver and other vital organs) only Zn uptake is increased since Cu is already overloaded.[1] It is clear that brain-Zn content changes during disease states and that brain Zn deficiency is possibly dynamically related to schizophrenia, alcoholism, Wilson's disease, and lead poisoning.

Zinc and Schizophrenias

The schizophrenias are biochemically numerous, so the simplistic term "schizophrenia" should be avoided. At least seven different biochemical imbalances can produce clinical symptoms that are indistinguishable by the so-called research diagnostic criteria for simplistic schizophrenia. As an example, Wilson's disease can be marked by psychosis and hallucinations. Oral zinc has an antagonistic effect on the reabsorption of Cu in the gastrointestinal tract and, for that reason, is considered valuable in the treatment of this disease.[32] We have already mentioned the work of Derrien and Benoit,[19] and Kimura and Kumura,[42] who suggested or found Zn to be involved in mental disease. In 1967 Pfeiffer and Iliev reported low-blood histamine levels in schizophrenic patients; histamine is stored with zinc.

A definite percentage of psychiatric patients have been found to have the chemical kryptopyrrole in their urine. Kryptopyrrole reacts avidly with all aldehyde chemicals, including pyridoxal.[50] The resulting kryptopyrrole-pyridoxal complex by chelating Zn produces a Zn deficiency as well as a severe pyridoxine deficiency. These patients, whom we have termed pyroluric, respond for the most part to vitamin B6 and Zn therapy.[52,54] Pyroluria is a form of schizophrenic porphyria similar to acute intermittent porphyria where both pyrroles and porphyrins are excreted in the urine in excess.[10] Both Zn and vitamin B6 are important cofactors in the pyrrole-porphyria-heme pathway.

Evans[22] found that rats absorb one and one-half times as much dietary Zn if given vitamin B6. Specifically, 71 percent of dietary Zn was absorbed when the animals were given 40 mg of the vitamin per kilogram of diet. Only 46 percent of the Zn was absorbed when 2 mg of vitamin B6 per kilogram were given.[23] This effect may be due to vitamin B6's role in the tryptophan-picolinic acid pathways.

Practical Aspects of Zinc Supplements

The physicians at the Princeton Brain Bio Center have had 15 years of experience in the use of trace element dietary supplements since Zn therapy was started in 1967. In 1968 we found in man that Zn plus Mn was more effective than Zn alone in eliminating Cu via the urinary pathway. Approximately, one half of the patients coming to the PBBC have a Cu overload as shown by blood serum or hair analysis. Molybdenum, an essential trace mineral, and occasionally D-penicillamine (Cuprimine) are used with Zn and Mn to control Cu overload. The Zn recommendations are based on our experience in 70,000 clinic visits of over 15,000 patients wherein the blood, Zn, Cu, (iron) Fe, and Mn were determined at each visit. In many patients blood aluminum, molybdenum, lead, and rubidium were also determined.

Oral Zn salts are readily and equally well absorbed.[68] The surgeons, pioneering in the use of adequate Zn for wound healing, used 50 mg Zn (as sulfate). The body needs only 15 mg of elemental Zn per day so this original 50 mg tablet is too large and may produce nausea and diarrhea. The use of Zn, 15 mg (as gluconate), should be standard. This lower dose seldom produces nausea if taken with food. For children, infants, and senile patients, a liquid preparation may be given. Immediate side effects of dietary Zn supplement may be occasional

nausea, more than normal sweating, intolerance to alcohol, and transient worsening of depression of hallucinations. All of these reactions respond to lessening of the dose or taking the 15 mg of Zn with food.

The immediate effect of Zn may be a decrease in serum iron level. With 15 mg of Zn this is rare and is usually self-corrective so that iron supplements are not needed. (No iron therapy unless serum iron level drops below 50 mcg percent!) Continued massive doses of Zn, up to 5,000 mg per day decreased both serum Cu levels and ceruloplasmin levels in one female patient.[57] This was corrected by the daily use of a high-potency multivitamin that contains 2 mg of Cu. Patients on Zn supplements may have more persistent visual after-images and the time for dark adaptation of the eyes may be prolonged.

The most insidious effect of excess Zn over a period of years is the reduction of blood Mn, 90 percent of which is contained in the erythrocytes. This produces macrocytosis when the blood Mn level falls to less than 8 ppb (normal 15 ppb). Low-blood Mn levels may accentuate depression, allergies, and seizure activity in epileptics. Manganese is poorly absorbed from the intestine and, while only 5 mg is needed per day, the patient may need as much as 300 mg of Mn as the gluconate to attain the normal blood level of 15 ppb. Zinc dietary supplements increase grand mal seizures in epileptics so Mn supplements should be started initially and Zn cautiously added one month later when the blood levels of Zn, Mn, and Cu are known.

We postulate that some part of the cerebral side effects of Zn supplementation are mediated by the mobilization of Cu from storage in liver and muscle. With Zn by mouth, the serum Cu may increase for a period of one to three months before falling to a normal level. With D-penicillamine therapy and Zn/Mn supplements this does not occur. In some instances such as severe paranoia, the prompt decision to start therapy with D-penicillamine plus Zn and Mn can be justified. The use of Zn and Mn with vitamin B6 makes D-penicillamine therapy safe because as a chelator D-penicillamine removes Cu, Zn, and Mn. The loss of taste with D-penicillamine is a sign of Zn deficiency.

704

Drug Flood Syndrome

Patients we have seen that take large doses of antipsychotics may get very sleepy when Zn and vitamin B6 are used in treatment. This is the effect of the neuroleptic on a brain made more normal and the dose of antipsychotic should be rapidly reduced. For example, 40 mg of Haloperidol can be reduced to 5–10 mg at bedtime. The patient's affect improves with the Zn and vitamin B6 so that the parents may suggest that the neuroleptic dose is too large.

Vitamin B6 (Pyridoxine) Toxicity

An occasional patient will show high-hair and high-serum Zn levels with elevated spermidine and low erythrocyte glutamic-oxaloacetic transaminase activity (both sensitive indicators of vitamin B6 status). We postulate that these patients have vitamin B6 deficiency and cannot utilize the Zn present until adequate vitamin B6 is provided. With vitamin B6 therapy, the high Zn level drops to normal. Doses of 1,000 mg of vitamin B6 each morning are well tolerated but oral vitamin B6 in doses of more than 2,000 mg may produce tingling or numbness of toes and fingers. This indicates the need for reduction in the vitamin B6 dosages. With lower doses of vitamin B6, the numbness is relieved.

The beneficial effect of Zn, Mn, and vitamin B6 in pyroluria is important since this defect extends through many diagnostic categories. The most urgent need is for daily supplements in those children now labeled mentally retarded, learning disabled, minimally brain damaged, autistic, dyslexic, and hyperactive. For this purpose some philanthropic foundation might wish to make available at cost (or free of charge), a simple supplement consisting of the daily need for Zn and Mn, namely 15 and 4 mg, respectively, plus 25 mg of vitamin B6. The patients could be used as their own controls and other vitamins could be used as placebo medication for the first two weeks of medication while the basic behavioral observations are being made.

Signs of Zinc Deficiency

In order to diagnose Zn deficiency of the brain, peripheral signs of Zn deficiency must be recognized. These are white spotted fingernails, stretch marks, nasal polyps, amennorhea (absence of menstrual periods), impotency, tinnitus, abdominal pain, stuttering, poor dental enamel, loss of taste, frequent infections, depression, insomnia, disperceptions, and hallucinations.

Signs of Zinc and Vitamin B6 Deficiency

Zinc is needed for conversion of pyridoxal to pyridoxal phosphate so adequate vitamin B6 should always be given with Zn. Patients without dream recall are vitamin-B6 deficient and vitamin B6 deficiency is the basic nutrition deficit in carpal tunnel syndrome and Chinese restaurant syndrome.[24] Double deficiency of Zn and vitamin B6, as in pyroluria, may cause the following: no dream recall, sweet breath and body odor, morning nausea, crowded upper incisors, splenic pain, pallor with itching in sunlight, constipation, achy knees, amennorhea, impotency, seizures, disperceptions, hallucinations, amnesia, paranoia, eosinophilia (high eosinophil count), lymphocytosis (high lymphocyte count), high bilirubin, and low-immune globulin A.[50] We have found a deficiency of Zn and B6 in all girl families we have treated also.

Summary—Zinc in Schizophrenia

The mauve factor (kryptopyrrole) depletes a patient of both Zn and vitamin B6 (pyridoxine) because the pyrrole combines with pyridoxal, and then with Zn, to produce a combined deficiency. These patients suffer from pyroluria, a familial disorder that occurs with stress. Pyroluria is treated by restoring the vitamin B6 and Zn so that this double deficiency is corrected. A dose of vitamin B6, which results in daily dream recall (a normal phenomenon), as well as a Zn-Mn supplement are given daily. One should increase the daily morning dose of vitamin B6 (up to 2,000 mg per day) until dream recall occurs.

With Zn, Mn, and vitamin B6 therapy, the pyroluric patient may start to respond in 24 hours and certainly some progress is noted within one week. However, total recovery may take three to four months. The biochemical imbalance and symptoms will usually recur within one to two weeks if the nutritional program is stopped.[51]

Pyroluria may occur together with other imbalances such as histapenia, histadelia, high Cu, or cerebral allergies and in these instances progress will be slower. Low-histamine patients are typically overstimulated with thoughts racing through their minds making normal ideation difficult. Low-histamine children are hyperactive while often healthy in other respects. Serum Cu levels in these patients are abnormally high. Since Cu is a brain stimulant and destroys histamine, the elevated serum (and presumably brain) Cu level probably accounts for many symptoms, including the low-blood histamine level.

The treatment program consists of the administration of Zn, Mn, vitamin C, niacin, vitamin B12, and folic acid. The rationale underlying the treatment is that folic acid in conjunction with vitamin B12 injections raises the blood histamine while lowering the degree of symptomatology. Zinc and Mn allow for the normal storage of histamine in both the basophils and the brain. With this treatment, the high-blood Cu is slowly reduced and symptoms are slowly relieved in several months' time. Zinc and Mn with vitamin C remove Cu from the tissues. The largest tissues of the body, namely the liver and muscles, are flushed of their Cu first so the serum Cu may rise to aggravate mental symptoms. If this occurs, then the dose of Zn should be reduced for a two-week period. Excess Cu may be acquired from commercial vitamins and minerals or drinking water flowing through copper pipes. Distilled water may occasionally be needed to reduce Cu intake.

David and others[18] find significant lead in the hyperactive child but at a level less than that of lead poisoning. We find similar levels of lead and high levels of Cu, which is also a central nervous system stimulant. We believe that with a high-Cu level, any lead level above the age of the child is suspect. These patients are also Zn and vitamin-B6 deficient. With adequate Zn and vitamin C, both the lead and Cu levels return to normal within a period of six months and the hyperactivity is decreased. These children frequently have an elevated serum uric acid level, which may indicate that the heavy metals are adversely affecting the kidneys. Excess Cu usually comes from the drinking water and lead exposure may be from air pollution (traffic), contact with the printed page, and other sources. Zinc deficiency occurs with faulty eating habits.

CONCLUSION

Nutrients at their best can be smart drugs that know exactly where to go and what to do. In contrast, other drugs are nonspecific and go everywhere, with the molecules wandering aimlessly, producing unwanted side actions. Nutrients at worst have no therapeutic effect and are either incorporated or excreted by the usual metabolic disposal systems. Drugs at worst can be rapidly fatal or chronically disabling, as in tardive dyskinesia. Nutrients are slow in relieving symptoms, but when effective the relief is more permanent. Drugs may have the impact of a bulldozer, so both the patient and the therapist know that the drug is working. The slow onset of action of nutrients makes rigid experimental design difficult. If the patient is used as his own control, the placebo must then be given initially rather than after the nutrient treatment.

The advantages of nutrient treatment are inherent in the accumulated knowledge needed to use the nutrient. Usually a study of the patient indicates that a specific defect might be present: sometimes this can be assayed by objective tests. If these tests indicate a deficiency, then the rigid statistical trials that are frequently applied to therapy become meaningless. Scientists discovered the therapeutic effect of the various B12 vitamins without a double-blind test because the objective tests were numerous and the biochemical insight was extensive. We hope that such biochemical tests will lead to better insight and treatment of the schizophrenias. Biological science can only give us progress reports: it is doubtful whether the final word will ever be spoken or written in our slow conquest of the schizophrenias.

REFERENCES

1. Aaseth J, Soli NE, Forre O. Increased brain uptake of copper and zinc in mice caused by diethyldithiocarbamate. *Acta Pharmacol, et Toxicol* 1979;45:41.

2. Barber GW, Spaeth GL. Successful treatment of homocystinuria with pyridoxine. *J Pediatr* 1969;75:463–478.

3. Barlow P. Hair metal analysis and its significance to certain diseases. Presented at the 2nd Annual Trace Minerals in Health Seminar, Boston, MA, Sept 8–9, 1979.

4. Borg DC, Cotzias GC. *The Clinical Significance of the Essential Biological Metals.* Springfield, IL: C.C. Thomas, 1972, 74.

5. Botez MI, Fontaine F, Botez T, et al. Folate-responsive neurological and mental disorders: report of 16 cases. *Cur Neurol* 1977;16:230–246.

6. Botez MI, Lambert B. Folate deficiency and restless legs syndrome in pregnancy. *N Engl J Med* 1977;297:670.

7. Botez T, Botez MI, Berube I, et al. Neuropsychological disorders responsive to folic acid therapy: a report of 39 cases. Exerpta Medica International Congress Series 1977;427:202.

8. Bowen HJM. Determination of trace elements in hair samples from normal and protein deficient children by activation analysis. *Sci Total Environ* 1972;1:75–78.

9. Bradford LD, Oner G, Lederis K. Effects of zinc deficiency on locomotor and stereotypic behavior in rats. *The Pharmacol* 23, 142, 1981.

10. Braverman E. Porphyrin metabolic pathways and their various applications to an understanding of some common human disorders. Proc. 2nd International Conference on Human Functioning, Biomedical Synergistics Institute, Inc., Wichita, Kansas, 1978.

11. Buell SJ, Fosmire GJ, Ollerich DA, et al. Effects of postnatal zinc deficiency on cerebellar and hippocampal development in the rat. *Experimental Neurology* 1977;55:199.

12. Bushwell PJ, Bowman RE. Reversal learning deficits in young monkeys exposed to lead. *Pharm Biochem and Behav* 1979;10:733.

13. Caldwell DF, Oberleas D, Prasad AS. Reproductive performance of chronic mildly zinc deficient rats and the effects on behavior of their offspring. *Nutrition Reports International* 1973;7:309.

14. Carney MWP. Folate-responsive schizophrenia. *Lancet* 1975;1:276.

15. Crawford IL, Connor JD. Zinc in maturing rat brain: hippocampal concentration and localization. *Journal of Neurochemistry* 1972;19:1451.

16. Cunnane SC, Horrobin DF. Parenteral linolenic and y-linolenic acids ameliorate the gross effects of zinc deficiency. Proceedings of the Society for Experimental Biology and Medicine 1980;164:583.

17. Czerniak, P, Haim DB. Phenothiazine derivatives and brain zinc. *Arch Neurol* 1971;24:555.

18. David O, McGann B, Hoffman S, et al. Low lead levels and mental retardation. *Lancet* 1976;25:1376–1379.

19. Derrien E, Benoit C. Notes et observations sur les urines et sur quelques organes d'une femme encrise de porphyrie aique. *Arch Soc Sci Med Biol Montpelier* 1929;8:456.

20. Dunn MF, Pattison SC, StromMC, et al. Comparison of the zinc binding domains in the 7S nerve growth factor and the zinc-insulin hexamer. *Biochem* 1980;19:718.

21. English WM. Report of the treatment with manganese chloride of 181 cases of schizophrenia, 33 of manic depression, and 16 other defects of psychoses at the Ontario Hospital, Brockville, Ontario. *Am J Psychiat* 1929;9:569–580.

22. Evans GW. Normal and abnormal zinc absorption in man and animals; the tryptophan connection. *Nutrition Reviews* 1980; 38:137.

23. Evans GW, Johnson EC. Growth-stimulating effect of picolinic acid added to rat diets. *Proceedings of the Society for Experimental Biology and Medicine* 1980;165:457.

24. Folkers K, Willis R, Takemura K, et al. Biochemical correlations of a deficiency of vitamin B-6, the carpal tunnel syndrome and the Chinese restaurant syndrome. *IRCS Med Sci* 1981;9: 444.

25. Foreman J, Mangor J. The action of lanthanum and manganese on anaphylactic histamine secretion. *Brit J Pharmacol* 1973;48:527–537.

26. Fosmire GJ, Al-Ubaidi Y, Sandstead HH. Some effects of postnatal zinc deficiency on developing rat brain. *Pediatric Research* 1975;9:89.

27. Gaskin G, Kress Y, Brosnan C, et al. Abnormal tubulin aggregates induced by zinc sulfate in organotypic cultures of nerve tissue. *Neuroscience* 1978;3:1117.

28. Halas ES, Sandstead HH. Some Effects of Prenatal Zinc Deficiency on Behavior of the Adult Rat. Pediatric Research 1975;9:94.

29. Helweg H. Treatment of dementia praecox with manganese: case. *Ugesk F. Laeger* 1928;90:227.

30. Henkin RI, Patten BM, Bronzert, DA. A syndrome of acute zinc loss. *Archives of Neurology* 1975;32:745.

31. Hesse G, Hesse KAF, Catalanotto FA. Behavioral characteristics of rats experiencing chronic zinc deficiency. *Physiology and Behavior* 1979;22:211; see also: Hesse GW. Chronic zinc deficiency alters neuronal function of hippocampla mossy fibers. *Science* 1979;205:1005, 1979.

32. Hoogenraad TU, Vandenhamer CJA, Koevoet R.et al. Oral zinc in Wilson's Disease. *Lancet* 1978;1262.

33. Hoskins RG. The manganese treatment of schizophrenic disorders. *J Nerv Ment Dis* 1934;79:59.

34. Hsu JM. Zinc deficiency and alterations of free amino acid levels in plasma, urine and skin extract. In: *Zinc Metabolism: Current Aspects in Health and Disease.* New York: Alan R. Liss, Inc, 1977.

35. Hurley LS, Wooley DE, Timiras PS. Threshold and pattern of electroshock seizure in ataxic manganese deficient rats. *Proc Soc Exp Biol Med* 1963;106:343–346.

36. Hurley LS, Shrader RE. Congenital malformations of the nervous system in zinc-deficient rats. In: *The International Review of Neurobiology* edited by CC Pfeiffer. New York: Academic Press, 1972, 7.

37. Irvine DG, Bayne W, Miyashita H. et al. Identification of kryptopyrrole in human urine and its relationship to psychosis. *Nature* 1969;224:811.

38. Jensen ON, Olesen OV. Folic acid and anticonvulsive drugs. *Arch Neurol* 1969;21:208–214.

39. Jonassen F. Histamine metabolism during the menstrual cycle. *Acta Obstet Gynecol Scand* 1976;55:297–304.

40. Kaz1mierczar N, Maslinski C. The mechanism of the inhibitory action of zinc on histamine release from mast cells. *Agents and Actions* 1974;4:203–204.

41. Keller R, Sorkin E. Selective incorporation of zinc into rat mast cells. *Experientia* 1970;26:30.

42. Kimura I, Kumura J. Preliminary reports on the metabolism of trace elements in neuro-psychiatric diseases. Part I. Zinc in schizophrenia, *Proc Jap Acad Sci* 1965;943.

43. Kunin RA. Manganese and niacin in the treatment of drug induced dyskinesias. *J Orthomolecular Psych* 1976;5(1):4–27.

44. McLardy T. Hippocampal zinc in chronic alcoholism and schizophrenia. *J Orthomolecular Psych* 1975:4:32.

45. Meltzer H, Elkun L, Moline RH. Serum enzyme changes in newly admitted psychiatric patients. Part I. *Arch Gen Psychiat* 1969;21:731–738.

46. Niklowitz WJ, Yeager DW. Interference of Pb with essential brain tissue, Cu, Fe and Zn as zinc and manganese in the schizophrenias main determinant in experimental tetraethyl-lead encephalopathy. *Life Sciences* 1973;13:897.

47. Pattison SE, Dunn MF. On the relationship of zinc ion to the structure and function of the 7S nerve growth factor protein. *Biochemistry* 1975;14:2733.

48. Pfeiffer CC. Blood histamine, basophil counts and trace elements in the schizophrenias. *Rev Can Biol* 1972;31:73–76.

49. Pfeiffer CC, Iliev V. A study of zinc deficiency and copper excess in the schizophrenias. In: *The International Review of Neurobiology* edited by CC Pfeiffer. New York: Academic Press, 1972, 141.

50. Pfeiffer CC. Observations on trace and toxic elements in hair and serum. *J Orthomolecular Psych* 1974;3(4):259–264.

51. Pfeiffer CC, Sohler A, Jenney EH, et al. Treatment of pyroluric schizophrenia (malvaria) with large doses of pyridoxine and a dietary supplement of zinc. *J Applied Nutrition* 1974;20:21–28.

52. Pfeiffer CC, Bacchi D. Copper, zinc, manganese, niacin and pyridoxine in the schizophrenias. *J Appl Nutr* 1975;27:9–39.

53. Pfeiffer CC. *Mental and Elemental Nutrients.* New Canaan, CT: Keats Publishing, 1975.

54. Pfeiffer CC. The schizophrenias '76. *Biological Psychiatry* 1976;11:773–775.

55. Pfeiffer CC. *Zinc and Other Micronutrients.* New Canaan, CT: Keats Publishing, 1978.

56. Pfeiffer CC, Braverman ER. Folic acid and vitamin B-12 therapy for the low-histamine, high-copper biotype of schizophrenia. In: *Folic Acid in Neurology, Psychiatry, and Internal Medicine* edited by M Botez and EN Reynolds. New York: Raven Press, 1979, 483–487.

57. Pfeiffer CC, Papaioannou R, Sohler A. Effect of chronic zinc intoxication on copper levels, blood formation and polyamines. *J Orthomolecular Psych* 1980;9:79–89.

58. Prasad AS. *Zinc Metabolism.* Springfield, IL: C.C. Thomas, 1966.

59. Prasad AS, Rabbani P, Abbash A. Experimental zinc deficiency in humans. *Ann Intern Med* 1978;89:483.

60. Reed GE. Use of manganese chloride in dementia praecox. *Canad M A J* 1929;21:96–149.

61. Reiter PJ. Behandlung von dementia praecox mit metallsalzen a.m. walbrim I. *Mangan Z Neur* 1927;108:464–480.

62. Rifkind JM, Heim JW. Interaction of zinc with hemoglobin: binding of zinc and the oxygen affinity. *Biochemistry* 1977;16:4438–4443.

63. Ruggles RL, Linquist PA. Zinc therapy in otology. *The Laryngoscope* 1976:LXXXVI:1688.

64. Ryan DE, Holzbecher J, Stuart DC. Trace elements in scalp-hair of persons with multiple sclerosis and of normal individuals. *Clin Chem* 1978;24(11):1996–2000.

65. Sandstead HH, Gillespie DD, Brady RN. Zinc deficiency: effect on brain of the suckling rat. *Pediat Res* 1972;6:119.

66. Sandstead HH, Fosmire GJ, Halas ES, et al. Zinc deficiency: effects on brain and behavior of rats and rhesus monkeys. *Teratology* 1977;16:229.

67. Schrijver, D. Die metallsalz behandlung der dementia praecox ab modum valbum. *Neurotherapie* 1928;10:6–12.

68. Sohler A, Pfeiffer CC. A direct method for the determination of manganese in whole blood: patients with seizure activity have low blood levels. *J Orthomolecular Psych* 1979;8(4):275–280.

69. Sohler A, Pfeiffer CC. Oral zinc in normal subjects: effect on serum copper, iron, calcium, and histidine levels. *J Orthomolecular Psych* 1980;9(1):6–10.

70. Staton MA, Donald AG, Green GB. Zinc Deficiency Presenting as Schizophrenia. *Curr Concepts Psychiatry* II, 1976.

71. Tanaka AY. Low manganese level may trigger epilepsy. *JAMA* 1977;238:1805.

72. Thompson RH, Todd JR. Muscle damage in chronic copper poisoning of sheep. *Res Vet Sci* 1974;16:96–97.

73. Tindinge G. Treatment of dementia praecox with salts of manganese. *Ugesk. F. Laeger* 1929;91:616.

74. Torok E. Serum diamine oxidase in pregnancy and trophoblastic tissue diseases. *J Clin Endocrinol Metab* 1970;30:59–65.

75. Underwood EJ. *Trace Elements in Human and Animal Nutrition.* New York: Academic Press, 1971.

76. Vasantha L. Niacin deficiency and histidine skin levels. *Indian J Med Res* 1970;58:1079.

77. Vasiliades J, Sahawneh T. Effect of diphenylhydantonin on serum copper, zinc, and magnesium. *Clin Chem* 1975;21:637.

78. Vinores S, Guroff G. Nerve growth factor: mechanism of action. *Ann Rev Biophys Bioeng* 1980;9:223.

79. Wallwork JC, Fosmire GJ, Sandstead HH. Effect of zinc deficiency on appetite and plasma amino acid concentrations in the rat. *Br J Nutr* 1981;45:127.

80. Wallwork J, Sandstead HH Effect of zinc deficiency on brain catecholamine concentrations in the rat. *Federal Proceedings* 1981;40:939.

81. Pfeiffer CC, Iliev V. A study of zinc deficiency and copper excess in the schizophrenias. In: *The International Review of Neurobiology* edited by CC Pfeiffer. New York: Academic Press, 1972, 141.

708

ORTHOMOLECULAR TREATMENT OF SCHIZOPHRENIA: AN APOLOGY AND EXPLANATION

by Abram Hoffer, MD, PhD, with Frances Fuller, RNCP

For many years we have advised physicians and psychiatrists about the therapeutic advantages of giving their schizophrenic patients niacin (vitamin B3) in the right doses as a part of the treatment they were already receiving. There were two general reactions: many psychiatrists became interested and spent one or more days with me. With one exception, they all became orthomolecular practitioners and many became the pioneers and leaders of this new field. However, very few doctors who did not visit me ever tried to follow the treatment, even though it has been described over and over in many papers and books. Why the difference?

One factor was that the psychiatric profession became corrupted by the observation that the powerful psychiatric drugs quickly controlled abnormal behavior. It was concluded this was the cure, and was all one needed to do—similar to giving an antibiotic to a patient with pneumonia or putting a cast on a broken bone; it would heal rapidly, and the psychosocial aspects of the doctor-patient relationship did not matter very much. Psychiatrists concluded the very rapid changes induced by the drugs were the same as a cure. One day you would be dealing with a very agitated, hospitalized patient, and the next day he or she would be tranquilized and apathetic, apparently much better. One enterprising psychiatrist installed a noise meter in one of the chronic wards of his mental hospital and recorded the level of noise before and after tranquilizing his patients on that ward. He provided objective evidence that the noise levels went way down. He assumed this meant patients were improved. All it showed is that they were less noisy.

What was not realized was that tranquilizing disturbed patients was not the same as curing them of the disease that had made them behave so badly in the first place. In the same way one can teach an autistic child new habits and ways of doing things, but it does not mean that their basic biochemical pathology is corrected. Depending upon these drugs as the treatment meant one could ignore all the other elements of a holistic treatment program—shelter, nourishing food, civility, and good care—that are part of any healthy doctor-patient relationship.

To give a bit of background, in the 1940s and 1950s psychiatric experience was usually gained in mental hospitals on patients for whom there was no treatment, and anything that would settle them was preferable to no treatment. A few doctors were more enterprising and were willing to use very harsh treatments such as insulin coma and electroconvulsive therapy (ECT) in order to help their patients; the results were not good, took a long time, and were unpredictable. Drugs appeared to settle all these issues. Discharging these patients—no better but tranquilized—became one of the new objectives of the mental hospitals. The clinical evidence that, while drugs are helpful, they are not and never will be curative was, and is, ignored. The word "cure," like the "N-word," is forbidden in modern psychiatry.

The doctors who did not visit me did not see the results that I and the doctors who visited me were seeing. They were therefore not impressed by anything I wrote. Over the last years of my practice in psychiatry, 40 medical students in their third or fourth year visited me and spent one or two days observing and interacting with me and my patients. They were completely surprised when they saw my recovered or recovering patients. During their training they had never seen even one schizophrenic patient who was as well.

We apologize because we did not understand that advising psychiatrists to add vitamins meant adding one new drug, so they could still ignore the other three essential elements of any good therapeutic program. Had we understood this, it might have been more effective to preach to

From the *J Orthomolecular Medicine* 2009;24(1):9–13.

doctors who were already practicing good therapy including those three elements. Most of the early pioneers around 1960 were trained as psychoanalysts: Allan Cott, David Hawkins, Jack Ward, Harvey Ross, and Moke Williams. They were accustomed to spending a lot of time with their patients.

The total dependence on drugs eliminates the basic three elements of good treatment for any disease: shelter, food, and treatment with civility and respect. These are the basic elements of the Moral Treatment of the Insane, the nonmedical approach to insanity practiced by the Quakers 150 years ago, which allowed nearly half of their psychotic guests to recover without drugs. No doctors or nurses were allowed into these treatment homes. We will not discuss shelter and food, as this should be so obvious: living on the streets or run-down slum areas, "dumpster diving" or eating modern hospital food is not good care. In this report we will concentrate on civility and care, and the doctor-patient relationship.

A second factor is that the journals usually read by psychiatrists refused to publish articles reporting positive orthomolecular findings. Many years ago an assistant editor of the *American Journal of Psychiatry* told me that he would never allow any of my papers to appear in his journal, no matter how good they were. He kept his word. But even worse is that MedLine, which is supposed to abstract and review scientific articles in the world scientific press, undertook a censoring function to keep orthomolecular reports out of medical awareness. It resolutely refused to abstract our journal, considering that *Readers' Digest* is more scientific. There are also no ads in the standard medical journals extolling the virtues of vitamins, whereas up to 50 percent of the pages of some medical journals carry very impressive drug ads. We think that many journals are in fact advertising sheets with a little content so they can call themselves medical journals. This stranglehold on the public dissemination of information has come to an end with Google and other Internet search devices. This journal can now be downloaded from Google. Perhaps it is time to say goodbye to MedLine.

Recovery Approach

We will describe a first interview with a schizophrenic patient and his mother in order to demonstrate our objective—recovery and how to achieve it. We believe patients must be taught something about their illness and must have hope that it can be treated successfully. We do not follow the usual mantra of modern psychiatry, which is: 1) you will never get well, 2) you will never be off drugs, and 3) you will never complete your education. We have seen too many examples of patients who have been given this advice and have recovered.

On November 13, 2007, John came with his mother from hundreds of miles away. Age 20, he was tall, good-looking, quiet, and his face was frozen in anxiety. His mother looked weary and fearful. John had been diagnosed schizophrenic, or schizo-affective, and was on parenteral drugs. On his own he had stopped taking olanzapine (Zyprexa) a month earlier with few withdrawal symptoms. When I asked how could we help him, he was very vague and spoke very softly. Fortunately, prior to his appointment, his mother had sent us a very good history of his illness.

I then opened up the topic of schizophrenia, telling him that I wished I had his genes but not that I wished to be sick. I emphasized that schizophrenia genes are good genes if you feed them properly, which meant giving his genes the vitamins he needed, especially niacin. Immediately, he woke up and became much more interested. I assume he thought I would once more make him tell me his history.

I then outlined why in our opinion schizophrenic genes are such good genes. On the physical side their possessors tend to be good looking (he was), they aged gracefully, hardly ever got arthritis and rarely got cancer. We told him that out of 5,000 schizophrenic patients I had seen, only ten had gotten cancer and they had all recovered with treatment that included vitamins. By this time he was wide awake. We then told him that, psychologically, possessors of these genes tend to be very intelligent, creative, and talented, and we described some of creative successful patients who had been treated. He told us he had received top marks in

Grade 12 but after that he deteriorated, was struggling in his second year of university, and could not even hold minor jobs. He previously loved to play classical guitar and had been an excellent athlete.

Why did we use this approach? We did it because the information we gave him is true, as anyone reading my books will realize, and, secondly, no one will ever recover without hope and a reason to live. The usual negative mantra of modern psychiatrists to their schizophrenic patients is correct, as they only use drugs.

The transformation in this young man in just a few minutes of discussion was amazing. He was now fully alert and taking part in the discussion. His mother now and then cried softly from relief and kept saying she should have brought him to see me a few years earlier. We also had to neutralize the word schizophrenia, so stigmatized and, of course, dead wrong. The term itself is meaningless, does not tell us anything about what is really wrong, and does not indicate the correct treatment. We told him that the correct term is pellagra and explained in detail what we meant.

What were we hoping to achieve? First, we had to start the process of giving him back his self-respect. He had been a very intelligent, creative young man and this had been taken away from him. He could again hold his head high, knowing that he had a biochemical disorder for which he was not to blame, and that this disorder, if treated properly, gave the possessor a whole set of highly desirable properties that most of us would like to have. Most people think that schizophrenic genes are bad genes. They are asked about them and a family history is taken, as if the whole family has been tainted. In our opinion there are no bad genes except for those that do not permit survival. If any individual has been well for even a short period of time, then the genes are not bad; they have been badly treated by not providing them with the essential nutrients in their environment, and by overwhelming them with the toxins with which our planet is now so overly loaded. If a brilliant scientist develops Alzheimer's disease at age 75, one cannot say that his or her genes were bad because they did so well for so many years. They have not been well treated (well fed) for about 20

years. With proper orthomolecular treatment, they would continue to serve as good genes.

Our second objective was to restore hope that the condition was treatable. Until now all he could look forward to was a life of chronic pain, medication, failure, and indifference from the psychiatric profession. The best way to restore hope was to tell him stories about other patients who were equally sick who had recovered; like the teenager with schizophrenia who was seen in 1973, now a professor at a famous university, or the teenaged girl practically on the streets, who recovered, married, raised her family, and then learned a new profession, which she is pursuing successfully. These stories inspire hope and are very therapeutic.

Treatment Approach

Then we asked about his diet and whether he had allergies. He did not think he had allergies but he did show some evidence of these including dark rings under his eyes, called allergy shiners, as well as a few white spots in his fingernails characteristic of dairy allergy. His mother told us that he drank a lot of milk when he was three years old, and, although he did not have many colds or earaches, he did suffer many episodes of strep throat. We talked with him about the need to rule out whether he had an allergy or not. We advised him to totally eliminate all dairy products for one month and gave him an instruction sheet to guide him. After the end of the month he would do a challenge test by eating a dairy product. To illustrate what I meant, I told him about a few patients I had seen and how they had responded. One particularly striking example was a young man, age 21, who complained he had been depressed all his life. After two weeks eliminating all dairy products he was normal, completely free of depression. He then ate some ice cream. Within two hours his depression had come back, and after another hour he was psychotic. He was very agitated all night, fell asleep in the morning, awakened after three hours, and has been well since he got off all dairy products.

Food allergies are trigger factors and have to be eliminated, as the constant inflammation of the gastrointestinal tract creates the "leaky gut" syndrome and prevents the absorption of nutrients, vitamins, and minerals from the small intestine. Milk intake is also associated with iron deficiency anemia and with zinc deficiency; being aware of this makes it easier for patients to accept that they will have to take nutrients in order to make up what they have been missing for many years.

Then we listed each of the nutrients John needed including the following recommendations:

• Niacin: 500 mg, three times daily, after meals for two weeks, and thereafter 1,000 mg, three times daily. This is a starting dose and one may have to go much higher depending upon the response. The most common minor and nonharmful side effect is the vasodilation or flush. Niacin itself is the best antiniacin-flush product and after a few days schizophrenic patients will have stopped flushing. The flush was discussed with him in detail so that he would not be surprised or frightened.

• Vitamin C: 1,000 mg, three times daily. This is a major antioxidant, antistress nutrient, and decreases the incidence of colds and the flu—a time when patients have an increased tendency to relapse.

• Vitamin-B complex: 100 mg of each major B vitamin daily to replace some of the other Bs that have not been absorbed well for several years.

• Vitamin D: 6,000 international units (IU) daily in winter.

• Omega-3 essential fatty acids (as fish oil): 1,000 mg, three times a day.

• Zinc citrate: 50 mg, daily. Dairy allergy often causes zinc deficiency and he had signs of deficiency.

John was advised to take all the pills together at the end of his meals. Finally, he was advised that if he had any reaction to any of the pills that worried him, he should immediately call us by phone or contact us by email. All questions are usually answered within 24 hours, The first part of the interview took about 30 minutes. The rest of the hour was open to questions from John and his mother. Every question was answered.

■ CONCLUSION

At the time I started in psychiatry, when no effective treatment was available, it was the fashion to prepare very long histories, almost brief biographies. The less that was known about causes and treatment, the more information was piled into the charts for the unfortunate secretaries to transcribe. This was based on the influential views of Adolf Meyer, an early 20th century psychiatrist, that everything was important. But with growing orthomolecular experience over the past 50 years it has become clear that most of the history is not essential, unless it is needed for legal reasons or to impress one's superiors while a student or resident. A brief history such as is taken by doctors not practicing psychiatry is adequate and should not take more than a few minutes. The only essential facts are when the problem started, what were the stresses (trigger factors), what was the treatment and response, and the present situation. Almost every schizophrenic patient I saw was referred by their general physicians, as I did not accept any non-referred patients. Almost all had failed to respond to previous multi-drug treatments or they would not have been referred. Usually the diagnosis was made by other doctors and psychiatrists and in most cases I agreed with it. Therefore, taking a history need not cut too much into the time needed for the real objective of the visit: to establish adequate treatment that will increase the patient's chance of becoming normal.

Orthomolecular treatment is sophisticated, effective, and safe and not time-consuming as many more patients can be seen. Patients need not be seen as frequently because they recover, in contrast to those given only drugs. The savings in time and money is enormous; there is nothing more economical than recovery. Unfortunately, because the medical profession has not endorsed orthomolecular treatment nor learned how to use it, patients are denied their chance for recovery and to take their place in a normal society. Sadly, it is a treatment for the people who can afford to travel long distances to get this treatment. It remains beyond the reach of the poor, who have to remain dependent upon the drugs-only therapy offered to them and enforced by government. A few patients recovered by following the regimen outlined in my books. Some of these cases are described in *Mental Health Regained*, published by the International Schizophrenia Foundation in 2007.

Postscript

December 1, 2007: John just emailed to tell us he was doing much better. According to him he has more energy, his sleeping patterns have returned to normal, his thoughts are much more organized and studying has been easier. He also said he is enjoying exercise and continues to hold athletic aspirations. John, who had been so vague about what was wrong with him, and somewhat withdrawn, especially during the early part of the consultation, made this email contact himself and was able to express clearly what was going right.

PHYSICIAN'S REPORT:
ORTHOMOLECULAR: THE OPTIMUM TREATMENT FOR SCHIZOPHRENIA
by Abram Hoffer, MD, PhD

Schizophrenic patients can get well and they deserve a chance to achieve this objective.

Today, I saw the following seven schizophrenic patients, one after the other: I had not selected them. The appointments were set up by my secretary and I did not know until this morning who I would be seeing.

Here are their case histories.

1. K. C., Born 1932, first seen September 1987

After seeing a psychiatrist for 2.5 years for her depression, K. C. she was confused about what treatment she should be following. She had heard of hypoglycemia. She first became depressed in 1953 following the birth of her first child. In 1962 she was given 4 ECT (electroconvulsive shock treatments) and following that took the antidepressant Nardil. Every time she went off this antidepressant her depression recurred. She was in hospital 10 days in 1985, again in January 1987 for 21 days. She told me she had been diagnosed manic-depressive because her first bout of depression had been preceded by a manic episode, but she had not had any since then. Her main complaint was fatigue to the point she could do only her housework and cooking. Anything more was impossible. She was also anxious and very worried about her weight, 135 pounds. Her best weight had been 120 pounds.

When I first saw her, she told me she had heard the voice of her son in 1986 for the 10 days she was in hospital, and again the next admission. She was worried about people staring at her. When very depressed she was also very paranoid, thinking the public was holding things back from her. Her memory and concentration were poor and she blocked a lot. I diagnosed her schizoaffective disorder.

She was started on a sugar-free diet with niacinamide (1,000 milligrams [mg]/3x per day), ascorbic acid (1,000 mg/3x per day), pyridoxine (250 mg/day), and zinc gluconate (100 mg/day), while continuing her Nardil (15 mg/3x per day), Haldol (4 mg at bedtime), and Serax (87.5 mg taken as needed). By December 1987 she was much better.

For the past few years she was been more or less well, developing a few symptoms when under severe pressure but usually able to deal with family pressures effectively. She is coping with her husband's retirement, with the need to move into a different home, but she does not require any more psychiatric attention than most of the patients I have seen with anxiety or depression. She is seen about four times each year for the nine years she has been under my care. She had her last of four admissions in 1987 and has not needed to go to hospital since then.

2. D. H., Born 1927, first seen June 1993

D. H. came to see me in June 1993 with his wife and brother. He had been seriously confused for the previous three months. I was not able to obtain the history from this patient as he was in a mental fog and seemed unaware of what was going on. His brother and wife gave me his history. He first became sick at age 27 and was admitted to hospital. Twenty-one years later, 1975, he became sick again and had needed repeated admissions from that time until his last one in 1986. His family did not know what medication he had been on, nor how long he had been in hospital on these admissions. At that time he had auditory hallucinations and was very paranoid. After his last discharge he was maintained on tranquilizer medication but in spite of this had begun to deteriorate again over the previous year and especially over the previous three months. He had about six series of ECT during his career as a chronic schizophrenic. He admitted he was hearing voices and believed that everyone was staring at him. He was very paranoid, believing there was a plot against him. He often spoke to his wife about the telephones being tapped. His memory and concentration were very poor. He also suffered mood swings. He weighed 250 pounds at five foot eleven.

I continued his medication as follows Thorazine (900 mg/day), lithium (900 mg/day), Trilafon (32 mg /day), Kemadrin (15 mg /day), L-thyroxine (200 micrograms [mcg]/day), and Adalat (20 mg/day). To this I added a sugar-free diet, niacin (1,000 mg/3x per day), and ascorbic acid (1,000 mg/3x per day).

By July 28, 1993, he had lost three pounds and his wife noted some evidence of his previous personality emerging. I decreased his Thorazine to 700 mg per day. On September 2, I decreased it further to 500 mg. He was more alive, more active, and more cheerful, but he still heard the same voices. On November 4, I increased his niacin to 1,500 mg/3x per day and decreased his Thorazine to 300 mg per day. By December 9, he had lost 13 pounds and his blood pressure had started to come down.

On January 19, 1994, he developed chills and fever from a bladder infection, was admitted to hospital in a confused state, and later was transferred to the psychiatric ward. There, they would not allow him to take any vitamins. He was discharged February 2, 1994. He had begun to deteriorate rapidly in hospital and was started on Risperdal. I saw him on February 10, 1994, stopped the Risperdal, decreased his lithium carbonate to 600 mg/day, Trilafon to 16 mg /day, and kept his Thorazine at 200 mg/day. On March 22, 1994, I increased his niacin to 2,000 mg/3x per day, and he was off lithium. By April 28 he weighed 223 pounds and was going on walks three times each week. On June 9, 1994, I reduced his Thorazine to 100 mg/day. A few weeks later he became nauseated and I increased it to 125 mg and added folic acid (5 mg/3x per day). On October 27, I decreased his Thorazine to 100 mg every second day. By December 15, 1994, he was still showing major improvement after each visit. His weight was 207 pounds.

In March 1995 I stopped all tranquilizers. He was nearly normal according to his wife and his brother, and I concurred. By June 15, he was symptom free. The voices were gone, his memory was much better, and he was on nutrients only. He was busy helping his wife. On September 14, 1995, he was well. He was cheerful, joked, had resumed painting with oils, something he had done before he became ill. His wife was delighted that she had back the husband she had known, who could now be a helpmate around their place and not just a burden. He is well, that is, free of signs and symptoms, gets on well with his family and with the community, and would be working if he had not been so badly damaged by his illness and inappropriate treatment he had received for such a long time. It was very exciting to see this chronic schizophrenic gradually come back to a full and productive life.

3. K. K., Born 1954, first seen July 1979

When I first saw K. K. in 1979, she complained that for the past year she had suffered from severe episodes of anxiety, which she had been able to control until one month before I saw her. Her physician gave her medication but it left her very tired and sleepy. She thought the doctor had given it to her to make her an addict. She told me she had taken LSD twice, the last time two years earlier. She denied any perceptual changes except hearing herself think occasionally. Her thinking was paranoid and she had been depressed in the past.

Her parents told me her personality had changed and she left home at age 18, quitting school two months before graduation from high school. She then went through a series of bad relationships with several men. She lived with one who abused her for two years and beat her. She had several miscarriages. Her behavior was strongly condemned by her parents and the church to which they belonged, and they had practically disowned her because they considered her a loose woman who could not be helped. At the time I did not think she was schizophrenic and suggested she continue with the program of nutrition and vitamins she was already taking.

I saw her again in February 1980 when she was depressed. This time she saw visual hallucinations in a picture hanging on the wall and heard voices. She had been admitted to hospital in December for 10 days and was started on Haldol. Because she had no money she had been unable to continue with her vitamin program from December. I rediagnosed her as schizophrenic and started her on niacinamide (1,000 mg/3x per day), ascorbic acid (1,000 mg/3x per day), pyridoxine (250 mg/day) and a zinc preparation (10 mg /3x per day) while continuing the Haldol (4 mg/day). By March 1980 she was less stiff and jerky, more alive, and had more initiative. In April her mother reported she was beginning to see her daughter's previous healthy personality emerge. September 2–29 she was in the hospital because her mother could not cope with her. She had had severe reactions to the Haldol, including spasms and limb tremor. She was discharged free of medication to stay with her sister. Her relationship with her parents was much better. They were beginning to see her as having been very sick, rather than very bad.

In April 1981 I started her on Elavil (25 mg) and Trilafon (2 mg at bedtime). By June she was only on the antidepressant plus her vitamins and she was normal. She was working.

In July 1982 she had a severe cold lasting several weeks and began to deteriorate. I admitted her to hospital July 15–22. She had been living with a man and she was pregnant. Her baby was born in January 1983. She continued to be seen at irregular intervals, usually requiring some adjustment in her medication.

For the five years beginning in 1980 I saw her 30 times, for the next five years 37 times, for the last five years 13 times, and for the last three years twice each year.

In 1986 I started her on Nozinan and gradually increased the dose until she was well on about 300 mg daily. July 24 1995, she accidently took an overdose. She had taken her bedtime medication, awakened during the night and took another 100 mg of Nozinan. She became frightened and called 911 and was admitted. When seen on September 14, she was well again. Her daughter was doing well and going to school. She had

been able to look after her child for many years with the kind and dedicated support of her parents and family. Whenever she was too tired, her child would move in with her parents for a few days to give her a rest.

I saw her daughter as a patient when she was nine years old. She had been experiencing auditory and visual hallucinations for two months. The voices varied from a mumble to calling her name. The voice would sometimes order her to "Come here," and she was very afraid of this. She located this voice either outside of her head or in her head. She also had shadow illusions and in shadows saw a person. She felt unreal as well. She was moody and irritable, cried a lot, but was a good student. I started her on a sugar-free, dairy-free diet with niacinamide (500 mg/3x per day) and ascorbic acid (500 mg/3x per day). Since then she has been well but has needed Elavil (25 mg at bedtime and taken as needed).

I consider the daughter well, that is, free of schizophrenic symptoms and signs, and getting on well with family and community. Her mother is much improved, a single mother on pension support. Her illness, the pregnancy, and later the need to bring up her child, prevented her from taking further training and from working. The need to remain on the high dose of tranquilizer prevents her from functioning at a fully normal level. I expect she will be working within a few years.

4. W. E., Born 1929, first seen October 1989

In 1987 W. E. was admitted to hospital with severe anxiety and paranoid ideas. He was diagnosed psychotic. For the year before he saw me he had been hearing voices, which he found comforting but which his wife found very disturbing. It was difficult to talk to him because he was very hard of hearing as well. He had been an alcoholic for 14 years but had been abstinent for the previous 10 years. I started him on niacin (1,000 mg/3x per day), ascorbic acid (1,000 mg/3x per day), folic acid (5 mg/2x per day), and thiamine (100 mg/3x per day), the last one because of his history of alcoholism.

Since then I have seen him on average eight visits each year for the past five years. Over the years he has become free of depression, his paranoid ideas have decreased, and the voices have become much less disturbing. At the last visit he told me that he believed he was now on top of the voices, that they were no longer dominating him as they had in the past. I see him more often than many of my patients because he has insight that he must not talk about his experiences to anyone else, and he finds great relief in being able to talk to me about them. I consider him much improved.

5. P. W., Born 1934, first seen October 1981

P. W.'s chief complaint when I first saw her was hearing voices. She had become sick for the first time at age 19, troubled by her auditory hallucinations. She was treated in Seattle, later in Vancouver in the mental hospital for one year, and received insulin coma and ECT. Six years later she was admitted for the second time for eight months and again in 1972 for four months. She had a fourth admission in 1977 for four months and two more in 1977 and 1979. The voices were always present and she was convinced that spirits were talking to her. For many years she had been given injectable tranquilizers, every two weeks. The first time she saw me she described her voices, saw visions, and could visualize spirits in her own mind. She was very suspicious, with blocking. Not surprisingly, her mood was depressed and she had made one suicide attempt in the past.

I started her on niacinamide (1,000 mg/3x per day), ascorbic acid (500 mg/3x per day), pyridoxine (250 mg/day), zinc sulfate (220 mg/day), and maintained her on the tranquilizer and the antidepressant. By October 1982 she was nearly normal. March 1983 the voices had returned. She had been off her tranquilizers for a while. She then resumed the drug and started a secretarial course. I added niacin (1,000 mg/3x per day) and kept her on Tofranil (75 mg at bedtime). She had to be admitted to the hospital October 7–12, and again October 18–26, 1984, because her thinking had become very bizarre and she was disoriented and agitated. There were no further recurrences.

She was well most of the time but would sometimes under stress hear voices again. She lived a normal life and traveled a lot. She was admitted August 23, discharged August 31, 1987, to readjust her medication, and readmitted the next day. After this discharge she was under the care of another psychiatrist until November 10, 1993, when she was referred to me again. During May 1993 her son was involved in a car accident. Her daughter went to Australia to look for work and she missed her terribly, and the voices had become very strong. She had been in the mental hospital May 25–October 6, 1993, and was given Resperidal but this was very toxic for her, and when I saw her she was on Trilafon (8 mg) and was well. The voices were in the far background.

On March 1994 her son married and she had found this stressful. She looked well, seldom heard her voices, and did volunteer work with schizophrenic patients. I added Zoloft, which did not help, and later Prozac, which did help. On December 19, 1994, she was symptom free. I stopped the Prozac.

On September 14, 1995, she was unhappy over a misinterpretation with her son but this was readily overcome. She was on Trilafon and the vitamin regimen. She had just returned from a visit with her daughter in Australia and was very happy that her daughter had found good employment and was happy there.

For the first five years under my care I saw her about four times each year. There were six visits in 1986, and 8 in 1987. When she came under care again I saw her twice in 1993, four times in 1994, and once in 1995. Before going on orthomolecular treatment she had had at least six, perhaps seven admissions, and had spent at least 28 months in the hospital. After starting on the program she was in for three brief admissions. After she went off the vitamin regimen she was again in the hospital for 4.5 months. Since going back on the program there have been no further admissions.

6. W. D., Born 1958, first seen November 1990

Nine years before I saw W. D., he was diagnosed schizophrenic on his first admission to the hospital for six weeks. He had two more admissions after that, the last in May of 1990. Seven years before seeing me he had started himself on inositol hexaniacinate (a flush-free preparation). He told me that under pressure he would hear voices. Sometimes he believed these voices were trying to trick him. He heard his own thoughts all the time and felt unreal. He was paranoid but was aware of it and was able to cope, and he still had to deal with episodes of depression. His dress was quite flamboyant and his language had an interesting schizophrenic flavor. I increased his inositol hexaniacinate to 1,000 mg/3x per day, adding ascorbic acid (500 mg /3x per day), vitamin B complex (50 mg/day), zinc citrate (50 mg/day), and continued him on his Moditen (5 mg/day). In December 1990 I advised him to start niacin as well.

In February 1991 he reported he usually took two trips each year to California to try and contact Hollywood stars and to get away from himself but he had realized this was impossible. In June 1991 he was better. The voices were gone but he still heard his own thoughts. On December 19, 1991, he had stopped the niacin and I advised him to start niacinamide (1,000 mg/3x per day) instead.

On October 13, 1992, he married a patient he had met while he had been in hospital. He had an incentive job and did volunteer work as a cook. The voices were still troublesome.

In November 1993 his marriage was working out well. He was still on small doses of tranquilizers. On November 15, 1994, his wife was hospitalized. She refused to take vitamins and did not want him to take any.

On June 15, 1995, he had a job. His wife was pregnant and he was happy about that. On September 14 he was still well and looking forward to his baby. I consider him much improved. He had no longer needed any admissions to the hospital.

7. S. O., Born 1973, first seen January 1992

S. O. became sick in 1989, consulted a psychologist, and was given psychotherapy plus an antidepressant and a tranquilizer. The drugs helped him to control his thinking but he did not feel well. He moved in with his parents and in September was started on long-acting injectable Haldol. When I saw him he could hear himself think and felt that these thoughts came from evil entities, mostly from the Devil. They instructed him to hurt himself and other people, but he never had done so. They also advised him to perform certain rituals without specifying what they were. He had violent difficult dreams where he found himself in a record shop surrounded by evil records. He sometimes was convinced people were staring at him and watching him. His thinking was paranoid, there was frequent blocking, and his memory and concentration were poor. Episodes of depression dogged him with suicide ideas.

I started on niacinamide (1,000 mg/3x per day), ascorbic acid (1,000 mg/3x per day), vitamin B complex (50 mg/day), while continuing his long-acting Haldol (75 mg) every three weeks. By March 1992 he was normal and making high grades with his studies. In the fall he entered university. On January 30, 1993, his Haldol dose was reduced to 30 mg every three weeks. In the summer he took summer school classes.

In April 1994 I added Zoloft 50 mg/day. One month later he was well. On September 14, 1995, he was still well. He was cheerful, told me he was completing his university training, taking five full courses. He expected to graduate in the spring. I see him about every six weeks.

Recap

Of the seven patients on long-term care, four are well and three are much improved. These seven fall within the normal range of our healthy population, but they may require continuing care even if it means one visit per year. I believe many of them are healthier than the average person since they are following the best principles of orthomolecular nutrition and are taking the supplements they need to stay well. My patients have to be protected from other psychiatrists. If I am not around, they will eventually go to other psychiatrists who will promptly remove the vitamins from their regimen, and they will resume their inexorable march downward into total disability.

I have given some detail of the therapeutic program I follow. It includes attention to nutrition to eliminate any foods that are harmful to the patient, usually sugar and foods to which they are allergic. It includes the nutrients, which are most helpful in the optimum dose ranges, which is determined by clinical experience, and it includes medication as long as it is necessary. The ultimate aim is to have patients well on nutrition and nutrients alone, or to need such low doses of drugs that they are not incapacitated by the toxic and side effects. To achieve this requires attention to detail and, above all, patience because chronic patients may need many years before they recover. Not every patient gets well, and this is a property shared with other diseases. But over 90 percent of early schizophrenic patients will recover within two years, and better than 50 percent will recover when they have been sick many years. These patients comprise only a small fraction of the 500 chronic schizophrenic patients under my care.

From the *J Orthomolecular Med* 1995;10(2):169–176.

ORTHOMOLECULAR PSYCHIATRIC TREATMENTS ARE PREFERABLE TO MAINSTREAM PSYCHIATRIC DRUGS: A RATIONAL ANALYSIS

by Jonathan E. Prousky, ND

Although *mainstream psychiatric drugs* (*MPDs*) can help to stabilize patients during mental episodes or breakdowns (e.g., first psychotic episode, disabling depression, and acute mania), there are rational reasons why clinicians may wish to consider using orthomolecular medicine to reduce patients' needs for MPDs and/or to facilitate the eventual reduction of doses to ameliorate side effects. MPDs might themselves be responsible for the protracted course of psychiatric illness and debility since recurrences and/or relapses might be attributable to the iatrogenic (treatment and/or doctor-induced) effects of medications.[1] In this paper, I will demonstrate why *orthomolecular psychiatric treatment* (*OPT*) is a safer and more effective treatment option than MPDs for the following reasons: 1) OPT utilizes optimal doses of substances that are normally present in the human body as opposed to MPDs, which are xenobiotics and are not normally present in the human body; 2) OPT supports and nourishes the mind (i.e., the brain) and body as opposed to MPDs, which induce abnormal brain states and produce worrisome and sometimes disabling psychologic and somatic side effects; and 3) OPT is not associated with physiological dependence, withdrawal symptoms, and significant long-term harm, whereas MPDs have been associated with dependence and can cause worrisome symptoms during withdrawal. They can also cause harm when vulnerable patients are experiencing symptoms and side effects during episodes of illness. In comparison to OPT, this paper asserts that MPDs are unnatural agents that induce abnormal brain states, produce iatrogenic symptoms, or even cause harm and have been associated with chronic long-term debility.

From the *J Orthomolecular Med* 2013;28(1):1–16.

Support for Orthomolecular Psychiatric Treatment

OPT Uses Optimum Doses of Naturally Occurring Substances to Correct Defective Enzyme-Catalyzed Reactions and Help to Restore Normal Brain Metabolism

Common sense dictates that orthomolecules, meaning micronutrients naturally and normally present in the human body such as vitamins, minerals, amino acids, and essential fatty acids, would be more health-promoting than synthetic prescription medications. OPT therapy provides the optimal molecular environment for the brain and other tissues by improving the patient's intake of essential nutrients, such as vitamins (and their metabolites), minerals, trace elements, macronutrients, as well as other naturally occurring metabolically active substances.

OPT should be preferable to using MPDs for the treatment of psychiatric disorders. Arguments in support of OPT have been previously published by Pauling and others.[2–4] Pauling argued that since the human race is characterized by genetic heterogeneity, enzyme concentrations in the tissues of individual patients can be expected to differ tremendously by factors of 2, 10, or even 100. It is therefore reasonable to consider that mental status changes might arise, in part, due to defective enzyme-catalyzed reactions, associated with biochemical individuality as well as deficiencies of precursors and suboptimal levels of enzyme cofactors. In a 2002 publication,[5] the need for large doses of orthomolecules was deemed necessary as a means to increase coenzyme concentrations and to correct defective enzymatic activity in 50 human genetic diseases. The authors of this study went further by stating that the "examples discussed here are likely to represent only a small fraction of the total number of defective enzymes that would be responsive to therapeutic vitamins." Therefore, it is reasonable to prescribe orthomolecules to psychiatric patients as a therapeutic treatment aimed at "normalizing" altered brain function resulting from deficiencies of essential nutrients and from defective enzyme-coenzyme reactions.

OPT Utilizes Naturally Occurring Substances That Offset Deficiencies in the Cerebral Spinal Fluid and/or in Other Tissues of the Body

Pauling also discussed the possibility that cerebrospinal fluid (CSF) concentrations of vital orthomolecules could be grossly diminished, while concentrations in the blood and lymph remained essentially normal.[2,3] He hypothesized that localized cerebral deficiencies might result from decreased rates of transfer (i.e., decreased permeability) of vital orthomolecules across the blood-brain barrier, increased rates of their destruction within the CSF, or from other (unknown) factors. Other authors have speculated that exposures to toxic chemicals (i.e., alcohol, industrial solvents, or halogenated hydrocarbons) might block the entry of specific orthomolecules into the brain, leading to CSF deficiencies.[6] This phenomenon of a localized cerebral deficiency has been described in reports documenting neuropsychiatric improvements from therapeutic vitamin B12 supplementation among subjects having normal vitamin B12 levels in the serum, but deficient levels within the CSF.[6,7] It is conceivable that the therapeutic administration of many orthomolecules might correct for micronutrient deficiencies within the CSF and therefore "normalize" altered brain function among patients with psychiatric disorders.

Even if one does not consider the relationship between nutrition and the "health" of the CSF, it is well-established that deficiencies of orthomolecules can lead to mental status changes resulting from many factors, such as poor diet and lifestyle habits,[8,9] concomitant disease (i.e., malabsorption), and prescription drugs (i.e., drug-induced nutrient depletions or compromised nutrition due to side effects like loss of appetite).[10] When micronutrient deficiencies arise they typically follow a fairly predictable course,[11] which invariably would impact the CSF and other tissues, and likely cause a deficiency or some perturbation within some or all of these compartments of the body. Following are the stages typical of a micronutrient deficiency:

• Stage 1: Micronutrient body stores begin to be depleted. Micronutrient urinary excretion decreases, while homeostatic mechanisms maintain a normal level of the micronutrient in the blood.

• Stage 2: Depletion is more marked. As the micronutrient urinary excretion declines, there is a corresponding drop in its concentration in the blood and other tissues. The result is a lowering of micronutrient metabolites and/or dysfunction of dependent enzymes. Occasionally, hormone concentrations will decrease and may be accompanied by observable physiological alterations.

IN BRIEF

Although mainstream psychiatric drugs (MPDs) can help to quickly stabilize patients having mental breakdowns or suicidal crises there are rational reasons for clinicians to consider orthomolecular psychiatric treatment (OPT). The practice of orthomolecular medicine encourages clinicians to diagnose accurately and recommend safer and more effective treatments than MPDs for the following reasons: 1) OPT utilizes substances that are normally present in the human body whereas MPDs are xenobiotics and not normally present in the human body; 2) OPT supports and nourishes the mind (i.e., the brain) and body opposed to MPDs that induce abnormal brain states and can produce worrisome, problematic, toxic, and sometimes even disabling psychologic and somatic side effects; and 3) OPT is not associated with physiological dependence, withdrawal symptoms, or significant long-term harm whereas MPDs are. Even if there are questions about the author's interpretation of published data or his personal biases, we should still be concerned and re-evaluate the current practice of placing vulnerable patients on MPDs for long periods of time. We need a mental health system that is life-affirming and not life-impeding, and open-minded and conscientious enough to seriously consider the recognized merits of OPT.

• Stage 3: Presence of morphological and/or functional disturbances. They are initially reversible, and then irreversible. Patients might present with nonspecific signs and symptoms. Unless they are adequately treated, death will eventually result.

Even though clinical symptoms can be recognizable at any point along this continuum (from Stages 1–3), they can be hidden to the untrained clinician who might not be cognizant that there is a relationship between common neuropsychiatric presentations (e.g., cognitive impairment, depression, psychosis, and even mania) and micronutrient inadequacy. Neuropsychiatric presentations might reflect long-latency deficiency disease states as a result of poor nutritional intakes for many years.[4] The following list highlights mental status changes associated with common micronutrient deficiencies.[12–14] Overall, the therapeutic administration of orthomolecules should have significant value in reversing many neuropsychiatric presentations when related to inadequate micronutrient status.

• Vitamin B-complex deficiencies (B1, B2, B3, B6, B12, and folic acid are the most common): Agitation, apathy, cognitive impairment, delirium, dementia, depression, dizziness, emotional lability, faintness, fatigue, insomnia, irritability, mania, memory impairment, mood swings, nervousness, pain sensitivity, psychosis, restless legs, rigidity, somnolence, and weakness.

• Vitamin D deficiency: Anxiety, depressed mood, insomnia, nervousness, and weakness.

• Mineral deficiencies (calcium and magnesium are the most common): Agitation, amnesia, apathy, behavioral disturbances, cognitive impairment, delirium, depression, dizziness, fatigue, hyperactivity, irritability, insomnia, nervousness, neurological problems, psychosis, restlessness, tremor, and weakness.

• Essential fatty acids deficiency: Alterations in thought and mood, anxiety, fatigue, and neurotic fears.

OPT Improves Short-Term (and Likely, Long-Term) Therapeutic Outcomes Among Patients with Mental Disorders

Decades of case reports have documented successful patient outcomes from using OPT either alone or in combination with MPD treatment for mood, thought, attention, and other mental disorders. Many published case reports document successful recoveries from the use of OPT, which include, for example: 1) fibromyalgia syndrome[15] (via micronutrients to offset mitochondrial myopathy); 2) schizophrenia[16] (via a low-carbohydrate, ketogenic diet that ameliorated the patient's psychotic symptoms as a result of gluten avoidance and/or modulation of the disease at a cellular level); and 3) recent onset of psychotic disorder, hypertension, and seizures in a 16-year-old patient[17] (via intramuscular injections of vitamin B12 as the only therapy administered).

In three review publications, the results of many short-term intervention trials (normally, around 12 weeks or less) demonstrate therapeutic benefits from single-orthomolecular and multiple-orthomolecular supplementation among patients having mental disorders.[4,18,19] In several of the reviewed intervention trials, patients provided with orthomolecules and MPDs fared better than patients given only MPDs.[20–26] A major criticism of OPT is the claimed dearth of clinical trials demonstrating benefits, yet these review articles clearly document successful short-term outcomes from using OPT in more than 80 intervention trials.

While rigorous long-term studies documenting the benefits from OPT are lacking, the therapeutic effects of OPT would likely sustain over time. Since the brain and body depend on a constant supply of micronutrients (i.e., achieved through dietary modifications and/or micronutrient supplementation), it seems plausible that the provision of optimal doses of OPT would facilitate improved mental and physical health over time. These effects would be cumulative, in that they would mitigate other risks of increased morbidity (e.g., nutrient insufficiency, hypertension, obesity, and immune dysfunction) and early mortality (e.g., diabetes, heart disease, and infectious disease)—for optimal nutrition is a sound and reasonable way to improve the quality (i.e., health span) and the duration (i.e., life span) of a person's existence.

For example, a depressed patient might be prescribed an optimal daily dose of 4,000 international units (IU) of vitamin D3 (cholecalciferol) by a clinician who uses OPT. While this intervention might positively impact depression by improving this patient's sense of well-being[27] (note: not all intervention trials have shown benefit on depression),[28] the addition of this amount of vitamin D3 would also reduce hypovitaminosis D-related ill health (i.e., many types of cancer, cardiovascular diseases, autoimmune diseases, diabetes types 1 and 2, specific bacterial and viral infections, and all-cause mortality rates)[29] and therefore improve the health and increase the life span of the depressed patient.

OPT Is Not Associated with Physiological Dependence, Withdrawal Symptoms, or Long-Term Harm

Our bodies demand a constant supply of micronutrients found in foods and through supplementation. If the body's needs are not met, the individual will suffer from the consequences of micronutrient insufficiency, and in more extreme cases, malnutrition. Based on these facts, the body is physiologically dependent on receiving a complete "sum" of micronutrients on a daily basis; otherwise, signs and symptoms of nutritional inadequacy will manifest and cause a myriad of physical and psychological perturbations. This healthy physiological dependency, described here, is not the same as the unhealthy physiological dependency that results from tapering down or stopping MPDs.

When patients have compromised micronutrient intake because of an insufficient diet, radical dietary changes, and/or stopping their micronutrient supplementation, they can present with a wide variety of neuropsychiatric manifestations when their depletion of certain micronutrients exceeds their individual thresholds (e.g., as in vitamin B12-deficienct mania,[30] obsessive-compulsive disorder,[31] and psychosis[32]). Their changed mental states, heretofore, can result from a "lack" of essential micronutrients and not from instability induced by the discontinuation of a MPD.

With respect to harm, the use of hugely excessive doses of micronutrients can cause worrisome symptoms, but usually any such harm is self-limited and will reverse itself soon after the micronutrient dosage is reduced or discontinued. Essentially, there are no risks of long-term harm associated with the use of micronutrients. To illustrate this, I offer several examples from the published literature. The first example involves a schizophrenic patient who developed hepatitis following large doses (9,000 mg/day) of niacinamide.[33] This patient had no evidence of clinical hepatitis when taking 2,000–3,000 mg per day of niacinamide but did develop clinical hepatitis when the dose was increased to 9,000 mg per day. The nausea and vomiting, as well as abnormal liver function tests, resolved after the patient discontinued the vitamin for three weeks.

The second example involves vitamin B6 (in the form of pyridoxine hydrochloride). Studies in dogs have shown neurotoxicity leading to peripheral neuropathy, with ataxia, muscle weakness, and loss of balance after having been administered 200 mg of vitamin B6 per kilogram (kg) of body weight for 40–75 days.[34] In dogs it has even been possible to have a more acute onset of swaying gait and ataxia within 9 days after taking 300 mg vitamin B6/kg body weight.[35] In humans, there are reports of sensory neuropathy following very large doses of vitamin B6. Seven patients in one report had ataxia and severe sensory nervous system dysfunction after taking 2,000–7,000 mg per day of vitamin B6 for several months.[36] Four of the patients were severely affected, but they all improved following cessation of the vitamin even though some patients did have residual nerve damage. Weakness was not part of their clinical presentation and the central nervous system was clinically spared.

In an experimental study of five human volunteers, daily doses of either 1,000 or 3,000 mg of vitamin B6 was given until laboratory and/or clinical abnormalities resulted.[37] Electrophysiological and clinical abnormalities occurred simultaneously in all subjects but occurred earlier in those taking higher daily doses of the vitamin. Upon stopping the vitamin, symptoms progressed for an additional two to three weeks before remitting. Most reports of sensory neuropathy following vitamin B6 therapy involve daily doses larger than 1,000 mg.[38] Review articles typically mention that safe daily doses are between 200–500 mg,[38,39] even though there are recent randomized trials showing no evidence of harm when large doses are used to treat medication-induced side effects (1,200 mg/day for 5 days among patients with acute neuroleptic-induced akathisia[40,41] and 1,200 mg/day for 12 weeks among patients with tardive dyskinesia[42]). These examples are representative of the relative safety of OMP since the negative effects caused by excessive doses of micronutrients are mostly reversible and are not associated with long-term impairment.

Another way to assess harm from OPT is to review data pertaining to mortality. The American Association of Poison Control Centers has been collecting data on the fatalities associated with numerous products (i.e., vitamin supplements, medications, household cleaning products, etc.) for decades. Only 13 deaths were linked to vitamins from 1983 to 2011,[43] but this data does not prove causality for it merely ascribes fatal outcomes to the use of vitamins.

QUALITY AND QUANTITY OF LIFE: TREATMENT TYPE MATTERS
by Jonathan Prousky, ND

Schizophrenia affects about 2 percent of the population. For those having this severe form of psychological distress, their entire world becomes unrecognizable, as does their sense of self. Such people might see things that are not there or they might hear voices from other people, outer space, the television, or even the Internet. Eventually, people experiencing this type of psychological distress get noticed by others because their social skills have eroded and they have become more immersed in their reality (an unreality) than the "real" world they disengaged from. The typical outcome is that these people become identified as mentally ill and are usually forcibly hospitalized or jailed and drugged. They are told that the only way forward is to take psychiatric drugs for the rest of their lives. What becomes of these people when they take these medications for the rest of their lives?

First, they become brain-damaged because the psychiatric drugs induce a generalized form of cognitive dysfunction that impairs the frontal lobes and the ability to think, reason, and make sound life choices.[1] Second, their course of illness is worsened as a result of the drug-induced brain-damaging effects. In other words, they have more psychotic episodes and fewer periods of remission as a result of the very drug treatments given to stabilize them.[2,3] Third, they develop neurological damage that makes them look as if they have mild or perhaps even severe Parkinson's diseases (called parkinsonism) because psychiatric medications damage the nervous system and suppress the emotions, creating an indifference to self and others as a result.[4] This destroys their passions, desires, libido, sexuality, and vitality—all sources of positive energy that make most people feel good about life. Fourth, these medications cause medical mayhem within the body, which amounts to obesity,[5] heart disease,[6,7] fatty liver,[8] blood sugar problems or diabetes,[9] and osteoarthritis (due to weight gain).[5] Lastly, the life spans of such people are dramatically shortened as a result of the psychiatric drugs, usually by some 1 to 25 years.[6,7,10–13]

What would happen if, instead of being drugged for life, such people had an opportunity to mostly use orthomolecular medicine? First, there would be no nervous system damage or brain-disabling effects, since orthomolecular medicine relies on natural substances normally present in the human body and brain (e.g., vitamins, minerals, amino acids, essential fatty acids, and hormones).[14] These natural substances sup-

722

Evidence Against MPDs

MPDs Are Xenobiotics That Induce Abnormal Brain States

The brain (and therefore, the mind) depends on a constant supply of nutrition, oxygen, and other naturally occurring substances to ensure their proper functioning. The proper functioning of the brain is not dependent on MPDs. These xenobiotic substances are not normally found in the brain and body. An emerging body of literature advocates for a drug-centered model of drug action as opposed to the outdated disease-centered model that espouses MPDs as correcting some known and well-validated disease process.[44]

For example, in the disease-centered model a depressed patient would be offered antidepressant medication as a means to correct some abnormal brain state (i.e., serotonin deficiency), which is then offset (i.e., helped) by the drug's action upon the underlying disease process (i.e., increasing serotonin within the central nervous system). In the drug-centered model, a depressed patient would be offered a medication to possibly induce a favorable "altered" mental state, which does not arise because the drug corrected some underlying disease process, but results from the consequences of being in a drug-induced altered state. This drug-centered model is a more accurate way to understand how MPDs function because the evidence

port the physiological and biochemical processes that the body and brain use to function normally.[14] Second, the course of illness would be less since people treated with orthomolecular medicine have a much less virulent course of mental illness and more functionality.[2,3] Third, these people would reap tremendous psychological and physical benefits since orthomolecular medicines can:

- Reduce symptoms of schizophrenia;[15–18]

- Moderate weight;[19]

- Improve blood sugar balance;[20]

- Slow joint deterioration;[21]

- Improve cardiovascular health;[22,23] and

- Protect the liver from damage.[24,25]

Fourth, orthomolecular medicine does not destroy peoples' energetic capacities or vitality but helps people to feel passionate, sexual, and vibrant throughout their lives. Lastly, orthomolecular medicine does not reduce life span and health span but extends both quality and quantity of life.[15]

Using orthomolecular medicine as the cornerstone of schizophrenia treatment not only makes a lot of sense but also can better the quality and quantity of life for the person with schizophrenia.

REFERENCES

1. Breggin PR. *Int J Risk Saf Med* 2011;23:193–200.

2. Harrow M. *Schizophr Bull* 2005;31:723–734.

3. Harrow M. *Schizophr Bull* 2013;39:962–965.

4. Moncrieff J. *J Hist Neurosci* 2013;22:30–46.

5. Citrome L. Schizophrenia, obesity, and antipsychotic medications. *Postgrad Med* 2008;120:18–33.

6. Straus SM. *Arch Intern Med* 2004;164:1293–1297.

7. Laursen TM. *Curr Opin Psychiatry* 2012;25:83–88.

8. Haberfellner EM. *J Clin Psychiatry* 2003;64:851.

9. Nasrallah HA. *Molecular Psychiatry* 2008;13:27–35.

10. Morgan MG. *Psychiatry Res* 2003;117:127–135.

11. Joukamaa M. *Br J Psychiatry* 2006;188:122–127.

12. Tenback D. *J Clin Psychopharmacol* 2012;32:31–35.

13. Tiihonen J. *Arch Gen Psychiatry* 2012;69:476–483.

14. Prousky J. *J Orthomol Med* 2013;28(1):17–32.

15. Ritsner MS. *J Clin Psychiatry* 2011;72:34

16. Wass C. *BMC Med*, 2011;9:40.

17. Sansone RA. *Innov Clin Neurosci* 2011;8:10–14.

18. Berk M. *Biol Psychiatry* 2008;64:361–368.

19. Whigham LD. *Am J Clin Nutr* 2007;85:1203–1211.

20. Nahas R. *Can Fam Physician* 2009;55:591–596.

21. Towheed TE. *J Rheumatol* 2007;34:1787–1790.

22. Ito MK. *Am J Manag Care* 2002; 8(12 Suppl):S315–S322.

23. Bays HE.? *Int J Clin Pract* 2009;63:151–159.

24. Hasegawa T. *Aliment Pharmacol Ther* 2001;15:1667–1672.

25. Yakaryilmaz F. *Intern Med J* 2007;37:229–235.

that mental disorders are associated with deficiencies or excesses of specific neurochemicals is inadequate[45] (e.g., proof is lacking for some of the major theories of mental illness, such as the monoamine hypothesis of depression[46] and the dopamine hypothesis of schizophrenia[47]).

Given the inherent problems with the disease-centered model of drug action, the obvious question arises: "What then do MPDs actually do?" Simply put, all MPDs are psychoactive and in being psychoactive they ". . . induce complex, varied, often unpredictable physical and mental states that patients typically experience as global, rather than distinct therapeutic effects and side effects."[44] Patients should be told that these drug-induced altered states might be useful, for some altered states might suppress unwanted manifestations of mental disorders; however, alternatively, these altered states might be harmful, for some altered states might induce unwanted or even unexpected physical and/or mental manifestations.[44,46] In reality, the alteration in mental state induced by MPDs is not natural, and the ability of MPDs to favorably impact symptoms of mental distress is largely unpredictable. Notwithstanding their potential benefit, it is not entirely clear if "therapeutic" drug effects are merely the result of a poorly understood science of drug-induced psychological toxicity.[48]

To further illustrate this, I offer an excerpt from psychiatrist Peter Breggin's book, *Brain Disabling Treatments in Psychiatry* (2008):

> The brain does not welcome psychiatric medications as nutrients. Instead, the brain reacts against them as toxic agents and attempts to overcome their disruptive impact. For example, when Prozac induces an excess of serotonin in the synaptic cleft, the brain compensates by reducing the output of serotonin at the nerve endings, by reducing the number of receptors in the synapse that can receive the serotonin, and by increasing the capacity of the transport system to remove serotonin from the synapse. Similarly, when antipsychotic drugs such as Risperdal, Zyprexa, or Haldol reduce reactivity in the dopaminergic system, the brain compensates, producing hyperactivity in the same system by increasing the number and sensitivity of

dopamine receptors. All of these compensatory reactions create new abnormalities in brain function, sometimes causing irreversible disorders, such as antipsychotic drug-induced tardive dyskinesia.[49]

MPDs are xenobiotic substances that do not support the brain; instead, they artificially affect biochemical and physiological processes within the human organism, creating a chemical imbalance or an abnormal brain state with the hope that this "altered" state affords patients with fewer disabling psychiatric symptoms and improved functionality.

MPDs Do Not Improve Therapeutic Outcomes Among Patients with Mental Disorders

When reviewing studies on all the major classes of psychotropic medication, many short-term studies (around 12 weeks or less) document beneficial responses from MPDs. However, none of this data sufficiently proves that MPDs help patients to live more fulfilling lives in the long-run. The results of these studies merely show that the psychoactive effects of MPDs moderate symptoms as per changes on specific clinical-rating scales.[44] Any psychoactive substance will moderate symptoms, but rarely do the clinical trials used to evaluate MPDs determine if these favorable changes in clinical-rating scales equate to an improved quality and quantity of life.

For example, MPDs with chemical properties that presumably "calm" an overexcited nervous system can moderate disturbances of agitation and overarousal, and therefore the clinical-rating scale will likewise demonstrate benefit. Does this benefit, however, really translate into better long-term functionality? In their chapter on the risks and benefits of psychiatric drugs, Sparks, Cohen, and Antonuccio stated: "Without longer follow-up, conclusions about effectiveness in real life cannot be determined [and the] initial effects of drug treatment must be weighed in terms of long-term tolerability and impact beyond symptom remission."[50]

When investigators have evaluated MPDs over periods of time longer than 12 weeks, many such trials have yielded negative results suggesting that tolerability and symptom remission do not sustain over time. A well-known example of this is the 6-

year $35 million National Institutes of Mental Health (NIMH)-funded study (i.e., Sequenced Treatment Alternatives to Relieve Depression, or STAR*D) that had data on almost 2,900 depressed participants (ages 18–75) and evaluated the impact of MPD augmentation or switching strategies, that is, either a different selective serotonin reuptake inhibitor (SSRI) or cognitive behavior therapy when a traditional regimen of a single SSRI had failed.[51] This study was unblinded and non-placebo-controlled and was designed to be naturalistic and emulate conditions experienced in everyday clinical practice. Among the participants who received the antidepressant citalopram (Celexa) (denoted as Level 1), 28 percent experienced side effects ranging from moderate to intolerable.[52] Among the participants who were augmented or switched (denoted as Level 2), 51 percent experienced side effects ranging from moderate to intolerable.[53] For all levels in this study, 24 percent dropped out due to MPD intolerability.[54] In addition, the 12-month follow-up data on participants who either remitted or responded showed a relapse rate of 58 percent.[55] The other finding from the STAR*D was that the average remission rate was 28 percent and 25 percent for Levels 1 and 2, respectively, and 14 percent and 13 percent for the remaining levels. None of these studies demonstrate "real" effectiveness since the typical placebo response in antidepressant trials is 30 percent.[58]

With respect to antipsychotic medication, the data on long-term outcomes is also disappointing. Many patients with either schizophrenia or bipolar disorder are often told that they will need antipsychotic medication for life; otherwise, their functionality will be severely impaired. These vulnerable patients are often pressured into feeling that they can never be normal unless they take medication for the duration of their life. In the NIMH-funded Clinical Antipsychotic Trials of Intervention Effectiveness (CATIE), the primary outcome measure was stoppage of MPD for any reason.[57] The reasoning for this primary outcome is that MPD compliance is very much associated with the patient's experience of side effects. Some 1,400 participants across 57 U.S. sites were included in this triple-blind study, meaning the clinicians, raters, and patients were unaware of

which MPD the patients were taking. In CATIE there was no placebo group, which allowed clinicians to decide upon therapeutic dosages, as well as including additional MPDs (excluding antipsychotic medication) if necessary. This was a real-world study since CATIE compared how well the second-generation antipsychotic medications compared to one another, and how well they compared to a first-generation antipsychotic medication such as perphenazine (Trilafon).

The results from CATIE showed that for the majority of patients, antipsychotic medication does not improve quality of life and induces objectionable side effects. Some 74 percent of CATIE patients stopped their MPD before 18 months due to a lack of efficacy and intolerable side effects (1,061 of the 1,432 patients who received at least one dose).[57] The investigators of this report also noted that this drop-out rate is similar to drop-out rates from prior antipsychotic drug trials.[57] For one-third of CATIE patients, psychosocial functioning improved only modestly at 12 months.[58] The range of moderate to adverse events was 42–69 percent, the hospitalization rates ranged from 11–20 percent, and weight gain of more than 7 percent happened in 14–36 percent of patients.[59] The CATIE investigators concluded that the superiority for SGAs was greatly overstated, and that aggressive marketing contributed to a false sense of effectiveness despite the absence of solid empirical evidence.[60]

With respect to the treatment of bipolar disorder, data once again from the NIMH does little to confirm long-term efficacy. In the NIMH-funded study, Systematic Treatment Enhancement Program for Bipolar Disorder (STEP-BD), the effectiveness of SGAs and anticonvulsants were determined among patients diagnosed with bipolar disorder.[61] This hybridized study collected longitudinal data from patients transitioning from naturalistic studies and randomized clinical trials. In one report encompassing data covering 24 months of the STEP-BD study, only 30 percent of patients experienced no recurrences of symptoms.[62] From 858 patients, some 416 (48.5 percent) experienced recurrences during two years of follow-up, with 298 (34.7 percent) developing depressive episodes compared to 118 (13.8 percent) that developed manic, hypomanic, or mixed episodes.[62] In another report on STEP-BD, the recovery rate was rather abysmal and determined to be just under 15 percent.[63] In another analysis that evaluated bipolar patients during periods of sustained and substantial remission, the degree of functional impairment as determined by the Work and Social Adjustment Scale was deemed to be significant.[64]

Thus, from trials funded by the NIMH, it can be seen that the long-term effectiveness of MPDs is significantly lacking. If we think even more broadly about the implications of MPD treatment, the work of Whitaker, as reported in a journal publication[45] and a book,[65] reveals even more disturbing long-term trends from MPD treatment. Whitaker reasoned that there has been a significant statistical rise in the percentage of Americans disabled by mental illness since 1955, which coincidentally began with the introduction of the antipsychotic chlorpromazine (Thorazine). Whitaker cites statistics from the U.S. Department of Health and Human Services, which has collected "patient care episodes" (i.e., an estimate of the number of people treated annually for mental illness) over the course of many decades. Whitaker's research focused on the years 1955–2000 and showed a nearly fourfold per-capita increase in patient care episodes (1,028 episodes per 100,000 population in 1955 compared to 3,806 per 100,000 population in 2000). He also reviewed data pertaining to the number of mentally ill people who were disabled or required some sort of disability payment (i.e., patients having received a disability payment from the Social Security Disability Insurance or the Supplemental Security Income programs). His analysis showed that in 1955 3.38 people per 1,000 population were disabled by mental illness, compared to 2003 in which the disability rate had risen to 19.69 people per 1,000 population.

The overarching problem, according to Whitaker, is that this rise in people being treated for mental illness, as well as those disabled by it, have markedly increased primarily as a result of the increased use of MPDs. It is no coincidence that there was a fortyfold increase in the combined sales of antidepressants and antipsychotics during this time period (from an estimated $500 million in 1986 to almost $20 billion in 2004). Additionally, Whitaker noted a substantive increase in roughly 2.4 million Americans designated as disabled from 1987 to 2003 (a marked acceleration beginning with the introduction of Prozac and other drugs), yielding some 410 people each day in the United States being designated as being "disabled" by their mental illness (i.e., requiring some form of social assistance).

MPDs Are Associated with Physiological Dependence, Withdrawal Symptoms, and Long-Term Harm

Pharmacological dependence is an expected and biological adaptation of the body becoming habituated to the presence of a psychotropic drug.[66] The mechanisms of withdrawal (i.e., overcoming pharmacological dependence) involve both "pharmacodynamic stress" and psychological reactions.[1] Since psychotropic drugs can induce unpredictable global reactions when used properly,[44,46] there are no reliable ways to predict how patients will overcome pharmacological dependence once their psychotropic drugs are tapered and eventually withdrawn. Every patient's withdrawal process is unique as is their susceptibility to developing withdrawal side effects.[67]

Moncrieff has identified and summarized the data pertaining to several important adverse outcomes caused by MPD withdrawal or reduction, and noted the following possibilities: 1) somatic discontinuation syndromes (also known as withdrawal or rebound reactions); 2) rapid onset psychosis (rebound psychosis, supersensitivity psychosis); and 3) psychological reaction and misattribution.[1] Somatic discontinuation syndromes refer to psychological and behavioral symptoms (e.g., anxiety, restlessness, and insomnia) resulting from withdrawal that might be misinterpreted as early distress signals of relapse. These problems may be associated with MPD withdrawal and patients can experience them to such a heightened degree that coming off their MPDs might be impossible. As such, patients might not be able to overcome their pharmacological dependence and end up taking MPDs for the duration of their lives.

A rapid-onset psychosis results shortly after discontinuing antipsychotic (i.e., neuroleptic) medication. This is believed to be an iatrogenic problem since patients without a psychiatric history have also reported this phenomenon. The onset is usually in a few days following discontinuation (e.g., resulting from clozapine due to its short half-life) and results in withdrawal reactions including auditory hallucinations, paranoid delusions, hostility, and sometimes visual hallucinations, grandiosity, and elation. With antipsychotic medications having longer half-lives, a withdrawal psychosis might be difficult to identify. Patients are normally managed as though their distress signals indicate a naturally occurring relapse instead of resulting from MPD withdrawal.

Another major adverse outcome facing patients on MPDs is that withdrawal symptoms might arise due to their psychological concerns or worries about discontinuing or reducing medication dosage. In other words, their expectations of psychiatric illness induce psychiatric illness. Since patients are normally told that they need their medications for life—they often believe this. If patients' doctors and other carers reinforce this notion, patients may become psychologically vulnerable to any decrease or stoppage of MPDs. Their psychological reactions can arise from fear and, if so, their ensuing clinical reactions to lowering or stopping their MPDs may be misattributed to having relapsed.

Above all, the regular use of MPDs produces a clinical syndrome akin to being addicted to illicit drugs such as cocaine and amphetamines. If we consider addiction to be a "state of being enslaved to a habit or practice or to something psychological or physically habit-forming, as narcotics, to such an extent that its cessation causes severe trauma" (dictionary.reference.com/browse/addiction), then there are few differences in the addictive process between that which results from illicit drug use and that which results from MPDs. In both instances, individuals become enslaved to what they are regularly consuming, they experience both physical (physiological) and psychological dependence and suffer tremendously when trying to stop. Most authorities on addiction now speak of this as a "brain disorder." If we are honest about what MPDs do to the brain, then understanding the addiction imposed by these drugs as

"There have been no deaths ever from niacin. The LD 50 (the dosage that would kill half of those taking it) for dogs is 6,000 milligrams per kilogram body weight. That is equivalent to half a pound of niacin per day for a human. No human takes 225,000 mg of niacin a day. They would be nauseous long before reaching a harmful dose. The top niacin dose ever was a 16-year-old severely schizophrenic girl who, in a suicide attempt, took 120 tablets (500 mg each) in one day. That is 60,000 mg of niacin. The 'voices' she had been hearing were gone immediately. She then took 3,000 mg a day to maintain wellness." — ABRAM HOFFER

resulting from a medication-induced brain disorder seems to be an appropriate way to understand the significance of the harm they can produce among increasing numbers of patients, especially patients who take MPDs chronically.

From a global perspective, prescription drugs result in far more deaths than vitamins, and likely other orthomolecules as well. In a meta-analysis of hospitalized patients, 106,000 patients had fatal adverse drug reactions (ADRs), making medications between the fourth and sixth leading cause of death in the United States in 1994.[68] Another report estimates that deaths due to ADRs from medications to be about 100,000 annually in the United States.[69] If we estimate the annual death rate due to medications in the United States from 1983 to 2011, then 2.8 million deaths can be attributed to medications compared to only 13 from vitamins during the same time period. The deaths attributed to other orthomolecules, such as amino acids, minerals, and essential fatty acids, would also be substantially lower than deaths attributed to medications.

If we look more specifically at MPD use and death (apart from medication use in general), a more devastating picture emerges about their potential for harm. While numerous studies have shown MPDs to be associated with increased disability (i.e., a reduced health span) due to many objectionable side effects (e.g., cardiometabolic risks associated with antidepressant and antipsychotic drugs[70]), the published literature is replete with studies showing significant long-term harm resulting from their use. Only several studies will be cited here to highlight the enormity of this problem. The use of neuroleptics (i.e., both the first- and second-generation antipsychotic medications) among schizophrenic patients (apart from lifestyle or other factors) when used alone or in combination with other medications is associated with reduced life spans.[71-74] Benzodiazepine medication is also associated with increased mortality among schizophrenic patients.[75] These results are even more disturbing since it is well-established that schizophrenic patients have a 10- to 25-year reduction in life expectancy compared to the general population.[76]

A short time ago I mentioned that the chronic use of MPDs induce a "brain disorder" in the context of addiction. Breggin has recently highlighted this issue more substantially in his article titled, "Psychiatric drug-induced chronic brain impairment: implications for long-term treatment with psychiatric medications."[77] Breggin mentions how all MPDs produce effects related to their specific mechanisms of action, but over time these initial specific effects change as the brain and body react to them, eventually causing more extensive changes to take place within the brain and in mental functioning. In proving his hypothesis, Breggin highlights the brain damage induced by long-term antipsychotic treatment. He mentions how these drugs shrink (atrophy) the brain, inhibit most mitochondrial enzyme systems, chronically block dopamine neurotransmission (resulting in death to the striatal neurons), and cause tardive dyskinesia with "associated impairment of cognitive and affective functioning." These brain changes, however, are not unique to the antipsychotic medications since all classes of MPDs, according to Breggin's research, cause mental dysfunction and atrophy of the brain following long-term exposure.

He asserts that the outcome of being chronically exposed to MPDs (especially, increasing doses over time) results in chronic brain impairment (CBI), which is very similar clinically to the effects arising from a closed-head injury due to trauma. He outlines the four major "symptom complexes" associated with CBI that significantly reduce quality of life, which include: 1) cognitive dysfunctions (short-term memory dysfunction, impaired ability to learn new material, inattention, and concentration problems); 2) apathy or loss of energy and vitality (indifference, fatigue, loss of creativity, lack of empathy, and loss of

TABLE 1. ORTHOMOLECULAR PSYCHIATRIC TREATMENT (OPT) VERSUS MAINSTREAM PSYCHIATRIC DRUGS (MPDS)	
OPT	**MPDS**
Orthomolecules are naturally occurring in the body and brain.	Xenobiotics are foreign to the body and brain.
OPT supports the proper functioning of the brain (and other tissues of the body) without disrupting biochemical and physiological processes resulting in improved or unchanged psychological function.	MPDs artificially alter the functioning of the brain (and other tissues of the body) and produce unpredictable brain-states that might help or harm psychological function.
Short-term intervention trials show efficacy.	Short-term intervention trials show efficacy.
Quality long-term trials are lacking, but there is a high probability that OPT will sustain both mental and physical health long-term.	Quality long-term trials lack efficacy, even though long-term use is associated with significant morbidity (i.e., decreased health span) and increased mortality (i.e., early death).
OPT is not associated with physiological dependence, withdrawal symptoms, and long-term harm.	MPDs are associated with physiological dependence, withdrawal symptoms, and long-term harm.

spontaneity); 3) emotional worsening or "affective dysregulation" (loss of empathy, heightened impatience, irritability, anger, frequent mood changes with depression and anxiety) with a gradual onset such that, over time, other people attribute these changes inappropriately to aging, stress, or to the mental illness itself; and 4) anosognosia (a lack of self-awareness of these symptoms of brain dysfunction).

Even though Breggin does mention several confounding factors that can cause or intensify CBI, his clinical experience has shown that nearly all patients on MPDs for many years develop some symptoms of CBI, with the most noticeable being short-term memory dysfunction and apathy. The apathy, according to Breggin, manifests as "a loss of interest in daily activities, hobbies, creative endeavors, and sometimes family and friends." The only way to recover from CBI is to slowly taper down and eventually stop taking MPDs. Breggin notes that recovery from CBI usually begins at the onset of the withdrawal process, but some patients unfortunately experience withdrawal years after stopping medication. Young children and teenagers can fully recover, even if they had been taking MPDs for years. By comparison, adults might experience persistent CBI problems, typically with memory, attention, and/or concentration, even though their lives will be much more fulfilling after stopping MPDs.

To enable patients to safely withdraw from MPDs, Breggin explains that a "person-centered" approach works best. This therapeutic process allows patients to be in charge of the withdrawal process and only proceed at a pace they are comfortable with. Also, providing psychotherapy during this process, but not insight therapy (e.g., working through childhood trauma), as well as encouraging patients to resume previous pleasurable hobbies (i.e., physical and/or mental activities) that they had neglected due to CBI, can significantly support the process of recovery.

■ CONCLUSION

The scope of harm induced by MPDs is immense. It is conceivable that psychiatrists risk substantial liability if they fail to obtain informed consent, if they do not fully inform their patients of the risks associated with MPD treatment, or if they overstate benefits.[78] Even if there are questions about my interpretation of this data or concerns about my personal biases, we should still be very concerned and reevaluate the current practice of placing patients on MPDs for long periods. Given the significant increase in the practice of MPD polypharmacy, and the fact that most combinations of MPDs are not supported by clinical trials and have unproven efficacy,[79] we need to seriously

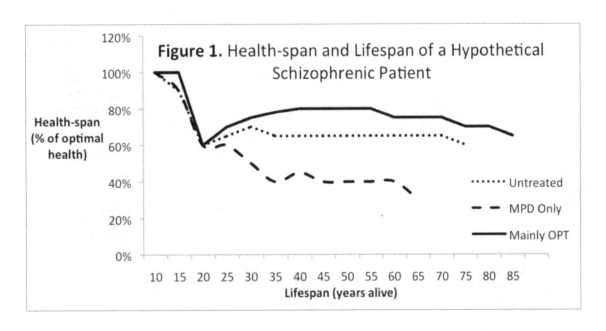

Figure 1. Health-span and Lifespan of a Hypothetical Schizophrenic Patient

consider the implications to the health span and life span of patients when MPD treatment is the only option provided. Orthomolecular psychiatric treatment is a rational and reasonable way to assist patients with mental disorders (see Table 1).

On the prior page, Figure 1 offers a hypothetical example of how a schizophrenic patient's future might be altered from either no treatment, MPD only, or mainly OPT. In all situations this patient's initial psychotic episode occurred around the age of 20. Following that episode, the likely differences in treatment outcomes are substantial, assuming the information contained in this paper is accurate.

When patients are given mainstream psychiatric drugs as a means to further their stability, the addition of orthomolecular psychiatric treatment could safely and easily integrate with standard treatment and allow carefully monitored patients to gradually reduce their medication while remaining mentally stable and physically healthy. We need a mental health system that is life-affirming and not life-impeding. We encourage open-minded and conscientious clinicians to review the extensive literature that documents six decades of research, development, progress, and success of orthomolecular medicine. Hopefully this will encourage mental health professionals to recognize and embrace the merits of orthomolecular psychiatric treatment.

REFERENCES

1. Moncrieff J. Why is it so difficult to stop psychiatric drug treatment? It may be nothing to do with the original problem. *Med Hypotheses* 2006;67:517–523.

2. Pauling L. Orthomolecular psychiatry: varying the concentrations of substances normally present in the human body may control mental disease. *Science* 1968;160:265–271.

3. Pauling L, Wyatt RJ, Klein DF, et al. On the orthomolecular environment of the mind: orthomolecular theory. *Am J Psychiatry* 1974;131:1251–1267.

4. Kaplan BJ, Crawford SG, Field CJ, et al. Vitamins, minerals, and mood. *Psychol Bull* 2007;133:747–760.

5. Ames BN, Elson-Schwab I, Silver EA. High-dose vitamin therapy stimulates variant enzymes with decreased coenzyme binding (increased Km): relevance to genetic diseases and polymorphisms. *Am J Clin Nutr* 2002;75:616–658.

6. van Tiggelen CJM, Peperkamp JPC, Tertoolen JFW. Vitamin B12 levels of cerebrospinal fluid in patients with organic mental disorders. *J Orthomolecular Psych* 1983;12:305–311.

7. van Tiggelen CJM, Peperkamp JPC, Tertoolen JFW. Assessment of vitamin B12 status in CSF. *Am J Psychiatry* 1984;141: 136–137.

8. Walsh R. Lifestyle and mental health. *Am Psychol* 2011;66:579–592.

9. Tsaluchidu S, Cocchi M, Tonello L, et al. Fatty acids and oxidative stress in psychiatric disorders. *BMC Psychiatry*, 2008;8 Suppl 1:S5.

10. Moss M: Drugs as anti-nutrients. *J Nutr Environ Med*, 2007;16:149–166.

11. Fidabza F. Biochemical assessment. In: *Encyclopedia of Human Nutrition* edited by MJ Sadler, JJ Strain, and B Caballero B. San Diego, CA: Academic Press, 1999;1364–1373.

12. Werbach MR. *Foundations of Nutritional Medicine.* Tarzana, CA: Third Line Press, Inc. 1997;1–78.

13, Werbach MR. *Nutritional Influences on Mental Illness.* Tarzana, CA: Third Line Press, Inc. 1991;335–343.

14. Rudin DO. The major psychoses and neuroses as omega-3 essential faty acid deficiency syndrome: substrate pellagra. *Biol Psychiatry* 1981;16:837–850.

15. Abdullah M, Vishwanath S, Elbalkhi A, et al. Mitochondrial myopathy presenting as fibromyalgia: a case report. *J Med Case Rep* 2012;6(1):55.

16. Kraft BD, Westman EC. Schizophrenia, gluten, and low-carbohydrate, ketogenic diets: a case report and review of the literature. *Nutr Metab (Lond)* 2009;6:10.

17. Dogan M, Ariyuca S, Peker E, et al. Psychotic disorder, hypertension and seizures associated with vitamin B12 deficiency: a case report. *Hum Exp Toxicol* 2012;31:410–413.

18. Lakhan SE, Vieira KF. Nutritional therapies for mental disorders. *Nutr J* 2008;7:2.

19. Lakhan SE, Vieira KF. Nutritional and herbal supplements for anxiety and anxiety-related disorders: systematic review. *Nutr J* 2010;9:42.

20. Pennington VM. Enhancement of psychotropic drugs by a vitamin supplement. *Psychosomatics* 1966;7:115–120.

21. McLeod MN, Gaynes BN, Golden RN. Chromium potentiation of antidepressant pharmacotherapy for dysthymic disorder in 5 patients. *J Clin Psychiatry* 1999;60:237–240.

22. Bell IR, Edman JS, Morrow FD, et al. Brief communication. Vitamin B1, B2, and B6 augmentation of tricyclic antidepressant treatment in geriatric depression with cognitive impairment. *J Am Coll Nutr* 1992;11:159–163.

23. Godfrey PS, Toone BK, Carney MW, et al. Enhancement of recovery from psychiatric illness by methylfolate. *Lancet,* 1990;336:392–395.

24. Coppen A, Bailey J. Enhancement of the antidepressant action of fluoxetine by folic acid: a randomised, placebo controlled trial. *J Affect Disord* 2000;60:121–130.

25. Lafleur DL, Pittenger C, Kelmendi B, et al. N-acetylcysteine augmentation in serotonin reuptake inhibitor refractory obsessive-compulsive disorder. *Psychopharmacology (Berl)*, 2006;184: 254–256.

26. Resler G, Lavie R, Campos J, et al. Effect of folic acid combined with fluoxetine in patients with major depression on plasma homocysteine and vitamin B12, and serotonin levels in lymphocytes. *Neuroimmunomodulation* 2008;15:145–152.

27. Kjaergaard M, Waterloo K, Wang CE, et al. Effect of vitamin D supplement on depression scores in people with low levels of serum 25 hydroxyvitamin D: nested case-control study and randomised clinical trial. *Br J Psychiatry* 2012;201:360–368.

28. Vieth R, Kimball S, Hu A, Walfish PG. Randomized comparison of the effects of the vitamin D3 adequate intake versus 100 mcg (4000 IU) per day on biochemical responses and the well-being of patients. *Nutr J* 2004;3:8.

29. Grant WB, Boucher BJ. Requirements for vitamin D across the life span. *Biol Res Nurs* 2011;13:120–133.

30. Goggans FC. A case of mania secondary to vitamin B12 deficiency. *Am J Psychiatry* 1984;141:300–301.

31. Sharma V, Biswas D: Cobalamin deficiency presenting as obsessive compulsive disorder: case report. *Gen Hosp Psychiatry* 2012;34(5):578.e7–8.

32. Tufan AE, Bilici R, Usta G, et al. Mood disorder with mixed, psychotic features due to vitamin B12 deficiency in an adolescent: case report. *Child Adolesc Psychiatry Ment Health* 2012;6(1):25.

33. Winter SL, Boyer JL. Hepatic toxicity from large doses of vitamin B3 (nicotinamide). *N Engl J Med* 1973;289:1180–1182.

34. Phillips WE, Mills JH, Charbonneau S, et al. Subacute toxicity of pyridoxine hydrochloride in the beagle dog. *Toxicol Appl Pharmacol* 1978;44:323–333.

35. Krinke G, Schaumburg HH, Spencer PS, et al. Pyridoxine megavitaminosis produces degeneration of peripheral sensory neurons(sensory neuronopathy) in the dog. *Neurotoxicology* 1981;2:13–24.

36. Schaumburg H, Kaplan J, Windebank A, et al. Sensory neuropathy from pyridoxine abuse. A new megavitamin syndrome. *N Engl J Med* 1983;309:445–448.

37. Berger AR, Schaumburg HH, Schroeder C, et al. Dose response, coasting, and differential fiber vulnerability in human toxic neuropathy: a prospective study of pyridoxine neurotoxicity. *Neurology* 1992;42:1367–1370.

38. Bender DA. Non-nutritional uses of vitamin B6. *Br J Nutr* 1999;81:7–20.

39. [No authors listed]. Vitamin B6 (pyridoxine and pyridoxal-5-phosphate)–monograph. *Altern Med Rev* 2001;6:87–92.

40. Lerner V, Bergman J, Statsenko N, et al. Vitamin B6 treatment in acute neuroleptic-induced akathisia: a randomized, double-blind, placebo-controlled study. *J Clin Psychiatry* 2004;65:1550–1554.

41. Miodownik C, Lerner V, Statsenko N, et al. Vitamin B6 versus mianserin and placebo in acute neuroleptic-induced akathisia: a randomized, double-blind, controlled study. *Clin Neuropharmacol* 2006;29:68–72.

42. Lerner V, Miodownik C, Kaptsan A, et al. Vitamin B6 treatment for tardive dyskinesia: a randomized, double-blind, placebo-controlled, crossover study. *J Clin Psychiatry* 2007;68:1648–1654.

43. American Association of Poison Control Centers. NPDS Annual Reports. *Retrieved from:* [www.aapcc.org/dnn/NPDS PoisonData/NPDSAnnualReports.aspx].

44. Moncrieff J, Cohen D. How do psychiatric drugs work? *BMJ* 2009;338:1535–1537.

45. Whitaker R. Anatomy of an epidemic: psychiatric drugs and the astonishing rise of mental illness in America. *Ethical Hum Psychol Psychiatry* 2005;7:23–35.

46. Moncrieff J, Cohen D. Do antidepressants cure or create abnormal brain states? *PLoS Med* 2006;3(7):e240.

47. Moncrieff J. A critique of the dopamine hypothesis of schizophrenia and psychosis. *Harv Rev Psychiatry* 2009;17:214–225.

48. Jacobs D, Cohen D. What is really known about the psychological alterations produced by psychiatric drugs? *Int J Risk Safety Med* 1999;12:37–47.

49. Breggin PR: *Brain-disabling treatments in psychiatry.* 2nd edition. New York: Springer Publishing Co, 2008;9.

50. Sparks JA, Duncan BL, Cohen D, et al. Psychiatric drugs and common factors: an evaluation of risks and benefits for clinical practice. In: *The Heart and Soul of Change: Delivering What Works in Therapy* edited by BL Duncan, SD Miller, BE Wampold BE, et al. 2nd ed. Washington, DC: American Psychological Association 2010;199–235.

51. STAR*D Investigators Group (Rush AJ, Fava M, Wisniewski SR, et al): Sequenced treatment alternatives to relieve depression (STAR*D): rationale and design. *Control Clin Trials* 2004;25:119–142.

52. Trivedi MH, Rush AJ, Wisniewski SR, et al. Evaluation of outcomes with citalopram for depression using measurement-based care in STAR*D: implications for clinical practice. *Am J Psychiatry* 2006;163:28–40.

53. Rush AJ, Trivedi MH, Wisniewski SR, et al. Bupropion-SR, sertraline, or venlafaxine-XR after failure of SSRIs for depression. *N Engl J Med* 2006;354:1231–1242.

54. Rush AJ, Trivedi MH, Wisniewski SR, et al. Acute and longer-term outcomes in depressed outpatients requiring one or several treatment steps: a STAR*D report. *Am J Psychiatry* 2006;163:1905–1917.

55. Trivedi MH, Fava M, Wisniewski SR, et al. Medication augmentation after the failure of SSRIs for depression. *N Engl J Med* 2006;354:1243–1252.

56. Thase ME, Jindal RD. Combining psychotherapy and psychopharmacology for treatment of mental disorders. In: *Handbook of Psychotherapy and Behavior Change* edited by MJ Lambert. 5th ed. New York: Wiley, 2004;743–766.

57. Clinical Antipsychotic Trials of Intervention Effectiveness (CATIE) Investigators (Lieberman JA, Stroup TS, McEvoy JP, et al). Effectiveness of antipsychotic drugs in patients with chronic schizophrenia. *N Engl J Med* 2005;353:1209–1223.

58. Swartz MS, Perkins DO, Stroup T, et al. Effects of antipsychotic medications on psychosocial functioning in patients with chronic schizophrenia: findings from the NIMH CATIE study. *Am J Psychiatry* 2007;164:428–436.

59. Stroup TS, Lieberman JA, McEvoy JP, et al. Effectiveness of olanzapine, quetiapine, and risperidone in patients with chronic schizophrenia after discontinuing perphenazine: a CATIE study. *Am J Psychiatry* 2007;164:415–427.

60. Lieberman JA: Comparative effectiveness of antipsychotic drugs. A commentary on: Cost Utility Of The Latest Antipsychotic Drugs In Schizophrenia Study (CUtLASS 1) and Clinical Antipsychotic Trials Of Intervention Effectiveness (CATIE). *Arch Gen Psychiatry* 2006;63:1069–1072.

61. Sachs GS, Thase ME, Otto MW, et al. Rationale, design, and methods of the systematic treatment enhancement program for bipolar disorder (STEP-BD). *Biol Psychiatry* 2003;53: 1028–1042.

62. Perlis RH, Ostacher MJ, Patel JK, et al. Predictors of recurrence in bipolar disorder: primary outcomes from the Systematic Treatment Enhancement Program for Bipolar Disorder (STEP-BD). *Am J Psychiatry* 2006;163:217–224.

63. Nierenberg AA, Ostacher MJ, Calabrese JR, et al. Treatment-resistant bipolar depression: a STEP-BD equipoise randomized effectiveness trial of antidepressant augmentation with lamotrigine, inositol, or risperidone. *Am J Psychiatry* 2006;163: 210–216.

64. Fagiolini A, Kupfer DJ, Masalehdan A, et al. Functional impairment in the remission phase of bipolar disorder. *Bipolar Disord,* 2005;7:281–285.

65. Whitaker R: *Anatomy of an Epidemic: Magic Bullets, Psychiatric Drugs, and the Astonishing Rise of Mental Illness in America.* New York: Broadway Paperbacks, 2010.

66. O'Brien CP. Benzodiazepine use, abuse, and dependence. *J Clin Psychiatry* 2005;66(Suppl 2):28–33.

67. Read J: *Coping with Coming Off: Mind's Research into the Experiences of People Trying to Come Off Psychiatric Drugs.* London, UK: Mind Publications, 2005.

68. Lazarou J, Pomeranz BH, Corey PN. Incidence of adverse drug reactions in hospitalized patients: a meta-analysis of prospective studies. *JAMA* 1998;279:1200–1205.

69. Shastry BS. Pharmacogenetics and the concept of individualized medicine. *Pharmacogenomics J* 2006;6:16–21.

70. Vieweg WVR, Hasnain M, Wood MA, et al. Cardiometabolic risks of antidepressant and antipsychotic drugs, Part 2. *Psychiatr Times* 2011(May):68–71.

71. Morgan MG, Scully PJ, Youssef HA, et al. Prospective analysis of premature mortality in schizophrenia in relation to health service engagement: a 7.5-year study within an epidemiologically complete, homogeneous population in rural Ireland. *Psychiatry Res* 2003;117:127–135.

72. Straus SM, Bleumink GS, Dieleman JP, et al. Antipsychotics and the risk of sudden cardiac death. *Arch Intern Med* 2004;164:1293–1297.

73. Joukamaa M, Heliövaara M, Knekt P, et al. Schizophrenia, neuroleptic medication and mortality. *Br J Psychiatry* 2006;188: 122–127.

74. Tenback D, Pijl B, Smeets H, et al. All-cause mortality and medication risk factors in schizophrenia: a prospective cohort study. *J Clin Psychopharmacol* 2012;32:31–35.

75. Tiihonen J, Suokas JT, Suvisaari JM, et al. Polypharmacy with antipsychotics, antidepressants, or benzodiazepines and mortality in schizophrenia. *Arch Gen Psychiatry* 2012;69:476–483.

76. Laursen TM, Munk-Olsen T, Vestergaard M. Life expectancy and cardiovascular mortality in persons with schizophrenia. *Curr Opin Psychiatry* 2012;25:83–88.

77. Breggin PR. Psychiatric drug-induced Chronic Brain Impairment (CBI): implications for long-term treatment with psychiatric medication. *Int J Risk Saf Med* 2011;23:193–200.

78. Gottstein JB: Psychiatrists' failure to inform: is there substantial financial exposure? *Ethical Hum Psychol Psychiatry* 2007;9:117–125.

79. Olfson M, Mojtabai R. National trends in psychotropic medication polypharmacy in office-based psychiatry. *Arch Gen Psychiatry* 2010;67:26–36.

CONTROLLED FASTING TREATMENT FOR SCHIZOPHRENIA
by Allan Cott, MD

The application of various modifications of fasting for its therapeutic value has been well documented during many different periods of our civilization. In the earliest eras of recorded civilization, humans found in fasting not only a method of treatment and prevention of some diseases but also a potent weapon for self-discipline and moral education. For this reason, the fast became an integral part of many religious doctrines and occupied the thinking of physicians and philosophers of ancient Greek, Tibetan, Indian, and Middle Eastern cultures.

Fasting vs. Starving

Fasting is not starving, and the synonymous use of the two indicates a lack of understanding of the principles of the fast or its meaning. The word "starvation" is derived from the Old English *sterofan*, a form of the Teutonic verb *sterb*, meaning to die. The word "fast" means to abstain from food. In modern usage, starvation is used to designate death from lack of food. Whenever fasting is mentioned to the average person and even to many professionals, the immediate response is to think of the dire consequences of going without food for even a few days. If "fasting" is used interchangeably with "starvation," the inevitable end result is conceived as death. Yet members of the professions and the press are guilty of confusing the use of the two terms and help to perpetuate the fear of fasting.

Experience with the fast makes the distinction between fasting and starvation quite simple and clear—as long as hunger is absent, one is fasting. When hunger returns, if one continues to abstain from food, he is starving. Only in this latter condition can death be the inevitable result. The confusion was compounded by the publication of the results of a study that was reported in *Scientific American* titled "The Physiology of Starvation."[1] It was described as a study to determine how the human body adapts to prolonged starvation, yet stated that their studies of fasting subjects indicated how best to utilize food when food is scarce and also how protein and calorie requirements are related. The article cites examples of "recent tests of total fasting" by obese individuals who have gone without food for as long as eight months. There are no recorded cases of patients treated by fasting in whom appetite did not spontaneously return within the usual 25-to-35-day period. Only occasionally does the period extend 40 to 42 days.

Starvation begins when one continues to abstain from food beyond the time when appetite returns. Throughout the article, the authors freely interchange "fast" for "starvation" when they report "fasts" that lasted from 210 to 249 days. The most misleading and frightening aspect of the article is a photo showing five "semi-starved volunteer subjects," resting in the sun, and the caption explains that their fast was only partial. There cannot be a partial fast since hunger does not cease during partial feeding—it ceases during a complete fast when only water is taken daily and then returns spontaneously. The subjects indeed resemble emaciated concentration camp victims who endured similar conditions of "partial feeding." Fasting patients never appear ill or emaciated. Their skin color becomes healthy and ruddy, muscle tone improves remarkably, especially in those patients who were sedentary, since three hours of exercise daily is a prerequisite throughout the period of fasting.

The authors of the article ask themselves a question, "Why is it that although a person can be stricken with this disease (kwashiorkor) when he or she eats a little food, it never shows up in total starvation when the person gets no protein intake at all?" Again, it is evident that they have substituted total starvation for total fast, since the answer to their question is obvious. If someone continues to eat small, insufficient amounts of food daily, the person does not get the benefits of the biochemical changes that take place during the

From the *J Orthomolecular Psychiatry* 1974;3(4):301–311.

fast. The edema that occurs in the victims of famine is never seen in fasting patients. The authors end their article with statistics compiled by Dr. Garfield Duncan of the University of Pennsylvania School of Medicine who fasted more than 1,300 obese patients without a fatality. Dr. Duncan limited the fasting period from 10 to 14 days with repeat fasts at varying intervals. Professor Yuri Serge Nikolayev, director of the Fasting Treatment Unit of Moscow Psychiatric Institute, has fasted many thousands of mentally ill patients for 25 to 30 days without fatalities.

Fasting as a Therapeutic Modality

It is only since the middle of the 19th century that investigation of fasting as a therapeutic modality was removed from the lore of folk medicine and became the principal method of treatment in clinics and sanatoriums in Switzerland, France, Germany, and to a lesser extent in the United States. Since then, the fasting experience has been the treatment of choice for many thousands of physically ill patients. It is used in internal medicine with excellent results in the treatment of metabolic disorders, allergic diseases, skin disorders, arthritis, ulcerative colitis, and cardiovascular disorders.

Fasting was first used 25 years ago as a treatment for mentally ill patients by Professor Nikolayev at the Moscow Psychiatric Institute. His experience now extends to over 6,000 patients, and the reported results are unusually encouraging with those patients who have failed to improve on all other treatment regimens. With the ever-increasing list of psychopharmacological drugs used for their psychotropic activity, there has concomitantly arisen an increasing number of patients resistant to those drugs. Many patients exhibit toxic and allergic complications during pharmacotherapy. For these patients, fasting treatment is a most valuable and potent alternative to decompensation and deterioration.

My experience with the use of fasting for the treatment of mentally ill patients began in 1970 with an invitation from Professor Nikolayev to come to the institute to observe his Therapeutic Fasting Unit and to discuss my work in orthomolecular treatment. The treatment incorporates the knowledge gained during 28 years of research and clinical experience by Professor Nikolayev and his staff. The treatment is conducted in an 80-bed unit in the Moscow Psychiatric Institute, a 3,000-bed psychiatric research center with a staff of 500 physicians.[2]

The fast consists of total abstinence from food for 25 to 30 days. The large majority of patients request voluntary admission to the unit. A small percentage of the patient population is transferred in from other units when all other conventional treatments have failed to produce improvement. All patients must agree to adhere to the required routine of the treatment and may leave the treatment on request. If the patient voluntarily breaks the fast, the treatment is ended. Hunger diminishes greatly by the end of the 2nd or 3rd day, and appetite is no longer felt by the 5th day. Throughout the fasting period the patients receive as much water as they desire but they must take a minimum of 1 liter (34 ounces) each day. They adhere to a regimen that includes outdoor walks and other exercise, breathing exercises, afternoon nap if desired, hydrotherapy procedures (baths and showers), daily cleansing enemas, and general massage. A minimum of three hours of exercise is required, but the patient may have two periods of exercise consisting of one and a half hours each.

Patients lose between 15 and 20 percent of their total body weight on a 30-day fast, but their clinical appearance is not that of a person who is starving. Their skin color is good and muscle and skin tone is healthy. The patients do not express any longing or desire for food. Because their prior experiences with treatment have been that of little or no improvement with frequent relapses, many patients request that their fasting period be extended to ensure the permanence of their improved state. When patients are discharged from hospital, they are advised to take prophylactic fasts of three to five days each month but not to exceed a total of 10 days in the first three months. After this period, three-to-five-day fasts (not to exceed 10 days in any month) are recommended. Fasting is terminated when the patient's appetite is restored, his tongue becomes clean, and his symptoms are alleviated. When feeding is begun, the patient remains in the hospital for the number of days equal to the length of the fast. Feeding is begun with a salt-free fruit, vegetable, and milk diet. The amount of food and its caloric value are gradually increased. Meat, eggs, and fish are excluded from the diet. Bread is not taken until the 6th or 7th day.

The treatment has been found to be effective in more than 70 percent of cases of schizophrenia of many years' duration. Forty-seven percent of patients followed for a period of six years maintained their improvement. Those patients who resume eating a full diet and break the diet prescribed relapse. The maximum effects of the treatment are seen two or three months after the recovery period is started and the diet followed closely.

Paranoid types do very well during the fast, but their improvement diminishes after feeding begins. I observed many patients who suffered from a form of schizophrenia called dysmorphobia, which is characterized by a fear of the escape of offending gases and odors from the body. The patient is convinced that everyone near him can hear the sounds and smell the odors. The syndrome generally includes delusions of cosmetic ugliness, small stature, and a variety of similar complaints. The resulting effect on behavior is similar to that of patients suffering from other forms of paranoid illness: fear of leaving his room and mingling with other people, fear that people are repelled by him, and then finding corroboration for this in his misperception of the ordinary changes in the facial expressions of people he passes in the street or on buses or trains. The results in treatment of these cases had in the past been extremely poor, but when treated with fasting the results are very good. The other types of schizophrenia do well throughout the fasting and recovery period. The manic phase of the manic-depressive illness is brought under control within five to seven days on the fast. Psychotropic drugs and antidepressants are used when necessary in the beginning of the fast.

Six Stages of Treatment

According to the clinical and laboratory data gathered from tests of secretory and vascular reflexes, food-conditioned reflex leukocytosis, electroencephalography (EEG), and other measurements, patients subjected to treatment pass through six consecutive stages: three of these belong to the fasting period and three to the recovery period.

Fasting Period

• *Stage 1* (days 1–3) of fasting is characterized by an initial hunger excitation. Conditioned and unconditioned secretory and vascular reflexes are sharply accentuated; food-conditioned reflex leukocytosis is considerably increased, and EEG shows intensified electrical activity in all leads with a prevalence of fast rhythms. Thus, excitative processes are increased, and the processes of active inhibition are relatively weakened.

• *Stage 2* (days 2–3 to days 7–12) is a stage of growing acidosis (excess acidity in the body). It is characterized by growing excitability of all systems concerned with nutrition, and by hypoglycemia and general psychomotor depression. The patient loses appetite, his tongue is covered with a white film, and his breath acquires the odor of acetone. Conditioned reflexes cannot be elicited, and unconditioned reflexes are greatly diminished. The EEG demonstrates a decrease in electrical activity, the food-conditioned reflex leukocytosis is sharply reduced. In this phase inhibition prevails over the excitative processes. This reduction in excitation extends to the cortex and produces a stage of inhibition similar to "passive" sleep caused by the blocking of stimuli. Stage 2 ends abruptly in an "acidotic crisis."

• *Stage 3* begins after a period of depression when the physical and mental condition of the patient suddenly improves, he feels stronger and is in a better mood. This marks the beginning of Stage 3; when acidosis diminishes. During this stage the tongue gradually loses its white coating, the odor of acetone disappears, the patient's complexion improves, and psychotic symptoms recede. Unconditioned secretory and vascular reflexes remain diminished, and conditioned reflexes, including reflex leukocytosis, are absent. By the end of Stage 3, however, when the tongue is completely cleared and appetite is restored, secretory and vascular reflexes increase.

Recovery Period

• *Stage 1* of the recovery period (1st, 2nd, 3rd to 5th days) of feeding is characterized by asthenia (weakness) and irritability. Unconditioned secretory and vascular reflexes are irregular, and there exists a pathological lability of the inhibitive processes.

• *Stage 2* of the recovery period is associated with a significant increase of excitability, an accentuation of secretory and vascular reflexes, the appearance of stable conditioned reflexes, and a marked rise of food-conditioned reflex leukocytosis.

• *Stage 3* is a stage of normalization. It is characterized by a steady improvement of the patient's physical and mental condition. Nutrition excitability is restored to normal, both conditioned and unconditioned reflexes are lowered, and food-conditioned reflex leukocytosis is reduced, yet these reflexes remain significantly above the control level. The EEG, as a rule, becomes normal only at a considerably later date.

Modes of Action

The enumerated stages of the controlled fasting treatment are to be regarded as a continuous sequence of events with each stage being a prerequisite for the development of the next. According to the degree in which the stages were manifested, as well as to the results of the fasting treatment, all patients are classified in three groups. Well-defined stages with a clear-cut "acidotic crisis" were associated with the best therapeutic effect. The unimproved cases revealed no appreciable changes either in their mental condition or in the dynamics of their nervous processes throughout the course of treatment. Professor Nikolayev states that the therapy seemingly has the following three modes of action:

1. While leading to acute exhaustion, fasting serves as a powerful stimulus to subsequent recuperation.

2. Fasting ensures rest for the digestive tract and the structures of the central nervous system, which receives digestive stimuli. This rest helps to normalize function.

3. Acidosis provoked by fasting and its compensation reflects a mobilization of detoxifying defense mechanisms that likely play an important role in the neutralization of toxins associated with the schizophrenic process. As acidosis decreases, the blood sugar level rises. The pH of the blood remains constant after acidosis decreases. Other parameters of the blood continue to remain constant. Insulin levels become normal. The biochemical dynamics during fasting are the same for mental illness and for normals.

Hematologic (blood) studies have shown that controlled fasting, far from causing any irreversible alterations in the blood, stimulates a striking intensification of regenerative, and consequently metabolic processes. Research into the biochemical dynamics of the fast reveals the vast changes stimulated in all the body systems. It has been proven that the fasting therapy mobilizes the proteins in the body, and this reaches a peak in seven days. When the recovery period begins, the protein level is found to be lower than at the beginning of the fast. Schizophrenics have a higher protein level than non-schizophrenics, and after the fast the protein level is normal. After three to six months, the schizophrenic's protein level tends to rise to the pre-fast level; therefore, they are put on recurrent short fasts to keep their protein levels at that of non-schizophrenics. Transaminase increases during the fast, up to the same level as that produced by noise, vibration, temperature, or heat. Cholesterol is increased during the 3rd to 5th day of the fast, decreases during the recovery period, and stabilizes at a normal level after two to three months. Bilirubin increases during the 3rd to 5th day of the fast and returns to normal during the 7th to 10th day.

The fast has a dangerous period during which thrombosis (blood clot) may occur in predisposed patients, and this period extends from the 7th to the 10th day. A similar danger period occurs during the 7th to the 12th day of the recovery period. Great care must be taken in those patients who have a history of thrombosis, and anticoagulants should be used. During these periods the prothrombin level (how fast blood clots) is elevated above the pre-fast level.

Glucose level falls from the 3rd to 12th day of the fast and returns to pre-fast levels by the 20th to 25th day. During the recovery period, the glucose level returns to normal. If a patient has hypoglycemia, his glucose-tolerance curve is normal at the end of the recovery period. Serotonin increases from the 5th to 7th day, and by the end of the fast the level is lower than it was in the pre-fasting period. A high concentration of serotonin in the pre-fasting stage was found in schizophrenic patients, a low concentration was found in neurotics. Both groups reach an optimum level during the fast, and after the fast each group slowly returns to pre-fasting levels. Histamine and heparin are both formed in the tissues that surround the blood vessels, and during the fast large amounts of heparin are formed, which lowers the histamine level.

Albumin levels in the blood are not greatly changed during the fast. When this was observed in groups of patients and related to the results achieved, three subgroups appeared. In one group, the albumin level rose during the fast, and in the second group the level dropped. Both of these groups achieved good results in the fast. In the third group, the albumin level remained stable, and this group achieved the least improvement. During the recovery period, each group returned to its pre-fast level. All catecholamines in the urine of ill people are found to be lower than in normals. During the fast, catecholamines increase and levels rise to that of normals. During the recovery period, catecholamines increase above pre-fast levels and are later maintained at normal levels.

Reintroduction of Food

During the recovery period feeding is begun slowly and with great care, as follows:

• *Day 1:* 500 grams (17.5 ounces) of fruit juice (half juice, half-boiled water), taken very slowly. A teaspoonful is put into the mouth and held, and when it disappears another spoonful is taken. An ideal way to begin is to extract the juice from an orange by sucking the orange and discarding the pulp.

• *Day 2:* 1 litre (34 ounces) of clear strained juice without water, taken slowly. The liquid is consumed in seven feedings taken at two-hour intervals. The juice may be varied daily.

• *Day 3:* 100 grams (3.5 ounces) of scraped apple (with skin) added to 150 grams (5 ounces) of yogurt or sour milk (kefir). The scraped apple is mixed with the yogurt, and the 250-gram mixture is divided into five portions and eaten every three hours. One orange is added to each of the five meals and is sucked as described above.

• *Day 4:* Same routine as on the 3rd day, but 50 grams (1.7 ounces) of carrot are added to each of the five meals. One orange is added to each meal.

• *Day 5:* Breakfast and lunch are the same as on the 4th day, but 150 grams (5 ounces) of vegetable salad are added to the lunch feeding. Three more meals are taken between lunch and bedtime, and 150 grams (5 ounces) of any juice are added to each of these three meals. The vegetable salad should contain some of every vegetable available.

• *Day 6:* Cottage cheese is added in very small quantities (100 grams, or 3.5 ounces, for the entire day). Four meals are eaten on this day and consist of the foods eaten on the previous days. Ten to 15 grams (up to 1 teaspoon) of honey are given with one of the meals. One small piece of dry brown bread may be taken during the day. One or two pieces of nut may be started and gradually increased.

• *Day 7:* A porridge of grits (ground hominy) is added to the above. The menu is increased gradually, and when the patient goes home he eats a diet of fruits, vegetables, and milk, sour milk, or yogurt, not to exceed 1 litre (34 ounces) each day. Not all patients can remain vegetarian, but they must not take meat for at least six months, and then in very small portions. Meals should be taken four times daily and later reduced to three. About 100 grams (3.5 ounces) of salad oiled with 10–15 grams (2–3 teaspoons) of sunflower oil may be taken. Butter may be started on the day 12 but should not exceed 30 grams (2 tablespoons) daily.

• *Day 10:* Starting on this day 25 grams (1 ounce) of sour cream may be taken to vary the bland taste of the diet.

• *Day 12 onward:* After day 12, oranges and apples should be taken in large quantities. Honey may be used daily for the sweet taste but should not exceed 1 teaspoonful daily.

Contraindications and Concerns

Contraindications for the use of the fasting treatment are: heart conditions (post-infarct condition, heart block, murmurs, history of thrombosis); tumors, sarcomas, etc.; bleeding ulcer; blood dyscrasias (abnormal materials); active pulmonary disease (if the condition is arrested, patient may be treated).

Indications for interrupting the fast are: development of an abnormal cardiac rhythm or permanently rapid pulse beat; gastric or intestinal spasm or symptoms of a surgical abdomen (if the spasm is functional, atropine may be used and the fast continued); cardiac asthma; persistence of hunger beyond the fifth day; unwillingness to exercise for a minimum period of three hours each day. Upper respiratory infections or colds are not indications for stopping the fast, since the experience has been that intercurrent infections most frequently clear more quickly during the fast.

Vital signs are checked daily and electrocardiographic tracings are made every other day during the danger period. Prior to starting the patient on the fast, a routine, thorough examination is done; this includes ECG, chest x-ray, complete blood and urine studies, and in elderly patients the examination should include urological studies.

Two Case Histories

The following cases from the Moscow Psychiatric Insitute are reported in detail because their history, mode of onset, and symptoms so closely parallel the cases we see.

22-Year-Old Disabled Male

The patient was a 22-year-old male who was on a full pension because his illness had so disabled him that he was unable to work. The family history was negative for mental illness. His early development was normal. His neurological organization was intact, his cognitive functions developed normally. His father was described as a jealous man with a temper; his mother as a soft, loving woman. The patient developed an interest in radio and began to collect transistors. At age 14 he experi-

enced his first breakdown, suffering from a "dissolution of his thoughts." He made a spontaneous recovery, continued in school, and in the 7th grade joined a society for First Aid because he had developed an interest in medicine.

Later, his interest focused on physiology and Pavlov's work. He became shy and embarrassed that people would laugh at this interest. His condition rapidly deteriorated. His memory began to fail, concentration was impaired, and he was unable to study. He left school and worked as a telephone technician. He became paranoid and complained to his superiors. He then left his job when, after a production meeting, it was decided that he was not being subjected to discrimination. He took other jobs and left them for the same reasons. He felt depressed and apathetic and believed that his friends looked at him peculiarly. Shortly afterward he was inducted into military service, where he experienced great fear and a crippling fatigue that made it impossible for him to do anything requiring physical effort. His apathy increased, he was unable to express his thoughts, and his vision blurred when he tried to read.

In 1968 he became violent and was hospitalized. He refused to eat and found that he felt better during three days of fasting. He did not improve with chlorpromazine treatment, was discharged from the Army, and admitted to the Moscow Psychiatric Institute. He was diagnosed with schizophrenia and started on the therapeutic fast. He was experiencing great fear, an inability to get out of bed in the mornings, and a feeling of extreme exhaustion. He complained that his thoughts streamed through his head without control. Concentration and comprehension were grossly impaired. Conversation was difficult, and he had suicidal thoughts and impulses; he wanted to kill himself by hanging. Improvement was felt after the 3rd day on the fast, at which time he reported that his head felt clear, his mood was even, he experienced an improvement in thinking, and he could communicate more easily.

He was examined with the aid of an interpreter during the latter part of his recovery period and expressed himself as follows:

I felt full of apathy, I was not concentrated and when reading I had to read a line over and over. When I spoke to people I couldn't remember what I said. I felt a complete weakness in my muscles. When I was punished by being isolated when I was in the Army, I refused to eat for three days and I found that I felt better. I then decided to fast or eat very little. I read about the fasting treatment in a magazine and applied to Professor Nikolayev for treatment after my discharge from the Army. From the 1st to the 5th day I had headache. On the 5th day my feelings of tension left and a feeling of indifference appeared. My feelings changed rapidly until the 18th day. On the 19th day I became restless and had to pace around the room. On the 20th day I felt that something changed in . . . inside and that there was something in my head and it had to come out. After that I felt better. On the 21st day I felt like I was covered with a sack. By the 22nd day I began to feel better. I felt the sun, the air, the forest, and I no longer felt alienated. The next day I felt like exploding and all my hostile feelings returned. The doctors felt that the return of these feelings was an indication that the fast should be stopped. The fast was terminated on the 27th day but I had a very poor appetite. My appetite gradually improved and my spirits improved. I felt joy for the first time in a long while.

27-Year-Old Polish Student

This patient's early development was normal, and he was robust and athletic. At age 15 he became excited and overactive, and his attitude toward his parents changed abruptly. He left his parents' home and went to live with his grandparents. He graduated from high school and shortly after became involved in a fight during which he suffered a stab wound of the kidney. During the period of hospitalization that followed, he had an episode of euphoria that continued after he was discharged. He believed that he was an important figure in the Polish Academy of Filmmakers and considered himself as highly talented in this art form. He was examined by a psychiatrist who advised hospitalization, but his mother rejected

> "For schizophrenics, the natural recovery rate is 50 percent. With orthomolecular medicine, the recovery rate is 90 percent. With drugs, it is 10 percent. If you use just drugs, you won't get well. This is because mental illness is usually biochemical illness. Mental illness is a disorder of brain dysfunction. Schizophrenia is vitamin B3 (niacin) dependency. Not a deficiency; a dependency. If schizophrenia strikes someone at age 25, he's finished—that is, if he or she is only given drugs. Patients are given drugs and released. The new mental hospital today is the streets."
>
> — ABRAM HOFFER

this advice. He entered Poznan University but found studying to be extremely difficult because of an inability to concentrate. His comprehension was very poor, and he was extremely depressed. He felt withdrawn and isolated, slept all day, and walked the streets of the city all night. His apathy increased, his general condition deteriorated, and he was diagnosed asthenic and given a leave of absence from school. He traveled to Moscow and was admitted to the Psychiatric Institute. On admission he was described as being well-oriented, and exhibiting circumstantial speech and feelings of unreality. He complained of weakness, poverty of ideation, poor memory, and quick exhaustion, most marked after reading. His facial expression was rigid, his speech was monotonous, and he found great difficulty in communicating. He felt hopeless and saw no future for himself. He was diagnosed "schizophrenia." He was treated with insulin shock therapy and his condition remained essentially unchanged.

He was seen in consultation by Professor Nikolayev and transferred to the Therapeutic Fasting Unit. On admission there he was oriented; spoke in a low, well-modulated voice; and appeared depressed. His primary complaints were apathy, fatigue, blank mind, and recurring periods of intense excitement (ranging from feeling agitated, perturbed, alarmed, or enraged to being over-wrought, ready to burst, or fly into a passion), and great ambivalence. His sleep pattern was disturbed, and capability for any work was drastically diminished. His fasting period lasted for 28 days.

The acidotic crisis began on the 7th day, and after that his spirits rose. Weakness appeared on the 7th and 8th days, and he found it difficult to continue the fast. He wanted to stay in bed all day. After the 8th day, his sugar level increased, the pH of his blood remained constant, and clinically he was markedly improved. On the 26th day, his appetite appeared, and on the 28th day he complained of generalized weakness. His tongue cleared, the fast was ended, and the recovery period was started. On the 5th day of recovery, he stated that he felt well, his head felt clear, his thinking was clear, and his concentration was markedly improved. On the 23rd day of recovery, he felt "greatly helped" but expressed concern that he might relapse and asked for a short prophylactic fast. Professor Nikolayev refused this, explaining that if he exercised daily, continued his hydrotherapy and diet, led a good life without drinking or smoking, he would not relapse. He was advised that he may do three- to five-day prophylactic fasts, but for not more than 10 days per month.

In an interview on the 23rd day of the recovery period, the patient described his experiences as follows:

Weakness appeared on the 2nd day, increased through the 6th or 7th day, and continued to the 10th day. (He distinguished between weakness and fatigue when I raised the question and described the crippling fatigue of schizophrenia which he suffered prior to the fasting treatment). For the next two days I felt very well and after that everything improved rapidly. When I began to drink juice during the recovery period, the world changed, colors became brighter, thinking became easier. I no longer feel the emptiness and my perception of the world has changed completely. I feel that I have a bright future. I do not want to return to school now, I want to live a normal, healthy life and I will decide later whether I will return to school.

On the 10th to the 14th day of the recovery period, the patient has an exacerbation of some of his symptoms. The experience has been that this occurs in the majority of patients and is related to the absorption of proteins in large quantities. Following this brief period, stabilization occurs and improvement continues.

Therapeutic Fasting Research Project Here at Home

I began using the controlled fasting treatment in a research project at the Gracie Square Hospital in New York City. A prerequisite for admission to the project must be the existence of a schizophrenic illness for a period of five years or longer and a history of failure in all prior treatments. A basic requirement is the full consent of the patient and his relatives. The treatment can be applied only in those cases where there is full awareness of illness and a desire to undergo this treatment, since it requires the patient's full cooperation.

The patient must be out of bed and remain active. The patient leaves the hospital daily to walk in the city, returning to rest in the afternoon. He is free to leave the hospital whenever he wishes. If the patient does not exercise by walking a minimum of three hours daily, weakness ensues, and the fast must then be arbitrarily broken.

If the patient willfully breaks the fast and eats, treatment is stopped, and the patient is discharged from the hospital. The patient must drink a minimum of 34 ounces of water daily but may drink more if he wants it. If the required amount of water is not consumed, the fast must be broken.

The daily cleansing enema and shower or bath are equally important parts of the required regimen. During the shower or bath, the patient stimulates the peripheral circulation by using a loofah straw mitt as a washcloth.

Those patients who are using medications are gradually withdrawn and usually by the end of the first week no longer require it. A patient whose fast recently ended on the 29th day was withdrawn from 500 milligrams (mg) of Thorazine, 20 mg of haloperidol (Haldol), and 10 mg of trifluoperazine (Stelazine) during the first week of his fast. He had been on these maintenance doses for one year.

Patients must give up smoking during the fast. If they cannot do so by the end of the first week of the fast, it may be necessary to break the fast and end the treatment. Most patients who smoke have success in giving up cigarettes even though they had tried and failed prior to entering the fasting program.

The entire period of the fasting is endured relatively easily, but during the recovery period complications occur that are directly related to the breaking of the diet. Overeating is the most common cause for these complications, which usually happen between the 5th and 10th day of the recovery period at which time protein intake is begun. The obvious prophylactic measure is strict adherence to the recovery diet, eating only the foods called for in the specified amounts. The education of the patient is extremely important, and this education must be followed up by frequent reminders to avoid overeating. Eating at each meal must stop before a feeling of fullness develops. In some patients the intake of protein foods produces a period of excitation, tension, or sleeplessness. Sleep medication and small doses of neuroleptic (antipsychotic) drugs may be used for several days. The symptoms dissipate in five to seven days.

Premature breaking of the recovery period may result in edema of the ankles or in the subcutaneous layer of the skin beneath the eye socket. However, this complication usually results from the use of table salt or the ingestion of many foods containing salt, such as bread, butter, cheese, nuts, and so on. The edema produces a feeling of lassitude, headache, and at times a bad mood. When the patient returns to strict observance of the diet with plentiful water intake, the edema clears rap-idly. Administration of a saline cathartic promotes disappearance of the edema.

■ CONCLUSION

In the study of Professor Nikolayev's mentioned earlier, statistics revealed that 70 percent of the 6,000 patients treated by controlled fasting achieved such significant improvement that they were restored to functioning. This represents an unparalleled achievement in the treatment of schizophrenia when one considers that these patients had an endless number of failures in all forms of therapy. They were all chronically ill and felt hopeless about their future. Most of them would never have functioned again. Many would have ended their lives, while the rest would have deteriorated and lived out the balance of their lives in the bleak back wards of a mental hospital.

My experience now extends over 35 cases of schizophrenia treated between July 1970 and April 1973, and to date 24 patients remain well. Three of these had to repeat the long fast nine months after the initial fast was completed, because they had precipitated relapse by breaking their diets. Four patients broke their diet and relapsed into psychosis and could not be fasted again. These patients were treated with antipsychotic drugs. Ten have remained well after two years. Two have remained well after four years. Three patients had to break the fast prematurely before the 15th day. One patient is not included in these statistics since he completed his fast at the time of this writing.

REFERENCES

1. Young VR, Scrimshaw Nevin S. The physiology of starvation. *Scientific American* 1971;225:14–21.

2. Cott A. Controlled fasting treatment of schizophrenia in the USSR. *Schizophrenia* 1971;3(1):1–10.

APPENDICES

APPENDIX 1

WHERE ARE THE BODIES?
THE SAFETY OF ANTIOXIDANTS AND MICRONUTRIENTS
by Andrew W. Saul, PhD

If vitamins are declared unsafe at low doses, they do not have to be tested for effectiveness at high doses. Some believe that nutrients are dangerous and that drugs, somehow, are not. It's a nice legend, but only a legend. Nutrient therapy is safe. According to national data collected by the American Association of Poison Control Centers (AAPCC) over a 30-year period, vitamin supplements are alleged to have caused the deaths of a total of 14 people in the United States (see Table 1). That is less than one-half a death per year.

TABLE 1: SUMMARY OF VITAMIN FATALITY DATA FROM ANNUAL REPORTS OF THE AMERICAN ASSOCIATION OF POISON CONTROL CENTERS		
2012: 1	2002: 1	1992: 0
2011: 2	2001: 0	1991: 2
2010: 0	2000: 0	1990: 1
2009: 0	1999: 0	1989: 0
2008: 0	1998: 0	1988: 0
2007: 0	1997: 0	1987: 1
2006: 1	1996: 0	1986: 0
2005: 0	1995: 0	1985: 0
2004: 2	1994: 0	1984: 0
2003: 2	1993: 1	1983: 0

*From www.aapcc.org/annual-reports

However, a new analysis of U.S. Poison Control Center annual report data indicates that there have, in fact, been no deaths whatsoever from vitamins . . . none at all, in the 30 years that such reports have been available.

The zeros are not due to a lack of reporting.

The AAPCC, which maintains the United States' national database of information from 57 poison control centers, has noted that vitamins are among the 16 most reported substances.

Even if these fatality figures are taken as correct, and even if they include intentional and accidental misuse, the number of alleged vitamin fatalities is strikingly low. In fact, in 20 of the 30 years, AAPCC reports that there was not one single death due to vitamins.

Still, the *Orthomolecular Medicine News Service* editorial board was curious.

Did 14 people really die from vitamins? And if so, how?

Vitamins Not the Cause of Death

In determining cause of death, AAPCC uses a 4-point scale called Relative Contribution to Fatality (RCF). A rating of:

1 means "Undoubtedly Responsible"

2 means "Probably Responsible"

3 means "Contributory"

4 means "Probably Not Responsible"

In examining poison control data for the year 2006, listing one vitamin death, it was seen that the vitamin's RCF was a 4. Since a score of 4 means "Probably Not Responsible," it negates the claim that a person died from a vitamin in 2006.

In other years with one or more of the remaining 13 alleged vitamin fatalities, the study of AAPCC reports reveals an absence of RCF ratings for vitamins.

If there is no Relative Contribution to Fatality at all, then the substance did not contribute to death at all.

Two people are alleged to have died from vitamin supplements in the year 2011.

Presentation at the Int. Wiener 1 Symposium Orthomolekulare Medizin, Vienna, Austria, Oct 23-25, 2013.

One death was allegedly due to vitamin C; the other supposedly because of "Other B-Vitamins."

The AAPCC report specifically indicates no deaths from niacin (vitamin B3) or pyridoxine (vitamin B6). That leaves folic acid, thiamine (vitamin B1), riboflavin (vitamin B2), biotin, pantothenic acid (vitamin B5), and cobalamin (B12) as the remaining B vitamins that could be blamed.

However, the safety record of these vitamins is extraordinarily good; no fatalities have been confirmed for any of them. Vitamin C is also an extraordinarily safe nutrient. No deaths have ever been confirmed from supplementation with vitamin C.

It was claimed that one person died from vitamin supplementation in the year 2012. That single alleged "death" was supposedly due to "Other B Vitamins." Yet, once again, the AAPCC report specifically indicates no deaths from niacin (vitamin B3) or pyridoxine (vitamin B6), and all the other B vitamins have never been known to cause death.

Vitamin Supplement Safety Confirmed by America's Largest Database

If there is insufficient information about the cause of death, which is needed to make a clear-cut declaration of cause, then subsequent assertions that vitamins cause deaths are not evidence-based. Although vitamin supplements have often been blamed for causing fatalities, there is no evidence to back up this allegation.

There have been zero confirmed deaths from vitamin supplements.

None at all in 30 years.

Well over half of the U.S. population takes daily nutritional supplements.

Even if each of those people took only one single tablet daily, that makes 165,000,000 individual doses per day, for a total of over 60 billion doses annually.

Since many people take far more than just one single vitamin or mineral tablet, actual consumption is considerably higher, and the safety of nutritional supplements is all the more remarkable.

Over 60 billion doses of vitamin and mineral supplements per year in the United States, and not a single fatality. Not one.

If vitamin and mineral supplements are allegedly so "dangerous," as the Food and Drug Administration (FDA), Codex (an international public health and consumer protection organization), and news media so often claim, then where are the bodies?

Where Are the Bodies?

Fifteen years ago, properly-prescribed pharmaceutical drugs, taken as directed, killed at least 80,000 people annually in the United States alone.[2] Some estimates place the yearly death toll from pharmaceuticals far higher, into the hundreds of thousands.[3]

Safety of Mineral Supplements

Minerals have an excellent safety record, but not quite as good as vitamins. Until iron supplements were put in childproof bottles, there were one or two fatalities per year attributed to iron poisoning from gross overdosing on supplemental iron. Deaths attributed to other supplemental minerals are very rare.

Mineral Supplement Safety Confirmed by America's Largest Database

In 2010, the AAPCC reports that three people died from non-supplement mineral poisoning: two from medical use of sodium and one from non-supplemental iron. On page 131, the AAPCC report specifically indicates that the iron fatality was not from a nutritional supplement.

In 2009, there were no deaths whatsoever from any dietary mineral supplement. However, two people died from non-nutritional mineral poisoning, one from a sodium salt, and one from an iron salt or iron. On page 1139, the AAPCC report specifically indicates that the iron fatality was not from a nutritional supplement.

One other person is alleged to have died from an "Unknown Dietary Supplement or Homeopathic Agent." This claim remains speculative, as no verification information was provided.

There were zero deaths in 2008 from any dietary mineral supplement. This includes iron. However, two children died as a result of the medical use of the antacid sodium bicarbonate. The other "Electrolyte and Mineral" category death was due to a man accidentally drinking sodium hydroxide, a highly toxic degreaser and drain-opener.

There were zero deaths in 2007 from any dietary mineral supplement, including iron.

There was one death from chronic overdose of magnesium hydroxide, commonly known as the laxative/antacid milk of magnesia.

It was inappropriately listed in the "Dietary Supplement" reporting category. Nutritional supplements do not contain magnesium hydroxide.

How Do You Make People Believe an Anti-Vitamin Scare?

It just takes lots of pharmaceutical industry cash.

Cash to Study Authors

Many of the authors of a highly publicized negative vitamin E paper have received substantial income from the pharmaceutical industry. The names are available on the last page of the paper (1556) in the "Conflict of Interest" section. A number of the study authors have received money from pharmaceutical companies, including Merck, Pfizer, Sanofi-Aventis, AstraZeneca, Abbott, GlaxoSmithKline, Janssen, Amgen, Firmagon, and Novartis.

You will not see the conflicts in the brief summary at the *Journal of the American Medical Association* (JAMA) website. The paper is Klein EA, Thompson Jr, IM, Tangen CM, et al. Vitamin E and the risk of prostate cancer: the Selenium and Vitamin E Cancer Prevention Trial (SELECT). JAMA 2011;306(14):1549–1556. http://jama.ama-assn.org/content/306/14/1549.

Advertising Revenue

Many popular magazines and almost all major medical journals receive income from the pharmaceutical industry. The only question is, How much?

Look in them all: *Readers Digest, JAMA, Time, American Association of Retired Persons (AARP), New England Journal of Medicine (NEJM), Lancet, Archives of Pediatrics, Prevention* magazine. Practically any major periodical is full of pharmaceutical advertising.

Count the number of pharmaceutical ads. The more space sold, the more revenue for the publication. If you try to find a periodical's advertisement revenue, you'll likely see that they don't disclose it.

Rigged Trials

Studies of the health benefits of vitamins and essential nutrients can be easily rigged by using:

• Low doses to guarantee failure;

• Biased interpretation to show a statistical increase in risk.

You can set up any study to fail. One way to ensure failure is to make a meaningless test. A meaningless test is assured:

• If you make the choice to use insufficient quantities of the substance to be investigated.

• If you shoot beans at a charging rhinoceros, you are not likely to influence the outcome.

• If you give every homeless person you meet on the street 20 cents, you could easily prove that money will not help alleviate poverty.

• If you give the Recommended Dietary Allowance (RDA) levels of vitamins, you do not expect therapeutic results.

One reason commonly offered to justify conducting low-dose studies is that high doses of vitamins are somehow dangerous. Nutritional supplementation is not dangerous. What is dangerous is failure to supplement. The battle over vitamin supplements has been going on for nearly 70 years. You can say one thing for vitamin critics: at least they are consistent. Consistently wrong, but consistent.

The oldest political trick in the book is to create doubt, then fear, and then conformity of action. The pharmaceutical industry knows this full well.

One does not waste time and money attacking something that does not work. Vitamin supplementation works well and works safely.

Bias in What Is Published, or Rejected for Publication

The largest and most popular medical journals receive very large income from pharmaceutical advertising. Peer-reviewed research indicates that this influences what they print, and even what study authors conclude from their data.[4]

Other research showed that more pharmaceutical company advertising results in a medical journal having more articles with "negative conclusions about dietary supplement safety." The authors stated, "The percentage of major articles concluding that supplements were unsafe was 4 percent in journals with fewest and 67 percent among those with the most pharmads (P = 0.02)." They concluded that "the impact of advertising on publications is real," and that "the ultimate impact of this bias on professional guidelines, health care, and health policy is a matter of great public concern."[5]

Censorship of What Is Indexed and Available to Doctors and the Public

There are nearly 6,000 journals indexed by the U.S. taxpayer-funded National Library of Medicine (NLM), and over 1 billion PubMed/Medline searches each year. (PubMed/Medline is the NLM's primary online database of references and abstracts, free to Internet users.) Not one of those searches found a single paper from the peer-reviewed *Journal of Orthomolecular Medicine*.[6] PubMed/Medline does, however, index material from *Time* magazine, *Consumer Reports*, and even *Reader's Digest*. (All accessed May 2014.) After nearly half a century of continuous, peer-reviewed publication, perhaps the *Journal of Orthomolecular Medicine* should be included by the world's largest public medical library.

It is ironic that critics of vitamins preferentially cite low-dose studies in an attempt to show lack of vitamin effectiveness, yet they cannot cite any double-blind, placebo-controlled studies of high doses that show vitamin dangers. This is because vitamins are effective at high doses, and vitamins are also safe at high doses. Yet it is probable that the main, persistent roadblock to widespread examination and utilization of nutrition therapeutics is the widespread belief that there simply must be dangers with vitamin and mineral supplements. The opposite is true. There is a long and extraordinarily safe track record of high-dose nutrient therapy, dating back to the early 1940s.

Postscript: As of June 1, 2014, the *Journal of Orthomolecular Medicine* is now indexed by PubMed. Well, at least some of it is. Actually, two papers are indexed[7]—and by PubMed only, not Medline. Admittedly, they are two mighty important studies, especially if someone in your family is battling cancer and wants to know more about using intravenous vitamin C therapy:

1. Schedule Dependence in Cancer Therapy: Intravenous Vitamin C and the Systemic Saturation Hypothesis. González MJ, Miranda Massari JR, Duconge J, et al. *J Orthomol Med*. 2012 Jan 1;27(1):9–12. PMID: 24860238 [PubMed]

2. Mitochondria, Energy and Cancer: The Relationship with Ascorbic Acid. González MJ, Rosario-Pérez G, Guzmán AM, et al. *J Orthomol Med*. 2010;25(1):29–38. PMID: 23565030 [PubMed]

But why index only two papers? After all, the *Journal of Orthomolecular Medicine* has been publishing research like this for 47 years. There are many hundreds of clinical nutrition papers that remain excluded by the NLM, the *taxpayer-funded* NLM.

REFERENCES

1. Bronstein AC, Spyker DA, Cantilena LR, et al. 2011 Annual Report of the American Association of Poison Control Centers' National Poison Data System (NPDS): 29th Annual Report. *Clin Toxicol* 2012;50(10):911–1164. The data discussed above can be found on p. 1134, Table 22B. Other reports are downloadable at no charge (along with previous years) at: www.aapcc.org/annual-reports.

2. Lazarou J, Pomeranz BH, Corey PN. Incidence of adverse drug reactions in hospitalized patients: a meta-analysis of prospective studies. *JAMA* 1998;279(15):1200–1205.

3. Null G, Dean C, Feldman M, et al. Death by medicine. *J Orthomolecular Med* 2005;20(1):21–34.

4. *Orthomolecular Medicine News Service.* Pharmaceutical advertising biases journals against vitamin supplements, Feb 5, 2009. Available at: http://orthomolecular.org/resources/omns/v05n02.shtml.

5. Kemper KJ, Hood KL. Does pharmaceutical advertising affect journal publication about dietary supplements? *BMC Complement Altern Med* 2008;8:11.

6. *Orthomolecular Medicine News Service.* NLM censors nutritional research, Jan 15, 2010. Available at: http://orthomolecular.org/resources /omns/v06n03.shtml. See also: How to fool all of the people all of the time, Jan 21, 2010. Available at: http://orthomolecular .org/resources/omns/v06n05.shtml.

7. U.S. National Library of Medicine. PubMed.com. Available at: www.ncbi.nlm.nih.gov/pubmed?term=%22J+Orthomol+Med%22[jour].

APPENDIX 2

TREATMENT SUMMARY: FREDERICK R. KLENNER'S OBSERVATIONS ON THE DOSE AND ADMINISTRATION OF VITAMIN C AS AN ANTITOXIN, ANTIBIOTIC, AND ANTIVIRAL.

Editor's note: Frederick R. Klenner, MD, found ascorbate to be an effective and nearly all-purpose antitoxin, antibiotic, and antiviral. One vitamin being useful for polio, pneumonia, measles, strep, and snakebite is counterintuitive. Yet Dr. Klenner reported success with these and nearly four dozen other diseases. Following is a treatment summary of his article in Part One of this book.

Severe Viral Diseases

Severe viral diseases can be deadly and must be treated heroically with intravenous and/or intramuscular injections of ascorbic acid. We recommend a dose schedule of from 350–700 milligrams (mg) per kilogram (kg) per body weight diluted to at least 18 cc of 5 percent dextrose water to each 1,000 mg of vitamin C. Ten thousand milligrams of ascorbic acid daily in divided doses is also given by mouth. In small children, 2,000 or 3,000 mg can be given intramuscularly, every two hours. An ice cap to the buttock will prevent soreness and induration.

Ascorbic acid in amounts under 400 mg per kg body weight can be administered intravenously with a syringe in dilutions of 5 cc to each 1,000 mg provided the ampule is buffered with sodium bicarbonate with sodium bisulfite added. As much as 12,000 mg can be given in this manner with a 50 cc syringe. Larger amounts must be diluted with bottle dextrose or saline solutions and run in by needle drip. This is true because amounts like 20,000–25,000 mg, which can be given with a 100 cc syringe, can suddenly dehydrate the cerebral cortex so as to produce convulsive movements of the legs. This represents a peculiar syndrome, symptomatic epilepsy, in which the patient is mentally clear and experiences no discomfort except that the lower extremities are in mild convulsion. This epileptiform-type seizure will continue for 20-plus minutes and then abruptly stop. Mild pressure on the knees will stop the seizure so long as pressure is maintained. If still within the time limit of the seizure, the spasm will reappear by simply withdrawing the hand pressure. I have seen this in two patients receiving 26,000 mg intravenously with a 100 cc syringe on the second injection. One patient had polio; the other malignant measles. Both were adults. I have duplicated this on myself to prove no aftereffects. Intramuscular injections are always 500 mg to 1 cc solution. With continuous intravenous injections of large amounts of ascorbic acid, at least 1,000 mg of calcium gluconate must be added to the fluids each day.

Multiple Uses

There are many other pathological conditions in which ascorbic acid plays an important part in recovery. To these might be added cardiovascular diseases, hypermenorrhea, peptic and duodenal ulcers, post-operative and radiation sickness, rheumatic fever, scarlet fever, poliomyelitis, encephalitis, viral hepatitis, acute and chronic pancreatitis, tularemia, whooping cough, and tuberculosis. In one case of scarlet fever in which penicillin and the sulfa drugs were showing no improvement, 50,000 mg of ascorbic acid given intravenously resulted in a dramatic drop in the fever curve to normal. Here the action of ascorbic acid was not only direct but also as a synergist. A similar situation was observed in a case of lobar pneumonia. In another case of purperal sepsis following a criminal abortion the initial dose of ascorbic acid was 1,200 mg per kg body weight and two subsequent injections were at the 600 mg level. Along with penicillin and sulfadiazine an admission temperature of 105.4°F was normal in nine hours. The patient made an uneventful recovery.

In one spectacular case of black widow spider bite in a 3-year-old child, in coma, 1,000 mg of calcium gluconate and 4,000 mg of ascorbic acid was administered intravenously when first seen in the office. Then, 4,000 mg of ascorbic acid was given every six hours using a 20 cc syringe. She was awake and well in 24 hours. Physical examination showed a comatose child with a rigid abdomen. The area about the umbilicus was red and indurated, suggesting a strangulated hernia. With a 4X lens, fang marks were in evidence. Thirty hours after starting the vitamin C therapy the child expelled a large amount of dark clotted blood. There was no other residual. A review of the literature confirmed that this individual has been the only one to survive with such findings; the others were reported at autopsy.

APPENDIX 3

THE RIORDAN INTRAVENOUS VITAMIN C (IVC) PROTOCOL FOR ADJUNCTIVE CANCER CARE: IVC AS A CHEMOTHERAPEUTIC AND BIOLOGICAL RESPONSE MODIFYING AGENT

by Hugh Riordan, MD, Neil Riordan, PhD, Joseph Casciari, PhD, James Jackson, PhD, Ron Hunninghake, MD, Nina Mikirova, PhD, and Paul R. Taylor

Grateful appreciation is expressed to the Riordan Clinic for permission to publish their complete intravenous vitamin C protocol.

Vitamin C (ascorbate, ascorbic acid) is a major water-soluble antioxidant that also increases extracellular collagen production and is important for proper immune cell functioning (Hoffman, 1985; Cameron, et al., 1979). It also plays key roles in L-carnitine synthesis, cholesterol metabolism, cytochrome P-450 activity, and neurotransmitter synthesis (Geeraert, 2012). The Riordan intravenous vitamin C (IVC) protocol involves the slow infusion of vitamin C at doses on the order of 0.1 to 1.0 grams (g) of ascorbate per kilogram (kg) body mass (Riordan, et al., 2003). IVC use has increased recently among integrative and orthomolecular medicine practitioners: a survey of roughly 300 practitioners conducted between 2006 and 2008 indicated that roughly 10,000 patients received IVC, at an average dose of 0.5 g/kg, without significant ill effects (Padayatty, et al., 2010). While IVC may have a variety of possible applications, such as combating infections (Padayatty, et al., 2010), treating rheumatoid arthritis (Mikirova, et al., 2012), it has generated the most interest for its potential use in adjunctive cancer care.

Vitamin C was first suggested as a tool for cancer treatment in the 1950s: its role in collagen production and protection led scientists to hypothesize that ascorbate replenishment would protect normal tissue from tumor invasiveness and metastasis (McCormick, 1959; Cameron, et al., 1979). Also, since cancer patients are often depleted of vitamin C (Hoffman, 1985; Riordan, et al., 2005), replenishment may improve immune system function and enhance patient health and well-being (Henson, et al., 1991). Cameron and Pauling observed fourfold survival times in terminal cancer patients treated with intravenous ascorbate infusions followed by oral supplementation (Cameron & Pauling, 1976). However, two randomized clinical trials with oral ascorbate alone conducted by the Mayo Clinic showed no benefit (Creagan, et al., 1979; Moertel, et al., 1985). Most research from that point on focused on intravenous ascorbate. The rationales for using intravenous ascorbate infusions to treat cancer, which are discussed in detail below, can be summarized as follows:

• Plasma ascorbate concentrations in the millimolar (mM) range can be safely achieved with IVC infusions.

• At mM concentrations, ascorbate is preferentially toxic to cancer cells in vitro and is able to inhibit angiogenesis in vitro and in vivo.

• Vitamin C can accumulate in tumors with significant tumor growth inhibition seen (in guinea pigs) at intra-tumor concentrations of 1 mM or higher.

• Published case studies report anticancer efficacy, improved patient well-being, and decreases in markers of inflammation and tumor growth.

• Phase I clinical studies indicate that IVC can be administered safely with relatively few adverse effects.

The Riordan Clinic has treated hundreds of cancer patients (Figure 1) using the Riordan protocol. At the same time, Riordan Clinic Research Institute (RCRI) has been researching the potential of intravenous vitamin C therapy for over thirty years. Our efforts have included in vitro studies, animal studies, pharmacokinetic analyses, and

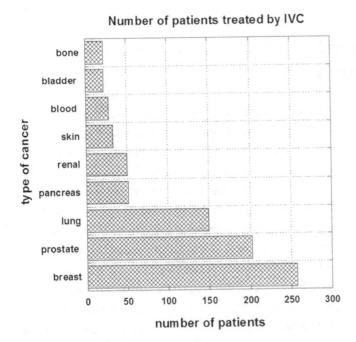

FIGURE 1. Types of cancers treated with IVC by the Riordan clinic.

jects were deficient in vitamin C (Mayland, et al., 2005). Deficiency (below 10 µM) was correlated with elevated CRP (C-reactive protein, an inflammation marker) levels and shorter survival times. Given the role of vitamin C in collagen production, immune system functioning, and antioxidant protection, it is not surprising that subjects depleted of ascorbate would fare poorly in mounting defenses against cancer. This also suggests that supplementation to replenish vitamin C stores might serve as adjunctive therapy for these patients.

When vitamin C is given by intravenous infusion, peak concentrations over 10 mM can be attained (Casciari, et al., 2001; Padayatty, et al., 2004) without significant adverse effects to the recipient. Figure 3 (page 753) shows plasma ascorbate concentrations attained via IVC infusion at the Riordan Clinic, while Figure 4 shows pharmacokinetic data for two subjects given 80-minute IVC infusions. These peak plasma concentrations are two orders of magnitude above what is observed with oral supplementation. This suggests that IVC may be more effective than oral supplementation in restoring depleted ascorbate stores in cancer patients. Physicians at the Riordan Clinic have observed that (a) peak plasma concentrations attained after IVC infusions tend to be lower in

clinical trials. The Riordan IVC protocol, along with the research results (by the RCRI and others) that have motivated its use, is described below.

Scientific Background

Pharmacokinetics

Vitamin C is water soluble and is limited in how well it can be absorbed when given orally. While ascorbate tends to accumulate in adrenal glands, the brain, and in some white blood cell types, plasma levels stay relatively low (Keith & Pelletier, 1974; Hornig, 1975; Ginter, et al., 1979; Kuether, et al., 1988). Data by Levine and coworkers indicate that plasma levels in healthy adults stayed below 100 micrometer microns (µM), even if 2.5 grams were taken when administered once daily by the oral route. (Levine, et al., 1996.)

Cancer patients tend to be depleted of vitamin C: 14 out of 22 terminal cancer patients in a phase I study we depleted of vitamin C, with 10 of those having zero detectable ascorbate in their plasma (Riordan, et al., 2005). This is shown in Figure 2. In a study of cancer patients in hospice care, Mayland and coworkers found that 30 percent of the sub-

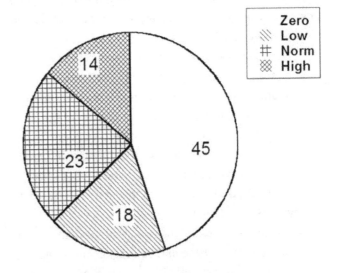

FIGURE 2. Distribution of pretreatment plasma ascorbate levels in terminal cancer patients: Depleted (< 10 µM), Low (10 to 30 µM), Normal (20 to 100 µM), and High (> 100 µM) (Riordan, et al., 2005).

THE RIORDAN CLINIC INTRAVENOUS VITAMIN C PROTOCOL AND BACKGROUND RESEARCH

The Riordan Clinic, which focuses on nutritional medicine, was founded in 1975 as the Center for the Improvement of Human Functioning under the leadership of Dr. Hugh Riordan, a medical doctor who practiced psychiatry.

Dr. Riordan originally focused on treating mentally ill patients through nutritional medicine. The value of vitamin C as a potential cancer treatment first came into light after an article published in 1976 by Ewan Cameron and Linus Pauling, in which the authors suggested an increased survival in cancer patients receiving intravenous vitamin C (IVC) treatments.

Dr. Riordan first became aware of this therapy in the early 1980s, when a 70-year-old patient suffering from metastatic renal cell carcinoma that had spread to his liver and lungs came to the clinic requesting IV ascorbate infusions. The patient had read Pauling's research, and Dr. Riordan was the only doctor in Wichita using IV vitamin C. Upon his request, he began IV vitamin C treatment, starting at 30 grams twice per week. Fifteen months after initial therapy, the patient's oncologist reported that the patient had no signs of progressive cancer. The patient remained cancer-free for 14 years.

Based on his experience, Dr. Riordan set a goal for a cancer research project. In 1989 Dr. Riordan announced the 11-year RECNAC (cancer spelled backward), a project devoted to finding of the non-toxic cancer treatment. The project manager of the research was Dr. Neil Riordan and the research group included many devoted scientists such as Dr. J. Casciari, Dr. J. Jackson, Dr. X. Meng, Dr. J. Zhong, P. Taylor, BS, Dr. N. Mikirova, and others.

The group validated the use of the IV vitamin C for cancer therapy. Using *in vitro* studies, more than 60 cell lines were tested for the toxicity to high dosages of ascorbate. It was demonstrated that at a high enough dose ascorbate can kill cancer cells while not affecting normal cells. The Riordan Clinic researchers were the first to demonstrate that selectively toxic plasma levels of ascorbate could be achieved in cancer patients (*Med Hypothesis*, 1995).

In 1997 the IVC treatment was patented by Drs. Neil Riordan and Hugh Riordan; the title of the patent is "Intravenous ascorbate as tumor cytotoxic chemotherapeutic agent." Other important results included: synergism between vitamin C and alpha-lipoic acid (*Br J Cancer*, 2001), protocol for reaching tumor cytotoxic blood levels of ascorbate in plasma (*P R Health Sci J*, 2003), inhibition of the angiogenesis by vitamin C (*J Transl Med*, 2008), effect of ascorbate on immune function, and Phase I trial of the safety of the proposed treatment.

In addition, it was found that IVC treatment improves the quality of life of advanced cancer patients, corrects deficiencies of vitamin C that often occur in cancer patients, and optimizes white blood cell concentrations of vitamin C. Analysis of the markers of inflammation in cancer patients showed that high-dose IVC treatment reduces inflammation in cancer patients. Treatment by IVC can improve response to radiation treatment and reduce the side effects of chemotherapy. In addition, the therapeutic effect of ascorbic acid can be enhanced by vitamin K3 and alpha-lipoic acid. Very important clinical trials inspired by the success of IVC at the Riordan Clinic were conducted at Thomas Jefferson University in Philadelphia.

Dr. Hugh Riordan's vision of treating and preventing ailments with a non-toxic nutritional approach led him to become one of the first doctors to use IV vitamin C as a treatment protocol in patients with terminal cancer. This vision led to original research at the clinic, as well as numerous articles, patents, a series of IVC symposiums, and health initiatives.

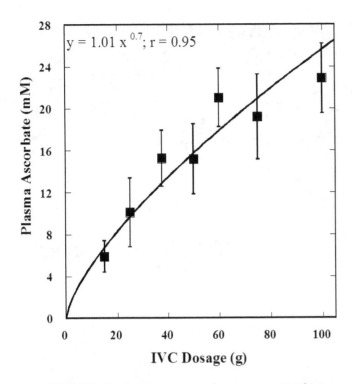

FIGURE 3. Peak plasma ascorbate concentrations (mM) versus IVC dose (grams) for 900 subjects given treatments at the Riordan Clinic.

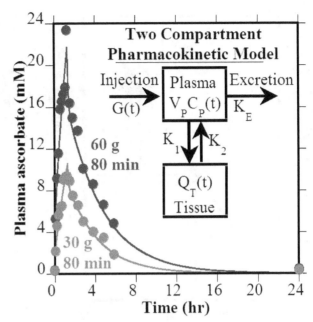

FIGURE 4. Vitamin C concentrations in plasma during and after an 80 min intravenous infusion of 60 (solid circles) or 30 (open circles) grams. The curves represent fits of the data to the two compartment pharmacokinetic model pictured in the figure inset, with K1, K2, and KE values of 0.31 min–1, 0.091 min–1, and 0.022 min–1 for the 60 gram infusion and 0.21 min–1, 0.060 min–1, and 0.027 min–1 for the 30 gram infusion. Invalid source specified.

cancer patients than in healthy volunteers, suggesting their depleted tissues act as a "sink" for the vitamin; and (b) in cancer patients given multiple IVC treatments, baseline plasma ascorbate concentrations tend to increase to normal levels slowly over time as reserves are restored with adequate IVC dosing.

In addition to providing ascorbate replenishment, IVC may allow oncologists to exploit some interesting anticancer properties, including high dose IVC's ability to induce tumor cell apoptosis, inhibit angiogenesis, and reduce inflammation. In vitro and in vivo data supporting these potential mechanisms of action, discussed below, suggest that they may be relevant at ascorbate concentrations on the order of 2 mM. As shown in Figures 3 and 4 (above), these concentrations are attainable in plasma using progressive dosing of IVC.

A 2-compartment model can be used to predict peak and "average" (over 24 hours) plasma ascorbate concentrations for an average-sized adult at a given IVC dose as shown in Figure 5 (page 754). This calculation suggests that a 50 gram, 1 hr. infusion would yield a peak plasma concentration of roughly 18 mM and an integral average of roughly 2.6 mM, a reasonable target for producing anticancer effects.

Peroxide-Based Cytotoxicity

Vitamin C, at normal physiological concentrations (0.1 mM), is a major water-soluble antioxidant (Geeraert, 2012). At concentrations on the order of 1 mM, however, continuous perfusion of ascorbate at doses that trigger "redox cycling" can cause a build-up of hydrogen peroxide, which is preferentially toxic toward tumor cells (Benade, et al., 1969; Riordan, et al., 1995; Casciari, et al., 2001;

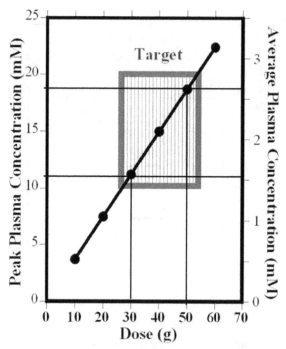

FIGURE 5. Target IVC dose based on attaining a high enough integral average ascorbate concentration (24 hr) for anticancer effects.

Chen, et al., 2005; Frei & Lawson, 2008), often leading to autophagy or apoptosis. To examine this cytotoxic effect in a three-dimensional model, the RCRI employed hollow-fiber in vitro solid tumors (HFST). Figure 6 (right) shows a histological section of colon cancer cells growing in this configuration. Dual staining annexin V and propidium iodide flow cytometry showed as significant increase in apoptosis, along with decreased surviving fractions, at ascorbate concentrations in the 1 mM to 10 mM range. Ascorbate concentrations required for toxicity in the HFST model (LC50 = 20 mM), with only two days incubation, were much higher than those typically observed in cell monolayers. The cytotoxic threshold could be reduced significantly (LC50 = 4 mM) by using ascorbate in combination with alpha-lipoic acid. Other reports suggest that ascorbate cytotoxicity against cancer cells can be increased by using it in combination with

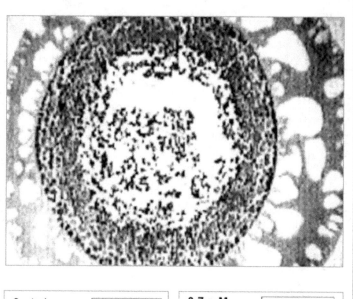

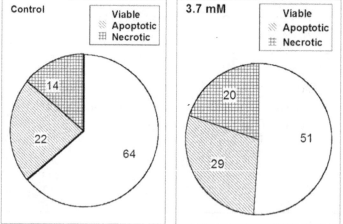

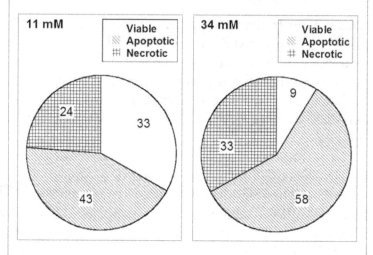

FIGURE 6. Histological cross section of an SW620 hollow fiber tumor (HFST) along with viable, apoptotic, and necrotic fractions after 2 days ascorbate treatment. Invalid source specified.

menadione (Verrax, et al., 2004) or copper containing compounds (Gonzalez, et al., 2002).

Studies from many laboratories in a variety of animal models, using hepatoma, pancreatic cancer, colon cancer, sarcoma, leukemia, prostate cancer, and mesothelioma, confirm that ascorbate concentrations sufficient for its cytotoxicity can be attained in vivo, and that treatments can reduce tumor growth (Chen, et al., 2008; Verrax & Calderon, 2009; Belin, et al., 2009; Yeom, et al., 2009; Du, et al., 2010; Pollard, et al., 2010). Figure 7 (right) shows data using the L-10 model in guinea pigs. L-10 tumor cells implanted subcutaneously metastasize to the lymph nodes. The overall tumor burden (primary plus metastases) was then determined after 30 days of tumor growth and 18 days of ascorbate therapy. Note that here the actual intra-tumor ascorbate concentrations were measured, and the correlation between tumor mass and tumor ascorbate concentration is strong regardless of the mode of ascorbate administration. The precentage of tumor growth inhibition, relative to controls, was roughly 50% at intra-tumor ascorbate concentrations of 1 mM tumor and roughly 65% once the intra-tumor ascorbate level went above 2 mM. The ascorbate dosage used in this study was 500 mg/kg/day. Our scientists also looked at survival times of BALP/C mice with S180 sarcomas. The results are shown in Figure 8 (right). The median survival time for the untreated mice was 35.7 days post implantation, while that for ascorbate treated mice (700 mg/kg/day) was 50.7 days. Of course, the efficacy observed in these animal studies may be due to some combination of direct cytotoxicity and other factors, such as angiogenesis inhibition (Yeom, et al., 2009) or other biological response modifications (Cameron, et al., 1979).

Angiogenesis Inhibition

Tumor angiogenesis is the process of new blood vessel growth toward and into a tumor. It is considered to be critical in tumor growth and metastasis. Reports in the literature suggest that ascorbate's effect on collagen synthesis can act to inhibit formation of new vascular tubules (Ashino, et al., 2003), that ascorbate can inhibit genes necessary for angiogenesis (Berlin, et al., 2009), and that

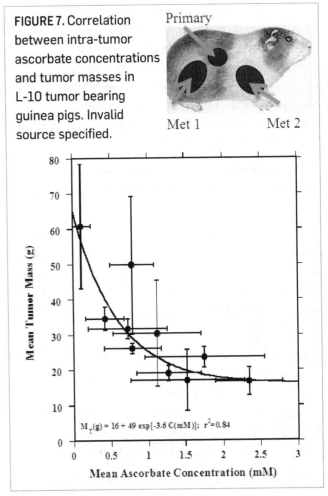

FIGURE 7. Correlation between intra-tumor ascorbate concentrations and tumor masses in L-10 tumor bearing guinea pigs. Invalid source specified.

$$M_T(g) = 16 + 49 \exp[-3.6\ C(mM)];\quad r^2 = 0.84$$

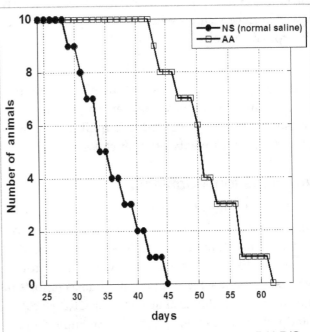

FIGURE 8. Survival time of sarcoma bearing BALP/C mice control and treated IP starting on day 12 with 700 mg/kg ascorbate.

it might influence angiogenesis through its effect on hypoxia inducable factor (Page, et al., 2007).

The Riordan Clinic researchers evaluated angiogenesis inhibition using four different experimental models. In all cases, there is an inhibitory effect on angiogenesis at ascorbate concentrations of 1 to 10 mM (Mikirova, et al., 2008; Mikirova, et al, 2012; see Figures 9A and 9B right).

• The growth of new micro-vessels from aortic rings ex vivo is inhibited by ascorbate at concentrations of 5 mM of more.

• Ascorbate inhibits endothelial cell tubule formation in Matrigel in vitro in a concentration-dependent fashion. Number of intact tubule loops was decreased by half at concentrations of 11 mM for endothelial progenitor cells and 17 mM for HUVEC cells.

• The rate at which endothelial cells can migrate on a petri dish to fill a gap between them was reduced when 5.7 mM ascorbate was added after the gap was created. The ascorbate also reduced ATP production in these endothelial cells by 20 percent but did not affect cell viability.

• For Matrigel plugs implanted subcutaneously in mice, the micro-vessel density we significantly lower in mice treated with 430 mg/kg every other day for two weeks.

In animal experiments and clinical case studies where high ascorbate doses show efficacy against tumors, this benefit may represent therapeutic synergism due to both angiogenesis inhibition as well as to direct cytotoxicity or other causes.

Inflammation Modulation

Analysis of clinical data from the Riordan Clinic suggests that inflammation is an issue for cancer patients, and that it can be lessened during IVC therapy (Mikirova, et al., 2012). C-reactive protein was used as a marker of inflammation, as reports in the literature indicate that elevated CRP is correlated with poor patient prognosis (St. Sauver, et al., 2009). Over 60 percent of analyzed Riordan Clinic cancer patients had CRP levels above 10 mg/L prior to IVC therapy. In 76 ± 13% of these subjects, IVC

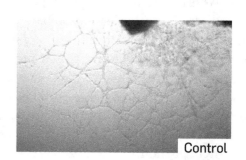
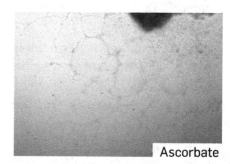

FIGURE 9A: Endothelial microvessel growth out of aortic rings: control versus ascorbate treated (5.7 mM, 4 days).

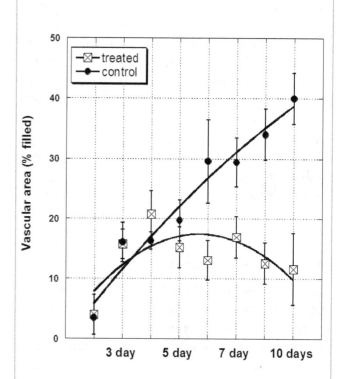

FIGURE 9B: Graph of vascular area near aortic ring as a function of time (Mikirova, et al., 2012).

reduced CRP levels. This improvement was more prevalent, 86 ± 13%, in subjects with elevated (above 10 mg/L) CRP. Comparisons of individual values before and after treatments are shown in Figure 10A (right).

Since many of the subjects in this database were prostate cancer patients, we examined prostate specific antigen (PSA) levels before and after therapy. This is shown in Figure 10B (right). Most of the prostate cancer patients showed reductions in PSA levels during the course of their IVC therapy. This was not true with other markers, as shown in Figure 10C (right). In some subjects, both tumor marker and CRP data were available both before and after IVC therapy. In those cases, there was a strong correlation (r2 = 0.62) between the change in tumor marker and the change in CRP during IVC therapy. This is consistent with observations from the literature showing a correlation between CRP levels and PSA levels in prostate cancer patients (Lin, et al., 2010).

The potential effect of IVC in reducing inflammation is also supported by cytokine data: serum concentrations of the pro-inflammatory cytokines IL-1α, IFN-γ, IL-8, IL-2, TNF-α and eotaxin were acutely reduced after a 50-gram ascorbate infusion, and in the case of the last three cytokines listed, reductions were maintained throughout the course of IVC therapy (Mikirova, et al., 2012).

Chemotherapy Controversy

The observations that ascorbate is an antioxidant and that it preferentially accumulates in tumors (Agus, et al., 1999) have raised fears that ascorbate supplementation would compromise the efficacy of chemotherapy (Raloff, 2000). In support of this, Heaney and coworkers found that tumor cells in vitro and xenografts in mice were more resistant to a variety of anticancer agents when the tumor cells were pretreated with dehydroascorbic acid (Heaney, et al., 2008). Questions have been raised, however, whether the experimental conditions used in the Heaney study are clinically or biochemically relevant, considering, among other issues, that dehydroascorbic acid rather than ascorbic acid was used (Espey, et al., 2009). It should also be noted that the goal of IVC is to attain mM intra-tumor concentrations (for the reasons described above) and thus the accumulation of ascorbate in tumors is considered an advantage.

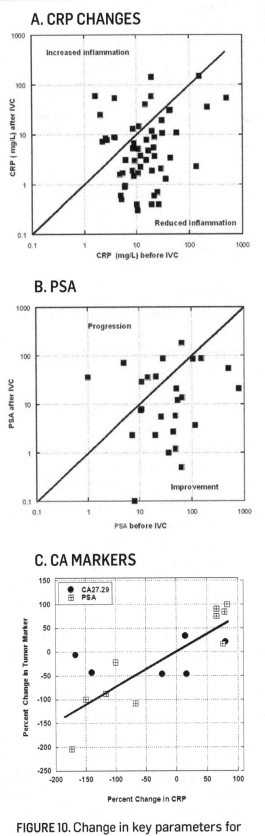

FIGURE 10. Change in key parameters for cancer patients at the Riordan Clinic after IVC therapy (Mikirova, et al., 2012)

A variety of laboratory studies suggest that, at high concentrations, ascorbate does not interfere with chemotherapy or irradiation and may enhance efficacy in some situations (Fujita, et al., 1982; Okunieff & Suit, 1987; Kurbacher, et al., 1996; Taper, et al., 1996; Fromberg, et al., 2011; Shinozaki, et al., 2011; Espey, et al., 2011). This is supported by meta-analyses of clinical studies involving cancer and vitamins; these studies conclude that antioxidant supplementation does not interfere with the toxicity of chemotherapeutic regimens (Simone, et al., 2007; Block, et al., 2008).

Clinical Data

Case Studies

The situation with intravenous ascorbate therapy is different from that with new chemotherapeutic agents in that Food and Drug Administration (FDA) approval was not strictly required in order for physicians to administer IVC. As a result, clinical investigations tended to run concurrently with laboratory research. Two early studies indicated that intravenous ascorbate therapy could increase survival times beyond expectations in cancer patients (Cameron & Pauling, 1976; Murata, et al., 1982). There have been several case studies published by the Riordan Clinic team (Jackson, et al., 1995; Riordan, et al., 1996; Riordan, et al., 1998) and collaborators (Drisko, et al., 2003; Padayatti, et al., 2006). While these case studies do not represent conclusive evidence in the same way that a well-designed Phase III study would, they are nonetheless of interest for comparing methodologies and motivating future research, in addition to being of monumental importance to the individuals who were their subjects. Some key case studies are summarized here:

A. A 51-year-old female with renal cell carcinoma (nuclear grade III/IV) and lung metastasis declined chemotherapy and instead chose to intravenous ascorbate at an initial dose of 15 grams. Her dose was increased to 65 grams after two weeks. She continued at this dose for ten months. Patient received no radiation or chemotherapy. The patient supplemented with thymus protein extract, N-acetylcysteine, niacinamide, beta-glucan, and thyroid extract. Seven

of eight lung masses resolved. Patient went four years without evidence of regression. Four years later, patient showed a new mass (consistent with small-cell lung cancer, not with recurrent renal carcinoma metastasis) and died shortly afterward (Padayatti, et al., 2006).

B. A 49-year-old male with a bladder tumor (invasive grade 3/3 papillary transitional cell carcinoma) and multiple satellite tumors declined chemotherapy and instead chose to receive intravenous ascorbate. He received 30 grams twice weekly for three months, followed by 30 grams monthly for four years. Patient supplementation included botanical extract, chondroitin sulfate, chromium picolinate, flax oil, glucosamine sulfate, alpha-lipoic acid, *lactobacillus acidophilus*, *L. rhamnosus*, and selenium. Nine years after the onset of therapy, patient is in good health with no signs of recurrence or metastasis (Padayatti, et al., 2006).

C. A 66-year-old woman with diffuse Stage III large B-cell lymphoma with a brisk mitotic rate and large left paraspinal mass (3.5–7 cm transverse and 11 cm craniocaudal) showing evidence of bone invasion agreed to a five-week course of radiation therapy but refused chemotherapy and instead chose to receive intravenous ascorbate concurrent with radiation. She received 15 grams twice weekly for two months, once per week for seven months, and then once every two–three months for one year. Patient supplementation included coenzyme Q10, magnesium, beta-carotene, parasidal, vitamin B and C supplements, Parex, and N-acetylcysteine. The original mass remained palpable after radiation therapy and a new mass appeared. Vitamin C therapy continued. Six weeks later, masses were not palpable. A new lymph mass was detected after four months, but the patient showed no clinical signs of lymphoma after one year. Ten years diagnosis, the patient remained in normal health (Padayatti, et al., 2006).

D. A 55-year-old woman with stage IIIC papillary adenocarcinoma of the ovary and an initial CA-125 of 999 underwent surgery followed by six cycles of chemotherapy (Paclitaxel, Paraplatin) combined with oral and parenteral ascorbate. Ascorbate infusion began at 15 grams twice weekly and increased to 60 grams twice weekly. Plasma ascorbate levels above 200 mg/dL were achieved during infusion. After six weeks, ascorbate treatment continued for one year, after which patient reduced infusions to once every two weeks. The patient also supplemented with vitamin E, coenzyme Q10, vitamin C, beta-carotene, and vitamin A. At the time of publication, she was over 40 months from initial diagnosis and remained on ascorbate infusions. All computed tomography (CT) and positron emission tomography (PET) scans were negative for disease, and her CA-125 levels remained normal (Drisko, et al., 2003).

E. A 60-year-old woman with stage IIIC adenocarcinoma of the ovary and an initial CA-125 of 81 underwent surgery followed by six cycles of chemotherapy (paclitaxel, carboplatin) with oral antioxidants. After six cycles of chemotherapy, patient began parenteral ascorbate infusions.

Ascorbate infusion began at 15 grams once weekly and increased to 60 grams twice weekly. Plasma ascorbate levels above 200 mg/dL were achieved during infusion. Treatment continued to date of publication. The patient supplemented with vitamin E, coenzyme Q10, vitamin C, beta-carotene, and vitamin A. Her CA-125 levels normalized after one course of chemotherapy. After the first cycle of chemotherapy, the patient was noted to have residual disease in the pelvis. At this point, she opted for intravenous ascorbate. Thirty months later, patient showed no evidence of recurrent disease and her CA-125 levels remained normal.

Note that these case studies involve a variety of cancer types, sometimes involve the use of IVC in conjunction with chemotherapy or irradiation, and usually involve the use of other nutritional supplements by the subject.

FIGURE 11.
BUN, creatinine, uric acid, and glucose levels in patients as a function of time from the onset of therapy (days). Normal range limits are indicated by horizontal dotted lines, while the onset of treatment is indicated by a vertical dashed line. Data from the 20 patients with the longest treatment times were selected for each graph. Invalid source specified.

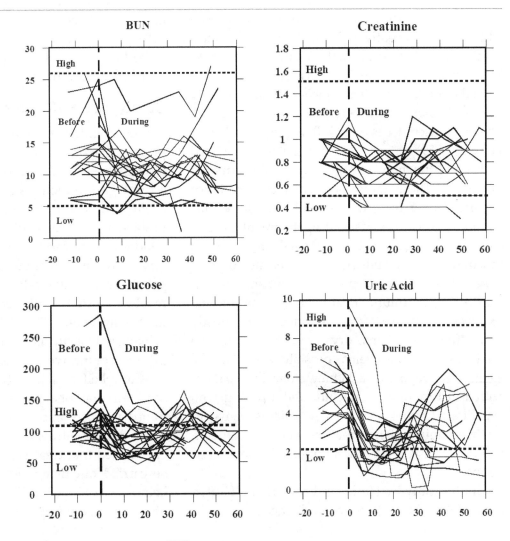

Several other clinical studies looked into the effect of vitamin C on quality of life in cancer patients. In a Korean study, IVC therapy significantly improved global quality of life scores, with benefits including less fatigue, reduction in nausea and vomiting, and improved appetite (Yeom, et al., 2007). In a recent German study, breast cancer patients receiving IVC along with standard therapy were compared to subjects receiving standard therapy alone (Vollbracht, et al., 2011). Patients given IVC benefited from less fatigue, reduction in nausea, improved appetite, reductions in depression and fewer sleep disorders. Overall intensity scores of symptoms during therapy and aftercare were twice as high in the control group as the IVC group. No side effects due to ascorbate were observed, nor were changes in tumor status compared to controls reported.

Phase I Clinical Trials

The safety of intravenous ascorbate has been addressed in recently published Phase I clinical studies (Riordan, et al., 2005; Hoffer, et al., 2008; Monti, et al., 2012). The first Phase I study was conducted with 24 terminal cancer patients (mostly liver and colorectal cancers) (Riordan, et al., 2005). The study used doses up to 710 mg/kg/day. Figure 11 (page 759) shows how parameters associated with renal function changed during the course of treatment. These indicators remained steady or decreased over time; this is significant since they would be expected to rise during treatment if ascorbate was having an acute detrimental effect on renal function. Blood chemistries suggested no compromise in renal function, and one patient showed stable disease, continuing treatment for an additional 48 weeks. Adverse effects reported were mostly minor (nausea, edema, dry mouth or skin). Two grade three adverse events "possibly related" to the agent were reported: a kidney stone in a patient with a history of renal calculus and a patient who experienced hypokalemia. These patients were generally vitamin C deficient at the start of treatment, and plasma ascorbate concentrations did not exceed 3.8 mM.

In the study by Hoffer and coworkers (Hoffer, et al., 2008), 24 subjects with advanced cancer or hematologic malignancy not amenable to standard therapy were given IVC at doses of 0.4 g/kg to 1.5 g/kg (equivalent to a range of 28 to 125 grams in a 70 kg adult) three times weekly. In this study, peak plasma concentrations in excess of 10 mM were obtained, and no serious side effects were reported. Subjects at higher doses maintained physical quality of life, but no objective anticancer response was reported. In the study by Monti and coworkers (Monti, et al., 2012), fourteen patients received IVC in addition to nucleoside analogue gemcitabine and the tyrosine-kinase inhibitor erlotinib. Observed adverse events were attributable to the chemotherapeutic agents, but not to the ascorbate, but no added efficacy due to the ascorbate was observed.

Thus far, Phase I studies indicate that IVC can be safely administered to terminal cancer patients at high doses (10 to 100 grams or more), but anticancer efficacy of the sort reported in case studies has not yet been observed. Of course, the terminal subjects used in Phase I studies would be expected to be the most difficult to treat. Phase II studies, with longer durations, are needed at this point.

Safety Issues Reported In Literature

Evidence indicates that patients who show no prior signs or history of renal malfunction are unlikely to suffer ill effects to their renal systems as a result of intravenous ascorbate (Riordan, et al., 2005). In cases where there are preexisting renal problems, however, caution is advised. In addition a kidney stone forming in one patient with a history of stone formation (Riordan, et al., 2005), a patient with bilateral urethral obstruction and renal insufficiency suffered acute oxalate neuropathy (Wong, et al., 1994). A full blood chemistry and urinalysis workup is thus recommended prior to the onset of intravenous ascorbate therapy.

Campbell and Jack (Campbell &. Jack, 1979) reported that one patient died due to massive tumor necrosis and hemorrhaging following an initial dose of intravenous ascorbate. It is thus recommended that treatment start at a low dose and be carried out using slow "drip" infusion. Fatal hemolysis can occur if a patient has glucose-6-phosphate dehydrogenase deficiency (G6PD). It is thus recommended that G6PD levels be assessed prior to the onset of therapy. The treatment is contraindicated in situations where increased fluids, sodium, or chelating may cause serious problems. These situations include congestive heart failure, edema, ascites, chronic hemodialysis, unusual iron overload, and inadequate hydration, or urine void volume (Rivers, 1987).

The Riordan IVC Protocol

Inclusion Criteria and Candidates

1. Candidates include those who have failed standard treatment regimens; those seeking to improve the effectiveness of their standard cancer therapy; those seeking to decrease the severity and carcinogenicity of side effects from standard cancer therapy; those attempting to prolong their remission with health-enhancing strategies; those declining standard treatment, yet wishing to pursue primary, alternative treatment.

2. Patient (guardian or legally recognized caregiver) must sign a consent-to-treat or release form for the IVC treatment. Patient should have no significant psychiatric disorder, end-stage congestive heart failure (CHF), or other uncontrolled comorbid conditions.

3. Obtain baseline and screening laboratory:

   a. Serum chemistry profile with electrolytes

   b. Complete blood count (CBC) with differential

   c. Red blood cell G6PD (must be normal)

   d. Complete urinalysis

4. In order to properly assess the patient's response to IVC therapy, obtain complete patient record information prior to beginning IVC therapy:

   a. Tumor type and staging, including operative reports, pathology reports, special procedure reports, and other staging information. (Re-staging may be necessary if relapse and symptom progression has occurred since diagnosis.)

   b. Appropriate tumor markers, CT, MRI, PET scans, bone scans, and x-ray imaging.

   c. Prior cancer treatments, the patient's response to each treatment type, including side effects.

   d. The patient's functional status with an Eastern Cooperative Oncology Group (ECOG) Performance Score.

   e. Patient weight.

Precautions and Side Effects

In the Riordan Clinic's experience giving over 40,000 onsite IVC treatments, the side effects of high-dose IVC are rare. However, there are precautions and potential side effects to consider.

1. The danger of diabetics on insulin incorrectly interpreting their glucometer finger stick has been found. It is important to notice to health-care workers using this protocol for the treatment of cancer in patients who are also diabetic: high-dose IVC at levels 15 grams and higher will cause a false positive on finger-stick blood glucose strips (electrochemical method) read on various glucometers (Jackson & Hunninghake, 2006). Depending on the dose, the false-positive glucose and occasionally "positive ketone" readings may last for eight hours after the infusion. Blood taken from a vein and run in a laboratory using the hexokinase serum glucose method is not affected! The electrochemical strip cannot distinguish between ascorbic acid and glucose at high levels. Oral vitamin C does not have this effect. Please alert any diabetic patients of this potential complication! Diabetics wishing to know their blood sugar must have blood drawn from a vein and run in the laboratory using the hexokinase glucose determination method.

2. Tumor necrosis or tumor lysis syndrome has been reported in one patient after high-dose IVC (Campbell & Jack, 1979). For this reason, the protocol always begins with a small 15 gram dose.

3. Acute oxalate nephropathy (kidney stones) was reported in one patient with renal insufficiency who received a 60 gram IVC. Adequate renal function, hydration, and urine voiding capacity must be documented prior to starting high-dose IVC therapy. In our experience, however, the incidence of calcium oxalate stones during or following IVC is negligible (Riordan, et al., 2005).

4. Hemolysis has been reported in patients with G6PD deficiency when given high-dose IVC (Campbell, et al., 1975). The G6PD level should be

assessed before beginning IVC. (At the Riordan Clinic, G6PD readings have yielded five cases of abnormally low levels. Subsequent IVC at 25 grams or less showed no hemolysis or adverse effects.)

5. IV-site irritation may occur at the infusion site when given in a vein and not a port. This can be caused by an infusion rate exceeding 1.0 gram/minute. The protocol suggests adding magnesium to reduce the incidence of vein irritation and spasm.

6. Due to the chelating effect of IVC, some patients may complain of shakiness due to low calcium or magnesium. An additional 1.0 mL of MgCl added to the IVC solution will usually resolve this. If severe, it can be treated with an IV push of 10 mLs of calcium gluconate, 1.0 mL per minute.

7. Eating before the IVC infusion is recommended to help reduce blood sugar fluctuations.

8. Given the amount of fluid used as a vehicle for the IVC, any condition that could be adversely affected by fluid or sodium overload (the IV ascorbate is buffered with sodium hydroxide and bicarbonate) is a relative contraindication (i.e. congestive heart failure, ascites, edema, etc.).

9. There have been some reports of iron overload with vitamin C therapy. We have treated one patient with hemochromatosis with high-dose IVC with no adverse effects or significant changes in the iron status.

10. As with any IV infusion, infiltration at the site is possible. This is usually not a problem with ports. Our nursing staff has found that using #23 butterfly needles with a shallow insertion is very reliable with rare infiltrations (depending upon the status of the patient's veins!).

11. IVC should only be given by slow intravenous drip at a rate of 0.5 grams per minute. (Rates up to 1.0 gram/minute are generally tolerable, but close observation is warranted. Patients can develop nausea, shakes, and chills.)

12. It should never be given as an IV push, as the osmolality at high doses may cause sclerosing of peripheral veins, nor should it be given intramuscularly or subcutaneously. Table 1 lists the calculated osmolality of various amounts of fluid

TABLE 1. RECOMMENDED DILUTION AND OSMOLARITY

ASCORBATE MASS(G) —> VOL†(CC) († 500 MG/ML STOCK)	DILUTE	MOSM/L
15 g —> 30 cc	250 mL Ringers	909
25 g —> 50 cc	250 mL H$_2$O	600
50 g —> 100 cc	500 mL H$_2$O	1097
75 g —> 150 cc	750ml H$_2$O	1088
100 g —> 200 cc	1000 ml H$_2$O	1085

volume. Our experience has found that an osmolality of less than 1,200 milliosmole (mOsm)/kg H2O is tolerated by most patients. A low infusion rate (0.5 grams IVC per minute) also reduces the tonicity, although up to 1.0 grams per minute can be used in order to achieve higher post-IVC saturation levels. (Pre- and post-serum osmolality measurements are advisable at this dose.)

13. We presently use a sodium ascorbate solution, MEGA-C-PLUS®, 500 mg/mL, pH range 5.5–7.0 from Merit Pharmaceuticals, Los Angeles, CA, 90065.

Administration of IVC

Having taken all precautions listed above and having obtained informed consent from the patient, the administering physician begins with a series of three consecutive IVC infusions at the 15, 25, and 50 gram dosages followed by post-IVC plasma vitamin C levels in order to determine the oxidative burden for that patient so that subsequent IVCs can be optimally dosed.

The initial three infusions are monitored with post-IVC infusion plasma vitamin C levels. As noted in Table 2 (below), research and experience has shown that a therapeutic goal of reaching a peak-plasma concentration of ~20 mM (350–400 mg/dL) is most efficacious. (No increased toxicity for post-IVC plasma vitamin C levels up to 780 mg/dL has been observed.) The first post-IVC plasma level following the 15-gram IVC has been shown to be clinically instructive: levels below 100 mg/dL correlate with higher levels of existent oxidative stress, presumably from higher tumor burden, chemo/radiation damage, hidden infection, or other oxidative insult, such as smoking.

Following the first three IVCs, the patient can be scheduled to continue either a 25- or 50-gram IVC dose (doctor's discretion) twice a week until the post-IVC plasma level results are available from the lab. If the initial 50-gram post-IVC level did not reach the therapeutic range of 350–400 mg/dL, another post-IVC vitamin C level should be obtained after the next scheduled 50 gram IVC. If the therapeutic range is achieved, the patient is continued on a 50 gram twice a week IVC schedule with monthly post-IVC determinations to assure continued efficacy. If the therapeutic range is still not achieved, the IVC dosage is increased to 75 grams of vitamin C per infusion for four infusions, at which time a subsequent post-IVC plasma level is obtained. If the patient remains in a sub-therapeutic range, the IVC dosage is increased to the 100 gram level.

If after four infusions the post-IVC dosage remains sub-therapeutic, the patient may have an occult infection, may be secretly smoking, or may have tumor progression. While these possibilities are being addressed, the clinician can elect to increase the 100-gram IVC frequency to three times per week. Higher infusion doses beyond 100 grams are not recommended without serum osmo-lality testing before and after infusions in order to properly adjust the infusion rate to maintain a near physiologic osmolality range.

If higher dosages are not tolerated, or there is tumor progression in spite of achieving the therapeutic range, lower dosages can still augment the biological benefits of IVC, including enhanced immune response, reduction in pain, increased appetite, and a greater sense of well-being.

Very small patients, such as children, and very large obese patients need special dosing. Small patients [less than] 110 lbs. with small tumor burdens and without infection may only require 25-gram vitamin C infusions 2x/week to maintain therapeutic range. Large patients > 220 lbs. or patients with large tumor burdens or infection are more likely to require 100-grams IVC infusions 3x/week. Post-IVC plasma levels serve as an excellent clinical guide to this special dosing.

In our experience, the majority of cancer patients require 50-gram IVC infusions 2–3x/week to maintain therapeutic IVC plasma levels. All patients reaching therapeutic range should still be monitored monthly with post-IVC plasma levels to ensure that these levels are maintained long term. We advise patients to orally supplement with at least 4 grams

TABLE 2. SCIENTIFIC RATIONALE

TREATMENT VOLUME OF ASCORBIC ACID	SOLUTION VOLUME		WITHDRAW FROM SOLUTION AND DISCARD	REMAINING SOLUTION	INJECT VOLUME OF AA INTO SOLUTION	INJECT VOLUME OF MgCL2 INTO SOLUTION	FINAL VOLUME	INFUSION RATE	TOTAL INFUSION TIME
	RINGER LACTATE	STERILE WATER							
15 grams (30cc)	250 cc		31cc	219 cc	30 cc	1 cc	250 cc	0.5-1.0 g/min	~ 0.5 h
25grams (50cc)	500cc		51cc	449cc	50cc	1cc	500cc	0.5-1.0 g/min	~ 1 h
50 grams (100cc)		500cc	102cc	398 cc	100 cc	2cc	500cc	0.5-1.0 g/min	~ 1.5 h
75 grams (150cc)		750cc	152cc	598cc	150cc	2cc	750cc	0.5-1.0 g/min	~ 2.5 h
100grams		1000cc	202cc	798cc	200cc	2cc	1000cc	0.5-1.0 g/min	~ 3.5 h

of vitamin C daily, especially on the days when no infusions are given, to help prevent a possible vitamin C "rebound effect." Oral alpha lipoic acid is also recommended on a case by case basis.

CONCLUSIONS

Vitamin C can be safely administered by intravenous infusion at maximum doses of 100 grams or less, provided the precautions outlined in this report are taken. At these doses, peak plasma ascorbate concentrations can exceed 20 mM.

There are several potential benefits to giving IVC to cancer patients that make it an ideal adjunctive care choice:

• Cancer patients are often depleted of vitamin C, and IVC provides an efficient means of restoring tissue stores.

• IVC has been shown to improve quality of life in cancer patients by a variety of metrics.

• IVC reduces inflammation (as measured by C-reactive protein levels) and reduces the production of pro-inflammatory cytokines.

• At high concentrations, ascorbate is preferentially toxic to tumor cells and is an angiogenesis inhibitor.

The next key step in researching the use of IVC for cancer would be Phase II studies, some of which are currently underway. IVC may also have a variety of other applications, such as combating infections, treating rheumatoid arthritis, and treating ADHD and other mental illnesses where inflammation may play a role.

REFERENCES

Agus, D., Vera, J. & Golde, D., 1999. Stromal cell oxidation: a mechanism by which tumors obtain vitamin C. *Cancer Res.*, Volume 59, pp. 4555–4558.

Ashino, H. et al., 2003. Novel function of ascorbic acid as an angiostatic factor. *Angiogenesis*, Volume 6, pp. 259–269.

Belin, S. et al., 2009. Antiproliferative effect of ascorbic acid is associated with inhibition of genes necessary to cell cycle progression. *PLoS ONE*, Volume 4, p. e4409.

Benade, L., Howard, T. & Burk, D., 1969. Synergistic killing of Ehrlich ascites carcinoma cells by ascorbate and 3-amino-1,2,4-triazole. *Oncology*, Volume 23, pp. 33–43.

Berlin, S. et al., 2009. Antiproliferative effect of ascorbic acid is associated with inhibition of genes necessary for cell cycle progression. *PLoS ONE*, Volume 4, pp. E44–0.

Block, K. et al., 2008. Impact of antioxidant supplementaion on chemotherapeutic toxicity: a systematic review of the evidence from randomized controlled trials. *Int J Cancer*, Volume 123, pp. 1227–1239.

Cameron, E. & Pauling, L., 1976. Supplemental ascorbate in the supportive treatment of cancer: Prolongation of survival times in terminal human cancer. *PNAS USA*, Volume 73, pp. 3685–3689.

Cameron, E., Pauling, L. & Leibovitz, B., 1979. Ascorbic acid and cancer, a review. *Cancer Res*, Volume 39, pp. 663–681.

Campbell, A. & Jack, T., 1979. Acute reactions to mega ascorbic acid therapy in malignant disease. *Scott Med J*, Volume 24, p. 151.

Campbell, G., Steinberg, M. & Bower, J., 1975. Letter: ascorbic acid induced hemolysis in a G-6-PD deficiency.. *Ann Intern Med*, Volume 82, p. 810.

Casciari, J., Riordan, H., Miranda-Massari, J. & Gonzalez, M., 2005. Effects of high dose of ascorbate administration on L-10 tumor growth in guinea pigs. *PRHSJ*, Volume 24, pp. 145–150.

Casciari, J., Riordan, N. S. T. M. X., Jackson, J. & Riordan, H., 2001. Cytotoxicity of ascorbate, lipoic acid, and other antioxidants in hollow fibre in vitro tumours. *Br. J. Cancer*, Volume 84, pp. 1544–1550.

Chen, Q. et al., 2008. Pharmaologic doses of ascorbate act as a prooxidant and decrease growth of aggressive tumor xenografts in mice. *PNAS USA*, Volume 105, pp. 11105–11109.

Chen, Q. et al., 2005. Pharmacologic ascorbic acid concentrations selectively kill cancer cells: action as a pro-drug to deliver hydrogen peroxide to tissues. *PNAS USA*, Volume 205, pp. 13604–13609.

Creagan, E. et al., 1979. Failure of high-dose vitamin C (ascorbic acid) therapy to benefit patients with advanced cancer: A controlled trial. *NEJM*, Volume 301, pp. 687–690.

Drisko, J., Chapman, J. & Hunter, V., 2003. The use of antioxidants with first-line chemotherapy in two cases of ovarian cancer. *Am J Coll Nutr*, Volume 22, pp. 118–123.

Du, J. et al., 2010. Mechanisms of ascorbate-induced cytotoxicity in pancreatic cancer. *Clin Cancer Res*, Volume 16, pp. 509–520.

Espey, M. et al., 2011. Pharmacologic ascorbate synergizes with gemcitabine in preclinical models of pancreatic cancer. *Free Radic Biol Med*, Volume 50, pp. 1610–1619.

Espey, M., Chen, Q. & Levine, M., 2009. Comment re: vitamin C antagonizes the cytotoxic effects of chemotherapy. *Cancer Research*, Volume 69, p. 8830.

Frei, B. & Lawson, S., 2008. Vitamin C and cancer revisited. *PNAC USA*, Volume 105, pp. 11037–11038.

Fromberg, A. et al., 2011. Ascorbate exerts anti-proliferative effects through cell cycle inhibition and sensitizes tumor cells toward cytostatic drugs.. *Cancer Chemother Pharmacol*, Volume 67, pp. 1157–1166.

Fujita, K. et al., 1982. Reduction of adriamycin toxicity by ascorbate in mice and guinea pigs. *Cancer Res*, Volume 309–316, p. 42.

Geeraert, L., 2012. *CAM-Cancer Consortium. Intravenous high-*

dose vitamin C. [Online] Available at: www.cam-cancer.ort/CAM-Summaries/Other-CAM/Intravenous-high-dose-vitamin-C.

Ginter, E., Bobeck, P. & Vargova, D., 1979. Tissue levels and optimal dosage of vitamin C in guinea pigs.. *Nutr Metab,* Volume 27, pp. 217–226.

Gonzalez, M. et al., 2002. Inhibition of human breast cancer carcinoma cell proliferation by ascorbate and copper.. *PRHSJ,* Volume 21, pp. 21–23.

Heaney, M. et al., 2008. Vitamin C antagonizes the cytotoxic effects of antineoplastic drugs. *Cancer Res.,* Volume 68, pp. 8031–8038.

Henson, D., Block, G. & Levine, M., 1991. Ascorbic acid: biological functions and relation to cancer. *JNCI,* Volume 83, pp. 547–550.

Hoffer, L. et al., 208. Phase I clinical trial of i.v. ascorbic acid in advanced malignancy. *Ann Oncol,* Volume 1969–1974, p. 19.

Hoffman, F., 1985. Micronutrient requirements of cancer patients. *Cancer,* 55(Supl. 1), pp. 145–150.

Hornig, D., 1975. Distribution of ascorbic acid metabolites and analogues in man and animals. *Ann NY Acad Sci,* Volume 258, pp. 103–118.

Jackson, J. & Hunninghake, R., 2006. False positive blood glucose readings after high-dose intravenous vitamin C. *J Ortho Med,* Volume 21, pp. 188–190.

Jackson, J., Riordan, H., Hunninghauke, R. & Riordan, N., 1995. High dose intravenous vitamin C and long time survival of a patient with cancer of the head and pancreas. *J Ortho Med,* Volume 10, pp. 87–88.

Keith, M. & Pelletier, O., 1974. Ascorbic acid concentrations in leukocytes and selected organs of guinea pigs in response to increasing ascorbic acid intake. *Am J Clin Nutr,* Volume 27, pp. 368–372.

Kuether, C., Telford, I. & Roe, J., 1988. The relation of the blood level of ascorbic acid to tissue concentrations of this vitamin and the histology of the incisor teeth in the guinea pig. *J Nutrition,* Volume 28, pp. 347–358.

Kurbacher, C. et al., 1996. Ascorbic acid (vitamin C) improves the antineoplastic activity of doxorubicin, cisplatin, and paclitaxel in human breast carcinoma cells in vitro. *Cancer Lett,* Volume 103, pp. 183–189.

Levine, M. et al., 1996. Vitamin C pharmacokinetics in healthy volunteers: evidence for a recommended dietary allowance. *PNAS USA,* Volume 93, pp. 3704–3709.

Lin, A., Chen, K., Chung, H. & Chang, S., 2010. The significance of plasma C-reactive protein in patients with elevated serum prostate-specific antigen levels. *Urological Sci,* Volume 21, pp. 88–92.

Mayland, C., Bennett, M. & Allan, K., 2005. Vitamin C deficiency in cancer patients. *Palliat Med,* Volume 19, pp. 17–20.

McCormick, W., 1959. Cancer: a collagen disease, secondary to nutrition deficiency. *Arch. Pediatr.,* Volume 76, pp. 166–171.

Mikirova, N., Casciari, J. & Riordan, N., 2012. Ascorbate inhibition of angiogenesis in aortic rings ex vivo and subcutaneous Matrigel plugs in vivo. *J Angiogenesis Res,* Volume 2, pp. 2–6.

Mikirova, N., Casciari, J., Taylor, P. & Rogers, A., 2012. Effect of high-dose intravenous vitamin C on inflammation in cancer patients. *J Trans Med,* Volume 10, pp. 189–199.

Mikirova, N., Ichim, T. & Riordan, N., 2008. Anti-angiogenic effect of high doses of ascorbic acid.. *J Transl Med,* Volume 6, p. 50.

Mikirova, N., Rogers, A., Casciari, J. & Taylor, P., 2012. Effects of high dose intravenous ascorbic acid on the level of inflammation in patients with rheumatoid arthritis. *Mod Res Inflamm,* Volume 1, pp. 26–32.

Moertel, C. et al., 1985. High-dose vitamin C versus placebo in the treatment of patients with advanced cancer who have no prior chemotherapy: a randomized double-blind comparison. *NEJM,* Volume 312, pp. 137–141.

Monti, D. et al., 2012. Phase I evaluation of intravenous ascorbic acid in combination with gemcitabine and erlotinib in patients with metastatic pancreatic cancer. *PLoS One,* Volume 7, p. e29794.

Murata, A., Morishige, F. & Yamaguchi, H., 1982. Prolongation of survival times of terminal cancer patients by administration of large doses of ascorbate. *Int J Vitam Res Suppl,* Volume 23, pp. 103–113.

Okunieff, P. & Suit, H., 1987. Toxicity, radiation sensitivity modification, and combined drug effects of ascorbic acid with misonidazole in vivo on FSaII murine firbosarcomas. *JNCI,* Volume 79, pp. 377–381.

Padayatti, S. et al., 2006. Intravenous vitamin C as a cancer therapy: three cases. *CMAJ,* Volume 174, pp. 937–942.

Padayatty, S. & Levine, M., 2000. Reevaluation of ascorbate in cancer treatment: emerging evidence, open minds and serendipity. *J Am Coll Nutr.,* Volume 19, pp. 423–425.

Padayatty, S. et al., 2010. Vitamin C: intravenous use by complementary and alternative medical practitioners and adverse effects. *PLoS ONE,* Volume 5, p. 11414.

Padayatty, S. et al., 2004. Vitamin C pharmacokinetics: implications for oral and intravenous use. *Ann. Intern. Med.,* Volume 140, pp. 533–537.

Page, E. et al., 2007. Hypoxia incudible factor-1 (alpha) stabilization in nonhypoxic conditions: role of oxidation and intracellular ascorbate depletion. *Mol Biol Cell,* Volume 19, pp. 86–94.

Pollard, H., Levine, M., Eidelman, O. & Pollard, M., 2010. Pharmacological ascorbic acid supresses syngenic tumor growth and metastases in hormone-refractory prostate cancer. *In Vivo,* Volume 2012, pp. 249–255.

Raloff, J., 2000. Antioxidants may help cancers thrive. *Science News,* Volume 157, p. 5.

Riordan, H. et al., 2005. A pilot clinical study of continuous intravenous ascorbate in terminal cancer patients. *PR Health Sci J,* Volume 24, pp. 269–276.

Riordan, H. et al., 2003. Intravenous ascorbic acid: protocol for its application and use. *PR Health Sci. J.,* Volume 22, pp. 225–232.

Riordan, H., Jackson, J., Riordan, N. & Schultz, M., 1998. High-dose intravenous vitamin C in the treatment of a patient with renal cell carcinoma of the kidney. *J Ortho Med,* Volume 13, pp. 72–73.

Riordan, N., JA, J. & Riordan, H., 1996. Intravenous vitamin C in a terminal cancer patient. *J Ortho Med,* Volume 11, pp. 80–82.

Riordan, N., Roirdan, H. & Meng, X., 1995. Intravenous ascorbate as a tumor cytotoxic chemotherapeutic agent. *Med Hypotheses,* Volume 44, pp. 207–213.

Rivers, J., 1987. Safety of high-level vitamin C ingestion. In: Third Conference on Ascorbic Acid. *Ann NY Acad Sci,* Volume 489, pp. 95–102.

Shinozaki, K. et al., 2011. Ascorbic acid enhances radiation-induced apoptosis in an HL60 human leukemia cell line. *J Ratiat Res,* Volume 52, pp. 229–237.

Simone, C., Simone, N. S. V. & CB, S., 2007. Antioxidants and other nutrients do not inferfere with chemotherapy or radiation therapy and can increase survival, part 1. *Atlern Ther Health Med,* Volume 13, pp. 22–28.

St. Sauver, J. et al., 2009. Associations betweeen C-reactive protein and benigh prosaic hyperplasia lower urinary tract outcomes in a population based cohort. *Am J Epidemiol,* Volume 169, pp. 1281–1290.

Taper, H., Keyeux, A. & Roberfroid, M., 1996. Potentiation of radiotherapy by nontoxic pretreatment with combined vitamins C and K3 in mice bearing solid transplantable tumor. *Anticancer Res,* Volume 16, pp. 499–503.

Verrax, J. et al., 2004. Ascorbate potentiates the cytotoxicity of menadione leading to an oxidative stress that kills cancer cells by a non-apoptotic capsase-3 independent form of cell death. *Apoptosis,* Volume 9, pp. 223–233.

Verrax, J. & Calderon, P., 2009. Pharmacologic concentrations of ascorbate are achieved by parenteral administration and exhibit antitumoral effects. *Free Radic Biol Med,* Volume 47, pp. 32–40.

Vollbracht, C. et al., 2011. Intravenous vitamin C administration improves quality of life in breast cancer patients during chemo-radiotherapy and aftercare: results of a retrospective, multicentre, epidemiological cohort study in Germany. *In Vivo,* Volume 82, pp. 983–990.

Wong, K. et al., 1994. Acute oxalate nephropathy after a massive intravenous dose of vitamin C. *Aust ZN J Med,* Volume 24, pp. 410–411.

Yeom, C., Jung, G. & Song, K., 2007. Changes of terminal cancer patients health-related quality of life after high dose vitamin C administration. *Korean Med Sci,* Volume 22, pp. 7–11.

Yeom, C. et al., 2009. High-dose concentration administration of ascorbic acid inhibits tumor growth in BALB/C mice implanted with sarcoma 180 cancer cells via the restriction of angiogenesis. *J Transl Med,* Volume 7, p. 70.

APPENDIX 4

RADIATION INJURY TREATMENT PROTOCOL
by Atsuo Yanagisawa, MD, Masashi Uwabu, MD, Burton E. Burkson, MD, Bradford S. Weeks, MD, Ronald Hunninghake, MD, Steven Hickey, PhD, and Thomas Levy, MD

JCIT PROTOCOL FOR PROTECTING AGAINST RADIATION-INDUCED INJURY

Recommendation 1. If environmental radioactivity becomes twofold higher than usual, women of childbearing age should take the following antioxidant supplements to keep optimal antioxidant reserve

SUPPLEMENT	DOSAGE
Vitamin C or Liposomal vitamin C	1,000–2,000 mg or 1,000 mg, 3–4 times daily or 2 times daily
Alpha-lipoic acid	100–200 mg, 2 times daily
Selenium	50–100 mcg, 2 times daily
Vitamin E	100–200 mg, 2 times daily

Plus other essential vitamins and minerals

Recommendation 2. If environmental radioactivity levels becomes more than fivefold higher than usual, people of all ages should take the following antioxidant supplements to keep maximum antioxidant reserve

Vitamin C or Liposomal vitamin C	2,000–3,000 mg or 1,000 mg, 3–4 times daily or 2 times daily
Alpha-lipoic acid	300 mg, 2 times daily
Selenium	200 mcg, 2 times daily
Vitamin E	200 mg, 2 times daily

Plus other essential vitamins and minerals

Recommendation 3. Dietary supplements to protect against radiation injury among workers in contaminated areas

Intravenous Vitamin C, containing sterile water (250 mL), 50% vitamin C (50mL), 20% Mg-chloride (5mL), B-complex 100 (1mL), 10% B6 (1mL), 1% B12 (1mL), and 25% dexpanthenol (1mL)	25,000 mg, administered before- and post-exposure
Liposomal Vitamin C	2,000 mg, 3 times daily
Alpha-lipoic acid	300 mg, 2 times daily
Selenium	200 mcg, 2 times daily
Vitamin E	200 mg, 2 times daily

Plus other essential vitamins and minerals

For more information, contact:
Japanese College of Intravenous Therapy (JCIT)
3–17–19–701 Shirokane, Minat-ku, Tokyo 108–0072
Phone: +81–3–6277–3318 Fax: +81–3–6277–4004
Email: info @iv-therapy.jp
Website: www.iv-therapy.jp

For Further Reading

Books on Nutrients

As *The Orthomolecular Treatment of Chronic Disease* does not contain a specific Nutrients section, we are providing this list of books that discuss nutrients in considerable detail. We also offer some comment. Omission from this list does not imply disapproval. These are the editor's recommendations and, in many cases, are books the editor has reviewed in the *Journal of Orthomolecular Medicine* (*JOM*). By way of disclaimer, we wish to state up front that a number of the most recent books in this list are published by Basic Health Publications, the publisher of the present volume. Some other titles are decades old but are historically important and still relevant today; we also include other recent works. Your personal investigation is encouraged to let the works speak for themselves.

Comprehensive Books

Gaby, Alan. *Nutritional Medicine*. Concord, NH: Fritz Perlberg, 2011. A recent major textbook providing thorough treatment of the subject expertly written by an orthomolecular medical doctor. This is a large and expensive volume, and for most readers may be more appropriate for library loan than for outright purchase.

Hoffer, Abram, and Andrew W. Saul. *Orthomolecular Medicine for Everyone: Megavitamin Therapeutics for Families and Physicians*. Laguna Beach, CA: Basic Health Publications, 2008. This book is an updated, expanded version of Dr. Hoffer's 1989 textbook *Orthomolecular Medicine for Physicians*, which has been out of print for some years.

Hoffer, Abram, and Jonathan Prousky. *Naturopathic Nutrition: A Guide to Nutrient-Rich Food & Nutritional Supplements for Optimum Health*. Toronto, ON: CCNM Press, 2006. Reviewed in *J Orthomolecular Med* 2007;22(1):52–53.

Hoffer, Abram, and Linus Pauling. *Healing Cancer: Complementary Vitamin & Drug Treatments*. Toronto, ON: CCNM Press, 2004. Patients on a strong nutritional program have far less nausea, and often experience little or no hair loss during chemotherapy. They experience reduced pain and swelling following radiation and have faster, uncomplicated healing after surgery. Supplements make a most positive contribution to the conventional treatment of cancer. Reviewed in *J Orthomolecular Med* 2007;22(2):93–94.

Murray, Michael T., and Joseph Pizzorno. *The Encyclopedia of Natural Medicine*. 3rd ed. New York: Atria Books, 2012.

Pauling, Linus. *How to Live Longer and Feel Better*. Rev. ed. Corvallis, OR: Oregon State University Press, 2006. Distilling thirty pages of references into logical, commonsense advice, Dr. Pauling covers vitamins and cancer, heart disease, aging, infectious diseases, vitamin safety, toxicity and side effects, medicines, doctors attitudes, nutrition history, vitamin biochemistry, and more—perhaps the strongest presentation ever written on the need for supplemental vitamins.

Werbach, Melvyn R. *Nutritional Influences on Illness*. 2nd ed. Tarzana, CA: Third Line Press, 1996, and *Textbook of Nutritional Medicine*, also published by Third Line Press, 1999. Both these books summarize thousands of nutritional studies, each in one expert paragraph or less. Both positive and negative findings are reported, earning this book the respect of almost all practitioners, both traditional and alternative. Organization is logical and simple: alphabetically by illness, followed by a listing of specific nutritional treatment recommendations for that illness.

CLASSICS OF ORTHOMOLECULAR MEDICINE

Cheraskin, Emanuel. *The Vitamin C Controversy: Questions and Answers.* Wichita, KS: Biocommunciations Press, 1988. Reviewed in *Townsend Letter for Doctors and Patients* 2001;217:142.

Cheraskin, Emanuel, and William M. Ringsdorf. *New Hope for Incurable Diseases.* New York: Exposition Press, 1971.

Cheraskin, Emanuel, and William M. Ringsdorf. *Psychodietetics* New York: Bantam Books, 1974. One of the most persuasive and readable books on megavitamin therapy for emotional illness. The authors put forward surprisingly effective cures for drug dependency, mental illness, senility, depression, anxiety, hyperactivity in children, alcoholism, and other ailments, supported by case histories and 290 medical references.

Cheraskin Emanuel, William M. Ringsdorf, and Emily Sisley. *The Vitamin C Connection: Getting Well and Staying Well with Vitamin C.* New York: Harpercollins, 1983.

Cleave, T. L. *The Saccharine Disease.* 2nd ed. New Canaan, CT: Keats Publishing, 1975. This book has nothing to do with the artificial sweetener known as saccharin. *The Saccharine Disease* refers to excess sugar consumption as a key cause of chronic disease in our time. Dr. Cleave, formerly a Surgeon Captain of the British Royal Navy, ascribes colitis, peptic ulcer, varicose veins, coronary heart disease, and diabetes to excess intake of simple carbohydrates.

Gerson, Max. *A Cancer Therapy: Results of Fifty Cases and the Cure of Advanced Cancer by Diet Therapy.* 6th ed. San Diego, CA: Gerson Institute, 2002.

Hawkins, David, and Linus Pauling. *Orthomolecular Psychiatry.* San Francisco: W.H. Freeman, 1973. Thirty-seven contributing authors in 30 articles provide abundant scientific basis for aggressive use of orthomolecular nutrition therapy, especially in psychosis. Complete, from case histories to biochemical mechanisms, *Orthomolecular Psychiatry* and its many hundreds of included references firmly establish very-high-dose vitamin therapy as the treatment of choice for schizophrenia, dementia, depression, obsessive-compulsive disorder, and related illnesses.

Hippchen, Leonard J. *Holistic Approaches to Offender Rehabilitation.* Springfield, IL: C.C. Thomas, 1982.

Hoffer, Abram. *Adventures in Psychiatry: The Scientific Memoirs of Abram Hoffer.* Alton, ON, Canada: KOS Publishing, 2005.

Hoffer, Abram and Humphry Osmond. *How to Live with Schizophrenia.* Rev ed. New York: Citadel Press, 1992.

Hoffer, Abram, and Morton Walker. *Orthomolecular Nutrition.* New Canaan, CT: Keats Publishing, 1978. A nontechnical book that capably guides the reader through discussions on hypoglycemia and sugar overconsumption, (saccharine disease), psychosomatic conditions, the failures of psychiatry, and many more topics.

Huemer, Richard P. *The Roots of Molecular Medicine: A Tribute to Linus Pauling.* New York: W.H. Freeman, 1986.

Illich, Ivan. *Limits to Medicine: Medical Nemesis, the Expropriation of Health.* Rev. ed. London: Marion Boyars Publishers, 1999. Illich speaks of doctors as "medical clergy" and their activities as disease-producing: iatrogenic. This means that the medical monopoly is making us sick. Illich provides solutions as well as enumerating problems.

Kaufman, William. (1943) *Common Forms of Niacinamide Deficiency Disease: Aniacin Amidosis.* New Haven, CT: Yale University Press. Very rare; interlibrary loan might be able to obtain one.

Kaufman, William. *The Common Form of Joint Dysfunction: Its Incidence and Treatment.* Brattleboro, VT: E.L. Hildreth & Co, 1949. Rare book.

Parsons, William B. *Cholesterol Control without Diet! The Niacin Solution.* Scottsdale, AZ: Lilac Press, 1998. This is the story of how the Mayo Clinic confirmed that niacin is the best way to lower LDL and triglycerides, and raise HDL.

Passwater, Richard. *Cancer and Its Nutritional Therapies.* New Canaan, CT: Keats Publishing, 1978.

Passwater, Richard. *The New Super-Nutrition.* Rev. ed. New York: Pocket Books, 1991. In this book, you learn how to find out, through guided experience, what amounts of vitamins you personally need to take for optimum health. No one prescriptive list is given; no "one-size-fits-all" approach is offered. Rather, Passwater builds a careful and documented case for megavitamin therapy and then shows how to increase your own vitamin intake until subjective and objective tests (which are described) show peak health has been reached.

Pauling, Linus. *Vitamin C, the Common Cold, and the Flu.* San Francisco: W.H. Freeman, 1976. An expansion of Pauling's *Vitamin C and the Common Cold* (1970). Pauling reexamined studies that originally concluded that vitamin C was of no benefit and showed that the authors failed to catch the statistical significance of their own work. Pauling also shows that animals, especially those most closely related to humans, either eat or make between 1,750 and 10,000 milligrams per human body weight per day. Even the U.S. government's Subcommittee on Animal Nutrition thinks that monkeys need a human body weight equivalent of 1,750 to 3,500 mg of vitamin C every day.

Pfeiffer, Carl C. *Mental Illness and Schizophrenia: The Nutrition Connection*. London: Thorsons Publishers, 1987.

Price, Weston A. *Nutrition and Physical Degeneration*. La Mesa, CA: Price-Pottenger Foundation, 1945. Dr. Weston Price traveled extensively back in the 1930s and studied firsthand the remote communities in Peru, Australia, coastal Scotland, Canada, Polynesia, Africa, New Zealand, and Alaska. After examining thousands of sets of teeth, he found perfect tooth and jaw development was the rule in native peoples, or at least until they started to eat "modern" foods such as white bread, sugar, and overcooked vegetables. Once they were "civilized," the native races began to suffer from a full array of diseases due, not to germs, but to diet.

Reed, Barbara. *Food, Teens and Behavior*. Manitowoc, WI: Natural Press, 1983. A parole officer who required a no-junk diet from her parolees speaks out about its success. Hard to find, but worth the search.

Riordan, Hugh D. *Medical Mavericks*. Wichita, KS: Biocommunications Press, Vol. 1 (1988); Vol. 2 (1989); Vol. 3 (1995). Review of Vol. 3 in the *J Orthomolecular Med* 2005;20(3):214–215.

Williams, Roger J. *Alcoholism: The Nutritional Approach*. Austin, TX: University of Texas Press, 1959.

Williams, Roger J. *Biochemical Individuality: The Basis for the Genetotrophic Concept*. Rev. ed. Austin, TX: University of Texas Press, 1973.

Williams, Roger J. *Nutrition Against Disease*. Rev. ed. New York: Bantam Books, 1973.

Williams, Roger J. *Nutrition and Alcoholism*. Norman, OK: University of Oklahoma Press, 1951.

Williams, Roger J. *Physicians' Handbook of Nutritional Science*. Springfield, IL: Charles C. Thomas, 1975.

Williams, Roger J. *The Prevention of Alcoholism Through Nutrition*. New York: Bantam Books, 1981.

Williams, Roger J. *The Wonderful World Within You*. 3rd ed. Wichita, KS: Biocommunciations Press, 1998.

Williams, Roger J., and Dwight K. Kalita. *A Physician's Handbook on Orthomolecular Medicine*. New Canaan,

CT: Keats Publishing, 1979. Here is presented an excellent collection of 29 papers by a variety of top nutritional physicians, including Abram Hoffer, Wilfrid Shute, Allan Cott, Carl Pfeiffer, Emanuel Cheraskin, and others. Editor R. J. Williams added to his already highly distinguished career by bringing great articles together, and several of the best are by him. Though aimed at physicians, there is every reason for everyone to obtain, and carefully read, a copy of this invaluable book.

"When you pick up a health or nutrition book and need to know really fast if it is any good or not, just check the index for 'Klenner' and three other key names: Cathcart, Stone, and Pauling. Robert F. Cathcart, an orthopedic surgeon, administered huge doses of vitamin C to tens of thousands of patients for decades, without generating a single kidney stone. Irwin Stone, the biochemist who first put Linus Pauling onto vitamin C, is the author of The Healing Factor: Vitamin C Against Disease. *Pauling cites Stone 13 times in his landmark book* How to Live Longer and Feel Better, *a recommendation if there ever was one. The importance of vitamin C's power against infectious and chronic disease is extraordinary. To me, omitting it is tantamount to deleting Shakespeare from an English Lit course."* —A.W.S.

BOOKS ON INDIVIDUAL NUTRIENTS

Vitamin A

There are strikingly few popular books on vitamin A. The general texts mentioned above are good references on this nutrient, along with the *User's Guide to Nutritional Supplements* (Basic Health Publications, 2003) by Jack Challem and the much shorter *User's Guide to Vitamins & Minerals* by Jack Challem and Liz Brown (Basic Health Publications, 2002).

Books on vegetable juicing are also relevant, as vegetable juices provide large amounts of carotene vitamin A precursor. One example among many is *Vegetable Juicing for Everyone* by Andrew W Saul and Helen Saul Case (Basic Health Publications, 2013).

B-Complex Vitamins

Aledjam, Henrietta. *The Sun Is My Enemy.* Boston, MA: Beacon Press, 1976. Niacin recovery from lupus.

Berkson, Burt, and Arthur J. Berkson. *User's Guide to B-Complex Vitamins.* Laguna Beach, CA: Basic Health Publications, 2005.

Carpenter, Kenneth J. *Beriberi, White Rice, and Vitamin B: A Disease, a Cause, and a Cure.* Berkeley and Los Angeles, CA: University of California Press, 2000.

Ellis, John M. *Free of Pain.* Dallas, TX: Southwest Publishing, 1983. An entire book on vitamin B6 (pyridoxine).

Ellis, John M., and James Presley. *Vitamin B6: The Doctor's Report.* New York: Harper & Row, 1973.

Ellis, John M., and Jean Pamplin. *Vitamin B6 Therapy: Nature's Versatile Healer.* New York: Avery Publishing, 1998.

Harrell, Ruth Flinn. Effect of Added Thiamine on Learning. Dissertation. New York: Bureau of Publications, Teachers College, Columbia University, 1943. Series: Contributions to education, no. 877.

Harrell, Ruth Flinn. Further Effects of Added Thiamin on Learning and Other Processes. New York: Bureau of Publications, Teachers College, Columbia University, 1947. Series: Contributions to education, no. 928.

Lonsdale, Derrick. *A Nutritional Guide to the Clinical Use of Vitamin B1.* Tacoma, WA: Life Sciences Press, 1988.

Hoffer, Abram. *Healing Children's Attention & Behavior Disorders: Complementary Nutritional and Psychological Treatments.* Toronto, ON: CCNM Press, 2004. Reviewed in *J Orthomolecular Med* 2006;21(4)229–230.

Hoffer, Abram. *Healing Schizophrenia: Complementary Vitamin & Drug Treatments.* Toronto, ON: CCNM Press, 2004. For a review, see *J Orthomolecular Med* 2006;21(1):59–60.

Hoffer, Abram. *Niacin Therapy in Psychiatry.* Springfield, IL: Charles S. Thomas, 1962.

Hoffer, Abram, and Linus Pauling. *Healing Cancer: Complementary Vitamin & Drug Treatments.* Toronto, ON: CCNM Press, 2004. Reviewed in *J Orthomolecular Med* 2007;22(2):93–94.

Hoffer, Abram, Andrew W. Saul, and Harold D. Foster. *Niacin: The Real Story.* Laguna Beach, CA: Basic Health Publications, 2012.

Pacholok, Sally M. *Could It Be* B12? *An Epidemic of Misdiagnoses.* 2nd ed. Fresno, CA: Linden Publishing, 2011.

Vonnegut, Mark. *Eden Express.* New York: Seven Stories Press, 2002. Niacin recovery from schizophrenia.

THE PIONEERING ORTHOMOLECULAR PUBLISHER

Nathan Keats, President of Keats Publishing, Inc., died February 3, 1995. His wife, An Keats, had preceded him in 1989. Both were pioneers in publishing a large variety of books dealing with the latest advances in orthomolecular medicine, in clinical ecology, and in nutrition. Their books provided one of the main literature bases for this new field in medicine. Almost every pioneer in the new medicine is represented among their stable of authors. Many of the more than 600 books that Keats has published were reviewed in the *Journal of Orthomolecular Medicine* over the decades, and most of the books reviewed occupy a prominent place in my personal library. The Keats' were my friends and colleagues, and they published the very books that any rapidly developing field must have. The Keats books were most helpful in changing the old and no longer useful vitamins-as-prevention paradigm, to the modern vitamins-as-treatment paradigm, which is sweeping into world mainstream medicine and at last into the medical schools of North America.

—ABRAM HOFFER

Vitamin C

Cameron, Ewan, and Linus Pauling. *Cancer and Vitamin C.* Rev. ed. Philadelphia: Camino Books, 1993. Now regarded as a classic of controversy, Cameron and Pauling's trail-blazing studies of megavitamin C therapy offer both education and hope in complementary cancer treatment. The book discusses successful vitamin C trials in Scotland, specific facts on vitamin C as an anticancer agent, and contains Dr. Cameron's instructions on administration of the vitamin, including dosage specifics.

Cass, Hyla. *User's Guide to Vitamin C.* Laguna Beach, CA: Basic Health Publications, 2002.

Cheraskin, Emanuel, William M. Ringsdorf, and Emily L. Sisley. *The Vitamin C Connection: Getting Well and Staying Well with Vitamin C.* New York: Harper & Row, 1983. An excellent guide to vitamin C therapy. Studies not supporting vitamin C are also included and thoroughly debunks many commonly held misconceptions about this versatile, safe, and effective vitamin.

Hickey, Steve, and Hilary Roberts. *Ascorbate: The Science of Vitamin C.* Morrisville, NC: Lulu Press, 2004. This book contains 575 references and is reviewed at www.doctoryourself.com/ascorbate.html.

Hickey, Steve, and Andrew W. Saul. *Vitamin C: The Real Story.* Laguna Beach, CA: Basic Health Publications, 2008. This book contains 387 references and is reviewed at www.doctoryourself.com/realstory.html.

Hickey, Steve, and Andrew W. Saul. *Vitamin C: The Real Story.* Laguna Beach, CA: Basic Health Publications, 2008.

Hickey, Steve, and Hilary Roberts. *Ascorbate: The Science of Vitamin C.* Morrisville, NC: Lulu Press, 2004.

Kalokerinos, Archie. *Every Second Child.* New Canaan, CT: Keats Publishing, 1981. A hard to find book.

Levy, Thomas E. *Curing the Incurable: Vitamin C, Infectious Diseases, and Toxins.* 3rd ed. West Greenwich, RI: Livon Books, 2009.

Levy, Thomas E. *Curing the Incurable: Vitamin C, Infectious Diseases, and Toxins.* 3rd ed. West Greenwich, RI: Livon Books, 2009.

Levy, Thomas E. *Stop America's #1 Killer: Reversible vitamin deficiency found to be the origin of all coronary heart disease.* West Greenwich, RI: Livon Books, 2006. (Dr. Levy is a board-certified cardiologist.) Reviewed in *J Orthomolecular Med* 2006;21(3):177–178. This book contains 60 pages of references.

Lewin, Sherry. *Vitamin C: Its Molecular Biology and Medical Potential.* Waltham, MA: Academic Press, 1976.

Smith, Lendon H. *Clinical Guide to the Use of Vitamin C: The Clinical Experiences of Frederick R. Klenner, M.D.* Tacoma, WA: Life Sciences Press, 1988. In just 57 pages, you can share a professional lifetime with one of the most innovative physicians of all time, Dr. Frederick Robert Klenner. He spent nearly 40 years successfully treating patients by administering enormous doses of vitamin C. "Vitamin C should be given to the patient while the doctors ponder the diagnosis," wrote Dr. Klenner. "I have never seen a patient that vitamin C would not benefit."

Stone, Irwin. *The Healing Factor: Vitamin C Against Disease.* New York: Grosset & Dunlap, 1972. It was Irwin Stone who first put Linus Pauling onto vitamin C. Stone thinks we humans have inherited a genetic trait to need but not manufacture the vitamin. Supported by over 50 pages of scientific references, learn about cures of infections (bacterial and viral), allergies, asthma, eye diseases, ulcers, poisoning, and the effects of smoking. Vitamin C's role in treating tetanus, glaucoma, cancer, heart disease, diabetes, fractures, shock, wounds, and pregnancy complications is also included. The complete text of Irwin Stone's book *The Healing Factor* is now posted for free reading at http://vitamincfoundation.org/stone.

Vitamin D

Holick, Michael, and Andrew Weil. *The Vitamin D Solution: A 3-Step Strategy to Cure Our Most Common Health Problems.* New York: Plume Publishing, 2011.

Keebler, Craig. *Know Your D: Optimizing Your Health With Vitamin D.* Mercer Island, WA: CreateSpace Publishing, 2010.

Madrid, Eric. *Vitamin D Prescription: The Healing Power of the Sun & How It Can Save Your Life.* Charleston, SC: BookSurge Publishing, 2009.

Mercola, Joseph, and Jeffry Herman. *Dark Deception: Discover the Truths About the Benefits of Sunlight Exposure.* Nashville, TN: Thomas Nelson, 2008.

Murray, Frank. *Sunshine and Vitamin D: A Comprehensive Guide to the Benefits of the "Sunshine Vitamin."* Basic Health Publications, 2008.

Rona, Zoltan. *Vitamin D: The Sunshine Vitamin.* Summertown, TN: Books Alive, 2013.

Vitamin E

Bailey, Herbert. *Vitamin E for a Healthy Heart and a Longer Life.* New York: Carroll & Graf, 1993.

Challem, Jack, and Melissa Block. *User's Guide to Antioxidant Supplements.* Laguna Beach, CA: Basic Health Publications, 2004.

Challem, Jack, and Melissa D. Smith. *User's Guide to Vitamin E.* Laguna Beach, CA: Basic Health Publications, 2002.

Shute, Evan. *Your Heart and Vitamin E.* London, Canada: Shute Foundation for Medical Research, 1961.

Shute, Wilfrid E. *The Complete Updated Vitamin E Book.* New Canaan, CT: Keats Publishing, 1975.

Shute, Wilfrid E. *Health Preserver: Defining the Versatility of Vitamin E.* Emmaus, PA: Rodale Press, 1977.

Shute, Wilfrid E. *Your Child and Vitamin E.* New Canaan, CT: Keats Publishing, 1979.

Shute, Wilfrid E., and Evan Shute. *Alpha Tocopherol (Vitamin E) in Cardiovascular Disease.* Toronto, ON: Ryerson Press, 1957.

Shute, Wilfrid E., with Harald J. Taub. *Vitamin E for Ailing and Healthy Hearts.* New York: Pyramid Books, 1969. Books written by Wilfrid E. Shute, MD, (or by his colleague and brother Evan) are the best reading there is on the therapeutic utility of vitamin E. The Shutes began vitamin E research in the late 1930s, and their books therefore encompass nearly 40 years of work. They remain the world's most experienced orthomolecular cardiologists, having treated tens of thousands of patients with vitamin E in high doses. This book succinctly presents dosages of E for angina, coronary occlusion, acute rheumatic fever, congenital heart diseases, thrombosis, and vascular disease. The Shutes enraged the medical profession by also successfully treating diabetes, kidney disease, ulcers, spontaneous abortion, menstrual problems, varicose veins, and burns.

Vitamin K

Rheaume-Bleue, Kate. *Vitamin K2 and the Calcium Paradox: How a Little-Known Vitamin Could Save Your Life.* New York: Harper, 2013. This vitamin is also discussed in most general books on nutrition.

MINERALS

Brownstein, David. *Iodine: Why You Need It, Why You Can't Live Without It.* 4th ed. West Bloomfield, MI: Medical Alternative Press, 2009.

Dean, Carolyn. *The Magnesium Miracle.* New York: Ballantine Books, 2006.

Fuchs, Nan Kathryn. *User's Guide to Calcium & Magnesium.* Laguna Beach, CA: Basic Health Publications, 2002.

Pfeiffer, Carl C. *Dr. Carl C. Pfeiffer's Updated Fact/Book on Zinc and Other Micro-Nutrients.* New Canaan, CT: Keats Publishing, 1978.

Pfeiffer, Carl C. *Mental and Elemental Nutrients.* New Canaan, CT: Keats Publishing, 1976.

Smith, Melissa D. *User's Guide to Chromium.* Laguna Beach, CA: Basic Health Publications, 2002.

AMINO ACIDS

Braverman, Eric, and Carl C. Pfeiffer. *The Healing Nutrients Within: Facts, Findings and New Research on Amino Acids.* New Canaan, CT: Keats Publishing, 1987.

Marshall, Keri. *User's Guide to Protein and Amino Acids.* Laguna Beach, CA: Basic Health Publications, 2005.

OTHER NUTRIENTS

Challem, Jack, and Marie Moneysmith. *User's Guide to Carotenoids & Flavonoids.* Laguna Beach, CA: Basic Health Publications, 2005.

Horrobin, David F. *Omega-6 Essential Fatty Acids.* New York: Alan R. Liss Inc, 1990.

Mindell, Earl. *User's Guide to Probiotics.* Laguna Beach, CA: Basic Health Publications, 2012.

Moneysmith, Marie. *User's Guide to Carnosine.* Laguna Beach, CA: Basic Health Publications, 2004.

Toews, Victoria Dolby. *User's Guide to Glucosamine & Chondroitin.* Laguna Beach, CA: Basic Health Publications, 2002.

Tweed, Vera. *User's Guide to Carnitine and Acetyl-L-Carnitine.* Laguna Beach, CA: Basic Health Publications, 2006.

Zucker, Martin. *User's Guide to Coenzyme Q10.* Laguna Beach, CA: Basic Health Publications, 2010.

NUTRITIONAL TREATMENT OF SPECIFIC DISEASES

Alcoholism and Drug Addiction

Challem, Jack. *The Food-Mood Solution: All-Natural Ways to Banish Anxiety, Depression, Anger, Stress, Overeating, and Alcohol and Drug Problems—and Feel Good Again.* Hoboken, NJ: John Wiley & Sons, 2007. Reviewed in *J Orthomolecular Med* 2008;23(2):106–107.

Hoffer, Abram, and Andrew W. Saul. *The Vitamin Cure for Alcoholism.* Laguna Beach, CA: Basic Health Publications, 2009. This brief book is about how to stop addictions to alcohol, caffeine, cigarettes, and drugs and also relieve depression using high-dose nutrition. So effective is this approach that Bill W., cofounder of Alcoholics Anonymous, strongly urged AA members to use vitamin therapy. Bill W. was a patient of Dr. Hoffer's.

Alzheimer's Disease

Newport, Mary. *Alzheimer's Disease: What If There Was a Cure?* 2nd ed. Laguna Beach, CA: Basic Health Publications, 2013.

Cancer

Gerson, Charlotte, with Beata Bishop. *Healing the Gerson Way: Defeating Cancer and Other Chronic Diseases.* 2nd ed. Carmel, CA: Totality Books, 2009. Reviewed in *J Orthomolecular Med* 2007;22(4):217–218.

Gonzalez, Michael, Jorge Miranda-Massari, and Andrew W. Saul. *I Have Cancer: What Should I Do? Your Orthomolecular Guide for Cancer Management.* Laguna Beach, CA: Basic Health Publications, 2009.

Hickey, Steve, and Hilary Roberts. *Cancer: Nutrition and Survival.* Morrisville, NC: Lulu Press, 2005. Reviewed in *J Orthomolecular Med* 2006;21(2):117–118.

Strauss, Howard D. *Dr. Max Gerson: Healing the Hopeless.* 2nd ed. Carmel, CA: Totality Books, 2009. Reviewed in *J Orthomolecular Med* 2002;17(2):122–124.

Cardiovascular Disease

Gerson, Charlotte. *Defeating Obesity, Diabetes, and High Blood Pressure: The Metabolic Syndrome.* Carmel, CA: Gerson Health Media, 2010. Reviewed in *J Orthomolecular Med* 2011; 26(1):42–43.

Janson, Michael. Review of *User's Guide to Heart-Healthy Supplements.* Laguna Beach, CA: Basic Health Publications, 2004. Reviewed in *J Orthomolecular Med* 2006;21(2):116–117.

Roberts, Hilary, and Steve Hickey. *The Vitamin Cure for Heart Disease.* Laguna Beach, CA: Basic Health Publications, 2011.

Shute, Evan. *The Vitamin E Story: The Medical Memoirs of Evan Shute.* Burlington, ON: Welch Publishing, 1985. Reviewed in *J Orthomolecular Med* 2002;17(3):179–181.

Depression and Anxiety

Challem, Jack. *The Food-Mood Solution: All-Natural Ways to Banish Anxiety, Depression, Anger, Stress, Overeating, and Alcohol and Drug Problems—and Feel Good Again.* Hoboken, NJ: John Wiley & Sons, 2007. Reviewed in *J Orthomolecular Med* 2008;23(2):106–107.

Jonsson, Bo H., and Andrew W. Saul. *The Vitamin Cure for Depression.* Laguna Beach, CA: Basic Health Publications, 2012.

Prousky, Jonathan. *Anxiety: Orthomolecular Diagnosis and Treatment.* Toronto, ON: CCNM Press 2007.

Eye Diseases

Smith, Robert G. *The Vitamin Cure for Eye Diseases.* Laguna Beach, CA: Basic Health Publications, 2012.

Fatigue

Challem, Jack. *No More Fatigue: Why You're So Tired and What You Can Do About It.* Hoboken, NJ: John Wiley & Sons, 2011. Reviewed in *J Orthomolecular Med* 2011;26(4):190–191.

Prousky, Jonathan. *The Vitamin Cure for Chronic Fatigue.* Laguna Beach, CA: Basic Health Publications, 2010.

HIV/AIDS

Brighthope, Ian, and Peter Fitzgerald. *The AIDS Fighters: The Role of Vitamin C and Other Immunity Building Nutrients.* New Canaan, CT: Keats Publishing, 1988.

Hyperactivity and Other Learning and Behavioral Disorders

Campbell, Ralph, and Andrew W. Saul. *The Vitamin Cure for Infant and Toddler Health Problems.* Laguna Beach, CA: Basic Health Publications, 2013.

Cott, Allan. *Dr. Cott's Help for Your Learning Disabled Child: The Orthomolecular Treatment.* New York: Times Books, 1985.

Hoffer, Abram. *Healing Children's Attention & Behavior Disorders: Complementary Nutritional & Psychological Treatments.* Toronto, ON: CCNM Press, 2004. Reviewed in *J Orthomolecular Med* 2006;21(4)229–230.

Santini, Linda. *Solving the Mystery of ADHD Naturally.* Battle Creek, MI: Acorn Publishers, 2005. Reviewed in *J Orthomolecular Med* 2005;20(4):281–282.

Radiation Sickness

Schechter, Steven. *Fighting Radiation and Chemical Pollutants with Foods, Herbs and Vitamins.* 2nd ed. Encinitas, CA: Vitality, Ink, 1990.

Schizophrenia and Other Mental Illness

Hoffer, Abram. *Healing Schizophrenia: Complementary Vitamin & Drug Treatments.* Naturopathic Healing Series, Professional Edition. Toronto, ON: CCNM Press, 2011. Reviewed in *J Orthomolecular Med* 2006;21(1):59–60.

Hoffer, Abram. *Orthomolecular Treatment for Schizophrenia.* New York: McGraw-Hill, 1999.

Hope, Carlene. *Recovery from the Hell of Schizophrenia.* Morrisville, NC: Lulu Press, 2005. Reviewed in *J Orthomolecular Med* 2006;21(1):58.

Other Conditions

Brighthope, Ian. *The Vitamin Cure for Diabetes.* Laguna Beach, CA: Basic Health Publications, 2012.

Campbell, Ralph, and Andrew W. Saul. *The Vitamin Cure for Children's Health Problems.* Laguna Beach, CA: Basic Health Publications, 2012.

Case, Helen Saul. *The Vitamin Cure for Women's Health Problems.* Laguna Beach, CA: Basic Health Publications, 2012.

Downing, Damien. *The Vitamin Cure for Allergies.* Laguna Beach, CA: Basic Health Publications, 2010.

Hickey, Steve. *The Vitamin Cure for Migraines.* Laguna Beach, CA: Basic Health Publications, 2010.

Hoffer, Abram, Andrew W. Saul, Steve Hickey. *Hospitals and Health: Your Orthomolecular Guide to a Shorter, Safer Hospital Stay.* Laguna Beach, CA: Basic Health Publications, 2011.

Hunninghake, Ronald. *User's Guide to Inflammation, Arthritis, and Aging.* Laguna Beach, CA: Basic Health Publications, 2005.

ADDITIONAL RECOMMENDED BOOKS, REVIEWED IN *JOM*

Angell, Marcia. *The Truth about the Drug Companies* by Marcia Angell. Reviewed in *J Orthomolecular Med* 2005; 20(2):120–122.

Challem, Jack. *Syndrome X: The Complete Nutritional Program to Prevent and Reverse Insulin Resistance.* Reviewed in *J Orthomolecular Med* 2003;18(1):49–51.

Dean, Carolyn. *Death by Modern Medicine.* Reviewed in *J Orthomolecular Med* 2006;21(1):60–61.

Friedman, Michael. *Fundamentals of Naturopathic Endocrinology: A Complementary and Alternative Medicine Guide.* Reviewed in *J Orthomolecular Med* 2007;22(2): 91–92.

Hoffer, Miriam. *Fueling Body, Mind and Spirit: A Balanced Approach to Healthy Eating.* Reviewed in *J Orthomolecular Med* 2004;19(3):186–187.

Levy, Thomas E. *Vitamin C, Infectious Diseases and Toxins.* Reviewed in *J Orthomolecular Med* 2003;18(2):117–118.

Schauss, Alexander G. *Obesity: Why Are Men Getting Pregnant?* Reviewed in *J Orthomolecular Med* 2008;23(2): 107–108.

Shames, Richard L., and Karilee H. Shames. *Thyroid Power.* Reviewed in *J Orthomolecular Med* 2004;19(2):116–118.

MISCELLANEOUS WORKS CITED IN TEXT

Abramson, Emanuel Maurice. *Body, Mind, & Sugar.* Whitefish, MT: Literary Licensing, 2012; originally published 1951.

Blank, Louis. *Alzheimer's Challenged and Conquered?* London: Foulsham, 1995.

Bland, Jeffrey. *Textbook of Functional Medicine.* 3rd ed. Gig Harbor, WA: Institute for Functional Medicine, 2010.

Boik, John. *Natural Compounds in Cancer Therapy: Promising Nontoxic Antitumor Agents from Plants & Other Natural Sources,* Princeton, MN: Oregon Medical Press, 2001.

Breggin, Peter. *Talking Back to Ritalin.* Rev. ed. Cambridge, MA: Da Capo Press, 2001.

Brownstein, David. *Iodine: Why You Need It, Why You Can't Live Without It.* West Bloomfield, MI. Alternative Press, 2009.

Cameron, Ewan. *Hyaluronidase and Cancer.* Philadelphia, PA: Elsevier, 1966.

Campbell, T. Colin. *The China Study.* Dallas, TX: BenBella Books, 2004.

Cheraskin, Emanuel. *Human Health and Homeostasis.* Birmingham, AL: Clayton College/Natural Reader Press, 1999.

———. *Psychodietetics: Food as the Key to Emotional Health.* Madison, WI: Madison Books, 1974.

———. *Vitamin C: Who Needs It?* Birmingham, AL: Atticus Press & Co, 1993.

Cleave, T. L. *The Saccharine Disease.* New Canaan, CT: Keats Publishing, 1975.

Cousens, Gabriel. *There Is a Cure for Diabetes.* Rev. ed. Berkeley, CA: North Atlantic Books, 2013.

Cousins, Norman. *An Anatomy of an Illness.* Rev. ed. New York: W.W. Norton & Co, 2005.

Davis, Adelle. *Let's Cook It Right.* New York: Signet Books, 1970; originally published in 1947.

———. *Let's Eat Right to Keep Fit.* New York: Signet Books, 1970; originally published in 1954.

———. *Let's Get Well.* New York: Signet Books, 1988; originally published in 1965.

———. *Let's Have Healthy Children.* New York: Signet Books, 1972; originally published in 1951.

Ernst, R. *Weakness Is a Crime: The Life of Bernard Macfadden* by R. Ernst. Syracuse, NY: Syracuse University Press, 1991.

Feist, Sister Theresa. *Schizophrenia Cured.* Toronto, ON: Canadian Schizophrenia Foundation, 1994.

Foster, Harold. *Health, Disease and the Environment.* Hoboken, NJ: John Wiley & Sons, 1992 ———. *Reducing Cancer Mortality: A Geographical Perspective.* Victoria, BC: University of Victoria Press, 1986.

———. *What Really Causes Schizophrenia.* Victoria, BC: Trafford Publishing, 2006.

Franklin, Jon. *Molecules of the Mind: The Brave New Science of Molecular Psychology.* New York: Atheneum, 1986.

Gaby, Alan. *Preventing and Reversing Osteoporosis.* Roseville, CA: Prima, 1994.

———. *The Doctor's Guide to Vitamin B6 (1984).* Emmaus, PA: Rodale Press, 1984.

———. *Nutritional Medicine.* Concord, NH: Fritz Perlberg, 2011.

Gaby, Alan, and Jonathan Wright, MD. *The Patient's Book of Natural Healing.* Roseville, CA: Prima, 1999.

Gordon, Gary, and Amy Yasko. *The Puzzle of Autism.* 2nd ed. Payson, AZ: Matrix Development Publishing, 2006.

Griffin, Edward. *World Without Cancer: The Story of Vitamin B17.* Rev. ed. Westlake Village, CA: American Media, 1997.

Hawkins, David. *The Eye of the Eye.* Rev. ed. Sedona, AZ: Veritas Publishing, 2010.

———. *I: Reality and Subjectivity.* Rev. ed. Carlsbad, CA: Hay House, 2014.

———. *Power vs. Force.* Rev. ed. Sedona, AZ: Veritas Publishing, 2013.

Hickey, Steve, and Hilary Roberts. *The Cancer Breakthrough.* Morrisville, NC: LuLu Press, 2007.

Hoffer, Abram. *Adventures in Psychiatry: A Scientific Memoir.* Ontario, CAN: KOS Publishing, 2005.

Hoffer, Abram, and Osmond Humphry with Fannie Hoffer Kahan. *New Hope for Alcoholics.* New Hyde Park, NY: University Books, 1968.

Hoffer, Abram, and Morton Walker. *Orthomolecular Nutrition.* New Canaan, CT: Keats Publishing, 1978.

Holick, Michael. *The UV Advantage.* New York: Ibooks, 2004.

Horrobin, David. *The Madness of Adam and Eve.* New York: Bantam Press, 2002.

Hunt, W. R. *Body Love: The Amazing Career of Bernard Macfadden.* Bowling Green, OH: Popular Press, 1989.

Kahan, Fannie Hoffer. *Brains and Bricks.* Regina, SK: White Cross Publications, 1965.

Kaufman, William. *The Common Form of Joint Dysfunction.* Brattleboro, VT: E.L. Hildreth 1949.

Kraut, Alan. *Goldberger's War: The Life and Work of a Public Health Crusader.* New York: Hill & Wang, 2003.

Kunin, Richard. *Mega-Nutrition.* New York: McGraw Hill, 1980.

———. *Mega-Nutrition for Women.* New York: McGraw Hill, 1983.

Lesser, Michael. *The Brain Chemistry Diet.* New York: Putnam, 2002.

———. *Fat and the Killer Diseases.* Parker House, 1991.

———. *Nutrition and Vitamin Therapy.* New York: Grove Press, 1979.

O'Malley, Martin. *Doctors.* New York: Paperjacks, 1988.

Ott, John. *Health and Light.* New York: Simon & Schuster, 1976.

Pauling, Linus. *Linus Pauling in His Own Words.* New York: Touchstone, 1995.

Pfeiffer, Carl C. *Dr. Pfeiffer's Total Nutrition: Nutritional Science and Cookery.* New York: Simon & Schuster, 1980.

———. *Neurobiology of the Trace Metals Zinc and Copper.* New York: Academy Press, 1972.

Quillin, Patrick. *Beating Cancer with Nutrition.* 4th ed. Carlsbad, CA: Nutrition Times Press, 2007.

Reading, Chris. *Trace Your Genes to Health.* 2nd ed. Ridgefield, CT: Vital Health Publishing, 2003.

———. *A Doctor in Orthomolecular Medicine.* Enhancement Books, 2012.

Rimland. Bernard. *Infantile Autism: The Syndrome and Its Implications for a Neural Theory of Behavior.* New York: Appleton-Century-Crofts, 1964.

Sanders, Marion. *The Crisis in American Medicine.* New York: Harper & Brothers, 1961.

Siegel Bernie. *Love, Medicine and Miracles.* New York: Harper & Row, 1986.

Simone, Charles B. *Cancer & Nutrition.* Garden City Park, NY: Avery, 1991.

Shute, Evan. *The Heart and Vitamin E.* London, ON: Shute Foundation for Medical Research, 1972.

Smith, Lendon, ed. *Clinical Guide to the Use of Vitamin C.* Tacoma, WA: Life Sciences Press, 1988.

Smith, Lendon. *Feed Your Kids Right.* New York: McGraw Hill, 1979.

———. *Foods for Healthy Kids.* New York: McGraw Hill, 1981.

Taube, Gary. *Good Calories, Bad Calories.* Rev. ed. New York: Anchor Books, 2008.

Warren, Tom. *Beating Alzheimer's: A Step Towards Unlocking the Mysteries of Brain Diseases.* Garden City Park, NY: Avery, 1991.

Williams, Roger. *An Introduction to Organic Chemistry.* 4th ed. Princeton, NJ: D. Van Nostrand Co, 1928.

———. *Free and Unequal.* Austin, TX: University of Texas Press, 1953.

———. *Nutrition Against Disease.* New York: Pitman Publishers, 1971.

———. *Nutrition and Alcoholism.* Norman, OK: University of Oklahoma Press, 1951.

———. *Physicians' Handbook of Nutritional Science.* Springfield, IL: C.C. Thomas, 1975.

Wright, Jonathan. *Dr. Wright's Book of Nutritional Therapy.* Emmaus, PA: Rodale Press, 1982.

———. *Dr. Wright's Guide to Healing with Nutrition.* New Canaan, CT: Keats Publishing, 1993.

Yudkin, John. *Sweet and Dangerous.* New York: Bantam Books, 1972.

ABOUT THE *JOURNAL OF ORTHOMOLECULAR MEDICINE* AND ITS DEVELOPMENT

In 1967, shortly after the formation of the Canadian Schizophrenia Foundation, and in the United States, the American Schizophrenia Association, Drs. Abram Hoffer, Humphry Osmond, and others published the first issue of a journal called the *Journal of Schizophrenia.* They had to create their own journals because it was impossible to obtain entry into the official journals of psychiatry and medicine. Before 1967, Dr. Hoffer had not found it difficult to publish reports in these journals, and by then he had about 150 articles and several books in the establishment press. The subsequent difficulty, therefore, did not arise from the quality and style of his writing since it has probably improved since then.

It was pretty obvious to those practicing nutritional psychiatry, later orthomolecular psychiatry, that it was the content of their material that was found to be not acceptable. This was proven by the attempt of the American Psychiatric Association (APA) to censor their work even several years after papers had been published. Dr. Hoffer and Dr. Osmond appeared before the Committee of Ethics of the APA to answer why they were publicizing a treatment not acceptable to standard psychiatry. According to Dr. Hoffer, one of the editors of the American Psychiatric Association's journal announced that he would never allow any article from the orthomolecular group to appear in his publication. Dr. Hoffer confirmed this to be the same person who chaired the task force that had condemned orthomolecular medicine out of hand.

This new journal was to become the forum available to practitioners of the new psychiatry, which official psychiatry found so unacceptable. The peer-reviewed journals effectively prevented any of these new ideas from appearing in their journals. As Dr. Hoffer has said, "Peer-reviewed journals do not protect the public from research reports of inferior quality, nor do they protect the public from dangerous ideas. They protect the establishment from ideas that run counter to their own."

After two years the title was shortened to *Schizophrenia* for three years. In 1972, the title was changed to the *Journal of Orthomolecular Psychiatry* to reflect the widening use of nutrition in the treatment of many physical and psychiatric disorders. Dr. Linus Pauling in 1968 had proposed the term orthomolecular psychiatry, which we recognized as the correct words to define the total interest in nutrition, clinical ecology, and the use of supplements. There were 14 volumes.

In 1986, as it became clear that nutritional therapy was widely applicable to both physical as well as mental disease, the publication underwent a final change to the more inclusive *Journal of Orthomolecular Medicine* (*JOM*) and is presently published as such today.

JOM has led the way in presenting, in advance of other medical journals, new health concerns and treatments including niacin therapy for schizophrenia and coronary disease; vitamin C for cancer; and the nutritional treatment of behavioral disorders, and drug and alcohol abuse. *JOM* was also the first medical journal to publish papers on the nutritional treatment of allergies, autism, and AIDS. *JOM* published pioneering research on candidiasis in 1978, mercury amalgam toxicity in 1982, and chronic fatigue syndrome in 1988. The journal has published over 100 papers on nutritional medicine and cancer, and over 400 articles on schizophrenia and other psychiatric illnesses. All the pioneers in orthomolecular medicine have reported their findings in this journal. It thus represents a unique source for these earlier and current studies, which provide a basis for the increasing growth of nutritional medicine.

The archives of *JOM* are posted online. Past issues from 1967 through 2009 are available for downloading, at no charge, at http://orthomolecular .org/library/jom/index.shtml. More recent issues are available by subscription.

ABOUT THE INTERNATIONAL SOCIETY FOR ORTHOMOLECULAR MEDICINE

The International Society for Orthomolecular Medicine (ISOM) held its inaugural meeting April 29, 1994, in Vancouver, Canada. The event brought together the many orthomolecular organizations already active worldwide.

ISOM's purpose is to further the advancement of orthomolecular medicine throughout the world, to raise awareness of this rapidly growing and cost-effective practice of health-care, and to unite the many and various groups already operating in this field. The society offers education to health professionals and the public on the benefits and practice of orthomolecular medicine through publications, conferences, and seminars.

The present membership includes groups active in Algeria, Australia, Austria, Belgium, Brazil, Canada, Denmark, France, Germany, India, Japan, Korea, Mexico, Netherlands, Spain, Switzerland, Taiwan, United Kingdom, and United States.

In 2012, Atsuo Yanagisawa from Japan was elected ISOM's president, a position he still maintains. Prior presidents include Gert Schuitemaker (1999–2009) from the Netherlands and Oslim Malina (1996–1999) from Brazil. ISOM was founded by Abram Hoffer, Steven Carter, and Jack Kay.

For more information on the ISOM, please contact:

International Society for Orthomolecular Medicine
16 Florence Avenue
Toronto, Ontario, Canada M2N 1E9
Phone: (416) 733–2117
Fax: (416) 733–2352
Email: centre@orthomed.org
Website: www.orthomed.org

Author Index

SUBJECT INDEX

AA. *See* Alcoholics Anonymous (AA).
Aascorbemia, 103–105
Abbey, Laraine, 441, 442
Abe, Hiroyuki, 161
 biography, 155
Abraham, Guy, 351
ACE inhibitors, 387
Acetaldehyde, 180, 181, 194
Acetylcholine, 215, 217, 226, 227, 228
Acetylcholinesterase, 227
Acetylcholinesterase-beta amyloid
 protein complexes, 215, 217
Acetyl-L-carnitine, 152, 226–227
Acetyltransferase, 215, 217
Acid rain, 212, 550
Acidosis, 735, 736
Acidotic crisis, 735, 736
Action for Healthy Kids (AFHK), 619
Acute myeloid leukemia (AML),
 289–295
Addis, Thomas, 14
Adele Davis Foundation, 137
Adenosine triphosphate (ATP), 455
Adenylyl cyclase, 216
ADHD. *See* Attention-deficit
 hyperactivity disorder (ADHD).
Adrenal glands, 657
Adrenaline, 185, 654, 658
Adrenochrome, 164, 644, 645, 658
Adrenolutin, 164, 644
Advertising
 food, 611
 pharmaceutical, 33, 54
Affective disorder, 424
Age-related macular degeneration
 (AMD). *See* Macular degeneration.
Aging, 28, 152, 212, 221–222, 506, 535
Agoraphobia
 allergies and, 458–459
 assessment of, 451–453
 case studies, 459–462
 vitamin B1 and, 457–458

vitamin B3 and, 451–462
AIDS. *See* HIV/AIDS.
ALA. *See* Alpha-lipoic acid (ALA).
Alanine aminotranferase (ALT), 537,
 538
Albumin, 737
Alcohol, 183, 197, 394
 chronic fatigue syndrome and, 537
 cravings for, 179, 181, 196, 198
 effect on gastrointestinal tract, 176
 effect on brain cells, 184–185
 effect on liver, 177
 effect on pancreas, 177–178
 food allergies and, 178–179
Alcoholic syndrome, 199
Alcoholics Anonymous (AA), 128,
 173, 194
Alcoholics, 175–176, 181, 558
 diet and, 177–178, 181, 186–188,
 197–199
 mental dysfunctions and, 178,
 179–180, 185, 186, 190–191
 personality and, 184, 185
 psychotic, 180, 187, 191
Alcoholism, 28, 173–199, 474
 diet and, 177–178, 179, 180, 181–182,
 183, 185, 186–188, 190, 192, 197–198
 heredity and, 179
 orthomolecular treatment, 186–188,
 191–193
 prevention, 195–199
 psychiatric aspects, 184, 190–191
 risk factors, 195–199
 terms of, 174
 treatment programs, 175, 191–193,
 622
 vitamin B-complex and, 183
 vitamin C and, 171, 177, 187, 485
 vitamins and, 35, 177, 178, 187, 188,
 191–192, 197, 398
"Alcoholism and Malnutrition"
 (Hillman), 175

Alkalosis, 187
Allen, Edgar V., 371, 372
Allergies and food intolerances, 29,
 178–179, 483–484, 486, 530,
 574–575, 579, 587, 652–653, 669,
 701, 711
 agoraphobia and, 458–459
 vitamin C and, 107
Alliance for Natural Health (ANH),
 257, 259
Allopathic medicine. *See* Medicine,
 Western.
Alpha blockers, 391
Alpha-linolenic acid, 218
Alpha-lipoic acid (ALA), 152, 257, 258,
 268, 277, 280, 332, 335, 336, 509,
 625, 635, 638
Alpha-Tocopherol, Beta-Carotene
 Cancer Prevention Study, 297, 303,
 311, 312, 313, 315, 316, 317, 319
*Alpha Tocopherol in Cardiovascular
 Disease* (Shute), 127
Alprazolam (Xanax), 487–488
ALS. *See* Amyotrophic lateral sclerosis
 (ALS).
Altschul, Rudolf, 371, 373, 374
Aluminum, 210–236, 655
Aluminum foil, 224
Aluminum maltolate, 214, 224
Alzheimer, Alois, 212
Alzheimer's Association, 204
Alzheimer's Challenged and Conquered
 (Blank), 225
Alzheimer's disease, 49, 201–236
 aging and, 221–222
 aluminum and, 210–236
 antagonist hypothesis, 211
 diet and, 209, 219
 education and, 222–224
 genetics and, 220
 head trauma and, 220–221
 preventive factors, 223

methadone and, 485

objections to megadose therapy, 62–63

oral, 258, 259, 261, 268, 281, 329–337, 347, 514

pharmacokinetics, 276, 282, 335

post-surgery blood plasma levels and, 74–75

pregnancy and, 72–74

psychiatry and, 64–66

radiation sickness/exposure and, 625, 627–628, 629–632, 633–635, 638

rebound effect in cancer, 250–251, 334

safety of, 238, 248, 253, 255, 265, 266, 332, 494, 496, 524

schizophrenia and, 241, 644, 646, 653–654, 660, 670, 700, 701, 706, 712

scurvy and, 62, 64, 67, 74–75, 90–93, 97–100

selective cytotoxicity of, 335, 348

shingles and, 38–39

studies, 82–89

synthesis of, 93, 468

systematic saturation hypothesis, 282–283

testing levels of, 68–69

urine and, 101–102

viruses and, 39, 69

water-soluble, 168

Vitamin C and Cancer (Richards), 247, 251, 252

Vitamin C and the Common Cold (Pauling), 9, 15, 82, 128, 153, 482

Vitamin C, the Common Cold, and the Flu (Pauling), 15

Vitamin C transporters, 92

Vitamin C: Who Needs It? (Cheraskin), 145

Vitamin Cure series (ed. by Saul), 165

Vitamin D, 18, 48, 65, 127–128, 163, 712, 720

Alzheimer's disease and, 212, 221

cancer and, 257, 343–344, 345, 353

learning and behavioral disorders and, 575

Vitamin D2, 13

Vitamin D3, 13

Vitamin E, 8, 13, 18–19, 27, 32, 34, 35, 36, 42, 48, 49, 118–119, 123, 127–129, 141, 361, 505, 560

Alzheimer's disease and, 204, 207, 208, 218–219, 220, 224, 228

blood pressure and, 400

cancer and, 293, 305–320

cardiovascular disease and, 357–358, 382, 389

drug addiction and, 467–468, 471

eye diseases and, 503, 506–507, 508, 509, 510, 511, 515–516, 517–518

heart disease and, 240

radiation sickness/exposure and, 625, 638

Vitamin K, 13, 353

Vitamin K3, 259, 261, 268, 335

Vitamins, 7, 59, 171, 237, 486

absorption and storage of, 177, 179

brand variations, 37–38

conditions that benefit from, 28

deficiencies, 29, 40–42, 525

dependencies, 29, 40–42, 204, 593, 601, 603, 642, 649

discoveries, 125–170

dosages, 35–36

fat-soluble, 34

media and, 48–49, 203–205, 257, 307, 552, 578–579, 603

multi-, with minerals, 48, 224, 275, 399, 507, 518, 552

megadoses, 1–3, 5–6, 8–9, 34–38, 136

precautions, 36

rebound effect, 41–42

safe upper levels, 43–47

safety of, 204, 238, 275, 721, 722, 727

side effects, 36

side effects, positive, 37

water-soluble, 34

Vitreous humor, 505

Vogel, Max J., 680

biography, 144

Volkow, Nora, 582–583

Vollmer, August, 475–475

Volstead Act (Alcohol Prohibition), 475

Wadsworth, Michael, 610

Wagner, E. S., 482

Walker, Morton, 26

Warburg, O., 593

Ward, Jack, 649, 710

Warfarin (Coumadin), 265

Warner, J. O., 579

Warnock, William, 263

Warren, Tom, 225

Water, 165, 384, 386, 388

Water supply, 210–211, 212, 213, 223, 224, 706

Weight loss, 393

Weiss, B., 605

Wellness and Nutrition Program, 618–619

Wernicke's encephalopathy, 187

Wernicke-Korsakoff syndrome, 180, 187

Western Electric Company Study, 296

Western New York Diet Study, 303

"What Killed Rebecca Riley" (TV segment), 569

What Really Causes AIDS (Foster), 543, 563, 565

Wheat-germ extract, fermented, 353

Whitaker, Julian, 354

Whitefish Central School, Montana, 619

Whittock, Donna, 619

Wikipedia, 552

Williams, Moke, 680, 684, 710

Williams, Robert R., 13

Williams, Roger J., 13, 64, 81, 127–128, 171, 176, 183, 184–185, 188, 196, 482, 516, 645, 696

biography, 134

Wilson, William Griffith, 128, 173, 193–194

biography, 134–135

Wilson's disease, 703

Wilson's temperature syndrome (WTS), 658

Wing, Steven, 637

Wolfe, Sidney M., 54

Women's Health Study, 309, 310

Wood, Rebecca, 203

World Health Organization, 114, 431

World without Cancer (Griffin), 350

Wrench, T. G., 139

Wright, C. R., 466

Wright, Jonathan V.

biography, 159–160

www.DoctorYourself.com, 164

Xanax. See Alprazolam (Xanax).

Yamaguchi, Dr., 128

Yanagisawa, Atsuo, xiii, 1, 627, 633

biography, 162–163

Yeast, 559

Yudkin, John, 25

Zeaxanthin, 506, 511

Zechmeister, László, 14

Zinc, 179, 180, 187, 190, 191, 208, 209, 211, 212–213, 216, 219, 224, 228, 509, 511, 519, 575, 605, 610, 705

schizophrenia and, 646, 652, 655, 656, 670, 696, 700–706, 712

Zinc citrate, 27

Zoloft. See Sertraline (Zoloft).

Zuckerkandl, Emile, 15

Zweifach, B. W., 70

ABOUT THE EDITOR

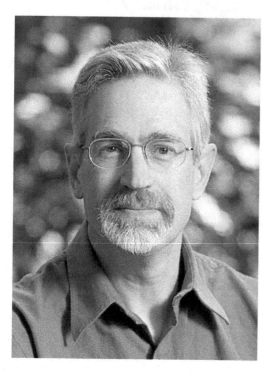

Andrew W. Saul, PhD, is founder and editor-in-chief of the *Orthomolecular Medicine News Service* and is on the editorial board of the *Journal of Orthomolecular Medicine.* He has published over 180 peer-reviewed articles and has written or coauthored twelve books, including four with Dr. Abram Hoffer. Those books have been translated into a number of languages, including Arabic, Chinese, Hindi, Italian, Japanese, Norwegian, and Spanish. Dr. Saul was on the faculty of the State University of New York for nine years and has twice won New York Empire State Fellowships for teachers. *Psychology Today* magazine named him one of seven natural health pioneers, and he is featured in the popular documentary movie *Food Matters.* In 2013, Dr. Saul was inducted into the Orthomolecular Medicine Hall of Fame and was appointed to the board of the Japanese College of Intravenous Therapy. His personal website is AndrewSaul.com, and his educational website is DoctorYourself.com, the largest non-commercial natural healing resource on the Internet.

CPSIA information can be obtained
at www.ICGtesting.com
Printed in the USA
JSHW021031301220
10596JS00003B/139